Consultations in Gastroenterology

Consultations in Gastroenterology

William J. Snape, Jr., M.D.
Clinical Professor of Medicine
University of California Los Angeles
Director, Bowel Disease and Motility Center
Memorial Medical Center, Long Beach, California

W.B. SAUNDERS COMPANY
A Division of Harcourt Brace & Company
Philadelphia   London   Toronto   Montreal   Sydney   Tokyo

W.B. SAUNDERS COMPANY

A Division of Harcourt Brace & Company

The Curtis Center
Independence Square West
Philadelphia, Pennsylvania 19106

Library of Congress Cataloging-in-Publication Data

Consultations in gastroenterology/[edited by] William J. Snape, Jr.
    p.   cm.
   ISBN 0-7216-4670-0
   1. Gastrointestinal system—Diseases. 2. Gastroenterology.
I. Snape, William J.
    [DNLM: 1. Gastrointestinal Diseases. WI 140 C759 1996]
RC801.C65   1996
616.3'3—dc20
DNLM/DLC   95-11486

CONSULTATIONS IN GASTROENTEROLOGY   ISBN   0-7216-4670-0

Copyright © 1996 by W.B. Saunders Company

All rights reserved. No part of this publication may be reproduced or transmitted in any form or by any means, electronic or mechanical, including photocopy, recording, or any information storage and retrieval system, without permission in writing from the publisher.

Printed in the United States of America

Last digit is the print number: 9   8   7   6   5   4   3   2   1

Contributors

NEZAM H. AFDHAL, M.D.
Associate Professor of Medicine, Boston University School of Medicine; Chief of Gastroenterology, Boston City Hospital, Boston, Massachusetts
Acalculous Cholecystitis

C. GREGORY ALBERS, M.D.
Attending Gastroenterologist, FHP Fountain Valley Medical Center, Fountain Valley, California
Endometriosis: A Gastroenterologist's Perspective

GIUSEPPE ALIPERTI, M.D.
Assistant Professor of Medicine and Director of Interventional Endoscopy, Washington University School of Medicine, St. Louis, Missouri
Gastric Ulcers

RAFAEL A. AMARAL, M.D.
Instructor in Medicine, Division of Gastroenterology, Milton S. Hershey Medical Center, The Pennsylvania State University, Hershey, Pennsylvania
Gastric Volvulus

JITRA ANURAS, M.D.
Professor, Department of Internal Medicine, Texas Tech School of Medicine; Attending Physician, University Medical Center, Lubbock, Texas
Chronic Intestinal Pseudoobstruction in Adults

SINN ANURAS, M.D.
Clinical Professor, Chulalongkorn University; Medical Director, Bumrungrad Hospital, Bangkok, Thailand
Chronic Intestinal Pseudoobstruction in Adults

MILES AUSLANDER, M.D.
Staff Gastroenterologist, Valley Presbyterian Hospital, Van Nuys, California
Gastric Outlet Obstruction

BRUCE R. BACON, M.D.
Professor of Internal Medicine and Director, Division of Gastroenterology and Hepatology, St. Louis University School of Medicine, St. Louis, Missouri
Hemochromatosis

VIJAYAN BALAN, M.B.B.S.
Gastroenterology Fellow, Mayo Medical School, Rochester, Minnesota
Hepatobiliary Complications of Ulcerative Colitis and Crohn's Disease; Primary Biliary Cirrhosis

ALAN R. BANK, M.D.
Consulting Gastroenterologist, West Boca Medical Center and Boca Raton Community Hospital, Boca Raton, Florida
Acute Lower Gastrointestinal Tract Bleeding

JAMIE S. BARKIN, M.D.
Professor of Medicine, University of Miami, Miami, Florida; Chief, Division of Gastroenterology, Mt. Sinai Medical Center, Miami Beach, Florida
Gastrointestinal Fistulas

JOYCE P. BARNETT, M.S., R.D./L.D.
Assistant Professor, Department of Clinical Nutrition, University of Texas Southwestern Medical Center at Dallas, Dallas, Texas
Obesity

PETER V. BARRETT, M.D.
Professor of Medicine, University of California Los Angeles School of Medicine, Los Angeles, California; Academic Chief of Medicine, St. Mary Medical Center, Long Beach, California
Disorders of Liver Function in Systemic Disease

WILLIAM M. BATTLE, M.D.
Clinical Assistant Professor of Medicine, University of Pennsylvania School of Medicine; Director of Gastrointestinal Endoscopy, Jeanes and Nazareth Hospitals, Philadelphia, Pennsylvania
Caustic Injury to the Upper Gastrointestinal Tract

JAMES M. BECKER, M.D.
James Utley Professor and Chairman of Surgery, Boston University School of Medicine; Surgeon-in-Chief, Boston University Medical Center Hospital, Boston, Massachusetts
Surgery for Peptic Ulcer Disease: For Whom and When

STANLEY B. BENJAMIN, M.D.
Professor of Medicine, Georgetown University; Chief, Gastroenterology, Georgetown University Hospital, Washington, D.C.
Acute Lower Gastrointestinal Tract Bleeding

CHARLES N. BERNSTEIN, M.D., F.R.C.P.C.
Assistant Professor of Medicine, Section of Gastroenterology, University of Manitoba; Staff Physician, Health Sciences Centre, Winnipeg, Manitoba, Canada
Variceal Bleeding

CONTRIBUTORS

LESLIE H. BERNSTEIN, M.D.
Professor of Medicine and Director of Gastroenterology, Albert Einstein College of Medicine and Montefiore Medical Center, Bronx, New York
Tropical Sprue: A Disappearing Enigma

LAURENCE BLENDIS, M.D., F.R.C.P., F.R.C.P.(C.)
Professor of Medicine, University of Toronto; Senior Physician, Toronto Hospital, Toronto, Ontario, Canada
Alcoholic Liver Disease

JOSEPH R. BLOOMER, M.D.
Professor of Medicine and Director of Gastroenterology, Hepatology and Nutrition, University of Minnesota Medical School; Attending Physician and Director of Watson Laboratory, University of Minnesota Hospital and Clinic, Minneapolis, Minnesota
Porphyria

GEORGE W. BO-LINN, M.D.
Chief, Division of Gastroenterology, St. John's Mercy Health System, St. Louis, Missouri
Protein-losing Gastroenteropathy

KENNETH L. BOWES, M.D., F.R.C.S.(C.)
Professor of Surgery, W.C. Mackenzie Health Sciences Centre, University of Alberta, Edmonton, Alberta, Canada
Toxic Megacolon

EUGENE MICHAEL BOZYMSKI, M.D.
Professor of Medicine, University of North Carolina School of Medicine; Chief of Endoscopy, Gastrointestinal Division, University of North Carolina Hospitals, Chapel Hill, North Carolina
Esophageal Infections

DONALD P. BRANNAN, M.D.
Gastroenterologist, Mississippi Baptist Medical Center, Jackson, Mississippi
Esophageal Infections

HANS A. BÜLLER, M.D., PH.D.
Faculty of Pediatrics, University of Amsterdam; Co-Director, Pediatric Gastroenterology, Academic Medical Center, Amsterdam, The Netherlands
Lactose Intolerance

ROBERT BURAKOFF, M.D.
Professor of Medicine, State University of New York at Stony Brook, Stony Brook, New York; Chief, Division of Gastroenterology, Hepatology, and Nutrition, Winthrop–University Hospital, Mineola, New York
Radiation Colitis

CAROL ANN BURKE, M.D.
Clinical Assistant Professor of Medicine, Pennsylvania State University, Hershey, Pennsylvania; Assistant Staff, Department of Gastroenterology, Cleveland Clinic Foundation, Cleveland, Ohio
Benign Tumors of the Small Bowel

MICHAEL CAMILLERI, M.D.
Professor of Medicine, Mayo Medical School; Consultant in Gastroenterology and Physiology and Biophysics, Mayo Clinic, Rochester, Minnesota
Dyspepsia

MARIA E. CAMILO, M.D., PH.D.
Professor of Medicine, University of Lisbon; Consultant in Gastroenterology, University Hospital of Santa Maria, Lisbon, Portugal
Vitamin Deficiency

JAMES J. CERDA, M.D.
Professor of Medicine and Chief, Nutrition Support, Division of Gastroenterology, Hepatology, and Nutrition, University of Florida College of Medicine, Gainesville, Florida
Blind Loop Syndrome

JOE M. CHEN, M.D.
Gastroenterology Fellow, University of California Los Angeles, Los Angeles, California
Choledocholithiasis

ROBERTO CHIPRUT, M.D.
Associate Clinical Professor of Medicine, University of California Los Angeles; Attending Physician, Cedars Sinai Medical Center, Los Angeles, California
Hepatic Granulomas

RAY E. CLOUSE, M.D.
Professor of Medicine, Washington University School of Medicine; Attending Physician, Barnes Hospital, St. Louis, Missouri
Motor Disorders of the Esophagus

MARK S. CODELLA, M.D.
Attending Physician in Gastroenterology, Jeanes and Nazareth Hospitals, Philadelphia, Pennsylvania
Caustic Injury to the Upper Gastrointestinal Tract

MANLEY COHEN, M.D.
Clinical Professor of Medicine, University of California Irvine, Irvine, California; formerly Chief of Education and Chief of Gastroenterology, currently Consulting Gastroenterologist, Long Beach Memorial Medical Center, Long Beach, California
Nausea and Vomiting

SIDNEY COHEN, M.D.
Professor and Chairman, Department of Medicine, Temple University School of Medicine; Assistant Vice President for the Health Sciences Center, Temple University Hospital, Philadelphia, Pennsylvania
Achalasia

ALLAN R. COOKE, M.D.
Professor of Medicine, University of Kansas Medical Center, Kansas City, Kansas
Malabsorption Syndromes

ALBERT J. CZAJA, M.D.
Professor of Medicine, Mayo Medical School; Consultant in Gastroenterology, Mayo Clinic, Rochester, Minnesota
Acute Hepatitis

MARTA L. DAVILA, M.D.
Assistant Professor of Clinical Medicine, University of California San Francisco; Attending Physician, Veterans Affairs Medical Center, San Francisco, California
Rectal Foreign Bodies

MARK H. DELEGGE, M.D.
Assistant Professor of Medicine and Assistant Director, Section of Nutrition, Medical College of Virginia Hospitals, Richmond, Virginia
Malnutrition

LAURIE D. DELEVE, M.D., PH.D.
Assistant Professor of Medicine, Division of Gastrointestinal and Liver Diseases, University of Southern California School of Medicine, Los Angeles, California
Drug- and Toxin-induced Liver Injury

PAUL J. DEMARTINO, M.D.
Gastroenterologist, Community Medical Center, Toms River, New Jersey
Diversion Colitis

TOM R. DEMEESTER, M.D.
Professor and Chairman, Department of Surgery, University of Southern California School of Medicine, Los Angeles, California
Hiatal Hernia

THOMAS J. DEVERS, M.D.
Assistant Clinical Professor of Medicine, University of Connecticut School of Medicine, Farmington, Connecticut; Associate Chief of Medicine and Senior Attending Gastroenterologist, New Britain General Hospital, New Britain, Connecticut
Bezoars

CHRISTIAN DE VIRGILIO, M.D.
Assistant Professor of Surgery, University of California Los Angeles School of Medicine, Los Angeles, California; Attending Surgeon, Division of Vascular Surgery, Harbor–University of California Los Angeles Medical Center, Torrance, California
Chronic Intestinal Ischemic Syndrome

GHISLAIN DEVROEDE, M.D.
Professor of Surgery, Faculte de Medicine, Université de Sherbrooke; Surgeon, Centre Hospitalier Universitaire de Sherbrooke, Sherbrooke, Quebec, Canada
Slow Transit Constipation

E. ROLLAND DICKSON, M.D.
Mary Lowell Leary Professor of Medicine, Mayo Medical School and Mayo Foundation; Professor of Medicine, Mayo Medical Center, Rochester, Minnesota
Primary Biliary Cirrhosis

GEORGE DICKSTEIN, M.D.
Instructor of Medicine, Boston University School of Medicine, Boston, Massachusetts; Director, Biliary Endoscopy, Deaconess–Waltham Hospital, Waltham, Massachusetts
Chronic Cholestatic Liver Disease

CARLO DILORENZO, M.D.
Associate Professor of Pediatrics, University of Pittsburgh; Associate Professor of Pediatrics, Division of Pediatric Gastroenterology, Children's Hospital of Pittsburgh, Pittsburgh, Pennsylvania
Foreign Bodies in Children

ANTHONY J. DIMARINO, JR., M.D.
Clinical Professor of Medicine, University of Pennsylvania; Chief, Division of Gastroenterology, Presbyterian Medical Center, Philadelphia, Pennsylvania
Diversion Colitis

ANDRE DUBOIS, M.D., PH.D.
Research Professor of Medicine and Surgery, Uniformed Services University of the Health Sciences, Bethesda, Maryland
Complications of Peptic Ulcer Disease

ELLEN C. EBERT, M.D.
Associate Professor of Medicine, Robert Wood Johnson Medical School and Gastroenterology Division, Department of Medicine, Robert Wood Johnson University Hospital, New Brunswick, New Jersey
Sclerosing Cholangitis

ATHENA ECONOMIDES, M.D.
Fellow in Training, University of California Los Angeles School of Medicine, Los Angeles, California
Foreign Bodies in Children

ARTHUR R. EULER, M.D.
Senior Director, Clinical Nutrition, Wyeth–Ayerst Research, Philadelphia, Pennsylvania
Gastrointestinal Tract Hemorrhage in Children

VIKTOR E. EYSSELEIN, M.D.
Associate Professor of Medicine, University of California Los Angeles School of Medicine, Los Angeles, California, and Harbor–University of California Los Angeles Medical Center, Torrance, California
Medical Management of Ulcerative Colitis

STEFANO FAGIUOLI, M.D.
Instructor and Transplant Physician, University of Padua, Padua, Italy
Liver Resection and Transplantation

FREDERICK FALLICK, M.D.
Clinical Assistant Professor of Medicine, New York Medical College, Valhalla, New York
Radiation Colitis

GIANRICO FARRUGIA, M.D.
Assistant Professor of Medicine and Physiology, Mayo Medical School; Senior Associate Consultant in Gastroenterology, Mayo Clinic, Rochester, Minnesota
Dyspepsia

KENNETH D. FINE, M.D.
Clinical Assistant Professor, University of Texas Southwestern Medical School; Associate Attending Physician, Internal Medicine, Gastroenterology, Baylor University Medical Center, Dallas, Texas
Diarrhea

ROBERT S. FISHER, M.D.
Professor of Medicine and Director, Functional Gastrointestinal Disease Center, Temple University School of Medicine; Chief, Gastroenterology Section, Temple University Hospital, Philadelphia, Pennsylvania
Gastroparesis

CONTRIBUTORS

PHILLIP R. FLESHNER, M.D.
Chief, Division of Colorectal Surgery, Cedars-Sinai Medical Center, Los Angeles, California
Anorectal Abscess

KENNETH D. FLORA, M.D.
Assistant Professor, Gastroenterology Division, Oregon Health Sciences University, Portland, Oregon
Clostridium difficile *Diarrhea*

ERIC W. FONKALSRUD, M.D.
Professor and Chief of Pediatric Surgery, University of California Los Angeles School of Medicine, Los Angeles, California
Complications of the Ileoanal Pullthrough Procedure and the Kock Continent Ileostomy

CHRIS E. FORSMARK, M.D.
Assistant Professor of Medicine and Chief, Diagnostic and Therapeutic Endoscopy, University of Florida College of Medicine, Gainesville, Florida
Chronic Pancreatitis

FRED C. FOWLER, M.D.
Attending Physician, University Hospital, Carolina Medical Center, and Presbyterian Hospital, Charlotte, North Carolina
Blind Loop Syndrome

STEVEN D. FREEDMAN, M.D., PH.D.
Assistant Professor of Medicine, Harvard Medical School; Associate Physician, Beth Israel Hospital, Boston, Massachusetts
Cancer of the Pancreas

MICHAEL W. FRIED, M.D.
Assistant Professor of Medicine, Division of Digestive Diseases, Emory University School of Medicine, Atlanta, Georgia
Ischemic Hepatitis

FRANK K. FRIEDENBERG, M.D.
Assistant Professor of Medicine, Temple University School of Medicine; Attending Physician, Division of Gastroenterology, Albert Einstein Medical Center, Philadelphia, Pennsylvania
Collagenous and Lymphocytic Colitis

DAVID L. GEIER, M.D.
Staff Physician, Smith-Glynn-Callaway Clinic, Springfield, Missouri
Hirschsprung's Disease

RALPH A. GIANNELLA, M.D.
Mark Brown Professor of Medicine and Director, Division of Digestive Diseases, University of Cincinnati College of Medicine, Cincinnati, Ohio
Invasive Pathogens

ROBERT G. GISH, M.D.
Assistant Clinical Professor, University of California Davis School of Medicine, Davis, California, and University of Nevada Reno School of Medicine, Reno, Nevada; Transplant Physician, California Pacific Medical Center, San Francisco, California
Short Bowel Syndrome

MICHAEL E. GLICK, M.D.
Instructor in Medicine, Harvard Medical School, Boston, Massachusetts; Gastroenterologist, Lahey Clinic Medical Center, Burlington, Massachusetts
Intestinal Obstruction

NORMAN D. GRACE, M.D.
Professor of Medicine, Tufts University School of Medicine; Chief of Gastroenterology, Faulkner Hospital, Boston, Massachusetts
Acute, Recurrent, and Chronic Appendicitis

RICHARD J. GRAND, M.D.
Professor of Pediatrics, Tufts University School of Medicine; Chief, Pediatric Gastroenterology and Nutrition, New England Medical Center, Boston, Massachusetts
Lactose Intolerance

LEOPOLDO GRAUER, M.D.
Assistant Professor of Medicine, University of Miami, Miami, Florida; Associate, Division of Gastroenterology, Mount Sinai Medical Center, Miami Beach, Florida
Gastrointestinal Fistulas

PERRY R. GRAY, M.D., F.R.C.S.C.
Assistant Professor of Surgery, University of Manitoba School of Medicine; Consultant, Intensive Care Unit, Director, Nutrition Support Service and Acute Care and Trauma Service, Health Sciences Center, Winnipeg, Manitoba, Canada
Fulminant Hepatic Failure

JACOB GREEN, M.D.
Associate Professor of Medicine, University of California Los Angeles School of Medicine; Director, Division of Nephrology, Cedars-Sinai Medical Center, Los Angeles, California
Hepatorenal Syndrome

JESSE GREEN, M.D.
Staff Physician and Gastroenterologist, St. Luke's Hospital and St. Elizabeth's Hospital, New York, New York, and Foxton Hospital, New Hartford, New York
Abdominal Abscesses

RICHARD L. GROTZ, M.D.
Clinical Instructor of Surgery, Tufts University School of Medicine, Boston, Massachusetts
Surgery for Ulcerative Colitis

SCOTT M. GRUNDY, M.D., PH.D.
Professor, Departments of Internal Medicine and Biochemistry, Chairman, Department of Clinical Nutrition, and Director, Center for Human Nutrition, University of Texas Southwestern Medical Center at Dallas, Dallas, Texas
Obesity

AHMET GURAKAR, M.D.
Staff Physician, Liver Transplant Medicine, Oklahoma Transplant Institute, Oklahoma City, Oklahoma
Liver Resection and Transplantation

DOUGLAS A. HALE, M.D.
Assistant Professor of Surgery, Uniformed Services University of the Health Sciences, Bethesda, Maryland; General Surgical Staff, Walter Reed Army Medical Center, Washington, D.C.
Complications of Peptic Ulcer Disease

RALPH R. HALL, M.D.
Associate Dean and Professor of Medicine, University of Missouri at Kansas City; Director of Medical Education, St. Lukes Hospital, Kansas City, Missouri
Carcinoid Tumors and Carcinoid Syndrome

KARL H. HANSON, M.D.
Clinical Associate Professor, University of Missouri Medical School at Kansas City; Staff Physician, St. Lukes Hospital, Kansas City, Missouri
Carcinoid Tumors and Carcinoid Syndrome

TAREK HASSANEIN, M.D.
Assistant Chief of Transplantation Medicine, Oklahoma Transplantation Institute, Baptist Medical Center of Oklahoma, Oklahoma City, Oklahoma
Liver Resection and Transplantation

J. EILEEN HAY, M.B., CH.B., F.R.C.P.
Assistant Professor of Medicine, Mayo Medical School; Consultant in Gastroenterology, Mayo Clinic, Rochester, Minnesota
Spontaneous Bacterial Peritonitis

JONATHAN R. HIATT, M.D.
Professor of Surgery, University of California Los Angeles School of Medicine; Director, Surgical Residency Program and Trauma Service, Cedars-Sinai Medical Center, Los Angeles, California
Anorectal Abscess

IVOR D. HILL, M.B., CH.B., M.D., F.C.P.
Professor of Pediatrics, University of Maryland School of Medicine; Clinical Director, Pediatric Gastroenterology and Nutrition, University of Maryland Hospital, Baltimore, Maryland
Hereditary Pancreatitis

CRAIG HILLEMEIER, M.D.
Professor of Pediatrics, Division of Pediatric Gastroenterology, University of Michigan Medical Center, Ann Arbor, Michigan
Gastroesophageal Reflux During Infancy and Childhood

CAROLYN J. HOLESKI, M.D., PH.D.
Fellow in Gastroenterology, Division of Gastrointestinal and Liver Diseases, University of Southern California School of Medicine, Los Angeles, California
Drug- and Toxin-induced Liver Injury

KEVIN J. HORGAN, M.B.
Assistant Professor, Department of Medicine, University of California Los Angeles School of Medicine, Los Angeles, California
Celiac Sprue

PAUL E. HYMAN, M.D.
Associate Clinical Professor of Pediatrics, University of California Los Angeles School of Medicine, Los Angeles, California; Director, Pediatric Gastrointestinal Motility Center, Children's Hospital of Orange County, Orange, California
Chronic Intestinal Pseudoobstruction in Childhood

ANDREW IPPOLITI, M.D.
Clinical Professor in Medicine/Gastroenterology, University of California Los Angeles Center for Health Sciences, Los Angeles, California
Gastroesophageal Reflux Disease

GERALD A. ISENBERG, M.D.
Assistant Clinical Professor of Surgery, Jefferson Medical College; Attending Surgeon, Thomas Jefferson University Hospital, Philadelphia, Pennsylvania
Anal Tumors

DANNY O. JACOBS, M.D., M.P.H.
Associate Professor of Surgery, Harvard Medical School; Associate Surgeon, Brigham and Women's Hospital, Boston, Massachusetts
Surgery for Peptic Ulcer Disease: For Whom and When

DENNIS M. JENSEN, M.D.
Professor of Medicine, University of California Los Angeles School of Medicine, Los Angeles, California
Gastrointestinal Tract Bleeding of Unknown Origin

ROBERT T. JENSEN, M.D.
Digestive Diseases Branch, National Institutes of Health, Bethesda, Maryland
Zollinger–Ellison Syndrome

ROME JUTABHA, M.D.
Assistant Professor of Medicine, Division of Digestive Diseases, University of California Los Angeles School of Medicine and Center for the Health Sciences; Staff Physician, West Los Angeles Veterans Administration Medical Center; Assistant Director, Center for Ulcer Research and Education (CURE) Clinic, Los Angeles, California
Gastrointestinal Tract Bleeding of Unknown Origin

MARSHALL M. KAPLAN, M.D.
Professor of Medicine, Tufts University School of Medicine; Chief, Division of Gastroenterology, New England Medical Center, Boston, Massachusetts
Chronic Cholestatic Liver Disease

FRANKLIN E. KASMIN, M.D.
Clinical Instructor, Mount Sinai School of Medicine; Attending Physician, Beth Israel Medical Center, New York, New York
Bile Duct Strictures

WILLIAM N. KATKOV, M.D.
Assistant Clinical Professor of Medicine, University of California Los Angeles School of Medicine, Los Angeles, California
Eosinophilic Gastroenteritis; Vascular Malformations of the Gastrointestinal Tract

CONTRIBUTORS

HERMAN KATTLOVE, M.D., M.P.H.
Assistant Clinical Professor of Medicine, University of California Los Angeles School of Medicine; National Medical Director, Salicknet, Inc., Los Angeles, California
Gastric Lymphoma

EMMET B. KEEFFE, M.D.
Professor of Medicine, Stanford University School of Medicine; Medical Director, Liver Transplant Program, and Chief of Clinical Gastroenterology, Stanford University Medical Center, Stanford, California
Short Bowel Syndrome; Hepatic Encephalopathy

KEITH A. KELLY, M.D.
Consultant in Surgery and Surgical Research, Mayo Clinic and Mayo Foundation, Mayo Clinic Scottsdale, Scottsdale, Arizona
Surgery for Ulcerative Colitis

PARDON R. KENNEY, M.D., M.M.SC.
Clinical Professor of Surgery, Tufts University School of Medicine; Chief of Surgery, Faulkner Hospital, Boston, Massachusetts
Acute, Recurrent, and Chronic Appendicitis

MYUNG-HWAN KIM, M.D., PH.D.
Senior Research Fellow, Division of Gastroenterology, Department of Medicine, University of Washington School of Medicine, Seattle, Washington
Cholelithiasis

DONALD F. KIRBY, M.D.
Associate Professor of Medicine and Chief, Section of Nutrition, Medical College of Virginia Hospitals, Richmond, Virginia
Malnutrition

KENNETH L. KOCH, M.D.
Professor of Medicine, Division of Gastroenterology, The Milton S. Hershey Medical Center, The Pennsylvania State University, Hershey, Pennsylvania
Gastric Volvulus

RAHUL KUVER, M.D.
Senior Fellow, Division of Gastroenterology, University of Washington School of Medicine, Seattle, Washington
Cholelithiasis

NICHOLAS F. LARUSSO, M.D.
Professor of Medicine and of Biochemistry and Molecular Biology, Mayo Medical School, Rochester, Minnesota
Hepatobiliary Complications of Ulcerative Colitis and Crohn's Disease

EMANUEL LEBENTHAL, M.D.
Professor, Hebrew University Medical School; Chairman, Department of Pediatrics, Hadassah University Hospital, Jerusalem, Israel
Hereditary Pancreatitis

SUM P. LEE, M.D., PH.D.
Professor of Medicine, Division of Gastroenterology, University of Washington School of Medicine, Seattle, Washington
Cholelithiasis

GLEN A. LEHMAN, M.D.
Professor of Medicine, Indiana University Medical Center, Indianapolis, Indiana
Tumors of the Gallbladder and Biliary Tract

FELIX W. LEUNG, M.D.
Associate Professor of Medicine in Residence, University of California Los Angeles School of Medicine, Los Angeles, California; Acting Director, Division of Gastroenterology, San Fernando Valley Program, Sepulveda Veterans Affairs Medical Center, Sepulveda, California, and Olive View Medical Center, Sylmar, California
Gastritis

JOSEPH W. LEUNG, M.D., F.R.C.P., F.A.C.G.
Professor of Medicine and Chief of Gastroenterology and Endoscopy, University of California Davis Medical Center, Sacramento, California
Acute Bacterial Cholangitis

GARY M. LEVINE, M.D.
Professor of Medicine, Temple University School of Medicine; Head, Division of Gastroenterology and Nutrition, Albert Einstein Medical Center, Philadelphia, Pennsylvania
Collagenous and Lymphocytic Colitis

MICHAEL LEVINSON, M.D.
Associate Professor of Medicine, University of Tennessee, Memphis, Tennessee
Intestinal Gas and Abdominal Bloating

ERIC D. LIBBY, M.D.
Assistant Professor of Medicine, Tufts University School of Medicine; Attending Physician, Division of Gastroenterology, New England Medical Center, Boston, Massachusetts
Acute Bacterial Cholangitis

KEITH D. LINDOR, M.D.
Associate Professor of Medicine, Mayo Medical Center, Rochester, Minnesota
Primary Biliary Cirrhosis

SIMON K. LO, M.D.
Associate Professor of Medicine, University of California Los Angeles School of Medicine, Los Angeles, California; Associate Chief of Gastroenterology and Director of Endoscopy, Harbor–University of California Los Angeles Medical Center, Torrance, California
Choledocholithiasis

WILLIAM B. LONG, M.D.
Associate Professor, University of Pennsylvania School of Medicine; Attending Physician, Hospital of the University of Pennsylvania, Philadelphia, Pennsylvania
Rapid Gastric Emptying

PETER F. MALET, M.D.
Associate Professor of Medicine, University of Pennsylvania School of Medicine; Chief, Gastroenterology Division, Veterans Affairs Medical Cen-

ter; Attending Physician, Hospital of the University of Pennsylvania, Philadelphia, Pennsylvania
Interferon Therapy for Chronic Viral Hepatitis B and C

JOHN R. MATHIAS, M.D.
Professor of Internal Medicine, The University of Texas Medical Branch at Galveston, Galveston, Texas
Toxigenic Diarrheas

RICHARD W. MCCALLUM, M.D.
Paul Janssen Professor of Medicine and Program Director, Division of Gastroenterology, Hepatology, and Nutrition, University of Virginia Health Sciences Center, Charlottesville, Virginia
Gastric Motor Disorders

JAMES H. MCKERROW, M.D., PH.D.
Professor of Pathology and Pharmaceutical Chemistry, Department of Pathology, University of California San Francisco; Chief of Pathology, Veterans Administration Hospital, San Francisco, California
Schistosomiasis

KENNETH R. MCQUAID, M.D.
Associate Professor of Clinical Medicine, University of California San Francisco; Director of Gastrointestinal Endoscopy, Veterans Affairs Medical Center, San Francisco, California
Rectal Foreign Bodies

MARK H. MELLOW, M.D.
Staff Physician, Baptist Medical Center; Associate Clinical Professor of Medicine, University of Oklahoma School of Medicine, Oklahoma City, Oklahoma
A Gastroenterologist's View of Chest Pain

CLIFFORD S. MELNYK, M.D.
Professor of Medicine and Head, Division of Gastroenterology, Oregon Health Sciences University, Portland, Oregon
Clostridium difficile *Diarrhea*

DAVID C. METZ, M.D.
Assistant Professor of Medicine and Co-Director, Gastrointestinal Physiology Laboratory, Division of Gastroenterology, University of Pennsylvania, and Hospital of the University of Pennsylvania, Philadelphia, Pennsylvania
Zollinger-Ellison Syndrome

PHILIP B. MINER, JR., M.D.
Professor of Medicine and Director, Division of Gastroenterology, University of Kansas Medical Center, Kansas City, Kansas
Hirschsprung's Disease

GERALD Y. MINUK, M.D., F.R.C.P.(C.)
Professor of Medicine and Pharmacology, University of Manitoba; Director, Liver Diseases Unit, Health Sciences Centre, Winnipeg, Manitoba, Canada
Fulminant Hepatic Failure

ROBERT K. MONTGOMERY, PH.D.
Associate Professor of Pediatrics, New England Medical Center and Tufts University School of Medicine; Assistant Professor (Joint Appointment), Department of Anatomy and Cellular Biology, Tufts University School of Medicine, Boston, Massachusetts
Lactose Intolerance

JOSEPH R. MURPHY, M.D.
Assistant Professor of Medicine, Uniformed Services University of the Health Sciences, Bethesda, Maryland; Assistant Chief, Gastroenterology Service, Walter Reed Army Medical Center, Washington, D.C.
Gastric Adenocarcinoma

VANDANA NEHRA, M.D.
Instructor of Medicine, Albert Einstein College of Medicine; Attending Physician in Gastroenterology, Bronx Municipal Hospital Center, Bronx, New York
Tropical Sprue: A Disappearing Enigma

DANIEL A. NG, M.D.
Fellow, Colon and Rectal Surgery, Ochsner Medical Foundation, New Orleans, Louisiana
Intestinal Obstruction

DAVID P. NUNES, M.B., M.R.C.P.I.
Assistant Professor of Medicine, Boston University School of Medicine and Section of Gastroenterology, Boston City Hospital, Boston, Massachusetts
Cholecystitis

CALVIN E. OLSON, M.D.
Practicing Gastroenterologist, Gould-Sutter Medical Foundation, Modesto, California
Pneumatosis Cystoides Intestinalis

ANN OUYANG, M.D.
Professor of Medicine, The Pennsylvania State University College of Medicine; Chief, Gastroenterology Division, The Milton S. Hershey Medical Center, Hershey, Pennsylvania
Solitary Ulcers of the Colon and Rectum

HENRY P. PARKMAN, M.D.
Assistant Professor of Medicine and Physiology, Temple University School of Medicine; Assistant Professor of Medicine and Director, Gastrointestinal Motility Laboratory, Temple University Hospital, Philadelphia, Pennsylvania
Achalasia; Gastroparesis

DILIP G. PATEL, F.R.C.P.(C.)
Associate Professor of Medicine, University of Ottawa; Active Attending Staff, Ottawa Civic Hospital, Ottawa, Ontario, Canada
Diverticular Disease of the Colon

JOHN H. PEMBERTON, M.D.
Professor of Surgery, Mayo Medical School; Consultant in Colon and Rectal Surgery and General Surgery, Mayo Clinic, Rochester, Minnesota
Surgery for Ulcerative Colitis

DAVID H. PERLMUTTER, M.D.
Professor of Pediatrics, Cell Biology and Physiology, Washington University School of Medicine; Director,

Division of Gastroenterology and Nutrition, Children's Hospital, St. Louis, Missouri
Alpha$_1$-Antitrypsin Deficiency

JEFFREY H. PETERS, M.D.
Assistant Professor of Surgery, University of Southern California School of Medicine; Chief, Division of General Surgery, University of Southern California University Hospital, Los Angeles, California
Hiatal Hernia

BRET T. PETERSEN, M.D.
Consultant in Gastroenterology and Assistant Professor of Medicine, Mayo Clinic and Mayo Graduate School of Medicine, Rochester, Minnesota
Chronic Cholecystitis

JOHN L. PETRINI, M.D.
Clinical Associate Professor of Medicine, University of Southern California, Los Angeles, California; Chief, Department of Gastroenterology, Sansum Medical Clinic, Santa Barbara, California
Acute Upper Gastrointestinal Tract Bleeding

CLAUS A. PIERACH, M.D.
Associate Professor of Medicine, University of Minnesota Medical School; Attending Physician, Abbott Northwestern Hospital, Minneapolis, Minnesota
Porphyria

EDWARD PIKEN, M.D.
Assistant Clinical Professor, Harbor General–University of California Los Angeles; Director of Gastroenterology, Torrance Memorial Hospital, Torrance, California
Pruritus Ani

HENRYK PLUTA, M.D.
Research Fellow, Department of Surgery, University of Alberta, Mackenzie Health Sciences Centre, Edmonton, Alberta, Canada
Toxic Megacolon

FRANK PROCACCINO, M.D.
Assistant Professor of Medicine, University of California Los Angeles School of Medicine, Los Angeles, California, and Harbor–Univeristy of California Los Angeles Department of Medicine, Torrance, California
Medical Management of Ulcerative Colitis

SOROYA M. RAHAMAN, M.D.
Brockton Hospital, Brockton, Massachusetts
Tumors of the Gallbladder and Biliary Tract

VONDA G. REEVES-DARBY, M.D.
Assistant Professor of Medicine, Division of Gastroenterology, Department of Internal Medicine, The University of Texas Medical Branch, Galveston, Texas
Toxigenic Diarrheas

JAMES C. REYNOLDS, M.D.
Associate Professor, University of Pittsburgh School of Medicine; Chief, Division of Gastroenterology and Hepatology, University of Pittsburgh Medical Center, Pittsburgh, Pennsylvania
Chronic Constipation

DAVID G. RIMER, M.D.
Clinical Professor of Medicine, University of California Los Angeles Center for the Health Sciences, Los Angeles, California
Obstructing Esophageal Disease

DAVID J. ROBERTS, M.D., M.C.
Lieutenant Commander, National Naval Medical Center, Bethesda, Maryland
Irritable Bowel Syndrome and Diarrhea

ARVEY I. ROGERS, M.D.
Professor of Medicine and Chief, Gastroenterology Division, University of Miami School of Medicine; Chief, Gastroenterology Section, Veterans Affairs Medical Center, Miami, Florida
Abdominal Abscesses

SUZANNE ROSE, M.D.
Assistant Professor of Medicine, University of Pittsburgh School of Medicine and University of Pittsburgh Medical Center, Pittsburgh, Pennsylvania
Fecal Incontinence

IRWIN H. ROSENBERG, M.D.
Professor of Medicine and Nutrition, Tufts University School of Medicine and School of Nutrition; Director, Jean Mayer United States Department of Agriculture Human Nutrition Research Center on Aging at Tufts University; Chief, Division of Clinical Nutrition, New England Medical Center, Boston, Massachusetts
Vitamin Deficiency

PHILIP ROSENTHAL, M.D.
Professor of Pediatrics and Surgery, Director of Pediatric Hepatology, and Medical Director, Pediatric Liver Transplant Program, University of California San Francisco Medical Center, San Francisco, California
Neonatal Hepatitis and Cholestasis

ROBIN D. ROTHSTEIN, M.D.
Assistant Professor of Medicine, University of Pennsylvania, Philadelphia, Pennsylvania
Rapid Gastric Emptying; Solitary Ulcers of the Colon and Rectum

ROBERT H. SCHAPIRO, M.D.
Associate Clinical Professor of Medicine, Harvard Medical School; Physician and Director of Gastrointestinal Endoscopy, Massachusetts General Hospital, Boston, Massachusetts
Eosinophilic Gastroenteritis

LAWRENCE R. SCHILLER, M.D.
Clinical Associate Professor of Internal Medicine, University of Texas Southwestern Medical School; Director, Gastrointestinal Physiology Laboratory, and Attending Physician, Baylor University Medical Center, Dallas, Texas
Diarrhea

MICHAEL L. SCHILSKY, M.D.
Assistant Professor of Medicine, Albert Einstein College of Medicine, Bronx, New York
Wilson's Disease

STEVEN D. SEAGREN, M.D.
Fellow, Gastroenterology, University of Nebraska Medical Center, Omaha, Nebraska
Hepatic Tumors

STEPHEN R. SEVERANCE, M.D.
Associate Clinical Professor of Medicine, University of California Irvine, Irvine, California; Gastroenterologist, Long Beach Memorial Hospital, Long Beach, California
Endometriosis: A Gastroenterologist's Perspective

REZA SHAKER, M.D.
Associate Professor of Medicine and Radiology and Assistant Professor of Surgery (Otolaryngology and Human Communications), Medical College of Wisconsin; Director, Medical College of Wisconsin Dysphagia Institute; Chief, Gastrointestinal Diagnostic Unit, Veterans Affairs Medical Center; Attending Physician, Froedtert Memorial Lutheran Hospital, Milwaukee, Wisconsin
Disorders of the Upper Sphincter and Proximal Esophagus

FERGUS SHANAHAN, M.D.
Professor of Medicine, National University of Ireland and Cork University Hospital, Cork, Ireland
Active Crohn's Disease

STUART SHERMAN, M.D.
Assistant Professor of Medicine, Indiana University School of Medicine, Indianapolis, Indiana
Choledochal Cysts

JEROME H. SIEGEL, M.D.
Assistant Clinical Professor of Medicine, Mount Sinai School of Medicine; Chief of Endoscopy, Beth Israel Medical Center, North Division, New York, New York
Bile Duct Strictures

ROBERT W. SJOGREN, M.D.
Assistant Professor of Medicine, Georgetown University School of Medicine, Washington, D.C.; Staff Gastroenterologist, Kaiser Permanente Medical Center, Falls Church, Virginia
Infectious Colitis

BENJAMIN N. SMITH, M.D.
Assistant Professor of Medicine, Tufts University School of Medicine; Attending Physician, Department of Gastroenterology, Faulkner Hospital, Boston, Massachusetts
Acute, Recurrent, and Chronic Appendicitis

THOMAS P. SOKOL, M.D.
Assistant Clinical Professor of Surgery, University of California Los Angeles; Chief of Division of Colon and Rectal Surgery, Cedars-Sinai Medical Center; Chief of Surgery, Century City Hospital, Los Angeles, California
Anal Fissure

MARSHALL SPARBERG, M.D.
Professor of Clinical Medicine, Northwestern University Medical School; Attending Physician, Northwestern Memorial Hospital, Chicago, Illinois
Nonneoplastic Polyps

MONROE H. SPECTOR, M.D.
Clinical Professor of Medicine, University of New Mexico School of Medicine; Attending Physician, Presbyterian and Saint Joseph's Hospitals, Albuquerque, New Mexico
Gastric Polyps

BRIAN SPIVACK, M.D.
Clinical Instructor, University of Southern California, Los Angeles, California; Staff Surgeon, Wilshire Oncology Medical Group, San Gabriel, California
Esophageal Tumors

BRUCE E. STABILE, M.D.
Professor of Surgery, University of California Los Angeles, Los Angeles, California; Chairman, Department of Surgery, Harbor–University of California Los Angeles Medical Center, Torrance, California
Chronic Intestinal Ischemic Syndrome

MICHAEL L. STEER, M.D.
Professor of Surgery, Harvard Medical School; Chief of General Surgery and Associate Surgeon-in-Chief, Beth Israel Hospital, Boston, Massachusetts
Cancer of the Pancreas

IRMIN STERNLIEB, M.D.
Professor of Medicine, Emeritus, National Center for the Study of Wilson's Disease, St. Lukes–Roosevelt Medical Center, New York, New York
Wilson's Disease

EUGENE SUN, M.D.
Associate Medical Director, Abbott Laboratories, Abbott Park, Illinois
Schistosomiasis

CHRISTINA M. SURAWICZ, M.D.
Associate Professor of Medicine, University of Washington School of Medicine; Chief, Division of Gastroenterology, Harborview Medical Center, Seattle, Washington
Infectious Proctitis in the Immunocompetent

R. SCOTT SYKES, M.D.
Medical Director, Glaxo, Incorporated, Research Triangle Park, North Carolina
Gastrointestinal Tract Hemorrhage in Children

W. GRANT THOMPSON, M.D., F.R.C.P.C.
Professor of Medicine, University of Ottawa; Chief of Division of Gastroenterology, Ottawa Civic Hospital, Ottawa, Ontario, Canada
Diverticular Disease of the Colon

RICHARD W. TOBIN, M.D.
Clinical Instructor, University of Washington and University Hospital, Seattle, Washington
Infectious Proctitis in the Immunocompetent

CONTRIBUTORS

EDWARD P. TOFFOLON, M.D.
Associate Clinical Professor of Medicine, University of Connecticut School of Medicine, Farmington, Connecticut; Chief of Gastroenterology, New Britain General Hospital, New Britain, Connecticut
Ascites

ANTHONY S. TORNAY, JR., M.D.
Co-Director, Gastrointestinal Laboratory, Eisenhower Medical Center, Rancho Mirage, California
Amebic Abscess

PHILLIP P. TOSKES, M.D.
Professor of Medicine and Vice Chairman for Clinical Affairs, Department of Medicine, and Chief, Division of Gastroenterology, Hepatology and Nutrition, University of Florida, Gainesville, Florida
Chronic Pancreatitis

MARK UHL, M.D.
Fellow in Gastroenterology, University of Kansas Medical Center, Kansas City, Kansas
Malabsorption Syndromes

JORGE E. VALENZUELA, M.D.
Emeritus Professor of Medicine, University of Southern California, Los Angeles, California; Gastroenterology Consultant, Clinica Los Condes, Santiago, Chile
Acute Pancreatitis

ROSALIND U. VAN STOLK, M.D.
Clinical Assistant Professor of Medicine, Pennsylvania State University, Hershey, Pennsylvania; Assistant Professor of Medicine, Ohio State University; Director, Center for Colon Polyps and Colon Cancer, Department of Gastroenterology, Cleveland Clinic Foundation, Cleveland, Ohio
Benign Tumors of the Small Bowel

DAVID H. VAN THIEL, M.D.
Medical Director of Transplantation, Baptist Medical Center of Oklahoma, Oklahoma City, Oklahoma
Liver Resection and Transplantation

ARNOLD WALD, M.D.
Professor of Medicine, University of Pittsburgh School of Medicine; Associate Chief, Division of Gastroenterology and Hepatology, University of Pittsburgh Medical Center, Pittsburgh, Pennsylvania
Fecal Incontinence

ALAIN WATIER, M.D., L.M.C.C., F.R.C.P.
Clinical Professor of Gastroenterology, Centre Hospitalier Universitaire de Sherbrooke; Faculte de Medicine, Université de Sherbrooke, Sherbrooke, Quebec, Canada
Slow Transit Constipation

IRVING WAXMAN, M.D.
Instructor in Medicine, Harvard Medical School; Director of Therapeutic Endoscopy, Beth Israel Hospital, Boston, Massachusetts
Cancer of the Pancreas

FREDERICK H. WEBER, M.D.
Attending Gastroenterologist, Memorial Medical Center, St. Joseph's Hospital, and Candler General Hospital, Savannah, Georgia
Gastric Motor Disorders

WILLIAM E. WHITEHEAD, PH.D.
Research Professor of Medicine, Adjunct Professor of Psychology, and Chief, Gastrointestinal Physiology Laboratory, University of North Carolina at Chapel Hill, Chapel Hill, North Carolina
Functional Abdominal Pain

JOHN W. WILEY, M.D.
Associate Professor of Internal Medicine, University of Michigan Medical Center, Ann Arbor, Michigan
Irritable Bowel Syndrome and Diarrhea

ROBERT F. WILLENBUCHER, M.D.
Assistant Professor of Medicine, University of California San Francisco School of Medicine; Director, Center for Inflammatory Bowel Disease, University of California San Francisco–Mount Zion Medical Center, San Francisco, California
Irritable Bowel Syndrome and Constipation

CHRISTOPHER WILLIAMS, M.D.
FHP of Utah, Incorporated, Salt Lake City, Utah
Chronic Constipation

RUSSELL A. WILLIAMS, M.D.
Professor and Vice Chairman, Director, Surgery Training Program, and Section Chief, Gastrointesinal Surgery, University of California Irvine, Irvine, California; Staff Surgeon, Vascular Surgery Section, Long Beach Veterans Administration Medical Center, Long Beach, California
Intestinal Obstruction

SAMUEL ERIC WILSON, M.D.
Professor of Surgery, University of California Irvine, Irvine, California; Chairman, Department of Surgery, University of California Irvine Medical Center, Orange, California
Esophageal Tumors

DAVID C. WOLF, M.D.
Assistant Professor of Medicine, Division of Liver Diseases, Department of Medicine, Mount Sinai School of Medicine, New York, New York
Invasive Pathogens

FLORENCE WONG, M.D., F.R.A.C.P.
Senior Research Fellow, The Toronto Hospital, Toronto, Ontario, Canada
Alcoholic Liver Disease

HARLAN I. WRIGHT, M.D.
Attending Physician in Transplantation Medicine, Hepatology, Oklahoma Transplant Institute, Baptist Medical Center, Oklahoma City, Oklahoma
Liver Resection and Transplantation

JOEL YAGER, M.D.
Professor of Psychiatry and Associate Chair for Education, University of California Los Angeles

School of Medicine; Director of Residency Education, University of California Los Angeles Neuropsychiatric Institute and Veterans Administration West Los Angeles Medical Center, Los Angeles, California
Eating Disorders

RUSSELL D. YANG, M.D., PH.D.
Assistant Professor of Medicine, University of Southern California School of Medicine; Co-Director, University of Southern California Center for Pancreatic and Biliary Diseases; Chief of Gastroenterology and Endoscopy, Los Angeles Veterans Administration Out-Patient Clinic; Attending Physician, Norris Cancer Hospital and University of Southern California and Los Angeles County Medical Center, Los Angeles, California
Acute Pancreatitis

ROBERT T. YAVORSKI, M.D.
Assistant Professor of Medicine, Uniformed Services University for the Health Sciences, Bethesda, Maryland; Staff Gastroenterologist, Walter Reed Army Medical Center, Washington, D.C.
Infectious Colitis

ROWEN K. ZETTERMAN, M.D.
Professor of Internal Medicine, University of Nebraska Medical Center, Omaha, Nebraska
Hepatic Tumors

GARY R. ZUCKERMAN, D.O.
Associate Professor of Medicine, Division of Gastroenterology, Washington University School of Medicine; Associate Physician and Director of Endoscopy, Digestive Disease Clinical Center, Barnes Hospital, St. Louis, Missouri
Gastric Ulcers

PLATE I

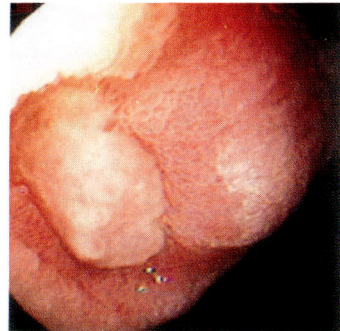

FIGURE 20–2. Benign ulcer with clean white base. Ulcers with this appearance rarely rebleed.

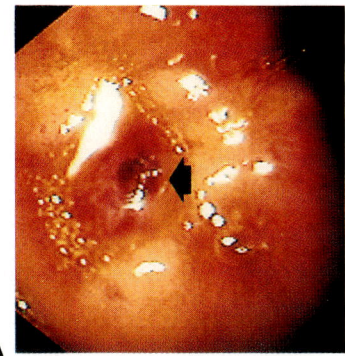
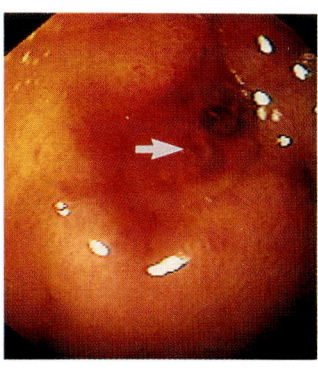

FIGURE 20–3. Benign ulcer with visible vessel. **A,** The ulcer has a small, red, raised area *(black arrow)*. **B,** After the clot is washed off the vessel, a small, circular vessel wall can be seen *(white arrow)*. The vessel subsequently rebled and required endoscopic cauterization for control.

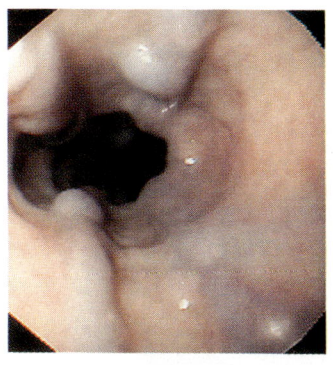
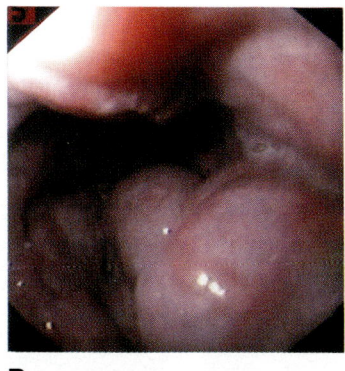
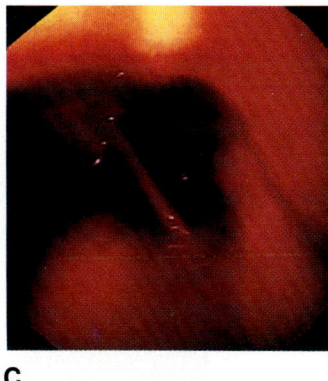

FIGURE 20–5. Varices. **A,** Grade II varices, without evidence of red color signs. The dilated submucosal vessels can be seen running longitudinally in the esophagus. **B,** Grade IV varices with near occlusion of the esophageal lumen with dilated submucosal veins and red color signs, which represent dilated mucosal vessels. **C,** Bleeding esophageal varix. This is the usual sight greeting endoscopists in active variceal hemorrhage.

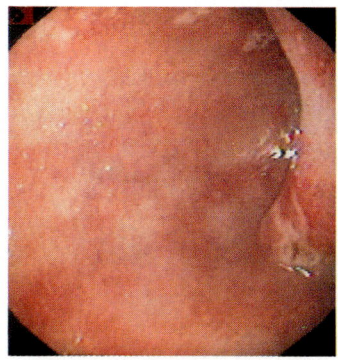
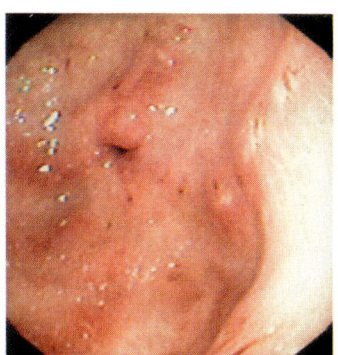

FIGURE 20–7. Nonsteroidal antiinflammatory drug (NSAID) erosions. **A,** Small prepyloric erosions can be seen extending radially from the pylorus. **B,** Antral view showing erosions from aspirin use.

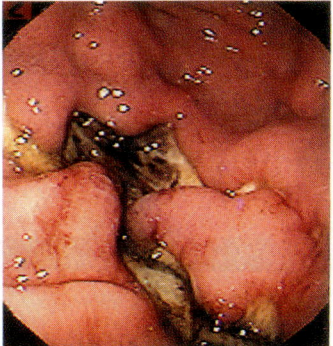

FIGURE 20–8. Stress ulceration. Large areas of the gastric mucosa have been ulcerated in this patient with head trauma. The ulcers have a white base with bloody residue that has been reduced by stomach acid to a black mucoid material.

PLATE II

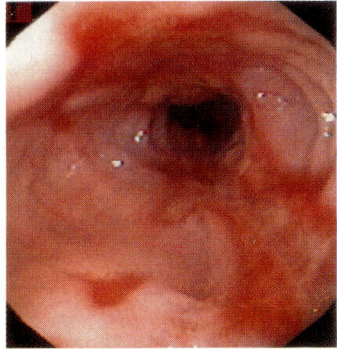
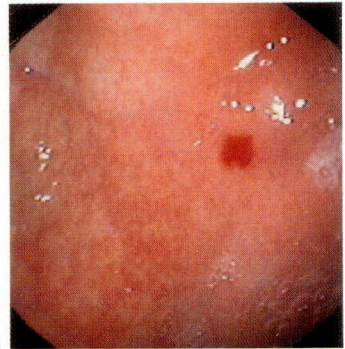
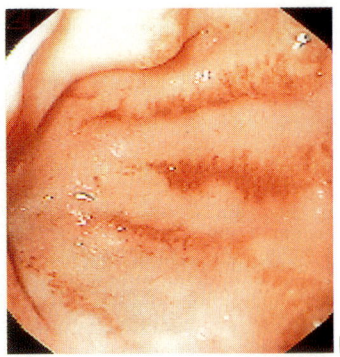

FIGURE 20-9. Peptic esophagitis. Two linear erosions are seen leading to a stricture in the distal esophagus in this patient with severe reflux disease.

FIGURE 20-10. A, Vascular ectasia. Small, cherry red lesions in the gastric mucosa are occasionally the source of significant hemorrhage. They are rarely a source of acute, severe bleeding and are more likely to be a source of chronic blood loss. **B,** Gastric antral vascular ectasia ("watermelon stomach"). These linear vascular lesions are a source of chronic blood loss from the antrum and can be eliminated by endoscopic cautery.

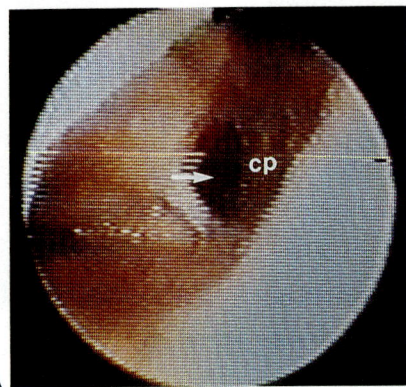
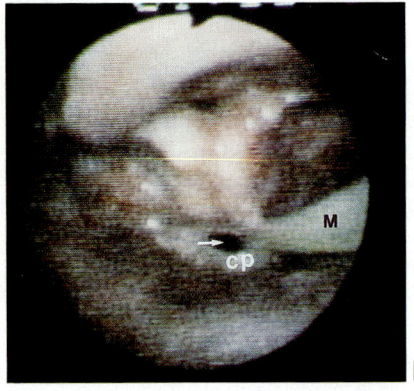

FIGURE 25-6. Still frame from videoendoscopic recordings of upper esophageal sphincter (UES) opening during swallowing **(A)** and belching **(B).** As seen, the UES opening *(arrow)* during swallowing is round, whereas during belching it is triangular. This difference in shape is believed to be due to the difference in the direction toward which the cricopharyngeal muscle is pulled open. cp = cricopharyngeal muscle, M = manometric catheter.

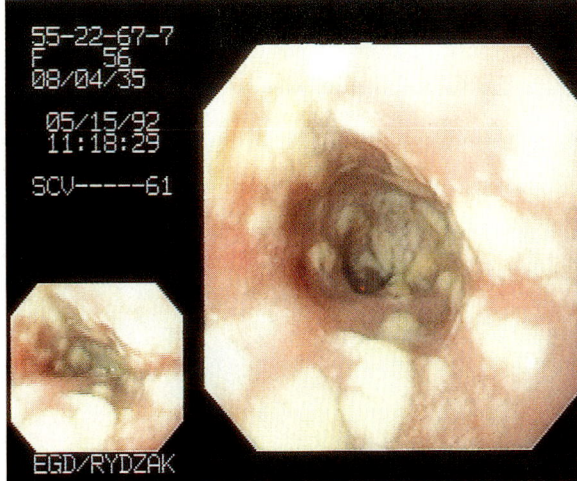
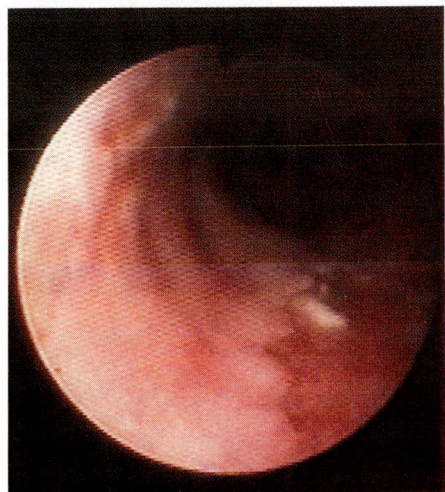

FIGURE 33-1. *Candida* esophagitis in a 26-year-old patient with AIDS.

FIGURE 33-2. Esophageal ulcer in a 22-year-old receiving chemotherapy for central nervous system malignancy.

PLATE III

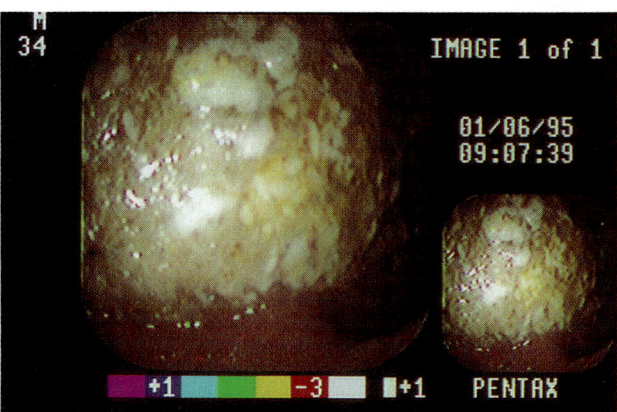

FIGURE 38–1. A phytobezoar seen 1 year after a Billroth I gastrectomy. It is composed of mucus and vegetable material and filled one third of the gastric pouch.

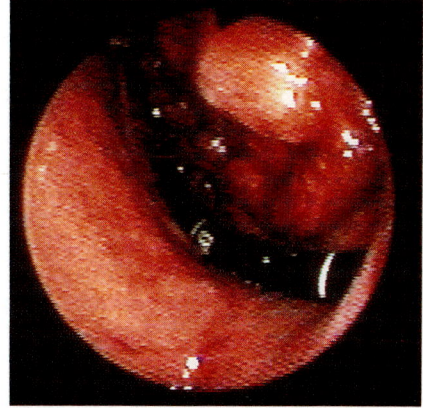

FIGURE 40–1. A retroflex view of a 5-cm mass in the cardia of the stomach with central ulceration, which on biopsy confirmed the diagnosis as adenocarcinoma.

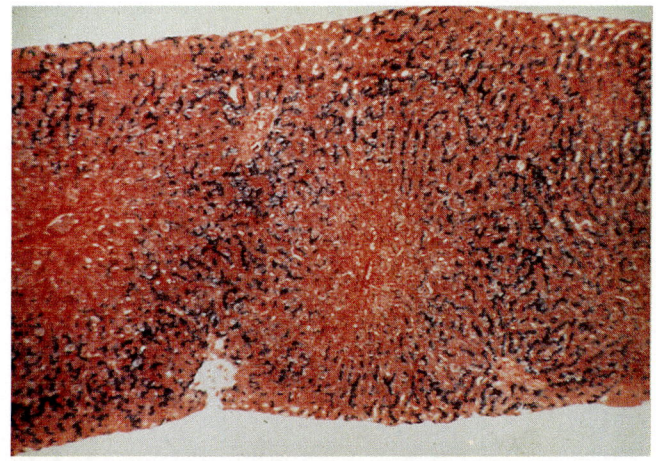

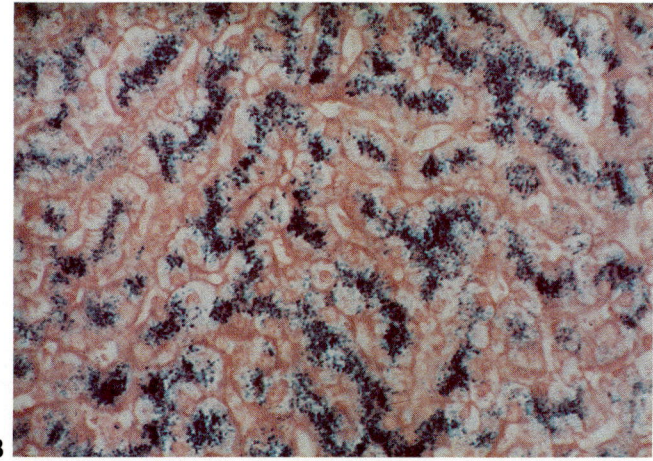

FIGURE 113–1. Liver biopsy in hereditary hemochromatosis. A 32-year-old white man presented with an elevated serum iron on routine screening. Transferrin saturation was 83%, and serum ferritin was 1485 µg/ml. **A,** A percutaneous liver biopsy was performed and shows increased stainable iron in a periportal distribution (lower power). **B,** At higher power, iron deposition is virtually all in parenchymal cells (Perls' Prussian blue stain). The hepatic iron concentration was 8355 µg/g with a calculated hepatic iron index of 4.66.

PLATE IV

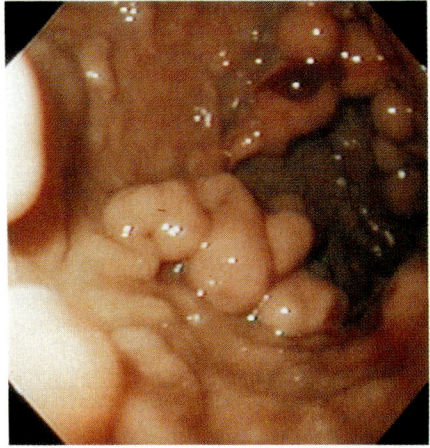

FIGURE 59–5. Multiple polypoid masses in the duodenum of a patient with Brunner's gland lesions. (Courtesy G. Falk, MD.)

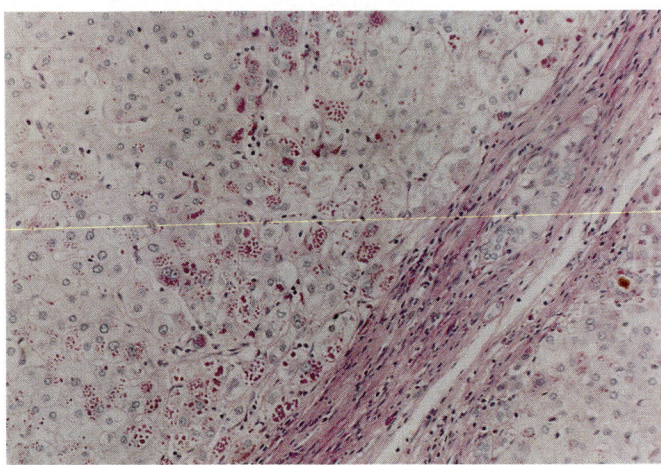

FIGURE 111–2. A, Photomicrograph of a liver biopsy in α_1AT deficiency (periodic acid–Schiff [PAS], diastase stain; magnification ×40) demonstrating PAS-positive, diastase-resistant globules in hepatocytes, especially periportal and adjacent to a broad band of fibrous tissues. (Courtesy Dr. C. Coffin, St. Louis, Mo.; reproduced with permission from Perlmutter DH. Alpha-1 AT deficiency. In: Suchy FJ, ed. *Liver Disease in Children*. St. Louis, Mo: Mosby–Year Book; 1994:697.)

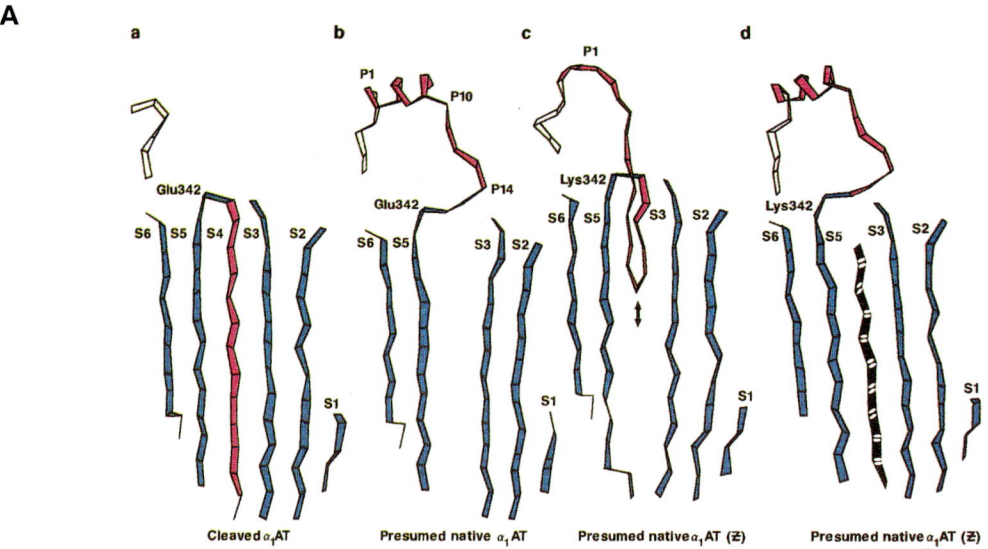

FIGURE 111–3. Schematic diagram of the A-sheet and reactive-site loop of α_1AT in **(a)** the cleaved conformation, in **(b)** presumed native conformation (based on the structure of ovalbumin), in **(c)** the presumed native conformation for the mutant (Z) α_1AT protein before insertion of synthetic peptide, and in **(d)** the presumed native (Z) α_1AT protein after insertion of the synthetic peptide. The reactive-site loop is shown in red, the β-helixes of the A-sheet in blue, the carboxyl terminal portion of the reactive-site loop in white, and a synthetic peptide that might insert into the gap in the A-sheet in black. (Adapted from Carrell RW, Evans DL, Stein PE. Mobile reactive centre of serpins and the control of thrombosis. *Nature*. 1991;353:576–578 and Lomas DA, Evans DL, Finch JJ, Carrell RW. The mechanism of Z alpha-1-antitrypsin accumulation in the liver. *Nature*. 1992;357:605–607 with permission.)

Preface

It has been an exciting experience to work on *Consultations in Gastroenterology*. Each chapter is written by an author who is an expert on the disease process covered. My aim when planning the book was to provide therapeutic advice on the broad field of gastrointestinal diseases. After reading each chapter many times, I believe the consultative authors succeeded by writing interesting and succinct commentaries on the treatment of gastrointestinal diseases.

The prospective reader of this volume may ask the importance of yet a new book covering gastroenterology. Patient therapy is the main thrust of this book. Pathogenesis and diagnosis are discussed only to bolster the rationale for successful therapy. It is my hope that this volume provides current treatment strategies for most if not all gastrointestinal diseases and symptom complexes encountered. Key references are included for the reader who requires in-depth discussion of disease pathogenesis or methods of diagnosis to treat the individual patient. The chapters are presented in an easy to read style, providing algorithms for therapy where appropriate. *Consultations in Gastroenterology* should fill the niche between multivolume encyclopedic reviews of disease processes and the "how-to" manuals for treatment.

It is important for the practicing physician to keep up with changes in therapy in the rapidly changing field of gastroenterology, since treatment strategies have changed for many diseases. Continuing hepatic inflammation from chronic hepatitis B and C can be stopped with interferon rather than corticosteroids. The parameters for liver transplantation, now part of the therapeutic armamentarium for end-stage cirrhosis, are updated. Healing of a duodenal ulcer requires eradication of *Helicobacter pylori* from the gastric mucosa as well as inhibition of acid production. These examples are just a few of the many changes that have occurred in the treatment of gastrointestinal diseases over the past 5 years.

The explosion of new information makes it difficult for the generalist to determine the best course of action. In light of this, *Consultations in Gastroenterology* is designed to sit by the generalist's hand and provide guidance for the care of the patient. The treatment protocols used by the experts in the care of different diseases of the gastrointestinal tract will direct the physician to the most efficient therapy. In an era of cost containment, effective treatment early in the patient's course of illness is not only the best therapy but also the least expensive.

This book would not have been possible without the editorial support of Richard Zorab and Andrea Cox of W.B. Saunders Company, who kept me and the chapter authors always moving forward. I thank my wife, Margie, for her support during the times that the editorial chores became consuming. Finally, I thank the authors who have provided the excellent reviews of current therapy.

William J. Snape, Jr., M.D.

Contents

Section I
GENERAL 1

1. **Obesity** 3
   Joyce P. Barnett and Scott M. Grundy
2. **Eating Disorders** 9
   Joel Yager
3. **Malnutrition** 16
   Donald F. Kirby and Mark H. DeLegge
4. **Vitamin Deficiency** 22
   Maria E. Camilo and Irwin H. Rosenberg
5. **Caustic Injury to the Upper Gastrointestinal Tract** 30
   William M. Battle and Mark S. Codella
6. **Rectal Foreign Bodies** 36
   Marta L. Davila and Kenneth R. McQuaid
7. **Foreign Bodies in Children** 41
   Carlo DiLorenzo and Athena Economides
8. **Nausea and Vomiting** 47
   Manley Cohen
9. **Dyspepsia** 57
   Gianrico Farrugia and Michael Camilleri
10. **Functional Abdominal Pain** 61
    William E. Whitehead
11. **Intestinal Gas and Abdominal Bloating** 70
    Michael Levinson
12. **Malabsorption Syndromes** 75
    Mark Uhl and Allan R. Cooke
13. **Protein-losing Gastroenteropathy** ... 84
    George W. Bo-Linn
14. **Diarrhea** 87
    Kenneth D. Fine and Lawrence R. Schiller
15. **Fecal Incontinence** 95
    Suzanne Rose and Arnold Wald
16. **Chronic Constipation** 100
    James C. Reynolds and Christopher Williams
17. **Intestinal Obstruction** 108
    Daniel A. Ng and Russell A. Williams
18. **Abdominal Abscesses** 117
    Arvey I. Rogers and Jesse Green
19. **Gastrointestinal Fistulas** 121
    Leopoldo Grauer and Jamie S. Barkin
20. **Acute Upper Gastrointestinal Tract Bleeding** 126
    John L. Petrini
21. **Acute Lower Gastrointestinal Tract Bleeding** 139
    Alan R. Bank and Stanley B. Benjamin
22. **Gastrointestinal Tract Hemorrhage in Children** 145
    Arthur R. Euler and R. Scott Sykes
23. **Gastrointestinal Tract Bleeding of Unknown Origin** 155
    Rome Jutabha and Dennis M. Jensen

Section II
ESOPHAGUS 169

24. **A Gastroenterologist's View of Chest Pain** 171
    Mark H. Mellow
25. **Disorders of the Upper Sphincter and Proximal Esophagus** 177
    Reza Shaker
26. **Achalasia** 186
    Henry P. Parkman and Sidney Cohen
27. **Motor Disorders of the Esophagus** . 193
    Ray E. Clouse
28. **Gastroesophageal Reflux Disease** .. 201
    Andrew Ippoliti
29. **Gastroesophageal Reflux During Infancy and Childhood** 207
    Craig Hillemeier
30. **Hiatal Hernia** 211
    Jeffrey H. Peters and Tom R. DeMeester

31 **Esophageal Tumors** 218
Brian Spivack and Samuel Eric Wilson

32 **Obstructing Esophageal Disease** . . . 224
David G. Rimer

33 **Esophageal Infections** 237
Donald P. Brannan and Eugene Michael Bozymski

SECTION III
STOMACH 245

34 **Gastric Motor Disorders** 247
Frederick H. Weber and Richard W. McCallum

35 **Rapid Gastric Emptying** 259
Robin D. Rothstein and William B. Long

36 **Gastric Outlet Obstruction** 264
Miles Auslander

37 **Gastroparesis** 269
Henry P. Parkman and Robert S. Fisher

38 **Bezoars** 280
Thomas J. Devers

39 **Gastric Volvulus** 283
Rafael A. Amaral and Kenneth L. Koch

40 **Gastric Adenocarcinoma** 289
Joseph R. Murphy

41 **Gastric Lymphoma** 296
Herman Kattlove

42 **Gastric Polyps** 300
Monroe H. Spector

43 **Carcinoid Tumors and Carcinoid Syndrome** 305
Ralph R. Hall and Karl H. Hanson

44 **Gastric Ulcers** 312
Gary R. Zuckerman and Giuseppe Aliperti

45 **Gastritis** 317
Felix W. Leung

46 **Zollinger-Ellison Syndrome** 322
David C. Metz and Robert T. Jensen

47 **Complications of Peptic Ulcer Disease** 335
Douglas A. Hale and Andre Dubois

48 **Surgery for Peptic Ulcer Disease: For Whom and When** 345
Danny O. Jacobs and James M. Becker

SECTION IV
INTESTINAL TRACT 357

49 **Eosinophilic Gastroenteritis** 359
William N. Katkov and Robert H. Schapiro

50 **Lactose Intolerance** 362
Richard J. Grand, Robert K. Montgomery, and Hans A. Büller

51 **Celiac Sprue** 367
Kevin J. Horgan

52 **Toxigenic Diarrheas** 372
Vonda G. Reeves-Darby and John R. Mathias

53 **Invasive Pathogens** 381
David C. Wolf and Ralph A. Giannella

54 **Schistosomiasis** 388
Eugene Sun and James H. McKerrow

55 **Tropical Sprue: A Disappearing Enigma** 394
Leslie H. Bernstein and Vandana Nehra

56 **Blind Loop Syndrome** 398
Fred C. Fowler and James J. Cerda

57 ***Clostridium difficile* Diarrhea** 403
Kenneth D. Flora and Clifford S. Melnyk

58 **Active Crohn's Disease** 408
Fergus Shanahan

59 **Benign Tumors of the Small Bowel** . 414
Carol Ann Burke and Rosalind U. van Stolk

60 **Vascular Malformations of the Gastrointestinal Tract** 424
William N. Katkov

61 **Radiation Colitis** 430
Frederick Fallick and Robert Burakoff

62 **Chronic Intestinal Ischemic Syndrome** 433
Christian de Virgilio and Bruce E. Stabile

63 **Chronic Intestinal Pseudoobstruction in Adults** 438
Sinn Anuras and Jitra Anuras

64 **Chronic Intestinal Pseudoobstruction in Childhood** . . . 448
Paul E. Hyman

65 **Short Bowel Syndrome** 457
Robert G. Gish and Emmet B. Keeffe

66 **Acute, Recurrent, and Chronic Appendicitis** 462
Benjamin N. Smith, Norman D. Grace, and Pardon R. Kenney

67 Hirschsprung's Disease 470
David L. Geier and Philip B. Miner, Jr.

68 Slow Transit Constipation 478
Alain Watier and Ghislain Devroede

69 Intestinal Obstruction 490
Michael E. Glick

70 Irritable Bowel Syndrome and Constipation 496
Robert F. Willenbucher

71 Irritable Bowel Syndrome and Diarrhea 502
David J. Roberts and John W. Wiley

72 Diverticular Disease of the Colon .. 510
Dilip G. Patel and W. Grant Thompson

73 Medical Management of Ulcerative Colitis 514
Frank Procaccino and Viktor E. Eysselein

74 Surgery for Ulcerative Colitis 524
Richard L. Grotz, John H. Pemberton, and Keith A. Kelly

75 Toxic Megacolon 534
Henryk Pluta and Kenneth L. Bowes

76 Infectious Colitis 537
Robert T. Yavorski and Robert W. Sjogren

77 Nonneoplastic Polyps 546
Marshall Sparberg

78 Complications of the Ileoanal Pullthrough Procedure and the Kock Continent Ileostomy 548
Eric W. Fonkalsrud

79 Anal Fissure 550
Thomas P. Sokol

80 Anorectal Abscess 560
Phillip R. Fleshner and Jonathan R. Hiatt

81 Pruritus Ani 567
Edward Piken

82 Anal Tumors 570
Gerald A. Isenberg

83 Endometriosis: A Gastroenterologist's Perspective . 573
Stephen R. Severance and C. Gregory Albers

84 Pneumatosis Cystoides Intestinalis . 580
Calvin E. Olson

85 Solitary Ulcers of the Colon and Rectum 584
Robin D. Rothstein and Ann Ouyang

86 Diversion Colitis 590
Paul J. DeMartino and Anthony J. DiMarino, Jr.

87 Collagenous and Lymphocytic Colitis 595
Frank K. Friedenberg and Gary M. Levine

88 Infectious Proctitis in the Immunocompetent 600
Richard W. Tobin and Christina M. Surawicz

Section V
PANCREAS 611

89 Hereditary Pancreatitis 613
Ivor D. Hill and Emanuel Lebenthal

90 Acute Pancreatitis 620
Russell D. Yang and Jorge E. Valenzuela

91 Chronic Pancreatitis 630
Chris E. Forsmark and Phillip P. Toskes

92 Cancer of the Pancreas 635
Irving Waxman, Steven D. Freedman, and Michael L. Steer

Section VI
HEPATOBILIARY TRACT 641

93 Drug- and Toxin-induced Liver Injury 643
Carolyn J. Holeski and Laurie D. DeLeve

94 Hepatic Encephalopathy 653
Emmet B. Keeffe

95 Acute Hepatitis 659
Albert J. Czaja

96 Interferon Therapy for Chronic Viral Hepatitis B and C 665
Peter F. Malet

97 Fulminant Hepatic Failure 675
Gerald Y. Minuk and Perry R. Gray

98 Ischemic Hepatitis 690
Michael W. Fried

99 Hepatorenal Syndrome 695
Jacob Green

100 Alcoholic Liver Disease 707
Florence Wong and Laurence Blendis

101 Variceal Bleeding 714
Charles N. Bernstein

102 Ascites 721
Edward P. Toffolon

103 Spontaneous Bacterial Peritonitis . . 724
J. Eileen Hay

104 Porphyria 731
Joseph R. Bloomer and Claus A. Pierach

105 Hepatobiliary Complications of Ulcerative Colitis and Crohn's Disease 741
Vijayan Balan and Nicholas F. LaRusso

106 Primary Biliary Cirrhosis 749
Vijayan Balan, E. Rolland Dickson, and Keith D. Lindor

107 Hepatic Granulomas 758
Roberto Chiprut

108 Amebic Abscess 768
Anthony S. Tornay, Jr.

109 Hepatic Tumors 771
Steven D. Seagren and Rowen K. Zetterman

110 Disorders of Liver Function in Systemic Disease 780
Peter V. Barrett

111 Alpha$_1$-Antitrypsin Deficiency 791
David H. Perlmutter

112 Wilson's Disease 802
Michael L. Schilsky and Irmin Sternlieb

113 Hemochromatosis 808
Bruce R. Bacon

114 Choledochal Cysts 814
Stuart Sherman

115 Liver Resection and Transplantation . 828
Stefano Fagiuoli, Ahmet Gurakar, Tarek Hassanein, Harlan I. Wright, and David H. Van Thiel

116 Neonatal Hepatitis and Cholestasis 842
Philip Rosenthal

117 Chronic Cholecystitis 848
Bret T. Petersen

118 Acalculous Cholecystitis 853
David P. Nunes and Nezam H. Afdhal

119 Cholelithiasis 858
Rahul Kuver, Myung-Hwan Kim, and Sum P. Lee

120 Chronic Cholestatic Liver Disease . . 864
George Dickstein and Marshall M. Kaplan

121 Acute Bacterial Cholangitis 877
Eric D. Libby and Joseph W. Leung

122 Choledocholithiasis 882
Simon K. Lo and Joe M. Chen

123 Sclerosing Cholangitis 891
Ellen C. Ebert

124 Bile Duct Strictures 895
Franklin E. Kasmin and Jerome H. Siegel

125 Tumors of the Gallbladder and Biliary Tract 902
Soroya M. Rahaman and Glen A. Lehman

Index 913

SECTION I

GENERAL

1
Obesity

JOYCE P. BARNETT and SCOTT M. GRUNDY

PREVALENCE

Obesity presents one of the great challenges in medicine. While relatively simple to identify, successful outcome in treatment remains elusive. One half of the women and one fourth of the men in the United States are on a diet at any given time, yet obesity is on the rise. Approximately 32% of men and 35% of women are overweight when acceptable weight is defined as a body mass index (BMI) of 20.7 to 27.8 kg/m^2 and 19.1 to 27.3 kg/m^2, respectively. Approximately 8% of men and 11% of women are severely overweight with morbid obesity affecting 1% of men and women. Obesity among American children is on the rise in both degree and prevalence. This trend is particularly alarming because it portends even greater demand for successful weight management in the future.

HEALTH RISKS

When evaluating potential risk for medical problems the degree of obesity and susceptibility to metabolic complications must be considered. Obesity is a risk factor for development of non–insulin-dependent diabetes mellitus (NIDDM), hypertension, dyslipidemias, and gallbladder disease (Table 1–1). As the degree of obesity increases, risk of complications also rises. Mortality is lowest with a BMI of 20 to 25 kg/m^2 and increases slightly with a BMI of 25 to 30 kg/m^2. Mortality from cardiovascular disease (CVD), diabetes mellitus (DM), and gallbladder disease increases significantly when BMI exceeds 30 kg/m^2. Increased susceptibility to metabolic complications is more likely in overweight individuals with a positive family history for these diseases. Accumulation of fat in the abdominal region significantly increases the risk for complications. Increased risk for development of some forms of cancer may also be linked to obesity.

ETIOLOGY

The cause of obesity can be easily identified as a state of positive energy balance, i.e., intake exceeds expenditure; however, a multitude of factors exert influence on this equation making the determination of cause anything but simple (Fig. 1–1). Energy imbalance may result from either excess intake or decreased expenditure but is more likely a combination of both. A small percentage of cases of obesity are the result of physiologic problems such as disorders of the hypothalamus or disturbances of the endocrine system, but the vast majority result from interaction of numerous factors exerting an exponential effect on weight (Fig. 1–2).

Genetic influence on development of obesity has long been suspected, and recent research supports the idea that it plays a role in predisposition to obesity. There is also some evidence that an individual's habitual physical activity level and response to overfeeding have significant genetic components. Distribution of body fat is definitely influenced by genetics.

Many theories related to *psychologic influences* in development of obesity have been proposed, but studies indicate that obese individuals are no more likely to have psychologic disturbances than the nonobese. There is some evidence that persons at risk for development of obesity respond more readily to external food cues. Anxiety-arousing situations have been shown to increase food intake in obese subjects,

TABLE 1–1. METABOLIC COMPLICATIONS OF OBESITY

Non-insulin-dependent diabetes mellitus (NIDDM)
Hypertension
Dyslipidemias
Gallbladder disease

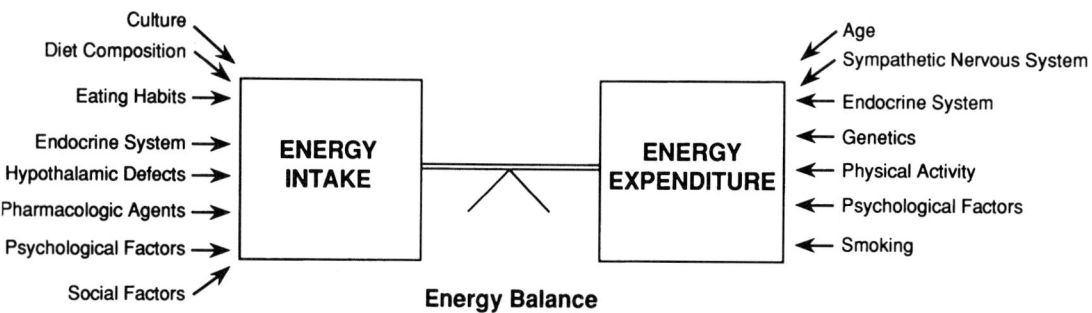

FIGURE 1-1. Factors influencing energy balance.

and obese patients often report eating more in response to anxiety or depression. An attitude of conscious restraint of food intake has been suggested as a factor in the cause of obesity. This attitude is influenced by physiologic cues that prompt a desire to eat and cognitively mediated processes inhibiting that desire. Periods of restrained eating during which the individual feels deprived are followed by loss of control and overeating.

Numerous *social, cultural,* and *environmental factors* may interact and influence development of obesity. Whereas society as a whole is obsessed with a "thin" body image, some groups equate power, authority, and good health with larger body size. Obesity is more prevalent in lower socioeconomic groups who cannot afford expensive, nutrient-dense, low-calorie foods. Cultural food preferences, as well as economic status, may influence the proportion of protein, fat, and carbohydrate in the diet. An abundance of highly palatable food and frequent social events increase food exposure for the susceptible person.

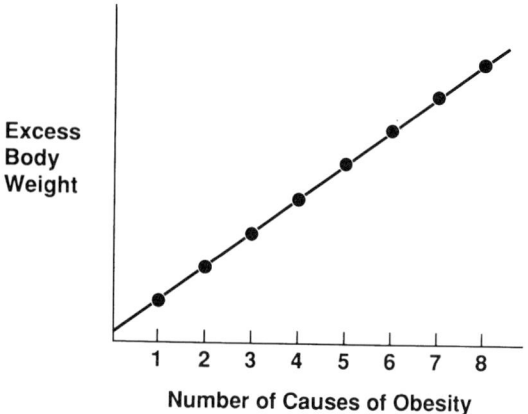

FIGURE 1-2. Exponential effect of factors on excess weight.

Eating habits may contribute to weight gain. A pattern of irregular meals, often consisting of one or two large meals per day has been associated with obesity. A higher fat intake is found in those who skip breakfast than in breakfast eaters. In studies evaluating metabolic effects, higher serum lipids and insulin secretion are found with decreased meal frequency. Large meals tend to promote fat storage in animals more than smaller, more frequent meals. Eating out frequently, especially at fast food restaurants, can lead to a diet higher in total calories and fat, contributing to caloric excess.

Composition of the diet may play a role in development of obesity. Percent of calories from fat has been implicated as a contributor to weight gain. Isocaloric diets with varying levels of fat do not affect caloric requirements, but in conditions of caloric excess, fat may be more efficiently metabolized and stored than protein or carbohydrate. In addition some studies demonstrate that the obese prefer calorically dense high-fat foods that also taste sweet.

A relative or absolute reduction in the activity of the *sympathetic nervous system* (SNS) is proposed as a contributor to the development of obesity. Neurotransmitters and hormones influenced by the SNS affect food intake and deposition of protein, fat, and carbohydrate through a feedback mechanism. The SNS also plays a role in activating the thermogenic systems of the body. When SNS activity is decreased, food intake increases leading to increased deposition of fat.

Certain *drugs* have been found to influence appetite and body weight. The tricyclic antidepressants increase craving for sweets. Steroid therapy is often accompanied by muscle wasting, an increase in body fat, and increased appetite. Chlorpromazine and cyproheptadine also increase food intake and contribute to weight gain.

Decreased energy expenditure may occur in a

number of situations. A familial tendency toward reduced metabolic rates is predictive of increased risk for obesity. Cessation of smoking often leads to weight gain. Intake may increase because food tastes better, but there is evidence that metabolic rate is somewhat lower in ex-smokers. Metabolic rate is reduced with aging because of decreased lean body mass, and physical activity often declines as well. Lack of physical activity has been identified as a contributing factor in the development of obesity, especially in children. Time spent watching television has been directly correlated with prevalence of obesity in adults and children. Physical activity may account for as much as 20% to 30% of total energy expenditure, but it may be much less in a sedentary individual. Because of the many labor-saving devices available in our environment, a conscious effort to expend energy is necessary for some to avoid weight gain. Weight gain often follows decreased activity resulting from a change in occupation, disabling injury, or chronic illness. Voluntary activity may be limited in severe depression promoting weight gain.

DIAGNOSIS

A diagnosis of obesity is often made when weight for height exceeds 20% of indexes such as the Metropolitan Life Tables or National Research Council standards. BMI (weight in kilograms divided by height in meters, squared) is an easy-to-calculate method for evaluating weight for height. The National Center for Health Statistics has defined the term *overweight* (in 20 to 29 year olds) as the 85th percentile, which corresponds to a BMI of 27.8 kg/m^2 in men and 27.3 kg/m^2 in women. The 95th percentile is defined as *severe overweight* and corresponds to a BMI of 31.1 and 32.3 kg/m^2 for men and women, respectively. Measurement of waist-hip ratio can be a useful diagnostic indicator of risk for CVD, DM, and hypertension. A waist-hip ratio >.95 in men and >.80 in women indicates increased risk. Skinfold measurements may be helpful in some situations to evaluate body composition and interpret distribution of fat, but these measurements can be difficult in obese patients.

THERAPY

TYPES OF TREATMENT

Most treatment regimens can lead to weight loss, but few achieve the goal of long-term maintenance of reduced weight. A review of advantages and disadvantages of the types of treatment available can help tailor treatment to patient need, increasing the likelihood of success.

Conservative management should be conducted by a multidisciplinary team and include at least three components: (1) a balanced reduced calorie diet (Table 1–2), (2) increased activity, and (3) behavior modification. This approach should be individualized to accommodate the lifestyle of and meet specific needs of the patient. Nutrition education may be needed to help with appropriate food selection. Some individuals may want a detailed meal plan and would therefore respond favorably to this approach. Others may find a meal plan too tedious to follow but would agree to try substituting lower calorie foods for certain high-calorie foods in their diets. Less focus on food and more attention to behavior change may be the best approach for the person who needs to increase activity. Individuals who exhibit restrained eating behavior or have a history of frequent dieting or skipping meals will need help to develop normal eating patterns. Most patients are able to identify at least some problem areas that contribute to their overweight condition and should be asked for input in planning treatment. A major advantage of conservative management is that it provides an opportunity to change dietary and exercise habits and minimizes loss of lean body mass. The patient can learn how to cope with

TABLE 1–2. GUIDELINES FOR BALANCED REDUCED-CALORIE DIETS

Determine appropriate calorie level:
  Evaluate current caloric intake.
  Estimate energy requirements.
  Subtract 500 kcal/d to lose ~0.45 kg (1 lb)/wk.
  Plan individualized meal pattern considering preferences and lifestyle.
  Weight loss should not exceed 0.45 to 0.90 kg (1 to 2 lb)/wk.
Determine protein requirements.
  Provide ~15% to 20% of calories from protein (or 1 to 1.5 g protein per kilogram desirable body weight).
Encourage low-fat food choices (~30% of calories from fat).
Encourage intake of complex carbohydrate foods (~50% to 55% of calories from carbohydrate).
Encourage moderate sodium intake (2500 to 3000 mg/d).
Provide vitamins and minerals to meet Recommended Dietary Allowances (RDA). (Meeting RDA on <1200 kcal/d is difficult without supplementation.)
Provide appropriate nutrition education.
Normalize eating habits by establishing set times to eat.

real life food situations, which may promote long-term weight control. A major drawback from the patient's point of view is that this is a slow process. The patient will need the help of trained professionals to develop and adhere to this approach. A follow-up plan for maintaining reduced body size should be included. Relapse prevention strategies and cognitive-behavioral treatment may help maintain reduced weight.

Very low calorie diets (VLCD) (<800 kcal/d) are used to facilitate rapid weight loss. These programs use a liquid formula, selected low-fat, high-protein foods, or a combination of formula and selected foods. Appropriate levels of high-biologic value protein (1.2 to 1.5 g/kg desirable body weight), vitamins, minerals, and fluid must be provided. Close supervision by a physician and dietitian with frequent monitoring of electrolytes is essential. Ideally the program should include exercise and behavior modification components. Follow-up is very important because of the propensity for rapid regain of weight following completion of the weight loss phase. Because of the monitoring required, these programs are expensive. This regimen is recommended for individuals who must lose large amounts of weight (BMI ≥ 32 kg/m^2) in a short period of time because of a medical problem. VLCD can be especially hazardous for the moderately overweight patient who needs to lose <13.5 kg (30 lb). Greater potential for excessive loss of lean body mass and potassium leads to increased risk of cardiac complications. Unsupervised use of VLCD or supervision by inadequately trained personnel also increases the risk of serious complications (Table 1–3).

Surgical treatment of obesity may be recommended for patients 45 kg (100 lb) or 100% above ideal body weight who have failed to lose weight with conventional methods and have serious comorbidity. Results depend on motivation and behavior change; therefore the patient should be committed to changing eating habits and lifestyle. The type of procedure used has evolved, with current surgery of choice being vertical banded gastroplasty or Roux-en-Y gastric bypass. With thorough multidisciplinary screening, operative and perioperative risks are relatively low when the procedure is performed by an experienced surgeon in a well-equipped facility. Ideal body weight is rarely attained, with maximum weight loss after gastroplasty and gastric bypass achieved 18 to 24 months postoperatively. The mean percentage of excess weight loss varies from 40% to 70%. Improvement is seen in patients with dyslipidemias, DM, sleep apnea, and hypertension, and most patients report improved quality of life. Potential for long-term complications depends on the type of procedure, is significant, and warrants lifetime follow-up by physician and dietitian (Table 1–4).

A number of *commercial and self-help weight loss programs* exist that may benefit some individuals. Self-help groups can provide social support needed to sustain weight reduction efforts. Degree of supervision and level of expertise and training of leaders vary and should be considered when evaluating these programs. There is little scientific data on long-term efficacy. Plans that make unrealistic claims of success or promote use of nutritionally unsound diets are unlikely to work and may be harmful. Cost of commercial programs can be prohibitive.

Pharmacologic therapy for weight control remains a controversial area. Some feel that appetite-suppressing drugs are placebos with potential harmful effects, whereas others view them as adjuncts to other forms of therapy. There is concern about risk of abuse. Phenylpropanolamine is the only over-the-counter drug available for weight control. It acts on the noradrenergic system and in studies has produced weight loss of ~0.25 kg/wk more than a placebo. Side effects are described as mild. Fenfluramine (a schedule IV drug) suppresses appetite by releasing and preventing reuptake of serotonin. It has facilitated weight loss in studies, but weight was regained when the drug was discontinued. Sched-

TABLE 1–3. MAJOR RISKS OF VERY LOW CALORIE DIET (VLCD)

Dehydration
Electrolyte imbalances
Cardiac arrhythmias
Inappropriate refeeding
Cholecystitis

TABLE 1–4. POTENTIAL LONG-TERM COMPLICATIONS OF SURGICAL TREATMENT

Protein-calorie malnutrition
Micronutrient deficiencies (especially vitamin B_{12}, folate, iron)
Significant malabsorption
Vomiting

ule II drugs (amphetamine, methamphetamine, and phenmetrazine) are not indicated for treatment of obesity. Thyroid hormone and growth hormone are not indicated for obesity treatment, and human chorionic gonadotropin is ineffective.

TREATMENT OF CONCOMITANT ILLNESS

Weight reduction should be considered a potential treatment when excess weight is contributing to illness, e.g., hypertension, glucose intolerance, and dyslipidemia. When a patient is unable to lose weight, or if progression to more severe complications is likely, appropriate treatment should be instituted to control the medical consequences of obesity. Blood pressure, blood glucose levels, serum lipids, etc. should be managed according to established guidelines.

GUIDELINES FOR TREATMENT OF OBESITY

In deciding to treat obesity several areas should be considered: (1) etiologic factors, (2) degree of risk for metabolic complications, (3) contraindicated situations, (4) likelihood of success, (5) psychologic and physical risks of weight loss, and (6) realistic goals for treatment. An evaluation of health status establishes a data base on which to develop a treatment plan (Table 1–5). The history will assist in evaluating etiologic factors and medical problems, as well as potential risks of treatment.

A multidisciplinary approach to obesity management is most likely to achieve a favorable outcome. After completion of the medical evaluation, referral to appropriate allied health professionals is helpful to facilitate comprehensive treatment. An accurate estimate of current intake and pattern of eating is crucial for planning (Table 1–5). Using this information, the dietitian can identify food-related etiologic factors, plan an individualized meal pattern, and offer suggestions for behavior change. An exercise physiologist may assist in developing an exercise plan for the patient with limitations on activity. Evaluation of anthropometric data and weight history is important in setting realistic goals (Table 1–5). A history of "dieting" (Table 1–6) and an exercise history (Table 1–6) can also be helpful. Weight loss may be contraindicated in some situations, and close supervision is required in high-risk cases. Weight loss in children can adversely affect linear growth. An acceptable approach for weight management in a child is to decrease caloric intake slightly to slow the rate of weight gain while allowing for continued linear growth. Pregnancy is not a time for weight loss. Current recommendations are for a weight gain of 7 to 11.5 kg (15 to 25 lb) in women with a prepregnancy BMI of 26 to 29 kg/m^2, with a minimum of 7 kg (15 lb) weight gain with BMI >29 kg/m^2. Any patient receiving medication for a chronic condition, especially patients over 65 years of age, should be monitored during active weight loss for adverse responses and to adjust medication requirements.

The likelihood of the patient's successful participation in a weight loss program should be evaluated. Certain personality traits have been identified as predictive of an inability to main-

TABLE 1–5. GUIDELINES FOR TREATMENT OF OBESITY

Evaluation of Health Status and Risks	*Components of Dietary History Evaluation*
Age	Quality and quantity of food consumed
Medical and family history	Frequency of meals, snacks, beverages
Presence of concomitant illnesses	Meals at home versus eating out
Glucose intolerance or diabetes	Methods of food preparation
Hypertension	Person who prepares meals
Cardiovascular disease	*Anthropometric Evaluation and Weight History*
Gout	Present weight
Dental status	Measured height
Limitations on physical activity	Body mass index (BMI)
Pregnancy, lactation	Waist-hip ratio
Alcohol or drug use	Desirable weight
Tobacco use	Usual weight
Current medications	Patient's preferred weight
Psychologic disturbances	Maximal adult (nonpregnant) weight
Eating disorders	Lowest weight maintained in adult life for at least 1 year
	Time of onset of excessive weight gain

TABLE 1–6. DIETING AND EXERCISE HISTORIES

Dieting History	*Exercise History*
Currently on prescribed diet? If so, what type?	Physical activity at work
Currently on weight reduction diet?	Physical activity at home
Ever tried to lose weight?	Limitations on physical activity
How was weight lost?	Past exercise experience, if any
How many "diets" followed?	Present exercise experience, if any
How much weight lost?	Frequency
How long was weight loss maintained?	Duration
How much was regained and in what time period?	Intensity

tain weight loss: anxiety, suspiciousness, monotony avoidance, and low degree of socialization. Other factors that impact emotional state (e.g., job stress, self-consciousness about weight, lack of social support, and type A behavior) are associated with minimal weight loss and poor retention in weight loss programs.

Realistic goals for weight loss are crucial. Unrealistic goals may be a contributor to the current high rate of treatment failure. A realistic goal weight may be quite different from ideal weight in standard tables. In conditions such as hypertension even small amounts of weight loss (2.25 to 4.5 kg [5 to 10 lb]) can improve status. Gradual weight loss accompanied by permanent changes in behavior for diet and exercise should be encouraged. Even though loss of 0.22 kg (½ lb)/wk seems almost too small to measure, this represents 11.7 kg (26 lb) in 1 year. Weight loss should not exceed 0.45 to 0.9 kg (1 to 2 lb)/wk, but will be in the range of 1.35 to 2.25 kg (3 to 5 lb)/wk if the VLCD approach is used. Drastic dietary changes that result in dramatic short-term weight loss are seldom sustained and may significantly decrease metabolic rate. Decreased metabolic rate hinders weight loss, and maintaining extreme reductions in intake long enough to lose the desired number of pounds is difficult. A pattern of chronic dieting with frequent cycles of loss and regain may be established, creating more stress than a static, but overweight, condition. Both the physician and patient must accept that obesity is a chronic condition that requires lifelong commitment for control.

Maintenance of reduced weight is probably the most challenging component of weight management. Permanent changes in eating habits are needed, as well as continued exercise. Several behavioral techniques have been identified that assist with weight maintenance, including self-monitoring with weekly or biweekly weighing and establishing a 2.25 kg (5-lb) limit for weight fluctuation. When the upper limit is reached, steps to decrease intake or increase activity must be implemented. Keeping a food diary can help monitor intake. Self-reward along with self-monitoring is even more effective. Lifestyle exercises, such as walking, that become routine are essential to weight maintenance. Strenuous exercise, like drastic dietary change, is unlikely to be continued; therefore, the patient needs to find an activity that he likes well enough to continue indefinitely.

Risks of Therapy

Psychologic risks may occur as a consequence of the weight loss process or as a result of repeated failure to maintain reduced weight. Depression can accompany weight loss. Obese individuals who lose significant weight may experience psychologic and physiologic changes similar to those seen in starvation, such as high rates of binge eating, depression, impaired concentration, preoccupation with food, and reduced caloric requirements. Eating disorders are on the rise, and attempts to lose weight may trigger anorexia nervosa or bulimia nervosa in some individuals. The psychologic consequences of repeated failure to maintain reduced weight are great, especially for those who undergo treatment in VLCD programs. They usually blame themselves for the failure, further eroding their self-esteem.

Some adverse consequences of body weight fluctuation have been reported in recent studies, including increased mortality. Frequent weight loss attempts could contribute to greater fluctuation in weight. Increased fat deposition and greater difficulty in losing weight are proposed consequences of repeated weight loss followed by rapid regain. Some studies support the idea that maintenance caloric requirements are reduced and tend to remain at lower-than-predicted levels following significant weight loss, but this has not been confirmed in all studies. Rapid weight loss may precipitate exacerbations of gout and cholecystitis.

CONCLUSION

Treatment of obesity should be based on thorough evaluation of patient needs and must incorporate realistic goals. It should promote increased physical activity, moderation in eating habits, and normalization of meal patterns. Treatment must be individualized and provide continued support, as for any chronic condition. With current lack of long-term success in weight control, prevention of obesity should be a primary concern. Although it is not possible to predict who will become obese, recognition of genetic tendencies toward obesity accompanied by a sedentary lifestyle would permit earlier intervention. An increase in physical activity and adoption of prudent eating habits could improve the individual's chances of maintaining a reasonable weight.

2

Eating Disorders

JOEL YAGER

Although cases consistent with anorexia nervosa and bulimia nervosa have been reported for centuries, including clinical descriptions of "anorexia mirabile" in sainted women who starved themselves in acts of piety, anorexia nervosa as we now recognize it was first described in the late 1870s, and bulimia (now bulimia nervosa) as we now think of it was described in the 1950s. Interest in the eating disorders has grown considerably over the past two decades as their prevalence has seemingly increased greatly in relation to ubiquitous pressures on women to be slim, stemming largely from popular media. Recent magazine articles have noted the scores of popular movie and television actresses who have struggled with, and in some instances succumbed to, eating disorders.

EPIDEMIOLOGY

The prevalence of eating disorders among college-aged women appears to be increasing, and may range from 1% to 3%, but the prevalence of these disorders elsewhere in the population is much lower. Bulimia nervosa is more common than anorexia nervosa. However, individual symptoms commonly associated with eating disorders are extremely prevalent, and they may even be seen in the majority of certain subgroups of the female population, as in select college sororities or among some groups of female athletes such as gymnasts. These include binge eating, restrictive and fad dieting, and purging by means of vomiting, laxative abuse, diuretic abuse, and hyperexercise among normal weight and even underweight individuals, and closely associated symptoms such as body image distortion, fear of being fat that is out of line with health concerns, and amphetamine and cocaine use for anorectic effects. About 90% to 95% of cases are girls or women.

DIAGNOSIS AND CLINICAL FEATURES

Current diagnostic criteria for anorexia nervosa and bulimia nervosa (American Psychiatric Association: *Diagnostic and Statistical Manual-IV*) are listed in Table 2–1. Currently under consideration as a new diagnosis is *binge eating disorder,* a condition that essentially mirrors bulimia nervosa but lacks purging, closely corresponding to what many would call *severe compulsive overeating.*

Eating disorders most typically first appear in the teenage and early adult years, but cases with later onset, and rarely earlier onset, have been reported. Anorexia nervosa tends to appear a few years before bulimia nervosa. Although previously associated primarily with the Euro-American upper and upper middle social classes, these disorders are now well represented among middle and lower middle class women including nonwhites as well.

Weight preoccupation is a primary symptom in both anorexia nervosa and bulimia nervosa. Many patients demonstrate both anorectic and bulimic behaviors. Anorexia nervosa appears in restrictor and bulimic subtypes; up to 50% of anorexia nervosa patients develop bulimic symptoms, significant numbers of initially bulimic patients develop anorectic symptoms, and restrictor and bulimic subtypes may occasionally alternate in the same patient so that some consider the disorders to occur along a continuum. Restrictors ("dieters") limit intake to as low as a few hundred kilocalories per day, limit food selection, and often demonstrate obsessive-compulsive symptoms regarding food, eating habits, exercise, and other matters. Bulimic subtypes suffer from frequent eating binges, usually purge, and are often self-destructive. In either subtype, patients may exercise for hours daily, and may demonstrate bizarre food preferences, social isolation, diminished sexual interest, and depression. Anorexia nervosa patients who purge but who do not objectively binge eat are often encountered ("vomiters and purgers"). Careful assessment of exactly what each patient means by a "binge" is imperative.

Patients with anorexia nervosa present with various degrees of malnutrition. Not infrequently such patients are brought for care against their own wishes, in spite of the fact that they may have already lost 30% to 40% of their weight. Many appear superficially healthy even with marked degrees of weight loss, but these superficial appearances are often deceiving, as cardiovascular and muscle reserves may be virtually gone.

The primary symptom complex of bulimia nervosa consists of repeated episodes of binge eating and purging. Patients binge eat large

TABLE 2–1. DIAGNOSTIC CRITERIA FOR EATING DISORDERS

Anorexia Nervosa
A. Refusal to maintain body weight over a minimal normal weight for age and height (e.g., weight loss leading to maintenance of body weight less than 85% of that expected; or a failure to make expected weight gain during period of growth, leading to body weight less than 85% of that expected).
B. Intense fear of gaining weight or becoming fat, even though underweight.
C. Disturbance in the way in which one's body weight or shape is experienced, undue influence of body weight or shape on self-evaluation, or denial of the seriousness of the current low body weight.
D. In postmenarcheal females, amenorrhea, i.e., the absence of at least three consecutive menstrual cycles. (A woman is considered to have amenorrhea if her periods occur only following hormone, e.g., estrogen, administration.)

Specify type:
Restricting Type: during the current episode of Anorexia Nervosa, the person has not regularly engaged in binge-eating or purging behavior (i.e., self-induced vomiting or the misuse of laxatives, diuretics, or enemas)
Binge-Eating/Purging Type: during the current episode of Anorexia Nervosa, the person has regularly engaged in binge-eating or purging behavior (i.e., self-induced vomiting or the misuse of laxatives, diuretics, or enemas)

Bulimia Nervosa
A. Recurrent episodes of binge eating. An episode of binge eating is characterized by both of the following:
  (1) eating, in a discrete period of time (e.g., within any 2-hour period), an amount of food that is definitely larger than most people would eat during a similar period of time and under similar circumstances
  (2) a sense of lack of control over eating during the episode (e.g., a feeling that one cannot stop eating or control what or how much one is eating)
B. Recurrent inappropriate compensatory behavior in order to prevent weight gain, such as self-induced vomiting; misuse of laxatives, diuretics, enemas, or other medications; fasting; or excessive exercise.
C. The binge eating and inappropriate compensatory behaviors both occur, on average, at least twice a week for 3 months.
D. Self-evaluation is unduly influenced by body shape and weight.
E. The disturbance does not occur exclusively during episodes of Anorexia Nervosa.

Specify type:
Purging Type: during the current episode of Bulimia Nervosa, the person has regularly engaged in self-induced vomiting or the misuse of laxatives, diuretics, or enemas
Nonpurging Type: during the current episode of Bulimia Nervosa, the person has used other inappropriate compensatory behaviors, such as fasting or excessive exercise, but has not regularly engaged in self-induced vomiting or the misuse of laxatives, diuretics, or enemas

Reprinted with permission from the *Diagnostic and Statistical Manual of Mental Disorders*—IV. Washington, DC: American Psychiatric Press Inc; 1994.

quantities of food in a very short time, usually at least 2000 kcal of high-calorie foods per binge, with some reporting more than 10,000 kcal per binge. When not binge eating, most patients with bulimia nervosa tend to eat highly restricted diets that contain fewer calories per day than they require for energy and weight maintenance. Such restriction causes hunger pangs, which in turn contributes to the likelihood of subsequent binges. Terrified by the quantities of food they consume, patients attempt to purge themselves of the ingested calories in every possible way. The majority, 80% or more, self-induce vomiting from several times per week to multiple times each day. About 30% to 40% use large quantities of laxatives—scores of stimulant laxatives each week are not uncommon—or diuretics. (Laxatives and diuretics are not very helpful for losing calories, but are highly effective in causing losses of fluid and electrolytes, thereby reducing weight quickly. However, patients who repeatedly dehydrate themselves with these agents are prone to rebound edema when they stop ingesting them.) Some patients exercise compulsively for hours each day. By the time they seek care, the majority of patients have been symptomatic for at least several years, with binge-purge cycles occurring as frequently as 8 to 10 times per day. The patients always feel as if their eating is out of control, and they feel so ashamed that they are often secretive about their problem.

ASSOCIATED MEDICAL FINDINGS

Patients who have concurrent anorexia nervosa and bulimia nervosa may have severe medical complications including all the sequelae of malnutrition, and such patients require careful assessment and management. Prepubertal patients experience growth arrest and may not grow to anticipated heights. Prolonged amenorrhea (more than 6 months) is associated with potentially irreversible osteopenia and a correspondingly increased rate of pathologic fractures. Infertility is common. With malnutrition hypothermia may be seen. Cardiac abnormalities range from benign arrhythmias to conduction defects and ventricular premature contractions leading to sudden cardiac death. Patients who purge suffer from dehydration, metabolic abnormalities including hypokalemia, hypochloremia, and hypomagnesemia. The chronic use of ipecac to induce vomiting may result in severe long-standing toxic myopathies, cardiomyopathy, and death.

Following are three common physical findings in bulimia nervosa:

1. "Chubby cheeks" due to edematous benign hyperplasia of overstimulated parotid and sublingual glands
2. Dental decay, most notably front teeth, due to erosion of enamel by gastric acid washes associated with vomitus
3. Scarring on the dorsum of the hands near the knuckles due to repeated abrasions from teeth occurring in the course of self-induced vomiting.

In addition to laboratory abnormalities in electrolytes and magnesium, laboratory findings may include low serum zinc; elevations in serum levels of amylase, cortisol, carotene, and cholesterol; abnormal liver function tests; elevated reverse T_3; and neutropenia with relative lymphocytosis.

GASTROINTESTINAL FINDINGS

The most common gastrointestinal findings are presented in Table 2–2. Esophageal and gastric irritation and bleeding due to vomiting may occur, and rare cases of death due to esophageal or gastric rupture have been reported. Damage to the haustral musculature of the large intestine

---

TABLE 2–2. COMMON GASTROINTESTINAL FINDINGS IN EATING DISORDERS

- Benign parotid hyperplasia in bulimia nervosa
- Mildly elevated serum amylase (25%–40%) in bulimia nervosa (salivary > pancreatic isoenzymes)
- Esophageal motor abnormalities in about one third of patients with bulimia nervosa (ranging from hypochalasia to vigorous chalasia and diffuse esophageal spasm)
- Mild lower esophagitis in about one quarter of daily vomiters
- Rare esophageal tears in bulimia nervosa
- Mucosal erythema of antrum, gastric body, or duodenum in about one quarter of patients with bulimia nervosa
- Delayed gastric emptying and gastrocecal transit in anorexia nervosa
- Possible delayed gastric emptying in bulimia nervosa
- Gastric distention in bulimia nervosa
- Irritable bowel syndrome
- Melanosis coli secondary to laxative abuse
- Impaired cecal peristalsis secondary to laxative abuse ("cathartic colon")

due to laxative abuse may result in chronic bowel dysfunction. In one series of 54 patients with diarrhea of unknown origin, all of whom denied laxative use, urine and fecal screens revealed that about 13% of these patients had been taking laxatives. Of these the large majority were women and most had a past psychiatric history. When chronic severe laxative or diuretic use is terminated abruptly, patients can experience significant bloating and edema, with rapid weight gains of 4.5 to 6.7 kg (10 to 15 lb) not uncommon.

CONCURRENT PSYCHIATRIC CONDITIONS

Many patients with anorexia nervosa and bulimia nervosa suffer from other psychiatric conditions together with the eating disorders. All malnourished patients exhibit some degree of irritability and emotional lability. Comorbid symptoms of major depression or dysthymia have been reported in 50% to 75% of patients with eating disorders. In anorexia nervosa, obsessive-compulsive disorder (OCD) may be found in about 10% to 13%, with lifetime prevalence of OCD in anorexia nervosa of about 25%. In bulimia nervosa increased rates have been reported for anxiety disorders (43%), chemical dependency disorders (34%), bipolar disorder (12%), and personality disorders (or at least substantial personality trait disturbances) (50% to 75%).

First-degree female relatives of patients with both anorexia nervosa and bulimia nervosa have increased incidence of these disorders. Additionally, families of patients with bulimia nervosa have increased incidence of substance abuse (particularly alcoholism), affective disorders, and obesity.

ETIOLOGY AND PATHOGENESIS

Theories regarding the etiology and pathogenesis of bulimia nervosa have implicated biologic, psychologic, family, and sociocultural factors.

A premorbid tendency toward being overweight or obese may be a contributing factor to bulimia nervosa. Furthermore, bulimic women require on average between 5% to 10% fewer calories per day than nonbulimic weight-matched normal women to maintain their weights.

The primary biologic influences in the pathogenesis of anorexia nervosa and bulimia nervosa are those related to hunger and starvation. Studies show that normal volunteers who have dieted to 25% below their usually healthy weights become irritable, food obsessed, depressed, socially isolated, and apathetic—symptoms very similar to those of patients with anorexia nervosa. Furthermore, they often hoard food and binge eat when food is presented. Current thinking also strongly suggests that hunger itself is the major stimulus for binge eating in both normal and low-weight bulimia nervosa patients. Many patients start to binge eat as "break through eating," primarily because they are not able to restrict their food intake to the degree that they desire.

Psychologic Factors

Currently popular theories relate the development of eating disorders to adolescents striving for self-esteem. For many young women self-esteem is closely tied to physical appearance, and in our society "slim is in" and chubbiness is scorned. Patients prone to develop anorexia nervosa are those whose initial personalities seem to be somewhat timid, anxious, avoidant of novelty, eager to please (especially parents), and, in turn, somewhat perfectionistic. When such patients are confronted by the difficult maturational tasks of adolescence such as separation from parents and sexual development, it is thought that usually healthy efforts to cope with these stresses fail and that the patients start to rely on more obsessionally focused attempts to perfect themselves through perfect control of their bodies via diet and exercise. These obsessional behaviors become autonomous, so that what might have initially started as something the patient desired then becomes an unrelenting compulsion.

Patients who develop bulimia nervosa tend premorbidly to be more emotionally sensitive, moody, and dramatic. They may have learned early in life to relieve states of tension and anxiety through food, as happens in many families, and to tend toward being overweight. When they strive to diet severely in adolescence but find themselves binge eating when hungry in spite of their best efforts at will power, the anxiety generated by the shame, guilt, and loss of self-control brought about by the eating binge is in turn relieved by purging. Patients may also become conditioned to seek the emotional states or sensations associated with certain physiologic events, e.g., those related to heightened arousal with binge eating, abdominal distention following a binge, or feelings of emptying or emptiness associated with purging.

FAMILY FACTORS

Families believed more likely to produce children with eating disorders include those in which familial depression, alcoholism, or eating disorders are more prevalent than in matched controls. Such families may exhibit "negative expressed emotion," a destructive pattern in which one or more family members, usually a parent, is unrelentingly critical of the patient, often blaming her for bringing on the disorder and for using it to harm everyone else in the family. These families are often weight preoccupied, with parents who are particularly weight and appearance conscious. Patients with bulimia nervosa are more likely to come from families where obesity is present.

SOCIAL AND CULTURAL FACTORS

Eating disorders have become more prevalent over the past several decades, mirroring society's changing attitudes about beauty and fashion as documented by steadily decreasing weights for height over the past two decades among fashion models, *Playboy* magazine centerfolds, and Miss America Beauty Pageant winners. These trends have paralleled the weights of many influential trend-setting women, including first ladies and women's magazine editors, and of other fashion influencers in our society.

PROGNOSIS

Anorexia Nervosa

Patients who have required hospitalization for anorexia nervosa have a mixed outcome—by about 5 years after presentation about 44% do well (weight restoration and resumption of menses), 25% do poorly regarding these criteria, 28% have intermediate outcome, and fewer than 5% are dead. For previously hospitalized patients anorexia nervosa carries a mortality as high as 5% to 10% within 10 years and nearly 20% after 20 years. Deaths occur from cardiac malnutrition and suicide in about equal proportions. Poorer prognosis is associated with initial lower minimum weight, failure to respond to previous treatment, premorbid disturbed family relationships, being married, and vomiting.

Furthermore, about two thirds continue to have persistent morbid food and weight preoccupations, up to 40% have bulimic symptoms, and many have dysthymia, social phobia, obsessive-compulsive symptoms, or substance abuse. However, the degree of chronicity is often significant, so that maintenance treatment programs are frequently necessary.

Bulimia Nervosa

Patients treated with a variety of psychosocial treatments improve; however, the number of patients that achieve full abstinence is highly variable, with the minority becoming fully abstinent. The overall short-term success rate for psychosocially or medication-treated patients varies, from about a 50% to 90% reduction in binging and purging, averaging at about a 70% reduction for those who complete treatment programs. Those treated as outpatients seem to have reasonably good maintenance of gains over follow-up periods of up to 6 years. Patients who function well and who have milder symptoms often have a better prognosis than those who function poorly and have disabling symptoms. In contrast, at 3 years of follow-up about 27% of hospitalized bulimics have a good outcome (binging and purging less than once per month), 40% have an intermediate outcome, and 33% have a poor outcome (daily binging and vomiting or ongoing cathartic-diuretic abuse). It is also well known that anorexia nervosa patients who purge are at much greater risk for developing serious medical complications. Very little is known about the prognosis of untreated bulimia nervosa. Over a 1- to 2-year period bulimics who were never treated have reported modest degrees of "spontaneous" improvement, with roughly 25% to 30% reductions in their overall levels of binging, purging, and laxative abuse.

ASSESSMENT AND MANAGEMENT

Physicians should play a major role in prevention, detection, and management of patients with eating disorders. Gastroenterologists are likely to see such patients with functional bowel complaints or in consultation for rare requests for general hospital management of the seriously malnourished patient who utterly refuses to eat.

1. Given the high prevalence of subclinical eating disorders, as well as of the full syndromes, physicians should maintain a high index of suspicion and be alert to excessive concerns about

dieting and appearance in female preteens, adolescents, and young adults, especially patients with functional bowel complaints and those seeking laxatives. These patients should be educated about healthy nutrition and the dangers of unrealistic appearance-oriented dieting and eating disorders. Physicians should routinely question young female patients about what they desire to weigh; their dietary, dieting, and exercise practices; and their use of laxatives.

2. Alerting symptoms include reports of unusual food preferences and eating behaviors, severely restrictive dieting or fasting, significant weight loss, compulsive eating, menstrual irregularities, functional bowel complaints, desires to weigh 10 to 15 lb less than reasonable for habitus, overconcern with weight or physical appearance, overuse of laxatives or diuretics, and mood disturbances. Alerting signs of self-induced vomiting include the physical findings described above.

3. Once an eating disorder is suspected, patients merit a full physical examination, screening laboratory tests (including electrolytes, complete blood count, thyroid, calcium, magnesium, and amylase studies), and, for the thin patient, an electrocardiogram. Occult laxative abuse may be detected by examining the stool for phenolphthalein.

4. Psychiatric consultation and referral: Most patients with serious eating disorders warrant consultation with a psychiatrist who is knowledgeable about eating disorders for guidance to the patient, family, and referring physician about the nature, severity, and prognosis of the disorder and regarding what treatment options are available. The physician and his team can expect specific guidelines for psychosocial and medical management.

Specific indications for mandatory consultation include failure of the patient to respond to attempts at management in the physician's setting with deteriorating status, severe depression with suicidal behavior, or marked family problems.

5. General treatment strategy: Physicians should work together with registered dieticians and psychiatrists or psychologists knowledgeable about eating disorders to see if the problems can be ameliorated in outpatient care. With motivated patients this multidisciplinary team approach can be highly successful. The general physician's role is to educate, counsel, refer, and monitor the patient's weight and laboratory tests. The primary goals are nutritional rehabilitation and helping the patient to correct distorted notions about weight and eating. An appropriate goal weight is one at which the patient resumes normal menstruation and ovulation. Primary physicians should also be able to prescribe and monitor a course of antidepressant medication for patients with bulimia nervosa and major depression associated with an eating disorder. Tricyclic antidepressants such as imipramine and desipramine (150 to 300 mg/d) and newer agents such as fluoxetine (20 to 60 mg/d) have been shown to be effective in decreasing binge eating and purging episodes in both depressed and nondepressed bulimic patients. These medications may also help anorexia nervosa patients, but tricyclic agents should be used with great caution in malnourished patients because of their cardiac effects. However, these medications do not by themselves constitute an adequate treatment program. Dietary management or counseling and individual or group counseling or psychotherapy, ordinarily using cognitive-behavioral and psychodynamic principles, should be employed concurrently. The extent to which the physician is willing or able to assume a more intense involvement with the psychologic and family issues varies considerably. As is true for many types of disorders, some self-help programs may be useful. Hospitalization is often necessary for the patient with anorexia nervosa who weighs 25% to 30% or more below recommended weight and, less frequently, for bulimia nervosa patients who have not responded to outpatient care.

6. Special issues of concern to gastroenterologists: Gastroenterologists may be called on to help wean patients from excessive laxative use. For outpatients, gradual withdrawal over a period of weeks to months is the recommended approach. Inpatients may be abruptly weaned. Substitutions for laxatives are made as necessary, in ascending order of case severity, with high-fiber diet, nonabsorbable bulk laxatives, lactulose, milk of magnesia, glycerin suppositories, mineral lubricants, and, as a last resort, enemas a few times each week. Potassium is replaced slowly. Salt restriction and occasionally diuretics may be necessary if fluid retention is marked.

In treating delayed gastric emptying and distension, anecdotal reports suggest that prokinetic agents may sometimes help.

Gastroenterologists may also be called on when all other treatments fail to arrange nasogastric or total parenteral nutrition feedings for life-threatening malnutrition. It should be noted that such interventions are needed only in extremely rare circumstances. Treatment plans must include close ongoing teamwork with mental health professionals knowledgeable in the care of patients with anorexia nervosa.

RUMINATION DISORDER

Rumination, an uncommon disorder occurring from infancy throughout adulthood, is classified among the eating disorders but bears little resemblance to anorexia nervosa or bulimia nervosa. The symptoms may occasionally be seen in bulimia nervosa or, more frequently, occur as a distinct and separate entity. Derived from the Latin "ruminare," meaning "to chew the cud," the disorder is characterized by postingestive regurgitation of food from the stomach to the mouth with subsequent rechewing and swallowing. The vomiting is usually effortless, is predominantly involuntary, and occurs without nausea. Except in infants where complications may be frequent, the disorder is generally benign, often embarrassing, and comes to the attention of the gastroenterologist only in severe cases in which malnutrition or hiatus hernia coexist. Medical complications, including aspiration pneumonia, are more common among mentally retarded patients with the disorder.

Current thinking suggests that rumination is a learned habit that may serve to relieve anxiety. The nature of biologic vulnerability is unknown. Although cases are rare prior to 3 months of age, earlier onsets have been reported. Infants and children may demonstrate a failure to thrive. The disorder has also been seen in families spanning several generations. Psychiatric disorders frequently coexist, including mood and personality disorders in addition to eating disorders.

Treatment of infants and children is usually multidisciplinary and includes nursing care with sensory stimulation of the infant, medical management that is essentially the same as for reflux (positioning, medications), and in extreme cases surgery. In adults behavioral therapies have been used most often, and a few case reports have suggested that paregoric or metoclopramide may be useful.

REFERENCES

1. Agras WS. *Eating Disorders: Management of Obesity, Bulimia and Anorexia Nervosa.* Oxford, England: Pergamon; 1987.
2. Andersen AE. *Practical Comprehensive Treatment of Anorexia Nervosa and Bulimia.* Baltimore, Md: Johns Hopkins University Press; 1985.
3. Andersen AE, ed. *Males with Eating Disorders.* New York, NY: Brunner/Mazel Inc; 1990.
4. Beumont PJV, Burrows GD, Casper RC, eds. *Handbook of Eating Disorders, Part I: Anorexia and Bulimia Nervosa.* New York, NY: Elsevier Science Publishing Co Inc; 1987.
5. Blinder BJ, Goodman S, Henderson P. Rumination. In: Karasu TB, ed. *Treatment of Psychiatric Disorders.* Washington, DC: American Psychiatric Press Inc; 1989:564–579.
6. Bytzer P, Stokholm M, Andersen I, et al. Prevalence of surreptitious laxative abuse in patients with diarrhoea of uncertain origin: a cost benefit analysis of a screening procedure. *Gut.* 1989;30:1379–1384.
7. Cuellar RE, Kaye WH, Hsu LK, et al. Upper gastrointestinal tract dysfunction in bulimia. *Dig Dis Sci.* 1988;33:1549–1553.
8. Garfinkel PE, Garner DM. *Anorexia Nervosa: A Multidimensional Perspective.* New York, NY: Brunner/Mazel Inc; 1982.
9. Garner DM, Garfinkel PE, eds. *Handbook of Psychotherapy for Anorexia Nervosa and Bulimia.* New York, NY: Guilford Press; 1985.
10. Garfinkel PE, Garner DM, eds. *The Role of Drug Treatments for Eating Disorders.* New York, NY: Brunner/Mazel Inc; 1987.
11. Gwirtsman HE. Laxative and emetic abuse in bulimia nervosa. In: Yager J, Gwirtsman H, Edelstein CK, eds. *Special Problems in Managing Eating Disorders.* Washington, DC: American Psychiatric Press Inc; 1991; 145–162.
12. Herzog DB, Copeland PM. Eating disorders. *N Engl J Med.* 1985;313:295–303.
13. Hsu LKG. *Eating Disorders.* New York, NY: Guilford Press; 1990.
14. Hutson WR, Wald A. Gastric emptying in patients with bulimia nervosa and anorexia nervosa. *Am J Gastroenterol.* 1990;85:41–46.
15. Johnson C, Connors ME: *The Etiology and Treatment of Bulimia Nervosa,* New York, NY: Basic Books Inc; 1987.
16. Kiss A, Bergmann H, Abatzi Th-A, et al. Oesophageal and gastric motor activity in patients with bulimia nervosa. *Gut.* 1990;31:259–265.
17. Kiss A, Wiesnagrotzki S, Abatzi Th-A, et al. Upper gastrointestinal endoscopy findings in patients with longstanding bulimia nervosa. *Gastrointest Endosc.* 1989;35:516–519.
18. Szmukler GI, Lichtenstein M, Young GP, et al. A serial study of gastric emptying in anorexia nervosa and bulimia. *Aust N Z J Med.* 1990;20:220–225.

3
Malnutrition

DONALD F. KIRBY and MARK H. DeLEGGE

Malnutrition is more prevalent in our "affluent" western society than most physicians realize. It can be seen in the families of migrant workers, the homeless, as well as pregnant teenagers. The first major hurdle in dealing with malnutrition is recognizing its existence in a variety of presentations. These patients are not always markedly underweight, and they can be either outpatients or hospitalized patients. Estimates over the years have ranged from one third to one half of hospitalized patients having one or more abnormalities in the commonly used indexes assessing nutrition. By definition malnutrition means imperfect nutrition or lack of proper nutrition. The human body requires approximately 40 nutrients for normal growth and maintenance. If the body cannot synthesize these nutrients or a deficiency state occurs with removal and disappears with reinstitution, then the nutrient is considered essential (Table 3–1).

Screening for malnutrition can be an easy task. Unfortunately, there is no single, ideal test that positively confirms a diagnosis of malnutrition. Inquiring about weight loss, diets less than 1000 kcal/d with less than 50 g protein, a serum albumin less than 3 g/dl, anergy to skin tests, and a global assessment of the physical appearance can be a simple office screen. Table 3–2 lists a more traditional approach to nutrition assessment and will be discussed in detail below.

MEDICAL HISTORY AND PHYSICAL EXAMINATION

A standard history and physical examination may facilitate categorization of malnutrition. Both overnutrition and undernutrition are examples of imperfect nutrition. *Overnutrition* is an excess of caloric intake or dangerous levels of certain nutrients (e.g., alcohol, vitamins, minerals), and this will be discussed later. *Undernutrition* is a lack of one or more of the essential nutrients, including energy. Undernutrition can be viewed as primary or secondary malnutrition. *Primary malnutrition* refers to being unable, either voluntarily or not, to ingest a proper diet. This may be due to economic difficulties, unavailability of foods during food shortages, and extremes in personal preferences or religious beliefs. *Secondary malnutrition* is caused by some disease process that influences one or more of the following processes: ingestion, digestion, absorption, or utilization of nutrients. Both forms of this type of malnutrition may be seen in a particular patient.

The gastrointestinal tract is a very integrated system. Any alteration of this system may lead to abnormal nutrient intake and utilization, and ultimately, malnutrition. Poor dentition leads to altered mastication of foods, often a problem for the elderly population. Swallowing dysfunction following a cerebral vascular accident may prohibit liquid or solid food intake. Esophageal and gastric motility disorders may lead to food retention, nausea, and vomiting. Small bowel disease, including vascular, inflammatory, or malignant processes, may reduce the bowel's absorptive capacity, resulting in malabsorption and malnutrition. Pancreatic and hepatobiliary diseases may inhibit proper food digestion and influence absorption. Finally, colonic disease processes, especially motility disorders, may cause an obstructive process, thus inhibiting overall "gut" function. A proper investigative approach to these patients is necessary to ascertain the most efficacious manner of feeding. This may be as simple as altering the consistency of food or as invasive as implanting a central venous catheter for total parenteral nutrition.

A weight history is an important part of the medical history. The physician should ask the patient's usual weight, ascertain the present weight, and compare these to the ideal weight as defined by standard height and weight tables. A patient who usually is overweight may present at

TABLE 3-1. REQUIRED NUTRIENTS

ESSENTIAL FUELS	VITAMINS	MACRONUTRIENTS†	MICRONUTRIENTS‡ (TRACE ELEMENTS)
Essential Amino Acids	Fat-soluble	Calcium	Chromium
Arginine	Vitamins A, D, E, K	Chloride	Cobalt
Isoleucine	Water-soluble	Magnesium	Copper
Lysine	Thiamine, vitamin B_1	Phosphorus	Iodine
Phenylalanine	Riboflavin, vitamin B_2	Potassium	Iron
Tryptophan	Niacin, vitamin B_3	Sodium	Manganese
Histidine	Pantothenic acid, vitamin B_5		Molybdenum
Leucine	Vitamin B_{12}		Selenium
Methionine	Ascorbic acid, vitamin C		Zinc
Threonine	Folic acid		
Valine	Biotin		
Essential Fatty Acids			
Linoleic acid			
Linolenic acid*			
Carbohydrates			
Glucose			

*May be essential in infants.
†Required in amounts >200 mg/d.
‡Required in amounts <100 mg/d.

his or her ideal body weight; knowledge of the usual weight provides an important clinical clue. The cause of the weight loss should also be considered in terms of primary or secondary causes before one embarks on a search for a malignancy, as is so often done in practice.

The physical examination may provide other important clues concerning a patient's nutritional status, especially micronutrient and macronutrient deficiency. Alopecia or "lackluster" hair may imply zinc deficiency. Keratomalacia or conjunctival xerosis may signify vitamin A deficiency. Stomatitis or cheilosis may indicate pyridoxine deficiency. Dry or scaling skin may be a sign of zinc or fatty acid deficiency. Paresthesias, mental confabulation, and congestive heart failure may be secondary to thiamine deficiency. Unfortunately, most clinical signs of nutrient abnormalities do not manifest until the patient has a marked deficiency. The physical examination may also provide a snapshot of a patient's overall nutritional status. Peripheral edema may signify body protein depletion; loss of subcutaneous fat tissue may result from caloric deficiency, whereas muscle wasting and muscle weakness may indicate protein and calorie malnutrition.

TABLE 3-2. STANDARD NUTRITION ASSESSMENT

1. Medical history and physical examination
    a. Weight history (ideal body weight versus usual body weight)
2. Diet history
3. Anthropometric measurements
    a. Midarm circumference
    b. Triceps skin fold, which indicates fat stores
    c. Midarm muscle circumference, which indicates protein stores
4. Biochemical tests
    a. Albumin
    b. Transferrin
    c. Retinol-binding protein
    d. Prealbumin
5. Immunologic assessment
    a. Skin tests
    b. Total lymphocyte count

DIETARY HISTORY

Unfortunately, most physicians are not trained to take a good dietary history. Without this information obvious problems from primary and secondary factors may be overlooked. If the physician lacks the skills to properly assess nutrient intake, then, in appropriate patients, a registered dietitian should be consulted. They can comment on the patient's past intake, monitor present intake via calorie counts, and counsel patients for future dietary needs.

A dietary history is also important in identifying behavior patterns that may have important medical consequences in certain patients. Megadose vitamin ingestion or adherence to fad diets or very low calorie diets that are unsupervised are examples where the patient may be influencing their medical condition without their knowledge or the physician's approval. Alcohol to excess also has its medical and social ramifications, as do other nontraditional ingestions.

ANTHROPOMETRIC MEASUREMENTS

Multiple anatomic sites have been used for anthropometric measurements as gauges of nutritional reserves; the sites that are most commonly used for nutrition assessment are the midarm circumference, triceps skin fold, and midarm muscle circumference. These measurements can be performed by a dietitian or taught to other ancillary staff. The triceps skin fold estimates fat stores, and the midarm muscle circumference correlates with protein stores. However, it must be remembered that there is no storage form for protein so that any use of muscle protein represents cannibalization of muscle to support the body's protein needs. There are published tables of normal values for these measurements. The anthropometric measurements are best used for initial categorization of body stores and following a patient over time (weeks to months), since these are insensitive measures of day-to-day nutritional changes.

BIOCHEMICAL TESTS

Many clinicians wrongly consider serum albumin levels as an indicator of a patient's nutritional status. Statistically, it is known that patients who have a low serum albumin and are anergic to skin test antigens have a higher operative morbidity and mortality compared with patients with normal values. It is now considered that the serum albumin is more indicative of the level of stress on the body. For example, a patient who has lost a significant amount of weight from an esophageal cancer may be able to mobilize his protein stores; here the albumin synthesis pathway in the liver usually works normally so that even though appearing malnourished, the patient's serum albumin is in the normal range. However, an overweight patient with a postoperative wound infection who "appears" to have adequate nutrition stores may have a low serum albumin reflective of that liver pathway being modulated in favor of acute phase protein synthesis as the body attempts to fight the infection. In addition, albumin has a long half-life (about 21 days), and it is not a sensitive tool for nutrition assessment. Transferrin, prealbumin, and retinol-binding protein have also been used because their half-lives are shorter, 7 days, 2 days, and 12 hours, respectively. These plasma proteins also have their limitations as nutritional markers and should not be the only "nutrition test," but must be put into perspective after reviewing all the nutrition assessment data.

IMMUNOLOGIC TESTS

Malnutrition affects the immune system by depressing neutrophil chemotaxis, neutrophil degranulation, total lymphocyte count (TLC), and skin reactivity to common antigens. Physicians often use the TLC as a marker of the immune system's function. The TLC is calculated by multiplying the percentage of lymphocytes in the peripheral blood smear times the reported total white blood count. A TLC >1500 is normal, whereas a TLC <800 is abnormal and indicative of an immunologic defect. However, other nonnutritional factors can influence the TLC including drug therapy, infection, severe physical stress, and neoplasm. Delayed cutaneous hypersensitivity is assessed by observing cutaneous response at 48 hours to intradermal injections of common antigens. Induration of 5 to 10 mm indicates a normal response, whereas a lesser or an anergic response may indicate an abnormality. Again, other nonnutritional factors similar to those that can affect the TLC may alter the cutaneous response. Thus, assessment of a patient's immune status as a marker of nutrition must be interpreted in the context of the patient's overall general disease status.

MAJOR CATEGORIES OF MALNUTRITION

Table 3–3 lists the major ways to utilize the information obtained from the nutrition assessment. Traditionally, when most physicians consider malnutrition, they envision an underweight patient with either a malignancy, end-stage acquired immunodeficiency syndrome (AIDS), or a devastating gastrointestinal disorder. However, this only describes a small portion of malnourished patients, but here the physical examination can be very revealing. With marasmus, or simple starvation, a patient has suffered from decreased

TABLE 3-3. NUTRITION ASSESSMENT FEATURES IN MALNUTRITION

	MARASMUS	KWASHIORKOR (IMMUNOREPRESSIVE MALNUTRITION)	MIXED MALNUTRITION
Nutritional intake	Decreased calorie intake	Decreased protein intake and stress	Decreased calorie and protein intakes plus stress
Time course to develop	Months to years	Weeks to months	Weeks
Physical examination	Cachetic, fat depletion, muscle wasting	May look well nourished	Cachetic, may have edema, giving more normal appearance
Anthropometric measurements			
Triceps skin fold	Depressed	Relatively preserved	Variable
Midarm circumference	Depressed	Relatively preserved	Variable
Weight for height	Depressed	Relatively preserved	Variable
Skin test responses	Normal or depressed	Depressed	Depressed
Visceral proteins			
Albumin	Relatively normal	Low	Low
Transferrin	Relatively normal	Low	Low
Total lymphocyte count	Relatively normal	Low	Low

Based in part on Silberman H. *Parenteral and Enteral Nutrition*. 2nd ed. Norwalk, Conn: Appleton & Lange; 1989:55 with permission.

nutrient intake for a prolonged period, usually weeks to months. The physical examination is good at detecting fat depletion and muscle wasting, and the patient may be so depleted as to be cachetic. Anthropometric measurements are generally depressed. Interestingly, without a significant "stressor," the response to skin test antigens and visceral protein levels are relatively normal. Low values in these two areas impart an even more serious condition termed *mixed malnutrition*. This refers to a patient who has serious nutritional deficits that would characterize them as marasmic, but with low serum proteins and low TLCs, this implies that there is also an immunologic defect. The morbidity and mortality of this group are particularly high.

The other major category has classically been referred to as kwashiorkor. This was originally characterized by a protein-deficient diet with some or even adequate caloric intake. Examples of this type of malnutrition can unfortunately still be seen in the famine-stricken children of Somalia or Ethiopia. A more accurate term for the ill, hospitalized patient is *immunorepressive malnutrition*. This describes a patient who may have near normal or even excess muscle and fat stores but who is unable to metabolically access them because of complex hormonal or cytokine alterations caused by severe illness. These patients may look well nourished but have strikingly low albumin levels and TLCs as gross indicators of metabolic and immunologic dysfunction.

TREATMENT OF UNDERNUTRITION

There are several ways to approach a malnourished patient, which include the following: diet alteration, use of nutritional supplements, drug therapy, enteral nutrition via tube, or parenteral nutrition. A single modality may be sufficient for some patients, but special circumstances may require the use of a combination of techniques to provide optimal rehabilitation.

Diet alteration may be as simple as dietary instruction to show a patient other methods of food preparation or foods to include. In extreme cases, such as celiac disease, this will require a rigorous education and follow-up to achieve maximal recovery from this gluten-sensitive enteropathy. Again, a registered dietitian can be a valuable consultant in this circumstance.

Nutritional supplements are generally considered either commercially available or easily prepared items that can be taken in addition to a meal or may even replace a meal, if given in the proper quantity. The supplements are usually in the form of liquids or puddings. These require less effort to prepare and to ingest. Their use is often limited by their taste and expense.

Drug therapy has been used to stimulate the appetite of malnourished patients. The following drugs have been used: amantadine for the elderly and dronabinol or megestrol acetate for AIDS and cancer patients. The data are early but encouraging for their use in selected patients.

Enteral nutrition via tube feeding may be re-

TABLE 3–4. OPTIONS IN ENTERAL ACCESS FOR TUBE FEEDING

1. Cervical pharyngostomy
2. Nasoenteric tubes
   a. Nasogastric
   b. Nasoduodenal
   c. Nasojejunal
3. Tube enterostomies
   a. Gastrostomies (surgical, endoscopic or radiologic)
   b. Jejunostomies (surgical, endoscopic or radiologic)

quired in patients who are either too ill to eat their caloric needs on their own or have an anatomic reason for being unable to ingest their calories. Tube feedings may also be used to supplement poor oral intake. Table 3–4 lists the options for enteral access. Options include cervical pharyngostomy, nasoenteric tubes (nasogastric, nasoduodenal, or nasojejunal), and tube enterostomies as either gastrostomies placed endoscopically, surgically, or radiologically or as jejunostomies placed by similar methods. Cervical pharyngostomy may be useful in patients with head and neck tumors or in patients who have had strokes with significant transfer dysphagia. Nasoenteric tubes are an appropriate short-term option but often are limited by frequent dislodgement of the tubes and the risk of aspiration. Tubes may be placed blindly or with endoscopic or fluoroscopic assistance. Percutaneous endoscopic gastrostomies (PEG) have replaced surgical placement in many hospitals, especially academic centers, because of the convenience of endoscopic placement. Jejunostomies are being placed more often during initial surgical procedures to facilitate early enteral feeding, particularly in trauma patients. They are also used for patients who do not tolerate gastric feedings or have a history of repeated episodes of aspiration. Local expertise plays a key role in choosing the method of placement of both gastrostomies and jejunostomies.

Parenteral nutrition, provided by either peripheral vein or central vein, may be necessary for a patient who has gastrointestinal tract malfunction or other limitations to using the gut. This is the most costly of the options, and the risks and benefits of this therapy must be carefully considered. In some patients who are markedly malnourished, a combination of parenteral nutrition and enteral nutrition may be indicated if the patient exhibits intolerance to enteral feeding. The patient may require slow tube feeding to rehabilitate the gastrointestinal tract, which is manifesting intolerance because of maldigestion. After tolerance is shown in an increasing fashion from the gastrointestinal tract, feedings can be advanced and dependence on parenteral nutrition reduced until the patient is tolerating a more regular diet.

MARASMUS

For the patient who has marasmus or simple starvation the provision of sufficient calories and protein is key. However, it is possible to overfeed an individual, and this can be associated with dire consequences seen as the refeeding syndrome. The refeeding syndrome is the combination of events that occur in a malnourished patient who is put into positive nitrogen balance too aggressively without adequate replacement of electrolytes, particularly potassium, phosphorus, and magnesium. Deficiency states from these electrolytes can manifest in these patients, and deaths from neuromuscular irritability and arrhythmias have been reported. Thus, calories should be slowly administered in these patients and electrolytes measured frequently. Laboratory abnormalities are particularly noticeable after initiating feedings between the third to fifth day of therapy in parenterally fed patients and the fifth through seventh day with enteral therapy.

IMMUNOREPRESSIVE NUTRITION

In patients with immunorepressive nutrition it is important to support their nutritional needs, but in certain disease states it may be difficult to meet their protein needs because of severe hypercatabolism. In this situation it is important to provide sufficient protein to approach their protein needs and to limit their losses without compromising the patient's fluid status or renal function from excess fluid or protein. Nitrogen balance studies and metabolic cart determinations, when available, can assist in selecting more appropriate targets for calories and protein. Overfeeding is also not indicated in this setting since it produces excess carbon dioxide production that may further stress patients with poor pulmonary reserve. Overfeeding can also be associated with hyperglycemia and development of fatty liver. The key issue is to assist the patients through the stressful period and allow them to finish their nutritional rehabilitation during their convalescence at home.

UTILITY OF NUTRITION SUPPORT TEAMS

Nutrition support teams may be found in many larger hospitals and are composed of physicians, nurses, dietitians, pharmacists, and often other health care professionals. In patients with complicated nutritional problems, the team can assist the primary physician, provide cost-effective nutrition support, and help to decrease the number of complications for enterally and parenterally fed patients.

OVERNUTRITION

Although often not considered as a form of malnutrition, overnutrition is actually the most prevalent type of malnutrition in the United States. It has been estimated that one third of men and two thirds of women weigh 20% or more above their ideal body weight and that there are 6 to 10 million Americans who are considered morbidly obese, the latter being defined as either ≥45 kg (100 lb) over their ideal body weight or more than twice their ideal body weight.

In addition, overnutrition was previously defined as not just obesity, but ingestion of excess nutrients or other items that could cause other medical problems. To avoid problems with ingestion of large doses of vitamins, herbal remedies, or over-the-counter medications, the physician must ask about these therapies during routine examinations. Some patients may wish to hide these alternative therapies from their physician, but more often the patient does not offer this information unless specifically asked. We shall not consider this area further.

TREATMENT OF OVERNUTRITION FROM OBESITY

The cornerstone of treatment of overnutrition from obesity involves adequate nutritional counseling. This may best be accomplished in concert with a registered dietitian to assist the patient in learning more about nutrition, stressing variety, balance, and moderation. The patient's economic, educational, and social circumstances must be considered to make any plan work. Patients may be unwilling to totally change their behavior, but they may be willing to modify it. For example, they may not stop megadose vitamin therapy, but may be willing to alter the doses or individual vitamins ingested to safer levels.

For the obese patient, weight strategies are generally divided into mild-moderately obese and morbidly obese categories. For patients with 9 to 45 kg (20 to 100 lb) of excess weight to lose, diet therapy, exercise, behavioral modification, and combination therapies may all play a role. These generally accepted therapies may result in a modest reduction (10%) of excess weight, but most patients regain the lost weight within 1 year. A good maintenance program is the most important feature of a successful weight loss program. Some patients have even found benefit with acupuncture, hypnosis, or other nontraditional approaches, but little data exist on the long-term outcome of these therapies.

The most common weight loss strategy is dietary change. Two levels of caloric restriction are currently used: (1) the low-calorie diet (LCD)—1000 to 1500 kcal/d, and (2) the very low calorie diet (VLCD)—800 kcal/d or less. The VLCD is generally supervised by a physician. The VLCD may provide more rapid weight loss initially, but by 5 years after treatment most patients have returned to pretreatment weight. The same results are usually found with the other therapies.

Currently drug therapy is not viewed in the proper perspective. There is certainly abuse potential with the amphetamine family of drugs, but other commonly used medications have no appreciable addictive potential. Unfortunately, these medications are only licensed for short-term use. However, obesity is a long-term disorder, just like hypertension, and perhaps treatment should be viewed this way. Trials using medications for extended periods are presently ongoing. Combination therapy may be slightly more effective, but only if long-term treatment and maintenance are incorporated.

Surgical intervention may be indicated for morbidly obese patients with medical complications from their obesity. The risks of surgical treatment of morbid obesity include a 0.5% mortality, thus potential benefits must outweigh the risks. Weight loss has been good in correcting type II diabetes mellitus, obstructive sleep apnea syndrome, pseudotumor cerebri, gastroesophageal reflux, and stress overflow urinary incontinence. Average weight loss of one half to two thirds of excess weight within 12 to 18 months is considered very satisfactory.

SUMMARY

Malnutrition, whether undernutrition or overnutrition, should be considered a major medical problem. However, even though it should seem like common sense, until more outcome-based studies are available to show clinicians the importance of early management of nutritional problems, nutrition science will continue to be considered a "soft" science that awaits hard documentation. Nutrition training must be more widely taught in medical schools and then continued throughout a physician's career with emphasis on a physician's individual practice requirements.

REFERENCES

1. Bray GA. Use and abuse of appetite-suppressant drugs in the treatment of obesity. *Ann Intern Med.* 1993;119(7 pt 2):707–713.
2. DeLegge MH, Kirby DF. Enteral nutrition overview, 1: enteral access devices. *Practical Gastroenterology.* 1991; 15:21–27.
3. Foxx-Orenstein A, Kirby DF. Malnutrition and refeeding. In: Kirby DF, Dudrick SJ, eds. *Practical Handbook of Nutrition in Clinical Practice.* Boca Raton, Fla: CRC Press; 1994:19–30.
4. Jeejeebhoy KN, Detsky AS, Baker JP. Assessment of nutritional status. *JPEN.* 1990;14:193S–195S.
5. Kirby DF, DeLegge MH. Nutritional assessment: the high and low tech tour. In: Kirby DF, Dudrick SJ, eds. *Practical Handbook of Nutrition in Clinical Practice.* Boca Raton, Fla: CRC Press; 1994:1–18.
6. Solomon SM, Kirby DF. The refeeding syndrome: a review. *JPEN.* 1990;14:90–97.
7. Sugerman HJ. Gastric surgery for morbid obesity. In: Cameron JL, ed. *Current Surgical Therapy.* 4th ed. St. Louis, Mo: Mosby Year Book; 1992:67–71.
8. Technology Assessment Conference Panel. Methods for voluntary weight loss and control: Technology Assessment Conference statement. *Ann Intern Med.* 1993;119(7 pt 2):764–770.

4

Vitamin Deficiency

MARIA E. CAMILO and IRWIN H. ROSENBERG

The gastrointestinal tract is a complex and extremely active metabolic organ. Its epithelial functions are directed primarily toward supporting digestion and delivery of ingested nutrients. These depend on the integrity of motility, brush border activity, transport, and intestinal vascular supply. The maintenance of adequate nutrition relies on the integration of the gastrointestinal tract with other organs. Secretion and motility are mainly influenced by primary autonomous intrinsic neurologic and hormonal systems. Pancreatic exocrine function aids in the digestion and absorption of food. Impairment of the intestinal immune system is implicated in the genesis of several diseases that affect gut function and nutritional status. The liver plays a major role in the metabolic homeostasis of nutrients. Before passage into the systemic circulation, most nutrients are first "processed" or stored in the liver, which in addition participates in intestinal function through secretion of bile. Biliary secretion carries nutrients and bile salts that will be subject to reabsorption by the small intestine; this is called the *enterohepatic cycle.* Failure of this cycle leads to fat malabsorption and specific nutrient deficiencies.

Nutritional deficiencies can occur whenever disease significantly impairs any of the above functions.

PATHOGENESIS OF VITAMIN DEFICIENCY IN GASTROINTESTINAL DISEASE

The causes of deficiency of water and fat-soluble vitamins are not identical. The difference is explicable by differences in requirements, distribution in foods, absorption, and metabolism.

The mechanisms that cause vitamin deficiency in gastrointestinal diseases are shown in Table 4–1; usually more than one mechanism is involved, leading to deficiency of more than one vitamin.

INADEQUATE FOOD INTAKE

Dietary assessment (including qualitative assessment) is mandatory in the evaluation of nutritional deficiencies.

Patients often decrease food intake because of anorexia, nausea, fever, or depression or to prevent symptoms associated with eating (nausea, vomiting, dysphagia, pain, gastrocolic reflex with diarrhea). In addition, patients who have diseases causing significant stenosis of the gastrointestinal tract are prone to progressive reduction of oral intake. Therapeutic regimens (e.g., radiation, cancer chemotherapy, many drugs) can cause protracted anorexia, nausea, and vomiting. Restrictive diets, whether they are from an established habit (e.g., vegetarian diets), self-imposed to attempt to reduce symptoms, or physician recommended, can increase the risk of a nutritional deficiency. Significant symptomatic benefits are rarely due solely to strict dietary restrictions, except in specific dietary intolerance such as lactase deficiency and celiac sprue. Whenever recommended, restrictions should be accompanied by other alterations in the diet or by supplements to prevent or correct deficiencies.

Decreased intake is more important for the water-soluble vitamins. Although widely distributed in animal and plant products, their availability may be decreased by factors such as food storage and processing, naturally occurring vitamin antagonists, or interfering nutrients (e.g., zinc and folate, vitamins C and B_{12}). A major contributing factor to diet-induced water-soluble vitamin deficiencies is their relatively high turnover rate with small body stores; hence, a continuous supply is necessary. There is uncertainty on the nutritional significance of vitamins synthesized by enteric bacteria (e.g., biotin, folate). There is some indirect evidence of utilization of bacterially synthesized folate, since sub-

TABLE 4–1. PATHOGENESIS OF VITAMIN DEFICIENCIES IN GASTROINTESTINAL DISEASE

Mechanism	Contributing Factors	Vitamins
Inadequate food intake	Anorexia, nausea, vomiting, dysphagia, pain, obstruction, depression	All vitamins
	Restrictive unbalanced diets	Folate, B_{12}, thiamine
	Alcohol	Water-soluble, folate,* thiamine,* A
Malabsorption	Intestinal disease	All vitamins, folate,* fat-soluble vitamins
	Interrupted enterohepatic circulation	A, D, E, B_{12}, folate
	Pancreatic insufficiency	Fat-soluble vitamins, B_{12}
	Bile salt deficiency	Fat-soluble vitamins, A,* D,* K*
	Gastric or intestinal resection or bypass	All vitamins, B_{12},* folate,* D,* A*
	Bacterial overgrowth	Fat-soluble vitamins, B_{12}
	Alcoholism	All vitamins, folate,* B_1*
Impaired storage and metabolism	Altered tissue utilization	A, B_6, folate
	Decreased liver storage	A, B_1, B_6, folate
	Intrahepatic metabolism	B_1, folate, A, D, K
Increased losses (urinary)	Catabolic states	B_2, C
	Alcoholism	Folate, C, B_6
Increased requirements	Inflammation, fever	Thiamine
	Cell renewal	Folate, B_{12}
	Pregnancy, hemolysis	Folate
Drugs	Interference with intake, absorption or metabolism	All vitamins, folate,* A,* D,* K*
	Mucosal toxicity	Folate

*Vitamins most affected.

jects with natural or drug-induced achlorhydria and bacterial overgrowth have normal or increased levels of serum folate, although folate malabsorption is present. Cobalamin is a major exception; it is only found in animal products, but its human body stores exceed the daily requirements by about 1000-fold. Therefore, dietary lack of cobalamin slowly leads to clinical deficiency and is only seen in the strictest vegetarians.

Multiple water-soluble vitamin deficiencies, usually including vitamin C, folic acid, and B complex vitamins, may result from inadequate food intake; isolated deficiencies are relatively uncommon.

In adults, decreased food intake is an uncommon cause of deficiency of fat-soluble vitamins. Most of them have large body stores (mainly in adipose tissue or liver) and low daily requirements. Diet-induced vitamin A deficiency is common in Third World children and has been reported in alcoholism. Endogenous vitamin D provides enough for daily needs under normal sunlight exposure except during winter months in northern latitudes; otherwise dietary vitamin D becomes essential. Diet-induced vitamin K biochemical deficiency has been reported; this may not be of clinical significance if bacteria synthesis contributes to daily requirements.

MALABSORPTION

Malabsorption is the major potential cause of vitamin deficiency in gastrointestinal disease (Table 4–1). Integrated motility and secretions from the mouth, stomach, small intestine, biliary tract, and pancreas enhance digestion and mucosal contact for ultimate absorption.

Water-soluble vitamins are predominantly absorbed by carrier-mediated processes at physiologic intakes. The maximum absorption occurs in the first 120 cm (4 ft) of intestine; vitamins actively transported are absorbed mainly in the jejunum. Folic acid is absorbed mainly in the upper intestine, although there is a potential for adaptive absorption in the lower intestine. Most of the absorption of cobalamin depends on binding to intrinsic factor and uptake occurs in the mid to distal ileum. Passive absorption in the jejunum and proximal ileum has only an efficiency of about 1%. The absorption of fat-soluble vitamins, dependent on the intraluminal presence of bile acids, parallels the absorption of fat. Folic acid, cobalamin, and vitamin A undergo a significant enterohepatic circulation, which has been described for vitamin D metabolites as well.

Diseases affecting a significant proportion of the total absorptive area of the small intestine are likely to produce multiple deficiencies, although sometimes there is a dominant presenting vitamin deficiency. Several drugs contribute to vitamin malabsorption either by direct mucosal toxicity (e.g., neomycin) or by interfering with absorption of specific nutrients (e.g., neomycin, H_2 blockers, cholestyramine, sulfasalazine). Acute and chronic infections involving the gastrointestinal tract may result in malabsorption, diarrhea, and malnutrition.

Malnutrition and Intestinal Function

Whether as a consequence of a disease or of inadequate nutrient intake, moderate malnutrition may be associated with a reduction in gastric, biliary, pancreatic, and intestinal secretions and mucosal enzyme content but with minimal degrees of malabsorption. With severe malnutrition, frank diarrhea and malabsorption are characteristic. Specific deficiencies of protein, vitamin B_{12}, folate, niacin, or minerals (calcium, potassium, magnesium, zinc) may further impair intestinal function.

IMPAIRED STORAGE AND METABOLISM

Altered tissue utilization usually results from disease or drug-nutrient interaction (e.g., methotrexate or alcohol versus folate). Liver disease, as well as drugs (e.g., cimetidine and vitamin D), may affect the intrahepatic conversion of the vitamin into the active metabolite. Liver storage is decreased in chronic liver disease.

INCREASED LOSSES AND INCREASED REQUIREMENTS

Increased losses or increased requirements are minor contributors to water-soluble vitamin deficiency (Table 4–1). Increased urinary losses have been reported in catabolic states and in alcoholism and can be drug induced (isoniazid and vitamin B_6; diuretics and thiamine). Increased requirements are associated with fever or inflammation and increased cell turnover, which are prominent in inflammatory bowel disease and acute pancreatitis.

DRUGS

Drug-induced vitamin deficiency may be acute or chronic. Acute forms are usually due to potent vitamin antagonists (methotrexate, triazinate), whereas chronic forms may develop because the drug may alter intake, synthesis, absorption, transport, storage, metabolism, or excretion of vitamins. Most frequently, drugs alter the absorption of vitamins by disrupting the intestinal or mucosal mechanisms of vitamin absorption. Drugs have little, if any, effect on the composition or flow of the hepatobiliary or pancreatic secretions, although they may sometimes interfere with the absorption and intrahepatic metabolism of vitamins. Demonstration that a drug is capable of inducing an adverse nutritional effect (Table 4-2) is not synonymous with risk. The highest risk of deficiency is associated with drugs that are vitamin antagonists, described for folic acid, vitamin B_6, and vitamin K. Other drugs may or may not cause a clinical state of deficiency, depending on circumstances. Susceptibility to drug-induced vitamin deficiency is greater during periods of increased requirements (i.e., during growth, pregnancy, or lactation or when other individual diet or disease variables may interact, concurrently or sequentially).

RECOGNITION OF VITAMIN DEFICIENCY

The likelihood of vitamin deficiencies must be addressed in a patient's clinical history and physical examination. However, clinical manifestations are late consequences, which reflect tissue organ changes that are sometimes irreversible.

The physician's awareness of the nutritional implications of gastrointestinal diseases demands a detailed evaluation of the possible deficiencies in each particular case. Vitamin status can be evaluated by biochemical or functional tests and clinical malnutrition manifestations (Table 4-3).

With the exception of vitamin B_{12}, plasma levels of water-soluble vitamins fall relatively early in the course of the deficiency. On the other hand, circulating levels of fat-soluble vitamins are maintained by the large body stores until late in the course of the deficiency; vitamin K is the exception.

TABLE 4-2. COMMON DRUGS THAT MAY CAUSE VITAMIN DEFICIENCIES

Drug Group	Drug	Vitamin
Antacids	Sodium bicarbonate	Folate
Anticonvulsants	Phenytoin, phenobarbital	D, K, folate
Antibiotics	Tetracycline	C
	Neomycin	A, B_{12}
Antibacterial agents	Boric acid	Riboflavin
	Trimethoprim*	Folate
	Isoniazid*	B_6,* D, niacin
	Cephalosporin	K
	Cycloserine*	B_6,* B_{12}, folate
Antiinflammatory agents	Sulfasalazine	Folate
	Aspirin	C, K, folate
	Colchicine	B_{12}
Anticancer drugs	Methotrexate*	Folate
Anticoagulants	Warfarin*	K
Antihypertensive agents	Hydralazine*	B_6
Antimalarials	Pyrimethamine*	Folate
Diuretics	Triamterene*	Folate
H_2 receptor antagonists	Cimetidine, ranitidine	B_{12}, D, folate
Hypocholesterolemic agents	Cholestyramine, colestipol	A, D, K, B_{12}, folate
Laxatives	Mineral oil	Carotene, A, D, K
Oral contraceptives	Phenolphthalein	D, thiamine, riboflavin, B_6, C, B_{12}, folate
Tranquilizers	Chlorpromazine	Riboflavin
Miscellaneous	Potassium chloride, metformin	B_{12}
	L-Dopa, penicillamine*	B_6

*Vitamin antagonists.

TABLE 4-3. DIAGNOSIS OF VITAMIN DEFICIENCY

Vitamin	Clinical Signs	Biochemical Test
Thiamine	Anorexia, mental confusion, muscle weakness or wasting, ataxia, peripheral paralysis, ophthalmoplegia, edema, tachycardia, enlarged heart	Red cell transketolase activity coefficient >1.25
Riboflavin	Seborrheic dermatitis (around the nose and mouth), angular stomatitis, cheilosis, corneal vascularization	Erythrocyte glutathione reductase activity coefficient >1.3
Niacin	Anorexia, glossitis, angular stomatitis, dermatosis, diarrhea, dementia	Urinary methyl nicotinamide <5.8 μmol/d
B_6	Dermatitis, cheilosis, glossitis, peripheral neuropathy, convulsions, anemia	Plasma pyridoxal-5-phosphate concentration <5 ng/ml
Biotin	Anorexia, dermatitis, paresthesias, muscle pain	Bioassay of circulating or urinary biotin <reference interval
Folate	Macrocytosis, megaloblastic anemia, glossitis	Serum folate <4 ng/ml, red blood cell folate <140 ng/ml, peripheral blood smear: hypersegmentation of the neutrophils
B_{12}	Megaloblastic anemia, paresthesias, diminution of vibration or position sense, mental changes, combined system degeneration	Serum B_{12} <200 pg/ml, Schilling test <8%
A	Anorexia, growth retardation, nervous and skin disorders, night blindness,* xerophthalmia (Bitot's spots-corneal ulceration), blindness	Plasma vitamin A <20 μg/dl
D	Children: rickets and growth failure Adults: muscular weakness, bone pain, bone fractures (osteomalacia)	Plasma 25(OH)D <10 ng/dl, 24 h urinary calcium <100 mg
K	Ecchymoses, bleeding	Plasma abnormal Prothrombin >20 ng/ml
E	Neuromuscular deficits, reduced red blood cell half-life, cerebellar ataxia	Plasma tocopherol: <0.8 mg/g lipid (adults), <0.6 mg/g lipid (children)

*Functional test.

GASTROINTESTINAL DISORDERS WITH MAJOR VITAMIN DEFICIENCIES

Patients with the following conditions are at risk of developing subclinical or clinical vitamin deficiencies, which need prevention or treatment.

POSTGASTRECTOMY STATE AND GASTRIC BYPASS

Patients who have undergone partial or total gastrectomy are prone to nutritional disturbances. Vitamin deficiencies may occur as a result of decreased food intake and secondary malabsorption (Table 4–1). The reported incidence of vitamin B_{12} deficiency has ranged from 14% to 57% and often does not develop until 6 to 15 years after surgery. Multiple mechanisms have been proposed: deficiency prior to surgery due to H_2 blocker therapy, deficient intrinsic factor activity, impaired acid or pepsin secretion producing deficient utilization of dietary vitamin B_{12}, bacterial overgrowth of the small intestine, and disturbed enterohepatic circulation (EHC). Concomitant iron deficiency may prevent the development of megaloblastosis or even macrocytosis.

Folate deficiency has been reported, although its pathogenesis is unclear: inadequate food intake, altered intestinal pH, and interactions between the metabolism of folate and of vitamin B_{12} may all be involved. Previous medication before surgery may be of interest as some antacids and H_2 blocker agents may induce folate deficiency.

Vitamin D deficiency bone disease (more often osteomalacia than osteoporosis) may occur 10 to 20 years after gastric surgery. Osteomalacia may be clinically silent or evident, with bone pain, radiologic abnormalities, low serum calcium and phosphorus, and elevated alkaline phosphatase. It is most common after subtotal gastrectomy and gastrojejunostomy (Billroth II) and less common after Billroth I or after vagotomy with drainage. The proposed mechanisms for vitamin D deficiency include decreased intake of milk and fatty foods and malabsorption due to rapid intestinal transit.

Thiamine deficiency presenting as beriberi or

Wernicke-Korsakoff syndrome and following gastrectomy in alcoholics has been reported. The major underlying factor is probably alcoholism, aggravated by poor dietary intake and eventually by other concurrent vitamin B deficiencies. In fact, riboflavin and niacin deficiencies have been reported after gastrectomy.

Vitamin B_{12}, folate, and vitamin D deficiencies have been reported after gastric bypass for obesity; they are more common and occur earlier.

Atrophic Gastritis

Vitamin B_{12} deficiency results from impaired absorption caused by lack of intrinsic factor, lack of acid pepsin digestion of cobalamin from the dietary protein, and binding of vitamin B_{12}, or production of vitamin B_{12} analogs by bacterial overgrowth. Drug-induced achlorhydria induces the same pattern of vitamin B_{12} malabsorption. A minority of patients with atrophic gastritis have pernicious anemia and lack of intrinsic factor. Impaired absorption of vitamins A and E and folate does occur as a consequence of increase intraluminal pH, but actual deficiencies are unlikely.

Small Bowel Resection or Bypass

Impaired absorption of vitamin B_{12} has been noted following ileal resection or bypass or whenever intraluminal overgrowth of bacteria develops.

Folate deficiency may result from inadequate dietary intake, vitamin B_{12} deficiency, or rapid intestinal transit. Whenever bacterial overgrowth is present, bacterial folate may contribute to circulating levels.

Osteomalacia may occur after jejunoileal bypass for morbid obesity or resection of jejunum, ileum, or both. The proposed major mechanisms include disturbances of bile acid metabolism or interruption of the enterohepatic circulation of bile salts, or both, bile acid deficiency due to bacterial contamination of the bypassed segment, and impaired intrahepatic hydroxylation of vitamin D whenever liver dysfunction develops as a consequence of the bypass. In addition, poor dietary intake of vitamin D, lack of exposure to sunlight, and cholestyramine therapy may contribute. The response to vitamin D is unpredictable. Cholestyramine may induce deficiencies of all fat-soluble vitamins, as well as vitamin B_{12} and folic acid.

Jejunoileal bypass can lead to vitamin A and E deficiencies, which appear to be caused by fat malabsorption unrelated to bacterial overgrowth. Both deficiencies have been reported together, and it is reported that in vitamin E deficiency vitamin A is poorly stored and metabolized in the liver.

Thiamine deficiency, presenting with neurologic symptoms, has been rarely reported after jejunoileal bypass or short bowel syndrome as a consequence of poor dietary intake.

Pyridoxine deficiency after jejunoileal bypass was reported once, apparently as a result of malabsorption, impaired storage, impaired intrahepatic metabolism, and increased vitamin requirements due to pregnancy.

Intestinal Malabsorption Syndromes

The intestinal malabsorption syndromes (Table 4–4) are mostly characterized by disorders of epithelial cell digestion or transport or by abnormalities of lymphatic transport or gastrointestinal motility. The specific consequences are determined by the total area involved, the severity of the underlying disorders, their pattern of distribution (diffuse or patchy), and the eventual concurrent parasitic or bacterial overgrowth. The latter increases the likelihood of impaired absorption of fat-soluble vitamins. In some malabsorption syndromes, vitamin deficiency may become more conspicuous as a consequence of decreased food intake and the interaction of drugs or micronutrient deficiencies (e.g., zinc). All the malabsorption syndromes with the exception of lymphangiectasia and abetalipoproteinemia are likely to result in water-soluble and fat-soluble deficiencies. Folate and vitamins B_{12}, A, D, and K are the more affected. Lymphangiectasia and abetalipoproteinemia only develop fat-soluble vitamin deficiencies. In the latter, vitamin E is predominantly affected, and replacement therapy may even require parenteral vitamin E.

In a number of endocrine disorders without intestinal disease (thyrotoxicosis, Addison's dis-

TABLE 4–4. INTESTINAL MALABSORPTION SYNDROMES

Celiac sprue	Radiation enteritis
Tropical sprue	Lymphangiectasia
Collagenous sprue	Eosinophylic gastroenteritis
Primary lymphoma	Hypogammaglobulinemia
Whipple's disease	Giardiasis
Amyloidosis	Opportunistic infections (AIDS)
Abetalipoproteinemia	

ease, diabetes mellitus), abnormalities of gastrointestinal motility with rapid intestinal transit and sometimes intestinal bacterial overgrowth may induce mild steatorrhea with a risk of fat-soluble vitamin deficiency.

Nutritional management of patients with malabsorption implies an individually tailored diet with the exclusion or reduction of some foodstuffs (gluten, milk, fat). The dietary measures may decrease the risk of vitamin deficiencies. Supplement therapy should be directed toward predicted deficiencies (B complex, folate, and fat-soluble vitamins).

CROHN'S DISEASE

A wide range of vitamin deficiencies may develop as a consequence of several pathophysiologic mechanisms (Table 4–1). Symptomatic periods usually induce a decreased food intake, sometimes on a background of self-imposed or iatrogenic dietary restrictions. Malabsorption due to inflammatory infiltration or resection may involve different areas, mostly the ileum, which will determine the vitamins most affected. This may be further complicated by bacterial overgrowth due to stenosis or fistulas and drug interaction (corticosteroids, sulfasalazine, cholestyramine). During active inflammation, catabolism will increase losses and requirements of water-soluble vitamins, which may already be diminished because of poor food intake. The clinical or functional consequences are dominated by the major vitamin deficiencies and are more serious in children. Folate malabsorption may result from intestinal disease, disturbed EHC, bacterial overgrowth, sulfasalazine, vitamin B_{12}, and folic acid deficiency itself. Vitamin B_{12} deficiency is mainly dependent on the involvement or resection of the ileum, although bacterial overgrowth, disturbance of EHC, and cholestyramine may play a role. All fat-soluble vitamins have been reported deficient as a result of bile salt deficiency or disturbed EHC (ileal disease or resection); bacterial overgrowth and cholestyramine are minor factors. Osteomalacia is a major concern; in addition to malabsorption of vitamin D, prolonged corticosteroid therapy results in chronic negative calcium balance. Measuring 25-hydroxyvitamin D levels may be the best way to screen patients at risk.

Mild vitamin K deficiency has been reported in ileitis or ileocolitis, with or without associated small bowel resection.

Replacement therapy should include multivitamins, folate and vitamins B_{12}, A, D, and rarely K.

ULCERATIVE COLITIS

In ulcerative colitis, spontaneous oral intake may be reduced, mainly during the exacerbation periods, and nutrient utilization increases because of catabolism, inflammation, and increased cell turnover. Thus, water-soluble vitamins may be affected. However, the major potential risk of vitamin deficiency comes from sulfasalazine, a drug used in life-long maintenance therapy; findings have been that 60% have low serum folate levels and 10% have macrocytosis. Both the intraluminal and the mucosal phase of folate absorption are impaired, as well as the intrahepatic metabolism. Ensuing folate deficiency may be further aggravated by the increased requirements and may contribute to cell dysplasia.

Vitamin K deficiency has been reported in some patients taking sulfasalazine or antibiotics; the mechanism is unknown, but impaired colonic function and absorption were suggested.

Patients with total colitis and backwash ileitis may be at risk for developing other vitamin deficiencies as in ileal disease. Among systemic complications, cirrhosis or more often primary sclerosing cholangitis may lead to deficiencies similar to those found in cirrhosis with or without cholestasis.

PANCREATIC EXOCRINE INSUFFICIENCY

Either chronic pancreatitis, pancreatic carcinoma, pancreatic resection, or cystic fibrosis may present significant steatorrhea as a consequence of deficient enzyme and bicarbonate output for intraluminal digestion of fat. Impaired vitamin B_{12} absorption is common, but deficiency is rare. Symptoms result from malabsorption of the fat-soluble vitamins A, D, E, and K.

CHOLESTATIC LIVER DISEASE

Primary or secondary biliary cirrhosis, biliary atresia, and sclerosing cholangitis have multiple disturbances in the EHC of bile acids, the end result of which is an intraluminal bile salt deficiency with ensuing fat and fat-soluble vitamin malabsorption. Signs of all fat-soluble vitamin deficiencies can occur because of malabsorption, disturbed intrahepatic metabolism of vitamins A and D, and further bile acid sequestration by cholestyramine (if used). Beyond aggravating fat malabsorption, this drug can induce vitamin B_{12} and dietary folate malabsorption. Osteomalacia is the major concern. Vitamin D deficiency is multifactorial; in addition to malabsorption, there is often poor nutritional intake, increased urinary excretion, and lack of exposure or response to sunlight. The present goal of therapy is the maintenance of normal serum levels of calcium, phosphorus, and 25-hydroxyvitamin D. The current approach is to give intramuscular injections of 100,000 IU of vitamin D_2 every 4 weeks or 50 to 100 µg of oral 25-hydroxycholecalciferol daily. The rare patient who still suffers from bone pain with documented osteomalacia should be treated with 15 to 30 µg of 1-25-dihydroxycholecalciferol as an intramuscular injection every 4 weeks. In already established hepatic osteomalacia, the response to vitamin D therapy is uncertain.

Once a chronic cholestatic liver disease is diagnosed, the provision of fat-soluble vitamins supplements is a standard procedure. In addition to vitamin D, the following should be administered: vitamin A, 100,000 IU, intramuscularly, every 4 weeks; vitamin K_1, 10 mg, intramuscularly, daily until the deficiency is corrected, then 10 mg every 4 weeks; and vitamin E: 20 mg/d orally.

CIRRHOSIS

Alcoholic cirrhosis is usually associated with vitamin deficiencies; water-soluble vitamins are more often affected. Impaired liver storage and intrahepatic metabolism contribute to the risk of deficiencies in folate, thiamine, and vitamins B_6, A, D, and maybe K and E. A diminished synthesis of bile acids may affect fat-soluble vitamin absorption.

Cirrhosis of other origins have less severe vitamin deficiencies, unless they are associated with cholestasis (see "Cholestatic liver disease").

In decompensated cirrhosis, drug therapy with diuretics (traimterene) or H_2 receptor antagonists may increase the risk of folate, vitamin B_{12}, or other vitamin deficiencies.

Replacement therapy is a common procedure and includes multivitamins and folate for alcoholic cirrhosis irrespective of the patient's actual alcohol intake. Vitamin D supplements must be considered whenever there is steatorrhea.

DIETARY MANAGEMENT AND VITAMIN THERAPY

Dietary intervention to improve vitamin bioavailability may involve an exclusion, restriction, or increase in the amount of a particular nutrient in the diet.

Major gastrointestinal disorders may lead to a variety of vitamin deficiencies, with different prophylactic or replacement needs. A possible approach for the treatment of established vitamin deficiencies is presented in Table 4–5.

For cyanocobalamin, 100 1g/d orally can maintain vitamin B_{12} levels in most patients,

TABLE 4–5. VITAMIN THERAPY IN GASTROINTESTINAL DISEASES

VITAMIN	ASSOCIATED CONDITIONS	PREPARATION AND DOSE
Folate	Chronic alcoholism, intestinal malabsorption syndromes, Crohn's disease, gastric or intestinal resection or bypass, cirrhosis, drugs (sulfasalazine, antiepileptic agents)	Pteroylglutamic acid 1 mg/d PO
Cobalamin*	Gastric or intestinal resection or bypass, achlorhydria, ileal disease, bacterial overgrowth (blind loop syndrome)	Cyanocobalamin 1000 µg/every 3 months IM
Other water-soluble vitamins	Decreased food intake, diffuse intestinal disease, chronic alcoholism, cirrhosis	Therapeutic multivitamin (5–10× RDA) 1–2× daily PO
A*	Short bowel syndrome, ileal disease, steatorrhea, chronic cholestasis, cystic fibrosis, celiac sprue, drugs (cholestyramine)	Vitamin A 10,000–20,000 IU/d PO
D*	Ileal disease, chronic cholestasis, cystic fibrosis, short bowel syndrome, cholestyramine, steatorrhea, gastric resection or bypass	25(OH)D 20–40 µg/d PO or vitamin D 100,000 IU/mo IM
E*	Short bowel syndrome, chronic cholestasis, cystic fibrosis, abetalipoproteinemia	α-tocopherol 100–200 IU/d PO
K*	Ileal disease or resection, drugs (cholestyramine, sulfasalazine, antibiotics), biliary obstruction	Vitamin K_1 5 mg/d PO

*See text.

even in the absence of intrinsic factor or ileal receptors; however, during oral therapy, monitoring vitamin B_{12} levels every 6 months is mandatory. On the other hand, in pernicious anemia the initial period of treatment requires intramuscular cyanocobalamin. Vitamin D_2, 2000 to 4000 IU/d orally, usually in liquid preparation, is used for prophylaxis or maintenance regimens; however, severe chronic cholestasis or malabsorption may require an intramuscular regimen or other oral forms with higher biologic and absorptive activity (25-hydroxycholecalciferol or 1-25-dihydroxycholecalciferol). In abetalipoproteinemia, as well as in other cases of severe fat malabsorption with clinical signs of vitamin E deficiency, there may be a need for the use of intramuscular vitamin E, either for repletion (50 mg [IU]/d for 1 week) or for maintenance (50 mg three times a week). In the setting of severe hypoprothrombinemia related to vitamin K deficiency, intravenous vitamin K_1 (10 mg) must be administered slowly over 10 minutes, once or twice, 8 hours apart. Chronic cholestatic disorders may need intramuscular vitamin K_1 (10 mg) and vitamin A (100,000 IU) every 4 weeks.

5

Caustic Injury to the Upper Gastrointestinal Tract

WILLIAM M. BATTLE and MARK S. CODELLA

CAUSTIC INGESTIONS

A number of household cleansing agents can cause a significant injury to the gastrointestinal tract when ingested. Caustic agents may include acid, alkali, bleaches, and detergents. Detergents containing phosphate and bleaches containing sodium hypochlorite are relatively harmless. On the other hand, drain cleaners containing sodium hydroxide or potassium hydroxide, decalcifiers containing formic acid, and granular detergents containing metasilicates are caustic. The ingestion of a caustic substance by an adult usually represents a suicide attempt, whereas caustic ingestion in a child is generally accidental. Over 12,000 cases of caustic ingestion occur yearly in the United States.

Strongly alkaline household cleansers, containing lye, are the most commonly ingested caustic agents, with highly concentrated acid solutions being involved in only a minority of cases in the United States. Prior to 1967, lye was available only in solid form, and when ingested, lye granules tended to adhere to the mucosa of the oropharynx and proximal esophagus with distal injury occurring only in a small number of cases. The adherent granules were frequently expectorated rapidly or the injury was diminished by swallowing water and diluting the remaining caustic substance. Proximal localized stricture formation was usually the major sequela. When drain cleansers in the form of concentrated liquid lye solutions were introduced to the household market in 1967, more serious clinical problems developed, such as extensive esophagogastric necrosis, tracheoesophageal fistula, esophagoaortic fistula, and nondilatable esophageal strictures. The odorless, colorless nature of liquid lye, along with its similar appearance to milk, adds to its potential for accidental ingestion. Its high viscosity causes it to remain in contact with tissue longer, leading to greater injury. As a result of laws adopted in the early 1970s, today's products are less concentrated but remain highly caustic, especially if ingested in large quantities.

Acids are commonly ingested caustics in India, the Middle East, Europe, and Latin America because of their easy availability as cleansing agents. The strong offensive odor and the immediate pain to the oropharynx, especially following ingestion of hydrochloric or sulfuric acid, usually limits the amount ingested, except in suicide attempts.

Although the original maxim was that alkali bite the esophagus and lick the stomach, whereas acid corrosives lick the esophagus and bite the stomach, recent radiologic and endoscopic studies suggest that the ingestion of either type of corrosive agent can inflict serious injury to the esophagus, stomach, and even duodenum.

PATHOPHYSIOLOGY OF ALKALI AND ACID INGESTION

Alkaline ingestion results in liquefaction necrosis, with initial superficial destruction of tissue secondary to saponification of lipoproteins. The corrosive agent then migrates into the deeper layers of tissue, eventually becoming diluted and neutralized by the destroyed tissue (Table 5–1). Polymorphonuclear leukocytes form at the edge of the injury as bacterial invasion and vascular thrombosis begin.

The pathologic course can be divided into four stages: necrosis, ulceration, granulation, and scar formation. During the first week, the esophagus becomes edematous and inflamed. Necrotic tissue is visible as a discolored membrane. As the acute inflammation subsides, the necrotic tissue sloughs. It is at this point that the esophagus is the weakest and most vulnerable to perforation, especially if manipulated endoscopically. The sloughed membrane leaves an ulcerated base, which is replaced with granulation tissue and collagen during the second week. As collagen fibers contract circumferentially and longitudinally during the third week, the esophagus shortens leading to stricture formation. Eighty percent of strictures will manifest themselves within 8 weeks, with 99% manifesting by 1 year.

Strictures will occur with an overall incidence of 10% to 20% in caustic ingestions. Various areas of the same esophagus may be in different states of repair at any one time.

Although lye affects the esophagus most extensively, by no means is the gastric mucosa spared. Indeed, the incidence of gastric involvement is grossly underestimated. Animal studies have shown that ingestion of liquid alkali results in pylorospasm followed by a seesaw, to-and-fro movement of caustic contents between esophagus and stomach for a total of 3 to 5 minutes. Cricopharyngeal spasm prevents reentry into the oropharynx. Ultimately, the pylorus relaxes allowing passage of the remainder of the caustic material into the duodenum. Esophageal atony probably contributes to the cessation of this physiologic response. Any form of esophageal dysmotility or exaggerated reflux prior to ingestion will only enhance esophageal exposure and propagate tissue destruction.

Esophageal burns are classified much like skin burns. First-degree burns involve superficial mucosal hyperemia, mucosal edema, and superficial sloughing of mucosa. Second-degree burns reflect deeper tissue damage with ulceration and exudate formation. Third-degree burns result in transmural injury of the esophagus and periesophageal tissue with resultant mediastinal, pleural, or peritoneal inflammation. A definite relationship is noted between the intensity of the burn and evolution of the pathologic damage such as the development of strictures. Strictures are most apt to occur where the caustic agent has had prolonged contact related to anatomic narrowing. This occurs most commonly in areas such as the cricopharyngeal region, the midesophagus, secondary to extrinsic compression from the aortic arch or left main stem bronchus, and in the region of the diaphragmatic hiatus.

Unlike alkali, acids cause a coagulative necrosis, forming an eschar and limiting the depth of penetration. Early estimates of esophageal burns

TABLE 5–1. PATHOPHYSIOLOGIC FEATURES OF ALKALI AND ACID INGESTION

Alkali Ingestion	*Acid Ingestion*
Usually accidental in children less than 5 years old	Less commonly ingested than alkali
Lye (drain cleaners)—chief ingestant and most harmful	Found in toilet bowl cleaners, deodorizers, antirust products, disinfectants
Result in liquefaction necrosis	Coagulation necrosis with superficial eschar
Full thickness involvement of mucosa to muscularis propria	Depth of penetration limited
Esophageal involvement greater than gastric involvement	Gastric involvement greater than esophageal involvement
10% to 20% incidence esophageal strictures	Presence of food determines extent of injury
2.6% incidence of squamous cell carcinoma of esophagus around 40 years after ingestion	Chronic antral scarring in up to 60% of cases

following acid ingestion were 6% to 20% because of the relative resistance of the squamous epithelium and the alkalinity of the esophagus. However, in countries where highly concentrated acids are found, the incidence of esophageal damage approaches 50%. The degree of stomach damage depends on whether the acid is ingested in the fed or unfed state. Like alkali, the degree of damage also depends on the quantity ingested, the concentration of the acid, and the contact time with the gastric mucosa. When acid is ingested on a full stomach, it travels along the lesser curvature to the pylorus with most of the caustic being diluted along the greater curvature by food. Significant damage is therefore confined to the antrum and pylorus. Pylorospasm contributes to antral pooling. Duodenal injury may be seen in approximately one third of all cases in this setting. When acid is ingested on an empty stomach, however, the stomach behaves like a funnel since the lesser curvature becomes almost vertical. Diffuse contact with the gastric mucosa results in extensive ulceration and damage to the lower one half to two thirds of the stomach. Only the fundus is spared. Pyloric obstruction, antral stenosis, or an hourglass deformity of the stomach resembling linitis plastica occurs in as many as 60% of patients weeks to months following the ingestion of strong acid.

Weak acids usually produce reversible mucosal injury in the distal esophagus or stomach, whereas stronger acids result in irreversible damage. As with alkali, signs and symptoms do not forecast the extent of the injury. Rarely will ammonia or bleach cause severe injury to the gastrointestinal tract. Most injuries are superficial, resulting in edema but without the risk of long-term complications. Strictures are uncommon. Ammonia may cause respiratory compromise if the tracheal mucosa becomes inflamed.

Button battery ingestions are becoming a more prevalent problem in our increasingly technologic society. These disks are commonly found in watches, calculators, computer games, and cameras. They house potassium hydroxide or sodium hydroxide, usually as a 45% solution, and when ingested, these solutions may leak spontaneously causing an alkaline injury. If the battery lodges in the esophagus, a severe local burn may develop leading to rapid tissue destruction related to liquefaction necrosis in addition to pressure necrosis. If the disk is lodged in a specific location for greater than 8 hours, the risk of perforation is greatly increased especially in the esophagus. Injury to the stomach is less severe owing to its acidic environment, fluid volume, and the protective nature of the gastric mucosa. A button battery impacted in the esophagus should always be considered an endoscopic emergency and removed as soon as possible. Once the battery has reached the stomach and intestine, it is not as great a hazard.

Management of Caustic Ingestion

Unfortunately the management of caustic injury to the upper gastrointestinal tract has been based mainly on animal studies and anecdotal patient reports. The literature is replete with uncontrolled and nonrandomized studies that have led to much controversy regarding what constitutes proper therapy. Recently there has been an attempt to approach the subject on a more scientific basis.

Emergency management should initially concentrate on resuscitative procedures, and diagnostic evaluation should be delayed. By the time the victim is admitted to the emergency room there are really no effective neutralization measures that can reduce the extent of the instantaneous necrosis produced by ingested caustic material. Emesis is contraindicated because it will reexpose the esophagus and perhaps oropharynx to further injury and may lead to aspiration of the caustic material, which further complicates the situation. As in any other trauma situation, attention should be given immediately to the assessment of airway status and hemodynamic stabilization. Endotracheal intubation or tracheostomy may be required urgently in patients who are in obvious respiratory distress. Clinical signs such as hoarseness, stridor, and aphonia reflect significant injury to upper airways and possible impending respiratory distress.

Injury to oropharynx and esophageal atony following damage to deep musculature and the nerves of Auerbach's and Meissner's plexi leads to recurrent salivation and drooling. Retrosternal chest pain, dysphagia, and odynophagia are all common symptoms that resolve as the acute inflammation subsides. Epigastric pain, emesis, and hematemesis may reflect gastric injury, whereas left shoulder pain implies fundic involvement.

After establishment of venous access, hypotension should be corrected with appropriate intravenous fluids. Attempts at gastric aspiration and lavage are of doubtful benefit because of instantaneous necrosis and the increased risk of inducing regurgitation or reflux. Theoretically neutralization can release large quantities of heat and could add thermal insult to caustic injury.

Following the above initial emergency measures, additional information should then be obtained from patient, family, or witness to the ingestion regarding the composition and quantity of material ingested. Several characteristics of the caustic agent including the type of agent ingested, its concentration, the quantity, and the duration of contact with the mucosa ultimately determine the extent and severity of the injury. X-ray examination of the neck, chest, and abdomen should be performed to rule out perforation or aspiration pneumonia. Obvious signs of mediastinal injury or peritonitis are indications for urgent surgery. Contrast studies are not very useful in assessing the degree of acute injury and should be reserved to follow the patient for the sequela of cicatrization of the esophagus and stomach or possible delayed perforation.

Once the patient is stabilized and if there is no indication for emergent surgery, then endoscopic evaluation should be performed. Early endoscopy is safe, reliable, and the most accurate diagnostic tool for the assessment of corrosive injury to the upper gastrointestinal tract and is crucial in management and predicting the prognosis.

Numerous studies have demonstrated that clinical symptoms and signs, oropharyngolaryngeal examination, and radiologic studies do not adequately predict the presence or severity of upper gastrointestinal tract burns from corrosive agents. All patients with a history of caustic ingestion should have endoscopic evaluation even if they are asymptomatic and in the absence of oropharyngeal burns.

With the availability of the new slim flexible pediatric panendoscope, the original concerns with the use of the rigid endoscopes regarding instrumental injury and perforation are no longer a major issue. However, extreme caution with termination of the examination is required when frank necrosis of the esophagus is encountered or complete obliteration of the esophageal lumen because of massive edema is encountered. *Contraindications to the performance of endoscopy in the setting of caustic ingestion include:*

- Perforation
- Shock
- Severe hypopharyngeal edema and necrosis
- Respiratory distress

Although endoscopy is generally performed in the first 12 to 24 hours and is safe up to 96 hours after the ingestion, it should be avoided in the subacute phase (5 to 15 days after corrosive ingestion) because of increased risk of perforation during the tissue sloughing stage, when the esophageal wall is at its thinnest. The management of caustic ingestion is summarized in Table 5–2.

Endoscopic grading (Table 5–3) of the caustic injury not only determines initial treatment but also allows the accurate prediction of early and late complications. It has recently been suggested that the traditional endoscopic classification be modified because prospective evaluation demonstrated different prognostic and therapeu-

TABLE 5–2. MANAGEMENT OF CAUSTIC INGESTION

1. Assess airway status and determine need for endotracheal intubation or tracheostomy.
2. Establish venous access and proceed with hemodynamic stabilization.
3. Do not administer emetics or attempt neutralization.
4. Obtain history regarding concentration and quantity of material ingested.
5. Plain x-ray films of neck, chest, and abdomen to assess for perforation or aspiration pneumonia. (Avoid contrast studies.)
6. In the absence of contraindications, perform early endoscopy with slim flexible panendoscope to establish grade of caustic injury.
7. Decide on emergent surgery based on the results of numbers 5 and 6.
8. Consider empiric use of antacids, H_2 blockers, or sucralfate suspension.
9. Although corticosteroids may be useful in certain subgroups of patients with moderate injury, they cannot be definitely recommended and may be hazardous.
10. Broad spectrum antibiotics should be given if steroids are administered, but otherwise they should be withheld until signs of infection occur.
11. Nutritional support with either small bore feeding tube or total parenteral nutrition.
12. Follow-up barium studies and dilation as needed.

TABLE 5–3. ENDOSCOPIC GRADING OF CAUSTIC INJURY

Grade	Findings
0	Normal examination
1	Edema and erythema
2A	Friability, hemorrhage, erosion, blisters, superficial ulceration, and whitish membranes
2B	Deep or circumferential ulceration
3A	Small areas of necrosis
3B	Extensive necrosis

tic implications for subgroups of patients with grade 2 and 3 injury (Table 5-4). Under this new classification, patients with grade 2A injury have friability, hemorrhagic inflammation, erosion, blisters, whitish membranous exudate and superficial ulcerations, whereas grade 2B reflects deep or circumferential ulcerations. Patients with grade 3A injury are characterized by small areas of necrosis (reflected by areas of brownish-black or grayish discoloration), and grade 3B connotes extensive necrosis. There has been some difference of opinion regarding the significance of blackish discoloration of the mucosa. Most authors believe it represents full thickness necrosis (mucosal gangrene); however, there is data to suggest that dark discoloration of the mucosa can represent only hematin formation due to effect of caustic on erythrocytes.

Patients with grade 0, 1, and 2A injury rarely develop complications and generally recover completely, whereas those with grade 2B injury have a 70% incidence of stricture formation. Patients with grade 3 injury are more prone to develop acute complications such as minor or major gastrointestinal bleeding, esophageal stricture, perforation, or esophageal-tracheal fistula formation. Twenty-five percent of grade 3A injury patients require surgery for late sequelae. Patients with grade 3B injury (extensive necrosis) develop acute complications 70% of the time with a 65% mortality, and the majority of the survivors require surgery for the sequelae of the severe injury. Obviously patients with circumferential ulceration (grade 2B) or necrosis (grade 3) are those at most risk for stricture formation and major morbidity and mortality.

Following the acute inflammation, a latent phase may last several weeks. This is accompanied by a resolution of symptoms in some patients which may lead the physician or patient to believe that the worst is over. However, the chronic phase then becomes manifest with recurrent dysphagia secondary to stricture formation. In a matter of a few days the symptoms may rapidly progress from just mild dysphagia to inability to handle secretions. Gastric outlet obstruction may be evidenced by anorexia, weight loss, early satiety, or recurrent emesis.

Unfortunately therapy to prevent stricture formation is controversial and unproven. Time-honored treatment has consisted of corticosteroids, antibiotics, and dilation. The basis of the corticosteroid treatment was a group of studies in animals showing that steroid administration within 48 hours of caustic injury and continued for 4 to 6 weeks inhibited fibrosis and granulation formation and thus reduced the incidence of stricture formation. Since animals treated with corticosteroids had an increased incidence of septic complications, antibiotics were added to decrease the incidence of fatal infections. There is no evidence that antibiotics alone, however, inhibit esophageal stricture formation. Based on the animal data, it became common practice to treat patients with mild-to-moderate esophageal burns (grade 1 and 2 injury) following caustic ingestion with corticosteroids and antibiotics. Numerous uncontrolled patient studies claimed efficacy for the corticosteroid-antibiotic combination, whereas others have questioned this approach and have cautioned against the administration of corticosteroids especially with grade 3 injury since, given in pharmacologic dosages, corticosteroids impair wound healing, depress the body's immune defense system, and mask signs and symptoms of infection and visceral perforation.

A recent prospective controlled evaluation of the use of steroids to prevent esophageal stricture in children following caustic ingestion failed to reveal any significant benefit. As in numerous other studies, the critical factor in stricture developments was the initial severity of the esophageal injury. Although present evidence does not exclude the possibility of benefit of corticosteroids in a subgroup of patients with moderate injury, the lack of proven efficacy and the potential

TABLE 5-4. PROGNOSIS AND MANAGEMENT BASED ON ENDOSCOPIC GRADING

Grade	
	Complication
0, 1, 2A	Usually none
2B, 3A	Gastrointestinal bleeding, esophageal and gastric strictures
3B	Gastrointestinal bleeding, stricture, perforation, fistula, death
	Management
0, 1	Minimal observation; discharged without treatment unless psychiatric referral is indicated
2A	Observe in the hospital; liquid diet; consider empiric use of antacids, H_2 blockers, or sucralfate suspension
2B, 3A	Observe in hospital (possibly ICU); keep NPO; administer IV H_2 blockers and provide nutritional support; empiric steroids and antibiotics cannot be recommended based on the present data
3B	Prompt surgical therapy

hazards in a patient with severe injury to the upper gastrointestinal tract following caustic ingestion suggest that corticosteroids are not indicated for stricture prophylaxis. In the absence of corticosteroids there is no rationale for prophylactic antibiotics, and they should be reserved until signs of infection have occurred.

Empiric use of antacids, H_2 blockers, and sucralfate suspension seem reasonable, but no control studies have been performed with any of these agents.

Alternative efforts to prevent stricture formation following caustic injury have been suggested. Several groups claim that esophageal stents inhibit stricture formation, but in the absence of randomized studies and with the potential to cause harm this cannot be recommended at the present time. Early prophylactic bougienage has been proposed, but the only clear benefit appears to be detection rather than prevention of stricture. Strictures begin to appear after 2 weeks, and the majority manifest themselves by 8 weeks. Dilations are usually begun around 2 to 3 weeks following the ingestion when stricture symptoms first appear. Various attempts to inhibit dense scar formation in experimental animals using agents such as collagenases, lathyrogens, N-acetylcysteine, and penicillamine have been reported; however, more animal and human experimentation is necessary before these agents can be recommended for routine clinical use. Total parenteral nutrition as a means of achieving positive nitrogen balance and allowing the inflamed gastrointestinal tract to rest without trauma of ingested food has also been recommended.

Surgical intervention is necessary for acute complications of caustic ingestion such as perforation, abscess, fistula formation, or for chronic stricture formation that is not amenable to bougienage. Aggressive surgical approach has been recommended in patients with endoscopic evidence of extensive esophagogastric necrosis, since delay in the diagnosis and treatment of transmural necrosis is the single most important factor contributing to significant mortality. A detailed discussion regarding the relative merits and risks of the various surgical procedures to manage the undilatable stricture is beyond the scope of this chapter. Options include an esophageal resection with replacement by stomach tissue, if it is uninjured, or by a long segment of colon or colonic bypass (retrosternal or presternal) leaving the strictured esophagus in situ. Alternatively gastric antral patch esophagoplasty has been recommended in selected patients to avoid the risks and difficulties associated with resection or bypass. Some authors favor resection since it abolishes the risk of esophageal carcinoma following caustic ingestion.

Squamous cell carcinoma of the esophagus occurs with an incidence of 2% to 3% following lye ingestion. The risk is 1000-fold greater than for the general population. There is a mean latency period of 40 years, and the most common site of development of carcinoma is the bronchial bifurcation. The prognosis of esophageal carcinoma following lye ingestion may be slightly better than usual because of the younger age of development, the earlier appearance of symptoms secondary to stricture of the esophagus, and the limitations of spread by scar tissue. Periodic endoscopic surveillance would be reasonable in patients with a previous history of lye ingestion. Although there have been occasional reports of gastric carcinoma after acid ingestion, there is no clear increased incidence.

REFERENCES

1. Anderson KD, Rouse TM, Randolph JG. A controlled trial of corticosteroids in children with corrosive injury of the esophagus. *N Engl J Med.* 1990;323:637–640.
2. Goldman LP, Weigert JM. Corrosive substance ingestion: a review. *Am J Gastroenterol.* 1984;79:85–90.
3. Kikendall JW. Caustic ingestion injuries. *Gastroenterol Clin North Am.* 1991;20:847–857.
4. Leape LL, Ashcraft KW, Scarpelli DG, Holder TM. Hazard to health—liquid lye. *N Engl J Med.* 1971;284:578–581.
5. Postlethwait RW. Chemical burns of the esophagus. *Surg Clin North Am.* 1983;63:915–924.
6. Spechler SJ. Caustic ingestion. In: Taylor MB, ed. *Gastrointestinal Emergencies.* Baltimore, Md: Williams & Wilkins; 1992:chap 2.
7. Zargar SA, Kochhar R, Mehta S, Mehta SK. The role of fiberoptic endoscopy in the management of corrosive ingestion and modified endoscopic classification of burns. *Gastrointest Endosc.* 1991;37:165–169.
8. Zargar SA, Kochhar R, Nagi B, Mehta S, Mehta SK. Ingestion of corrosive acids. *Gastroenterology.* 1989;702–707.
9. Zargar SA, Kochhar R, Nagi B, Mehta S, Mehta SK. Ingestion of strong corrosive alkalis: spectrum of injury to upper gastrointestinal tract and natural history. *Am J Gastroenterol.* 1992;87:337–341.

6
Rectal Foreign Bodies

MARTA L. DAVILA and KENNETH R. McQUAID

Foreign bodies of the rectum are being encountered with increased frequency in the emergency facilities of both large metropolitan hospitals and small community clinics. In over two thirds of cases, they can be removed safely and expeditiously in the outpatient setting.[2,9] The remainder of cases require hospital admission with transanal removal under general or spinal anesthesia or, rarely, laparotomy.

The subject of rectal foreign bodies is the frequent source of amusement and ribaldry among physicians. On reviewing a list of various rectal foreign bodies reported in the world's literature, one cannot help being struck by their variety of shapes and sizes (Table 6–1). Indeed, it has been stated that the nature of these objects is limited "only by the capacity of the rectum and the bounds of the human imagination."[5] Their oddity notwithstanding, rectal foreign bodies may present difficult therapeutic problems and occasionally have life-threatening consequences. It therefore behooves the emergency room physician, general internist, gastroenterologist, and surgeon to understand the principles of outpatient management of patients with rectal foreign bodies and the indications for surgical consultation and hospital admission.

The circumstances under which foreign bodies may be introduced into the rectum include:

1. Diagnostic or therapeutic mishap; e.g., thermometer, enema tip, irrigation catheter, etc.[7]
2. Criminal sexual assault.
3. Intentional insertion for illicit purposes, e.g., drug smuggling.
4. Anal eroticism (self-inserted or with participation of a partner), e.g., vibrators, plastic phalluses, fruits, vegetables, bottles, sticks, etc.[3]
5. Accidental or intentional oral ingestion, e.g., toothpicks, pins, glass, etc.[13]

PRESENTATION

Rectal foreign bodies most commonly occur in the setting of self-introduction for anal erotic gratification. The overwhelming majority of patients are young to middle-aged males. Although the problem of rectal foreign bodies is commonly presumed to be limited to male homosexuals, this may not be the case. Sexual preferences are not usually reported in the literature and may be unreliable because of embarrassment or a desire to protect a third party. It is known that a significant number of heterosexual men and women and lesbian women also practice anal sexual stimulation.[9] It has been hypothesized that the greater curvature of the male pelvic sacral hollow may increase the propensity for a foreign object to become impacted with the lower end of the object resting on the hollow.

Many patients will freely divulge to the physician the circumstances surrounding the foreign body impaction, thereby obviating any diagnostic dilemma. Others may be reluctant to disclose that they have a rectal foreign body or may con-

TABLE 6–1. COLLECTED DATA ON RECOVERED RECTAL FOREIGN BODIES

OBJECT	NUMBER
Rubber phalluses	27
Vibrators	24
Bottles or jars	19
Sharp objects	14
Vegetables (carrot, zucchini, cucumber, corn cob)	6
Metal can	5
Light bulb	4
Sachets of heroin	3
Bones	3
Wax candle	2
Others: brush, bottle top, cement, toothpick, pen, screwdriver, bicycle hand grip	1 of each

Data from references 2, 5, 7, 12.

coct fantastic stories to account for its presence. Still others may report various rectal or abdominal symptoms but withhold information about the presence of a foreign body. A professional, nonjudgmental demeanor on the part of the physician is required. Most patients seek medical attention within 24 hours of insertion; however, some seek medical attention days later after unsuccessful attempts to extract the object themselves manually or with enemas.

Cases of sexual assault are relatively rare; nevertheless a careful history should be taken in all cases of rectal foreign bodies in an effort to determine whether a crime may have been committed. If suspected, appropriate documentation of evidence and consultation with police and rape counselors is indicated.

Foreign body ingestion is most likely to occur in children, denture wearers, the mentally impaired, and prisoners. These cases may pose a diagnostic challenge to the physician because the patient may not realize that he swallowed a foreign body. Furthermore, days to weeks may pass between the ingestion and the onset of rectal or anal symptomatology, resulting in patients forgetting that they swallowed an object or failing to make the association between the remote ingestion and their current symptoms. Patients who have the acute onset of rectal symptoms or rectal abscess should be asked about accidental foreign body ingestions.

By whatever method of introduction, rectal foreign bodies may cause symptoms of rectal or anal pain, fullness, obstruction, hematochezia, or rectal discharge. Perforations may occur but are surprisingly uncommon. Perforations are not restricted to sharp objects but also relate to the forcefulness of penetration. Above the peritoneal reflection, perforations result in obvious signs of peritonitis and are a surgical emergency. Perforations below the reflection may be much more insidious with pain, fever, and sepsis developing over hours to days.

MANAGEMENT

INITIAL APPROACH

Management begins with a detailed history that should include the number and type of objects introduced, the length of time that has elapsed since its insertion, whether it was inserted by the patient or a partner, and whether it was inserted voluntarily. Any efforts by the patient to extract the object should be determined. The patient should be asked about the presence of fever, abdominal pain, anal discomfort, rectal fullness or pain, constipation, and bleeding.

The physical examination should concentrate on the abdomen, anus, and rectum with a particular emphasis on peritoneal signs. The foreign body is often palpable in the lower abdomen. Anal examination should include an assessment of tone and careful inspection for any evidence of sphincteric disruption. Digital rectal examination is vital to determine whether the object is palpable in the lower rectum and to determine its orientation.

Prior to any therapeutic intervention, biplane abdominal radiographs should be performed to elucidate the number, shape, orientation, and location of the foreign body. Perforation above the peritoneal reflection is usually evident from the physical examination and is confirmed on x-ray examination by the presence of free intraabdominal air. A water-soluble contrast enema should be obtained in a patient who has a suspected perforation based on physical examination but negative plain abdominal roentgenography.

After confirming the identity and location of the rectal foreign body, a therapeutic approach to its safe and expeditious removal can be planned. The suggestion of perforation on physical examination or abdominal roentgenography precludes endoscopic approaches to foreign object removal and requires emergent surgical intervention (outlined below). In all other patients, the initial approach depends on the location of the foreign body. On the basis of physical examination and plain abdominal x-ray examination, rectal foreign bodies may be classified in the following manner[1,7]:

- *Low lying:* objects located in the rectal ampulla and usually *palpable* on digital examination.
- *High lying:* objects located at or proximal to rectosigmoid junction.

LOW-LYING OBJECTS

Over two thirds of rectal foreign bodies are low lying in location. Although these objects are inserted by patients with (apparent) relative ease, physician retrieval can be fraught with difficulties. A variety of factors may hinder removal.[6] The anal sphincter may be in spasm. The rectal mucosa is often edematous and blood or mucus may obscure visualization. The object may impact in the sacral hollow away from the anus. Certain characteristics of the objects also pose particular problems. For example, smooth round hard objects are difficult to grasp. Tapered objects generally have the widest end oriented caudally. Organic matter may be quite friable. Finally, negative pressure may develop above the foreign body as it is retracted, resulting in a suction effect. Notwithstanding these difficulties, the majority of low-lying rectal foreign bodies, with ingenuity and persistence, can be removed transanally in the outpatient setting.[2,7,9]

In preparing for a transanal retrieval of a foreign body, it is helpful to keep some basic principles in mind:

1. Based on the size and shape of the object, decide whether the object can be removed manually or requires assistance with anoscopy or proctosigmoidoscopy (see below).
2. Manual extraction or flexible sigmoidoscopy can be performed in the left lateral or lithotomy positions; rigid sigmoidoscopy in the prone jack knife or left lateral position. If retrieval is unsuccessful in one position, another should be tried.
3. Obtain adequate relaxation of the patient and of the anal sphincter. Anxious patients may require intravenous conscious sedation. Many patients have an anal sphincter that is lax enough to allow several fingers to be inserted to remove the object. If the patient experiences significant discomfort with such manipulations, however, local anesthesia of the anal sphincter is necessary (see below).
4. Enemas should not be administered because they can push the object higher into the rectum.
5. If proctosigmoidoscopy is required, care should be taken not to push the object higher into the rectum.
6. Instruments used in extraction should never be inserted blindly into the rectum but only under guidance with anoscopy or proctoscopy; objects should be removed under direct visualization.
7. The "suction effect" described above may be overcome by the insertion of a venting device, such as a 24 Fr. Foley catheter or endotracheal tube, beyond the foreign body.[8]
8. After removal of the foreign object, proctosigmoidoscopy must be performed to look for evidence of significant bowel wall injury.

Smaller, blunt low-lying objects can usually be removed blindly by grasping the object directly with gloved fingers after adequate sedation and manual anal dilation of the anus are achieved.[15] However, small sharp low-lying objects should be removed through an operative anoscope or proctoscope under direct visualization to avoid iatrogenic injury to the rectum or anus.[12] Particular caution should be taken with glass objects to avoid breaking them during retrieval.

With larger foreign bodies, it may be difficult to achieve a secure digital grip for successful retrieval. In these cases proctosigmoidoscopy (rigid or flexible) is necessary to facilitate grasping the object with sundry instruments. The rigid sigmoidoscope has been employed most frequently. Given its size, a variety of instruments can be passed through it to grasp or ensnare the object. Snares, forceps, clamps, and uterine tenacula have been used most successfully. Flexible sigmoidoscopes are not readily available in most emergency facilities; hence their utility is not as well established. Large snares and foreign body forceps may be useful during flexible sigmoidoscopy.

There are as many ingenious techniques used for removing foreign bodies as there are foreign bodies themselves. In most cases, the above approaches will be successful. Sometimes more creative methods must be employed. Large hollow objects may be removed by inflating a Foley catheter balloon, a Sengstaken-Blakemore tube, or an endoscopic dilation balloon within them, allowing for better traction.[11] Open containers with their mouths directed caudally can be filled with plaster of Paris around a tongue blade or piece of gauze; after the plaster sets the object can be removed with steady traction. Other novel extraction methods have included suction darts and "Crazy Glue."

If the patient is uncooperative, if dilation of the anus is inadequate, or when dealing with larger rectal objects, local anesthesia is strongly recommended. Local anal block can be achieved by using lidocaine or bupivacaine (0.5%) with epinephrine (1:200,000). A continuous wheal is raised around the anal verge with a 30-gauge needle. Approximately 8 to 15 ml are used in this phase. Subsequently a 22-gauge, 1½-inch needle is inserted submucosally in all four quadrants (2.5 ml in each quadrant) while the finger is maintained in the rectum to guide the needle.[4,9] With this technique, complete relaxation of the sphincter is consistently obtained. Should further dilation be necessary, Parks anal retractors or vaginal wall retractors may aid in anal dilation and in shortening the anal canal.[9,14]

The overwhelming majority of low-lying rectal foreign bodies can be removed successfully in the outpatient setting using the above approach.[2,5,9,15] If the object cannot be removed within a reasonable period of time and with adequate patient comfort, the patient should be admitted and brought to the operating room for extraction of the object under spinal or general anesthesia. With the patient in the lithotomy position attempts are again made to retrieve the object transanally using manual manipulation or the previously mentioned surgical or obstetrical devices. Under general anesthesia, the entire hand can be inserted into the rectum, allowing more vigorous manipulation and bimanual pressure on the anterior abdominal wall. Successful extraction of low-lying rectal objects is virtually always achieved without the need for laparotomy.[5]

Proctosigmoidoscopy should be performed in all patients after removal of the foreign body to assure no missed foreign bodies and to look for evidence of significant anal or rectal injury.[7] Not unexpectedly, small mucosal lacerations and abrasions can be seen on examination but are of little consequence. It was previously held that all patients with rectal foreign bodies should be admitted for 24 hours observation to look for evidence of delayed perforation or perirectal suppuration.[7] More recently, it is felt that patients who have an uncomplicated outpatient extraction and no abnormal findings after post-extraction proctosigmoidoscopy may be safely observed as outpatients.[2,4,5,12] Patients who have persistent pain or bleeding after extraction or who have deep lacerations evident on proctosigmoidoscopy should be admitted for at least 24 hours' observation.[2,4,12] The majority of cases of bleeding and rectal lacerations will resolve with expectant management.[2,5] Anal sphincteric injuries are surprisingly uncommon from the insertion of rectal foreign bodies. If such injuries are present, however, prompt surgical repair is warranted.[2,5,12]

HIGH-LYING OBJECTS

Approximately one quarter of rectal foreign bodies are not palpable on digital examination and are classified as "high lying."[7] High-lying foreign bodies cannot be readily removed in the outpatient setting and therefore require hospital admission.[9,15] In managing these patients, the goal is to convert the object from a high-lying to a low-lying position to facilitate a transanal extraction. Provided the patient is reasonably comfortable, most patients can be sedated, given nothing by mouth, and observed for 12 to 24 hours. In the majority of cases, the object will descend on its own into the rectum, permitting transanal removal by one of the previously described methods.[2,12]

Patients in whom the object does not descend after a waiting period require an examination under spinal or general anesthesia. An attempt is made to deliver the object into the rectal ampulla with bimanual manipulation or proctosigmoidoscopy with some means of traction.[7] If these techniques are unsuccessful, laparotomy is performed with blind, external manipulation of the foreign body into the rectum followed by transanal removal.[3,5,7] This is successful in virtually all patients; rarely is an actual colotomy necessary.[2,5,9,12] In the two largest series of rectal foreign bodies that have been reported to date, laparotomy was required in less than 2% of all patients.[2,12]

COLORECTAL PERFORATIONS

Patients with evidence of perforations require urgent hospital admission and therapy. Intravenous fluids and broad spectrum antibiotics are administered routinely. Perforations above the peritoneal reflection are usually obvious on physical examination and plain abdominal roentgenography. If there is any doubt, a water-soluble contrast enema examination should be performed. In patients with established perforations, emergency laparotomy is required. When the peritoneal cavity is entered, the laceration is identified, and the damaged segment is repaired. Although customary surgical practice would be to resect or exteriorize the damaged segment, the low level of injury in most cases precludes this. Because gross fecal contamination is usually present, an end-sigmoid colostomy with either a distal mucous fistula or a Hartmann procedure is recommended for fecal diversion.[5] Other surgeons feel that a diverting loop colostomy is sufficient in most patients.[2]

Perforations below the peritoneal reflection may develop signs of sepsis, pelvic cellulitis, perirectal abscess, or perivesicular abscess if unrecognized or if treatment is delayed.[2] Management of these patients can be extremely difficult. Antibiotics are given in all cases. In most cases, laparotomy with diverting colostomy is necessary to prevent further pelvic soilage. Patients with established infection at the time of presentation also require presacral drainage; however, patients in whom perforation is recognized and treated early may respond to conservative management.[5] Treatment must be individualized.

Removal of Foreign Bodies Located Above the Rectum

Since the advent of colonoscopy with flexible fiber optic or video endoscopes, there has been a growing body of literature reporting the removal of selected foreign bodies located above the rectum by means of these instruments. Over 80% of these foreign bodies were swallowed by the patient, either intentionally or accidentally. To reach the colon the object must traverse several anatomic constrictions including the esophagus, pylorus, duodenal sweep, and ligament of Treitz. Thereafter, the most common sites of lodgment are the ileocecal valve, the sigmoid colon, and the rectum.[10,13] Despite these anatomic pitfalls, approximately 90% of foreign objects that traverse the stomach will pass through the remainder of the gut uneventfully.

Objects that are long, slender, and pointed are most apt to become impacted during their passage and pose the greatest risk of perforation. Fortunately, these items are the most amenable to colonoscopic removal. Pins, needles, chicken bones, toothpicks, ball-point pens, dental instruments and dentures have been most commonly reported.[13] Polypectomy snares, biopsy forceps, foreign body forceps, and baskets are often helpful in their removal.

The following steps should be followed in the management of patients with ingested foreign bodies in the colon[10,13]:

1. Obtain initial plain abdominal radiographs to document location, shape, size, and number of objects present, as well as to rule out perforation.
2. Serial abdominal films should be done to follow the progression of the object. During this waiting period, the patient should be placed on a high-fiber diet, Metamucil, and mineral oil to aid in the safe transport of the object through the colon.
3. If an object in the colon fails to progress over a 48-hour period or the patient develops bleeding or obstruction without an evident perforation, colonoscopic extraction should be attempted.
4. Objects on the left side of the colon may be approached after bowel cleansing with enemas. Previous reports have cautioned against the use of cathartics for fear of exacerbating an impaction or precipitating a perforation. This concern notwithstanding, it is difficult and dangerous to attempt an extraction in an unprepared colon. A cleansing with an oral polyethylene-based solution (Golytely) is recommended.
5. If colonoscopic retrieval fails, laparotomy is indicated.

SUMMARY

Rectal and colonic foreign bodies are being encountered with increased frequency. Their management may pose a recurrent challenge to the practicing emergency room physician, gastroenterologist, and surgeon.

Most foreign bodies will be found in the rectum, accessible to removal manually or through an anoscope or proctosigmoidoscope. The initial approach to the patient is largely dependent on whether the object is low-lying or high-lying.

Most low-lying objects can be removed in the outpatient setting. Every effort should be made to extract these rectal objects transanally. Local anesthesia may be helpful to achieve sufficient relaxation of the anal sphincter. After all rectal foreign body extractions, proctosigmoidoscopy is required to rule out significant mucosal injury.

Patients with high-lying objects or low-lying objects that cannot be readily removed in the emergency room setting warrant inpatient management. Many high-lying objects will descend into the lower rectum during a period of observation and may be removed transanally. The majority of difficult high-lying or low-lying foreign bodies can be removed manually or with proctosigmoidoscopy under spinal or general anesthesia. Laparotomy is reserved for those cases where all other attempts have failed.

In cases involving the ingestion of sharp objects that have lodged in the colon, the initial approach should be a period of observation. If the object does not progress through the colon, colonoscopic removal is indicated.

REFERENCES

1. Abcarian H, Lowe R. Colon and rectal trauma. *Surg Clin North Am.* 1978;58:519–537.
2. Barone JE, Yee J, Nealon TF. Management of foreign bodies and trauma of the rectum. *Surg Gynecol Obstet.* 1983;156:453–457.
3. Busch D, Starling J. Rectal foreign bodies: case reports and a comprehensive review of the world's literature. *Surgery.* 1986;100:512–519.
4. Busch RA, Owen WF. Trauma and other noninfectious problems in homosexual men. *Med Clin North Am.* 1986;70:549–566.

5. Couch CJ, Eric T, Watt A. Rectal foreign bodies. *Med J Aust.* 1986;144:512–515.
6. Crass RA, Tranbaugh RF, Kudsk KA, Trunkey DA. Colorectal foreign bodies and perforation. *Am J Surg.* 1981;142:85–88.
7. Eftaiha M, Hambrick E, Abcarian H. Principles of management of colorectal foreign bodies. *Arch Surg.* 1977;112:691–695.
8. Garber HI, Rubin RJ, Eisenstat TE. Removal of a glass foreign body from the rectum. *Dis Colon Rectum.* 1981;24:323.
9. Geist R. Sexually related trauma. *Emerg Med Clin North Am.* 1988;6:439–466.
10. Hacker JE, Cattau EL. Management of gastrointestinal foreign bodies. *Am Fam Physician.* 1986;34:101–108.
11. Hughes JP, Marice HP, Gathright JB. Methods of removing a hollow object from the rectum. *Dis Colon Rectum.* 1976;19:44–45.
12. Kingsley AN, Abcarian H. Colorectal foreign bodies, management update. *Dis Colon Rectum.* 1985;28:941–944.
13. Rocklin MS, Apelgren KN. Colonoscopic extraction of foreign bodies from the rectum. *Am Surgeon.* 1989;55:119–123.
14. Sohn N, Weinstein MA. Office removal of foreign bodies in the rectum. *Surg Gynecol Obstet.* 1978;146:209–210.
15. Wigle RL. Emergency department management of retained rectal foreign bodies. *Am J Emerg Med.* 1988;6:385–389.

7

Foreign Bodies in Children

CARLO DiLORENZO and ATHENA ECONOMIDES

Swallowed foreign bodies are common in children. Children put objects in their mouths to explore and learn about their environment. Some are given inappropriate foods to eat, toys to play with, or both. In addition, older children tend to eat, play, laugh, walk, and climb simultaneously, not concentrating on chewing or swallowing. As a consequence, 80% of all gastrointestinal foreign bodies occur in children ages 2 weeks to 16 years; 50% are ingested by children less than 2 years of age, and 30% are ingested by children under 1 year of age.[1] There are subgroups of children at greater risk for complications after swallowing foreign bodies. Conditions such as vascular compression (such as in double aortic arch or vascular ring), strictures or stenoses whether congenital or acquired from repaired tracheoesophageal fistulae, reflux esophagitis, or caustic ingestion and altered mental status may make complications from swallowed foreign bodies more likely. These conditions may be already known or may not be found until after the foreign body is diagnosed.[2]

Invariably, the types of foreign bodies swallowed by children prompting medical attention tend to be inedible objects and most commonly are coins. This is different from adults who usually swallow boluses of food that get lodged. In some series, coins accounted for as much as 80% of all foreign bodies.[1]

The location of the foreign body along the gastrointestinal tract is important both in terms of symptoms and treatment. Foreign bodies lodge in any natural or acquired point of stricture or curve (Fig. 7–1). However, impaction is the exception, not the rule. In children, 80% of the foreign bodies that are swallowed pass through the esophagus without sequelae, and 90% of the foreign bodies that have reached the stomach will pass through the intestines without trouble.[1] The constrictor muscles of the pharynx can force even large and irregularly shaped objects downward. On the other hand, the esophagus is the least distensible or adaptable structure of the gastrointestinal tract. These two factors contribute to the frequent impaction of foreign bodies in the esophagus. Of the esophageal foreign bodies, 80% come to rest just below the cricopharyngeal muscle, which corresponds to the fourth cervical vertebrae. Foreign bodies may also become lodged in the middle and lower third of the esophagus, at the level of the aortic arch and the gastroesophageal junction, respectively.[3] Foreign bodies infrequently lodge in the

42   GENERAL

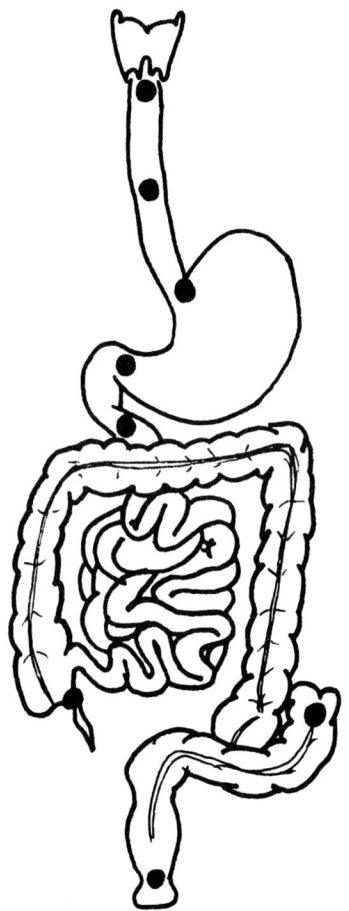

FIGURE 7–1. Anatomic areas in the gastrointestinal tract where foreign objects may arrest after ingestion.

pylorus, the ligament of Treitz, the ileocecal region, and the anus.

SIGNS AND SYMPTOMS

Most children with swallowed foreign bodies in the gastrointestinal tract are asymptomatic and have normal physical examinations at presentation.

Pharyngeal foreign bodies can sometimes be palpable by a gloved index finger, or they may be localized by the subjective feeling of being "caught in the throat." A scratch produced by the foreign body in this area will produce the same symptoms as the foreign body itself.[4] Most commonly, it is the esophageal foreign body that gives some signs and symptoms that should not be missed. Children may drool and refuse to eat. They may gag or vomit. They may complain of pain or discomfort with swallowing. One should always attempt to test oral intake in the emergency room. Large esophageal bodies can impinge on the trachea, causing symptoms such as stridor, cough, or wheezing. If the foreign body is high in the cervical esophagus, it may markedly impede swallowing. The child may have recurrent aspiration of saliva or food. Pain radiating to the sternum or back may indicate perforation or mediastinitis. In contrast to the esophagus, where symptoms of obstruction and danger of perforation demand expedient action, foreign bodies in the stomach and intestine usually cause few, if any, symptoms.

DIAGNOSIS

The patient with a history of ingestion of an inedible substance places the physician in the position of having to prove or disprove the presence of a retained foreign body. In children, 44% to 83% of swallowed foreign bodies in the gastrointestinal tract are witnessed or self-reported.[5] These statistics indicate that at least half of all ingestions may be prevented. Forty percent of children seek medical treatment within 24 hours of ingestion, 50% within the first week, and 10% later than 30 days.[2]

A large percentage of esophageal foreign bodies are radiopaque. Some radiolucent objects, such as aluminum pull tabs, plastic toys, and chicken and fish bones may be visualized by xeroradiography. Whenever there is a suspicion of a foreign body ingestion, one should perform radiographic examination, because 17% to 44% of the children who have esophageal foreign bodies are asymptomatic.[5–7] Radiographs are indicated in the following cases[6]: history of coin ingestion regardless of symptoms; new onset of wheezing in a preschool-aged child; localized neck pain without historical or physical explanation; signs of esophageal obstruction such as drooling, vomiting, inability to swallow solid food, or dysphagia; suspected bronchiolitis during atypical time of year; wheezing not responsive to bronchodilators. Plain films of the neck with soft tissue technique may reveal the foreign body in the hypopharynx, nasopharynx, glottis and epiglottis, cervical esophagus, or posterior pharyngeal wall. Widening of the retropharyngeal soft tissues, air in the soft tissues, or both, when present, may indicate perforation with abscess formation. Chest radiographs differentiate a coin in the esophagus from one in the trachea. The anteroposterior film shows the edge of the coin if it is in the trachea and shows the flat surface if it lies in the esophagus. In the lateral films, the flat surface is seen if the coin lies in the trachea, and the edge of it is seen if it is in the esophagus. Thus, in a child with stridor or respiratory distress one can diagnose the position of the object. Contrast studies should not be routinely used. If the patient complains of dysphagia or odynophagia, a barium swallow may show an "incidental" esophageal foreign body, or, in the case of radiolucent foreign bodies, a barium-coated cotton ball can outline the shape of the object. However, the contrast agents can also obscure the foreign body and delay intervention.

A metal detector reveals the presence of metallic objects by measuring the change in conductance of a coil placed near a metallic mass. An inexpensive hand-held metal detector was used in 28 patients with the presumptive diagnosis of metallic foreign bodies.[8] Every case was correctly diagnosed by the metal detectors. This diagnostic tool does not distinguish tracheal from esophageal foreign bodies and therefore could be recommended only as a screening tool prior to radiographs.

Finally, endoscopy has dramatically changed the diagnosis and management of swallowed foreign bodies by allowing identification of their exact location and allowing their removal.

SWALLOWED FOREIGN BODIES

The management of swallowed foreign bodies in children is the topic of much controversy. A "wait-and-see" attitude is frequently practiced in adults, but in children, observation should be restricted to those cases where the ingestion was witnessed, the patient is asymptomatic, and the foreign body is in the stomach or the duodenum, is small and blunt enough to traverse the post-esophageal sites of impaction, and is progressing as assessed by radiologic follow-up.[9] Therefore, in the case of coins, marbles, or toys without sharp edges, with a diameter less than 20 mm, and location anywhere but the esophagus, parents are instructed to strain or crush the stools until the object is identified and to return for immediate evaluation should symptoms of obstruction, perforation, or peritonitis develop. The position and progress of such objects are evaluated radiographically, at weekly intervals, until they pass. Removal should not be considered before 2 weeks have gone by without progress.

Special diets and laxatives have been recommended occasionally for speeding the passage of the foreign body via the bowel.[3] However, the most important part of expectant management is to reassure the parents that as long as the child remains asymptomatic there is no cause for alarm. The child instead should be given a regular diet, because normal bowel contents will carry the object along.

Medical management has little, if any, role in the management of foreign bodies in pediatrics. Ipecac, papain, and gas-forming agents, such as tartaric and sodium bicarbonate have all been used with some success and considerable risk for perforation. Therefore, they are no longer recommended. Medications, such as glucagon and diazepam, that decrease lower esophageal sphincter (LES) pressure and have little effect on esophageal peristasis have been recommended in some adult patients for objects, especially food boluses, that are impacted in the distal esophagus. Care must be taken to avoid rapid infusion of glucagon, producing nausea and vomiting that can lead to perforation in an obstructed esophagus.

The Foley balloon catheter technique has been frequently used for the removal of blunt, smooth foreign bodies. There is consensus for using the Foley balloon technique in the following cases: the foreign body must be a coin, must be a single coin without other possible radiolucent foreign body, and must have been swallowed within 24 hours from Foley removal. The technique is contraindicated for all foreign bodies other than coins and in patients with respiratory distress, complete esophageal obstruction, or inability to cooperate. Relative contraindications are previous history of esophageal foreign bodies, esophageal disease, and surgery. Also, if the lateral chest x-ray examination suggests a widening of the tracheoesophageal interface, as often is the case with children less than 18 months old, the Foley balloon catheter should not be used.[1] A Foley balloon catheter is introduced into the esophagus via the nasopharynx, or the mouth, and the balloon is passed beyond the foreign body. The balloon is then inflated with 3 to 5 ml of barium or gastrografin and under fluoroscopy gently withdrawn, pulling the object along with it. This procedure should be performed with the patient in a steep, head-down position. Suction apparatus must be available because children may vomit during the procedure and are at risk from aspiration. Once the foreign body has been removed, patients are observed for 2 hours and allowed to go home. The advantages of the Foley balloon catheter extraction are its low cost and the avoidance of endoscopy, general anesthesia, and endotracheal intubation. This technique is a safe and effective procedure. In the hands of experienced personnel and in adherence to the above indications, several series have reported a greater than 90% success rate.[10]

Esophageal bougienage has been recently recommended for coins lodged in the esophagus, with the same indications as in Foley removal.[11] In this method, a supple tube is passed via the esophagus, and it advances the coin distally into the stomach, where the majority of coins are expected to pass through the remainder of the gastrointestinal tract without sequelae. The procedure is typically performed in the emergency department with the patient in an upright position. This technique has been used in a large series with excellent results.

For foreign bodies other than coins such as fish bones or toy jackstones at the level of the hypopharynx or cricopharyngeal muscle, the rigid laryngoscope and a surgical grasping clamp should be used. The rigid esophagoscope has a protective lip under which sharp foreign bodies can be directed and safely removed. The patient should be intubated and under general anesthesia to protect the airway. After the foreign body has been removed, the esophagus should be reentered to make sure that there is no second foreign body. The complications experienced by patients undergoing rigid endoscopy are mostly related to endotracheal intubation or preexisting respiratory conditions and only rarely are associated with long-term morbidity.[9]

Flexible endoscopy, under sedation or general anesthesia, allows removal of most foreign bodies from the lower part of the esophagus, stomach, and proximal duodenum. The use of increasingly smaller endoscopes and imaginative retrieving devices makes flexible endoscopy in experienced hands a safe and successful technique. Because of the difficulty visualizing the upper third of the esophagus with flexible endoscopy, this technique should be reserved for retrieving objects below this point.

Less than 1% of intestinal foreign bodies require surgery.[3] However, when the objects fail to pass, are unlikely to pass spontaneously, cause symptoms of perforation, or have failed endoscopic retrieval, exploratory laparotomy is the only method of extraction. Even within surgical procedures, many ingenious ways for foreign body removal have been described. Removal of foreign bodies through an appendicostomy that also included an appendectomy has been reported.[12]

There are some foreign bodies that require emergent removal regardless of their location. Toothpicks, pins, nails, needles, razors, and even dental retainers are among the sharp-pointed objects that should be removed immediately to prevent perforation. Needles (Fig. 7–2) especially should be removed regardless of location, length, or age of the patient, because a perfora-

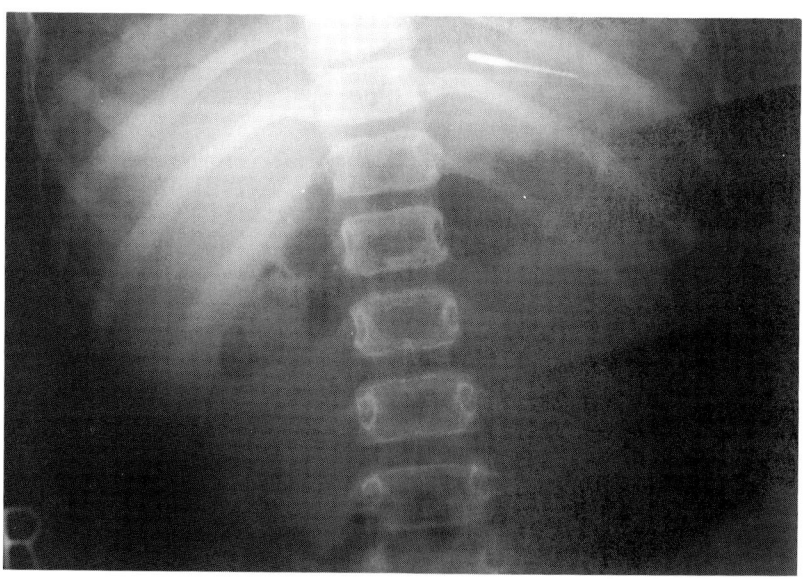

FIGURE 7–2. Anteroposterior chest film showing a sharp needle in the stomach of a 9-year-old boy.

tion from a needle may initially cause minimal symptoms.[13] Razor blades are removed through a rigid endoscope if lodged in the esophagus and through laparotomy and gastrotomy if lodged in the stomach or duodenum. Toothpicks are notorious for causing bowel perforation and vasculoenteric fistulas, and one death has been reported.[14] Safety pins in the proximal esophagus should be pushed into the stomach and removed using the flexible endoscope through an overtube. Open safety pins in the stomach may also be pulled out by the hinge through a flexible endoscope and an overtube. If an open safety pin is beyond the stomach, then its progress through the gastrointestinal tract should be followed daily with abdominal radiographs, so that it may be removed by laparotomy if not progressing. Objects longer than 5 cm or wider than 2 cm are unlikely to pass through the pylorus, especially in children under 2 years of age. Therefore, they warrant removal.[1,3] Long objects especially must be removed because they tend to pass in a flip-flop manner through the gastrointestinal tract and may cause perforations.

Thanks to a national registry for button battery ingestions, a great deal of information has become available as to the proper management for button batteries.[15] Pressure necrosis, direct flow current, mercury toxicity, and alkali electrolyte leakage are the mechanisms causing harm. Batteries lodged in the esophagus require emergent removal. Burns due to esophageal impaction have occurred as early as 4 hours after ingestion, and perforation has occurred as soon as 6 hours after ingestion. Batteries should be removed under direct visualization, and endoscopic removal of esophageal batteries is highly successful. Batteries that have passed beyond the esophagus need not be retrieved unless the patient manifests signs or symptoms of injury to the gastrointestinal tract, such as hematochezia, abdominal pain, or tenderness. If the battery is larger than 15 mm in diameter and has not passed the pylorus in 48 hours, it is unlikely to pass and should be removed. Finally, if a mercury-containing battery, which may fragment and release mercury, is ingested, then levels of mercury in the blood and urine should be obtained and chelation therapy should be initiated in toxic symptomatic patients. A mercury-containing battery should be removed if the cell is observed to split in the gastrointestinal tract or radiopaque droplets are evident in the gut.

An algorithm for management of swallowed foreign bodies is proposed in Figure 7–3. Following the removal of an esophageal foreign body, one should diligently watch for signs and symptoms of perforation, such as fever, tachy-

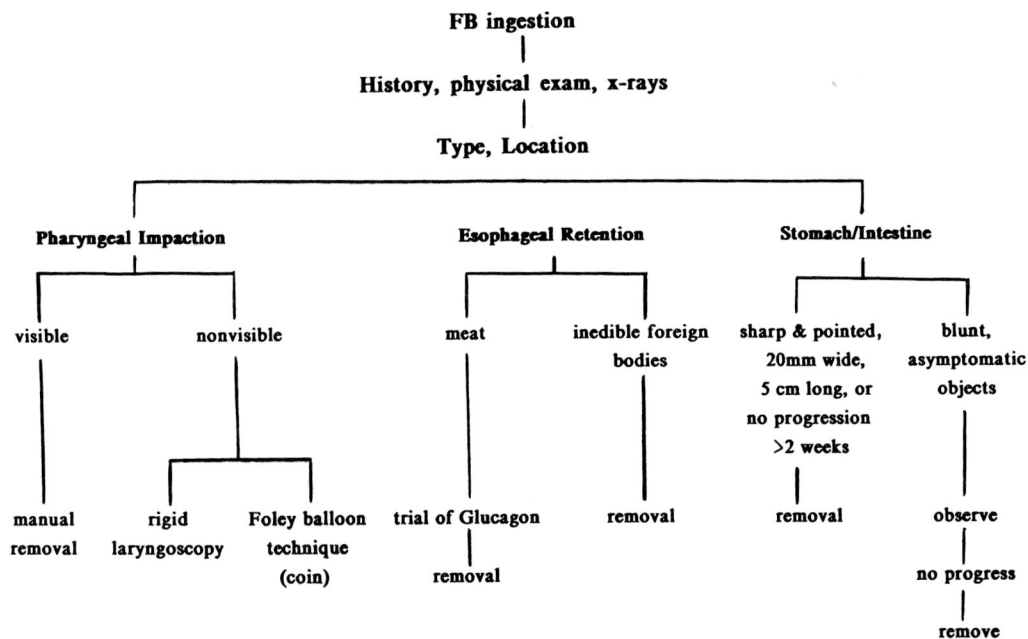

FIGURE 7–3. Algorithm for the management of swallowed foreign bodies in pediatrics.

TABLE 7–1. COMPLICATIONS OF ESOPHAGEAL AND POSTESOPHAGEAL FOREIGN BODIES

Esophageal Foreign Bodies
Edema, granulation, erosion, ulcer
Perforation, pneumomediastinum
Airway obstruction, aspiration pneumonia
Acquired esophageal pouch
Pseudodiverticuli
Tracheoesophageal fistula, aortoesophageal fistula
Stricture
Malnutrition and weight loss

Postesophageal Foreign Bodies
Pressure necrosis, ulcer
Infection
Hemorrhage
Obstruction
Perforation
Peritonitis

---

cardia, shortness of breath, chest and abdominal pain, and crepitations in the neck. Table 7–1 describes the complications associated with foreign bodies that are not removed.

RECTAL FOREIGN BODIES

Rectal foreign bodies can occur in infants, small children, and adolescents. A broken thermometer is the most common rectal foreign body in small children. Colorectal foreign bodies as a result of ingestions are usually diagnosed only after they have caused complications, and the history is likely to be elicited only with great difficulty because of the time lapsed since the event. Rectal foreign bodies are so rare in the older pediatric population that they may indicate sexual abuse and warrant a full workup for abuse.[16] Without a guiding history, it is very difficult to diagnose a rectal foreign body. The physical examination is in general unrewarding. With a digital examination one may palpate the object, but more likely not. Instead, it is most likely that the object will be detected on a plain x-ray examination of the abdomen. If x-ray examination shows no abnormal findings, then a contrast study or sigmoidoscopy can be performed to localize the foreign body. Small objects in the rectum can occasionally be hooked by the examining finger and withdrawn. More often a proctoscope or vaginal speculum must be inserted, and the end of the foreign body visualized and grasped by ring forceps through the speculum. In children, removal under general anesthesia is preferred because it allows for psychologically atraumatic removal, as well as inspection of the canal for injuries and repair of any damage. Following the removal of the object, sigmoidoscopy should be performed to ensure the integrity of the bowel wall.

REFERENCES

1. Webb W. Management of foreign bodies in the upper gastrointestinal tract. *Gastroenterology.* 1988;94:204–216.
2. Kenna M, Bluestone C. Foreign body in the air and food passages. *Pediatr Rev.* 1988;10:25–31.
3. Gryboski JD. Traumatic injury of the esophagus. In: Walker A, Duric PR, Hamilton JR, Walker-Smith JA, Watkins JB, eds. *Pediatric Gastrointestinal Disease.* Philadelphia, Pa: BC Decker Inc; 1991;371–378.
4. Paul RI, Jaffe DM. Sharp object ingestions in children: illustrative cases and literature review. *Ped Em Care.* 1988;4:245–248.
5. Economides A, Berkowitz C, Little C. Foreign bodies and orifices: where do children put things? *AJOC.* 1992;4:557. Abstract.
6. Savitt D, Watson S. Delayed diagnoses of coin ingestion in children. *Am J Emerg Med.* 1988;6:378–381.
7. Schunk J, Corneli H, Bolte R. Pediatric coin ingestions. *Am J Dis Child.* 1989;143:546–548.
8. Arena L, Baker SR. Use of a metal detector to identify ingested metallic foreign bodies. *AJR.* 1990;155:803–804.
9. Crysdale W. Esophageal foreign bodies in children: 15 year review of 484 cases. *Ann Otol Rhinol Laryngol.* 1991;100:320–324.
10. Nixon GW. Foley catheter method of esophageal foreign body removal: extension of application. *AJR.* 1979;132:441–442.
11. Bonadio WA, Jona JZ, Glicklick M, Cohen R. Esophageal bouginage technique for coin ingestion in children. *J Pediatr Surg.* 1988;23:917–918.
12. Mizrahi S, Eyal I, Shtamler B. Foreign body removal through an appendicostomy. *Dis Colon Rectum.* 1990;33:902.
13. Holinger LD. Management of sharp and penetrating foreign bodies of the upper aerodigestive tract. *Ann Otol Rhinol Laryngol.* 1990;99:684–688.
14. Bec M, Citron M, Vannix RS, et al. Delayed death from ingestion of a toothpick. *N Engl J Med.* 1989;320:673.
15. Litovitz T, Schmitz B. Ingestion of cylindrical and button batteries: an analysis of 2382 cases. *Pediatrics.* 1992;89:747–757.
16. Busch DB, Starling Jr. Rectal foreign body: case reports and a comprehensive review of the literature. *Surgery.* 1986;100:512–518.

8
Nausea and Vomiting
MANLEY COHEN

The ancient Romans after a banquet would retire to the vomitorium and there stimulate their tympanum with a feather to induce vomiting. Here the cure is obvious—remove all feathers from anyone's reach! Similarly, vomiting after drinking an emetic made from button-snake root was part of the festival of first fruits of the North American Creek Indians, and the Seminole Indians of Florida would annually "quaff a nauseous 'Black Drink' which acts as an emetic and purgative," after which they are sufficiently purified to eat the new green corn.[2] Here again the cure for vomiting is obvious—change the religious rites and do not drink the emetic. Rational management of patients with nausea and vomiting is rarely so easy because it is only possible when the underlying cause can be treated. So diagnosis, as always, is paramount. Unfortunately even when the diagnosis is clear, such as when it is due to cancer chemotherapeutic agents, the motion of a ship, or even morning sickness of pregnancy, treatment may be less than optimal. Symptomatic treatment for nausea, which originally meant seasickness from the Greek *nausus* (ship), can sometimes be merely avoiding sea, car, or plane travel, taking dimenhydrinate (Dramamine), or placing a scopolamine patch before the trip. If nausea is due to digitalis overdosage, withholding the offending drug may be all that is required. More often the diagnosis is not clearcut.

Nausea is the unpleasant subjective sensation associated with the urge to vomit, often felt in the back of the throat and epigastrium. Some patients, especially from England, say they are *bilious,* which has been defined as a condition associated with a sickish feeling, lack of appetite, indigestion, bad taste in the mouth, commonly thought to be due to a "sluggish liver," queasiness, and revulsion. *Retching,* or dry heaves, is spasmodic contraction of those muscles associated with vomiting without expelling any gastric content. *Rumination* is the effortless regurgitation of food within minutes of ingestion without nausea or dysphagia or spasmodic muscle contractions. *Esophageal regurgitation* is seen with Zenker's diverticulum, epiphrenic diverticulum, or obstruction caused by achalasia, stricture, gastroesophageal reflux disease, and esophageal cancer. *Vomiting* is the forceful expulsion of upper gastrointestinal contents via the mouth, with spasmodic muscular contractions of the abdomen and chest.

The patient with difficult chronic nausea, especially one who complains of having a "bad taste," usually suffers from depression, and can be difficult to evaluate and treat. Serendipity sometimes helps:

A 70-year-old widow, DB, was brought by her daughter, complaining that for 2 years she had had nausea and a "bad taste." Her local physician of many years had "done a few tests" and sent her to "some specialists" and prescribed some antidepressants. The daughter now wanted a "thorough evaluation" and a second (or fifth) opinion. There was no weight loss, change in bowel habit, anorexia, vomiting, or any other symptom I could elicit, and my examination was as negative as those before me. Initial screening blood and urine tests were also negative (see checklist Table 8–1). The nausea and bad taste were a "real problem," and I told the patient and daughter that I thought she had dysgeusia and nausea and that I had no better explanation than depression. We tried Entex LA (phenylpropanolamine [75 mg] with guaifenesin [400 mg]) every 12 hours for 2 weeks in case she had postnasal drip, and then zinc supplements, which did not help. After 4 weeks she volunteered that she enjoyed square dancing every Friday night, so she seemed hardly depressed. I embarked on what I told them would be an extensive evaluation, which might turn out to be negative. Chest x-ray and abdominal sonography failed to show any abnormality or pancreatic or hepatic pathology. Radiographic upper gastrointestinal studies and endoscopy with duodenal, gastric, and esophageal biopsy were all negative. But a barium enema showed a transverse colonic constricting but nonobstructing carcinoma, confirmed by colonoscopy to the cecum with biopsy. No other neoplasms were found. I thought this was an incidental finding. This small, moderately differentiated adenocarcinoma, without nodal metastases, was resected with complete resolution of both nausea and bad taste, with recurrence of neither symptom over the past 5 years of follow-up.

This is a most unusual case, in my experience, but demonstrates how little we still know about the cause(s) of chronic nausea.

Vomiting is only a little better understood. The physiology of vomiting has been recently reviewed.[11] The vomiting "center" (or centers) in the lateral reticular formation of the medulla has been well defined. It lies close to the respiratory center and those nuclei concerned with defecation and salivation; and the chemoreceptor trigger zone in the area postrema, where the blood-brain barrier is modified, in the region of the fourth ventricle. Since vomiting is often preceded by nausea, some believe that nausea results from low-level stimulation of the vomiting center. Perhaps in some with "queasiness" this is so, but nausea is not always a forme fruste of vomiting. Often it is a symptom of depression. Nausea without vomiting may be initiated by something in the brain—seeing, smelling, or hearing nauseating things—or a response to a metabolic problem rather than from visceral (gut) problems, which most often result in vomiting as well.

WHY DOES VOMITING OCCUR?

The obvious answer to this metaphysical teleologic question, that we vomit to expel contaminated food from the upper gastrointestinal tract and that nausea may prevent further ingestion of such toxins, has little basis in observed data. Indeed, nausea usually precedes vomiting, doubtless to give one time to reach the bathroom and prevent soiling of the Persian rug. The deleterious effects of vomiting and retching, which include mechanical and metabolic consequences (Table 8–2), are far more obvious than any beneficial effects. The protective and survival benefits of vomiting have yet to be demonstrated to sailors in a storm, passengers trying to enjoy a cruise, pregnant mothers, postoperative patients recovering from anesthesia, and cancer patients receiving life-prolonging medication. Indeed, the psychologic impact of nausea and vomiting associated with cancer chemotherapy may outdo any good the chemotherapy may otherwise be achieving and merely make the patient's remaining life more miserable. It is easy to understand the need for a respiratory center, thermoregulatory center, and many of the other "centers" in the region of the fourth ventricle, but the raison d'être of the vomiting center remains a mystery.

At least 17 neurotransmitters have been identified in the brain areas associated with vomiting, but the four currently considered most important are dopaminergic, cholinergic, histaminic, and serotoninergic. How they all interact is unknown.

TABLE 8–1. CHECKLIST OF TESTS FOR NAUSEA AND VOMITING

1. Perform screening tests:
    a. Pregnancy test in females
    b. Complete blood count
    c. Urinalysis
    d. Chemistry panel with electrolytes
    e. C-reactive protein
    f. Sedimentation rate
    g. Serology for syphilis
    h. Serum ferritin
    i. Highly sensitive thyroid stimulating hormone
    j. Amylase and lipase
    k. X-ray examination (after pregnancy excluded)
        (1) Chest
        (2) Abdomen
2. Go back and take another detailed history.
3. Listen to the patient and have a close relative present.
4. Reexamine the patient.
5. Consider neurologic or endocrine evaluation.
6. Consider a formal search for abnormalities in the abdomen.

TABLE 8–2. SOME COMPLICATIONS OF NAUSEA AND VOMITING

1. Mechanical effects
    a. Mallory-Weiss mucosal tears of the esophagus with bleeding
    b. Boerhaave syndrome of transesophageal perforation and mediastinitis
    c. Rib fracture
    d. Gastric herniation
    e. Wound dehiscence (rupture of suture line)
    f. Intraocular bleeding
    g. Aspiration of vomitus and pneumonia
2. Metabolic consequences
    a. Anorexia
    b. Dehydration
    c. Alkalosis
3. Psychologic effects in chemotherapy

TABLE 8-3. SOME CAUSES OF VOMITING

1. Cerebral
   a. Emotional (seeing, hearing, smelling, or tasting nauseating things or thinking of them)
   b. Tumors and other space-occupying lesions and raised intracranial pressure
   c. Pain from any cause
2. Medulla
   a. Afferent from viscera
   b. Directly from drugs affecting the chemoreceptor trigger zone by metabolic effects:
      (1) Chemotherapeutic agents
      (2) Narcotics
      (3) Anticholinergics
      (4) Antibiotics
      (5) Levodopa
      (6) Digoxin
      (7) Ipecac including surreptitious use
3. Labyrinthine disorders:
   a. Ménière's disease
   b. Labyrinthitis
   c. Motion sickness
4. Sinusitis and postnasal drip (often difficult to diagnose)
5. Tracheobronchial and lung disease
6. Cardiac problems
7. Gastritis and gastric stasis; some drugs that may delay gastric emptying include
   a. Opiates
   b. Anticholinergics
   c. Phenothiazines
   d. Levodopa
   e. β-Agonists
   f. Progesterone
   g. Aluminum antacids
   h. Nicotine
   i. Potassium salts
   j. Alcohol
8. Hepatic and biliary disease
9. Pancreatic disorders
10. Renal colic and failure (azotemia)
11. Small or large bowel obstruction or stasis
12. Pregnancy
13. Use of general anesthetics causing postoperative nausea and vomiting
14. Use of drugs that regularly induce nausea and vomiting:
    a. Ipecac
    b. Many cancer chemotherapeutic drugs
    c. Cardiac glycosides (The first clue to digitalis overdosage may be nausea and vomiting.)
    d. Levodopa and other dopamine receptor agonists such as bromocriptine
    e. Ergot alkaloids
    f. Muscarinic and nicotinic receptor antagonists and anticholinesterases such as tacrine and physostigmine used in Alzheimer's disease
    g. Opiates
    h. Peptides and amino acids affecting the chemoreceptor trigger zone
       (1) Angiotensin
       (2) Glutamic acid
       (3) Neurotensin
       (4) Peptide YY
       (5) Substance P
       (6) Vasoactive intestinal peptide
    i. Theophylline
    j. Aminoglycoside antibiotics from vestibular damage

Following are the three major "causes" of vomiting (Table 8–3 and Fig. 8–1):

1. *Chemical causes* (via the chemoreceptor trigger zone) include drugs, especially morphine, peptides, and those produced by some tumors, urea, and hypercalcemia.
2. *Central nervous system causes* include emotion, particularly anxiety, raised intracranial pressure, and vestibular causes (seasickness and vertigo).
3. *Mechanical or obstructive causes* include true obstruction and stasis and even constipation.

HOW DOES VOMITING OCCUR?

How vomiting occurs is somewhat better understood than why it occurs, but much still needs to be learned about the chemical mediators and nerve pathways. Afferents to the vomiting center arise from at least four sites:

1. Abdominal splanchnic and vagal nerves
2. Vestibulolabyrinthine receptors
3. Cerebral cortex
4. The chemoreceptor trigger zone in the area postrema in the region of the fourth ventricle. It is outside the blood-brain barrier and is exposed to emetic chemostimuli of
   a. Endogenous type, such as
      (1) Hormones in vomiting of pregnancy
      (2) Metabolic products of renal failure
   b. Exogenous agents, such as
      (1) Digitalis
      (2) Morphine
      (3) Anticancer drugs

The efferent motor output of cranial nerves V, VII, and IX and the vagus and sympathetic nu-

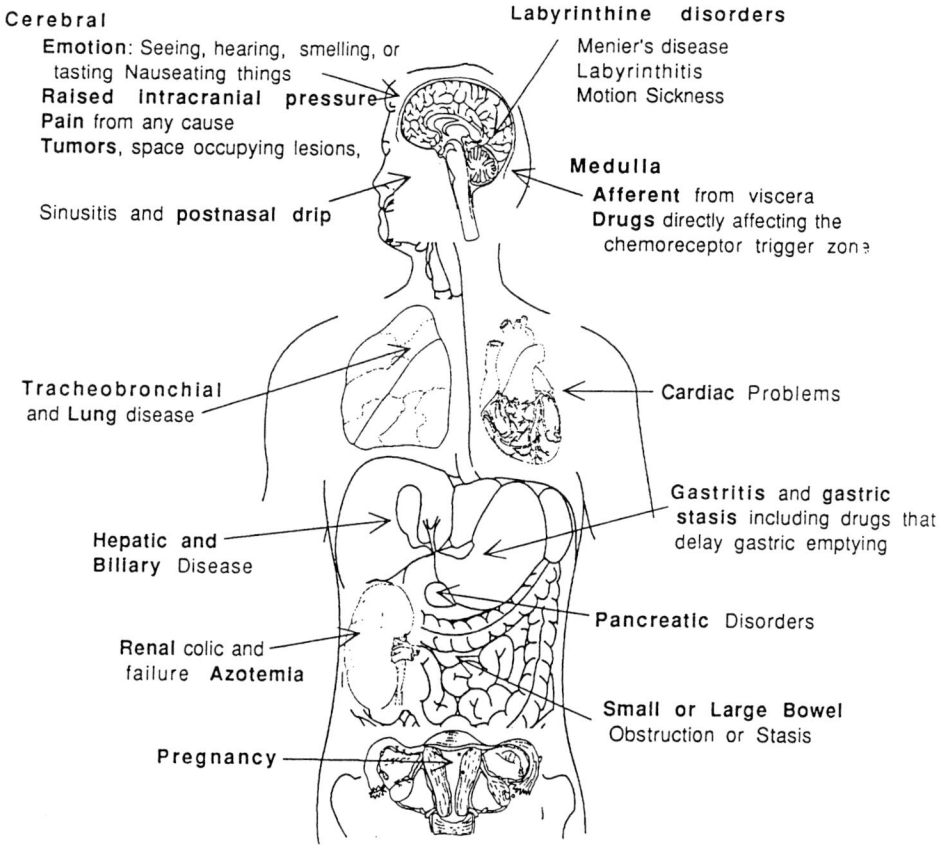

FIGURE 8–1. Some causes of vomiting. (Modified from Haubrich WS. Nausea and vomiting. In: Berk JE, Haubrich WS. *Gastrointestinal Symptoms, Clinical Interpretation.* Philadelphia, Pa: BC Decker; 1991.)

clei produce the prodromal salivation, licking, and chewing components, the complex contraction of the diaphragm and intercostal and abdominal muscles associated with reverse peristalsis, and the cardiovascular responses seen in vomiting, which is the forceful expulsion of upper gastrointestinal contents via the mouth.

CLINICAL APPROACH IN GENERAL

Nausea alone, vomiting alone, or nausea followed by vomiting are all fairly nonspecific. Although symptomatic therapy is available, it should be used only when one knows the cause or after initial evaluation to prevent giving pregnant patients potentially teratogenic drugs or obscuring the symptoms of, for example, bowel obstruction. Table 8–4 provides checklists for evaluating patients presenting with nausea and vomiting. Rarely is it necessary to give symptomatic treatment for violent retching and vomiting of unknown cause only to prevent the complications listed in Table 8–2. Sometimes it is necessary to sedate a vomiting patient to provide relief. One usually knows the cause of such violent vomiting, and then more rational treatment is often possible.

In chronic nausea, and especially if the patient also complains of a "bad taste," a Minnesota multiphasic personality inventory (MMPI) or similar questionnaire may be quite helpful, particularly if it discloses abnormality in the hypochondriasis, depression, and hysteria scales. But depressed patients can have organic disease, in which case the MMPI is not helpful. Furthermore, in places like Southern California with its large immigrant population, many of whom do

TABLE 8-4. CHECKLISTS FOR NAUSEA AND VOMITING AS A PRESENTING SYMPTOM

All women of childbearing age should be assumed to be pregnant until proven otherwise. This will prevent dangerous radiographic studies and administration of potential teratogenic medications.

Nausea
1. Onset
2. Duration
3. Time of day
4. Frequency
    a. Episodic after a large meal
    b. Continuous
5. Severity: weight loss suggests malignancy
6. Timing in relation to food: anorexia nervosa or bulimia
7. Time of day: morning sickness of pregnancy or raised intracranial pressure
8. Long history of diabetes suggesting gastroparesis
9. Past surgery, especially abdominal
10. Drug and medication history: anyone else in the house taking any medication? Ipecac? Digitalis? Morphine?
11. Associated pain: is the vomiting from drugs to control the pain?
    a. Abdominal pain of
        (1) Gastric origin
        (2) Biliary origin
        (3) Renal origin
        (4) Pancreatic origin
    b. Headache with intracranial pathology
12. History of psychiatric problems: remove all feathers from the vomitorium—see text
13. Previous hospitalizations for medical, psychiatric, or surgical reasons
14. Preceding cough
15. Chronic sinusitis and postnasal drip
16. Do you want to talk about AIDS?
17. Do you have any other concerns, legal, financial, personal, or family, that might be affecting your health?

Vomiting
1. Vomiting without preceding nausea: suspect increased intracranial pressure or in infants, hypertrophic pyloric stenosis
2. With preceding nausea, see nausea checklist also
3. With preceding abdominal rumbling
4. Vomitus
    a. Volume
    b. Food particles
    c. Bile (green or yellow)
    d. Color
    e. Blood
    f. Odor (retained gastric content, feculent may suggest gastrocolic fistula)
5. Postvomiting symptoms
    a. Relief after vomiting
    b. Cramps and diarrhea
6. Examination
    a. General
    b. Dehydrated
    c. Malnourished
    d. Neurologic and funduscopic
    e. Abdominal
        (1) Scars
        (2) Distension
        (3) Masses
        (4) Tenderness
        (5) Organomegaly
        (6) Succussion splash
        (7) Fecal occult blood (and vomitus)
    f. Anything to suggest
        (1) Hyperthyroidism
        (2) Addison's disease
        (3) Uremia
        (4) Hyperparathyroidism
7. Go back and take another detailed history

---

not speak English, the MMPI is often not helpful. Nevertheless, if the MMPI is abnormal, one may be able to persuade the unwilling patient to seek psychiatric or counseling help. Sometimes psychiatric hospitalization alone is helpful.[12]

The peasants of Perche, in France, labour under the impression that a prolonged fit of vomiting is brought about by the patient's stomach becoming unhooked, as they call it, and so falling down. Accordingly, a practitioner is called in to restore the organ to its proper place. After hearing the symptoms he at once throws himself into the most horrible contortions, for the purpose of unhooking his own stomach. Having succeeded in the effort, he next hooks it up again in another series of contortions and grimaces, while the patient experiences a corresponding relief. Fee five francs.[2]

Such practitioners are rarely available here. However, psychotherapists and practitioners of acupuncture and transdermal electrical nerve stimulation (TENS) have achieved good results in some patients who vomit.[1,10,12]

Unpleasant emotions can induce vomiting. In his 1943 book *Nervousness Indigestion and Pain* (Harper, NY, pp. 8 and 9), Alvarez describes "a nervous young woman [who] on receiving a menacing letter from the income tax collector took to her bed and vomited day and night for a week.... I appeased Uncle Samuel with $3.85, which ... shows that much good medicine does not come out of bottles." Another woman vomited for 2 weeks when she learned her mother had gastric cancer, and a famous opera singer vomits for hours before each performance. Men also vomit from nervousness, and Alvarez describes both a salesman and the head of an advertising firm with these problems. The executive frequently had to telephone and delay meetings because of his nervous nausea. Disgust causes nausea, and women are described who vomited after intercourse with an unloved husband.

Less understandable are those who vomit when overjoyed or pleasurably excited. Alvarez describes men and women who vomit from happiness on returning to loved ones after a trip, and "girls who had to get out of the car to vomit while on their way happily to a dance." One young woman "confessed that when her future husband proposed to her in a restaurant she promptly vomited." Another had to rush to the toilet when her husband-to-be slipped a diamond ring on her finger.

Psychologic factors play just as important a role in curing vomiting, as demonstrated by many of the cures that have been recommended. Most interesting is the use of ipecac, a powerful emetic, to cure vomiting.

Psychologic factors cannot be overstressed. Ipecac also stimulates gastric muscle contraction. Yet when its administration was accompanied by a strong suggestion that it would stop nausea and was given by nasogastric tube so that its bitter taste was not recognized, it decreased not only nausea but also gastric motility in experimental subjects. This demonstrates that placebo reactions can override pharmacologic responses.[16]

If the cause seems obvious after taking a history and performing a physical examination, the next question is whether the cause can be treated. Stop the digitalis in digitalis overdose, and treat the gastric outlet obstruction with nasogastric suction and endoscopic balloon dilation or surgery. If the cause cannot immediately be treated (chemotherapeutic drug–induced vomiting, vomiting of pregnancy, or seasickness on a cruise), symptomatic therapy may be indicated. Then the question is which therapy to use. I generally use only the first six drugs listed in Table 8–5 but may consider the additional drugs listed. As more drugs become available, I may add to my armamentarium and hopefully delete some!

"The election of the adequate antiemetic drug

TABLE 8–5. SYMPTOMATIC THERAPY FOR NAUSEA AND VOMITING

1. Give no drug until pregnancy has been excluded.
2. Doses given are high; side effects should be monitored; and doses should be reduced as soon as possible.
3. Avoid metoclopramide if obstruction is suspected.
4. In chronic nausea of unknown cause, give no drug therapy initially and consider antidepressants later.
5. Cisapride, recently approved for other uses, may replace metoclopramide.*

Four Useful Drugs

Metoclopramide (Reglan)	1–3 mg/kg IV q2h
	10 mg PO 30 min a.c. and at h.s.
Dimenhydrinate (Dramamine)	50 mg PO or IV q4h
Prochlorperazine (Compazine)	5–10 mg PO q4h
	5–10 mg IM q4h
	0–40 mg IV q3h
	25 mg suppository q4h
Lorazepam (Ativan)	1.5 mg/m^2 IV q4h (or PO dose)

Two Special-use Drugs

Scopolamine (Transderm scop)	1 patch behind the ear q3d while *traveling;* watch for side effects; avoid with glaucoma; do not exceed dose
Ondansetron (Zofran)	0.15 mg/kg 15 min before and 4 and 8 h after *chemotherapy*

CTZ = chemoreceptor trigger zone, MMPI = Minnesota Multiphasic Personality Inventory.

*An updated list of frequently prescribed antiemetics approved by the US Food and Drug Administration (FDA) is published monthly by Prescribing Reference, Inc., NY, which lists "commonly prescribed pharmaceutical products currently available on prescription as well as certain over the counter products." Its usefulness lies in that newly approved products are listed there rapidly after introduction. It lists indications, contraindications, precautions, interactions, and side effects more concisely than in the *Physicians' Desk Reference (PDR)*, which is published annually, but entries are less complete. Like the *PDR* it does not list unapproved uses for approved drugs. Thus, for example, it does not list Ativan and droperidol as antiemetics, because they are not approved for this use. Whether it is necessary to obtain informed consent for this use of an approved drug for an unapproved use has to be considered in each individual patient.

†Many drugs listed are not yet available even for research studies. They are listed because they may become available, and their classification here may aid understanding. Because the dosage and use of some of the drugs listed may not be approved by the US FDA for the indication mentioned, the package insert must be consulted. If used in an unapproved dose or for unapproved uses, informed consent and open communication with the patient and family is mandatory.

TABLE 8–5. SYMPTOMATIC THERAPY FOR NAUSEA AND VOMITING *Continued*

Additional Drugs†

Dopamine Receptor Antagonists (Antidopaminergics)
1. Benzamides
    a. Metoclopramide (Reglan)
    b. Domperidone (Motilium)
    c. Cisapride (Propulsid)
    d. Trimethobenzamide (Tigan)
    e. Alizapride
    f. Clebopride
    g. Levosulpiride
2. Phenothiazines
    a. Chlorpromazine (Thorazine)
    b. Prochlorperazine (Compazine)
    c. Perphenazine (Trilafon)
    d. Thiethylperazine (Torecan)
    e. Promethazine (Phenergan)
3. Butyrophenones
    a. Haloperidol (Haldol)
    b. Droperidol (Inapsine)

Histamine H_1-Receptor Antagonists (Antihistamines)
1. Piperazine derivatives
    a. Cyclizine (Marezine)
    b. Chlorcyclizine
    c. Cinnarizine
    d. Meclizine (Antivert, Bonine)
2. Ethanolamine derivatives
    a. Diphenhydramine (Benadryl)
    b. Dimenhydrinate (Dramamine)
    c. Doxylamine
3. Promethazine (Phenergan)

Muscarinic Receptor Antagonists (Anticholinergics)
1. Scopolamine (hyoscine) (Transderm-scop)
2. Atropine
3. Trihexyphenidyl (benzhexol) (Artane)
4. Benztropine (Cogentin)

Serotonin ($5HT_3$)-Receptor Antagonists (Antiserotonins)
1. Ondansetron (Zofran)
2. Bemesetron
3. Granisetron (Kytril)
4. Renzapride
5. Tropisetron
6. Zacopride
7. Batanopride, ICS 205-930, MDL 72222, RG-12915, . . .

Cannabinoids
1. Nabilone
2. Levonantradol
3. Dronabinol (Marinol)

Steroids
1. Dexamethasone
2. Methylprednisolone

Ephedrine

Combination Drug Therapy
1. Subtherapeutic doses of droperidol, which blocks D_2 and H_1 receptors, scopolamine, which blocks muscarinic cholinergic and H_1 receptors, and metoclopramide, which blocks dopamine D_2 and H_1 receptors, worked as well as full doses of droperidol and with fewer side effects.[8]

Miscellaneous
1. Psychiatric hospitalization.[12] Even with abnormal MMPI results and clinically significant psychiatric disorders, the patients did not accept a psychologic explanation for their nausea, although while in hospital most of these patients experienced symptomatic improvement of their chronic nausea.
2. Acupuncture at the P6 right wrist point.[1] Unproven efficacy.
3. Psychotherapy by reciprocal inhibition, neurolinguistic programming, etc.
4. Transdermal electric nerve stimulation in combination with drugs. Electrodes are placed above the nose, on one mastoid, and on the epigastrium.[10] Unproven efficacy.
5. Give ipecac, a powerful emetic, by nasogastric tube to mask its bitter taste, accompanied by a strong suggestion that it will stop the nausea. This worked in human experimental subjects[16] but is not recommended.

Surgical Ablation of the Vomiting Center[4]
1. Five patients with intractable severe vomiting, caused by conversion reaction or primary or metastatic brain tumor, had surgically induced lesions placed in the CTZ, with both relief of vomiting and failure to respond to apomorphine by vomiting. The lack of subsequent reports of CTZ surgical ablation helping nausea by these or any other workers is disappointing.

in each clinical situation is not easy because the precise mechanism involved in vomiting is unknown in the majority of situations."[5] Since nausea and vomiting, like fever, are so nonspecific, in many cases it is hard to choose the appropriate drug. For example, the $5HT_3$-receptor antagonist ondansetron may help chemotherapy-induced vomiting but does not help motion-induced emesis. Dimenhydrinate, its derivative dimenhydramine, and scopolamine are useful in motion sickness. So people who routinely get car-, air-, or seasick may be helped with a scopolamine patch or a dimenhydrinate tablet.

DELAYED GASTRIC EMPTYING

Delayed gastric emptying is caused by mechanical or gastroparetic disorders. *Mechanical causes* can usually be diagnosed by a good history and appropriate imaging and endoscopic techniques. If there is no suggestion of dysphagia caused by an esophageal problem, endoscopy is usually done first; I routinely biopsy the stomach and duodenum in these cases—giardiasis is sometimes diagnosed in the duodenal biopsy—and if the patient has *Helicobacter* gastritis, it is worth treating. Gastric, pancreatic, or rarely duodenal adenocarcinoma in a patient with Gardner's or Peutz-Jeghers syndrome, strictures at the site of prior surgery, and duodenal Crohn's disease may be causing delayed gastric emptying. A contrast study of the gastrointestinal tract or a computerized tomographic (CT) scan may be the next step. *Gastroparesis* has been divided into primary and secondary causes.[7] The *secondary causes* include chronic postsurgical gastroparesis and systemic diseases including metabolic (e.g., diabetic), neurologic, myopathic, and connective tissue disorders, and psychiatric disorders. The *primary disorders* include hollow viscus myopathy and neuropathy syndromes. However, despite the fact that gastroparesis is present in 80% of patients with anorexia nervosa, motility studies and transcutaneous electrogastrography, although useful research tools, are rarely clinically indicated in most patients with gastroparesis except for research purposes. Radiographic studies generally suffice, but if these are unhelpful, then a radionuclide study of solid-meal gastric emptying may help to confirm delayed gastric emptying. Diabetes, scleroderma, and postsurgical gastroparesis are the most frequent causes, and if they are severe, nutritional support (intravenous hyperalimentation or feeding jejunostomy) may be required. Laparoscopic jejunostomy with full-thickness, small-bowel biopsy to look for a defect in the myenteric plexus or smooth muscle to diagnose one of the primary disorders is currently fashionable but rarely necessary, because these conditions are rare. Treatment depends on the cause. Surgery or endoscopic balloon dilation is used for obstruction; and prokinetic agents including erythromycin, cisapride, metoclopramide, domperidone, naloxone, leuprolide, and proglumide, and even gastric electrical pacing with surgically placed serosal electrodes are experimental considerations (Table 8–6).

NAUSEA AND VOMITING OF PREGNANCY

Morning sickness should be treated with reassurance. If vomiting is severe as in hyperemesis gravidarum with dehydration, fluid replacement and prochlorperazine or metoclopramide may be required, although there is no drug approved by the US Food and Drug Administration for vomiting of pregnancy. Obviously, causes other than pregnancy should be looked for even in pregnant women; if the vomiting is severe, a sonogram to look for a hydatidiform mole or multiple pregnancy may be indicated.

MOTION SICKNESS

Individuals prone to vomiting caused by motion sickness frequently respond to a scopolamine patch behind the ear and antihistamines, especially dimenhydrinate (Dramamine). Suggestible subjects may respond to the acupressure of a Sea Band, but there is no scientific evidence to support this.

POSTOPERATIVE NAUSEA AND VOMITING

Postoperative nausea and vomiting can occur in 8% to 92% of patients, is usually treated by the anesthesiologist, is poorly understood, and has been recently reviewed in the US[15] and British[11] literature. It is multifactorial in origin, reflecting the patient's personality, anesthetic used, type of surgery, premedication, and amount of postoperative pain. Perioperative gastric aspiration

---

TABLE 8–6. EXPERIMENTAL THERAPY FOR GASTROPARESIS: DIABETIC IDIOPATHIC, POSTSURGICAL

Prokinetic Agents
1. Erythromycin IV or PO
2. Cisapride
3. Metoclopramide
4. Domperidone
5. Naloxone
6. Leuprolide acetate, a gonadotropin-releasing-hormone antagonist
7. Proglumide, a cholecystokinin-receptor antagonist

Electrical Pacing:
Surgical Placement of Electrodes on the Serosal Surface of the Stomach

does not prevent it, probably aggravates it,[14] and should not be done unless required for other reasons. Prevention should be attempted if possible. If that fails, ondansetron or granisetron is the current fashionable treatment. If one antiemetic does not work, another with a different mechanism of action should be tried (Table 8–5). Since postoperative vomiting is multifactorial, it may be a good plan to combine different agents that work at different sites, and by using lower doses one might reduce the incidence of side effects.[8] Pain should be controlled and the patient sedated enough to prevent mechanical complications (Table 8–2) but not enough to risk aspiration of vomitus and pneumonia.

CHEMOTHERAPY-INDUCED VOMITING

Besseler in 1910 wrote that "when nausea is a symptom of some definite form of disease, the treatment is that of the primary affection." Though he wrote that before we poisoned people with chemotherapy, his remarks are as true now as then. Martin in 1992 described myths about chemotherapy-induced vomiting. The old ones were that emesis was a minor problem and an inevitable consequence of treatment and that antiemetics had little value. The new myths are that we can control emesis with currently available antiemetics, and so chemotherapy-induced vomiting is not an important problem for cancer patients. The emetic potential of chemotherapeutic agents differs (Table 8–7), and drug dosage is another variable. In addition sociologic and psychologic factors play a role so that prior exposure to alcohol, labyrinth stimulation (seasickness), vomiting of pregnancy, prior nausea from drugs, and patient anxiety, which cannot be quantitated even if the patient verbalizes it, are all important factors. At this stage we are still only beginning to understand these relationships. Nausea itself is almost impossible to quantify. Vomiting is more objective; the number of times the patient vomits can be counted, and the duration of the vomiting episode timed.

Chemotherapeutic-induced vomiting is common, and a management approach is required, but this must be understood in a historical perspective. In 1908 Osler discussed nausea due to achylia gastrica, appendicitis, phlegmonous and toxic gastritis, volvulus of the omentum, as well as nausea nervosa, nervous gastralgia, and splanchnoptosis. Many of these conditions are no longer recognized 80 years later or have different names. I have seen only one case of phlegmonous gastritis that was recognized antemortem and the patient saved by gastrectomy. Nausea and vomiting were not the main presenting features. Pain was. "Gastralgia is usually considered a neurosis of the vagus, and there are five types—of gastric origin, central origin, neurotic origin, constitutional origin and reflex origin." In any case gastralgia is associated with pain, and pain and nausea are differently approached than nausea alone.

Splanchnoptosis, enteroptosis, and Glénard's disease are all conditions of hypostasis, which at the turn of the century were thought pathologic and possible causes of nausea, vomiting, and other symptoms that Glénard cured by having

TABLE 8–7. RELATIVE POTENTIAL OF CHEMOTHERAPEUTIC AGENTS TO INDUCE EMESIS

HIGH POTENTIAL (>90%)	HIGH POTENTIAL (60% TO 90%)	MODERATE POTENTIAL (30% TO 60%)	LOW POTENTIAL (10% TO 30%)
Cisplatin	Carmustine	L-Asparaginase	Bleomycin
Cytarabine (high dose)	Cyclophosphamide	5-Azacytidine	Cytarabine (standard dose)
Dacarbazine	Dactinomycin	Daunorubicin	Etoposide
Mechlorethamine	Lomustine	Doxorubicin	Hydroxyurea
Streptozotocin	Methotrexate ($\geq$200 mg)	Fluorouracil	Melphalan
	Mithramycin	Hexamethylmelamine	6-Mercaptopurine
	Procarbazine	Mitomycin C	Methotrexate ($\leq$200 mg)
	Semustine		Teniposide
			Thiotepa
			Vinblastine
			Vincristine

Reproduced with permission from Graves T. Emesis as a complication of cancer chemotherapy: pathophysiology, importance and treatment. *Pharmacotherapy.* 1992;12(4):337–345.

his patients "take the waters at Vichy" after his paper in 1885. Even in 1908 Osler felt that "too many disorders have been ascribed to 'gastroptosis'." We are in the same situation in the 1990s, and any discussion of nausea needs to have the caution that we understand little about it still. In the 1990s, instead of learning about hypostasis, we spend great effort classifying the three kinds of vomiting that occur after chemotherapeutic drugs.[3]

1. *Acute nausea and vomiting* begins within 2 hours of drug administration, peaks in 4 to 10 hours, and resolves in 12 to 24 hours. This is the most common syndrome. The episodes are frequent and severe.
2. *Delayed nausea and vomiting* occurs 1 to 5 days after chemotherapy administration, with peak frequency between 48 and 72 hours. It is less severe but lasts longer than the acute type.
3. *Anticipatory nausea and vomiting* is a conditioned reflex associated with poor control of emesis during prior chemotherapy treatments. Agents with a distinct odor, taste, or even the sight of the intravenous administration equipment may elicit an emetic episode prior to actual therapy, and its mechanism is even more poorly understood than the mechanism of vomiting in most other conditions. Speculation and theories abound, and those interested in metaphysics can review the large literature on the subject. Suggestible patients can be treated with *acupuncture* and Chinese herbs and even *TENS*, but these have little place in scientific medicine at this time except for research centers. I personally do not discourage those of my patients who ask to see an acupuncturist, although I do try to have them see a (behavioral) psychotherapist first, sometimes with good results. Modern practitioners of psychotherapy by reciprocal inhibition or other techniques such as neurolinguistic programming do sometimes help as much and sometimes more than any medication.

Chemotherapeutic drugs are classified as having a very high (>90%), high (60% to 90%), moderate (30% to 60%), or low (10% to 30%) potential for causing acute nausea and vomiting (Table 8-7). Drug dosage also is important.

At this time drug treatment of this serious condition is with ondansetron or granisetron and metoclopramide or cisapride and combinations of drugs. Graves points out that the quality of life is decreased in 30% of patients with cancer by iatrogenically induced nausea and vomiting and that in addition the iatrogenic psychosocial effects of these drugs can lead to loss of jobs, curtailment of social life, and interference of performance of daily living activities. "Patients who experience severe drug induced nausea and vomiting often value quality of life over potentially curative but very toxic treatments."[3]

REFERENCES

1. Dundee JW, McMillan C. Positive evidence for P6 acupuncture antiemesis. *Postgrad Med J.* 1991;67:417–422.
2. Frazer JG. *The Golden Bough: A Study in Magic and Religion.* New York, NY: Macmillan; 1922:19, 562–563.
3. Graves T. Emesis as a complication of cancer chemotherapy: pathophysiology, importance and treatment. *Pharmacotherapy.* 1992;12(4):337–345.
4. Lindstrom PA, Brizee KR. Relief of intractable vomiting from surgical lesions in the area postrema. *J Neurosurg.* 1962;19:228–236.
5. Marin J, Ibañez MC, Arribas S. Therapeutic management of nausea and vomiting (Review). *Gen Pharmacol.* 1990;21(1):1–10.
6. Martin M. Myths and realities of anti-emetic treatment. *Br J Cancer.* 1992;19:S46–S51.
7. McCallum RW, Kendall BJ. Treatment options for chronic nausea and vomiting. *Contemporary Internal Medicine.* 1993;5:62–69.
8. Michaloudis D, O'Keeffe N, O'Sullivan K, Healy TEJ. Postoperative nausea and vomiting: a comparison of anti-emetic drugs used alone or in combination. *J R Soc Med.* 1993;86:137–138.
9. Mitchelson F. Pharmacologic agents affecting emesis, a review in 2 parts. *Drugs.* 1992;43(3):295–315, 43(4):443–463.
10. Saller R, Hellenbrecht D, Bühring M, Hess H. Enhancement of the antiemetic action of metoclopramide against cisplatin-induced emesis by transdermal electrical nerve stimulation. *J Clin Pharm.* 1986;26:115–119.
11. Smith G, Rowbotham DJ, eds. Supplement on postoperative nausea and vomiting. *Br J Anaesth.* 1992;69(suppl 1):1S–68S.
12. Swanson DW, Swenson WM, Huizenga KA, Melson SJ. Persistent nausea without organic cause. *Mayo Clinic Proc.* 1976;51:257–262.
13. Tortorice PV. Management of chemotherapy-induced nausea and vomiting. *Pharmacotherapy.* 1990;10(2):129–145.
14. Trepanier CA. Perioperative gastric aspiration increases postoperative nausea and vomiting in outpatients. *Can J Anaesth.* 1993;40:325–328.
15. Watcha MF, White PF. Postoperative nausea and vomiting: etiology, treatment and prevention. *Anaesthesiology.* 1992;77:162–184.
16. Wolf S. Effects of suggestions and conditioning on the action of chemical agents in human subjects: the pharmacology of placebo. *J Clin Invest.* 1950;29:100–109.

9
Dyspepsia

GIANRICO FARRUGIA and MICHAEL CAMILLERI

DEFINITION

Dyspepsia is defined as a group of episodic or persistent symptoms that include abdominal pain or discomfort, nausea, early satiety, and bloating and are referable to the upper gastrointestinal tract. Functional dyspepsia implies that the symptoms are unrelated to demonstrable mucosal or biochemical disease and that clinical investigations have been carried out to exclude these diseases. Functional dyspepsia is common; based on questionnaire data, its prevalence is estimated at 10% to 20% in the general population. It is a significant component of the group of diseases termed *functional gastrointestinal diseases*, which includes the irritable bowel syndrome and accounts for up to 50% of all gastrointestinal outpatient referrals.

Several disorders present with similar symptoms and need to be excluded before a diagnosis of functional dyspepsia can be made. These include cholelithiasis, acid peptic disease, gastric erosions, gastrointestinal reflux disease, chronic pancreatitis, gastric and pancreatic malignancy, and secondary motility disorders. Less commonly, similar symptoms result from malabsorption syndromes such as celiac sprue, metabolic disorders, ischemic heart disease, and collagen vascular disorders (Table 9–1). Thus, a careful history and examination, as well as upper endoscopy and ultrasound are indicated for patients with chronic dyspeptic symptoms, especially in those over 40 years of age. The nature of the presenting symptoms may point toward further investigation, e.g., right upper quadrant pain may suggest biliary colic and pain that wakes the patient at night and can be sharply localized to a small area of the upper abdomen suggests peptic ulcer disease. In contrast prominent heartburn suggests gastroesophageal reflux. Nausea, early satiety, bloating, and belching suggest a disturbance of motor function, and with the presence of such symptoms a gastric emptying test is appropriate.

SYMPTOMATIC CATEGORIES

It has been proposed that among patients with functional dyspepsia, symptoms can be used to identify distinct subgroups. The proposed subgroups included: those with symptoms suggestive of classic peptic ulcer disease (ulcerlike dyspepsia), those with symptoms suggestive of dysmotility (stasis dyspepsia), and those with symptoms suggestive of gastrointestinal reflux (refluxlike dyspepsia). Other patients had symptoms that did not fit in any of these categories (nonspecific dyspepsia). Although these subgroups initially gained general acceptance, there is little evidence to support this classification. Based on symptom questionnaires the most common subgroup in epidemiologic studies was ulcerlike dyspepsia (64%); but 43% of the subjects with dyspepsia could be classified into more than one subgroup. Others in secondary and tertiary referral centers have found that symptom subgroups were not associated with the presumed abnormality of function on formal testing. Therefore it appears that categorizing subgroups on the basis of symptoms alone may not be useful in tailoring the investigation and treatment of dyspepsia.

MECHANISMS

ALTERED GASTROINTESTINAL MOTILITY

A subgroup of patients with functional dyspepsia have abnormal gastric motor function. When gastric emptying is restored to normal by pro-

TABLE 9–1. CONDITIONS THAT MUST BE CONSIDERED IN PATIENTS WITH SUSPECTED FUNCTIONAL DYSPEPSIA

Common
Cholelithiasis
Acid peptic disease
Erosions
Gastrointestinal reflux disease
Chronic pancreatitis
Malignancy, gastric or pancreatic
Motility disturbances

Rare
Drugs
Malabsorption
Metabolic disorders
Ischemic heart disease
Collagen vascular disease

kinetic agents, there is a parallel resolution of dyspeptic symptoms. Ten trials using cisapride as the prokinetic agent, in patients with documented impairment of gastric emptying and symptoms similar to those of dysmotility such as epigastric pain, early satiety, heartburn, belching, and postprandial belching, showed a relief of symptoms supporting the concept that abnormal motility was responsible for the dyspepsia. Although this data is suggestive of an idiopathic disturbance of motility in patients with functional dyspepsia, disordered motility is only present in about 50% of patients and, even when present, does not always temporally correlate with symptoms. It is therefore difficult to establish a causal relationship between motor abnormalities and symptoms.

Little is known about the mechanisms resulting in disordered gastrointestinal motor function (Fig. 9–1). Among functional dyspepsia patients with slow transit, there is evidence of a disturbance in extrinsic neural control of the gut. In contrast, in dyspeptic patients with normal transit, there was a greater perception of luminal stimuli, suggesting an alteration in afferent function (see below).

Identification of the subgroup of patients with impaired motor function may select those patients more likely to respond to prokinetic agents. Ultrasonography and impedance (applied potential) tomography have been used to assess motor function; however, they measure liquid transit, which is often normal in functional dyspepsia. A simple, cost-effective, sensitive, noninvasive test for upper gut dysmotility is a scintigraphically measured gastric and small bowel transit time, which may help select those patients most likely to respond to treatment.

INCREASED VISCERAL PERCEPTION

In recent years, several groups have explored the alterations in visceral afferent function shown by the increased perception of intraluminal stimuli in patients with functional dyspepsia. In dyspeptic patients with normal transit the distention threshold volume necessary for perception in the proximal jejunum was smaller than in healthy controls; the peristaltic reflex response to that distention in these patients was also diminished (Fig. 9–2). In the stomach the perception of an intragastric balloon occurs at lower pressure and volumes of distention in patients as compared with controls. Although central perception is enhanced, intestino-intestinal reflexes are not exaggerated, and the increased perception does not result in any greater changes in autonomic or stress hormone responses than in healthy controls. Thus, in dyspepsia, sensory pathways appear to be normal, but perception is enhanced, without excessive stimulation of autonomic stress responses.

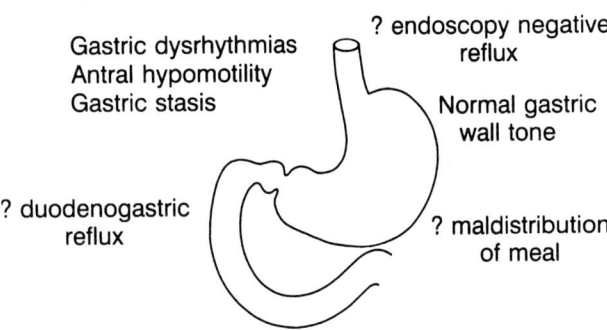

FIGURE 9–1. The proven and controversial (indicated by ?) motor dysfunction reported in patients with functional dyspepsia.

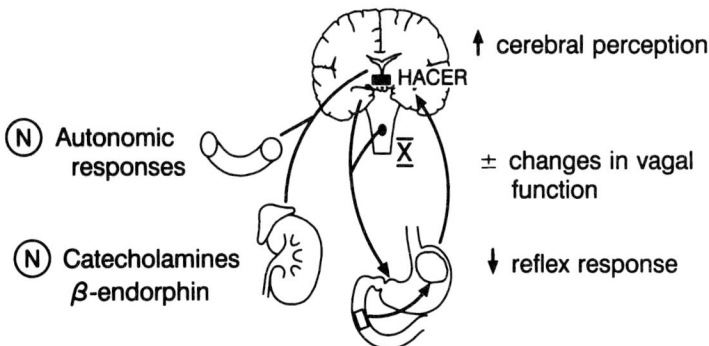

FIGURE 9–2. Sensory and autonomic alterations in functional dyspepsia. Note the increased central perception of visceral stimuli, that is, unassociated with any evidence of exaggerated catecholamine, b-endorphin, or autonomic responses. Some evidence also suggests that patients with altered motor function have impaired efferent vagal function. The significance of reported reduction in viscerovisceral reflex responses is unclear. *HACER* = hypothalamic area for control of emotional responses.

HELICOBACTER PYLORI

Several studies have shown that despite appearing endoscopically normal, mucosa can be inflamed on histologic examination. Gastritis, both endoscopically and histologically determined, is commonly blamed as a cause of functional dyspepsia, despite a lack of data to support this hypothesis. *Helicobacter pylori* is a common cause of histologically confirmed inflammation, and therefore a causative role has been proposed for this organism in patients with dyspepsia and *H. pylori*. *H. pylori* is detected in approximately 40% to 50% of patients with functional dyspepsia; this figure is not different from the prevalence anticipated in an age-matched, nondiseased group. Inflamed mucosa is asymptomatic in many patients, and therefore a cause and effect relationship between *H. pylori* and functional dyspepsia is not established. In five recent trials using bismuth to eradicate the organism, three showed an improvement in symptoms, while two did not. In patients with gastric stasis there does not appear to be an increased incidence of *H. pylori* infection. At present there is inadequate evidence to justify treatment of *H. pylori* if it were detected in functional dyspepsia patients. More studies are necessary to determine whether and to what extent *H. pylori* is a cause of functional dyspepsia.

GASTRIC ACID

Dyspepsia was previously thought to be associated with an increased risk of subsequent ulcer formation, and patients with dyspepsia were thought to be abnormally sensitive to their gastric acid concentration. This has led to the treatment of many dyspeptic patients with H_2 blockers. Available data now show that patients with functional dyspepsia do not secrete more acid and are not more sensitive to gastric acid than controls. Patients who benefit from H_2 blockers and antacids may have organic diseases such as esophagitis or peptic ulcer rather than dyspepsia. Thus, in these patients a 24-hour pH reflux test may be indicated, particularly in those with prominent heartburn.

DIETARY, STRESS, PSYCHOLOGIC AND ENVIRONMENTAL FACTORS

Psychologic profiles in patients with functional dyspepsia have shown more anxiety, neuroticism, and depression than healthy subjects, but personality scores are no different from other patients with organic or functional chronic abdominal pain. Increased age, male gender, unmarried status, and social incongruity are associated with an increased frequency and severity of symptoms but are not associated with health care-seeking behavior. Alcohol, coffee, and analgesic use are not associated with an increased incidence of dyspepsia.

Although it does not appear that psychiatric disease or psychologic problems are a cause of dyspepsia, such illnesses may manifest symptoms suggestive of functional dyspepsia. Depression is common among gastroenterology outpatients, and its symptoms should be sought, particularly in those who have predominant chronic abdominal pain. Well-structured studies of hypnotherapy and psychotherapy are warranted, and trials with the newer antidepressants that are devoid of anticholinergic side effects are awaited in carefully selected patients.

DIAGNOSIS

The detailed history should include a search for indicators of biliary colic, peptic ulceration, and reflux (see above). Also indicators for depression, anxiety, or psychologic disturbance should be sought at the first interview. Physical examination may reveal a succussion splash in the abdomen in those with significantly disturbed gastric emptying. Rarely, neurologic evaluation will identify pupillary, sweating, or blood pressure disturbances consistent with an autonomic neuropathy affecting gastrointestinal motility.

Hematology and biochemistry screens are usually normal. When abnormal, they indicate the need to exclude diseases affecting the upper gut mucosa. Endoscopy is essential to exclude mucosal disease, and imaging of the biliary tract and pancreas is most conveniently achieved by ultrasonography (Fig. 9–3). There is at present not enough data to mandate a search for *H. pylori*. Therefore it is reasonable to look for this organism in research studies, but not necessarily in clinical practice. In patients with prominent heartburn, an esophageal pH test (e.g., Bernstein or preferably 24-hour pH monitoring) is indicated.

In patients with a negative endoscopy, a gastric emptying test is necessary. Identification of delayed gastric emptying should lead to a trial of prokinetic agents. If gastric emptying is not delayed, some would suggest a search for *H. pylori* and attempted eradication with a bismuth compound and antibiotics; however, this is controversial.

In those patients with indicators of psychologic or psychiatric disorder during the first interview or on formal personality inventory, a psychiatric evaluation, or a therapeutic trial with fluoxetine or trazodone is indicated.

TREATMENT

Figure 9–4 shows an approach to management of patients with functional dyspepsia that is based on identifying the etiologic mechanism. Clearly, this approach follows exclusion of ulceration, biliary tract, or pancreatic disease. For delayed gastric emptying, small, more frequent meals, with reduced fat and nondigestible fiber content and use of liquid supplements may be helpful. Prokinetic agents are the mainstay of treatment. The prokinetics of choice in the long term are cisapride (10 to 20 mg tid and qhs), domperidone (10 to 30 mg tid), or metoclopramide (10 to 20 mg tid): each agent is administered 30 minutes before the three main meals. Analogs of erythromycin, which appears to act on the motilin receptor in the gut, may be available in the future. Psychologic disturbances re-

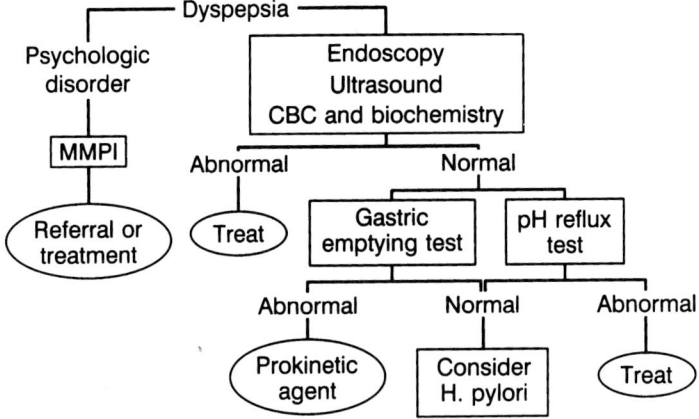

FIGURE 9–3. Management algorithm for functional dyspepsia. *CBC* = complete blood count, *MMPI* = Minnesota Multiphasic Personality Inventory.

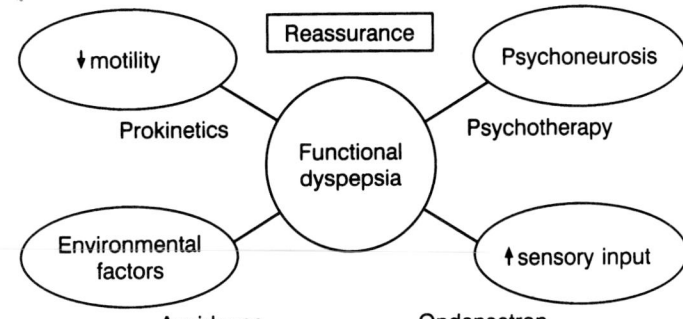

FIGURE 9-4. Treatment of functional dyspepsia. Selected by associated mechanism.

quire specific treatment, including the use of antidepressants without anticholinergic side effects such as fluoxetine or trazodone.

In the future, when there are no indicators for structural disease, psychologic disturbance, or abnormal gastric emptying, there may be a role for $5HT_3$ antagonists. Ondansetron, a $5HT_3$ antagonist, is thought to reduce visceral afferent sensation and stimulation of the vomiting center, as shown by its inhibition of cisplatin-induced vomiting.

In patients with unexplained vomiting antiemetics may be useful. It should, however, be kept in mind that a substantial proportion of patients need only reassurance that their symptoms are not due to a "serious" medical problem, and, therefore, this form of psychotherapy should be liberally prescribed.

REFERENCES

1. Camilleri M, Malagelada JR, Kao PC, Zinsmeister AR. Gastric and autonomic responses to stress in functional dyspepsia. *Dig Dis Sci.* 1986;31:1169–1177.
2. Greydanus MP, Vassallo M, Camilleri M, Nelson DK, Hanson RB, Thomforde GM. Neurohormonal factors in functional dyspepsia: insights on pathophysiologic mechanisms. *Gastroenterology.* 1991;100:1311–1318.
3. Heading RC. Definitions of dyspepsia. *Scand J Gastroenterol.* 1991;26(suppl 182):1–6.
4. Lemann M, Dederding JP, Jian B, Franchisseur C, Rambaud JC, Jian R. Abnormal perception of visceral pain in response to gastric distention in chronic idiopathic dyspepsia: the irritable stomach syndrome. *Dig Dis Sci.* 1991; 36:1249–1254.
5. Nyren O, Adami HO, Bates S, et al. Absence of therapeutic benefits from antacids or cimetidine in nonulcer dyspepsia. *N Engl J Med.* 1986;314:339–343.
6. Talley NJ, Zinsmeister AR, Schleck CD, Melton LJ. Dyspepsia and dyspepsia subgroups: a population-based study. *Gastroenterology.* 1992;102:1259–1268.

10

Functional Abdominal Pain

WILLIAM E. WHITEHEAD

Functional abdominal pain is one of the most common reasons for consulting a physician, accounting for approximately 40% of visits to gastroenterologists.[38] Of the several types of functional abdominal pain now recognized (Table 10-1), irritable bowel syndrome (IBS) has been the most thoroughly investigated. IBS accounts for 2.4 to 3.5 million outpatient visits per year, for 2.2 million prescriptions for medication,[47] and for an average of 13.4 disability days per year.[12] IBS is associated with a threefold increase in the prevalence of hysterectomy and other types of abdominal surgery.[23,61]

The pathophysiology of this type of pain is by definition unknown; treatment is empiric and is frequently unsuccessful. However, several recent

TABLE 10–1. FUNCTIONAL ABDOMINAL PAIN SYNDROMES

Functional dyspepsia[56]
Irritable bowel syndrome[57]
Functional abdominal pain syndrome[57]
Functional biliary pain[8]
  Gallbladder dysfunction
  Dysfunction of Oddi's sphincter
Functional anorectal pain[64]
  Levator ani syndrome
  Proctalgia fugax

---

advances have been made in the refinement of diagnostic criteria, the investigation of possible pathophysiology, and the evaluation of treatments by controlled trials. As a result, treatment outcomes have improved, and more rational guidelines for treatment can now be offered.

SUBTYPES

Several subtypes of functional abdominal pain are now recognized (Table 10–1), and multinational committees of experts have developed research diagnostic criteria and have summarized treatment recommendations for each.[56,57,64]

PHYSIOLOGIC MECHANISMS FOR SYMPTOMS

Both abnormal motility[24,26,49] and increased sensitivity to distension of the bowel[45,62] have been suggested as mechanisms for functional abdominal pain. It is likely that these mechanisms interact: nonpropulsive contractions may temporarily increase the amount of pressure in isolated segments of bowel, although there is no overall increase in the amount of gas or stool in the whole bowel.[30,37]

Investigators have shown that patients with irritable bowel syndrome have increased sensitivity to distension of the rectum,[28,59] sigmoid colon,[45,62] distal ileum,[25] and duodenum,[27] and that patients with functional dyspepsia have increased sensitivity to distension of the stomach.[5,33] Patients with these functional pain syndromes show increased sensitivity not only to painful intensities of stimulation but also to weak distensions associated with sensations in the rectum of flatus and urge to defecate[44] and in the stomach with sensations of bloating.[5]

This enhanced sensitivity to distension does not appear to be due to a psychologic tendency to exaggerate the painfulness of any aversive sensation since patients with IBS do not have lower pain thresholds for nongastrointestinal aversive stimuli,[62,7] and pain thresholds are not correlated with psychologic measures of neuroticism.[62] Thus, the weight of evidence suggests that increased sensitivity to distension is an important component of the physiologic mechanism for functional abdominal pain.

PSYCHOLOGIC FACTORS

The majority of patients with functional abdominal pain who consult physicians have abnormally high levels of psychologic distress,[55,60] and more than half meet criteria for a psychiatric diagnosis.[36,60] The psychologic symptoms and psychiatric diagnoses most frequently found include depression, somatization (i.e., a tendency to report multiple somatic symptoms in the absence of evidence for a disease process), and anxiety.

The consistency with which psychologic symptoms are seen in medical clinic patients with functional abdominal pain has led some to conclude that functional abdominal pain is a psychiatric disorder.[31] However, when subjects who have functional abdominal pain but have not consulted physicians are identified from community studies, they have no more symptoms of psychologic distress than the rest of the population.[10,58] This suggests that psychologic symptoms do not cause functional abdominal pain syndromes but do influence which patients with these pain syndromes will consult physicians; only 20% to 50% of patients with irritable bowel syndrome consult a physician.

Another psychologic factor that is important to the understanding of functional abdominal pain syndromes is stress; up to 88% of patients with irritable bowel syndrome, for example, report that stress is associated with an exacerbation of their abdominal pain.[48] Research confirms that stressful life events contribute to exacerbations of bowel symptoms, although the magnitude of the effect is much smaller than patients believe.[63] Specific stressors that have been identified as important to the development of IBS include the loss of a parent during childhood[34] and a history of sexual or physical abuse.[11]

DIAGNOSTIC EVALUATION

The diagnostic assessment of these patients is guided by (1) exclusion of alternative disease explanations for the symptoms, (2) determining that the patient satisfies positive diagnostic criteria for a functional disorder, and (3) testing for comorbid psychiatric disorders.

Exclusion of Other Diseases

Following is a list of the most common diseases that should be excluded:

- Peptic ulcer disease
- Inflammatory bowel disease
- Chronic intestinal pseudoobstruction
- Mechanical obstruction
- Diverticulitis
- Parasitic or infectious causes

In most cases, relatively few tests are required as most of these candidate disorders can be ruled out on the basis of the history and physical examination. However, hematologic tests for an infection, tests of stools for blood, and sigmoidoscopy for lower bowel symptoms should be routine. Recent evidence suggests that these simple tests, when combined with a careful history, enable the physician to exclude an alternative disease explanation for recurring abdominal pain with 95% confidence.[18,21,54]

Positive Diagnostic Criteria

Multinational committees of experts have developed by consensus symptom criteria to be used for the diagnosis of dyspepsia,[56] functional bowel disorders,[57] and functional anorectal disorders.[64] These criteria are listed in Table 10–2. In some instances these criteria are very restrictive and may exclude many patients in whom the clinician feels a diagnosis of a functional pain syndrome is warranted; the diagnostic criteria allow for this by creating categories for nonspecific functional dyspepsia, nonspecific functional bowel disorder, and nonspecific functional

---

TABLE 10–2. SYMPTOM CRITERIA FOR DIAGNOSIS OF COMMON FUNCTIONAL ABDOMINAL PAIN SYNDROMES

Functional Dyspepsia
1. Chronic or recurrent abdominal pain or discomfort centered in the upper abdomen; a duration of ≥1 month with symptoms 25% of the time (i.e., on 7 days or more) is recommended for the purposes of research.
2. No clinical, biochemical, endoscopic, or ultrasonographic evidence of any known organic disease that is likely to explain the symptoms (i.e., acid-peptic or neoplastic disease of stomach, esophagus, or duodenum or disease of the pancreas or hepatobiliary system) and no history of major gastric or intestinal surgery. Patients with a *past* history of *documented* chronic peptic ulcer disease should not be classified as having functional dyspepsia at least until the relationship between these entities is clarified.[56]

Irritable Bowel Syndrome
At least 3 months of continuous or recurrent symptoms of
1. Abdominal pain or discomfort that is
   a. Relieved with defecation,
   b. Associated with a change in frequency of stool, or
   c. Associated with a change in consistency of stool
2. Two or more of the following, at least a quarter of occasions or days:
   a. Altered stool frequency
   b. Altered stool form (lumpy, hard or loose, watery stool)
   c. Altered stool passage (straining, urgency, or feeling of incomplete evacuation)
   d. Passage of mucus
   e. Bloating or feeling of abdominal distension[57]

Functional Abdominal Pain Syndrome
1. Frequently recurrent or continuous abdominal pain for at least 6 months
2. Incomplete or no relationship of pain with physiologic events (e.g., eating, defecation, or menses)
3. Some loss of daily functioning
4. No evidence for organic disease to explain the pain and insufficient criteria for other functional gastrointestinal disorders that would explain the abdominal pain.[57]

Levator Ani Syndrome
1. Chronic or recurrent rectal pain or aching for at least 3 months. Confidence in the diagnosis is substantially increased if posterior traction on the puborectalis reveals tight levator ani muscles and tenderness or pain.[64]

Proctalgia Fugax
1. Recurrent episodes of midline pain localized to the lower rectum for at least 3 months
2. Episodes last from seconds to minutes
3. There is no anorectal pain between episodes
4. There is no evidence of anorectal disease.[64]

anorectal disorder. It should be noted that these diagnostic criteria were based on the consensus of experts whose views were informed by available empiric research, but where empiric research was lacking, the criteria took into account clinical experience. Empiric validation of many of these diagnostic criteria has not yet been reported.

Assessment of Comorbid Psychiatric Conditions

A high proportion of patients with functional abdominal pain have psychiatric disorders severe enough to warrant referral for treatment, although it does not appear that the psychiatric symptoms cause the gastrointestinal symptoms. It is recommended that clinicians screen for psychiatric disorders early in the assessment process using a standard psychometric test such as the Psychiatric Symptom Checklist 90R.[9] Having the patient complete a psychologic test as a routine part of intake rather than after a negative evaluation for disease will reduce the tendency of patients to view such tests as a rejection by the physician.

TREATMENT

Education and Reassurance

The development of good rapport with the patient, followed by education and reassurance, is the most important element in successful management of functional abdominal pain syndromes. Its efficacy has not been directly evaluated because it is considered to be inherent in a good doctor-patient relationship. However, the fact that one third of patients with IBS consult alternative medicine practitioners, apparently because these providers spend more time listening sympathetically to the patient,[51] attests both to the importance that patients attach to these factors and to the deficiencies of many physicians in this regard.

Conveying sympathy and interest in the distress and fear that patients with functional abdominal pain experience is critical to establishing a trusting doctor-patient relationship, but it is difficult for many physicians because it is at odds with their training. Physicians are trained in hospitals where time and resources are prioritized in terms of how potentially fatal the patient's injuries or illness may be; the worried well and the minimally ill are viewed as a low priority or a nuisance. Dealing effectively with patients who have functional abdominal pain (in an outpatient setting) requires that the doctor see the illness from the patient's perspective.

Appropriate education includes teaching the patient that functional abdominal pain syndromes are chronic, recurring disorders and that occasional recurrences of symptoms do not mean that the diagnosis or the treatment was incorrect. Explaining the role of stress and diet is also helpful as it makes the natural history of the disorder more understandable to the patient and increases the patient's control. Reassurance that the symptoms are not indications of cancer, inflammatory bowel disease, or peptic ulcer and that the symptoms are not progressive or life threatening is also helpful. This reassurance can take the form of reviewing with the patient what alternative diagnoses were considered and the evidence that led to rejecting them. Each visit should be ended with the offer of a follow-up appointment; periodic visits are appropriate for chronic disorders, and they convey to the patient that the physician has a continuing interest in them.

Conservative management often combines education and reassurance with encouragement to increase the amount of fiber in the diet and prescription of an antispasmodic drug to be taken as needed. However, neither dietary fiber nor antispasmodics appear to be very effective (see below). Nevertheless, conservative measures such as these are all that is needed for an estimated 68% of patients with functional abdominal pain syndromes.[18]

DIETARY MANAGEMENT

Increased dietary fiber is often prescribed for patients with IBS, but there is little evidence that it is beneficial. IBS patients do not habitually consume less dietary fiber than the rest of the population,[20] and augmented dietary fiber is no more effective than placebo for reducing the symptoms of abdominal pain and diarrhea.[6] In adequate amounts, dietary fiber does ameliorate colonic inertia-type constipation, however, and on this basis it can be recommended when abdominal pain is combined with this type of constipation.

Idiosyncratic food intolerances or food allergies are believed by some to account for half[40] to two thirds[22] of patients with diarrhea-predominant IBS. Diagnosis is usually made by placing the patient on a highly restricted, bland diet and, if symptoms decrease or disappear, reintroducing foods one at a time. Nanda and colleagues[40] reported that 91 of 199 IBS patients improved on an exclusionary diet and that 90 of 91 were still improved 1 year later (only 72 of whom were still following a restricted diet). The most common food intolerance was lactose, which was present in one third of patients. The status of idiosyncratic food intolerance other than lactose remains controversial, although it is very popular with patients. Most clinicians find that the best approach is to tolerate patients experimenting with their diets so long as it does not lead them to adopt a highly restrictive or unhealthy diet.

DRUG THERAPY

Anticholinergic Compounds

Dicyclomine hydrochloride (Bentyl) and hyoscyamine sulfate (Levsin) are the anticholinergic drugs most widely prescribed for functional abdominal pain in the United States. Early trials[42] showed that dicyclomine was more effective than placebo for reducing abdominal pain and global measures of bowel dysfunction. However, 50% to 67% of patients develop significant side effects such as dry mouth and blurred vision at doses (e.g., 160 mg) that are adequate to reduce symptoms of IBS.[43] Other anticholinergic compounds with fewer side effects are under investigation, and some are marketed in Europe.

Opiate Analogs

The antidiarrheal agent loperamide (Imodium), at an individually titrated dose averaging 4 mg/d, is effective for symptoms of urgency, excessive stool frequency, and loose stool consistency. Pain may also be reduced.[32] Loperamide does not cross the blood-brain barrier and therefore does not cause addiction. Another opiate analog, diphenoxylate (Lomotil), is also effective for diarrhea-predominant IBS, but it is less desirable than loperamide because it does cross the blood-brain barrier and can produce euphoria; for this reason it is supplied in combination with atropine to reduce the potential for abuse. For both opiate analogs, careful titration of the dose is required because of a tendency to cause constipation.

Antidepressants

Several controlled trials (Table 10–3) show tricyclic antidepressants to be more effective than placebo for reducing abdominal pain and diarrhea. However, they do not benefit patients with constipation. No data have been reported on the benefits of the newer antidepressant compound fluoxetine (Prozac) for patients with functional abdominal pain.

It is unclear whether the benefits of antidepressants are related to their antidepressant action or to their anticholinergic action. The fact that these compounds are often effective at doses that are subclinical for the management of depression, and that they are effective in groups of patients who were unselected for the presence of depression, suggests that the benefits are related to the anticholinergic properties of these compounds.

Tranquilizers

Tranquilizers are sometimes prescribed for patients with functional abdominal pain because

TABLE 10–3. CONTROLLED TRIALS OF ANTIDEPRESSANTS FOR FUNCTIONAL ABDOMINAL PAIN

Drug	Dose	Effectiveness	Reference
Amitriptyline	50 mg	14 patients studied; self-rated severity tended to decrease ($p<.08$).	Steinhart, et al[52]
Desipramine	150 mg h.s.	28 patients; diarrhea and pain improved significantly, but constipation did not	Greenbaum, et al[15]
Desipramine	150 mg h.s.	IBS-constipation and IBS-diarrhea patients pooled; no effect on pain or stool frequency	Heefner, et al[19]
Trimipramine	50 mg or divided	428 patients; pain, nausea, and reflux decreased	Myren, et al[39]
Nortriptyline (combined with 1.5 mg fluphenazine)	30 mg h.s.	38 patients; pain and diarrhea decreased, but constipation did not	Lancaster-Smith[29]
Fluoxetine		No published trial as yet	

many of these patients are anxious and most report that their symptoms are exacerbated by stress. However, controlled trials suggest that tranquilizers' therapeutic benefit is small.[1,46] Because they are also addictive, tranquilizers are not recommended for abdominal pain syndromes, which tend to be chronic or recurring.

BEHAVIORAL AND PSYCHOLOGIC TREATMENT

Although abdominal pain and bowel symptoms do not seem to be caused by psychologic symptoms,[10,58] psychologically based treatment may nevertheless contribute to the management of these patients for the following reasons. Such treatment may reduce the frequency with which the patient experiences psychologic stress, and psychologic stress is known to trigger abdominal pain and altered bowel habits in both healthy subjects and patients with IBS. Psychologic treatment may also reduce psychologic symptoms that occur as comorbid conditions in patients who also have IBS or other functional abdominal pain syndromes.

PSYCHOTHERAPY

Two large, controlled studies support the benefits of brief psychotherapy for patients with IBS. Svedlund and colleagues[53] recruited 101 patients (out of 119 consecutive patients approached) and randomly assigned half of them to receive psychodynamic psychotherapy. This therapy aimed at identifying conflicts and stressors in the patient's life and teaching more appropriate ways of coping. The control patients received standard medical therapy. Only two patients dropped out of the trial. By the end of 3 months of treatment (average of 7.4 hours of contact with a psychiatrist), the psychotherapy group had improved more on abdominal pain and altered bowel habits than had the controls. At follow-up 1 year later, the difference between the psychotherapy group and the controls was further increased.

A second psychotherapy study[16] was similar in design and outcome. Guthrie and colleagues randomly assigned 102 patients to two groups, one of which participated in discussions with the psychiatrist of current problems in living with the aim of teaching more effective ways of coping with stress and conflict. In addition, the psychotherapy patients were taught exercises to help them relax and were encouraged to use these exercises daily. The controls received standard medical care consisting of fiber supplements and antispasmodics but no psychotropic medications. At the end of 3 months of treatment (seven sessions), the psychotherapy group showed significantly less pain, diarrhea, anxiety, and depression than the controls, although there were no differences for symptoms of constipation or bloating. These improvements were well maintained at follow-up 1 year later. Thus, individual psychotherapy is beneficial for patients who have failed to respond to conservative medical management. Patients are more likely to benefit if they are anxious or depressed. Psychotherapy requires referral to a psychologist or psychiatrist.

HYPNOTHERAPY

Whorwell and colleagues[65-67] reported on the basis of an experience with over 200 IBS patients that hypnosis is an effective treatment for functional abdominal pain. In their first report, they randomly assigned patients to receive hypnotherapy or a control treatment that combined a placebo tablet with half-hour discussions of the role of emotion and stress in bowel symptoms. Hypnosis consisted of suggestions to relax striated muscles and suggestions to use imagery to relax the smooth muscle of the gastrointestinal tract. Half-hour clinic sessions were supplemented with daily practice of autohypnosis using taped instructions. By the end of 4 weeks, the hypnosis group showed greater reductions in abdominal pain and altered bowel habits. In their larger but uncontrolled study, Whorwell[65] reported that 85% of patients benefited and that results were well sustained for 1 year provided the patient returned for an additional hypnosis session every 3 months. His group also reported that patients over age 50 and patients with significant amounts of anxiety or depression benefited less, a finding that contrasts with Guthrie's report[16] that anxious and depressed patients were more likely to benefit from psychotherapy.

An independent research group[17] has replicated Whorwell's work. Harvey and colleagues[17] found that a somewhat lower proportion benefited from hypnosis (61%), but this was still superior to control values. Like Whorwell, they found that older and more anxious patients were less likely to benefit. Harvey's study extended Whorwell's work by showing that hypnotherapy provided in groups was as effective as individual hypnotherapy, making this a more cost-effective approach to treatment. Hypnosis requires special training and is normally performed by clinical psychologists or psychiatrists. However, Whorwell and several other gastroenterologists have learned to provide hypnotherapy.

COGNITIVE BEHAVIOR THERAPY

Cognitive behavior therapy represents an alternative approach to teaching stress management skills in patients with IBS. Its essential ingredient is to teach patients to recognize that their depression or anxiety is not spontaneous but occurs in response to self-defeating or negative thoughts such as "I am worthless" or "I always fail in situations like this." Patients are taught to recognize these thoughts and to substitute more positive thoughts when negative thoughts are detected. Generally, attempts to modify habitual ways of thinking are combined with teaching the patient techniques for controlling stress or anxiety. As practiced by Blanchard's group, which has published most extensively on this form of treatment, stress management involves teaching the patient progressive muscle relaxation techniques and using biofeedback training. Progressive muscle relaxation training uses standard exercises of tensing and relaxing major skeletal muscle groups to teach patients to recognize muscle tension and to voluntarily relax quickly. Biofeedback as used in this type of therapy involves using electronic feedback to teach patients to warm their hands through changes in blood flow or teaching them to relax the muscles of the forehead.

Blanchard and colleagues[3,41,50] report that two thirds of patients treated by this technique show at least a 50% reduction in symptoms of abdominal pain and altered bowel habits. In a similar study of a multicomponent behavior therapy treatment, Lynch and Zamble[35] also found that treated patients showed greater reductions in bowel symptoms than patients waiting for treatment. This form of treatment also requires referral to a specialist.

PROGRESSIVE MUSCLE RELAXATION TRAINING

An element common to many of the psychologic interventions described above is progressive muscle relaxation training, and there are indications that relaxation training alone is beneficial for patients with IBS. Bennett and Wilkinson[2] compared a stress management treatment, which consisted of one lecture on how stress and diet affect IBS plus eight sessions in which relaxation training was taught, with a medical treatment, which included an antidepressant-anxiolytic combination in addition to a bulking agent and an antispasmodic. The relaxation group received no medications. The two groups showed similar reductions in bowel symptoms, but the relaxation group showed greater improvements in anxiety. In a follow-up study Rumsey, a colleague of Wilkinson, showed that relaxation training provided in a group format was more effective than a similar medical control treatment for reducing abdominal pain, bloating, and psychologic symptoms of depression and anxiety. These studies are important because they suggest that a form of stress management training that can be provided by a gastroenterologist or nurse after minimal training is also effective.

ASCERTAINMENT BIAS AND PLACEBO EFFECTS

The studies reviewed above provide persuasive evidence that psychologic treatments are effective. However, in research on the evaluation of psychologic treatment, it is difficult to develop research designs that provide adequate protection against ascertainment bias and placebo effects. With respect to ascertainment bias, the psychotherapy studies[16,53] involved recruiting from a consecutive series of patients in a medical clinic, and the refusal rate was low, providing some assurance that the patients were representative of the patients seen by most gastroenterologists. However, in the cognitive behavior therapy trials,[3,35,41,50] one can have less confidence in the representativeness of the patients; in one study the refusal rate was 63% and in other trials the refusal rate was unknown. Similarly, the patients studied by Whorwell[65,66] appear to have been self-selected for their interest in hypnosis as a treatment for bowel symptoms.

It has been particularly difficult to exclude expectancy effects in trials of psychologic treatments. In most instances, the investigators recruited from among patients who had failed to benefit from standard medical management, but standard medical care was nevertheless used as the control. In other cases, a treated group was compared with patients who were waiting for an opportunity to begin treatment (a negative placebo group since people generally do not expect to get better while waiting to begin treatment). In the one study where a persuasive placebo treatment was designed,[4] the placebo group did as well as the active treatment group. Although these are serious methodologic concerns, the persistence of treatment effects for 1 year or more after treatment ends[50,53,67] suggests that placebo effects cannot account for all the benefits associated with psychologic treatment.

No studies have been published on the effectiveness of psychologic treatments for functional abdominal pain syndromes other than IBS.

SUMMARY AND RECOMMENDATIONS

Functional abdominal pain syndromes appear to have a physiologic basis related to increased sensitivity to distension of the gastrointestinal tract and perhaps to altered motility. Psychologic symptoms do not seem to cause these disorders but may influence which patients seek treatment and how they respond to treatment.

Because comorbid psychiatric disorders are common in patients with functional abdominal pain, a screening test for psychologic dysfunction should be a routine part of the assessment. It should not be postponed until a negative physical evaluation raises the index of suspicion.

The first line of treatment for functional abdominal pain is conservative treatment based on (1) establishing a trusting relationship with the patient, (2) providing education about the natural history of the disorder and factors such as diet and stress that are likely to influence it, and (3) reassuring the patient that they do not have cancer or other life-threatening conditions. Such conservative management is all that is required for 68% of patients with functional abdominal pain.

In patients who fail to respond to conservative management, tricyclic antidepressants may provide the most cost-effective second line of treatment. Psychotherapy, cognitive behavior therapy, and hypnotherapy may be more helpful than antidepressants alone, but because these treatments are costly and require referral to a specialist, it is recommended that they be reserved for patients who fail to respond to antidepressants.

REFERENCES

1. Baume P, Cuthbert J. The effect of medazepam in relieving symptoms of functional gastrointestinal distress. *Aust N Z J Med.* 1973;3:457–460.
2. Bennett P, Wilkinson S. A comparison of psychological and medical treatment of the irritable bowel syndrome. *Br J Clin Psych.* 1985;24:215–216.
3. Blanchard EB, Schwartz SP. Adaptation of a multicomponent treatment for irritable bowel syndrome to a small-group format. *Biofeedback Self Regul.* 1987;12:63–69.
4. Blanchard EB, Schwarz SP, Suls JM, et al. Two controlled evaluations of multicomponent psychological treatment of irritable bowel syndrome. *Behav Res Ther.* 1992;30:175–189.
5. Bradette M, Pare P, Douville P, Morin A. Visceral perception in health and functional dyspepsia: crossover study of gastric distension with placebo and domperidone. *Dig Dis Sci.* 1991;36:52–58.
6. Cann PA, Read NW, Holdsworth CD. What is the benefit of coarse wheat bran in patients with irritable bowel syndrome? *Gut.* 1984;25:168–173.
7. Cook IJ, van Eeden A, Collins SM. Patients with irritable bowel syndrome have greater pain tolerance than normal subjects. *Gastroenterology.* 1987;93:727–733.
8. Corazziari E, Funch-Jensen P, Hogan WJ, Tanaka M, Toouli J. Functional disorders of the biliary tract. *Gastroenterology International.* In press.
9. Derogatis LI. *The SCL–90R. Administration, scoring, and procedures manual, II.* Towson, Md: Clinical Psychometric Research; 1983.
10. Drossman DA, McKee DC, Sandler RS, et al. Psychosocial factors in the irritable bowel syndrome: a multivariate study of patients and nonpatients with irritable bowel syndrome. *Gastroenterology.* 1988;95:701–708.
11. Drossman DA, Leserman J, Nachman G, et al. Sexual and physical abuse in women with functional or organic gastrointestinal disorders. *Ann Intern Med.* 1990;113:828–833.
12. Drossman DA, Li Z, Andruzzi E, et al. US householder survey of functional GI disorders: prevalence, sociodemography and health impact. *Dig Dis Sci.* In press.
13. Drossman DA, Sandler RS, McKee DC, Lovitz AJ. Bowel patterns among subjects not seeking health care. *Gastroenterology.* 1982;83:529–534.
14. Everhart JE, Renault PF. Irritable bowel syndrome in office-based practice in the United States. *Gastroenterology.* 1991;100:998–1005.
15. Greenbaum DS, Mayle JE, Vanegeren LE, et al. Effects of desipramine on irritable bowel syndrome compared with atropine and placebo. *Dig Dis Sci.* 1987;32:257–266.
16. Guthrie E, Creed F, Dawson D, Tomenson B. A controlled trial of psychological treatment for the irritable bowel syndrome. *Gastroenterology.* 1991;100:450–457.
17. Harvey RF, Hinton RA, Gunary RM, Barry RE. Individual and group hypnotherapy in treatment of refractory irritable bowel syndrome. *Lancet.* 1989;i:424–425.
18. Harvey RF, Mauad EC, Brown AM. Prognosis in the irritable bowel syndrome: a 5-year prospective study. *Lancet.* 1987;i:963–965.
19. Heefner JD, Wilder RM, Wilson ID. Irritable colon and depression. *Psychosomatics.* 1978;19:540–547.
20. Hillman LC, Stace NH, Fisher A, Pomare EW. Dietary intakes and stool characteristics of patients with the irritable bowel syndrome. *Am J Clin Nutr.* 1982;36:626–629.
21. Holmes M, Salter RH. Irritable bowel syndrome: a safe diagnosis? *Br Med J.* 1982;285:1533–1534.
22. Jones VA, McLaughlan P, Shorthouse M, Workman E, Hunter JO. Food intolerance: a major factor in the pathogenesis of irritable bowel syndrome. *Lancet.* 1982;ii:1115–1117.

23. Keeling PWN, Fielding JR. The irritable bowel syndrome: a review of 50 consecutive cases. *J Ir Coll Phy Surg.* 1975;4:91–94.
24. Kellow JE, Phillips SF. Altered small bowel motility in irritable bowel syndrome is correlated with symptoms. *Gastroenterology.* 1987;92:1885–1893.
25. Kellow JE, Phillips SF, Miller LJ, Zinsmeister AR. Dysmotility of the small intestine in irritable bowel syndrome. *Gut.* 1988;29:1236–1243.
26. Kellow JE, Gill RC, Wingate DL. Prolonged ambulant recordings of small bowel motility demonstrate abnormalities in the irritable bowel syndrome. *Gastroenterology.* 1990;98:1208–1218.
27. Kellow JE, Eckersley GM, Jones MP. Enhanced perception of physiological intestinal motility in the irritable bowel syndrome. *Gastroenterology.* 1991;101:1621–1627.
28. Kullman G, Fielding JF. Rectal distensibility in the irritable bowel syndrome. *Ir Med J.* 1981;74:140–142.
29. Lancaster-Smith MJ, Prout BM, Pinto T, Anderson JA, Schiff AA. Influence of drug treatment on the irritable bowel syndrome and its interaction with psychoneurotic morbidity. *Acta Psychiatr Scand.* 1982;66:33–41.
30. Lasser RB, Bond JH, Levitt MD. The role of intestinal gas in functional abdominal pain. *N Engl J Med.* 1975;293:524–526.
31. Latimer P, Sarna S, Campbell D, Latimer M, Waterfall W, Daniel EE. Colonic motor and myoelectric activity: a comparative study of normal subjects, psychoneurotic patients, and patients with irritable bowel syndrome. *Gastroenterology.* 1981;80:893–901.
32. Lavo B, Stenstam M, Nielsen AL. Loperamide in treatment of irritable bowel syndrome: a double-blind placebo controlled study. *Scand J Gastroenterol (Suppl).* 1987;130:77–80.
33. Lemann M, Dederding JP, Flourie B, Franchisseur C, Rambaud JC, Jian R. Abnormal perception of visceral pain in response to gastric distension in chronic idiopathic dyspepsia: the irritable stomach syndrome. *Dig Dis Sci.* 1991;36:1249–1254.
34. Lowman BC, Drossman DA, Cramer EM, McKee DC. Recollection of childhood events in adults with irritable bowel syndrome. *J Clin Gastroenterol.* 1987;9:324–330.
35. Lynch PM, Zamble E. A controlled behavioral treatment study of irritable bowel syndrome. *Behav Res Therapy.* 1989;20:509–523.
36. Magni G, di Mario F, Bernasconi G, Mastropaolo G. DSM-III diagnoses associated with dyspepsia of unknown cause. *Am J Psychiatry.* 1987;144:1222–1223.
37. Maxton DG, Martin DF, Whorwell PJ, Godfrey M. Abdominal distension in female patients with irritable bowel syndrome: exploration of possible mechanisms. *Gut.* 1991;32:662–664.
38. Mitchell CM, Drossman DA. Survey of the AGA membership relating to patients with functional gastrointestinal disorders. *Gastroenterology.* 1987;92:1282–1284.
39. Myren J, Lovland B, Larssen SE, et al. A double-blind study of the effect of trimipramine in patients with the irritable bowel syndrome. *Scand J Gastroenterol.* 1984;19:835–843.
40. Nanda R, James R, Smith H, Dudley CRK, Jewell DP. Food intolerance and the irritable bowel syndrome. *Gut.* 1989;30:1099–1104.
41. Neff DF, Blanchard EB. A multi-component treatment for irritable bowel syndrome. *Behav Res Therapy.* 1987;18:70–83.
42. Page JG, Dirnberger GM. Treatment of the irritable bowel syndrome with Bentyl (dicyclomine hydrochloride). *J Clin Gastroenterol.* 1981;3:153–156.
43. *Physicians' Desk Reference, 47th Edition.* Montvale, NJ: Medical Economics Co Inc; 1993:1363–1364.
44. Prior A, Maxton DG, Whorwell PJ. Anorectal manometry in irritable bowel syndrome: differences between diarrhoea and constipation predominant subjects. *Gut.* 1990;31:458–462.
45. Ritchie J. Pain from distention of the pelvic colon by inflating a balloon in the irritable colon syndrome. *Gut.* 1973;14:125–132.
46. Ritchie JA, Truelove SC. Comparison of various treatments for irritable bowel syndrome. *Br Med J.* 1980;281:1317–1319.
47. Sandler RS. Epidemiology of irritable bowel syndrome in the United States. *Gastroenterology.* 1990;99:409–415.
48. Sandler RS, Drossman DA, Nathan HP, McKee DC. Symptom complaints and health care seeking behavior in subjects with bowel dysfunction. *Gastroenterology.* 1984;87:314–318.
49. Sarna SK. Physiology and pathophysiology of colonic motor activity: part two of two. *Dig Dis Sci.* 1991;36:998–1018.
50. Schwarz SP, Blanchard EB, Neff DB. Behavioral treatment of irritable bowel syndrome: a 1-year follow-up study. *Biofeedback Self Regul.* 1986;11:189–190.
51. Smart HL, Mayberry JF, Atkinson M. Alternative medicine consultations and remedies in patients with the irritable bowel syndrome. *Gut.* 1986;27:826–828.
52. Steinhart MJ, Wong PY, Zarr ML. Therapeutic usefulness of amitriptyline in spastic colon syndrome. *Int J Psychiatry Med.* 1981/82;11:45–57.
53. Svedlund J, Sjodin I, Ottosson JO, Dotevall G. Controlled study of psychotherapy in irritable bowel syndrome. *Lancet.* 1983;ii:589–592.
54. Svendsen JH, Munck LK, Andersen JR. Irritable bowel syndrome: prognosis and diagnostic safety: a 5-year follow-up study. *Scand J Gastroenterol.* 1985;20:415–418.
55. Talley NJ, Fung LH, Gilligan IJ, McNeil D, Piper DW. Association of anxiety, neuroticism, and depression with dyspepsia of unknown cause: a case-control study. *Gastroenterology.* 1986;90:886–892.
56. Talley NJ, Colin-Jones D, Koch KL, Koch M, Nyren O, Stanghellini V. Functional dyspepsia: a classification with guidelines for diagnosis and management. *Gastroenterology International.* 1991;4:145–160.
57. Thompson WG, Creed F, Drossman DA, Heaton KW, Mazzacca G. Functional bowel disease and functional abdominal pain. *Gastroenterology International.* 1992;5:75–91.
58. Whitehead WE, Bosmajian L, Zonderman A, Costa P, Schuster MM. Symptoms of psychologic distress associated with irritable bowel syndrome: a comparison of community and medical clinic samples. *Gastroenterology.* 1988;95:709–714.
59. Whitehead WE, Engel BT, Schuster MM. Irritable bowel syndrome: physiological and psychological differences between diarrhea-predominant and constipation-predominant patients. *Dig Dis Sci.* 1980;25:404–413.
60. Whitehead WE, Enck P, Anthony JC, Schuster MM. Psychopathology in patients with irritable bowel syndrome. In: Singer MV, Goebell H, eds. *Nerves and the Gastrointestinal Tract (Falk Symposium 50).* Boston Mass: MTP Press, 1989:465–476.
61. Whitehead WE, Cheskin LJ, Heller BR, et al. Evidence for exacerbation of irritable bowel syndrome during menses. *Gastroenterology.* 1990;98:1485–1489.
62. Whitehead WE, Holtkotter B, Enck P, et al. Tolerance for rectosigmoid distention in irritable bowel syndrome. *Gastroenterology.* 1990;98:1187–1192.

63. Whitehead WE, Crowell MD, Robinson JC, Heller BR, Schuster MM. Effects of stressful life events on bowel symptoms: subjects with irritable bowel syndrome compared with subjects without bowel dysfunction. *Gut.* 1992;33:825–830.
64. Whitehead WE, Devroede G, Habib FI, Meunier P, Wald A. Functional disorders of the anorectum. *Gastroenterology International.* 1992;5:92–108.
65. Whorwell PJ. Hypnotherapy in irritable bowel syndrome. *Lancet.* 1989;i:622.
66. Whorwell PJ, Prior A, Faragher EB. Controlled trial of hypnotherapy in the treatment of severe refractory irritable-bowel syndrome. *Lancet.* 1984;ii:1232–1234.
67. Whorwell PJ, Prior A, Colgan SM. Hypnotherapy in severe irritable bowel syndrome: further experience. *Gut.* 1987;28:423–425.

11

Intestinal Gas and Abdominal Bloating

MICHAEL LEVINSON

The irritable bowel syndrome (IBS) refers to a well-recognized symptom complex arising from the interactions among the digestive tract, the psyche, and the luminal factors (Fig. 11–1). One of the classic symptoms of IBS[1] is abdominal distension, which the patient usually attributes to excessive bowel gas. The first thing to do is to have the patient clarify what he means by a gas problem. Is the patient referring to belching, bloating, and distension or the excessive passage of flatus? In this chapter, we will only deal with the pathophysiology and treatment of bloating and gas. The approach to the average patient with these complaints remains predominantly based on clinical appraisal, a tentative diagnosis, exclusion of organic disease, and a therapeutic trial that partly confirms the diagnosis.[2] However, some patients have intractable symptoms and require further evaluation. In these cases, the predominant unresolved symptom in this chapter, gas and distension, provides the focal point for a second tier of evaluations and therapeutic trials.[3] This second tier of tests should confirm the presence and assess the severity of the disorder of digestive function and provide the basis for therapeutic trials to correct that abnormal function. Thus, an understanding of the pathophysiologic mechanisms resulting in the patient's symptoms is paramount to optimize therapy.

BLOATING AND DISTENSION

By far, the most common gaseous complaint is bloating and distension, which the patient attributes to excessive bowel gas. The classic study is by Lasser, Bond, and Levitt[4] using rapid perfusion of the gut with argon and measuring the gas washed out at the rectum. The study showed that patients with bloating had the same volume of bowel gas as did normal controls, about 200 ml. This observation is supported by x-ray examination, which seldom shows excessive intestinal gas in patients who complain of bloating. However, patients with bloating had much more discomfort during argon infusion than did the controls. Many of these patients developed such severe pain that the gas infusion had to be discontinued. There also was a tendency for more of the infused argon to reflux back into the stomach of patients with bloating as compared with controls. Thus, the basic problem of bloating and distension has nothing to do with excessive bowel gas; rather, these subjects are suffering from an irritable small bowel. The intestine in these subjects does not seem to propel gas (or liquids) in a well-coordinated fashion[5,6] and, as a result, the patient senses that the gut is overdistended and perceives pain not felt in healthy controls.[7] Psychologic factors including acute stress[8] and overt psychiatric disease, i.e., depres-

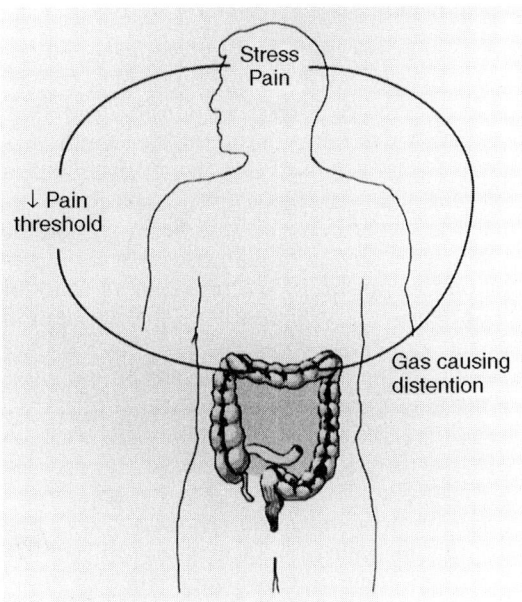

FIGURE 11–1. Interactions among digestive tract, the psyche, and luminal factors give rise to irritable bowel syndrome complex.

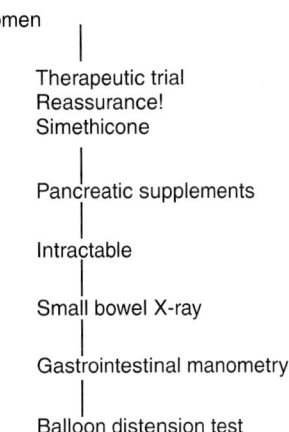

FIGURE 11–2. Management of patient with bloating.

sion,[9] significantly alter gastrointestinal motor dysfunction. Alvarez noted over 50 years ago that the psyche is a major player that interacts with other putative mechanisms in IBS.[10] The latest problem associated with IBS is physical and sexual abuse leading to psychologic distress,[10] and when the confidence of the patient has been obtained it must be asked about.

The evaluation required for the patient with bloating and distension is dependent on a number of factors, including age, sex, and the duration of the problem (Fig. 11–2). Organic disease of the gut, particularly carcinoma of the colon and Crohn's disease, can present with bloating and distension. Thus, colon cancer must be ruled out in patients over 40 years of age, particularly when there is a short history and a positive family history of polyps or colon cancer. In younger patients, Crohn's disease must be ruled out. The presence of unexplained weight loss, nocturnal pain, blood in the stool, or diarrhea (especially nocturnal and associated with weight loss) must also be evaluated. A plain film of the abdomen is extremely helpful. If a normal gas pattern is seen, it helps explain the symptoms to the patient. On the other hand, if a lot of gas is seen or an abnormal pattern, an early obstruction, Crohn's disease, or intestinal pseudo-obstruction may be found.

TREATMENT

Unfortunately, there is no proven effective therapy.[11] The most important part of the therapy is reassurance to the patient that this abdominal distress is not life threatening. The patient also must be relieved of his or her cancer phobia. Each patient is treated individually, but with the preliminary studies ordered above, the patient can be reassured. The next step is to explain the problem to the patient. The disordered motility and the gut's misperception of these events leads to "gaslike" feelings and distension. In many patients seen for the first time, this reassurance and explanation may be highly effective. However, in patients seen by many different physicians, especially if gastroenterologists, it will not be enough. It is also unlikely that any therapy will be dramatically effective in this subgroup of patients. These patients may be considered intractable and require the next tier of studies,[3] gastrointestinal manometry[12] and balloon distension test.[13]

After reassurance and explanation, a careful

dietary history should be obtained looking for lactose or fructose intolerance, wheat intolerance, and the excessive use of weight reduction diets using sorbitol-based sweeteners. Hence, a diet eliminating these foodstuffs should be tried. Increasing fiber in these patients would only aggravate the condition because fiber increases gas production in the colon, especially in these patients, making the problem worse. There are few controlled trials of drugs in patients with bloating. Anticholinergics show little benefit and actually increase bloating and distension. Simethicone and pancreatic supplements are ineffective, but safe, and may play a harmless placebo role as the physician is developing a good physician-patient relationship. Because of the abnormal motility, metoclopramide may be of benefit, as demonstrated in one small study of this syndrome.[14] The bottom line in the bloated, distended patient is the initial visit and the physician's reassurance and concern for the patient, which is the most effective form of therapy in the majority of patients.

FLATUS

A surprisingly difficult problem in flatulent patients is the determination as to whether the patient truly is abnormal or merely perceives himself as abnormal with regard to the flatus passage. Sutalf and Levitt[15] found that healthy 25- to 35-year-old men passed gas about 14 ± 4.5 (LSD) times per day. The upper limit of normal is 23 gas passages a day. A simple method is to have the patient record each passage of gas, a flatulent gram. An abnormal pattern of flatulence usually leads to some abnormality. Levitt[16] believes that frequency in most instances equals volume of gas passed.

PHYSIOLOGY AND PATHOPHYSIOLOGY

The volume, composition, and frequency of flatus are determined by several variables, including age, heredity, stress, antibiotics, and diet. The quantity of flatus produced by normal individuals eating a typical diet ranges from 400 to 1600 ml/d (14 flatus passes).[16] Composition varies markedly because of age, heredity, colonic fermentation, and air swallowing. Methane production has not been detected before 2 years of age. After age 2 years, 30% of the population that has methane-producing bacteria will have methane in the gas. Five simple odorless gases are the major components of flatus (Fig. 11–3). The odor associated with flatus is imparted by skatole, hydrogen sulfide, indole, volatile amines, and short-chain fatty acids. Substances are detectable by smell in concentrations as low as one part per 100 million.[17] Diet clearly affects gas production. In a study by Steggerdan,[18] five normal men were fed a diet in which 56% of the calories were derived from beans. The mean flatus excretion rate in these subjects increased from 15 to 176 ml/h. Fermentation of indigestible polysaccharides by colonic bacteria resulted in dramatic increases in hydrogen production and flatus passage. In beans, raffinose and stachyose have been implicated as the major oligosaccharides that provide substrate for colonic bacteria.

Air swallowing can be a major source of gastrointestinal gas. Eating, stress, ill-fitting dentures, cigarette smoking, and gum chewing are all associated with increased air swallowing, up to 70% in one study.[19] Postprandial bloating secondary to air swallowing is exacerbated by fat ingestion, which is known to delay gastric emptying.[20]

Compared with colonic fermentation and air swallowing, diffusion of gas from the tissues and bloodstream to the bowel is a relatively minor

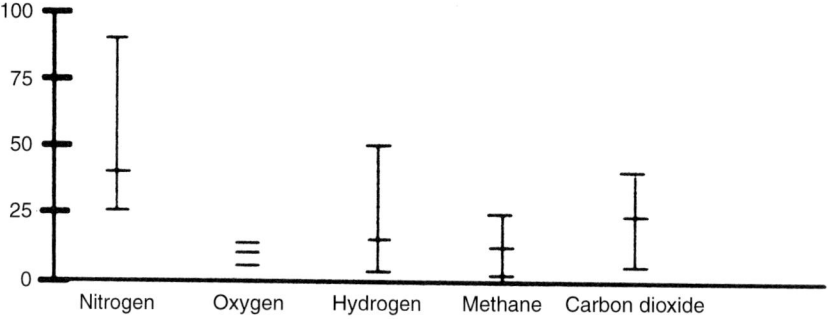

FIGURE 11–3. Composition of intestinal gas.

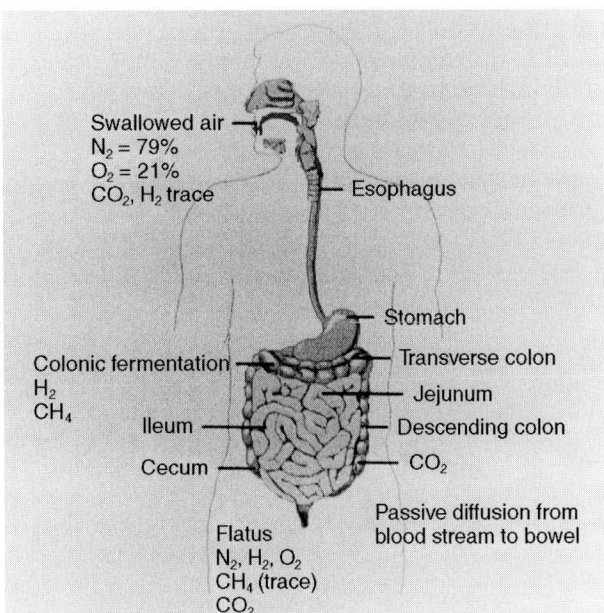

FIGURE 11–4. Sources of gastrointestinal gas: swallowed air, colonic fermentation, and passive diffusion from bloodstream to bowel.

contributor to flatus volume unless the patient is a mountain climber or an astronaut (Fig. 11–4).

TREATMENT

If the patient is passing gas only 14 times a day, or especially if less than 23 times a day, the patient should be reassured that he or she is normal. For those who are truly passing excess flatus, first the diet should be manipulated with a sorbitol-, lactose-, and legume-free diet for several weeks and a record of flatus kept. Avoidance of chewing gum, cigarette smoking, and carbonated beverages should also be stressed. If the patient does not respond at this early stage, he will usually not respond to therapy.[11] At this time, especially if the patient has lived in or traveled to an endemic area for *Giardia*, evaluating for the presence of *Giardia* is indicated. Evaluation for malabsorption and maldigestion should proceed, and if findings are negative, the physician may proceed with therapeutic drug trials (Fig. 11–5). Simethicone is harmless and is worth a trial, but it has not been control effective[21]; it appears to turn little gas bubbles to big gas bubbles. Activated charcoal has been tried with varying success.[21,22] In patients who have responded well to it, charcoal may absorb gas, absorb fermentable products, and inhibit gas-forming bacteria. However, activated charcoal will effectively reduce flatus and odor and is

Careful history and physical examination
|
Limited screening tests but include stools for ova and parasites, especially Giardia
|
Have patients keep record of how many times and when they pass gas "flatulentgram"
|
No excessive gas, reassure
|
Dietary history especially for carbohydrate intolerance: beans, fatty food intolerance (malabsorption)
|
Elimination diet: avoid chewing gum, cigarette smoking, and carbonated beverages
|
Intractable
|
Evaluate for malabsorption and maldigestion if negative
|
Simethicone
|
No response, prescribe activated charcoal (especially good for foul-smelling gas)

FIGURE 11–5. Management of the flatulent patient.

worth a trial in that regard. An innovative approach to the problem of gas production is the introduction of oral microbial a-galactosidases in an effort to produce in vivo assisted digestion of oligosaccharidases. The agent is "beanase" enzyme and is marketed as *Beano.* A few drops of beanase mixed with mashed black beans reduces breath hydrogen production in a dose-related fashion when compared with a placebo. A progressive reduction in flatulence was demonstrated, but bloating and fullness were not ameliorated.[23] The evaluation and treatment of a flatulent, bloated, distended patient remains a challenge. Most patients will do well with tender loving care, but that small minority of patients, the intractable patients, will cause the physician many sleepless nights.

REFERENCES

1. Manning AP, Thompson WG, Heaton KW, Morris AF. Towards a positive diagnosis of the irritable bowel. *Br Med J.* 1978;2:653–654.
2. Thompason WG, Dotevall G, Drossman DA, Heaton KW, Kraus W. Irritable bowel syndrome: guidelines for the diagnosis. *Gastroenterol International.* 1989;2:92–95.
3. Camilleri M, Prather C. The irritable bowel syndrome: mechanisms and a practical approach to management. *Ann Intern Med.* 1992;116:1001–1008.
4. Lasser RB, Bond JH, Levitt MD. The role of intestinal gas in functional abdominal pain. *N Engl J Med.* 1975;293:524–526.
5. Horrovitz L, Farrar JT. Intraluminal small intestinal pressure in normal patients and in patients with functional gastrointestinal disorders. *Gastroenterology.* 1962;42:455–464.
6. Kellow JE, Phillips SF. Altered small bowel motility in irritable bowel syndrome is correlated with symptoms. *Gastroenterology.* 1987;92:1885–1893.
7. Mayer EA, Raybould HE. Role of visceral afferent mechanisms in functional bowel disorders. *Gastroenterology.* 1990;99:688–704.
8. Almy TP, Tulin M. Alterations in man under stress: experimental production of changes stimulating the irritable colon. *Gastroenterology.* 1947;8:616–626.
9. Tally NJ, Camilleri M, Orkin BA, Kramlinger KG. Effect of cyclical unipolar depression on upper gastrointestinal motility and sleep. *Gastroenterology.* 1989:775–777.
10. Drossman DA, Leserman J, et al. Sexual and physical abuse in women with functional or organic gastrointestinal disorders. *Ann Intern Med.* 1990;113:828–833.
11. Klein KB. Controlled treatment trials in irritable bowel syndrome: a critique. *Gastroenterology.* 1988;84:26–29.
12. Malagelada JR, Camilleri M, Stanghellini V. *Manometric Diagnosis of Gastrointestinal Motility Disorders.* New York, NY: Thieme Medical Publishers Inc; 1986.
13. Swarbrick ET, Hegarty JE, Batt L, Williams CB, Dawson AM. Site of pain from the irritable bowel. *Lancet.* 1980;2:443–446.
14. Johnson AG. Controlled trial of metoclopramide in the treatment of flatulent dyspepsia. *Br Med J.* 1971;2:25–26.
15. Sutalf LO, Levitt MD. Follow up of the flatulent patient. *Dig Dis Sci.* 1979;24:652–654.
16. Levitt MD. Volume and composition of human intestinal gas determined by means of an intestinal washout technique. *N Engl J Med.* 1971;284:1394.
17. Levitt MD, Bond JH Jr. Volume composition and source of intestinal gas. *Gastroenterology.* 1970;59:921–929.
18. Steggerda FR. Gastrointestinal gas following food consumption. *Ann NY Acad Sci.* 1960:150–157.
19. Rider JA, Moeller HC. Use of silicone in the treatment of intestinal gas and bloating. *JAMA.* 1960;174:2052–2054.
20. Polish E, Kadish U. Influence of food composition on the retention of gas in the stomach. *Ann NY Acad Sci.* 1968;150:67–74.
21. Jain NK, Patel VP, Pitchumoni CS. Activated charcoal, simethicone, and intestinal gas: double blind study. *Ann Intern Med.* 1986;105:61–62.
22. Hall GH Jr, Thompson H, Strother A. Effects of orally administered activated charcoal on intestinal gas. *Ann J Gastroenterol.* 1981;75:192–196.
23. Friedman G. Treatment of irritable bowel syndrome. *Gastroenterol Clin North Am.* 1991;20:330.
24. Danholf IE. Clinical gas syndromes: a pathophysiologic approach. *Ann NY Acad Sci.* 1968;150:127–140.

12
Malabsorption Syndromes

MARK UHL and ALLAN R. COOKE

Malabsorption means failure to absorb one or more dietary constituents, often because of a defect in the mucosa of the small intestine, e.g., celiac disease, lactase deficiency. Malabsorption should be distinguished from maldigestion, which results from abnormal luminal events, e.g., deficiency of pancreatic enzymes, bile salts, etc. Commonly, the result of malabsorption or maldigestion is diarrhea with increased fat in the stool, which is foul smelling and porridgelike in appearance; i.e., the patient has steatorrhea. On further study, these patients usually have malabsorption of other nutrients as well. The term *malabsorption syndrome,* for convenience, will be used to denote malabsorption as well as maldigestion.

The absorption of most nutrients in the gastrointestinal tract is fairly site specific. Iron and calcium are mainly absorbed in the duodenum, whereas folate absorption occurs in the jejunum. Vitamin B_{12} and bile salts are actively absorbed in the terminal ileum. Water and electrolytes are absorbed throughout the small and large intestine, so that disease in any segment may lead to electrolyte abnormalities or dehydration.

CLINICAL PRESENTATION

Common symptoms of the malabsorption syndrome include diarrhea, weight loss, flatulence, and bloating. Generally, the physical examination will reveal nonspecific signs, such as generalized wasting and loss of muscle mass. Table 12–1 illustrates the common manifestations and pathophysiology of nutrient deficiencies in the malabsorption syndrome.

The initial laboratory investigation should include a complete blood count with a mean corpuscular volume. Even in a nonanemic patient, serum iron, ferritin, vitamin B_{12}, and folate levels should be obtained, as deficiencies in these substances may not be sufficient enough to cause anemia. As a result of the large storage capacity for vitamin B_{12} by the liver, a cobalamin deficiency may be a late finding in malabsorption. A routine chemistry profile should be obtained, with special attention to the electrolytes and evidence of chronic liver dysfunction. Assessment of levels of fat-soluble vitamins can be made either directly or indirectly. An elevated prothrombin time indicates a vitamin K deficiency, either from malabsorption or liver disease. Carotene is a vitamin A precursor obtained only through the diet. Vitamin D levels are indirectly reflected by the serum calcium.

GENERAL REMARKS

Normal stool weights are 200 to 300 g/d (about 200 to 300 ml). The diarrhea of malabsorption is osmotic, and generally, volume is less than 1 L/d (small volume) and is reduced by fasting. These values distinguish it from secretory diarrhea, which has a larger volume (greater than 1 L/d) and does not respond to fasting.

The hallmark of malabsorption is steatorrhea with diarrhea, but approximately 10% of patients may have isolated steatorrhea without diarrhea. Steatorrhea is defined as greater than 6 g/d of fat in the stool in subjects taking at least 100 g/d of fat in their diet. The initial screening test is a qualitative examination of the stool for undigested meat fibers and neutral fats. The presence of muscle fibers tends to favor pancreatic insufficiency. A properly performed Sudan III stain for neutral fat is 80% to 90% sensitive in detecting *significant* steatorrhea. However, a negative test does not exclude steatorrhea, and a full 72-hour stool collection should be undertaken. This is considered the "gold standard" for detecting steatorrhea. Fecal fat concentration >9.5% strongly suggests pancreatic insufficiency.

TABLE 12–1. PATHOPHYSIOLOGIC BASIS FOR SYMPTOMS AND SIGNS IN MALABSORPTIVE DISORDERS

Organ System	Symptom or Sign	Pathophysiology
Gastrointestinal	Generalized malnutrition and weight loss	Malabsorption of fat, carbohydrate and protein leads to loss of calories
	Diarrhea	Impaired absorption or increased secretion of water and electrolytes; unabsorbed dihydroxy bile acids and fatty acids lead to decreased absorption of water and electrolytes; excess load of fluid and electrolytes presented to the colon may exceed its absorptive capacity
	Flatus	Bacterial fermentation of unabsorbed carbohydrate
	Glossitis, cheilosis, stomatitis	Deficiency of iron, vitamin B_{12}, folate, and other vitamins
Genitourinary	Nocturia	Delayed absorption of water, hypokalemia
	Azotemia, hypotension	Fluid and electrolyte depletion
	Amenorrhea, decreased libido	Protein depletion and "caloric starvation" lead to secondary hypopituitarism
Hematopoietic	Anemia	Impaired absorption of iron, vitamin B_{12}, and folic acid
	Hemorrhagic phenomena	Vitamin K malabsorption leads to hypoprothrombinemia
Musculoskeletal	Bone pain	Protein depletion leads to impaired bone formation, which leads to osteoporosis
		Calcium malabsorption leads to demineralization of bone, which leads to osteomalacia
	Osteoarthropathy	Cause uncertain
	Tetany, paresthesias	Calcium malabsorption leads to hypocalcemia; magnesium malabsorption leads to hypomagnesemia
	Weakness	Anemia; electrolyte depletion (hypokalemia)
Nervous system	Night blindness	Impaired absorption of vitamin A leads to vitamin A deficiency
	Xerophthalmia	Vitamin A deficiency
	Peripheral neuropathy	Vitamin B_{12}, thiamine deficiency
Skin	Eczema	Cause uncertain
	Purpura	Vitamin K deficiency
	Follicular hyperkeratosis and dermatitis	Deficiency of vitamin A, zinc, essential fatty acids, and other vitamins

Adapted from Greenberger NJ, Isselbacher KJ: Disorders of absorption. In: *Harrison's Principles of Internal Medicine.* 12th ed., New York, NY: McGraw-Hill Book Co; 1991:1059.

Before embarking on an extensive workup of patients with malabsorption syndrome, a general review of the causes is appropriate because the workup can be targeted more specifically. Four organs are responsible for causing the malabsorption syndrome. These are the stomach, liver, pancreas, and small intestine (Table 12–2).

SPECIFIC ORGAN SYSTEMS

The following is an outline for evaluating each organ system involved in the malabsorption syndrome. Specific tests for evaluating both structure and function are discussed. Tests to distinguish maldigestion from malabsorption are given in Table 12–3.

STOMACH

Gastric surgical operations, particularly gastrectomy, result in maldigestion because of rapid emptying of large food particles, dilution of pancreatic enzymes and bile salts, poor mixing, and rapid small bowel transit. Zollinger-Ellison syndrome (gastrinoma) causes steatorrhea by the large amounts of acid inactivating pancreatic enzymes, by damage to jejunal mucosa, and by gastrin inhibiting electrolyte transport.

STRUCTURE. Structure is ascertained by the type of operation, upper endoscopy and barium studies.

FUNCTION. Rapid emptying is confirmed by a radionuclide-labeled meal (gastric emptying time).

LIVER

Hepatobiliary disease causes steatorrhoea by failure to excrete bile salts or, in rare circumstances, failure to make bile salts. The common diseases of the liver causing malabsorption are primary biliary cirrhosis (PBC) or sclerosing cholangitis (primary or secondary).

TABLE 12-2. SITE SPECIFIC CAUSES FOR MALABSORPTION

Stomach
1. Postgastrectomy causes (Billroth I and II)
2. Pyloroplasty
3. Zollinger-Ellison syndrome
4. Achlorhydria

Liver: Chronic Bile Salt Deficiency
1. Primary biliary cirrhosis and primary sclerosing cholangitis
2. Depleted bile salt pool as a result of ileal disease or resection
3. Unconjugated bile salts as a result of bacterial overgrowth

Pancreas: Pancreatic Exocrine Insufficiency
1. Chronic pancreatitis
   a. Alcoholic
   b. Hereditary
   c. Trauma
   d. Idiopathic
2. Cystic fibrosis
3. Neoplasm
4. Severe protein and caloric deprivation (Kwashiorkor)
5. Postsurgical causes: Whipple procedure, pancreatectomy
6. Hemochromatosis
7. Others: trypsinogen deficiency, enterokinase deficiency, Shwachman's syndrome

Small Bowel Disease
1. Celiac disease
2. Crohn's disease
3. Whipple's disease
4. Lactase deficiency
5. Eosinophilic gastroenteritis
6. Tropical sprue
7. Short bowel syndrome
8. Bacterial overgrowth
9. AIDS
10. Lymphangiectasia
11. Abetalipoproteinemia
12. Radiation enteritis
13. Diabetes mellitus
14. Ischemia
15. Motility disorders
16. Infectious causes
17. Lymphoma

TABLE 12-3. EVALUATION OF MALABSORPTION

Test	Maldigestion	Malabsorption
Stool fat (qualitative, quantitative)	Increased	Increased
D-Xylose	Normal, except bacterial overgrowth	Abnormal
Secretin and CCK test	Abnormal in chronic pancreatic disease	Normal
Peroral biopsy	Normal	Often abnormal
Breath H_2 (after 50 g lactose)	Normal	Abnormal
Lactulose breath test	Early H_2 peak in bacterial overgrowth	Normal
Schilling test (vitamin B_{12} absorption)	Abnormal in bacterial overgrowth and pancreatic insufficiency	Abnormal in extensive ileal disease
Small bowel x-ray examination	Pancreatic Ca^{2+}; otherwise normal	May show mucosal disease
ERCP	May show pancreatic or hepatobiliary disease	Normal
Serum iron	Normal	Often abnormal
Serum albumin	Normal	Often abnormal
Serum folate	Normal	Often abnormal
Serum calcium	Usually normal	Often abnormal
Serum carotene	Usually normal	Often abnormal
Prothrombin time	Usually normal	Often abnormal

CCK = cholecystokinin, ERCP = endoscopic retrograde cholangiopancreatography.

STRUCTURE. The anatomy of the bile ducts is determined by sonography, computed axial tomography (CAT) scan, endoscopic retrograde cholangiopancreatography (ERCP), and liver biopsy.

FUNCTION. Function is determined by liver function tests, antimitochondrial antibody assay, and studies of bile salt production and turnover. This latter study is rarely needed.

PANCREAS

STRUCTURE. An upright plain x-ray of the abdomen is often obtained in a patient with suspected malabsorption syndrome to rule out pancreatic calcification, but this is rarely helpful in early disease. Ultrasonography is useful to rule out anatomic abnormalities in the pancreas or biliary system. A computed tomography (CT) scan of the abdomen may also demonstrate pancreatic calcification or mass lesions. The most sensitive test for chronic pancreatitis is ERCP, which outlines pancreatic ductal structure and evaluates mass lesions.

FUNCTION. Pancreatic exocrine function can be assessed in a number of ways. The most sensitive test is the secretin stimulation test sometimes combined with cholecystokinin. This test involves intubating the small intestine and administering intravenous secretin (1 U/kg). The duodenal aspirate should normally contain >1.8 ml/kg/h with a bicarbonate concentration of >80 mEq/L. Pancreatic insufficiency is diagnosed when volumes are low and bicarbonate concentration is <60 mEq/L. The disadvantage of this test is the need for intubation.

A less sensitive screening method to assess pancreatic exocrine function is the bentiromide (Chymex) test. In this test, patients ingest 500 mg of N-benzoyl-L-tyrosyl-*p*-aminobenzoic acid (BZ-ty-PABA). The compound is cleaved intraluminally by chymotrypsin, and the PABA is then absorbed and excreted in the urine. A 6-hour urine specimen should contain greater than 50% of the dose. Sensitivity of the Chymex test ranges from 60% to 90%. Remember in all tests using oral ingestion and urine collections to check the "be sures". "Be sure" the patient took the dose and did not vomit after ingestion; that gastric emptying is normal; that renal function is normal, and that urine collection is complete. The D-xylose test (see below) is used in conjunction with the bentiromide test to ensure that absorption is intact.

SMALL INTESTINE

STRUCTURE. Radiographic and endoscopic studies are used to evaluate small bowel structural abnormalities. A small bowel enteroclysis may reveal mucosal abnormalities, wall edema, strictures, fistulas, blind loops, or diverticula. Enteroclysis is preferred to an upper gastrointestinal series (UGI) with small bowel follow through. Routine upper endoscopy or enteroscopy allows direct visualization and biopsy of the intestinal mucosa. Endoscopy has mostly replaced the Rubin tube for obtaining biopsies. Small bowel biopsy results are often diagnostic and specific but can miss a patchy lesion. The usefulness of a biopsy is summarized in Table 12–4.

FUNCTION. Mucosal function is assessed by the D-xylose absorption test. After an oral dose of 25 g, the compound is measured in a 5-hour urine specimen or a 1-hour serum specimen. Urine levels less than 4.5 g or 1-hour serum levels less than 30 mg/dl indicate malabsorption, secondary to a mucosal defect. False positives may result from incomplete urine collection, renal failure, ascites, or bacterial overgrowth.

The Schilling test for vitamin B_{12} absorption may be abnormal with a diseased or resected terminal ileum.

An unusual but important cause of malabsorption is bacterial overgrowth. Definitive diagnosis is made by small bowel culture, but the diagnosis is likely (even without a positive culture) if the patient's condition improves with a course of broad spectrum antibiotics.

Various breath tests are also employed in delineating the cause of malabsorption. Lactose malabsorption is tested with the lactose breath test. Since undigested carbohydrates are the source of hydrogen and carbon dioxide production by colonic bacteria, a rise in either of these gases after lactose ingestion indicates malabsorption. After an overnight fast, a baseline sample of expelled air is obtained. Lactose (2 g/kg in a 20% solution) is then given orally. Breath samples are then taken every 30 minutes for 3 hours. A rise of 10 ppm hydrogen is considered abnormal. Similarly, bacteria in the upper intestine may hydrolyze lactulose and give an early H_2 peak in the lactulose breath test.

MANAGEMENT OF MALABSORPTION SYNDROME

NUTRIENT REPLACEMENT

The first step in the management of patients with steatorrhea is a low-fat diet. Reduced fat intake generally will reduce steatorrhea of any origin. Increased calories should be given as complex carbohydrates, as these have less osmotic effect in the bowel lumen. Vitamins and minerals are replaced individually or with multivitamin preparations. Typical doses are shown in Table 12–5. Patients with severe steatorrhea may require fat replacement with short- and medium-chain triglycerides; these are 6- to 12-carbon fatty acids, which do not require bile salts for absorption, are absorbed directly into the portal system (ver-

TABLE 12-4. DIAGNOSTIC RELIABILITY OF PERORAL SMALL INTESTINAL BIOPSY RESULTS

Diagnostic Histologic Findings; Diffuse Lesions; Should Be Present in Endoscopic Biopsy Specimens

Whipple's disease	PAS-positive lamina propria macrophages
Mycobacterium avium-intracellular	Acid-fast lamina propria macrophages
Abetalipoproteinemia	Vacuolated, lipid-laden enterocytes with normal architecture
Agammaglobulinemia	Spruelike histology with *Giardia*

Abnormal, but Not Diagnostic, Histologic Findings; Diffuse Lesions; Should Be Present in Endoscopic Biopsy Specimens

Celiac, refractory, and tropical sprue	Varying degrees of villus atrophy and crypt hyperplasia with lamina propria inflammation
Viral enteritis	Same as mild-moderate sprue
Bacterial overgrowth	Same as mild-moderate sprue
Severe, prolonged folate and vitamin B_{12} deficiency	Same as sprue, reduced mitoses in crypts

Diagnostic Histologic Findings; Patchy Distribution; Therefore May Be Missed in Endoscopic Biopsy Specimens

Lymphoma	Villi widened and lamina propria filled with malignant lymphoma cells
Lymphangiectasia	Dilated lymphatics in lamina propria and submucosa
Eosinophilic enteritis	Lamina propria infiltrated with eosinophils and neutrophils; mucosa normal to flat
Mastocytosis	Lamina propria infiltrated with mast cells, eosinophils and neutrophils; mucosa normal to flat
Amyloidosis	Amyloid in lamina propria and submucosa with Congo red stain; normal mucosa and architecture
Crohn's disease	Varying inflammation and ulceration with subepithelial granulomas
Giardiasis, Coccodia, strongyloidiasis	Mucosa normal to flat with *Giardia*, *Cryptosporidium*, or *Strongyloides* on surfaces of villi or crypts; *Eimeria*, *Isospora*, or *Microsporidia* within enterocytes

Abnormal but Not Diagnostic Histologic Findings; Patchy Distribution; May Be Missed in Endoscopic Biopsy Specimens

Acute radiation enteritis, enteropathy of dermatitis herpetiformis	Spruelike lesion of varying severity

PAS = periodic acid-Schiff stain.
From Yamada T, ed. *Textbook of Gastroenterology.* Philadelphia, Pa: JB Lippincott; 1991. Modified from Trier JS. Intestinal malabsorption: differentiation of cause. *Hosp Pract.* 1988;23:195; Trier JS. Diagnostic value of peroral biopsy of the proximal small intestine. *N Engl J Med.* 1971;285:1470.

TABLE 12-5. DOSAGES OF COMMONLY USED NUTRIENT AND VITAMIN SUPPLEMENTS

NUTRIENT	ROUTE	DOSAGE
Calcium	PO	500–2500 mg elemental Ca^{2+}/d
Magnesium	PO	Magnesium oxide 400 mg t.i.d.
Iron	PO	Iron sulfate 325 mg t.i.d., between meals
Folate	PO	1 mg PO q.d.
Vitamin B_{12}	IM	1000 μg/d × 3 d, then 1000 μg q3mo
Zinc	PO	Zinc sulfate 220 mg q.d. to t.i.d. or MVI
Vitamin K	SQ/PO	Phytonadione 10 mg SQ or 5 mg PO
Vitamin E	PO	300 mg/d d-α-tocopherol
Vitamin D	PO	25–150,000 U/d ergocalciferol
Vitamin A	PO	10–20,000 U/d
Vitamin B_1 (thiamine)	PO	100 mg/d
Vitamin B_2 (riboflavin)	PO	5 mg b.i.d. or MVI
Vitamin B_3 (niacin)	PO	MVI
Vitamin B_6 (pyridoxine)	PO	50–150 mg/d or MVI
MCT	PO	15 ml q.i.d.

MCT = medium-chain triglycerides, MVI = multivitamins.

sus the lymphatics for long-chain fats), and have a high caloric content (115 kcal/tbsp). They facilitate absorption of fat-soluble vitamins but their poor palatability and tendency to produce diarrhea at high doses limit their use.

SPECIFIC CAUSES OF MALABSORPTION SYNDROME

The following is a discussion of specific causes of the malabsorption syndrome. The diagnostic tests and treatment options for each disorder will be listed.

STOMACH

Postsurgical Cause

Usually, surgery as the cause of symptoms is apparent from the history. Symptoms compatible with the dumping syndrome may predominate.

TESTS. Upper endoscopy, UGI series, gastric emptying time.

TREATMENT. Frequent small meals, avoid simple sugars, high-fiber diet, H_2 blockers, antidiarrheals, calcium and iron supplementation, antibiotics if bacterial overgrowth is suspected.

Zollinger-Ellison Syndrome

Zollinger-Ellison syndrome is a well-recognized but unusual cause of steatorrhea. Peptic ulceration with diarrhea is a good clinical clue to the diagnosis, which is confirmed by an elevated serum gastrin level and a positive secretin-gastrin test.

TESTS. Upper endoscopy, serum gastrin, secretin-gastrin test, CT scan, arteriography.

TREATMENT. Omeprazole 20 to 120 mg/d, to keep basal acid output below 10 mEq/h; surgical resection of tumor when possible.

LIVER

Cholestatic Liver Disease

Cholestatic liver disease can either be solely intrahepatic, e.g., PBC, or intrahepatic and extrahepatic, e.g., primary sclerosing cholangitis (PSC). Rarely, tumors of the biliary system are found with malabsorption.

TESTS. Sonogram, ERCP, liver biopsy, CT scan, antimitochondrial antibody.

TREATMENT. Treat underlying cause; cholestyramine 4 g tid for pruritus; vitamin D; ursodeoxycholic acid, 10 to 15 mg/kg/d (PBC); methotrexate 0.25 mg/kg/w (PSC); biliary drainage (PSC); liver transplantation.

PANCREAS

Chronic Pancreatitis

A variety of diseases can result in chronic pancreatitis and pancreatic insufficiency. The most common cause is chronic alcoholism. Other causes are listed in Table 12–2. Maldigestion from pancreatic amylase deficiency is rare because of the excessive production of this enzyme. Deficiencies of lipase and proteases result in the maldigestion, but steatorrhea does not occur until lipase values are reduced to 10% of their normal values. Chronic abdominal pain complicates chronic pancreatitis and may be the most difficult symptom to treat. Diabetes mellitus can also occur.

TESTS. Secretin test, bentiromide (Chymex) test, ERCP.

TREATMENT. Low-fat diet. Pancreatic enzyme replacement therapy (to ensure at least 28,000 U of lipase per meal) should be given. Various enzyme preparations are listed in Table 12–6. Therapy with antacids and H_2 antagonists or omeprazole will help to reduce enzyme breakdown by acid. An elemental diet or total parenteral nutrition (TPN) may be required in severe cases of malnutrition.

Cystic Fibrosis

Cystic fibrosis should be considered in children or young adults with malabsorption and recurrent pulmonary infections.

TESTS. Sweat chloride test.
TREATMENT. Pancreatic enzymes.

Miscellaneous

Pancreatic Carcinoma

Patients with pancreatic carcinoma usually succumb to their tumor burden before pancreatic insufficiency develops. However, exocrine insufficiency may result from ductal obstruction, gland replacement by tumor, or resection.

TESTS. Sonogram, CT scan, ERCP.
TREATMENT. Surgical resection (Whipple procedure, i.e., pancreatoduodenectomy), stent placement by ERCP, enzyme replacement.

Kwashiorkor

Severe protein-calorie deprivation may lead to pancreatic exocrine insufficiency.

TESTS. Clinical history.
TREATMENT. Caloric and protein replacement, pancreatic enzymes.

TABLE 12-6. COMMERCIAL PANCREATIC ENZYME SUPPLEMENTS

	STRENGTH IN USP UNITS*			
PRODUCT	LIPASE	AMYLASE	PROTEASE	PREPARATIONS
Creon	8,000	30,000	13,000	EC
Viokase	8,000	30,000	30,000	Tablets
Viokase Powder	16,800	70,000	70,000	†
Pancrease MT-4	4,000	12,000	12,000	EC
Pancrease MT-10	10,000	30,000	30,000	EC
Pancrease MT-16	16,000	48,000	48,000	EC
Cotazyme	8,000	30,000	30,000	Capsules
Cotazyme-S	8,000	30,000	30,000	EC

*Source: *Physicians' Desk Reference.* 45th ed. Oradell, NJ: Medical Economics Books; 1991.
†Each 1/4 teaspoonful.
EC = enteric coated microspheres.

Deficiency of Trypsinogen or Enterokinase

TESTS. Low levels of duodenal trypsin, chymotrypsin, and carboxypeptidase, which normalize with the addition of exogenous enterokinase or trypsin. A negative sweat chloride test is also required.

TREATMENT. Pancreatic enzyme supplementation.

SMALL INTESTINE

Gluten-Sensitive Enteropathy

Celiac disease is characterized by damage to the mucosa of the small intestine caused by an intolerance of gluten. This protein is found in wheat, rye, barley, and oats but not corn or rice. Mucosal biopsy specimens in celiac disease reveal villous flattening with crypt hyperplasia. Patients typically show marked improvement when gluten-containing foods are removed from the diet. They may also have secondary lactose intolerance, caused by low levels of lactase.

TESTS. Small bowel biopsy, small bowel radiographs, improvement with gluten-free diet.

TREATMENT. Gluten-free diet. Foods that should be avoided are shown in Table 12–7. Patients may tolerate lactose products when the mucosa normalizes. Occasionally, patients with proven celiac disease fail to respond to the gluten-free diet and may have refractory sprue or intestinal lymphoma. Prednisone may be helpful in up to 50% of patients with refractory sprue.

Crohn's Disease

Steatorrhea occurs when there is extensive disease or extensive resection of the small bowel. Vitamin B_{12} and bile salt malabsorption are common, secondary to the diseased or resected terminal ileum. Disease or resection of less than 100 cm of terminal ileum characteristically results in a choleraic diarrhea. Involvement of greater than 100 cm results in bile acid deficiency, with steatorrhea.

TESTS. Colonoscopy to terminal ileum with biopsy specimens demonstrating characteristic granulomatous inflammatory lesions; small bowel radiographs.

TREATMENT. 5-Aminosalicylic acid products (sulfasalazine 2 to 4 g/d, olsalazine, mesalamine), corticosteroids, metronidazole, immunosuppressant therapy. Cholestyramine (up to four 4-g packets/d) may be useful in controlling choleraic diarrhea. However, administration of cholestyramine may exacerbate steatorrhea as a result of bile salt deficiency (greater than 100 cm of terminal ileum involved).

Whipple's Disease

Whipple's disease is systemic bacterial illness that usually affects middle-aged men and is characterized by diarrhea, arthralgias, weight loss, fever, lymphadenopathy, and skin pigmentation. The disease usually involves the intestine, mesentery, heart, and brain. Mucosal biopsy specimens reveal macrophages that stain positive with periodic acid-Schiff (PAS). The disease is due to small rod-shaped Gram-positive actinomycete *(Tropheryma whippelli)*.

TESTS. Peroral small bowel biopsy, radiographs.

TREATMENT. Parenteral penicillin and streptomycin for 10 days, followed by trimethoprim-sulfamethoxazole (Bactrim) twice daily for 1 year.

TABLE 12-7. GUIDELINES FOR GLUTEN-FREE DIETS

Food Categories	Foods to Avoid
Milk	Malted milk, some commercial chocolate drinks, some nondairy creamers
Meat	Prepared meats that contain wheat, rye, oats, or barley such as some sausages, frankfurters, bologna, luncheon meats, meat loaf
Cheeses	Any cheese containing oat gum as an ingredient
Eggs	Eggs in sauce made from gluten-containing ingredients
Potato or other starch	Regular noodles, spaghetti, macaroni, most packaged rice mixes
Vegetables	Creamed vegetables, vegetables canned in sauce, some canned baked beans
Fruits	Thickened or prepared fruits, some pie fillings
Breads	All breads containing wheat, rye, oats, or barley; bran; graham; wheat germ; malt; kaska; bulgur; buckwheat; millet
Flours and thickening agents	Wheat starch; all flours containing wheat, rye, oats, or barley
Beverages	Cereal beverages; alcoholic beverages distilled from grains such as gin, whiskey, beer, and others

From Shils ME, Young VR. *Modern Nutrition in Health and Disease.* Philadelphia, Pa: Lea & Febiger; 1988.

Lactase Deficiency

The prevalence of primary lactase deficiency varies from 15% of Caucasians to nearly 90% of Asians and Blacks. Secondary lactase deficiency results from mucosal damage from other processes, e.g., celiac disease.

TESTS. Clinical history, lactose breath hydrogen test.

TREATMENT. Minimizing lactose intake; over-the-counter lactase preparations. Yogurt is usually well tolerated.

Eosinophilic Gastroenteritis

Eosinophilic gastroenteritis is commonly associated with several food intolerances, systemic allergic reactions, peripheral eosinophilia. Small bowel biopsy specimens reveal marked infiltration of the mucosa by eosinophils.

TESTS. Small bowel biopsy, peripheral eosinophil count.

TREATMENT. Periodic courses of corticosteroids or chronic low-dose steroids are usually necessary.

Tropical Sprue

This bacterial-mediated disease should be suspected in any patient presenting with malabsorption who has visited the tropics. Mucosal biopsy specimens reveal crypt lengthening, villous flattening, and chronic inflammation.

TESTS. Radiographs, small bowel biopsy.

TREATMENT. Tetracycline 250 mg qid and folate 5 mg/d for up to 6 months.

Short Bowel Syndrome

Massive resection of the small intestine may be the result of an ischemic event, Crohn's disease, neoplasm, or radiation enteritis. The remaining intestine can adapt to losses up to 40%. Complications are most common with loss of the duodenum, upper jejunum, or terminal ileum. Diarrhea and hyperacidity are common complications following massive intestinal resection. Other complications are oxalate stones, gallstones, and bacterial overgrowth.

TESTS. Medical and surgical history, enteroclysis, small bowel transit time (rapid).

TREATMENT. Low-fat diet, antidiarrheals, H_2 antagonists, omeprazole, medium-chain triglycerides, octreotide (Sandostatin), TPN.

Bacterial Overgrowth

Bacterial overgrowth results in deconjugation of bile salts and thus maldigestion of fats. It is commonly seen in surgically created blind loops and resection of the ileocecal valve. However, bacterial overgrowth may also complicate radiation enteritis, Crohn's disease, and motility disorders such as scleroderma or small bowel diverticulosis.

TESTS. Culture of upper intestinal secretions, breath tests, abnormal Schilling test that corrects with antibiotics.

TREATMENT. Broad spectrum antibiotics (metronidazole, tetracycline) for 2 weeks.

Acquired Immunodeficiency Syndrome (AIDS)

Malabsorption frequently is the result of opportunistic infections. Other patients may have malabsorption secondary to "idiopathic AIDS enteropathy."

TESTS. Stool for culture, acid-fast stain, analysis for ova and parasites.

TREATMENT. Treat infections, antidiarrheals.

TABLE 12-8. TREATMENT SUMMARY FOR MAJOR MALABSORPTION SYNDROMES

DISEASE	TREATMENT
Stomach	
Postsurgical disorders	Frequent small meals, antidiarrheals; high-fiber diet, avoid simple sugars; H_2 blockers, Ca^{2+}, Fe^{2+} supplementation; treat bacterial overgrowth
Zollinger-Ellison syndrome	Resection of gastrinoma, omeprazole 20–120 mg/d
Liver	
Cholestatic liver disease	Relieve biliary obstruction, cholestyramine 4 g t.i.d. for pruritus, ursodeoxycholic acid, 10–15 mg/d (PBC), methotrexate 0.25 mg/kg/wk (PSC), vitamin D, liver transplantation
Pancreatic Disease	
Pancreatic insufficiency	Pancreatic enzymes, low-fat diet, fat-soluble vitamins, H_2 blockers
Intestinal Mucosal Disease	
Celiac disease	Gluten-free diet; prednisone (refractory disease)
Crohn's disease	5-Aminosalicylic acid products, steroids, azathioprine (Imuran), metronidazole; if bile salt deficiency, low-fat diet, fat-soluble vitamins
Whipple's disease	Parenteral penicillin plus streptomycin $\times$ 10 d, sulfamethoxazole-trimethoprim (Bactrim) b.i.d. $\times$ 1 y, folate 1 mg q.d. $\times$ 1 y
Lactase deficiency	Low-lactose intake; lactase enzyme replacement (OTC)
Eosinophilic gastroenteritis	Steroid bolus or long-term low-dose steroids
Tropical sprue	Tetracycline or Bactrim, folate 5 mg/d
Short bowel syndrome	Antidiarrheals, possibly low-fat diet, H_2 blockers, omeprazole, TPN, octreotide (Sandostatin), vitamin B_{12}; treat bile salt deficiency
Bacterial overgrowth	Broad spectrum antibiotics $\times$ 2 wk, prokinetics (Reglan 10 mg q.i.d. or erythromycin 200 mg t.i.d.) for motility disorders, possible surgical correction
AIDS enteropathy	Treat underlying infection, antidiarrheals
Lymphangiectasia	Medium-chain triglycerides, low-fat diet; treat underlying disease
Abetalipoproteinemia	Vitamins E, A, and K; medium-chain triglycerides
Radiation enteritis	Antidiarrheals, cholestyramine, trial of antibiotics
Diabetic diarrhea	Antidiarrheals, octreotide, clonidine

AIDS = acquired immunodeficiency syndrome, PBC = primary biliary cirrhosis, PSC = primary sclerosing cholangitis, OTC = over the counter.

TABLE 12-9. ANTIDIARRHEAL AGENTS

DRUG	DOSE
Opiates	
Loperamide (Imodium)*	2–4 mg initially, then 2 mg PO q4h up to 16 mg/d
Diphenoxylate-atropine (Lomotil)†	2 tablets PO 6 hours prn
Deodorized tincture of opium	10 drops in water t.i.d.
Codeine	30–60 mg PO t.i.d.
Paregoric	1–2 tsp PO q.i.d.
Probantheline (Probanthine)	15 mg ac and 30 mg at hs
Cholestyramine (Questran)	4 g packet; 1 packet PO q.d. to q.i.d.
Bismuth subsalicylate (Pepto Bismol)	2 tablets PO prn; up to 8 tablets per day
Psyllium (Metamucil)	1 tsp q.d. to q.i.d.
Octreotide (Sandostatin)	50–200 μg SQ t.i.d.
Clonidine	0.3–1 mg PO q.d.

*Poor central nervous system penetration; low toxicity.
†Atropine toxicity may result.

Lymphangiectasia

Intestinal lymphangiectasia is characterized by hypoalbuminemia, steatorrhea, lymphopenia, and dilated lacteals in small intestine biopsy specimens. The syndrome results from obstruction of lymphatics, either primary (congenital) or secondary (tuberculosis, constrictive pericarditis, sarcoidosis, lymphoma).

TESTS. Small bowel biopsy, CT scan of the abdomen to rule out secondary causes of obstruction, small bowel x-ray examination.

TREATMENT. Medium-chain triglycerides; treat any underlying cause.

Abetalipoproteinemia

Abetalipoproteinemia is an autosomal recessive disease with fat malabsorption, acanthocytotic erythrocytes, and progressive neurologic disease.

TEST. Small bowel biopsy.

TREATMENT. Fat-soluble vitamin replacement, especially vitamin E, medium-chain triglycerides.

Miscellaneous

Other causes of malabsorption include radiation enteritis, diabetes mellitus, and ischemia.

TESTS. Pertinent history, small bowel biopsy in selected cases.

TREATMENT. Predominantly antidiarrheal agents, although octreotide and clonidine have been shown to be effective in refractory cases of diabetic diarrhea.

Other causes of malabsorption are listed in Table 12–2.

In Table 12–8, we have summarized the treatments for various disorders causing malabsorption. Table 12–9 lists several antidiarrheal agents that are commonly used and their usual dosage.

REFERENCES

1. Brasitus TA, Sitrin MD. Intestinal malabsorption syndromes. *Annu Rev Med.* 1990;41:339–347.
2. Craig RM, Atkinson AJ. D-Xylose testing: a review. *Gastroenterology.* 1988;95:223–231.
3. Fisher RL, ed. Malabsorption and nutritional status and support. *Gastroenterol Clin North Am.* 1989;18:467–512, 543–565, 589–601.
4. Gilinsky NH. Pancreatic function testing. *Postgrad Med.* 1989;86:165–172.
5. Kirsch M. Bacterial overgrowth. *Am J Gastroenterol.* 1990;85:231–237.
6. Niederau C, Grendell JH. Diagnosis of chronic pancreatitis. *Gastroenterology.* 1985;88:1973–1995.
7. Ogbonnaya KI, Arem R. Diabetic diarrhea. *Arch Intern Med.* 1990;150:262–267.
8. Schjonsby H. Vitamin B_{12} absorption and malabsorption. *Gut.* 1989;30:1686–1691.
9. Trier JS. Intestinal malabsorption: differentiation of cause. *Hosp Practice.* 1988;23:195–211.
10. Winter HS. Breath tests as a diagnostic technique for malabsorption. *Pediatr Ann.* 1987;16:258–262.
11. Yamada T, ed. *Textbook of Gastroenterology.* Philadelphia, Pa: JB Lippincott Co; 1991:Chap 48, 69, 89.

Acknowledgments

We would like to thank Amy Stehli for typing this manuscript.

13
Protein-losing Gastroenteropathy

GEORGE W. BO-LINN

Protein-losing gastroenteropathy (PLGE) is not a single disease. Rather, it refers to a variety of diseases characterized by an excessive protein loss into the gastrointestinal (GI) tract that results in hypoproteinemia. In normal individuals, the GI tract absorbs >95% of total luminal protein (approximately 100 g dietary protein, 30 g digestive enzymes, and 30 g sloughed enterocytes) daily. Dietary and endogenous proteins are hydrolyzed equally well, but a few proteins such as intrinsic factor, immunoglobulin A (IgA) secretory component, and a-1-antitrypsin are relatively resistant to digestion. The hydrolytic resistance of a-1-antitrypsin explains its usefulness as a measure of serum protein loss into the GI tract.

In patients with PLGE, hypoproteinemia develops because the enteric loss of serum proteins overwhelms the capacity of the GI tract to reabsorb enough protein and constituent amino acids to permit adequate resynthesis. Although albumin synthesis in patients with PLGE ranges from normal to slightly increased, the total body albumin pool and half-life of albumin are diminished.[1] Concentrations of serum proteins that have a relatively limited synthetic rate and a

CAUSES OF PLGE

The excessive loss of serum protein into the GI tract usually results from one or more of the following factors: intestinal lymphatic obstruction, ulcerative mucosal GI disease, or nonulcerative mucosal disease.

INTESTINAL LYMPHATIC OBSTRUCTION

Plasma cannot be reabsorbed from the interstitial space of the enterocytes when the flow of lymph from the GI tract is impaired as a result of lymphatic obstruction or congestion from increased systemic venous pressure on the liver. Thus, protein-rich plasma and lymph are lost into the intestinal lumen.

Congenital intestinal lymphangiectasia, also known as Milroy's disease, primarily affects children and young adults. Patients usually have chronic, dependent edema caused by marked hypoproteinemia.[2] Occasionally, they may exhibit asymmetric edema of an extremity as a result of localized lymphatic obstruction. GI symptoms may include diarrhea, steatorrhea, abdominal distension, nausea, and vomiting.

Patients with Milroy's disease also exhibit hypoalbuminemia, hypoimmunoglobulinemia, and lymphocytopenia. In spite of low concentrations of IgA, IgM, IgG, and T cells, they rarely suffer from opportunistic infections. Small bowel barium radiographs reveal nonspecific nodular folds and retained secretions. Jejunal biopsy specimens often demonstrate characteristic dilated lacteal vessels. Lymphangiography confirms the malformed, hypoplastic lymphatic channels.

Acquired intestinal lymphangiectasia occurs when a disease obstructs mesenteric lymphatic drainage. Diseases associated with intestinal lymphatic obstruction are listed in Table 13–1. Cardiac diseases that increase right ventricular pressure may elevate systemic venous pressure enough to obstruct intestinal lymphatic flow. Most patients with PLGE that results from cardiac disease have constrictive pericarditis, but other associated cardiac diseases are also listed in Table 13–1. Ascites, marked hypoalbuminemia, hypogammaglobulinemia, and lymphocytopenia also usually occur.

long circulating half-life, such as immunoglobulins or fibrinogen, decrease rapidly but rarely fall to clinically significant levels.

TABLE 13–1. DISEASES ASSOCIATED WITH PROTEIN-LOSING GASTROENTEROPATHY

Diseases Associated with Intestinal Lymphatic Obstruction
Congenital intestinal lymphangiectasia
Acquired mesenteric lymphatic obstruction
  Abdominal tuberculosis
  Abdominal sarcoidosis
  Pancreatic cancer
  Chronic pancreatitis
  Lymphoma
  Lymphenteric fistula
  Retroperitoneal fibrosis, carcinoma
  Retroperitoneal surgery
  Crohn's disease
  Whipple's disease
Cardiac diseases
  Congestive heart failure
  Constrictive pericarditis
  Fontan procedure
  Interatrial septal defect
  Pulmonary hypertension
  Pulmonic valvular stenosis
  Tricuspid valvular regurgitation

Nonulcerative Gastrointestinal Diseases
Hypertrophic gastropathies
  Giant hypertrophic gastropathy (Ménétrier's disease)
  Hypertrophic hypersecretory gastropathy
Intestinal bacterial overgrowth
Parasitic infections: malaria, giardiasis, schistosomiasis, strongyloidiasis, cryptosporidiosis, capillariasis, hookworms
Viral enteritides: cytomegalovirus, human immunodeficiency virus, rotavirus
Allergic enteritis
Eosinophilic gastroenteritis
Gluten-sensitive enteropathy (celiac sprue)
Tropical sprue
Connective tissue diseases: rheumatoid arthritis, mixed connective tissue disease, systemic sclerosis, systemic lupus erythematosus
Neoplasms: lymphoma, neurofibromatosis, neuroblastoma, mesenteric mesenchymoma, histiocytosis, juvenile gastrointestinal polyposis
Whipple's disease
Postmeasles diarrhea
Microscopic colitis
Collagenous colitis
Acquired immune deficiency syndrome
Amyloidosis
Lymphocytic gastritis
Endometriosis
Henoch-Schönlein purpura

Ulcerative Mucosal Diseases
Acute graft-versus-host disease
α-Chain disease
Carcinoid syndrome
Crohn's disease
Erosive gastritis or colitis
Idiopathic ulcerative jejunoileitis
Neoplasia (esophageal, gastric, or colonic)
Pseudomembranous colitis
Ulcerative colitis
Waldenström's macroglobulinemia

ULCERATIVE MUCOSAL DISEASES

Erosions and ulcerations destroy the integrity of the mucosal lining of the GI tract and result in the loss of protein-rich plasma via the denuded mucosal capillaries and lymphatic channels into the intestinal lumen. Cancers that cause PLGE usually involve substantial portions of the GI tract. Patients with cancer or severe chronic disease may also have decreased hepatic protein synthesis, which exacerbates hypoproteinemia. In Table 13–1, ulcerative diseases that can cause PLGE are listed.

NONULCERATIVE MUCOSAL DISEASES

Hypertrophic gastropathy refers to a variety of rare, poorly defined diseases that produce enlarged gastric folds in the body and in the fundus of the stomach and hypertrophy of the gastric mucosa. This term also refers to giant hypertrophic gastritis (Ménétrier's disease), to hypertrophic, hypersecretory gastropathy, and to the gastric appearance induced by Zollinger-Ellison syndrome.

Ménétrier's disease is characterized by a thickened gastric mucosa of hyperplastic mucus gland cells that have replaced the normal fundic parietal and chief cells. These abnormalities are thought to cause plasma proteins to "weep" into the gastric lumen after disrupted intercellular and paracellular permeability has been disrupted. Submucosal lymphangiectasia, which has also been noted in Ménétrier's disease, suggests that obstructed lymphatics may contribute to PLGE. Patients with hypertrophic gastropathy may have no specific GI symptoms other than dyspepsia and mild diarrhea.

Allergic gastroenteropathy occurs very rarely in adults. Intolerance to certain food items rather than a true immunologically mediated allergy is almost always the more accurate diagnosis. However, in children and infants PLGE can occur as an allergic response to certain dietary constituents. b-Lactoglobulin in milk has been identified as the antigen in some patients. Patients with allergic gastroenteropathy usually have a personal or family history of allergic conditions such as eczema or allergic rhinitis.

Patients with various connective tissue diseases have been reported as having PLGE. The mechanism of protein loss in these patients is poorly defined, although an immunologically mediated response has been postulated.[3]

DIAGNOSIS OF PLGE

PLGE should be suspected when hypoalbuminemia occurs without significant renal or hepatic disease. Patients with PLGE, hypoalbuminemia, and lymphocytopenia usually have intestinal lymphangiectasia. To confirm enteric protein loss, the fecal a-1-antitrypsin clearance should be measured. Measurements of radiolabeled proteins and albumin clearance are accurate but are more difficult to perform because of the expense and potential hazards of radioactive material and the inconvenience of prolonged stool and urine collections. a-1-Antitrypsin is a glycoprotein with a molecular weight similar to that of albumin. It is resistant to hydrolysis in the intestinal tract and is normally present in low fecal concentrations. The assay can usually be completed in 1 day and serves as an excellent measure of albumin loss into the GI tract.

Clearance (ml/d) can be calculated as follows: $C = FW/S$ where C is clearance, F is the fecal concentration in mg/100 g dry fecal weight, W is the dry fecal weight in g/d, and S is the serum concentration in mg/dl. In patients who do not have diarrhea, a value >24 ml/d represents excessive enteric protein loss. In patients with diarrhea, a value >56 ml/d is abnormal because diarrhea apparently increases a-1-antitrypsin clearance.[4] False-positive results may be found in infants less than 1 week of age because residual meconium contains a-1-antitrypsin. Bloody diarrhea can also produce a false-positive result.[4] A false-negative result can occur in patients whose protein losses are in the stomach, because a-1-antitrypsin is degraded at a pH <3.

When the patient has been diagnosed as having PLGE, appropriate studies should be performed to identify the primary disease. If the disease is not evident after a thorough initial investigation, then the patient should undergo barium studies of the entire GI tract and perhaps endoscopy and biopsy of the mucosa. If those studies are nondiagnostic, then the patient should be examined for lymphatic obstruction via an abdominal computed tomography (CT) scan. In the adult, a pedal lymphangiogram is usually unnecessary. If an underlying cardiac disease is suspected, the patient should undergo cardiac ultrasonography before invasive procedures such as cardiac catheterization are considered.

TREATMENT OF PLGE

Patients with PLGE should first be treated for the underlying disease. If the primary disease can be treated, then the PLGE usually improves or resolves. Unfortunately, patients with PLGE usually do not have a primary disease that is as treatable as is constrictive pericarditis via pericardiectomy.

Treatment for patients with primary or acquired intestinal lymphangiectasia may include elevating edematous extremities and wearing elastic support hose for dependent edema. These patients should be vigilant about treating swollen extremities to avoid injury and should seek prompt, aggressive treatment for infections. Diuretics are rarely helpful. However, eating a low-fat diet may decrease enteric protein loss. Medium-chain triglyceride oil (C 6:0 to C 12:0) should be substituted in the diet for long-chain triglycerides (LCG), which increase intestinal lymphatic flow.

Patients with mucosal disease should receive treatment for the primary disease in addition to vigorous correction of nutritional deficiency. Fat-soluble vitamin supplements may be necessary if significant steatorrhea exists. Treatment of patients with Ménétrier's disease should be individualized according to the severity of their symptoms and hypoproteinemia. Medications including histamine H_2 antagonists, proton pump inhibitors, octreotide, anticholinergics, and corticosteroids are occasionally helpful.[5] Partial gastric resection may be necessary for patients with Ménétrier's disease and severe PLGE.

REFERENCES

1. Brasitus TA. Protein-losing gastroenteropathy. In: Sleisinger MH, Fordtran JS, eds. *Gastrointestinal Disease: Pathophysiology, Diagnosis, and Management.* 5th ed. Philadelphia, Pa: WB Saunders Co; 1994:1027.
2. Fox U, Lucani G. Disorders of the intestinal lymphatic system. *Lymphology.* 1993;26(2):61.
3. Tsutsumi A, Sugiyama T, Matsumura R, et al. Protein losing enteropathy associated with collagen diseases. *Ann Rheum Dis.* 1991;50:178.
4. Strygler B, Nicar MJ, Santangelo WC, et al. Alpha 1-antitrypsin excretion in stool in normal subjects and in patients with gastrointestinal disorders. *Gastroenterology.* 1990;99:1380.
5. Yeaton P, Frierson HF Jr. Octreotide reduces enteral protein losses in Ménétrier's disease. *Am J Gastroenterol.* 1993;88(1):95.

14
Diarrhea

KENNETH D. FINE and LAWRENCE R. SCHILLER

GENERAL APPROACH

Diarrhea is a common symptom and usually is successfully treated by patients with altered diets or over-the-counter remedies. Patients seek medical evaluation of diarrhea when they are concerned that their stools have been too liquid or too frequent for more than a few days or if they develop fever, prostration, or rectal bleeding.

Because the number of conditions that cause diarrhea is large, it is useful to classify the diarrheal illness in some way that limits the number of potential causes and diagnostic tests that need to be considered. Several classification schemes can be used, such as duration of illness (acute versus chronic), population at risk (e.g., travelers to third world countries, patients with acquired immunodeficiency syndrome [AIDS]), severity (large versus small volume), pathophysiologic findings (osmotic versus secretory), or by specific etiologic class (infectious, inflammatory, abnormal motility, etc.). The first two ways of classifying diarrhea (by duration and by population at risk) require only a basic history and are therefore most useful initially.

The key to the appropriate evaluation of a patient with diarrhea is the *medical history,* which must be thorough and specific. The diarrhea should be characterized as to its duration, frequency, volume (in general terms), relation to meals or fasting, occurrence during the day versus the night, consistency, quality (e.g., excessively foul, floats, hard to flush, color), and content (e.g., blood, mucus, pus, oil droplets, or food particles). Etiologic factors involving significant colonic inflammation (e.g., infectious or idiopathic colitis) cause frequent small volume stools, usually with blood, pus, or mucus; urgency is common, and fecal incontinence may result. (The physician should always inquire about fecal incontinence, since it is almost never reported voluntarily.) In contrast, diarrhea resulting from secretion by the small intestine, such as that which occurs with toxigenic bacteria (e.g., *Escherichia coli* or *Vibrio cholerae*) or vipoma, causes voluminous watery stools without blood, pus, or mucus. Excessively foul stools containing oil droplets or food particles, indicate that malabsorption or a gastrocolic fistula may be present. Nocturnal diarrhea, especially with fecal incontinence, strongly suggests an organic disease, such as diabetic enteropathy, rather than a functional problem, such as irritable bowel syndrome. Associated symptoms, such as abdominal pain, flatulence, gaseous distension, bloating, cramps, tenesmus, fever, and weight loss, should be sought.

The physician also should explore previous medical problems, surgeries, and family history. All prescription and over-the-counter medications taken by the patient must be discussed, since many drugs cause diarrhea as a side effect.[1] Magnesium-containing products, such as antacids or mineral supplements, are especially frequent causes of medication-induced diarrhea.[2] A course of antibiotics in the preceding few months should be considered a risk factor for *Clostridium difficile*–induced pseudomembranous enterocolitis.

The possible influence of psychologic stress should also be investigated. Diarrhea made worse by stress, accompanied by pain or alternating with constipation suggests a diagnosis of irritable bowel syndrome. Diarrhea in the setting of attempted weight loss or a fixation on body image should raise the possibility of laxative abuse associated with anorexia or bulimia nervosa.[3]

A thorough dietary history is also important. The physician should ask about changes in diet or special diets. Consumption of poorly absorbed carbohydrates, such as sorbitol, mannitol, fructose, and lactose, can lead to excessive gas production by the colon and diarrhea[4]; therefore, intake of fruits, vegetables, bran, some sugar-free foods, artificial sweeteners and milk products should be estimated.

A careful social history should be obtained. Diarrhea during or soon after foreign travel to Mexico or other third world countries makes traveler's diarrhea likely.[5] The social history also should include the type of residential area (i.e., urban or rural), living conditions, sources of drinking water, occupation, sexual preference and activity, and use of illicit drugs or alcohol. Patients living in rural settings may be exposed to farm animals with bacterial infections, such as *Salmonella* and *Brucella*. These patients may also drink untreated well water or raw milk, which can cause infectious diarrhea or epidemic chronic diarrhea.[6,7] Health care–related employment may be a risk factor for enteric infections and factitious diarrhea. The physician also should ask discreetly, but directly about sexual activity. Anal intercourse is associated with proctitis due to gonorrhea, herpes simplex, *Chlamydia,* syphilis, and amebiasis. In addition, unprotected sexual activity as well as intravenous drug use are risk factors for AIDS, which is associated with a multitude of causes of diarrhea (see Table 14–1).

In patients with acute diarrhea the *physical examination* is usually more helpful in determining the severity of illness than its cause. Volume status should be assessed, and fever and signs of

TABLE 14–1. CAUSES OF DIARRHEA IN PATIENTS WITH AIDS

1. Infections
   a. Bacteria
      (1) *Campylobacter*
      (2) *Salmonella*
   b. Fungi
      (1) *Candida*
      (2) *Cryptococcus*
      (3) *Histoplasma*
   c. Mycobacteria
      (1) *Mycobacterium avium intracellulare*
   d. Parasites or protozoa
      (1) *Cryptosporidium*
      (2) *Entamoeba*
      (3) *Giardia*
      (4) *Isospora*
      (5) *Microsporidia (Enterocytozoon)*
   e. Viruses
      (1) Adenovirus
      (2) Cytomegalovirus
      (3) Herpes simplex
2. AIDS enteropathy
3. Intestinal lymphoma

toxicity should be noted. Particular attention must be given to the examination of the abdomen for the presence and quality of bowel sounds, distension, and tenderness. In this setting the anorectal examination mainly serves the purpose of obtaining a stool sample for detection of gross or occult blood.

In patients with chronic diarrhea all aspects of the physical examination mentioned above apply. In addition, clues to the underlying cause may be found; these include the presence of bruits, masses, organomegaly, fissures or fistulae, fecal impaction, and diminished anal sphincter tone. Characteristic skin changes are associated with systemic mastocytosis, glucagonoma, Addison's disease, amyloidosis, carcinoid syndrome, Degos' disease, and celiac disease. Hepatosplenomegaly, bilateral carpal tunnel syndrome, and orthostatic hypotension may be present in amyloidosis. A thyroid nodule may be palpated in medullary carcinoma of the thyroid or hyperthyroidism due to a functioning adenoma; thyromegaly and exophthalmos occur in Graves' disease. A right-sided heart murmur may be the only physical finding present in the carcinoid syndrome. Peripheral or lumbosacral arthritis can occur with inflammatory bowel disease, Whipple's disease, collagenous colitis, and some cases of bacillary dysentery. Lymphadenopathy may be a diagnostic clue in patients with AIDS or lymphoma. Finally, signs of peripheral vascular disease, with or without an abdominal bruit, should point to intestinal ischemia as a possible cause of diarrhea.

ACUTE DIARRHEA

Acute diarrhea is defined as diarrhea that has been present for less than 4 weeks. Although chronic diarrhea may initially present as an "acute" process, for our purposes this discussion of acute diarrhea will be limited to those etiologic factors that usually run their courses within a 4-week period (see Table 14–2). Inherent in the approach to acute diarrhea is the fact that most cases will resolve in a matter of weeks without treatment; thus, the aim of evaluation is to identify those conditions that need special attention from the treating physician.

Patients requiring diagnostic and therapeutic intervention are those with moderate-to-severe volume depletion, with fever or other signs of toxicity, with bloody diarrhea, or with diarrhea lasting more than a few days. In these patients a complete blood count should be done to look for anemia, hemoconcentration, or an abnormal

TABLE 14–2. CAUSES OF ACUTE DIARRHEA

1. Infections
    a. Bacterial
        (1) *Campylobacter* species
        (2) *Clostridium difficile*
        (3) *Escherichia coli*
        (4) *Salmonella enteritidis*
        (5) *Shigella* species
    b. Parasitic
        (1) *Entamoeba hystolytica*
        (2) *Giardia lamblia*
    c. Viral
        (1) Adenovirus
        (2) Norwalk virus
        (3) Rotavirus
        (4) Others
2. Food poisoning
    a. *Bacillus cereus*
    b. *Clostridium perfringens*
    c. *Salmonella* species
    d. *Staphylococcus aureus*
    e. *Vibrio* species
3. Medications
    a. Antacids
    b. Antiarrhythmics
    c. Antibiotics
    d. Antineoplastics
    e. Antihypertensives
    f. Cholinergic agents
    g. Laxatives
    h. Lactulose
    i. Magnesium supplements
    j. Nonsteroidal antiinflammatory drugs
    k. Potassium supplements
    l. Prostaglandins
    m. Others
4. Ingestion of poorly absorbed sugars
    a. Fructose
    b. Lactose (in selected individuals)
    c. Mannitol
    d. Sorbitol

white blood cell count or differential. Lymphocytosis usually indicates a viral cause, whereas neutrophilia or the presence of immature white blood cells or both suggest an inflammatory or bacillary cause. Neutropenia can occur in salmonellosis. Serum electrolytes and renal function should be assessed. When signs of toxicity or fever are present or when diarrhea has been present for more than 1 week, a stool sample should be sent for culture, and examined for white blood cells, ova, and parasites. Hospitalized patients, residents of nursing homes, or those treated with antibiotics in the preceding several months should have stool analyzed for *C. difficile* toxin.

Proctoscopy or flexible sigmoidoscopy should be considered in toxic patients, bleeding patients, or those with persistent acute diarrhea. Sigmoidoscopy is performed in these settings for the diagnosis of colitis. Findings of particular interest include multiple, punched-out ulcers with normal intervening mucosa (as seen in amebiasis) and pseudomembranes (as seen in antibiotic-associated diarrhea due to *C. difficile*). Mucosal biopsies can be obtained,[8] and a fresh stool sample can be collected, if the patient is unable to pass one on demand. Plain films of the abdomen are worthwhile in toxic, hospitalized patients and can help confirm the diagnosis of colitis or detect ileus or megacolon.

Therapy for acute diarrhea consists mainly of volume and electrolyte repletion, antibiotics, or nonspecific antidiarrheal agents. In severely ill and volume-depleted patients the initial phase of volume and electrolyte repletion should be done intravenously. Oral rehydration solutions are an alternative for less volume-depleted patients or situations where intravenous fluids are not available.[9] When signs of toxicity, fever, leukocytosis with a "left shift," or toxic megacolon are present in a patient with acute diarrhea, empiric antibiotic therapy (with a quinolone or trimethoprim-sulfamethoxazole) should be started to treat the common causes of bacillary dysentery. The major exception to this recommendation is when a patient has antibiotic-associated pseudomembranous colitis; oral treatment with vancomycin or metronidazole should be instituted to suppress *C. difficile*. In the absence of significant toxicity, high fever, or megacolon, nonspecific antidiarrheals, such as loperamide, diphenoxylate-atropine, or codeine may be used to reduce stool frequency and output.

CHRONIC DIARRHEA

When diarrhea persists for more than 4 weeks, it can be designated as *chronic*. This time frame excludes most infectious causes of diarrhea and self-limited conditions and allows the physician to formulate a different differential diagnosis than when diarrhea presents acutely. Table 14–3 lists some of the diagnoses that need to be considered.

One diagnosis that should be applied reluctantly to patients with chronic diarrhea is irritable bowel syndrome. Patients in whom pain is not the predominant symptom should not be given this label, especially when diarrhea is continuous and does not alternate with constipation.[10] All too often patients with chronic con-

TABLE 14–3. CAUSES OF CHRONIC DIARRHEA

1. Fecal incontinence
2. Iatrogenic diarrhea
   a. After surgery
      (1) Vagotomy, gastrectomy
      (2) Cholecystectomy
      (3) Ileocolonic resection
   b. After abdominopelvic radiation therapy
   c. Drug-induced diarrhea
3. Laxative abuse
4. Systemic diseases
   a. Endocrinopathies
      (1) Hyperthyroidism
      (2) Addison's disease
      (3) Diabetes mellitus
      (4) Hypoparathyroidism
   b. Heavy metal poisoning
   c. Circulatory problems
      (1) Congestive heart failure
      (2) Constrictive pericarditis
      (3) Vasculitis
      (4) Chronic mesenteric ischemia
   d. Amyloidosis
   e. Immune deficiencies
      (1) AIDS
      (2) Immunoglobulin deficiencies
   f. Neurological diseases
5. Chronic infections
   a. Bacterial
      (1) *Aeromonas*
      (2) *Pleisiomonas*
      (3) Tuberculosis
      (4) Yersiniosis
   b. Parasitic
      (1) *Giardia*
      (2) *Strongyloides*
   c. ?Epidemic chronic diarrhea (Brainerd diarrhea)
6. Inflammatory bowel disease
   a. Crohn's disease
   b. Ulcerative colitis
   c. Microscopic (lymphocytic) colitis
   d. Collagenous colitis
   e. Eosinophilic gastroenteritis
   f. Ulcerative jejunitis
   g. Diverticulitis of the colon
7. Malignancies
   a. Villous adenoma of the rectum
   b. Colorectal cancer
   c. Lymphoma
   d. Carcinoid tumors
   e. Vipoma
   f. Gastrinoma
   g. Medullary carcinoma of thyroid
8. Maldigestion or malabsorption
   a. Generalized
      (1) Mucosal disease of small intestine
      (2) Pancreatic exocrine insufficiency
   b. Limited
      (1) Bacterial overgrowth in small bowel
      (2) Carbohydrate malabsorption
      (3) Bile acid malabsorption
9. Chronic idiopathic diarrhea

tinuous diarrhea are labeled as having irritable bowel syndrome, and correctable causes of diarrhea are overlooked. When patients present with continuous diarrhea or are otherwise atypical for irritable bowel syndrome (e.g., first symptoms in middle age or later, failure to respond to fiber supplements or anticholinergics), a thorough evaluation is mandatory.

This evaluation should include a careful history, physical examination, selected laboratory tests, including analysis of stool, and thoughtfully conducted radiographic and endoscopic studies. In some patients, specific absorption tests may be necessary. Table 14–4 summarizes tests that may need to be done to evaluate chronic diarrhea.

A careful history is necessary to differentiate *fecal incontinence* as the primary cause of the complaint of diarrhea from incontinence as a result of chronic diarrhea. If stools are frequently passed involuntarily and are small in amount, it is likely that incontinence is primary. On the other hand, if passage of liquid stool is habitual, but uncontrolled passage of stool is infrequent and only occurs in the setting of urgency, then incontinence probably is not the cause of the complaint of diarrhea. Measurement of stool weight can also be helpful; normal stool weights ($<$250 g/24 h) suggest that incontinence is the primary problem, whereas higher stool weights suggest a fundamental problem with intestinal fluid absorption. If a history of fecal incontinence is elicited, a careful physical examination and anorectal manometry can help to define the pathophysiology of this symptom and to direct treatment. Therapeutic options include stimulating defecation at intervals to keep the rectum free of stool, antidiarrheal drugs such as loperamide, biofeedback training, and surgery.[11]

History is also of great value in recognizing *iatrogenic diarrhea*. This category includes diarrhea induced by surgery (such as gastrectomy, cholecystectomy, and intestinal resection), diarrhea as a side effect of drug therapy, and diarrhea after abdominal or pelvic irradiation. Patients do not always associate these therapeutic interventions with diarrhea because the onset of diarrhea may be remote from the intervention. For instance, gastrectomy can lead not only to diarrhea due to dumping syndrome immediately after surgery but also to diarrhea due to bacterial overgrowth years later. It is essential to ask patients about previous treatments to make these associations.

Diarrhea after gastric surgery can have several mechanisms. Vagotomy, gastric resection, or gastric drainage can be complicated by the dumping syndrome because of rapid, unregulated gastric emptying. This can usually be appreciated by history alone; formal gastric emptying studies are necessary only when the diagnosis is in doubt. Dietary manipulation, anticholinergic drugs, or opiate antidiarrheal drugs are helpful in most cases. In refractory cases of dumping syndrome, the somatostatin analog, octreotide, has been useful.[12] In addition to dumping syndrome, gastric surgery can produce diarrhea by inducing maldigestion and malabsorption, by allowing for bacterial overgrowth, and by unmasking celiac disease. Fecal fat excretion may need to be measured, and tests for bacterial overgrowth and celiac disease may be required (see below).

Cholecystectomy may be associated with diarrhea also.[13] In some patients, bile acid malabsorption seems to be important, since diarrhea abates with cholestyramine treatment.[14] In others, the mechanism is less certain, and the association is less clear. An empiric trial of cholestyramine or another bile acid sequestrant (e.g., aluminum hydroxide) may be reasonable in patients who have diarrhea soon after cholecystectomy. If this fails, further evaluation of diarrhea is necessary.

TABLE 14–4. TESTS THAT MAY BE DONE IN THE EVALUATION OF CHRONIC DIARRHEA

1. Personal history and epidemiology, physical examination
2. Complete blood count
3. Serum electrolyte and glucose concentrations
4. Liver function tests, thyroid function tests
5. Plasma gastrin, calcitonin, and VIP levels
6. Urinary 5-HIAA excretion
7. Stool examination for ova and parasites
8. Stool occult blood test, stool leukocytes
9. Stool cultures, *Clostridium difficile* toxin
10. Quantitative stool collection for weight, fat
11. Stool electrolyte concentrations, pH
12. Stool chymotrypsin concentration
13. Stool and urine laxative screening
14. Schilling test with intrinsic factor
15. Quantitative culture of jejunal fluid
16. Upper gastrointestinal and small bowel radiograms
17. Upper gastrointestinal endoscopy, small bowel biopsy
18. Colonoscopy with multiple biopsies
19. Abdominal and pelvic sonography or computed tomography

5-HIAA = 5-hydroxyindoleacetic acid, VIP = vasoactive intestinal polypeptide.

Ileocolic resection can also be associated with chronic diarrhea.[15] Although distal ileal resection is regularly associated with bile acid malabsorption, this may not be the mechanism of diarrhea in some of these patients. With extensive ileal resection, steatorrhea or the loss of absorptive surface itself may be the primary cause of diarrhea. Patients with diarrhea after ileocolic resection should be given an empiric trial of cholestyramine, but, if unresponsive, they may need large doses of opiate antidiarrheals for control. If diarrhea starts long after the resection, an evaluation for recurrent disease (e.g., Crohn's disease) or complicating factors is wise.

Radiation therapy can cause diarrhea both simultaneously with treatment and also years later. Radiation can induce ileal dysfunction and altered rectal compliance, which may lead to frequency, urgency, or frank incontinence. Stool weight is usually moderate unless there are superimposed problems. Treatment with cholestyramine or opiates can be helpful.

Many drugs have diarrhea as a side effect (Table 14-2), and therefore a careful drug history (including over-the-counter drugs) is essential when interviewing a patient with chronic diarrhea. Proof of the association requires stopping the suspect drug, producing improvement, and then causing diarrhea with rechallenge. Management involves discontinuing the drug or reducing its dose. Antidiarrheal drugs rarely should be used to treat drug-induced diarrhea.

Laxative abuse is another form of drug-induced diarrhea, but in this instance deception is part of the patient's interaction with the physician.[3,16] Because of this, laxative abuse needs to be considered in every patient who has chronic diarrhea.[17] History can still be useful in identifying patients more likely to be abusing laxatives. Four stereotypes should be looked for:

1. Anorexic or bulimic patient who uses laxatives to treat perceived obesity
2. Malingering patient with a secondary gain from illness
3. Munchausen patient for whom being ill is an aim in itself
4. Victims of poisoning with laxatives, usually dependent children with a hovering parent.

Most laxatives can be detected by analysis of stool, and physicians should have a low threshold for ordering laxative screening for patients with chronic diarrhea,[17] especially when they fit into one of the stereotypes above or if diarrhea has been difficult to diagnose or treat. In general, once laxative abuse has been found and confirmed, patients should be confronted with the findings and a psychiatric evaluation should be conducted.

The next group of conditions to consider are *systemic diseases* that have diarrhea as a manifestation. These include endocrinopathies, such as hyperthyroidism, Addison's disease, diabetes, and hypoparathyroidism; heavy metal poisoning; circulatory problems, such as congestive heart failure, constrictive pericarditis, vasculitis, and chronic mesenteric ischemia; amyloidosis; immune deficiencies, such as AIDS and immunoglobulin deficiencies; and neurologic diseases, such as dysautonomia. These conditions can be detected by careful questioning, physical examination, and laboratory tests. Treatment of the underlying condition will usually mitigate diarrhea.

With systemic diseases excluded, attention can be directed to intestinal problems. Certain *chronic infections* should be excluded next. These include bacterial infections, such as *Aeromonas* and *Pleisiomonas,* which may require special culture techniques; parasitic infections with *Giardia* or *Strongyloides,* which may require duodenoscopic biopsy for diagnosis, if not discovered by stool examination; and granulomatous infections, such as tuberculosis or yersiniosis. In addition, chronic diarrhea sometimes occurs in the setting of a point-source outbreak, so-called epidemic chronic diarrhea (Brainerd diarrhea). Although this epidemiology suggests an infectious cause, no pathogen has been identified and no antibiotic therapy has been helpful.[6,7,18]

Inflammatory bowel disease should be considered in all patients with chronic diarrhea. Crohn's disease and ulcerative colitis are common causes of diarrhea and must be excluded by appropriate sigmoidoscopic (or colonoscopic) and radiographic findings. Less common forms of inflammatory bowel disease can be important causes of chronic diarrhea. Microscopic (lymphocytic) colitis and collagenous colitis are characterized by abnormal histologic features in biopsy specimens, but no gross abnormalities are found by colonoscopy.[19-22] They tend to affect older patients, are not associated with rectal bleeding or intense abdominal pain, and do not develop into ulcerative colitis or Crohn's disease. Microscopic colitis and collagenous colitis respond to nonspecific antidiarrheals and often to antiinflammatory agents, such as sulfasalazine or prednisone. Two rare forms of inflammatory bowel disease are eosinophilic gastroenteritis and ulcerative jejunitis, which usually present as malabsorption syndrome. Diverticulitis is another form of colonic inflammation that can be associated with diarrhea; this occurs more often in the setting of an acute exacerbation, but occasionally it can be chronic.

Several *malignancies* can cause chronic diarrhea. These include villous adenoma of the rectum, colon cancer, lymphoma, carcinoid tumors and various hormone-secreting tumors, such as vipoma, gastrinoma, glucagonoma, and medullary carcinoma of the thyroid. Villous adenoma and colon cancer can be discovered by colonoscopy or barium enema. Lymphomas that cause chronic diarrhea usually involve the small intestine and can usually be found by radiography (small bowel studies and computed tomography [CT] scans). Carcinoid tumors and other hormone-secreting tumors can be diagnosed by finding the tumors on CT scan or by finding elevated levels of circulating humoral mediators (such as vasoactive intestinal polypeptide [VIP], gastrin, glucagon, or calcitonin) or metabolic products (such as urinary 5-hydroxyindoleacetic acid [5-HIAA] excretion). These secretory tumors are rare, and care must be taken not to overinterpret elevated blood levels of these hormones, because false-positives are more common than true-positives.

When the patient has dramatic and continuing weight loss in the setting of chronic diarrhea, attention should focus on the possibility of *maldigestion or malabsorption*. The problem with absorption may be limited to only one class of nutrients, such as carbohydrate or fat, or it may be generalized. Evidence of malabsorption syndrome is usually only found in patients with generalized malabsorption due to mucosal disease of the small intestine or pancreatic exocrine insufficiency. More limited forms of malabsorption such as lactase deficiency or bile acid malabsorption usually present with only excess gas or diarrhea and not a broader constellation of symptoms.

The key to diagnosing malabsorption is a quantitative stool collection. Patients need not be on a set intake of fat, but calorie and fat intake should be monitored so that the efficiency of absorption can be calculated (i.e., the percent of intake that is not excreted). It is now clear that diarrhea can cause an elevation of fat excretion, and so minor degrees of "steatorrhea" (<14 g/d) are not necessarily indicative of serious malabsorption.[23] Carbohydrate[24] and protein losses can be measured as well, but these measurements have not gained widespread clinical acceptance. Carbohydrate malabsorption can be recognized by acid stools (pH <5.3) and the presence of an osmotic gap in stool water (calculated by doubling the sum of fecal sodium plus potassium concentrations and subtracting this from 290, the osmolality of stool water within the body; values >50 mOsm/kg suggest osmotic diarrhea).[25]

If steatorrhea is present, the differential diagnosis includes mucosal diseases of the small intestine, such as celiac sprue, Whipple's disease, or lymphangiectasia; bacterial overgrowth in the small intestine; and pancreatic exocrine insufficiency. Biopsy of the small intestine, quantitative culture of small bowel contents, Schilling test with intrinsic factor, breath hydrogen testing after a glucose load (and more exotic breath tests), and stool chymotrypsin concentration may help sort out these possibilities. Formal pancreatic exocrine function studies are rarely needed, and a well-conducted empiric trial of pancreatic enzyme replacement therapy may be performed instead. This should include high doses of a potent supplement and quantitation of stool fat before and after therapy. Treatment of maldigestion and malabsorption depends on the underlying cause of the problem and is dealt with elsewhere.

One malabsorption problem that may not be associated with steatorrhea or carbohydrate malabsorption is *bile acid malabsorption* due to ileal dysfunction. This usually presents as a secretory diarrhea due to inhibition of absorption or stimulation of secretion in the colon by unabsorbed bile acids. Although many patients with chronic diarrhea will have evidence of bile acid malabsorption, particularly when measured by sensitive tests, few develop high enough concentrations of bile acid in stool water to produce a secretory diarrhea by this mechanism. In most cases, bile acid malabsorption is an epiphenomenon to the diarrhea itself.[26,27] Since measurement of aqueous phase bile acid concentration is not readily available, empiric trials of a bile acid sequestering agent, such as cholestyramine, are worthwhile in patients with chronic secretory diarrheas. These trials are not often successful, however, and should be halted if no objective effect is apparent.

When all the preceding diagnoses have been excluded, but diarrhea continues, the patient can be said to have *chronic idiopathic diarrhea*.[20,28] In most of these cases, stool analysis is consistent with a secretory diarrhea, and diarrhea continues during a fast. Nevertheless, when intestinal absorption has been measured by perfusion studies, it may be largely intact. There is no proven explanation for this dichotomy. Clinically, these patients may develop hypokalemia and salt depletion, but diarrhea is usually moderate in amount (about 500 g/d). Empiric therapy with potent antidiarrheals, such as deodorized tincture of opium (5 to 20 drops before meals and at bedtime), can control diarrhea in some of these patients. A recent follow-up study suggests that diarrhea spontaneously abates after an average of 15 months in patients with chronic idiopathic diarrhea, and therefore attempts to diagnose or treat these patients with surgery should be avoided.[28]

REFERENCES

1. *Physicians' Desk Reference: Drug Interactions and Side Effects Index.* 45th ed. Oradell, NJ: Medical Economics Books; 1991:1085–1087.
2. Fine KD, Santa Ana CA, Fordtran JS. Diagnosis of magnesium-induced diarrhea. *N Engl J Med.* 1991;324:1012–1017.
3. Fine KD, Krejs GJ, Fordtran JS. Diarrhea. In: Sleisenger MH, Fordtran JS, eds. *Gastrointestinal Disease: Pathophysiology, Diagnosis, Management.* 5th ed. Philadelphia, Pa: WB Saunders Co; 1993:1043–1072.
4. Caspary WF. Diarrhea associated with carbohydrate malabsorption. *Clin Gastroenterol.* 1986;15:631–655.
5. Gorbach SL, Edelman R, eds. Traveler's diarrhea: National Institutes of Health consensus development conference. *Rev Infect Dis.* 1986;8(suppl 2):S109–S233.
6. Parsonnet J, Trock SC, Bopp CA, et al. Chronic diarrhea associated with drinking untreated water. *Ann Intern Med.* 1989;110:985–991.
7. Osterholm MT, MacDonald KL, White KE, et al. An outbreak of a newly recognized chronic diarrhea syndrome associated with raw milk consumption. *JAMA.* 1986;256:484–490.
8. Nostrant TT, Kumar NB, Appelman HD. Histopathology differentiates acute self-limited colitis from ulcerative colitis. *Gastroenterology.* 1987;92:319–328.
9. Casteel HB, Fiedorek SC. Oral rehydration therapy. *Pediatr Clin North Am.* 1990;37:295–311.
10. Drossman DA, Thompson WG. The irritable bowel syndrome: review and a graduated multicomponent treatment approach. *Ann Intern Med.* 1992;116:1009–1016.
11. Schiller LR. Fecal incontinence. In: Sleisenger MH, Fordtran JS, eds. *Gastrointestinal Diseases: Pathophysiology, Diagnosis, Treatment.* 5th ed. Philadelphia, Pa: WB Saunders Co, 1993:934–953.
12. Geer RJ, Richards WO, O'Dorisio TM, et al. Efficacy of octreotide acetate in treatment of severe postgastrectomy dumping syndrome. *Ann Surg.* 1990;212:678–687.
13. Hutcheon DF, Bayless TM, Gadacz TR. Postcholecystectomy diarrhea. *JAMA* 1979;241:823.
14. Arlow FL, Dekovich AA, Priest RJ, Beher WT. Bile acid-mediated postcholecystectomy diarrhea. *Arch Intern Med.* 1987;147:1327–1329.
15. Arrambide KA, Santa Ana CA, Schiller LR, Little KH, Santangelo WC, Fordtran JS. Loss of absorptive capacity for sodium chloride as a cause of diarrhea following partial ileal and right colon resection. *Dig Dis Sci.* 1989;34:193–201.
16. Morris AI, Turnberg LA. Surreptitious laxative abuse. *Gastroenterology.* 1979;77:780–786.
17. Bytzer P, Stokholm M, Andersen I, Klitgaard NA, Schaffalitzky De Muckadell OB. Prevalence of surreptitious laxative abuse in patients with diarrhoea of uncertain origin: a cost benefit analysis of a screening procedure. *Gut.* 1989;30:1379–1384.
18. Janda RC, Conklin JL, Mitros FA, Parsonnet J. Multifocal colitis associated with an epidemic of chronic diarrhea. *Gastroenterology.* 1991;100:458–464.
19. Lindstrom CG. "Collagenous colitis" with watery diarrhea: a new entity? *Pathol Eur.* 1976;11:87–89.
20. Read NW, Krejs GJ, Read MG, Santa Ana CA, Morawski SG, Fordtran JS. Chronic diarrhea of unknown origin. *Gastroenterology.* 1980;78:264–271.
21. Giardiello FM, Lazenby AJ, Bayless TM, et al. Lymphocytic (microscopic) colitis: clinicopathologic study of 18 patients and comparison to collagenous colitis. *Dig Dis Sci.* 1989;34:1730–1738.
22. Sylwestrowicz T, Kelly JK, Hwang WS, Shaffer EA. Collagenous colitis and microscopic colitis: the watery diarrhea-colitis syndrome. *Am J Gastroenterol.* 1989;84:763–768.
23. Fine KD, Fordtran JS. The effect of diarrhea on fecal fat excretion. *Gastroenterology.* 1992;102:1936–1939.
24. Hammer HF, Fine KD, Santa Ana CA, Porter JL, Schiller LR, Fordtran JS. Carbohydrate malabsorption: its measurement and its contribution to diarrhea. *J Clin Invest.* 1990;86:1936–1944.
25. Eherer AJ, Fordtran JS. Fecal osmotic gap and pH in experimental diarrhea of various causes. *Gastroenterology.* 1992;103:545–551.
26. Schiller LR, Hogan RB, Morawski SG, et al. The incidence and significance of bile acid malabsorption in patients with chronic idiopathic diarrhea. *Gastroenterology.* 1987;92:151–160.
27. Schiller LR, Bilhartz LE, Santa Ana CA, Fordtran JS. Comparison of endogenous and radiolabeled bile acid excretion in patients with idiopathic chronic diarrhea. *Gastroenterology.* 1990;98:1036–1043.
28. Afzalpurkar RG, Schiller LR, Little KH, Santangelo WC, Fordtran JS. The self-limited nature of chronic idiopathic diarrhea. *N Engl J Med.* 1992;327:1849–1852.

15
Fecal Incontinence
SUZANNE ROSE and ARNOLD WALD

Fecal incontinence, defined as the involuntary passage of stool after toilet training, is a socially limiting and embarrassing problem affecting all age groups. Since many patients are reluctant to disclose this problem to their families and physicians, and physicians are not aware that effective therapy may be available, significant numbers of patients may needlessly suffer from this condition.

Although fecal incontinence may occasionally occur in otherwise healthy individuals with acute diarrhea, chronic fecal incontinence is often due to a neurologic or muscular disorder affecting critical continence mechanisms. When patients seek medical attention because of this complaint, diagnostic studies to investigate the cause of incontinence may suggest effective treatment modalities to allow patients to resume normal productive lives.

ANORECTAL PHYSIOLOGY

The main task of the anorectum is storage of fecal material until elimination can take place at a socially acceptable time and place. The rectum serves as a reservoir, whereas the external anal sphincter, internal anal sphincter, and selected pelvic floor muscles help to control continence and elimination. Continence is maintained by a number of interacting mechanisms: ability to sense impending defecation and to differentiate gas, liquid, and solid stool; intact neuromuscular activity; and motivation to maintain continence.

The external anal sphincter (EAS) consists of three bundles of striated muscle surrounding the anal canal. This sphincter is partially contracted at rest but is capable of voluntary phasic and sustained contractions. The efferent innervation is from S-2, S-3, and S-4 of the spinal cord via the pudendal nerves. Increased abdominal pressure, as occurs with coughing and lifting, will increase the tonic pressure of the EAS. Scratching the perianal skin will elicit phasic contraction of the EAS, which is referred to as the "anal wink." Inhibition of the EAS during defecation facilitates the passage of stool. Voluntary responses of the EAS, which depend on afferent and efferent pathways from the rectum to the cerebral cortex, are also important for maintaining continence.

The puborectalis muscle (PRM) is a striated muscle that forms a sling around the anorectal junction to maintain a sharp angle between the rectum and anal canal. The significance of the anorectal angle in maintaining continence is somewhat controversial. The PRM receives efferent innervation from S-3 and S-4 of the spinal cord and, like the EAS, can be contracted by voluntary effort, which further narrows the anorectal angle. The strength of contraction of the PRM can be assessed by placing an examining finger over the posterior rim of the rectum and asking the patient to squeeze.

The internal anal sphincter (IAS) is a smooth muscle that receives its innervation from the enteric nervous system. This muscle is tonically contracted in the normal resting state and accounts for about 80% of resting tone of the anal canal. The IAS is inhibited during defecation and transiently relaxes in response to rectal distension.

PATHOPHYSIOLOGY OF FECAL INCONTINENCE

Although in some patients no associated risk factors or underlying diseases are identified as the cause of fecal incontinence, in others there may be a history of trauma, surgery, or neurogenic diseases. Abnormalities of continence mechanisms may include one or more of the following: impairment of rectal sensation, abnormal rectal compliance, and dysfunction of the anal sphincters or PRM (Table 15–1).

TABLE 15–1. ANORECTAL ABNORMALITIES ASSOCIATED WITH FECAL INCONTINENCE

CATEGORIES	RESERVOIR	SPHINCTERS	SENSATION
Anal trauma	N	A	N
Idiopathic	N	A	N
Diabetes	N	A	A
Proctitis	A	N	N
Neurogenic	N	A	A
Encopresis	N	N	A

A = abnormal most or all of the time, N = normal most or all of the time.

IMPAIRED RECTAL SENSATION

Perirectal stretch receptors can be activated by rectal filling to elicit a sensation of fullness or an urge to defecate. Impairment of this ability to sense rectal filling may contribute to incontinence in some patients since the normal warning that defecation is imminent is lost or blunted.

Physically and mentally impaired geriatric patients and children with encopresis may have decreased sensation as a result of megarectum associated with fecal impaction. Symptoms may persist after bowel cleansing and disimpaction. Neurologic conditions often associated with abnormal sensation include meningomyelocele, multiple sclerosis, insulin-dependent diabetes mellitus, and spinal cord injuries.

ABNORMAL RECTAL COMPLIANCE

Viscoelasticity of the rectum is due to the longitudinal muscle layer that allows for storage of fecal wastes until defecation should take place. Neurologically mediated factors may also contribute. Because of this elasticity, it is possible to distend a balloon in the rectum with volumes exceeding those possible in the sigmoid colon. Fecal impaction with "overflow diarrhea" is a frequent cause of incontinence in the institutionalized geriatric patient with megarectum. These patients may also have impaired rectal sensation. Likewise, most children with fecal incontinence have constipation and overflow soiling, which often is in association with megarectum.

Disorders that decrease compliance impair the storage function of the rectum and may also result in incontinence. These include inflammatory conditions affecting the rectum such as radiation and ulcerative proctitis, as well as ischemia and rectal surgery.

ANAL SPHINCTER DYSFUNCTION

Decreased resting or squeeze pressures in the anal canal can lead to incontinence; this may result from anal trauma or surgery and can occur in patients with meningomyelocele, multiple sclerosis, and diabetes mellitus.[1,2]

Schiller et al described decreased resting anal sphincter pressures in greater than 50% of diabetic patients with fecal incontinence, a finding confirmed by other studies.[3] Abnormalities of external sphincter function have also been observed, including decreased contractile strength and elevated thresholds of phasic contraction of the EAS in response to rectal distension.

Idiopathic fecal incontinence occurs primarily in middle-aged or elderly women. Denervation of the puborectalis muscle or the EAS has been demonstrated in many of these patients associated with pudendal neuropathy, perhaps by traction injury, as evidenced by electrophysiologic studies. This is thought to be due to repetitive and excessive pelvic floor descent during defecation over a long period of time. A similar phenomenon may occur in multiparous women with obstetric injury. Many of these patients have perineal descent and widening of the anorectal angle, indicating weakening of the striated muscles of the pelvic floor.

EFFECTS OF DIARRHEA

Only rarely does fecal incontinence occur with diarrhea in the absence of abnormal continence mechanisms. However, some individuals may have incontinence during an acute diarrheal illness. Diarrhea will stress normal continence mechanisms since liquid stool is more difficult to perceive and retain than is solid.

The causes of diarrhea in diabetic patients with incontinence are multifactorial. Suggested contributing factors include autonomic dysfunction, bacterial overgrowth, ingestion of hexitols that may cause an osmotic diarrhea, and pancreatic insufficiency. Diarrhea commonly occurs approximately 10 years after the diagnosis of diabetes is established. Incontinence may begin concomitantly or may follow some time later. Nocturnal incontinence without warning is characteristic in these patients. Diarrhea in incontinent diabetic patients is rarely of high volume, but several studies indicate that one or more abnormalities of continence are present in the vast majority of these patients.[1,3]

DIAGNOSTIC STUDIES

HISTORY AND PHYSICAL EXAMINATION

It is important to characterize stool patterns and to determine the frequency, duration, and pattern of incontinence. Inquiry should be made about daytime and nocturnal soiling and associated symptoms such as urgency, lack of warning, diarrhea, constipation, and straining. Possible contributory factors should be noted including previous anorectal surgery or trauma, childbirth involving forceps delivery or significant lacerations, inflammatory bowel disease, diabetes mellitus, multiple sclerosis or other neurologic conditions, and medications and dietary factors that may affect the stool. Psychosocial testing may be useful in some patients, especially children and occasionally the elderly.

The physical examination should include careful inspection of the perianal area. The perianal skin should be lightly scratched to elicit the anocutaneous reflex. Digital examination of the rectum will detect fecal impaction and assess the resting tone and squeeze pressures, although the latter may correlate poorly with manometric measurements in less-experienced hands. The strength of contraction of the PRM should also be assessed.

Initial studies may include sigmoidoscopy with possible biopsy to rule out mucosal inflammation, neoplasm, or ischemic changes. The rectum should be examined for the presence of solitary rectal ulcers. The evaluation of patients with chronic diarrhea should include stool studies to characterize the nature of the diarrhea. These may include quantitative 24- to 72-hour stool samples for volume with measurement of stool electrolytes, osmolality, and fat to determine if high-volume diarrhea is osmotic or secretory in nature.

ANORECTAL MANOMETRY

Anorectal manometry can quantitate resting and squeeze anal pressures, internal sphincter relaxation, rectal sensation, and compliance. After preparation with one or two enemas, a perfused catheter is inserted into the rectum. Resting and maximal anal sphincter pressures are then determined by station pull-through technique. The volume to inhibit IAS tone is assessed by successively inflating the rectal balloon at the end of the catheter until resting pressure is completely suppressed.

Rectal compliance may be measured using a catheter with a cylindrical balloon that is placed into the rectum and incrementally inflated with air. Allowances are made for pressures within the balloon by subtracting pressures when the balloon is inflated with the same volume ex vivo.

DEFECOGRAPHY AND PROCTOGRAPHY

Anorectal radiographs have been used to evaluate some patients with fecal incontinence. Lateral views of the anorectum filled with barium provide information about the anorectal angle and the location of the anorectal angle relative to the pelvic floor. Defecography involves rapid-sequence radiographs or video during evacuation of barium paste while the patient is sitting on a radiolucent commode. The patient may be evaluated at rest, with squeeze, and with defecation of the barium paste. An estimation of the anorectal angle and change of the angle with squeeze effort can be made. These studies have potential limitations but also offer a qualitative assessment of the PRM and assessment of adequacy of rectal emptying. The role of such studies in evaluating patients with fecal soiling and defecatory disorders is unclear at the present time.

ANORECTAL ELECTROMYOGRAPHY

Anorectal electromyography (EMG) can determine if there is an abnormality of striated muscle and whether it is associated with damage to the pudendal nerve. EMG studies of the PRM and EAS in idiopathic fecal incontinence indicate that these patients often have evidence of denervation injury to these muscles.

EMG involves placing a needle electrode percutaneously into the EAS or PRM to analyze the motor unit potentials of these muscles. A surface electrode has also been used to evaluate the EAS; although there are concerns about this technique, it does offer the advantage of a painless examination. The conduction velocity of the distal pudendal nerve can also be determined by stimulating the nerve on digital examination with an electrode attached to a glove. These studies are available in many centers but largely remain a research tool.

TREATMENT

Three modalities, alone or in combination, have proved useful in the treatment of fecal incontinence. These are dietary modification and pharmacologic intervention, biofeedback, and surgery.

DIET AND PHARMACOLOGIC AGENTS

Dietary modifications may be helpful to the patient with chronic diarrhea. These consist of exclusion of lactose-containing foods in patients with lactose intolerance, fructose-containing foods in fructose intolerance, and elimination of hexitol-containing foods that may cause an osmotic diarrhea (Table 15–2). Magnesium-containing antacids should be avoided as they may cause diarrhea. Fiber supplements may help some patients, perhaps by increasing the consistency of the stool, although this remains unproven.

Opiate derivatives such as loperamide or diphenoxylate with atropine may reduce fecal incontinence associated with diarrhea. Improvement may be due to decreased stool volume and frequency, a more formed fecal consistency, or a direct effect on anorectal function. One study has shown that codeine and loperamide were more effective than diphenoxylate with atropine in reducing soiling in patients with chronic diarrhea.[4] Another concluded that loperamide may increase anal sphincter pressures in addition to increasing stool consistency and decreasing stool volume.[5] Loperamide together with a low-fiber diet may be effective in the treatment of neurogenic incontinence, perhaps by decreasing stool frequency and volume and increasing stool consistency. Weekly enemas or a bisacodyl suppository promote colonic evacuation to prevent impaction in these conditions.

Phosphate enemas (4.5 oz or more) or warm tap water enemas (1 qt administered by a bag drip) may be used to treat fecal incontinence associated with megarectum. In elderly or physically immobilized patients, enemas should be given once or twice daily until there is no stool left in the rectal vault and colon. Occasionally, it is necessary to use a mineral oil enema to soften a hard impaction. When evacuation is complete, enemas should be given on a regular intermittent basis, perhaps with bisacodyl suppositories, to maintain colonic evacuation and prevent further impactions.

The management of children with encopresis starts with colonic and rectal evacuation. Initially, enemas should be employed to accomplish this task. Once evacuation is attained, lactulose or mineral oil may be given on a daily basis orally in a sufficient dose to produce soft yet formed stools daily. This therapy should be combined with a bowel retraining behavioral program. The child should sit on the toilet 20 minutes after a meal with his legs supported by a stepstool. This is done to take advantage of the gastrocolic reflex. A calendar is kept to record the patterns of defecation and soiling. The patient should receive positive reinforcement and punishment should be avoided. Office visits should be frequent for assessment of progress. Formal psychotherapy should be considered if behavioral problems are perceived, especially in patients who do not respond to treatment or those who have incontinence without constipation or fecal impaction. Tapering and eventual discontinuation of the lactulose can take place 6 to 12 months after continence has been achieved.

BIOFEEDBACK

Biofeedback is an operant conditioning technique based on the work of Engel et al[6] which may be an effective treatment for incontinence. It requires sufficient motivation, comprehension of and ability to follow directions, some degree of rectal sensation, and the capacity to generate a squeeze pressure (Table 15–3).

One method uses a three-balloon manometer. Patients are instructed to watch the recording of the sphincteric responses on a visual display. The rectal balloon is inflated with volumes of air and the patient learns to recognize this as rectal distension (sensory discrimination). The smallest volume of distension sensed by the patient is de-

TABLE 15–2. SUBSTANCES HIGH IN FRUCTOSE AND SORBITOL

FRUCTOSE	SORBITOL
Apple juice	Apple juice
Pear juice	Pear juice
Soft drinks	Sugar-free gum
Grape juice	Sugar-free candy
Cranberry juice	Some antacids
	Some elixirs

TABLE 15–3. INDICATIONS FOR AND CONTRAINDICATIONS TO BIOFEEDBACK IN FECAL INCONTINENCE

INDICATIONS	CONTRAINDICATIONS
Anal sphincter weakness	Dementia
Obstetric damage	Spinal cord injuries
Idiopathic	Absent rectal sensation
Diabetes mellitus	Poor motivation
Meningomyelocele (few)	Impaired rectal storage

termined, and then progressively smaller distension volumes are administered to try to lower the threshold of sensation. The volume is progressively decreased until no further improvement occurs.

The patient is also taught to increase pressures on the external sphincter balloon by squeezing the muscle in response to rectal distension while using visual feedback from the manometric recording. This process is then repeated without the visual cues using decreasing volumes of distension until the threshold of sensation is reached. Patients are instructed to practice contracting the EAS and to use the technique when sensing rectal distension or urgency. Most adult patients respond after a single session with follow-up sessions rarely necessary.

Other methods involve using a pneumatic device or an intraanal plug. Although these techniques do not attempt to synchronize sphincter contraction with rectal distension, they appear to be successful. They offer the advantages of use by the patient at home with less supervised technician time and reduced use of the hospital setting.

None of the biofeedback techniques have been studied by controlled protocols but the encouraging reports from multiple centers are helpful. Controlled studies of biofeedback are necessary to evaluate this treatment modality. All biofeedback techniques offer the possibility of improvement without risk to the patient.

SURGERY

In general, surgery should be considered only after medical, pharmacologic, and biofeedback techniques have failed. The one exception is gross rectal prolapse, since surgical resuspension restores continence in approximately half these patients.

The large number of surgical procedures advocated for fecal incontinence suggests that no single technique is best for all cases. Obstetric injuries, trauma, and acute disruption of the sphincter are best managed by direct primary repair. Most repairs, however, are performed at a time remote from any identifiable injury or in the absence of an identifiable cause. Surgical approaches include restoration of the anorectal angle by repair of the puborectalis and pubococcygeus muscles. Anal encirclement procedures, artificial sphincter implantation, and muscle transpositions have also been described.

Approximately 80% of patients will regain continence of solid stool after sphincter repair with poorer results with liquid stool. Since poor surgical results are associated with a neuropathy of the pelvic floor, preoperative EMG and nerve conduction studies may help to identify those patients who may have limited success with this operation.

Postanal repair has been used to treat patients with a poorly functioning but anatomically intact sphincter. The levator ani, PRM, and EAS are plicated posteriorly to restore the anorectal angle and tighten the anal canal. Early studies from the United Kingdom reported that continence was satisfactory in 80% of patients,[7] but recent studies indicate less satisfactory results. An anterior repair has been described in one study as showing a satisfactory outcome in 62% of patients with idiopathic fecal incontinence and 71% of patients with fecal incontinence caused by trauma.[8]

Anal encirclement uses a silver wire or, more recently, a Silastic sling or rod to mechanically tighten the anus to provide a passive barrier to the passage of feces. These procedures often are unsatisfactory with frequent complications including infection, impaction, and erosion of the encircling material.

An implantable artificial sphincter consisting of an inflatable cuff filled with fluid from a balloon controlled by a subcutaneous pump has been described. This is inserted in the anal canal and may be complicated by infection and sepsis or erosion of the prosthetic cuff through the anal canal.

Skeletal muscle transpositions using the gluteus maximus, gracilis, or palmaris longus muscles have been performed for fecal incontinence. Transposition of the gracilis muscle was first described in 1952,[9] in which the gracilis muscle is mobilized to preserve the proximal attachments and maintain the neurovascular supply. An implantable nerve stimulator may be used to achieve sustained contraction.

ALTERNATIVE THERAPIES

Several plugs made of polyurethane sponge and wrapped in a water-soluble coat have been described. The plug is inserted into the anal canal and with dissolution of the water-soluble coat, the plug expands to act as a physical barrier to the passage of fecal material.

Colostomy is reserved for failures of medical, biofeedback, and surgical techniques. Colostomy has been advocated for patients with immobility who suffer from severe skin breakdown and complications including sepsis related to fecal incontinence.

CONCLUSION

Fecal incontinence can be a distressing and devastating symptom that may result from a number of disease processes that affect the anorectum and pelvic floor. It is important to understand the pathophysiology of incontinence and to recognize specific abnormalities using objective tests of anorectal function. Treatment can be chosen from a number of modalities to improve function and quality of life.

REFERENCES

1. Caruana BJ, Wald A, Hinds JP, et al. Anorectal sensory and motor function in neurogenic fecal incontinence. *Gastroenterology.* 1991;100:465–470.
2. Wald A, Tunuguntla AK. Anorectal sensorimotor dysfunction in fecal incontinence and diabetes mellitus: modification with biofeedback therapy. *N Engl J Med.* 1984;310:1282–1287.
3. Schiller LR, Santa Ana CA, Schmulen AC, et al. Pathogenesis of fecal incontinence in diabetes mellitus, evidence for internal-anal-sphincter dysfunction. *N Engl J Med.* 1982;307:1666–1671.
4. Palmer KR, Corbett CL, Holdsworth CD. Double-blind cross-over study comparing loperamide codeine and diphenoxylate in the treatment of chronic diarrhea. *Gastroenterology.* 1980;79:1272–1275.
5. Read M, Read NW, Barber DC, et al. Effects of loperamide on anal sphincter function in patients complaining of chronic diarrhea and fecal incontinence and urgency. *Dig Dis Sci.* 1982;27:807–814.
6. Engel BT, Nikoomanesh P, Schuster MM. Operant conditioning of rectosphincteric responses in the treatment of fecal incontinence. *N Engl J Med.* 1974;190:646–649.
7. Browning GGP, Parks AG. Postanal repair for neuropathic faecal incontinence: correlation of clinical results and anal canal pressures. *Br J Surg.* 1983;70:101–104.
8. Miller R, Orrom WJ, Cornes H, et al. Anterior sphincter plication and levatorplasty in the treatment of faecal incontinence. *Br J Surg.* 1989;76:1058–1060.
9. Pickrell KL, Broadbent TR, Masters FW, et al. Construction of a rectal sphincter and restoration of anal continence by transplanting the gracilis muscle; report of four cases in children. *Ann Surg.* 1952;135:853–862.

16

Chronic Constipation

JAMES C. REYNOLDS and CHRISTOPHER WILLIAMS

Motility disorders of the colon are among the most common entities for which patients seek medical attention, representing a significant diagnostic and therapeutic challenge for the clinician, as well as a formidable economic burden on society in health care dollars and employee absenteeism.[1] Functional bowel disorders are responsible for over 40% of office visits to the gastroenterologist and affect 8% to 17% of the general population with no age constraints.[2–4] The presenting signs and symptoms are often indistinct and rarely pinpoint a specific cause or pathophysiologic mechanism, with abdominal pain being the most common symptom and altered stool frequency or consistency the most common consequence. Manifestations range from a mild intermittent nuisance to a life-threatening condition or complication.

Constipation may result from primary disorders of the large intestine or result from a more generalized process. The major primary functional colonic causes of constipation are idiopathic constipation, impaired rectoanal inhibitory reflex (RAIR), or adult Hirschsprung's disease spastic pelvic floor syndrome, the irritable bowel syndrome (IBS), acute and chronic intestinal pseudoobstruction, and diverticulosis.

Systemic diseases that may impair colonic motility (i.e., secondary motility disorders) include collagen vascular diseases, infectious diseases, inherited neuromuscular disorders, metabolic diseases, neuropathic disorders, and pregnancy (see Table 16–1). A number of medications also affect colonic motility and may result in constipation, including anticholinergic, antineoplastic, cardiovascular, cation-containing, central nervous system (CNS), and opiate analgesics (see Table 16–1). A complete medication history should be taken for each patient with constipation, including all prescription and over-the-counter medications. The patient's functional disorder may completely abate with removal of an offending medication.

Patients with constipation should undergo a thorough history and physical examination (including neurologic evaluation), laboratory studies (including those related to specific secondary causes of abnormal motility), and flexible sigmoidoscopy. Evaluation of the entire colon with either barium enema or colonoscopy to rule out mucosal or structural lesions, should be considered in most patients with new onset of constipation and in all patients over age 35 or with a family history of colonic neoplasms. In addition to excluding a structural problem, a thorough evaluation should distinguish between primary and secondary colonic motility abnormalities. A thorough evaluation may also reveal complications of the patient's underlying motility disorder such as diverticular disease, stercoral ulcers, rectal prolapse, rectal fissures, melanosis coli, or hemorrhoids before they become overtly evident through bleeding, infection, or perforation.

Because of the wide variability in the cause of constipation, the key to optimal treatment is elucidation of the mechanisms underlying the al-

TABLE 16–1. CAUSES OF COLONIC MOTILITY DISORDERS: SYSTEMIC AND MEDICATION

Systemic Causes	*Constipating Medications*
Collagen vascular disease	Anticholinergic medications
Scleroderma	Antihistamines
Mixed connective tissue disease	Antispasmodics
Amyloidosis	Antidepressants (tricyclics, MAOIs)
Infectious diseases	Antipsychotics (phenothiazines)
Chagas disease	Antineoplastic agents
Metabolic diseases	Vinca alkaloids
Thyroid disease	Cardiovascular medications
Disorders of calcium metabolism	Calcium-channel blockers
Parathyroid disease	Ganglionic blockers
Malignancies	b-Adrenergic antagonists
Porphyria	Clonidine
Inherited neuromuscular diseases	Diuretics (hypokalemia)
Familial visceral myopathy	Cation-containing drugs
Familial autonomic neuropathy	Calcium, iron, barium
Neurofibromatosis	Antacids (magnesium, aluminum, calcium)
Neuropathic disorders	Sucralfate
Diabetes mellitus	Central nervous system medications
Multiple sclerosis	Anticonvulsants
Spinal cord disease	Antiparkinsonian drugs (anticholinergic effect)
Disk disease	Opiates
Tumor	Other
Trauma	Prokinetic agents
Familial and sporadic visceral myopathies or neuropathies	Oral hypoglycemics
	Colchicine
Muscular dystrophy	Prostaglandin analogs and inhibitors (NSAIDs, misoprostol)
Neurofibromatosis	Cholestyramine
Paraneoplastic syndromes	
Pregnancy	

MAOI = monoamine oxidase inhibitor, NSAIDs = nonsteroidal antiinflammatory drugs.

tered colonic motility, which will result in development of a more specific and efficacious treatment plan. Since our current understanding of the specific pathophysiology of disordered colonic function is limited, current treatment modalities are largely symptomatic rather than disease specific, being rather crude means of enhancing or impairing bowel storage function.

With this in mind, therapy generally consists of alterations of diet, lifestyle, and medications, though certain conditions in selected patients may require chronic medical therapy or even surgery. In every case, the regimen should be tailored to the patient's presentation, including consideration of the duration and severity of symptoms and the extent of physiologic impairment. Therapeutic safety and efficacy should always be the primary goal. A majority of patients improve considerably with the addition of bulk to their fiber-deficient diet.[5-8] As noted above, if the patient is taking medications known to adversely affect motility, these should be discontinued, whenever possible. Often, substitutions can be made that will benefit the colonic motility (e.g., nonsteroidal antiinflammatory drugs [NSAIDs] for narcotic analgesics, or a less-constipating serotonin-antagonist antidepressant like trazodone or fluoxetine for anticholinergic-predominant tricyclics). Magnesium-containing antacids or an H_2 receptor antagonist can be substituted for aluminum-containing antacids or sucralfate in patients with constipation. As colonic transit time has been shown to accelerate with moderate exercise, the addition of an exercise program appropriate for the patient's age and cardiovascular status may have a direct positive effect. Exercise may also improve stress-induced effects on motility and enhance the patient's sense of well being.[9]

In developing a treatment plan for the patient with constipation, the clinician must consider the predisposing factors, underlying pathophysiologic mechanisms, safety and efficacy of the therapeutic options, and degree of impairment to the patient's quality of life attributable to the constipation. Recommendation to reduce excessive stress and establish a time of day to relax and gently attempt a bowel movement is often recommended. Although these measures can often be beneficial, further intervention is often necessary to regulate the bowels. The ideal agent should, in addition to promoting colonic evacuation, have the following characteristics:

1. Efficacy for both acute decompensation and chronic symptoms
2. Promotion of return to normal bowel function and reduction of dependency on further treatment
3. Reduction of accompanying bloating and pain
4. A favorable safety profile
5. A cost acceptable for chronic use

The best approach to patients with minimal symptoms is to withhold unproven, ineffective, or potentially harmful agents.

An ever-increasing number of products with several distinct mechanisms of action have been advocated for use alone or in combination for treatment of chronic constipation.[10] As the list of available agents continues to grow, selecting a proper medication may seem unnecessarily confusing. Selection and application of a specific therapy is based on understanding its mechanisms of action, knowing the particular clinical characteristics of the patients constipation, and tailoring therapy to the individual's needs. Certain agents that are occasionally useful for treatment of IBS, such as those containing anticholinergic compounds or phenobarbital, have no defined role for treatment of constipation and may actually be harmful. Several broad categories of agents used to treat constipation will be discussed in further detail: (1) dietary fiber, (2) laxatives and cathartics, (3) prokinetic agents, and (4) enemas. In addition, endoscopic and surgical interventions will be reviewed.

DIETARY FIBER

Enhancement of dietary fiber intake in conjunction with adequate fluid intake is the cornerstone of the medical management of constipating disorders. Several epidemiologic studies have suggested that inadequate dietary fiber intake is a major cause of colonic pathologic conditions, including constipation.[5,11] Burkitt and colleagues[5] have shown that colon cancer, diverticulosis, and other disorders endemic to the United States occur very rarely in people living in countries in which dietary fiber intake results in up to 500 g of stool daily (versus 100 g/d in Western countries). Constipation is quite rare in these countries, with individuals often passing several large bowel movements per day. Addition of fiber to the diet of persons with milder forms of constipation increases the bulk and frequency of stools and may alleviate associated discomfort.[6,8,11–13] Adding 10 to 15 g of fiber to the diet, either in the form of supplements or additional high-fiber foods, will benefit many patients with constipation. This regimen may be used chronically without adverse effect. The patient should be led to understand that the ingested fiber is not a medication, but the addition of a natural substance in which their diet is deficient. A high-fiber diet, therefore, should be initiated in most patients with constipation.[8,10]

Several important limitations to the use of fiber must be appreciated. It is important to note that a high-fiber diet not be initiated if the colon remains impacted with stool or when obstructive symptoms are present. Fiber should be used with caution in patients with a diffuse gastrointestinal motility disorder accompanied by severe gastroparesis or absence of migrating motor complexes (MMCs), as bezoars have been reported to occur in this situation. Patients should also be instructed that they may experience increased symptoms of bloating and gas with introduction of fiber into the diet, but that these side effects will dissipate over 1 to 2 weeks. Fiber diets may lead to excessive colonic gas in selected patients. A reduction in beans, broccoli, cauliflower, and cabbage may be necessary.

LAXATIVES AND CATHARTICS

Most laxatives and cathartics work to facilitate defecation through a net increase in the water content of the stool or promotion of propagating contractions. The water content of the stool is increased by osmotic trapping of solute, inhibition of absorption, stimulation of secretion, or adsorption of water to hydrophilic substances. Contact laxatives may increase stool water content by increasing mucosal permeability, perhaps through direct damage to the epithelium or intercellular junctions.[14] Motility is enhanced by direct irritation of intramural sensory nerves, reflex-induced contractions in response to stretch receptor stimulation in the presence of increased bulk, and increased frequency of mass movements that propel intraluminal contents from the right colon. Transit may also be improved through laxative-induced increase of substances which promote gut motility, such as cholecystokinin, prostaglandins, vasoactive intestinal polypeptide, and cyclic AMP. The ability to design the most effective therapies will be enhanced by a greater insight into the specific mechanisms by which these agents work. A detailed explanation of the mechanism of action of these agents is beyond the scope of this article and has been reviewed elsewhere.[10]

Although laxatives are still among the most potent drugs available to treat constipation, routine daily use of these agents should be strongly discouraged and considered potentially harmful. Patients with impactions and severe constipation may have severe pain induced by potent laxatives, whose mode of action develops pressure proximal to the point of relative obstruction. Available data suggest that the safety of these agents must be questioned when used on a long-term basis for a condition that is a chronic, daily problem. Melanosis coli, a striking black discoloration of the colonic mucosa, has been correlated with the chronic use of anthraquinone cathartics and may be related to increased endothelial permeability produced by irritant laxatives.[15] The long-term health implications of this lesion are not certain, but the discoloration can persist for years after the laxative is discontinued. Histologic data from animals and man suggest that the chronic use of some laxatives may also result in damage to the intrinsic enteric nervous system (in particular, the myenteric plexus) of the colon.[16,17] These and other observations have led to the following warning in the package insert of several popular irritant laxatives: "Frequent or prolonged use of this or any other laxative may result in dependence on laxatives."

The term *cathartic colon* has been coined to describe the colonic dysfunction associated with chronic laxative use with the implication that the laxative use was causally related to development of the colonic disturbance.[17–19] Since most patients suffered from constipation prior to the use of laxatives, this causal relationship has been questioned. Laxatives have been used inappropriately, however, by patients with a normal frequency of bowel movements to reduce caloric intake and control weight. This variant of bulimia can result in a marked disruption of a previously normal bowel habit.[18] Patients with these eating disorders may also develop gastroparesis, even in the absence of laxative abuse. The contribution of malnutrition, thyroid disturbances, and fiber deprivation to the acquisition of motility disorders by these patients must be considered.

The available data indicating adverse effects from prolonged use of irritant laxatives strongly suggests that further studies are needed to evaluate their safety and efficacy when used for chronic treatment of constipation. The possibility that the physician may be recommending a treatment that could worsen the underlying condition conflicts with the first dictum of medicine, to "do no harm." Until the safety of these agents is established, the use of irritant laxatives should be restricted to patients with acute symptoms. The judicious use of a cathartic or purgative once every 2 to 3 weeks, however, may be safely recommended to avoid the development of impactions and reduce the intraluminal diameter to a degree that will permit the circular muscle to generate more effective contractions. Alternating various laxatives reduces the likelihood of developing potential adverse effects that could accompany the use of a single agent over a prolonged period.

Other agents effective in the acute setting must also be used with caution in patients with chronic disease. Mineral oil may bind to fat-soluble vitamins, inhibiting their absorption. Its use is not infrequently complicated by soiling or incontinence. As with other medicinal oils, when taken at bedtime it may be aspirated with development of lipoid pneumonia.

Although questions exist as to the safety of the more potent laxatives, the efficacy of stool softeners is even less certain. Docusate sodium and related surface-acting compounds are thought to act by increasing the water content of the stool. Although the mechanisms of action were evaluated in animal models many years ago, this extremely popular agent was evaluated in a double-blind controlled study in man only recently. Two studies were unable to demonstrate any improvement by docusate in stool water content, colonic transit, after time, or any other objective measures of efficacy using currently recommended doses compared with placebo.[21]

Osmotic laxatives provide a safe, gentle, and effective treatment for the vast majority of patients with constipation. Magnesium salts, lactulose, and polyethylene glycol-based electrolyte-balanced solutions are the most widely used osmotic laxatives. Although manganese citrate can result in effective bowel cleansing, it is often associated with abdominal bloating and cramping. Magnesium hydroxide solutions are more gentle and better tolerated.

Polyethylene glycol saline lavage solutions (GoLytely, Nulyte, CoLyte, and others) are particularly effective in patients with refractory constipation and are generally well tolerated for intermittent purging. Patients with cardiac or renal insufficiency should be monitored for evidence of fluid overload or electrolyte abnormalities.[20] The chronic use of magnesium-containing laxatives, particularly in the presence of renal insufficiency, may lead to hypermagnesemia with resulting muscle weakness, sedation, mental status changes, and electrocardiogram (ECG) abnormalities. Lactulose is another relatively safe osmotic laxative, even with chronic use in the elderly. Lactulose is frequently associated with bloating and increased flatulence, however, and was shown to be only marginally beneficial relative to placebo in a recent review.[22]

PROKINETIC AGENTS

Prokinetic medications enhance normal, neurally mediated propulsive contractions of the bowel and are thus intuitively more appealing than the use of agents whose efficacy is the result of irritation of local nerves or alteration of the integrity of mucosal barriers. Cholinomimetics such as bethanechol have been used to promote bowel contractility with variable success. The stimulation of muscarinic receptors would be expected to enhance contractile amplitude and reduce the stimulus threshold for peristaltic reflexes. Cholinesterase inhibitors (e.g., neostigmine) have been recommended for the same reasons, and are often associated with fewer systemic side effects.[23] Although cholinomimetics can increase contractive amplitude, they do not increase the frequency or characteristic of peristaltic contraction and thus are not true "prokinetic" agents. Furthermore, their efficacy in chronic constipation has been questioned.

Prokinetic agents represent the newest class of medications that enhance the intrinsic motor functions of the gut.[24] Metoclopramide, the prototypical prokinetic agent, is useful in the treatment of gastroparesis and gastroesophageal reflux disease. Motility is enhanced by promotion of acetylcholine release from enteric nerves and blockade of dopamine receptors. Although metoclopramide induces colonic contractions, it is rarely useful in the treatment of constipated patients except when upper intestinal symptoms predominate. The use and dosage of metoclopramide are limited because athetoid movements, tremors, or sedation are seen in up to 20% of patients; it must be used with particular care in the elderly. Second- and third-generation prokinetic agents, such as domperidone and cisapride, promise to have fewer side effects and be more applicable to the full gamut of bowel motility disorders.[24,25] In preliminary studies, cisapride has been found to be effective in managing some patients who were intractable to other treatments.

Endogenous opioid compounds have been shown to be among the most abundant neurotransmitters in the gut and contribute to the mechanisms that mediate the gastrocolic reflex. Kreek et al[26] were able to reverse chronic severe constipation in two patients by the intravenous infusion of the opioid antagonist naloxone. Long-acting oral opioid antagonists (e.g., naltrexone) are presently being investigated for possible future application in the treatment of chronic constipation.

The efficacy of other putative prokinetic agents including macrolides, the somatostatin analog sandostatin, and leuprolide is currently being investigated for use in chronic severe constipation.

USE OF ENEMAS

Enemas containing a variety of agents have been effective in the treatment of chronic constipation. A retention enema of mildly warm tap water is the safest and easiest to use. Although normal patients often obtain an effective elimination with an enema volume of 250 ml, chronically constipated patients may require four times this volume. Reassurance must be given to the patient who may become anxious when unable to eliminate the enema fluid; this is a hallmark of the patient with severe disease and is a strong argument against the use of more irritant laxative mixtures such as soapsuds. The latter has been reported to cause a chemically induced colitis. Although messy, mineral oil enemas may be necessary for the patient with a particularly inspissated stool. When all else fails, a milk and molasses enema is almost always effective and is surprisingly well tolerated.

SURGICAL APPROACHES TO CHRONIC CONSTIPATION

Certain constipating disorders may be successfully dealt with endoscopically or surgically if conservative medical management fails. These include acute colonic pseudoobstruction (Ogilvie's syndrome), impaired RAIR or adult Hirschsprung's disease, and chronic, debilitating constipation due to delayed transit that is unresponsive or refractory to medical treatment.

Impaired RAIR or an adult variant of Hirschsprung's disease is present in 8% to 10% of patients with severe constipation.[27,28] For these patients, posterior anal sphincter myomectomy may provide treatment.[27–31] Every patient with chronic severe constipation should undergo anorectal manometry to exclude isolated RAIR dysfunction. The diagnosis of impaired RAIR, or short segment Hirschsprung's disease, must be made with caution in patients with chronic constipation, particularly in the presence of rectal distension. A falsely abnormal test may occur if the volume of insufflation in the rectal balloon is insufficient. Of patients with unequivocal evidence of anal sphincter dysfunction (with or without aganglionosis), treated with a limited posterior myotomy, excellent outcome can be expected.[27,29,31] The indiscriminate use of surgical anal myomectomy for all patients with chronic severe constipation, however, is only beneficial in one third of patients and will result in complications such as incontinence of stool in another third.[28] Children over 10 years of age and adults rarely require the more extensive Soave or Duhamel procedures required in children with classic Hirschsprung's disease.[28,31,32] Patients with functional rectal obstruction at the level of the pelvic floor ("spastic pelvic floor syndrome" or "anismus") rarely respond well to surgical attempts at correction through ablation of the rectal sling, but they may be amenable to biofeedback training.[33,34]

The role of colectomy in patients with idiopathic chronic severe constipation is not clear. It is essential that a thorough physiologic investigation be performed prior to surgery to select patients who can reasonably be expected to benefit.[35,39] Early in this century, colectomy was performed for "autointoxication" and other vague maladies thought to result from "stasis" (constipation) at a time when the procedure involved a high mortality.[33] At present, there is some consensus of opinion regarding the futility of a limited colonic resection, as the result is often complicated by a high rate of anastomotic leaks.[40,41] The procedure of choice for patients with incapacitating chronic constipation associated with documented colonic inertia or delayed colonic transit is a subtotal colectomy with ileorectal anastomosis.[35–41] In properly selected patients with normal preoperative gastroesophageal and small bowel function, this procedure produces excellent results with minimal diarrhea that usually improves with time. Mortality associated with the procedure is about 2%, with a complication rate of greater than 20%. However, lower morbidity and mortality may be obtained with scrupulous preoperative colonic cleansing with enemas and several gallons of polyethylene glycol purgative (GoLytely or CoLyte). Patient satisfaction with the procedure has generally been high (90% to 100%).[35,37,39] Less satisfactory results are obtained in patients with evidence of widespread motility disorders (e.g., esophageal spasm, lower esophageal sphincter [LES] dysfunction, gastroparesis, or megaduodenum).[40-42]

TREATMENT OF ACUTE COLONIC PSEUDOOBSTRUCTION

Ogilvie's syndrome, characterized clinically by abdominal distension, decreased bowel sounds, and tympany, is usually associated with radiographic segmental colonic distension greater than 9 cm. There are a variety of predisposing factors, the most common of which include medications, surgery, serious infection, neurologic disorders, obstructive lung disease (and particularly mechanical ventilation), cardiac disease, metabolic derangement, and hip fracture. Mechanical obstruction should be considered and ruled out with a water-soluble contrast enema or colonoscopy. Conservative treatment with placement of nasogastric and rectal tubes, metabolic corrections, and discontinuation of possible offending medications have been reported successful in up to 70% of patients, with recurrence in one third who initially respond.[43-47] The diameter of segmental dilation should be closely monitored by abdominal film every 8 to 12 hours for the first few days.[43] The potential for perforation and abdominal catastrophe must be recognized, especially when cecal diameter exceeds 9 to 12 cm or left colon diameter exceeds 10 cm. Distension to this degree or beyond require elective decompression.

Surgical decompression by tube cecostomy was previously considered the treatment of choice, although it may be associated with greater than 20% mortality.[45-47] Kukora and Dent[45] were the first to report effective colonoscopic decompression of acute colonic pseudoobstruction in 1977. Subsequently, this approach has become accepted as an alternative to surgical decompression in the nonperforated colon.[46-51] However, the unprepped colon filled with thick, viscid fecal material makes the procedure quite difficult and potentially risky; air insufflation should be minimized. Some advocate gentle preparation of the colon with repeated saline enemas prior to an attempt at decompression to significantly improve visibility.[45,46,48] Complications are relatively rare with appropriate caution, although mortality for the procedure of 2% to 5% is characteristically reported.[45-47,50] Cecal perforation is the most common major complication. Advancement to the cecum is not necessary as adequate decompression may be achieved with the tip of the endoscope at the hepatic flexure.[46,51] Prolonged decompression may be achieved via endoscopic placement of a long vented decompression tube, although such tubes require regular irrigation and often become clogged with stool and fail (they may continue to provide some wicking action for decompression).[50,51] Successful decompression is obtained in up to 80% of patients after initial colonoscopy, although recurrence occurs in up to 15% of patients.[46,51] Repeat colonoscopy may be attempted, although the 10% to 15% of refractory cases should have surgical cecostomy without delay. Successful laparoscopic cecostomy has recently been reported.[52]

If clinical signs of cecal ischemia or perforation are found, laparotomy should be performed via vertical incision with selection of definitive procedure based on the state of the cecum.[51] The mortality for patients treated surgically is 30% versus 14% for those treated conservatively; perforation increases mortality to 40% to 50% despite therapy.[51] Surgery for chronic idiopathic pseudoobstruction should be avoided, as it rarely leads to any substantial improvement in this chronic, progressive disease; in addition, fluid management following colectomy with ileostomy may be difficult.

To summarize, the treatment regimen selected for a particular patient with constipation should be based on the findings of a logical diagnostic evaluation intended to identify the underlying factors contributing to the constipation. All patients should adhere to a high intake of fiber and fluids. Laxatives, purgatives, and enemas should be used judiciously on an intermittent basis. Newer approaches involve the use of nonabsorbable saline cathartics, third-generation prokinetic agents, and oral opioid antagonists. If medical therapy fails, surgery can provide dramatic and highly effective therapy in patients carefully selected on the basis of a complete intestinal physiologic evaluation.

REFERENCES

1. Reynolds JC. Motility disorders of the colon. In: Yamada T, ed. *Textbook of Gastroenterology.* Philadelphia, Pa: JB Lippincott Co; 1991:1715.
2. Greenbaum DS, Mayle JE, Vanegeren LE, et al. Effect of desipramine on irritable bowel syndrome compared with atropine and placebo. *Dig Dis Sci.* 1987;32:257.
3. Whitehead WE, Engel BT, Schuster MM. Irritable bowel syndrome. *Dig Dis Sci.* 1980;25:404.
4. Drossman DA, Powell DW, Sessions JT. The irritable bowel syndrome. *Gastroenterology.* 1977;73:811.

5. Burkitt DP, Walker ARP, Painter NS. Effect of dietary fiber on stools and transit-times, and its role in the causation of disease. *Lancet.* 1972;2:1408.
6. Tucker DM, Sandstead HH, Logan GM Jr, et al. Dietary fiber and personality factors as determinants of stool output. *Gastroenterology.* 1981;81:879.
7. Graham DY, Moser SE, Estes MK, et al. The effect of bran on bowel function in constipation. *Gastroenterology.* 1982;77:599.
8. Freeman HJ, Spiller GA, Kim YS. A double blind study of the effect of purified cellulose dietary fiber on 1,1 dimethyl hydrazine-induced rat colonic neoplasia. *Cancer Res.* 1978;38:2912.
9. Moses FM. The effect of exercise on the gastrointestinal tract. *Sports Med.* 1990;9:159.
10. Brunton LL. Laxatives. In: Gillman AG, Goodman LS, Gilman A, eds. *The Pharmacological Basis of Therapeutics,* 7th ed. New York, NY: Macmillan Publishing Co Inc; 1985:994.
11. Burkitt D. Fiber as protective against gastrointestinal diseases. *Gastroenterology.* 1984;79:249.
12. Bueno L, Praddaude F, Fioramonti J, et al. Effect of dietary fiber on gastrointestinal and jejunal transit time in dogs. *Gastroenterology.* 1981;80:701.
13. Slavin JL, Levine AS. Dietary fiber and gastrointestinal disease. Part 1. What is fiber and how much should I take? Part 2. How to use fiber to treat disease. *Pract Gastroenterol.* 1986;10:19.
14. Morehouse JL, Specian RD, Stewart JJ, et al. Translocation of indigenous bacteria from the gastrointestinal tract of mice after oral ricinoleic acid treatment. *Gastroenterology.* 1986;91:673.
15. Balzs M. Melanosis coli: ultrastructural study of 45 patients. *Dis Colon Rectum.* 1986;29:839.
16. Smith B. Effect of irritant purgatives on the myenteric plexus in man and the mouse. *Gut.* 1968;9:139.
17. Koch TR, Carney JA, Go L, et al. Idiopathic chronic constipation is associated with decreased colonic vasoactive intestinal peptide. *Gastroenterology.* 1988;94:300.
18. Harris RT. Bulimarexia and related serious eating disorders with medical complication. *Ann Intern Med.* 1983;99:800.
19. Plum GE, Weber HM, Sauer WG. Prolonged cathartic abuse resulting in roentgen evidence suggestive of enterocolitis. *Roentgenology.* 1960;83:919.
20. Andorsky RI, Goldner F. Colonic lavage solution (polyethylene glycol electrolyte lavage solution) as a treatment for chronic constipation: a double-blind, placebo-controlled study. *Am J Gastroenterol.* 1990;85:261.
21. Chapman RW, Sillery J, Fontana DD, et al. Effect of oral diocytl sodium sulfosuccinate on intake-output studies of human small and large intestine. *Gastroenterology.* 1985;89:489.
22. Kot TV, Pettit-Young NA. Lactulose in the management of constipation: a current review. *Ann Pharmacother.* 1992;26:1277.
23. Smith JL. Sir Arbuthnot Lane, chronic intestinal stasis, and autointoxication. *Ann Intern Med.* 1982;96:365.
24. Reynolds JC. Prokinetic agents: a key in the future of gastroenterology. *Gastroenterol Clin North Am.* 1989;18:37.
25. Krevsky B, Mauer AH, Malmud LS, Fisher RS. Cisapride accelerates colonic transit in constipated patients with colonic inertia. *Am J Gastroenterol.* 1989;84:882.
26. Kreek MJ, Hahn EF, Schaefer RA, et al. Naloxone: a specific opioid antagonist, reverses chronic idiopathic constipation. *Lancet.* 1983;1:262.
27. Reynolds JC, Ouyang A, Lee CA, et al. Chronic severe constipation: prospective studies in twenty-five consecutive patients. *Gastroenterology.* 1987;92:414.
28. Martelli H, Devroede G, Arhan P, et al. Mechanisms of idiopathic constipation: outlet obstruction. *Gastroenterology.* 1978;75:623.
29. Udassin R, Nissan S, Lernau O, et al. The mild form of Hirschsprung's disease (short segment). *Ann Surg.* 1981;3:767.
30. Harrison MW, Dietz DM, Campbell JR, et al. Diagnosis and management of Hirschsprung's disease. *Am J Surg.* 1986;152:49.
31. McCready RA, Beart RW. Adult Hirschsprung's disease: results of surgical treatment at Mayo Clinic. *Dis Colon Rectum.* 1980;23:401.
32. Orr JD, Anderson JR, Scobie WG. The treatment of Hirschsprung's disease. *J R Coll Surg Edinb.* 1981;26:153.
33. Bleijenberg G, Kuijpers HC. Treatment of the spastic pelvis floor syndrome with biofeedback. *Dis Colon Rectum.* 1987;30:108.
34. Roe AM, Bartolo DCC, Reed NW, et al. Diagnosis and surgical management of intractable constipation. *Br J Surg.* 1986;73:854.
35. Wexner SD, Daniel N, Jagelman DG. Colectomy for constipation: physiological investigation is the key to success. *Dis Colon Rectum.* 1991;34:851.
36. Fleshman JW, Fry RD, Kodner IJ. The surgical management of constipation. *Bailliere's Clin Gastroenterol.* 1992;6:145.
37. Pemberton JH, Rath DM, Ilstrup DM. Evaluation and surgical treatment of severe chronic constipation. *Ann Surg.* 1991;214:403.
38. Coremans GE. Surgical constipation of severe chronic non-Hirschsprung constipation. *Hepatogastroenterology.* 1990;37:588.
39. Beck DE, Jagelman DG, Fazio VW. The surgery of idiopathic constipation. *Gastroenterol Clin North Am.* 1987;16:143.
40. Belliveau P, Goldberg SM, Rothenberger DA, et al. Idiopathic acquired megacolon: the value of subtotal colectomy. *Dis Colon Rectum.* 1982;25:118.
41. McCready RA, Beart RJ Jr. The surgical treatment of incapacitating constipation associated with idiopathic megacolon. *Mayo Clin Proc.* 1979;54:779.
42. Schuffler MD, Rohrmann CA, Chaffee RG, et al. Chronic intestinal pseudoobstruction: a report of 27 cases and review of the literature. *Medicine.* 1981;60:173.
43. Anuras S, Shirazi SS. Colonic pseudoobstruction. *Am J Gastroenterol.* 1984;79:525.
44. Nanni C, Garbini A, Luchetti P, et al. Ogilvie's syndrome (acute chronic pseudoobstruction): review of the literature (October 1948 to March 1980) and report of four additional cases. *Dis Colon Rectum.* 1982;25:157.
45. Kukora JS, Dent TL. Colonoscopic decompression of massive nonobstructive cecal dilation. *Arch Surg.* 1977;112:512.
46. Strodel WE, Nostrant RR, Eckhauser FE, et al. Therapeutic and diagnostic colonoscopy in non-obstructive colonic dilation. *Ann Surg.* 1983;197:416.
47. Nivatvongs S, Vermeulen FD, Fant DT, et al. Colonoscopic decompression of acute pseudoobstruction of the colon. *Ann Surg.* 1982;196:598.
48. Bode WE, Beart RW, Spencer RJ, et al. Colonoscopic decompression for acute pseudoobstruction of the colon (Ogilvie's syndrome): report of 22 cases and review of the literature. *Am J Surg.* 1984;147:243.

49. Fausel CS, Goff JS. Nonoperative management of acute idiopathic colonic pseudoobstruction (Ogilvie's syndrome). *West J Med.* 1985;143:50.
50. Nano D, Prindiville T, Pauly M, et al. Colonoscopic therapy of acute pseudoobstruction of the colon. *Gastroenterology.* 1987;82:145.
51. Dorudi S, Berry AR, Kettlewell MGW. Acute colonic pseudo-obstruction. *Br J Surg.* 1992;79:99.
52. Duh Q, Way LW. Diagnostic laparoscopy and laparoscopic cecostomy for colonic pseudo-obstruction. *Dis Colon Rectum.* 1993;36:65.

17

Intestinal Obstruction

DANIEL A. NG and RUSSELL A. WILLIAMS

Since the early 1900s several significant advances have improved the management of complete intestinal obstruction. In 1912, Hartwell and Hoguet demonstrated that fluid resuscitation was vital in the management of bowel obstruction. In the 1930s, nasogastric and intestinal tubes were found to decrease distension and subsequent progression of intestinal obstruction. In the 1940s through 1950s, antibiotics were used to improve survival in patients with bowel obstruction. Finally, improvements in technology in both anesthesia and surgery have reduced mortality from 50% to 10% in the past century. Nevertheless, for patients with strangulated intestine the high mortality remains.[1,2]

The key principles in the management of intestinal obstruction are prompt recognition, early resuscitation, and expedient, appropriate intervention.

DEFINITION

Intestinal obstruction occurs when there is an interference with the normal aboral progression of intestinal contents by a *physical* barrier, i.e., a mechanical intestinal obstruction. This is in contrast to "ileus," which is a failure of caudad progression of bowel contents because of disordered propulsive motility, i.e., "paralytic ileus." Causes of ileus, or nonmechanical "obstruction" range from neuromuscular deficiencies (megacolon) and systemic derangements (electrolyte abnormalities) to local factors (retroperitoneal hematoma, pneumonia, spinal fracture). The enigmatic entity, Ogilvie's syndrome, or "pseudo-obstruction" also falls within this category.[1]

INCIDENCE[2]

Mechanical intestinal obstruction is a common disorder seen by surgeons and accounts for 20% of patients admitted to the hospital with an acute abdomen. Eighty percent of all intestinal obstructions are caused by postoperative and postinflammatory adhesions, groin hernias, and neoplasias, in order of decreasing frequency. The actual frequency varies with the location of the obstruction and the age of the patient, facts important in diagnosing the cause of an obstruction. When small bowel is obstructed, the primary cause is adhesions (50%), followed by hernias and neoplasms (15% each).

Notably, bowel obstruction secondary to hernias presents more frequently with strangulation, hence the need for aggressive management of hernia-related bowel obstruction. However, the number of bowel obstructions in hernias has decreased as the result of most hernias being repaired electively.

Colon cancer is the leading cause of large bowel obstruction (60%), whereas diverticular disease and volvulus each account for 15% of large bowel obstruction. The remainder are due to hernias, stricture from inflammatory disease (Crohn's disease, ulcerative colitis), carcinomatosis, foreign body, and intussusception.

In evaluating intestinal obstruction the patient's age is important. In the younger population, groin hernias are the most common cause of obstruction, but intussusception, malrotation, pyloric stenosis, and congenital atresias and stenosis are particularly more likely in this age group. Colon carcinoma and diverticular disease are the most frequent causes in the elderly, an important observation because of the increasing elderly population.

TYPES OF INTESTINAL OBSTRUCTIONS[1]

Intestinal obstruction is commonly classified by the mechanism of the obstruction:

1. Obturation of the intestinal lumen
2. Encroachment by an intrinsic intestinal wall lesion
3. Extrinsic lesions
4. Volvulus

OBTURATION OF THE LUMEN

In the pediatric population, occlusion of the lumen by meconium or intussuscepted loops of intestine are important. In children, the diagnosis of intussusception is based on a history of passing bloody stools ("currant jelly stool"), intermittent waves of pain during which the child draws up his entire body in flexion, and radiologic studies (barium or air enema). A Meckel's diverticulum or a segment of intestinal lymphoid hyperplasia is frequently the "lead point." In the older population, gallstones, feces, and bezoars may act as bowel occluders. The classic finding in "gallstone ileus" is air in the biliary tree secondary to a cholecystoduodenal fistula (Fig. 17–1). Bezoars are most common in psychiatric and developmentally delayed patients.

ENCROACHMENT BY INTRINSIC INTESTINAL WALL LESIONS

The intestinal tract can also be occluded by lesions of the intestinal wall. Adult patients tend to present with more indolent symptoms because the obstruction is the result of either a slow-growing tumor or a chronic inflammatory process such as Crohn's disease or ulcerative colitis, which leads to a stricture. In contrast, in the pediatric population, symptoms may be present

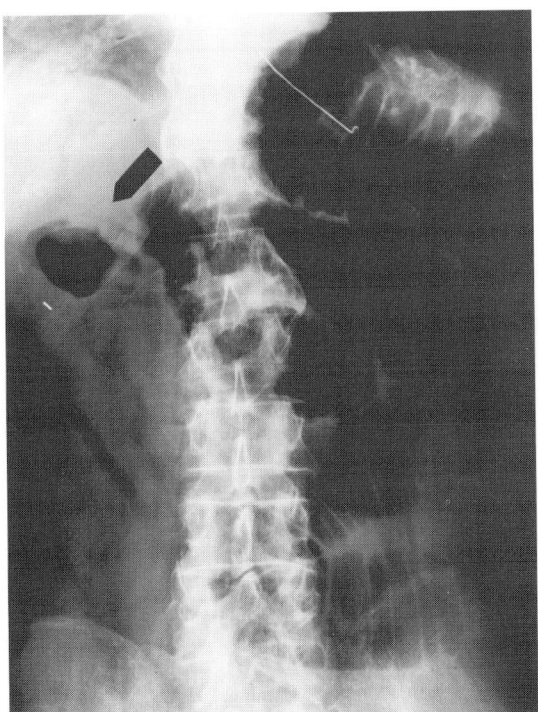
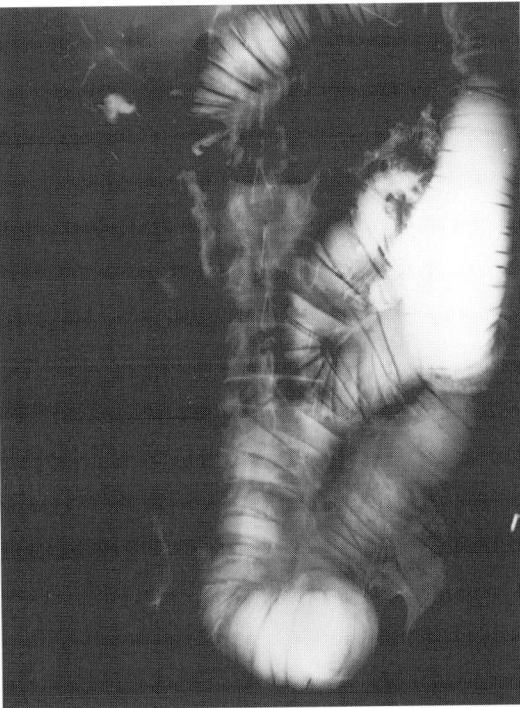

FIGURE 17–1. Gallstone ileus shows air in biliary tree on plain radiographs (**A**) and contrast in biliary tree and filling defect in colon on contrast study (**B**).

at birth; these lesions are congenital and include intestinal atresia, stenosis or duplications, Meckel's diverticula, and imperforate anus.

EXTRINSIC LESIONS

Lesions extrinsic to the intestinal tract can cause obstruction by compression or binding and angulation of the intestine. Adhesive bands, either postoperative or postinflammatory, e.g., following cholecystitis, pancreatitis or trauma, can cause kinking and narrowing of the bowel lumen (Fig. 17–2). In addition, there may be compromise of the intestinal vascular supply leading subsequently to ischemia and perforation.

Hernias and mesenteric defects, which may be either congenital, traumatic, or iatrogenic in origin, account for a large percentage of intestinal strangulation obstruction (Fig. 17–3). Metastatic cancer and abscesses will cause compression of the intestine, and this compressive effect can be seen on contrast studies.

VOLVULUS

Twisting of the intestinal tract, or volvulus, accounts for 3% to 7% of all intestinal obstruction. Malrotation and twisting about congenital or adhesive bands cause volvulus of the small intestine more frequently in the pediatric population.[3] Cecal volvulus and sigmoid volvulus are common entities described in the elderly population, accounting for 45% and 50% of colonic volvulus, respectively. Sigmoid volvulus is more common in those over 60 years of age. Volvulus is a closed loop obstruction, and interruption of the blood supply occurs early so that gangrene is a frequent finding (10% of sigmoid volvulus, 33% of cecal volvulus) (Fig. 17–4). The gangrenous bowel frequently perforates, a complication that accounts for the high mortality.

PATHOPHYSIOLOGY[2]

In simple small bowel obstruction (i.e., nonstrangulated obstruction of the small intestine), key events include fluid and electrolyte losses, intestinal distension, and altered intestinal motility.

In a patient with small bowel obstruction, one of the most important physiologic derangements is fluid and electrolyte loss. Patients become hypovolemic and develop hemoconcentration and oliguria. With bowel obstruction there is an

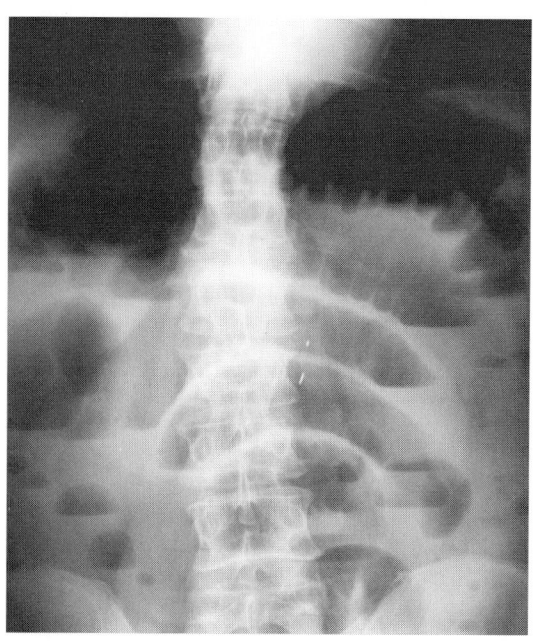

FIGURE 17–2. Small bowel obstruction secondary to adhesions. The classic ladder pattern and scattered air fluid levels are shown.

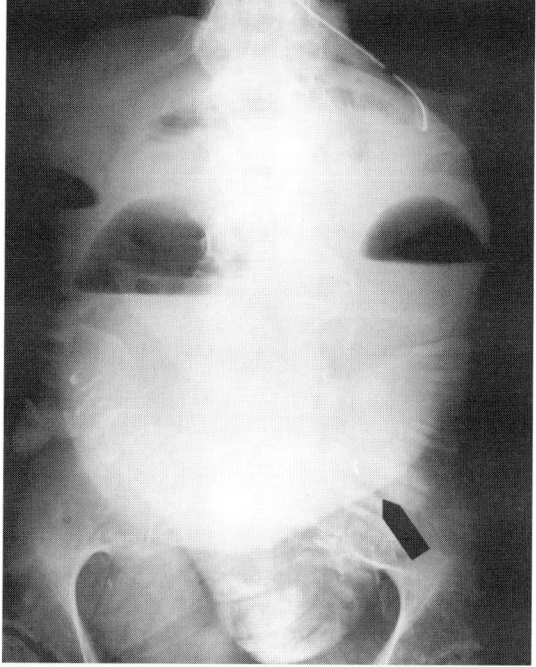

FIGURE 17–3. Patient is a 69-year-old man with a large umbilical hernia and incarcerated loop of small intestine.

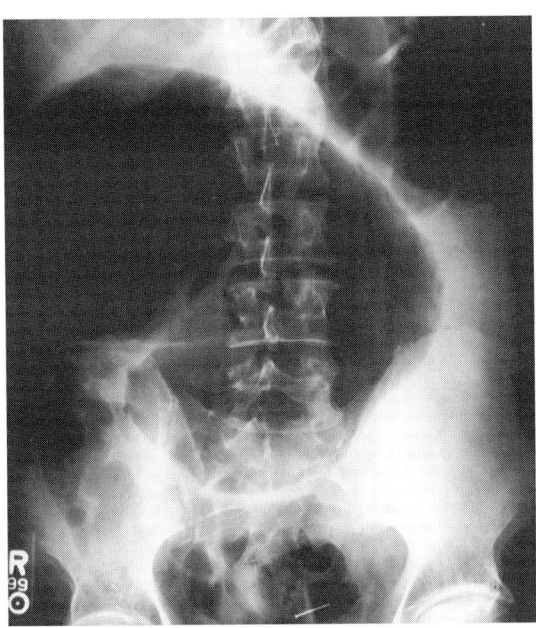 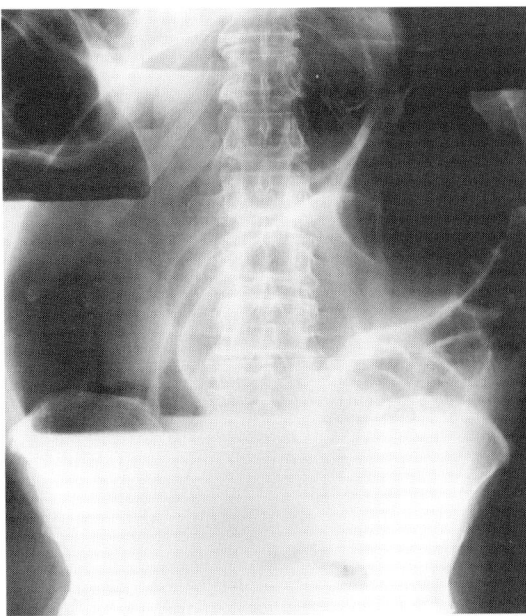

FIGURE 17-4. A, Sigmoid volvulus. 80-year-old man with constipation and lower abdominal pain. The distended colon (coffee bean) points toward the right upper quadrant contrast with cecal volvulus. **B,** Cecal volvulus. The "coffee bean" is seen in the left upper quadrant

accumulation of fluid in the lumen proximal to the obstruction.

Fluids and electrolytes that are normally absorbed distal to the obstruction are lost during vomiting and nasogastric suctioning, and additional fluid losses are incurred as a result of increased secretion of fluid into the bowel lumen. Bowel distension, which occurs with obstruction, is a stimulus for increased bowel secretory activity. Prostaglandins are a possible mediator in the process.

Distension of the intestine with a raised intraluminal pressure results in venous obstruction with compromise of bowel wall perfusion and subsequent ischemia. Accompanying this there is bowel wall edema and "third spacing" with transfer of fluid from the vascular space into the bowel wall and the lumen and across the serosa into the peritoneal cavity. More distal lesions have less fluid losses.

With small bowel obstruction, there is accumulation of gas proximal to the blockage, which is predominantly nitrogen from swallowed air, since the carbon dioxide is absorbed readily. Also, intestinal stasis and bacterial fermentation lead to organic gas production. The end result is increased distension of the intestine and stimulation of increased fluid secretion.

Finally, in simple small bowel obstruction, motility is altered. Proximal to the obstruction, motility increases, reflected in the so-called "hyperactive bowel sounds." The more proximal the obstruction, the more frequent the contraction (every 3 to 5 minutes in a proximal bowel obstruction and every 10 to 15 minutes in a distal obstruction). These increased waves of motor activity are often associated with pain. In contrast, distal to the obstruction the motility decreases via an intestinal reflex.

With small intestinal obstruction complicated by strangulation,[2] in addition to the foregoing pathophysiologic derangements, bowel viability is a major concern. Strangulation obstruction of the intestine is associated most frequently with obstruction due to hernias, volvulus, and adhesions. In all these entities there is compression or twisting of the vessels with blockage of venous return, which leads to extravasation of fluid and blood into the intestinal wall and lumen. Diffusion of bacterial exotoxins and endotoxins systemically and locally further compromise the hemodynamic stability of the patient.

A persistently distended bowel is associated with an increased intraluminal pressure that also interferes with venous return. Bowel wall ischemia is followed by necrosis and ultimately intestinal perforation with gross spillage of luminal contents into the free peritoneal cavity.

One subset of strangulation obstruction is the "closed loop obstruction" such as occurs with volvulus. The afferent and efferent limbs of the involved length of bowel are blocked, leading to a rapid rise in intraluminal pressure, venous occlusion, the early development of gangrene, and perforation, often before the patient becomes markedly disturbed hemodynamically.

Large bowel obstruction presents with less acute symptoms than small bowel obstruction does. Electrolyte and fluid derangements are less marked because the primary function of the colon is "storage of fecal material." Strangulation of the colon is less common unless, of course, volvulus is involved. However, with a competent ileocecal valve and a distal colonic obstruction, there is the potential for a closed loop obstruction with increased risk of perforation.

The cecum is the most distensible portion of the colon, and in accord with LaPlace's law distension results in the tension being greatest in the cecal wall; hence, the risk of rupture is highest here. Despite the indolent, more slowly progressive course of a large bowel obstruction, perforation, particularly of the cecum, is a potentially lethal consequence.

DIAGNOSIS

In managing the patient with "an acute abdomen," obstruction must always be a consideration. Answers to the following questions are needed.

1. Is an obstruction present?
2. It is complete or "partial"?
3. Where is the obstruction?
4. What is the cause of the obstruction?
5. Is there strangulation or perforation?
6. What is the general condition of the patient?
7. Is an operation required?

HISTORY AND PHYSICAL EXAMINATION[1]

A detailed history is critical in the diagnosis of a patient with intestinal obstruction. Not only are the severity and progression of the symptoms important, but also knowledge of any prior operations, prior episodes of obstruction, and other medical conditions is essential. In reviewing the most common causes of obstruction, the duration of symptoms with hernia and adhesion-related obstructions is much shorter than when the obstruction is secondary to a neoplastic process (1 to 3 days versus several days to weeks, respectively).

Pain is the predominant symptom described by most patients. This is especially true in patients with adhesions and hernias. Pain is described as crampy (from hyperperistalsis), diffuse, and "coming in waves." The more proximal the obstruction, the shorter the intervals of quiescence. Jejunal obstruction tends to be associated with epigastric pain; ileal obstruction, with periumbilical pain; colonic obstruction, with infraumbilical pain; and rectosigmoid obstruction, with perineal pain. This observation corresponds with the distribution of afferent sympathetic fibers. The pain may subside after the intestine becomes markedly distended, which leads to the ominous physical finding of "the quiet abdomen." *Beware* that "ileus" may have similar symptoms, and the two entities must not be confused! Continuous severe pain should raise the question of strangulation.

Vomiting is common, and the frequency and quality of emesis varies according to the time of presentation of the obstruction and the location of the obstruction. Early in the course, vomiting is frequent. If the obstruction is proximal, the frequency remains high, especially with continued attempted oral intake.

In distal obstruction, the number of episodes decrease, and the quality of the emesis may be described as "feculent" and thick. The material is not actually feces, but luminal contents that have undergone bacterial fermentation. In colonic obstruction, vomiting is less frequent and does little to decompress the intestine.

Finally, obstipation and distension are frequent complaints in patients with intestinal obstruction. Obstipation, failure to pass gas or feces, is characteristic of complete obstruction. Early in the course, the patient may pass flatus or feces distal to the obstruction. However, with time, passage of contents diminishes. Diarrheal stools are more characteristic of partial obstruction as liquid luminal contents may be forced through a partially obstructed segment. The failure to pass gas may be correlated with "no air in the colon" seen on plain abdominal radiographs. Remember, however, that with postoperative ileus, it is common that patients do not pass luminal contents.

In intestinal obstruction, the physical examination is often helpful, not only in determining the cause (for example, a loop of intestine obstructed in an inguinal hernia) but also in the assessment of the patient's overall condition. Patients who appear ill and toxic, and who are hypotensive and orthostatic may well have strangulation.

On abdominal examination, bowel sounds may range from the borborygmi of an early obstruction, the "silent abdomen" of an impending abdominal catastrophe, to the loud high-pitched metabolic rushes during peristalsis. This is in contrast to the "hypoactive bowel sounds" of paralytic ileus. At times the peristalsis of loops of intestine is seen through the abdominal wall.

An abdominal mass should raise the suspicion of volvulus, hernias, abscesses, neoplasm, or intussusception. The scars of surgical incisions are an important finding in assessing the patient with an acute abdomen. Rectal examination is noted for blood, a finding that may be associated with intestinal ischemia or neoplasia. Finally, a common finding late in the course of obstruction is a distended and tympanic abdomen.

LABORATORY FINDINGS[2,4]

With prolonged vomiting, alkalosis, hypochloreia, uremia, and hemoconcentration may be detected. Specific gravity of urine is elevated and oliguria is the rule. In patients who have progressed to bowel ischemia and shock, acidosis secondary to ketosis and lactic acidosis from poor peripheral perfusion presents an ominous finding. Respiratory acidosis is another late finding in the patient with severe distension who suffers respiratory embarrassment.

White blood cell counts in the 15,000/mm^3 range with a moderate left shift are common. Progression to strangulation may be accompanied by an increase in white cell count to 25,000 with a marked shift. Mesenteric vascular occlusion of the intestine yields levels as high as 40,000 to 60,000.

RADIOLOGIC STUDIES[2]

In most circumstances, the plain abdominal films are helpful. However, in some instances they are nondiagnostic, equivocal, and nonspecific. In one series, the diagnosis of midbowel obstruction was made on the basis of plain films in only approximately 50% of patients with obstruction secondary to adhesions, hernias, and neoplasms. In this series the abdominal film in patients with obstruction was interpreted as normal in 15% and as equivocal in 30%. Nevertheless, certain radiologic findings are pathognomonic for bowel obstruction, and radiologic studies are very helpful in the management.

An "acute abdomen series" should include an upright chest film and supine and upright abdominal films. The chest radiograph is examined for infiltrates, abnormalities of the cardiac silhouette, effusions, and the presence of pneumoperitoneum under the diaphragm. In the patient with a small bowel obstruction the loops of intestine appear in a "ladder pattern" or "stacked coins" array. Air fluid levels are commonly found, although these are nonspecific.

The normal diameter of the small bowel should not exceed 3 cm. The characteristic appearance of dilated small intestine as discussed above represents the mucosal folds of the small intestine, the valvulae conniventes, which are most prominent in the proximal jejunum. On radiographs these folds traverse the entire diameter of the lumen. The dilated loops of the small bowel are found more centrally in the abdomen, and often the diameter of dilated loops of small intestine exceeds 4 cm. In contrast, in large bowel obstruction, the colonic haustra, which do not traverse the entire diameter of the intestine, appear on radiographs as incomplete folds, and the colon gas pattern is found commonly along the "perimeter" of the abdomen.

With a competent ileocecal valve and colon obstruction, little small bowel distension is noted. Absence of air in the colon may indicate long-standing small bowel obstruction.

The characteristic pattern of ileus on plain film is the nondescript "scattered gas pattern" with gas throughout the small and large intestine and occasional air fluid levels.

If there is a suspicion of large bowel obstruction, a contrast enema can be important both in demonstrating the site of obstruction and its cause. With intussusception in children and occasionally with volvulus, a contrast enema can be used to reduce the intussusception or volvulus. The success rate for enema reduction of intussusception is about 75% in most centers with a recurrence rate of 5% which is equivalent to the recurrence rate of operation. Thus, in this condition the test can be both therapeutic and diagnostic.[6]

There are also disadvantages to contrast enema, including the risk of perforating an acutely inflamed segment of colon (such as in diverticulitis) or perforating a markedly distended gangrenous segment of bowel particularly if the hydrophilic contrast agent, gastrografin, is used. Also, a partial obstruction can be converted to a complete obstruction secondary to inspissated barium. Certainly, these complications are uncommon but must be appreciated prior to the study.

There is debate regarding the type of contrast to use, barium versus diatrizoate meglumine (gastrografin). The argument against the use of barium is if perforation were to occur, the chemical peritonitis secondary to barium worsens the overall mortality. Also, barium concretions can worsen an obstruction. Gastrografin in some patients has a cathartic effect if given orally, and defecation induced by gastrografin rules out bowel obstruction. However, gastrografin is strongly hydrophilic, and in a partially closed loop this may result in bowel perforation.[5]

The "upper gastrointestinal series with small bowel follow through" remains a controversy in terms of the indications for usage and its potential dangers. Although there are some who advocate the use of an upper gastrointestinal series to distinguish a complete bowel obstruction from a partial obstruction or postoperative ileus, a better study for demonstrating this is enteroclysis. With this method, a long intestinal tube is passed into the proximal small bowel. Under fluoroscopy a large bolus of contrast is administered, follow-up films are obtained in rapid succession, and the site of obstruction is usually more clearly visualized. The long intestinal tube can also be left for suction and drainage. There are those who avoid instillation of contrast above an obstruction because of the danger of exacerbating the obstruction. This is controversial.

Diagnosis of obstruction, biopsy of intraluminal lesions, and even decompression of a volvulus can be performed via endoscopy. Proctosigmoidoscopy can be used for decompression of a volvulus and pseudoobstruction with the aid of a rectal tube passed with colonoscopic guidance. An experienced endoscopist is extremely important in the management of colonic obstruction since overinsufflation of air in an obstructed segment may lead to colonic perforation.[7]

MANAGEMENT

Once the diagnosis of complete intestinal obstruction has been established, management is straightforward. This includes resuscitation, intestinal decompression, and appropriate operative intervention to relieve the obstruction. Administration of preoperative antibiotics is also important once the diagnosis is established. Difficulty arises in cases in which the diagnosis is unclear. Examples of this include distinguishing complete intestinal obstruction from partial obstruction or distinguishing postoperative small intestinal obstruction from ileus.

FLUID RESUSCITATION[1,8]

Patients with intestinal obstruction are dehydrated with hypovolemia and hemoconcentration. If the patient has had protracted vomiting, and consequently, large amounts of acidic fluid loss, normal saline with dextrose can be used for resuscitation. Otherwise, lactated Ringer's solution with dextrose is a suitable fluid. Once the patient is urinating adequately (0.5 to 1 ml/kg/h) and if the potassium level is low, potassium supplementation is administered.

Broad spectrum antibiotics are administered especially if strangulation is suspected. Ischemia and distension result in transmigration of bacteria into the portal blood and peritoneal cavity from the overgrown luminal bacterial flora. The volume of fluid needed to completely resuscitate the patient depends on the patient's duration of symptoms, current central venous pressure, vital sign examination, and urine output.[1,9]

If the patient is in shock and if strangulation is suspected, a central venous catheter or Swan Ganz catheter may be needed to assist in resuscitation particularly in elderly patients with poor cardiac reserve. A Foley catheter allows for close urinary output monitoring. A baseline hematocrit is helpful since it reflects the degree of hemoconcentration. If long-term bowel inactivity is anticipated, parenteral nutrition is needed particularly in patients who have little nutritional reserve.

Intestinal intubation is a valuable adjunct in the management of intestinal obstruction. Its intended role is to decompress the intestine and prevent further distension; however, nasogastric suctioning prevents vomiting by primarily relieving the stomach and not the small bowel of fluid and swallowed air. This is important and in most instances, nasogastric intubation provides adequate decompression. In some cases, a long intestinal tube, if successfully placed, can assist in decompressing a dilated small intestine. However, these long tubes (e.g., Miller-Abbot) are often difficult to pass relying on peristalsis for advancement, and multiple attempts at placement may delay definitive therapy.

There are several conditions in which nasal-intestinal intubation should be considered definitive treatment: postoperative ileus, partial small bowel obstruction, and obstruction secondary to an inflammatory process that is amenable to medications (e.g., Crohn's disease, ulcerative colitis, peptic ulcer disease). Pediatric intussusception and sigmoid volvulus may be treated by rectal intubation in conjunction with other maneuvers.

OPERATIVE MANAGEMENT

Once resuscitation and intestinal decompression are achieved, the need for and timing of an operation are considered. The shorter the duration of obstruction (less than 24 hours), the smaller the magnitude of the fluid and electrolyte derangement and the sooner the surgery can be performed. Obstruction secondary to hernias tends to present with a shorter time course; these patients are at higher risk for strangulation; thus, earlier intervention is required. Operative mortality is less than 1% in patients with early obstruction.[1]

Other situations in which early operative intervention is imperative include patients with strangulated bowel. Despite all current resuscitatory efforts, overall mortality still remains high in cases of strangulation obstruction (25% to 30%). Antibiotics administration is important in patients with strangulated intestine to reduce septic complications due to transmigration of bowel bacteria.[10]

The patient who has obstruction but no history of abdominal operations is less likely to have adhesions as a cause of the obstruction and may require earlier intervention. Finally, once intestinal intubation and resuscitation have been initiated, early operation is indicated if the patient does not improve or worsens as manifested by tachycardia, fevers, leukocytosis, hemodynamic instability, or peritoneal signs.

The choice of operation will depend on the cause of the obstruction and can be categorized into five groups:

1. Creation of an enterotomy to remove a foreign body (gallstone, bezoars)
2. Resection of a portion of intestine with or without reanastomosis[11] (strictured areas and devitalized small intestine)
3. Bypass of strictured areas (if resection is difficult)
4. Creation of a proximal stoma to decompress the system (carcinomatosis, cecal volvulus cecostomy)
5. Other procedures that do not require violating the intestinal wall such as lysis of adhesions, reduction of volvulus, hernias, or intussusception[12]

The need to resect the bowel depends on its viability. This can be judged principally by the return of color, pulsation, and peristalsis once the strangulated segment is released. Fluorescein stain or ultrasonic Doppler has been used as an aid to determine viability. If long segments of intestine are involved and there is a risk that resection will be severely crippling, a second-look operation can be planned in 24 to 48 hours with the hope that relief of the obstruction and fluid resuscitation can restore bowel that appeared of dubious viability at the initial procedure.[5]

Postoperatively, patient management involves fluid and electrolyte resuscitation and close follow-up. "Third spacing" is the rule and not the exception. Return of bowel function varies according to the duration of preoperative symptoms, length of operation, amount of intestinal strangulation, and degree of inflammation. Generally, small intestinal function returns in 24 to 36 hours; stomach, in 48 hours; and colon, in 3 to 5 days.

NONOPERATIVE MANAGEMENT

There are several conditions in which nonoperative management for bowel obstruction is the correct treatment. With pediatric intussusception, reduction with enemas should be attempted at least two or three times before deciding to operate. There is some debate whether to use air or barium, but most institutions use barium. Some radiologists prefer air because it better fills any space in which it is instilled, affording a more effective pressure column in the bowel. Also, were perforation to occur, air is inert and is not associated with the intense peritonitis barium incites. Finally, there is less radiation exposure when air is used.[6] In contrast, with adult intussusception, operative intervention is recommended because typically the lead point is a tumor or other lesion.

With sigmoid volvulus, initial management, as in other forms of obstruction, is resuscitation and nasogastric intubation. In addition to decompression from above, the sigmoid volvulus can be decompressed and actually reduced with colonoscopically guided placement of a rectal tube. This maneuver allows elective resection in several days under more optimal conditions, when the bowel wall edema subsides and antibiotics have been administered. The definitive treatment for sigmoid volvulus is eventual sigmoid resection (excision of redundant sigmoid colon) to avoid a recurrence.[3,7]

Patients with a history of chronic small bowel obstruction relieved by intestinal intubation can be managed without surgery if they show no signs of strangulation, peritonitis, or hemodynamic instability. However, if after 12 to 36 hours there is no improvement or if symptoms worsen, surgery should be considered.[13,14] With posttraumatic obstruction due to a jejunal or duodenal hematoma, a waiting period of 10 to 14 days with parenteral intubation has been proposed, with good results, as the hematoma reabsorbs.[15]

Early postoperative small bowel obstruction, within 2 weeks of surgery, is managed initially by nasogastric intubation, parenteral nutrition, and resuscitation. The timing of nonoperative management varies from 48 hours to as long as 10 days. The rationale is that the cause is likely postoperative ileus or is due to fibrinous rather than fibrous adhesions, which will usually spontaneously lyse. Fibrous adhesions are not likely to have formed in such a short period of time. However, as in any other obstruction, should bowel viability be in question or the patient worsen, surgery is required.[16]

OTHER ENTITIES

It is often difficult to distinguish between ileus and obstruction, whether the ileus be adynamic (absence or decrease in neuromuscular activity), spastic (common in heavy metal poisoning), or vascular occlusion. Postoperative ileus is common and has a well-defined course so that any deviation from this should raise the question of other conditions. Any source of inflammation (e.g., pancreatitis or an intraabdominal abscess) can give rise to an ileus. A retroperitoneal process such as a hematoma, ureteral stone, or spinal fracture can also give rise to an ileus, and electrolyte disturbances and medications including narcotics, anticholinergics, and anticoagulants can also cause bowel inactivity.

Ogilvie's syndrome (or pseudoobstruction) can cause confusion because it presents as a large bowel obstruction. Its cause is unknown, but associated conditions include pancreatitis, sepsis, pregnancy, and renal failure. Pseudoobstruction can be associated with massive cecal dilation and perforation with an associated mortality of 50%. The risk of perforation increases with a cecal diameter greater than 10 cm. Regardless of the size, initial decompression via colonoscopy usually affords adequate relief of bowel wall tension, and colonoscopy can be used to rule out complete obstruction. Failure to decompress the intestine or recurrent episodes of pseudoobstruction necessitate operative intervention such as a tube cecostomy.

CONCLUSION

Intestinal obstruction is an entity that should be appreciated by all clinicians. Initial management involves fluid resuscitation and intestinal tube decompression, and in cases of suspected strangulation, prompt operative intervention is needed. With chronic obstruction or a long duration of symptoms, delayed operation is prudent provided there is no evidence of strangulation.

REFERENCES

1. Jones RS. Intestinal obstruction. In: Sabiston DC, ed. *Textbook of Surgery.* 14th ed. Philadelphia, Pa: WB Saunders; 1991:835–842.
2. Schwartz SI. Manifestations of gastrointestinal disease. In: Schwartz SI, ed. *Principles of Surgery.* 5th ed. 1989:1061–1102.
3. Smith SD, Golladay ES, Wagner C, Seibert JJ. Sigmoid volvulus in childhood. *South Med J.* 1990;83(7):778–781.
4. Asbun HJ, Pempinello C, Halasz NA. Small bowel obstruction and its management. *Int Surg.* 1989;74:23–27.
5. Yeo CJ. Obstruction of the large bowel. In: Cameron, ed. *Current Surgical Therapy,* 3rd ed. 1989:125–127.
6. Palder SB, Ein SH, Stringer DA, Alton D. Intussusception: barium or air? *Onc Ped Surg.* 1991;26(3):271–275.
7. Wyman A, Zeiderman M. Maintaining decompression of sigmoid volvulus. *SGYNO.* 1989;169(3):265.
8. Mucha P. Small bowel obstruction. In: Ameroniz, ed. *Current Surgical Therapy.* 3rd ed. 1989:71–77.
9. Byrne JJ. Intestinal obstruction. *Postgrad Med.* 1990;87(6):217–222.
10. Halevy A, Levi J, Ordu R. Emergency subtotal colectomy. *Ann Surg.* 1989;210(2):220–223.
11. Tan SG, Narribian R, Rauff A, Ngoi SS, Goh HS. Primary resection and anastomosis in obstructed descending colon due to cancer. *Arch Surg.* 1991;126:748–751.
12. Ellis CN, Boggs HW Jr, Slagle GW, Cole PA. Small bowel obstruction after colon resection for benign and malignant diseases. *Dis Colon Rectum* 1991;34(5):367–371.
13. Akgur FM, Tanyez FC, Buyukpamukcu N, Hicsonniez A. Adhesive small bowel obstruction in children: the place and predictors of success for conservative treatment. *Ped Surg.* July 1991;26(1):37–41.
14. Fahri PJ, Rosemurgy A. Reoperation for small intestinal obstruction. *Surg Clin North Am.* 1991;71(1):131–146.
15. Czyrko C, Weltz C, Markowitz R, O'Neill JA. Blunt abdominal trauma resulting in intestinal obstruction: when to operate? *J Trauma.* 1990;30(12):1567–1571.
16. Pickleman J, Lee RM. The management of patients with suspected early postoperative small bowel obstruction. *Ann Surg.* 1989;1210(2):216–219.

18
Abdominal Abscesses

ARVEY I. ROGERS and JESSE GREEN

For purposes of the following discussion, *abscess* will be defined as a collection of pus; and *abdominal* will include intraperitoneal and retroperitoneal sites. Abscesses within viscera (i.e., liver, gallbladder, pancreas) will not be considered.

Common sites for the occurrence of abscesses include both right and left subphrenic spaces, the pelvis, and infrahepatic space. These share certain clinical features and present distinguishing features as well.[1]

DEVELOPMENT OF ABSCESSES

Abscesses usually occur as a consequence of conditions that alter transmural permeability of a viscus either by direct wall disruption (i.e., trauma, perforation, anastomotic leaks postoperatively) or by inflammation or infection of the viscus.[2] The lymphatics of the peritoneal membrane and the diaphragm are capable of absorbing bacteria and particulate matter. Cellular and immunologic mechanisms are recruited to kill bacteria contaminating the peritoneal cavity. When these mechanisms fail for a variety of reasons, localization of infection takes place by the elaboration of fibrin and the absence of fibrinolytic activity. Once the process is localized, an abscess forms that perpetuates the growth of anaerobic bacteria; progressive wall thickness precludes abscess resolution by factors that cannot enter the abscess cavity.[3]

ORGANISMS USUALLY RESPONSIBLE

Anaerobic cocci, *Bacteroides, Clostridium, Enterobacter, Enterococcus, Escherichia coli, Klebsiella,* and *Proteus* are the organisms usually cultured from abscess cavities. Saprophytic organisms such as *Candida albicans, Pseudomonas,* and *Serratia marcescens* may occur in immunocompromised patients. Infections that complicate distal small bowel or colonic diseases that are populated by great quantities of anaerobic and aerobic bacteria are usually more serious, because the proximal small intestine is characterized by low bacterial counts, more often aerobic, and the usually acidic stomach is relatively sterile. *E. coli* is the dominant aerobe and *Bacteroides fragilis,* the dominant anaerobe, found in intraabdominal and retroperitoneal abscesses.[2]

CHARACTERISTIC CLINICAL MANIFESTATIONS

The principal local manifestations include fever and abdominal pain, accompanied often by abdominal distension and ileus. Profound endotoxemia or bacteremia may result in septic shock.[4,5] Infrequently, adult respiratory distress syndrome or unexplained renal failure may be remote organ consequences of unsuspected intraperitoneal or retroperitoneal abscesses.[6] Shoulder pain or hiccups should suggest subphrenic abscess in the appropriate clinical setting. Symptoms of urinary urgency or frequency or worsening of abdominal pain on bladder emptying may be experienced when the abscess abuts on the bladder. Pain in the right hip region or pain that worsens when a person is assuming a full upright posture suggests the abscess is proximal to or within the right psoas muscle. Diarrhea could suggest a pericolitis involving the sigmoid colon region.

Bowel sounds may or may not be altered over a moderately distended, sometimes diffusely tender abdomen. Abdominal palpation over or near an abscess will evoke localized tenderness. A pelvic abscess may be palpated during rectal or pelvic examination.

The white blood cell (WBC) count is usually moderately to markedly elevated. Localized sepsis is indicated by (1) worsening of glycemic control in a known diabetic patient or (2) the new onset of hyperglycemia unexplained by high-dose steroid therapy or inadequate insulin coverage of large intravenous glucose loads via hyperalimentation, whether or not the patient is febrile. Jaundice may be caused by many factors in the setting of suspected sepsis, but an abscess compressing the common bile duct should be considered when it is encountered. It should be recalled that abnormalities of the liver biochemical profile may be a consequence of sepsis alone.

SUBPHRENIC ABSCESSES

The majority of subphrenic abscesses are a consequence of intraabdominal surgery. Four subphrenic spaces have been characterized anatomically in which abscesses may develop. They are suprahepatic and subhepatic on the right; and combined subphrenic and subhepatic on the left. Two thirds of the abscesses occur on the right with a small percentage occurring bilaterally. Upper gut pathology is responsible for 30% to 40%; disorders or surgery of the biliary tract, 20% to 30%; and appendicitis and appendectomy, 10% to 15%. The remainder of abscesses are caused by trauma and radical surgical procedures.[1]

These abscesses may present in a more chronic setting characterized by general poor health, anorexia, low-grade fever, and pleural effusion. A pleural effusion suggests the possibility of a subphrenic abscess. Upper back, shoulder, or pleuritic pain may suggest a subphrenic location. A raised diaphragm or otherwise unexplained unilateral basal atelectasis also should suggest a subphrenic abscess.[1,7]

CONFIRMING THE DIAGNOSIS

Once suspected, an abdominal abscess can be confirmed by one of several diagnostic imaging techniques. In general, chest and abdominal roentgenograms are nonspecific. During the past decade, refinements in computed tomography (CT scan), ultrasound (US), and nuclear medicine techniques have markedly improved diagnostic accuracy.[8] Abdominal CT scanning has become the preferred method of diagnosing abdominal abscesses for several reasons. Most importantly, this modality has a sensitivity of 95% to 100% and is not compromised by overlying bowel gas.

Oral and intravenous (IV) contrast-enhanced CT scans are essential to ensure a high-quality study and improve sensitivity. The use of oral contrast enables the radiologist to differentiate the abscess, which may contain air bubbles, from intestinal loops (Fig. 18–1A). Subdiaphragmatic, retroperitoneal and midabdominal abscesses are best visualized by CT scanning in comparison with other techniques. (Fig. 18–1B). The major disadvantages of CT scanning include its higher cost and use of ionizing radiation. Furthermore, a mature abscess may exhibit so-called ring enhancement with IV contrast. The most common appearance, however, is a round or oval mass of homogenous density with a thin wall. Although CT scanning can accurately localize an intraabdominal abscess, it cannot distinguish between infected and noninfected fluid. Therefore, a fine needle aspiration frequently becomes an important part of the diagnostic workup.

Abdominal US is best for evaluating the right upper quadrant (RUQ), retroperitoneum, and pelvis.[9] Its accuracy ranges from 57% to 96%. It is especially useful in critically ill patients who cannot be transported to the CT scanner. Because it lacks ionizing radiation, it is an attractive alternative in pregnant women. A major drawback is that its use is frequently confounded by overlying bowel gas. Unlike CT scanning, its effectiveness is determined by the individual performing the examination, and it is also much more time consuming. Despite these caveats, the less costly US can be particularly helpful in following lesions identified previously on CT scans or in guiding the percutaneous drainage of such an abscess.[9]

Nuclear imaging is most useful in identifying an abscess that is difficult to pinpoint by clinical examination (Fig. 18–2).[10] It can then direct further diagnostic studies to a particular focus. In one method, a radioactive substance is injected intravenously and is sequestered by the lung, liver, and spleen but not by the abscess. This results in the appearance of a "cold spot" on the scan. Alternatively, radiolabeled WBCs (e.g., indium or gallium) are reinjected into the patient. These cells are then recruited to an inflammatory site resulting in a "hot spot." Because nuclear medicine studies invariably require correlation with a more specific technique such as CT or US to confirm an abscess, their use in this arena has become increasingly limited.

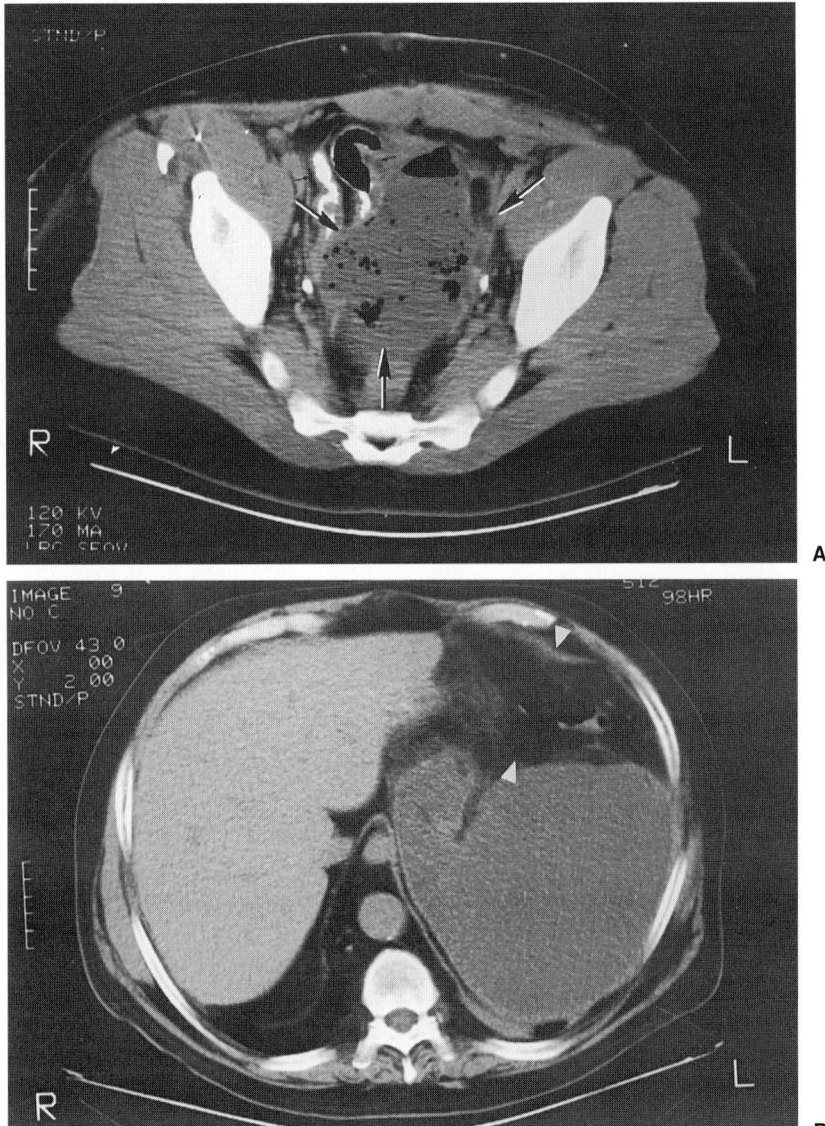

FIGURE 18–1. A, An interloop abscess is demonstrated in the midportion of the pelvis. Air bubbles indicative of gas formation by bacteria in the abscess are apparent; an air-fluid level is present as well. Thickening of the bowel wall is evident in contrast and air-filled loops of small intestine affected by Crohn's inflammatory bowel disease (arrows). **B,** A large subphrenic abscess is delineated by *two arrows.* Its cause was a perforated sigmoid colon diverticulum. (Courtesy of J. Casillas, MD, Department of Radiology, University of Miami.)

Unless otherwise indicated, when an abdominal abscess is suspected by history, physical examination, and laboratory data, the recommended approach is to begin with a contrast-enhanced CT scan of the abdomen and pelvis. If localized, diagnostic drainage is then warranted. If CT scanning is inconclusive, most authors recommend proceeding to exploratory laparotomy rather than attempting other modalities.

TREATMENT OPTIONS

The cornerstone of the effective treatment of an abdominal abscess is adequate drainage of the purulent contents. Antibiotic treatment is therefore adjunctive. Without drainage, mortality approaches 90%.[11]

Drainage can be accomplished either percutaneously or surgically.[12] Percutaneous drainage is

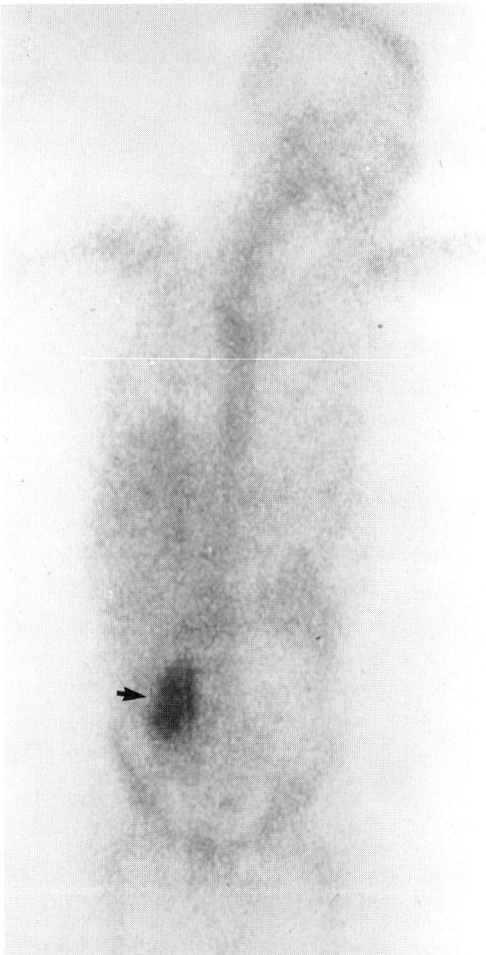

FIGURE 18–2. This whole body (anterior view) nuclear scintiscan utilizing gallium 67 citrate reveals a focal uptake of the isotope in the right lower abdominal quadrant consistent with the ultimately diagnosed periappendiceal abscess. (Courtesy of A. Serafini, MD, Department of Nuclear Medicine, University of Miami.)

performed with a fine, flexible needle using either CT or US guidance. It may conveniently be performed at the time of the initial diagnostic study. Successful percutaneous drainage requires a carefully planned, direct route to avoid entering a viscus or a large vessel. Failure to aspirate purulent material does not exclude an abscess, and additional attempts should be made if feasible. If pus is aspirated, a drainage catheter should then be placed. If the patient's clinical response improves (i.e., defervescence and decreased WBC count) within 1 to 2 days and there is minimal or no purulent drainage, the drainage catheter should be discontinued. Continuous drainage sets the stage for complex cavity infection by catheter contamination. If the patient fails to respond clinically with continued catheter drainage, the catheter should be repositioned. Persistent drainage with lack of a clinical response would then suggest a fistula between the bowel and the abscess that may require surgical intervention. On the other hand, cessation of drainage in the setting of a poor clinical response despite repositioning of the catheter should prompt surgical intervention. When percutaneous drainage is successful, the overall efficacy for abscess ablation is 90%.

Surgical drainage is indicated when there is an unfavorable response to percutaneous drainage or if percutaneous drainage cannot be performed safely (e.g., the abscess is surrounded by loops of bowel). An exploratory laparotomy (i.e., intraperitoneal approach) is preferable to the transperitoneal approach, which has largely been supplanted by the equally efficacious percutaneous technique. Laparotomy and drainage of the abscess are followed by placement of a large bore surgical drain. As the purulent drainage decreases, abscess resolution can be measured by injecting contrast via the drainage tube. When drainage ceases and the abscess cavity has decreased in size, the drainage tube is then removed.

Antibiotic therapy should be initiated once an abscess has been diagnosed, prior to percutaneous or surgical intervention. Accordingly, initial treatment is almost always empiric as the precise organism has not been identified. The initial antibiotic should inhibit gram-negative enteric organisms, obligate anaerobes, and gram-positive cocci (particularly the enterococcus). Traditionally, ampicillin, an aminoglycoside such as gentamicin, and metronidazole (or clindamycin) have been used to broadly inhibit these groups of organisms. The monobactam, aztreonam, harbors excellent bactericidal activity against gram-negative enteric organisms and can replace ampicillin in patients who are allergic to the penicillins. It is also useful for patients with renal insufficiency in whom an aminoglycoside could both worsen renal function and lead to ototoxicity because of impaired excretion. Second-generation cephalosporins have been substituted for ampicillin with equal efficacy. The duration of antibiotic therapy is dictated by the patient's clinical response. In general, a 1- to 2-week course is required. It is important to observe for complications of prolonged antibiotic use such as emergence of resistant strains, pseudomembranous colitis, and gastrointestinal candidiasis.

The general medical condition of the patient with an abdominal abscess must also be closely monitored. Complications of sepsis include disseminated intravascular coagulation (DIC), adult respiratory distress syndrome (ARDS), acute tubular necrosis (ATN), decreased systemic vascular resistance with shock, and hyperbilirubinemia. These conditions must be recognized and promptly corrected with the appropriate supportive measures, preferably in an intensive care setting. Partial or complete mechanical bowel obstruction caused by the abscess can occur during any phase of the illness and can readily be recognized on plain films of the abdomen. This complication can be managed conservatively with nasogastric suction, but it frequently requires surgical correction.

REFERENCES

1. Bernstein SA, Rogers AI. Diaphragm, peritoneum, mesentery, omentum. In: Dietschy JM, ed. *Disorders of the Gastrointestinal Tract. Disorders of the Liver. Nutritional Disorders.* New York, NY: Grune & Stratton; 1976:348.
2. Pellegrini CA, Gordon RL. Abdominal abscesses and gastrointestinal fistulas. In: Sleisenger MH, Fordtran JS, eds. *Gastrointestinal Disease: Pathophysiology, Diagnosis, Management,* 5th ed. Philadelphia, Pa: WB Saunders Co; 1993:1962, chap 98.
3. Styrt B, Gorbach SL. Recent developments in the understanding of the pathogenesis and treatment of anaerobic infections. *N Engl J Med.* 1989;321:240.
4. Hau T, Haaga JR, Aeder MI. Pathophysiology, diagnosis, and treatment of abdominal abscesses. *Curr Prob Surg.* 1984;21:1–82.
5. Whitman DH. World progress in surgery: intraabdominal infections. *World J Surg.* 1990;14:145.
6. Mustard RA, Bohmen JM, Rosati C, et al. Pneumonia complicating abdominal sepsis. *Arch Surg.* 1991;126:170.
7. Halasz NA. Subphrenic abscesses: myths and facts. *JAMA.* 1970;214:724.
8. Haaga JR. Imaging intra-abdominal abscesses and nonoperative drainage procedures. *World J Surg.* 1990;14:204.
9. Carroll B, Silverman PM, Goodwin DA, McDougall IR. Ultrasonography and indium III white blood cell scanning for the detection of intra-abdominal abscesses. *Radiology.* 1981;140:155.
10. Pellegrini CA, Gordon RL. Abdominal abscesses and gastrointestinal fistulas. In: Sleisenger MH, Fordtran JS, eds. *Gastrointestinal Disease, II.* 5th ed. Philadelphia, Pa: WB Saunders Co; 1993:1962.
11. Datz FL, Luers P, Baker WJ, Christian PE. Improved detection of upper abdominal abscesses by combination of 99m to sulfur colloid and indium III in leukocyte scanning. *Am J Radiol.* 1985;144:319.
12. Aeder MI, Wellman JL, Haaga JR, Hau J. Role of surgical and percutaneous drainage in the treatment of abdominal abscesses. *Arch Surg.* 1983;118:273.

19

Gastrointestinal Fistulas

LEOPOLDO GRAUER and JAMIE S. BARKIN

A fistula is defined as an abnormal communication between two epithelialized surfaces. Overall, a fistula is described by the anatomic feature and the organ(s) involved.

In this chapter, we will discuss the factors that favor development of fistulas, their sequelae, and therapy.

ETIOLOGY

Fistulas of the gastrointestinal tract are either acquired or congenital. Among the congenital defects, esophageal atresia with tracheoesophageal fistulas and rectovaginal fistulas are the most common.

Acquired fistulas result from a variety of conditions; however, the majority result from previous surgical procedures,[1–3] appears within 2 weeks after surgery, but may take a few months to be discovered.[1,4] The factors that contribute to the occurrence of postoperative fistulas include unrecognized surgical bowel penetration, anastomosis leakage, and devascularized bowel.

Spontaneous fistulas occur most commonly as a result of a variety of underlying causes including inflammatory bowel disease (most frequently Crohn's disease, radiation, cancer, diverticulitis, peptic ulcer disease, gallbladder diseases, and pancreatic disorders).[5,6] Trauma to the abdomen (blunt or penetrating) is also a major cause for intestinal fistulas.

CLASSIFICATION

Fistulas are classified according to their anatomic features and amount of daily discharge. These characteristics influence the final outcome and guide the proper treatment (Table 19–1).

If there is communication between the gut and the body surface, an external fistula is present. Conversely, when the bowel communicates directly or via an abscess with another viscus, an internal fistula is present. Overall, external fistulas are more likely to require surgical treatment than internal fistulas. However, internal fistulas that involve the urinary or reproductive systems or bypass a large portion of bowel also require surgical treatment.

An important factor that influences fistula healing is the presence or absence of obstruction distal to the bowel wall defect. Whenever distal obstruction is present, an uninterrupted, preferential flow of intestinal contents through the fistula occurs, thus preventing spontaneous healing. Therefore, maintenance of intestinal continuity, which allows distal progression of intestinal contents through the gastrointestinal tract, is important for spontaneous fistula closure. A lateral fistula arises perpendicular to the bowel wall, resulting in only partial diversion of intraluminal contents through the fistula. Conversely, an end fistula is present when there is loss of intestinal continuity beyond the fistula and the fistula functions as a colostomy. These fistulas are usually complex and require surgical intervention.

A simple fistula communicates directly to the skin or another organ, whereas complicated fistulas are defined as multiple fistulas involving more than one viscus. The volume of fistula output is a useful but variable method to classify fistulas. In general, a low-output fistula discharges less than 500 ml/d. A fistula that discharges more than 500 ml of fluid daily is said to be of high output and usually is located in the proximal gastrointestinal tract (e.g., stomach, duodenum, or jejunum). High-output fistulas are more difficult to treat and carry a worse prognosis.[7,8]

SEQUELAE AND PROGNOSTIC FACTORS

Multiple problems may result as a consequence of fistula formations, all of which should be aggressively treated prior to embarking on any surgical therapy.[2] The exteriorization of enteric contents produces fluid and electrolyte losses and skin excoriation. Internal fistulas, on the other hand, contaminate sterile bowel and may produce malabsorption by bypass of portions of the gut and by bacterial contamination. The overgrowth of sterile bowel with an inoculum of colonic bacteria of 10^9 counts of anaerobic bacteria produces diarrhea and malassimilation similar to gastrocolonic fistulas.

Overall, electrolyte imbalance, sepsis, and malnutrition are associated with high mortality in enterocutaneous fistulas. Mortality secondary to a fistula has markedly decreased when these abnormalities are corrected early and adequately. Rapid control of sepsis is of paramount importance to achieve this goal. It remains the single most important factor contributing to mortality in these patients.[6,13] Fortunately, early recognition and evolving therapies have decreased the mortality of enterocutaneous fistulas from an average of 50% to less than 20%.[1,6–9]

The probability of fistula closure and the mortality associated with a fistula is related to anatomic and physiologic factors (Table 19–2). Athanassiades and others[5] found that the most common causes for lack of medical success were:

1. Presence of intestinal obstruction distal to the fistula
2. Loss of bowel continuity
3. Active underlying bowel disease (e.g., Crohn's disease, postradiation, malignancy)[10,11]
4. Eversion of bowel mucosa with mucocutaneous continuity
5. Epithelialization of the fistulous tract
6. Bowel wall opening larger than 1 cm
7. Presence of a foreign body

TABLE 19–1. CLASSIFICATION OF GASTROINTESTINAL FISTULAS

- External versus internal
- Complicated versus simple
- Low versus high output
- Lateral versus end
- Congenital versus acquired

TABLE 19–2. FACTORS ASSOCIATED WITH POOR FISTULA CLOSURE AND PROGNOSIS

- Intestinal obstruction
- Active underlying bowel disease (Crohn's disease, malignancy, radiation)
- High output (>500 ml/24 h)
- Epithelialization of the fistula tract
- Proximal small bowel location
- Eversion or bowel wall opening larger than 1 cm
- Age >50 years
- Malnutrition

Large abdominal wall defects and a short fistulous tract are not likely to heal spontaneously, and they carry a higher mortality.[12] Increased mortality has also been observed in relation to age.[10,13] In one study, the mortality in patients over the age of 70 years was 76% compared with 39% for those below the age of 70 years. This was confirmed by Levy who found a progressive increase of mortality from 35% up to 45% in patients 50 years and older, compared with 20% in patients under 50 years.[13]

Other important factors that influence the healing of a fistula are its location, its output, and the patient's nutritional status. Proximal jejunal fistulas have an overall mortality of 37.8% compared with 17.5% for ileal fistulas.[7] This increased mortality of proximal fistulas is probably secondary to their large volume of fluid losses, delay in closure, and predisposition for infection. A number of studies have shown an increased mortality associated with high-output fistulas compared with patients with low-output fistulas.[1,6,7] Edmunds[1] reported a mortality of 54% versus 16% in patients with high- versus low-output fistulas, and Coutsoftides and Fazio[7] found a mortality of 30% in high-output fistulas versus 5% in low output.

The presence of malnutrition will interfere with the healing process of a fistula. Coutsoftides and Fazio[7] found that malnutrition defined as loss of more than 15% of body weight, anemia with a hemoglobin less than 10 g/dl, and hypoalbuminemia significantly increases mortality. This deleterious effect of poor nutritional status on mortality has been confirmed by several studies.[2,3,7] Therefore, nutritional support is essential for management of patients with external fistulas to prevent and treat malnutrition in an effort to promote healing.

MANAGEMENT

Rapid deterioration of patients with a fistula may occur if its complications are not recognized and managed aggressively. Some fistulas may manifest insidiously with small amounts of discharge, whereas others may manifest with copious discharge, hypotension, and fever.[3] Chapman and others[2] summarized the caveats that must be avoided in the management of these patients:

When the fistula appears, there is a tendency to do nothing at first, see how bad it is going to be and, by the time the full impact of the catastrophe has struck, the patient is septic, anemic, nutritionally depleted, often severely dehydrated and has extensive breakdown of the skin.

Gastrointestinal fistulas may require either medical or surgical therapy or a combination of the two modalities. The medical treatment includes nasogastric suction, fluid replacement, antibiotics, percutaneous abscess drainage, and enteral or parenteral nutrition. The surgical management consists of abscess drainage, fistula closure, obstruction relief and revision, and remaking of anastomosis. The management of these patients can be divided into three phases: (1) stabilization, (2) investigation, and (3) definitive therapy.[3]

STABILIZATION PHASE

During this early period, the following activities are conducted: fluid resuscitation, sepsis control, skin care, nutrition support, and correction of electrolyte abnormalities. Volume replacement must include fistulas output. Thus, the total volume administered includes measured losses of urinary and nasogastric secretions, insensible losses, fistula output, and daily requirements. A nasogastric tube is suggested for patients with high enterocutaneous fistulas to have a better control of high fistula output. A central intravenous catheter should be placed to provide long-term fluid and parenteral nutrition. Control of sepsis is mandatory in these patients. Multiorganism sepsis is not uncommon and is the consequence of disruption of bowel integrity. Bacteroides, enterococci, and coliforms are the most common organisms involved. The presence of an active infectious process (abscess formation and infected necrotic tissue) prevents fistula healing and therefore must be treated. Broad spectrum antibiotics are used when indicated by clinical and laboratory findings. Control of an external fistula drainage is necessary to protect the skin from the effects of the effluence and quantification of fluid output. Insertion of a soft catheter into the fistula, attached to low intermittent suction permits this goal. The fistula opening should be covered with stomatoadhesive and skin karaya paste applied to the borders to prevent any leakage.[14]

Malnutrition is an important factor influencing the fistula outcome. External fistulas, especially those with an output of more than 500 ml/d, affect the patient's nutritional status. Lack of oral intake and associated hypermetabolic state are the other factors that increase this deficit. Overall, correction of nutritional status, although questioned,[6,15] has been shown to improve fistula closure and decrease mortality.[3,16,17]

The associated hypercatabolic state with sepsis requires large caloric intake, which can be provided by enteral feeding or total parenteral nutrition (TPN). Enteral nutrition is possible for patients with low-output fistulas or fistulas located distally in the ileum or colon. To be effective, enteral nutrition must be infused proximal or distal to the disrupted bowel.[18] Parenteral nutrition is mandatory in patients with high-output fistulas who are unable to use their enteral route.

Chapman and others[2] found that the administration of optimal versus suboptimal amounts of calories made a significant difference in mortality. The mortality rate in patients receiving 2500 kcal/d or more was 12% in contrast to 58% in patients receiving less than 1600. Sheldon et al[3] found similar results in 51 patients and MacFayden et al[15] reported a mortality of 6.5% in patients receiving between 2000 and 5000 kcal via TPN.[17]

However, the beneficial effect of TPN on fistula mortality is unclear, and most likely its major contribution is the prevention of malnutrition, with its favorable physiologic effects.[6,15] Soeters et al,[6] in a review of 404 patients with external gastrointestinal fistulas, concluded that although fistula closure rate improved from 10% to 35% with TPN, there was no change in mortality. Reber et al,[13] in a review of 186 patients, found that the fistula-related mortality and spontaneous closure rates were unchanged. This difference in opinion regarding the import of TPN on mortality is probably due to the inhomogeneous population of patients.

Somatostatin, a tetradecapeptide known for its inhibitory effects on gastrointestinal secretions, has been used as an adjunctive therapy for fistula closure.[19,20] Geerdsen et al,[21] in a small cohort study of patients, demonstrated decreased fistula closure time and hospital stay in patients treated with somatostatin. Penderzoli et al[22] compared healing rates in patients with external fistulas who were treated with either TPN alone, TPN and somatostatin, TPN and calcitonin, or TPN and glucagon. No significant difference among these treatments was observed in the percentage of fistula closures, ranging from 85% to 100% in these regimens. However, in patients treated with TPN plus somatostatin, the fistulas closed within a shorter period of time. This shortened healing time was confirmed in a recent multicenter trial of 40 patients from Spain.[23] The usual dose used in these trials was 250 1g/h; however, alternate intermittent subcutaneous doses may also be given.

INVESTIGATION PHASE

The anatomy of a fistula, its underlying pathology, and the presence of bowel obstruction or abscess formation must be precisely defined prior to surgical intervention. These factors will determine the type and timing of therapeutic intervention. The investigative modalities include endoscopic studies and radiologic imaging luminal studies with orally or intrarectal administration of contrast. Small bowel follow-through or barium enema are needed to evaluate bowel integrity. A fistulogram is an inexpensive and often very informative study performed by inserting a small catheter into the skin opening of the fistula and injecting water-soluble contrast. This procedure often helps to determine the anatomic extent of the fistula and defines its complexity. New endoscopic techniques may be useful as diagnostic and therapeutic modalities. Fistuloscopy with a small choledochoscope has been useful in determining the extent of the inflammatory process, the precise placement of drainage catheters into complex abscesses, and the removal of foreign bodies (i.e., suture material and necrotic tissue).[24,25] Abdominal computed tomography is the most reliable technique for evaluating extraluminal pathology contributing to or resulting from fistula formation. It is especially useful for diagnosis of abdominal abscesses and for guidance of percutaneous drainage.[26]

DEFINITIVE THERAPY

Definitive surgical therapy is usually only performed after a trial of medical treatment. Fortunately spontaneous fistula closure occurs in the majority of patients after an average of 30 days.[2,3,10,17,21,22] Early surgical intervention is indicated whenever poor medical response is anticipated, as in the presence of severe intraabdominal sepsis, bowel obstruction distal to the fistula, visualization of intestinal mucosa or disease process, or loss of bowel continuity. Once sepsis is eliminated and nutritional support is adequate, external fistulas should begin to close. Internal fistulas rarely require surgery unless fever, diarrhea, or obstruction is present. If after 8 weeks of continuous medical treatment the fistula has not closed, surgical intervention is indicated. This time will allow for any peritoneal reaction to subside and underlying infection, malnutrition, and electrolyte imbalance to be corrected.

The definitive operation of choice is resection of the segment of bowel containing the fistula followed by end-to-end anastomosis. If this is not possible, bypass operations with fistula exclusion or exteriorization of bowel proximal to the fistula is desirable.[1,3,7] Obviously, if an associated abscess cavity is found, it should be evacuated and properly drained. Fistulas located in the second portion of the duodenum are treated with the serosal patch technique.

Healing of biliary fistulas without surgery has been accomplished with endoscopic techniques. External biliary fistulas, usually the result of surgery, can be treated endoscopically with the insertion of a biliary stent through the ampulla of Vater or by papillotomy. These techniques eliminate or decrease the high-pressure ampullary zone, allowing for biliary drainage into the duodenum as opposed to through the fistula. Feretis et al[27] achieved a success rate of 90% in 14 patients managed with these techniques. Goldin et al,[28] in a study of 5 patients with intrahepatic and common bile duct leaks, found no evidence of leakage 1 year after the successful placement of a temporary biliary stent. Unconventional treatments with fast-hardening amino acid solutions and fibrin tissue sealant injected into the fistula have been used with encouraging results in a limited number of patients; however, their role is undetermined.[24,29,30]

In summary, gastrointestinal fistulas are usually the consequence of a surgical procedure. Their location and output, as well as the presence of infection and other associated morbid conditions, are important considerations for successful management of patients with gastrointestinal fistulas. Early recognition and therapy of electrolyte imbalance, sepsis, and malnutrition are critical factors in the management of these patients.

REFERENCES

1. Edmunds LH, Williams GM, Welch CE. External fistulas arising from the gastrointestinal tract. *Ann Surg.* 1960;152:445–466.
2. Chapman R, Foran R, Dunphy JE. Management of intestinal fistulas. *Am J Surg.* 1964;108:157–162.
3. Sheldon GF, Gardiner BN, Way LW, Dunphy JE. Management of gastrointestinal fistulas. *Surg Gynecol Obstet.* 1971;133:385–389.
4. Allardyce DB. Management of small bowel fistulas. *Ann Surg.* 1983;145:593–595.
5. Athanassiades S, Notis P, Tountas C. Fistulas of the gastrointestinal tract: experience with eighty-one cases. *Am J Surg.* 1975;130:26–28.
6. Soeters PB, Ebeid AM, Fischer JE. Review of 404 patients with gastrointestinal fistulas: impact of parenteral nutrition. *Ann Surg.* 1979;190:189–202.
7. Coutsoftides T, Fazio VW. Small intestine cutaneous fistulas. *Surg Gynecol Obstet.* 1979;149:333–336.
8. Fischer JE. The pathophysiology of enterocutaneous fistulas. *World J Surg.* 1983;7:446–450.
9. McIntyre PB, Ritchie JK, Hawley PR, et al. Management of enterocutaneous fistulas: a review of 132 cases. *Br J Surg.* 1984;71:293–296.
10. Schein M, Decker GAG. Gastrointestinal fistulas associated with large abdominal wall defects: experience with 43 patients. *Br J Surg.* 1990;77:97–100.
11. Levy E, Frileux P, Cugnenc PH, Honiger J, Ollivier JM, Parc R. High output external fistulae of the small bowel: management with continuous enteral nutrition. *Br J Surg.* 1989;76:676–679.
12. Rombeau J, Rolandelli R. Enteral and parenteral nutrition in patients with enteric fistulas. *Surg Clin North Am.* 1987;67(3):551–568.
13. Reber HA, Roberts C, Way LW, Dunphy JE. Management of external gastrointestinal fistulas. *Ann Surg.* 1978;188:460–465.
14. Sitges-Serra A, Jaurrieta E, Sitges-Creus A. Management of postoperative enterocutaneous fistulas: the roles of parenteral nutrition and surgery. *Br J Surg.* 1982;69:147–150.
15. MacFayden B, Dudrick SJ, Ruberg RL. Management of gastrointestinal fistulas with parenteral hyperalimentation. *Surgery.* 1973;74:100–104.
16. Hollender LF, Meyer C, Avet D, Zeyer B. Postoperative fistulas of the small intestine: therapeutic principles. *World J Surg.* 1983;7:474–480.
17. Knighton D, Burns K, Nyhus L. The use of stomadhesive in the care of the skin of enterocutaneous fistula. *Surg Gynecol Obstet.* 1976;143:449–451.
18. Ali SD, Leffall LD. Management of external fistulas of the gastrointestinal tract. *Am J Surg.* 1972;123:535–537.
19. Konturek SJ. Somatostatin and gastrointestinal secretions. *Scand J Gastroenterol.* 1976;11:11–14.
20. Grosman I, Simon D. Potential gastrointestinal uses of somatostatin and its synthetic analogue octreotide. *Am J Gastroenterol.* 1990;85:1061–1072.
21. Geerdsen JP, Pedersen VM, Kjaergard HK. Small bowel fistulas treated with somatostatin: preliminary results. *Surgery.* 1986;100:811–813.

22. Penderzoli P, Bassi C, Falconi M, Albrigo R, Vantini I, Micciolio R. Conservative treatment of external pancreatic fistulas with parenteral nutrition alone or in combination with continuous intravenous infusion of somatostatin, glucagon or calcitonin. *Surg Gynecol Obstet.* 1986;163:428–431.
23. Torres AJ, Landa JI, Moreno-Azcoita M, et al. Somatostatin in the management of gastrointestinal fistulas, a multicenter trial. *Arch Surg.* 1992;127:97–99.
24. Yamakawa T, Suzuki T, Kobayashi S, et al. Fistuloscopy for the management of postoperative intra-abdominal abscesses. *Endoscopy.* 1992;24:218–221.
25. Nakagawa K, Momono S, Sasaki Y, Furusawa A, Ujiie K. Endoscopy examination for fistula. *Endoscopy.* 1990;22:208–210.
26. Van Sonnemberg E, D'Agostino H, Casola G, et al. Percutaneous abscess drainage: current concepts. *Radiology.* 1991;181:617–626.
27. Feretis C, Kekis B, Bliouras N, et al. Postoperative external and internal biliary fistulas, unassociated with distal bile duct obstruction: endoscopic treatment. *Endoscopy.* 1990;22:211–213.
28. Goldin E, Katz E, Wengrower D, et al. Treatment of fistulas of the biliary tract by endoscopic insertion of endoprostheses. *Surg Gynecol Obstet.* 1990;170:418–423.
29. Cadoni S, Ottonello R, Maxia G, et al. Endoscopic treatment of a duodenocutaneous fistula with fibrin tissue sealant (Tissucol). *Endoscopy.* 1990;22:194–195.
30. Marone G, Santoro M, Torre V. Successful endoscopic treatment of GI tract fistulas with a fast-hardening amino acid solution. *Endoscopy.* 1989;21:47–49.

20
Acute Upper Gastrointestinal Tract Bleeding

JOHN L. PETRINI

Upper gastrointestinal (UGI) tract bleeding is a life-threatening emergency requiring immediate attention and evaluation, with effective treatment based on accurate diagnosis. Although many patients have minimal or self-limited bleeding, significant hemorrhage is common, and mortality is approximately 10%, a figure that has not changed in seven decades.

Studies of patients with UGI tract hemorrhage, based on relatively fixed populations with single-source medical services in Great Britain, have suggested that the annual rate of hospital admissions for UGI tract bleeding is approximately 50 per 100,000, which would represent approximately 130,000 people in the United States. Information derived from US hospital admissions for bleeding peptic ulcer alone suggests a somewhat higher incidence of between 50 and 150 per 100,000 or roughly 250,000 people per year. This data underestimates the magnitude of the problem, as individuals who suffer UGI tract bleeding while in the hospital for another reason are not included. Despite reduction in the number of hospital admissions for peptic ulcer disease with changing medical therapy and the introduction of H_2 receptor antagonists, admissions for bleeding ulcer have not changed.

Although mortality has not appreciably changed since the first report by Bulmer in 1927, there has been a shift toward advancing age for both bleeding and a fatal outcome from UGI tract bleeding. Advances in diagnosis, resuscitation, surgery, and endoscopic therapy have improved the chances of survival from the bleeding episode, but underlying physical condition, nutritional status, and other medical illnesses still place the elderly at increased risk. It is clear that few patients succumb to the bleeding itself, as most bleeding subsides with falling intravascular pressure. However, the consequences of prolonged hypotension, impaired perfusion of tissues, transfusions of crystalloids and blood products, and therapeutic interventions may still impart significant consequences to those with underlying poor health. UGI tract bleeding should be evaluated and treated within the context of the clinical situation and individualized to meet each patient's unique medical condition (Fig. 20–1).

This chapter confines itself to UGI tract bleeding that occurs within the area from the proximal esophagus to the ligament of Treitz. Bleeding site or the lesion responsible for UGI tract bleeding has been shown to be remarkably similar in studies on unselected patients. Peptic ulcer accounts for 40% to 50% of bleeding, with varices, gastritis, esophagitis, Mallory-Weiss lesion, vascular ectasia, tumors, and others, such as Dieulafoy's lesion, accounting for the majority of the remaining identified sites of bleeding. Selected patient populations will have differing incidences of bleeding sites, and these differences will often indicate the course of action that will maximize outcome from acute UGI tract hemorrhage (see Table 20–1).

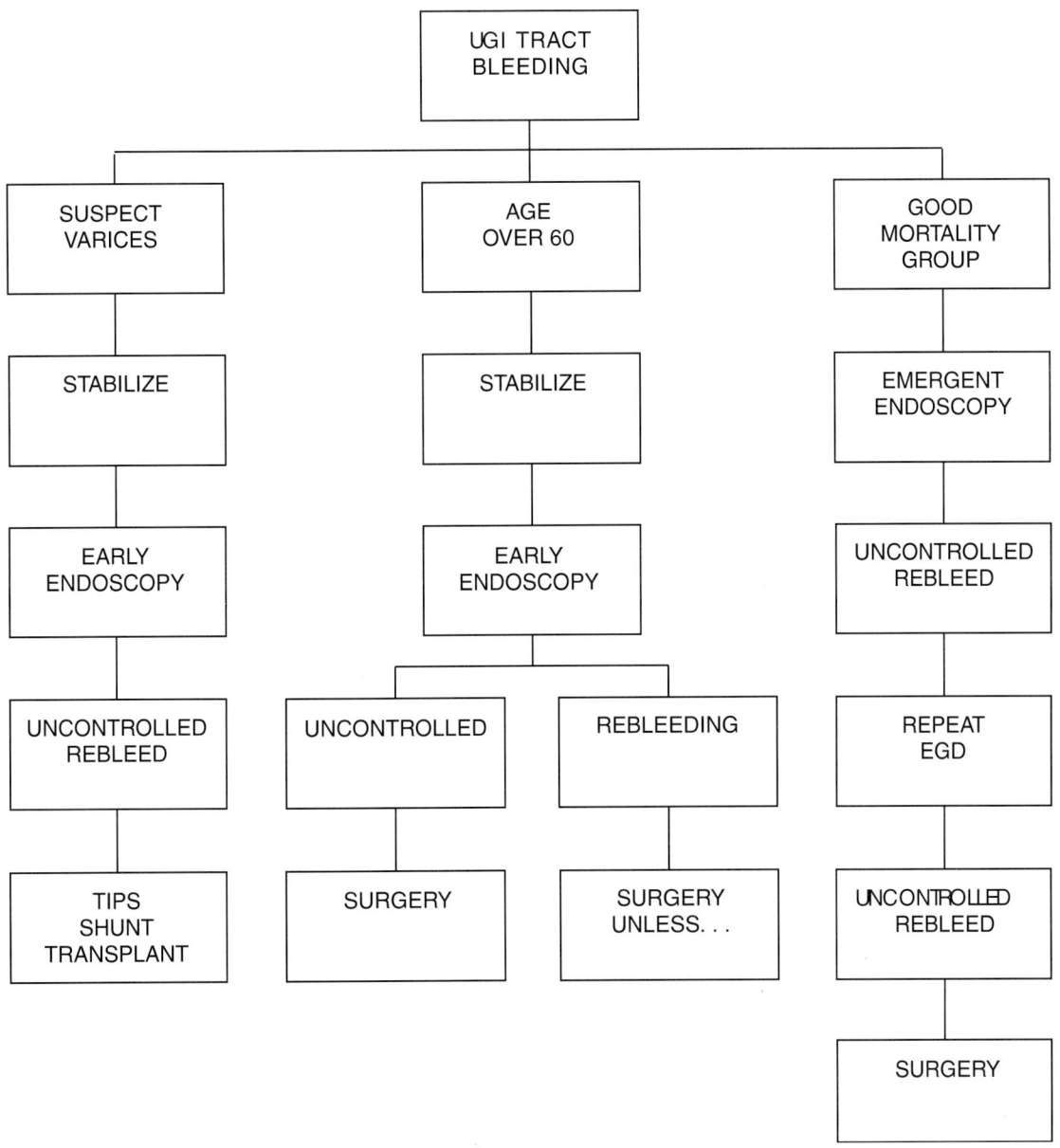

FIGURE 20–1. Evaluation and treatment of UGI tract bleeding. *EGD* = esophagogastroduodenoscopy, *TIPS* = transjugular intrahepatic portosystemic shunt, *UGI* = upper gastrointestinal.

TABLE 20–1. SOURCE OF BLEEDING FROM THE UGI TRACT

SOURCE	ASGE SURVEY*	LOS ANGELES COUNTY HOSPITAL†
Duodenal ulcer	22%	27%
Gastric erosions	22%	3%
Gastric ulcer	20%	13%
Varices	10%	31%
Mallory-Weiss lesion	7%	13%
Peptic esophagitis	6%	2%
Erosive duodenitis	6%	
Neoplasm	2%	1%
Vascular ectasia	<1%	1%
Dieulafoy's lesion	<1%	
Aortoenteric fistula	<1%	
Unknown or other	3–5%	8%

*Data from Gilbert, Silverstein, Tedesco, et al. *Gastrointest Endosc.* 1981;27:94–102.
†Data from Laine. *Aliment Pharmacol Ther.* 1993;7:207–232.

CLINICAL PRESENTATION

While the initial manifestations of UGI tract bleeding are usually hypotension, tachycardia, diaphoresis, and increased activity of the bowel, patients most often become aware of the bleeding when they experience melena or hematemesis. An estimate of the severity of bleeding and subsequent mortality can be based on the clinical presentation. Patients who vomit red blood are bleeding more rapidly than patients with coffee-ground hematemesis, and patients with maroon stool are bleeding more rapidly than patients with melena. These criteria also correlate with morbidity and mortality, with patients vomiting bright red blood or passing maroon stool more likely to require transfusion, experience rebleeding, require surgery, and have a fatal outcome. A survey of members of the American Society for Gastrointestinal Endoscopy published in 1981 correlated mortality with the findings at presentation. In patients with clear nasogastric aspirate and black stools, mortality was 5%; with coffee-ground aspirate and black stools, 8%; with fresh blood aspirate and black stool, 12%; with red or maroon stool, 18%; and those with fresh blood aspirate and red or maroon stool, 29%. Other presenting findings suggesting more severe hemorrhage include hypotension on admission, bleeding requiring more than 6 U in 24 hours to maintain pressure, bleeding that occurs while hospitalized for another illness, history of liver disease, previous episodes of UGI tract bleeding, and the use of nonsteroidal antiinflammatory drugs (NSAIDs) or underlying coagulopathy.

The initial assessment of patients with UGI tract bleeding includes immediate measurement of vital signs, including orthostatic blood pressure and pulse, along with a careful, directed history and physical examination. Patients manifest orthostatic hypotension for some time before a drop in hemoglobin or hematocrit is apparent, because of initial contraction of blood volume with bleeding prior to hemodilution. Orthostasis or supine hypotension on admission to a medical facility is correlated with significant hemorrhage. A nasogastric tube is a valuable adjunct to assessment of active bleeding, but the lack of blood return does not eliminate the UGI tract as the source of bleeding. Brown or black particulate matter (coffee-grounds) suggests limited hemorrhage or bleeding that is currently inactive, whereas fresh blood is indicative of rapid or active bleeding. Placing a nasogastric tube is a better diagnostic than therapeutic tool, as the role of lavage for treatment has never been established, and small nasogastric tubes will not clear the stomach of significant blood clots. A large bore (Ewald) tube is required in most instances to remove large volumes of retained or clotted blood for better visualization of the gastric mucosa at endoscopy.

Since 75% to 85% of bleeding stops spontaneously, factors associated with prolonged bleeding, increased mortality, or rebleeding should be sought. These factors will help direct the timing and extent of intervention and further evaluation (see Table 20–2).

The stability of the patient is established by resuscitation using fluids administered through 16- or 18-gauge intravenous cannulas, as all bleeding can theoretically be managed with adequate blood replacement until definitive control of the bleeding is obtained. The number of intravenous access sites and rates of fluid replacement must be tailored carefully to each clinical situation, but two sites are usually required for significant bleeding, both for volume replacement and administration of medications. Since patients have decreased oxygen-carrying capacity with reduction in hemoglobin, supplemental nasal cannula oxygen is appropriate, particularly if the patient is elderly or has underlying cardiac or pulmonary disease. Patients should be transfused to an appropriate level. For young, healthy patients a hemoglobin of 8 g/dl might be easily tolerated, whereas an elderly patient with coronary artery disease or peripheral vascular disease might need a hemoglobin of 10 g/dl or more to be com-

TABLE 20-2. FACTORS ASSOCIATED WITH A GREATER LIKELIHOOD OF REBLEEDING (AND GREATER MORTALITY)

- Large volume blood loss at admission:
    Transfusion of greater than 6 U
    Persistent hypotension
- Coagulopathy, including use of NSAIDs
- History of previous UGI tract bleeding
- Stigmata of liver disease
- Age greater than 60 years
- Other major system medical problems (cardiac, pulmonary, renal, neurologic)
- Bleeding that occurs while hospitalized for another problem
- Stigmata of recent hemorrhage at endoscopy:
    Active bleeding
    Visible vessel
    Adherent clot

NSAIDs = nonsteroidal antiinflammatory drugs, UGI = upper gastrointestinal.

fortable. If patients have an underlying coagulopathy or have received large doses of NSAIDs, transfusions of fresh-frozen plasma or platelets may be helpful to slow or stop bleeding. Measurement of urine output is an important parameter to ascertain adequate intravascular volume. Care must be taken to prevent excess fluid transfusion in patients with cardiac, pulmonary, renal, and hepatic disease to avoid congestive heart failure and increased portal pressure. For most patients with significant hemorrhage, management in an intensive care unit is essential.

Once the patient is hemodynamically stable, an appropriate diagnostic and therapeutic plan can be established. Although numerous diagnostic modalities are available for the evaluation of patients with UGI tract bleeding, UGI tract endoscopy performed within the first 12 hours after admission is the diagnostic procedure of choice. Factors that suggest a higher risk of rebleeding, including the possibility of variceal hemorrhage, should prompt earlier endoscopy. One special consideration is the patient with previous aortic graft, as the initial presentation of aortoenteric fistula may be mild or "herald" bleeding. These patients should be evaluated at once, as the next episode of bleeding may be exsanguinating, and early surgical intervention is required.

Endoscopy provides not only excellent visualization of the UGI tract, it can permit assessment of multiple potential sites of bleeding, as well as offer therapeutic modalities to control bleeding. It is contraindicated when the patient is unable to safely undergo the examination or in the presence of a perforated ulcer. If perforation is suspected, plain films of the abdomen should be obtained prior to endoscopy. Patients with severe bleeding or esophageal bleeding (varices, sclerotherapy-induced ulcers in the esophagus, or Mallory-Weiss lesion) and those with an impaired gag reflex may be unable to protect their airway during endoscopy, and endotracheal intubation should be considered before endoscopy is attempted. Although complications in patients undergoing elective or diagnostic endoscopy are uncommon, emergency endoscopy carries a higher risk of cardiopulmonary complications, such as aspiration and arrhythmia, as well as perforation and reactivation of bleeding.

Contrast UGI tract series is not only less likely to reveal the bleeding site, but residual barium may interfere with angiography and endoscopy if they are subsequently needed. Angiography and tagged red blood cell studies are of use during the active bleeding phase, which may be intermittent, and are not likely to reveal the active bleeding site at rates less than 0.5 ml/min.

The utility and superiority of endoscopy in diagnosing the site of UGI tract bleeding have been established in numerous studies. Only recently, however, have improvements in outcome and survival been demonstrated with a variety of endoscopic techniques to control the bleeding lesion. Emergency endoscopy in the bleeding patient is one of the most difficult endoscopic procedures, and it should be performed by a skilled endoscopist who is ready to treat any bleeding lesion appropriate for endoscopic therapy at the time of the initial endoscopy. Although diagnostic endoscopy is usually an outpatient procedure performed with minimal intravenous sedation, emergency endoscopy in a bleeding patient may be performed with no sedation or may require protection of the patient's airway with an endotracheal tube and general anesthesia. Endoscopy should not delay surgery for patients with exsanguinating hemorrhage, and a "team management" approach with gastroenterologist and surgeon both involved early in the patient's hospitalization is advantageous.

The type of bleeding lesion (e.g., ulcer, varix, tumor) has properties that may offer therapeutic advantages to one or more forms of therapy. These lesions are discussed in the sections that follow. In general, an initial attempt at endoscopic hemostasis is preferable to surgery and is less expensive than radiographic approaches. In addition, the therapy can be brought to the patient at the bedside rather than requiring the patient be moved to the radiology suite, usually at some distance from the support services provided in the intensive care unit (ICU).

THERAPY FOR SPECIFIC BLEEDING LESIONS

BLEEDING PEPTIC ULCER

The initial endoscopic assessment of bleeding from gastric or duodenal ulcer should include the size, location, and appearance of the ulcer. Large ulcers, gastric ulcers (especially those high on the lesser curvature), duodenal ulcers located on the posteroinferior wall, and ulcers with active bleeding, visible vessel, or adherent clot are more likely to rebleed and require surgical therapy if bleeding cannot be arrested. If patients are older or have multiple medical problems, there is evidence that early surgical intervention in these cases may reduce the mortality associated with either the operation or consequences of bleeding.

Most bleeding from ulcers is mild, usually from small mucosal blood vessels, and does not require any endoscopic or surgical therapy. Patients with this type of bleeding will present with melena and a mild drop in hemoglobin levels. At endoscopy, the ulcer will appear with a white base without visible vessel or adherent clot (Fig. 20–2, see Color Plate I). These ulcers require no endoscopic therapy and are managed as if they have not bled, including correction of any underlying coagulopathy.

In contrast, bleeding from deeper submucosal or muscularis propria vessels that have been exposed or eroded by ulceration may present with melena, but it is more common to present with maroon stool, hematemesis, and shock. If spontaneous cessation of bleeding occurs, the usual progression is for a large, soft clot to form over the exposed vessel, gradual contraction to a firm stable clot, with ultimate healing of the vessel wall and repair of the overlying tissue. In 20% to 30% of cases, however, the bleeding may recur, and intervention is required to prevent continued hemorrhage and ongoing transfusion (Fig. 20–3, see Color Plate I).

Endoscopic criteria to define ulcers more likely to continue bleeding or rebleeding have been established. While the rebleeding rate for ulcers with a clean, white base is around 1%, the incidence of continued bleeding or rebleeding from ulcers with active spurting vessels is 50% or higher, from ulcers with a protruding visible vessel in the ulcer base is about 40%, and from ulcers with an adherent clot is around 20%. For patients with lesions at high risk for rebleeding, endoscopic hemostasis appears to reduce the rate of rebleeding, subsequent transfusions, hospital stay, need for surgical intervention, and mortality. If these criteria are interpreted in the context of the clinical presentation and the patient's condition, it is possible to reduce morbidity and mortality from bleeding ulcers. An elderly patient with a large gastric ulcer presenting with orthostasis, requiring multiple transfusions, and failing one attempt at endoscopic hemostasis would probably be better served by a surgical approach to hemostasis rather than repeated endoscopic attempts.

The types of endoscopic therapy available to treat bleeding ulcers include thermal (lasers, heat probe, multipolar or bicap probe, monopolar probe) and nonthermal (injection therapy, hemoclip, and topical fibrin or cyanoacrylate glue) treatments. A National Institutes of Health (NIH) Consensus Conference evaluating UGI tract bleeding therapies has recommended that multipolar probe and heat probe are safe and effective for endoscopic treatment of bleeding ulcers in patients who have a high likelihood of rebleeding. Although lasers and monopolar probe are effective, their safety has been an issue, and they are not recommended at this time. More recent data clearly support the use of injection therapy (saline, saline with epinephrine or ethanol) in and around the bleeding vessel to control bleeding from ulcers, whether used alone or in combination with thermal devices. Injection offers high efficacy (approximately 95%) combined with low cost and may ultimately be the treatment of choice. Two trials were recently conducted comparing injection alone to injection plus heat probe and multipolar probe alone to multipolar probe plus injection. Control of bleeding was similar in both studies, and there were no significant differences in the need for surgery and mortality. There is no clear consensus on which therapy is superior, whether a single treatment is better than two or more treatment sessions, or if combination treatments offer improved control of bleeding.

Angiography may be used to define the bleeding lesion, but it is primarily of value in the active bleeding phase. Angiography is more expensive and removes the patient from the ICU, often at a time when the patient is most unstable. It is usually reserved for those patients in whom endoscopy has failed to define or control the bleeding lesion and who are poor candidates for surgical intervention. In these patients, angiography may not only help isolate the bleeding site; control of bleeding may be attempted via injection of gelfoam or wire coils into the arterial supply to the lesion.

The need for surgical intervention in the treatment of a bleeding peptic ulcer has been markedly reduced by less invasive therapies, but it remains the definitive treatment for a small number of patients. The efficacy of medical ulcer treatment, combined with new information about *Helicobacter pylori* and its role in ulcer disease, makes a limited approach (ulcer resection or oversew of the bleeding vessel) more reasonable. The previous surgical approach (primarily vagotomy and pyloroplasty, with oversew of the ulcer for duodenal ulcers, and resection of gastric ulcers) may be in flux, as definitive ulcer therapy has been associated with a substantial morbidity.

Emergency surgery in clinically unstable patients has a higher mortality than elective surgery. Therefore, the decision to operate to control UGI tract bleeding is made based on clinical parameters as much as unremitting hemorrhage. Studies comparing early surgery (bleeding requiring 4 U transfused within the first 24 hours) versus surgery performed only after multiple transfusions (12 U in the first 48 hours or 16 U in 72 hours) demonstrate reduced mortality in the early surgical group in elderly patients but not in those less than 60 years of age. Parameters that suggest continued bleeding (patients with coagulopathy, recent use of NSAIDs, multiple medical problems, previous UGI tract bleeding, large ulcers, and a failed attempt at endoscopic therapy) should prompt early surgical intervention if the patient is elderly and otherwise a candidate for surgery. For young individuals the need to control bleeding surgically can be delayed while a second attempt at endoscopic control is made without increasing surgical mortality. Large vessels (greater than 2 mm) have been particularly resistant to endoscopic therapy and are probably best handled with surgical oversew.

Medical therapy for ulcers has a limited role in active bleeding. There is a theoretic advantage supporting the use of H_2 receptor antagonists or antacids to raise the pH of the stomach to 5 or more, in that an acid environment enhances clot dissolution and instability. However, studies have failed to demonstrate any convincing evidence that even potent suppression of acid has reduced the rate of rebleeding in patients with bleeding from peptic ulcers. It is appropriate to begin treatment to heal the ulcer as soon as possible; if therapy with an intravenous H_2 receptor antagonist is contemplated until the patient is able to tolerate oral medications, a continuous infusion will maintain pH at a higher level than intermittent boluses. However, the expense and lack of efficacy of intravenous therapy in preventing rebleeding make this practice questionable.

Once bleeding is controlled and the patient is stable for 12 to 24 hours, oral intake may resume, and the diet may be advanced as tolerated. Although there are no hard figures to support the continuing role of hospitalization, patients should remain under observation for 48 to 72 hours after the cessation of bleeding. Antiulcer medication should be given to complete a full course of healing, usually 8 to 12 weeks. If present, *Helicobacter pylori* should be eradicated, as there is some evidence to indicate reduction in future bleeding in patients after treatment clears the infection. The risk of subsequent bleeding episodes following one episode of UGI tract bleeding is reported to be as high as 30%.

VARICEAL HEMORRHAGE

The management of esophageal or gastric variceal hemorrhage is complicated and variable (Fig. 20-4). Suspected variceal bleeding (patients with stigmata of liver disease, such as spider angiomas, splenomegaly, ascites, and jaundice, as well as those with previous variceal hemorrhage) is initially treated with the same assessment and resuscitation as peptic ulcer. Because of the higher mortality and greater likelihood of rebleeding associated with variceal hemorrhage, early endoscopic intervention is critical. In addition, the spectrum of therapies is more dependent on the underlying cause of variceal hemorrhage, and each patient must be treated with two purposes in mind: initial control of hemorrhage and prevention of rebleeding (see Table 20-3).

Variceal hemorrhage results from portal hypertension, although splenic vein thrombosis and splenomegaly can cause sufficient pressure in the submucosal gastric and esophageal veins to precipitate the formation and rupture of varices. The bleeding occurs from mucosal or submucosal veins that are in direct continuity with the deeper veins external to the esophageal muscularis by perforating veins. Although the risk of bleeding cannot be directly correlated with portal pressure, studies have demonstrated that a portal pressure gradient (the difference between portal and systemic venous systems) of 10 to 12 mm Hg or greater is reached before variceal hemorrhage occurs, and pressures below this

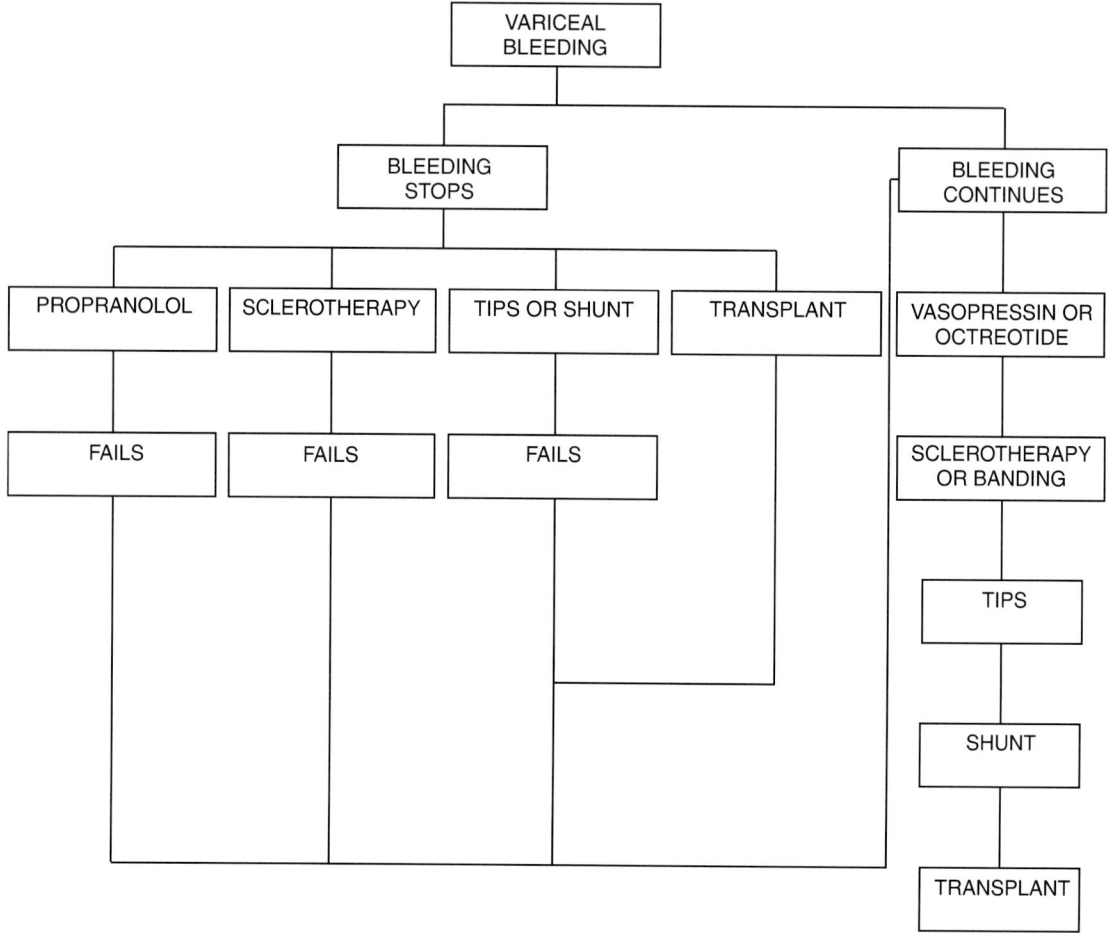

FIGURE 20–4. Management of variceal hemorrhage.

level are not associated with bleeding. This fact allows therapy to be directed at the portal pressure independent of the varices themselves. Portal pressure can be reduced with pharmacologic methods (vasopressin, β-blockers, or octreotide) or with shunting (either surgical or transjugular intrahepatic portosystemic shunt [TIPS]). Direct methods to deal with the variceal hemorrhage include compression tubes, esophageal variceal sclerotherapy or band ligation, and esophageal transection and aim at controlling the bleeding site rather than reducing portal pressure. In the case of end-stage cirrhosis, definitive therapy to reduce portal pressure involves replacing the liver with a normal one (hepatic transplantation). In each clinical situation, the appropriate therapy to prevent rebleeding is determined by the underlying liver disease and the patient's overall status.

The mortality from variceal hemorrhage is related to the degree of hepatic function. Variceal hemorrhage usually occurs in the setting of end-stage liver failure, but it may be seen in patients with relatively good liver function who have inflammatory changes that increase portal pressure. These patients may have nearly normal prothrombin time and normal albumin on admission, in contrast to the reduced synthetic function of the end-stage cirrhotic patient. Alcoholic cirrhosis with a component of alcoholic hepatitis may present with evidence of severe liver impairment and portal hypertension, yet it may be fairly reversible with cessation of alcohol. Primary biliary cirrhosis, sclerosing cholangitis, and schistosomiasis are other examples of liver disease where portal hypertension may be out of proportion to liver cell dysfunction. The 1-year survival of patients with bleeding esophageal varices is 40%. In the setting of compensated cirrhosis, variceal hemorrhage should also bring to mind the possibility of a complicating hepatoma.

TABLE 20–3. TREATMENT OF ESOPHAGEAL VARICEAL HEMORRHAGE

Pharmacologic
Vasopressin
Vasopressin plus nitroglycerine
Octreotide
β-Blockers

Compression Tubes
Sengstaken-Blakemore
Linton
Minnesota tube

Endoscopic
Injection sclerotherapy
Band ligation

Radiographic
Selective vasopressin infusion
Transjugular intrahepatic portosystemic shunt (TIPS)

Surgical
Esophageal transection
Esophageal transection with splenectomy (Sugiura procedure)
Selective shunts (e.g., distal splenorenal)
Nonselective shunts (e.g., end-to-end portocaval)
Hepatic transplantation

If variceal hemorrhage is suspected, early endoscopy is indicated; this assumes the patient can be evaluated safely, and empiric therapy to reduce portal pressure with vasopressin or octreotide may be necessary to suppress bleeding initially to permit endoscopy. Vasopressin may be administered via continuous infusion of 0.1 to 0.6 U/min, and it may reduce portal pressure by vasoconstriction of the splanchnic circulation. Bolus infusions prior to starting a continuous infusion have been associated with more complications and do not appear to improve efficacy. The use of cutaneous, sublingual, or intravenous nitroglycerine to reduce systemic vascular resistance has been shown to improve cardiac output, improve peripheral circulation, and further reduce portal pressure in patients given vasopressin and should be considered as part of vasopressin therapy. It should be noted that studies convincingly demonstrating the efficacy of vasopressin infusions in reducing bleeding and improving mortality are not available. Octreotide, a long-acting somatostatin analog, has been shown to improve variceal hemorrhage in some studies by reducing splanchnic blood flow, but the data are not consistently favorable, and the drug is considerably more expensive than vasopressin.

In contrast to the empiric use of vasopressin or octreotide, mechanical devices used to control bleeding (Sengstaken-Blakemore, Linton, or Minnesota tube) have significant complications associated with their use and should not be passed empirically. The data on these devices suggest that control of bleeding is better with endoscopic treatment and that even emergency portocaval shunting may be associated with fewer complications. The use of mechanical devices has been markedly reduced over the last decade as safe, more effective procedures to control variceal hemorrhage have been developed.

Endoscopic evaluation will usually reveal the presence of varices, unless the splanchnic circulation has been so volume depleted that the vessels are not obvious. The presence of varices does not mean that bleeding will occur, and from 25% to 50% of patients with varices bleed from another source. Endoscopic criteria suggesting a greater likelihood of bleeding from esophageal varices include the presence of large varices and red color signs (wales, hematocystic spots, cherry red spots), which probably represent small mucosal vessels in continuity with the submucosal and deep venous systems (Fig. 20–5, see Color Plate I).

The finding of gastric varices alone suggests splenic vein thrombosis or previous sclerotherapy of the esophageal varices. Gastric variceal hemorrhage may be more difficult to approach endoscopically, except at the cardia or gastroesophageal junction. Gastric varices may be missed on initial examination because of the normally large folds of the fundus.

Endoscopic treatment of varices includes sclerotherapy and band ligation. Esophageal variceal sclerotherapy was used initially in 1936 but was not embraced enthusiastically until studies in the early 1980s began to demonstrate good initial control of bleeding and, with eradication of the varices, prevention of rebleeding. Injections are placed either into the varix (intravariceal) or alongside the vessels (paravariceal). In either case, the goal is eradication of the mucosal and submucosal veins but not sclerosis of the deep system, which shunts the blood from the high-pressure portal system to the systemic circulation. In practicality, either technique overlaps with the other, and combined paravariceal and intravariceal injections are common. Sclerotherapy is usually begun in the acute bleeding phase and stops variceal hemorrhage in more than 90% of cases. Rebleeding is common, however, until the varices are eradicated. Most endoscopists repeat variceal injections at regular intervals until the varices are obliterated. Complications of variceal sclerotherapy are fairly common and include bacteremia, fever, pleural effusions, chest pain, ulceration of the esophagus, motility disturbances, dysphagia, and rarely thrombosis of distant vessels.

Banding of esophageal varices is a relatively new technique modeled after hemorrhoidal banding. An overtube is used to gain repeated access to the esophagus, and a sleeve is placed over the instrument that enables a rubber band to be released onto the varix after it is aspirated into the overtube. The varices then thrombose, and the necrosed area within the band is sloughed after a few days. The varices are systematically banded until they are obliterated. Initial comparison studies suggest that this technique is as efficacious as sclerotherapy and is associated with fewer complications, but the device is not yet approved for use in the United States.

If endoscopic methods fail to control bleeding, additional measures to reduce portal pressure are then employed. These include the TIPS and surgical shunts. TIPS initially offers a far less invasive approach to reduction in portal pressure, as the shunt is placed intravascularly in the hepatic parenchyma under fluoroscopic control. Using a transjugular approach, a communication is established between branches of the portal and hepatic veins, and the communication is dilated with balloons. A wire mesh stent is then placed between the two veins and allowed to expand or is dilated to a size necessary to reduce the portal gradient to less than 10 mm Hg. The shunts were viewed initially with great enthusiasm, as they reduced the need for general anesthesia and a prolonged postoperative recovery period. Their use has been tempered, however, as further experience has demonstrated relatively poor long-term patency and a higher level of encephalopathy than initially noted. It is an extremely useful tool, however, to control bleeding in the short term while awaiting liver transplantation and for those patients with some element of reversibility of their liver disease, such as alcoholic hepatitis (Fig. 20–6).

Surgical decompression of the portal circulation had been the last resort prior to recent advances in hepatic transplantation. The more effective shunts (end-to-end portocaval, end-to-side portocaval) had a relatively high early postoperative mortality and long-term encephalopathy but low incidence of rebleeding. Operations that preserve liver blood flow and reduce the risk of encephalopathy, such as distal splenorenal shunt, trade fewer complications for less efficacy at preventing rebleeding. There are studies using emergency shunting as primary therapy for bleeding esophageal varices, with shunts performed within 8 hours of admission, showing excellent survival and elimination of further bleeding. These studies, however, are from one center, and other studies comparing shunt surgery to variceal sclerotherapy are less favorable, particularly in the high risk or Child's class C group. The most reasonable approach seems to be initial control of bleeding with sclerotherapy, if possible, and salvage shunt surgery for those whose bleeding continues or recurs despite sclerotherapy.

Liver transplantation offers the only long-term solution to those patients with end-stage liver disease and complications of portal hypertension or liver cell failure. Patients who are candidates for liver transplantation and present with variceal hemorrhage are usually managed with temporizing endoscopic therapy or TIPS but referred for transplantation as soon as possible. Surgical shunts in these patients have a relatively high mortality and may complicate subsequent transplantation.

The use of β-blockers (propranolol, atenolol, nadolol) has been shown to reduce portal pressure when given in doses that suppress baseline blood pressure and pulse by 25% or more. Initial studies showed β-blockers to be efficacious in preventing rebleeding in alcoholic patients, and subsequent studies confirm this finding. However, there are no long-term studies that demonstrate improved survival in patients treated with β-blockers over placebo.

EROSIVE GASTRITIS

The diagnosis of *gastritis* is used by many endoscopists to describe the endoscopic appearance of edema, submucosal hemorrhages, and erosions in the gastric lining, typically induced by NSAIDs. Histologically, *gastritis* is defined as inflammatory infiltration of the mucosa, as in the antral gastritis associated with *Helicobacter pylori* or the fundic gastritis associated with the autoimmune gastritis or pernicious anemia. It is also used to describe the inflammation associated with gastric atrophy. Patients with these types of gastritis rarely bleed, and most UGI tract bleeding from "gastritis" is from erosions in the antrum, better termed erosive gastritis. These erosions are nearly always associated with the use of NSAIDs (Fig. 20–7, see Color Plate I). Superficial erosions in the antrum may account for up to 23% of patients presenting with UGI tract bleeding. Erosions are shallow ulcerations,

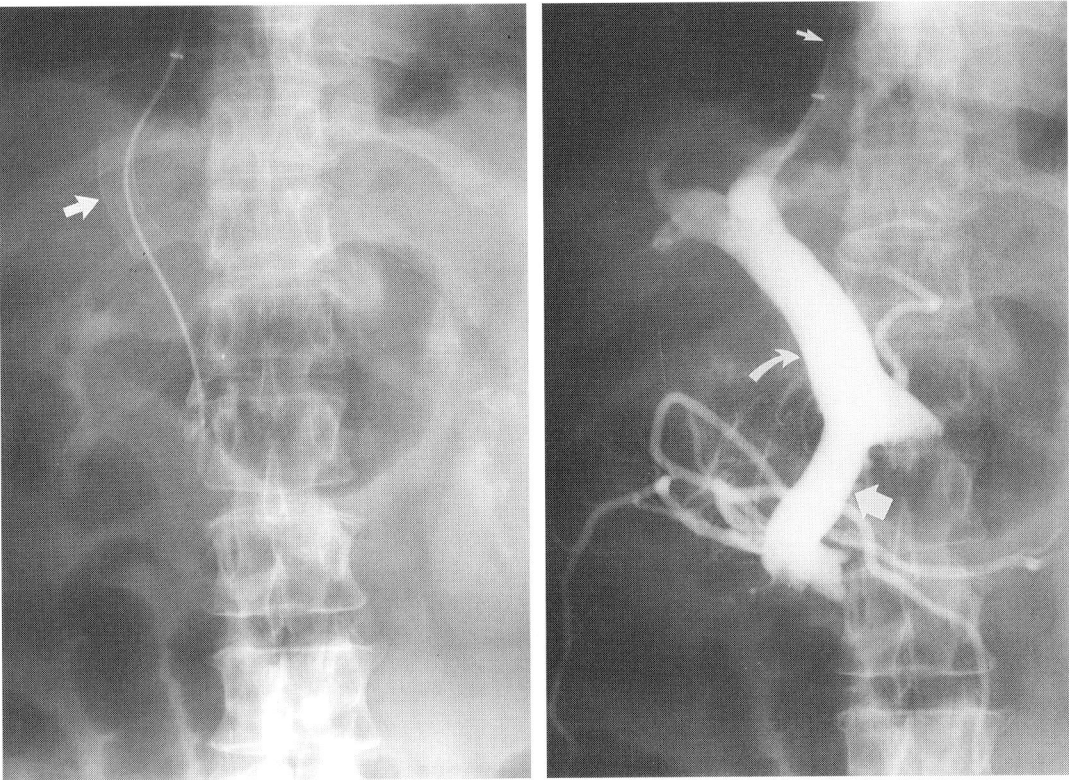

FIGURE 20-6. Transjugular intrahepatic portosystemic shunt (TIPS). **A,** The expandable wire stent is shown here in place *(white arrow)*, communicating the hepatic and portal venous systems. A catheter is shown entering the portal circulation from the inferior vena cava. **B,** Injection into the portal system showing the superior mesenteric vein *(large white arrow)*, the portal vein *(curved white arrow)*, and the inferior vena cava *(small white arrow)*. The TIPS allowed decompression of the portal system and has eliminated variceal hemorrhage in this patient.

pathologically confined to the mucosa above the muscularis mucosa, which should prevent major vessel bleeding as the vessels are normally submucosal. In practicality, endoscopists are not able to differentiate between erosions and small ulcers at endoscopy.

The formation of antral erosions is clearly linked to the use of NSAIDs, and most bleeding from these erosions is self-limited. Endoscopic therapy is not usually needed. Correction of any underlying coagulopathy early in the hospitalization is important to halt persistent blood loss and the need for intervention. In contrast, major stress, such as head trauma, significant burns, and admission to an ICU may induce erosions or ulcerations in the proximal stomach. These erosions may be substantially different and may present with major hemorrhage that is difficult to control. Large ulcerations may be seen in the fundus and body of the stomach; although endoscopic therapy can be effective, angiographic placement of Gelfoam or coils in feeding arteries may be required. Stress ulcerations are occasionally refractory to nonsurgical management; although vagotomy and pyloroplasty with oversew of bleeding points is the operative procedure of choice, at the extreme, total gastrectomy may be required to control bleeding. Prevention of erosive gastritis in the ICU setting with antacids, H_2 receptor antagonists, and other medications is widely practiced and reasonably well supported by the literature (Fig. 20–8, see Color Plate I).

Acute ethanol ingestion also causes a "gastritis," but the injury pattern is classically described as edema and submucosal hemorrhages without erosions. The bleeding that occurs is usually self-limited and does not require endoscopic therapy. Removing the patient from access to alcohol is usually sufficient to correct the lesion.

Portal Hypertensive Gastropathy

Endoscopists also used *gastritis* to describe the erythema, edema, and friability of portal hypertensive gastropathy or congestive gastropathy. This is one of the additional bleeding lesions in portal hypertension and may become more prominent after esophageal varices are obliterated by sclerotherapy. Bleeding is usually mild, unless the liver disease has progressed to the point of severe coagulopathy. Endoscopic or angiographic therapy is usually not required, but infusions of vasopressin or octreotide may control acute bleeding. Prevention of rebleeding is usually accomplished with β-blockers, shunt procedures, or hepatic transplantation.

Mallory-Weiss Tear

Mallory-Weiss tear is the eponym applied to a tear in the gastric mucosa at or near the gastroesophageal junction. The lesion is most common in alcoholics, although it may be seen in any vomiting situation, including the retching that sometimes accompanies endoscopy. The tear appears to occur with either large, transient high-pressure gradients between the thorax and abdomen that develop with retching, thereby overstretching the tissues of the gastroesophageal junction when herniating into the chest, or with trauma to the gastric mucosa from intussusception into the esophagus with retching. This lesion is not to be confused with a true perforation of the esophagus or Boerhaave's syndrome, which can occur with vomiting, originally described as self-induced. Patients with Boerhaave's syndrome present with chest pain and sepsis and have a much worse prognosis.

Patients with Mallory-Weiss tear usually present with hematemesis and signs of mild to moderate bleeding. Melena is not common, occurring in about 10% of cases. Classically, patients present with initial episodes of vomiting without hematemesis, but more recent literature suggests that this pattern is seen only about half the time, with blood or coffee-grounds noted with the first emesis in the remaining cases.

Bleeding from Mallory-Weiss tear is self-limited in over 90% of cases, with only about 40% requiring transfusion. Resuscitation and supportive care are usually sufficient to manage patients with this lesion. If patients require endoscopic therapy, it is successful in about 80% of cases, and only about 2% of Mallory-Weiss tears ultimately require surgery. Initial control can be attempted with vasopressin, endoscopic thermal coagulation, angiographic embolization, or large volume (Linton) gastric balloons. All have been reported to control bleeding but mostly in uncontrolled studies or case reports. There is one controlled study demonstrating the efficacy of the multipolar probe in controlling hemorrhage.

Peptic Esophagitis

Bleeding from the esophagus occurs with erosion or ulceration of the mucosa, usually in response to acid or peptic reflux (Fig. 20–9, see Color Plate II). Bleeding from ulceration is also seen in Barrett's epithelium, a metaplastic change in the lining from squamous to gastric-type tissue. Acute hemorrhage may also be seen from the gastric mucosa in severe prolapse from a large hiatal hernia or paraesophageal hernia, but these more commonly present with chronic occult-blood-positive stool or iron deficiency anemia.

Bleeding from the esophagus commonly presents with hematemesis of coffee-ground material with occult-blood-positive stool and is rarely severe except in the setting of coagulopathy or NSAID use. The finding of a deep ulcer in the esophagus suggests Barrett's epithelium or ulceration from medications such as aspirin, iron, tetracycline, or quinidine. If bleeding is significant and unremitting, endoscopic measures to control bleeding (injection and thermal devices) can be beneficial. Other therapeutic options, including angiographic embolization, Sengstaken-Blakemore tube, and surgery, are rarely required.

Chronic blood loss from large hiatal or paraesophageal hernias is not amenable to endoscopic or angiographic therapies, and surgical correction of the underlying defect is appropriate.

Neoplasm

Tumors of the UGI tract commonly bleed but usually in a slow, chronic fashion. In rare instances, major bleeding will occur from tumors in the esophagus or stomach, representing about 2% of the cases reported by the membership of the American Society of Gastrointestinal Endoscopists (ASGE). Although these tumors are most commonly squamous cell carcinoma in the esophagus and adenocarcinoma in the cardia and stomach, a variety of other tumors, including lymphoma, leiomyomas, sarcomas, carcinoid tumors, and other rare neoplasms, can present with UGI tract bleeding. Bleeding in the setting of malignancy usually occurs when necrosis of tumor exposes large vessels. Patients who present with severe bleeding can be approached with therapy similar to peptic ulcer to initially control bleeding, with the exception that laser therapy may offer a greater role in tumor treatment than in other types of bleeding. Although initial control is possible with injection (saline, saline plus epinephrine, or ethanol), thermal devices, or laser therapy, control is usually temporary. Long-term management of the tumor with appropriate therapy (chemotherapy, radiation, or surgery) is usually required to prevent subsequent hemorrhage.

Vascular Ectasia

Small arteriovenous communications in the mucosa of the gastrointestinal (GI) tract are commonly referred to as arteriovenous malformations (AVMs), vascular ectasias, telangiectasias, vascular malformations, or angiodysplasia. They are responsible for a small number of patients who present with UGI tract bleeding, may be present anywhere in the GI tract, but are most common in the fundus, duodenum, and cecum. Most patients with these lesions are elderly and have no apparent cause for the lesion. There is a higher incidence of valvular heart disease in patients with vascular ectasia, but whether this relationship is causal or coincidental is unknown. Similar lesions are present in the GI tract in patients with renal failure, but such lesions are more extensive. A genetic disorder, hereditary hemorrhagic telangiectasia or Rendu-Osler-Weber syndrome, has identical lesions but in far greater numbers than the idiopathic variant; such lesions may also be present on the fingers and mucus membranes or in the liver, central nervous system, and other organs. Patients with vascular ectasias may present with acute UGI tract hemorrhage, but chronic blood loss is more common.

The lesions are usually identified at endoscopy and are described as small, flat, red spots or spiderlike lesions on the mucosa, occasionally with a white halo around the red area (Fig. 20–10A, see Color Plate II). They are friable and bleed freely when manipulated or biopsied. They are sometimes difficult to identify, especially when patients have been sedated with meperidine, which may cause the arteriole supply to constrict. Other vascular lesions are described, some that may involve large areas of the mucosa such as antral vascular ectasia. These lesions also have chronic blood loss more common as a presenting sign (Fig. 20–10B, see Color Plate II).

Once the lesions are identified, endoscopic therapy with thermal devices can destroy the ectatic lesion. Laser therapy with neodymium-yttrium-aluminum-garnet (Nd-YAG) or argon laser has also been associated with reduction in blood loss from vascular ectasia. Control of the bleeding from accessible lesions is only part of the long-term solution, as lesions may be present beyond the reach of fiberoptic instruments. Even if all of the vascular ectasias are eradicated, new ones may form and cause recurrent bleeding. One group has reported long-term reduction in transfusion requirements with combination estrogen-progesterone therapy in doses of 0.05 mg ethinyl estradiol and 1 mg norethindrone. Another recent case report suggested that aminocaproic acid might offer some resistance to rebleeding. Either therapy may reduce the bleeding from vascular ectasia sufficiently to allow oral iron replacement to be effective at maintaining adequate red cell mass.

Dieulafoy's Lesion

Dieulafoy's lesion refers to a large submucosal artery that ruptures through the mucosa, usually is present in the cardia or upper body of the stomach, but also is found in the duodenum, jejunum, and right colon. It is thought to be a congenital variant, and is also known as cirsoid aneurysm, caliber-persistent artery, or exulceratio simplex. It is an unusual but significant cause of UGI tract bleeding, presenting with hematemesis and melena in most cases, along with orthostatic changes. The lesion may be difficult to see endoscopically, as there is no associated mucosal defect or ulcer; it is often missed at first endoscopy unless actively bleeding. Once identified, treatment consists of endoscopic thermal or injection therapy with fairly good results in uncontrolled studies. About 5% of patients fail endoscopic control and can be managed with attempts at angiographic control or surgery to oversew the lesion.

Aortoenteric Fistula

Although communications between the GI tract and a previously repaired aortic aneurysm is a rare cause of UGI tract bleeding, it should be high on the list of differential diagnostic possibilities in any patient with a previously repaired aneurysm. A fistula may develop from an aneurysm that has not been repaired (primary fistula) but is more common to occur after surgical repair of the aneurysm. Two major theories have been proposed to explain the formation of a fistula. One proposes fixation of the bowel to the repaired site and subsequent pulsatile trauma leading to pressure necrosis of the bowel with breakdown of the mucosa, erosion into the muscularis, and ultimately to erosion into the repaired graft. The second theory assumes that the repair is complicated by a low-grade infection at the suture line and the development of a pseudoaneurysm. This pseudoaneurysm then leads to pressure necrosis of the adjacent bowel with necrosis of the mucosa and later the muscularis with ultimate communication between the bowel and the pseudoaneurysm. In either scenario the necrosis of the mucosa is associated with "herald" bleeding that presents as mild to moderate UGI tract bleeding. If not recognized and corrected, the second bleeding episode is often an exsanguinating communication between the aorta and bowel. The usual site of communication is the third portion of the duodenum because of its proximity to the aorta. However, aortoenteric fistula may occur anywhere in the GI tract.

A high index of suspicion often directs the physician to this lesion and permits early surgical intervention. Part of the difficulty in managing aortoenteric fistulas is to identify their presence, which may be impossible preoperatively. Erosion of the aortic graft into the duodenum is visible endoscopically, provided the endoscopist advances the instrument into the third or fourth portion of the duodenum. Angiographic studies often fail to demonstrate the lesion, but pseudoaneurysm of the graft can be sometimes seen. Computed tomography (CT) scan may show the bowel in close proximity to the graft, and if extraluminal air is seen in the adjacent graft or aneurysm, the diagnosis is confirmed. Endoscopic or angiographic treatment of aortoenteric fistulas is not appropriate or effective, and the threshold for surgical intervention in patients with previous aortic aneurysm resection should be low.

Miscellaneous Lesions

There are a variety of less common lesions in the UGI tract that can account for bleeding. In addition to the mucosal lesions induced by NSAIDs, other medications including corticosteroids, anticoagulants, and slow-release potassium chloride tablets can precipitate bleeding. A number of other bleeding lesions, including splenic artery aneurysm, vasculitis, hemangiomas, fistulas, diverticula, and benign polyps have also been reported.

The biliary tree and pancreas are rare sites of UGI tract hemorrhage, usually from tumors of the liver, bile ducts, or pancreas or from splenic artery aneurysm. These lesions are suspected when blood is seen exiting from the ampulla of Vater, and can be confirmed angiographically. Tumors bleeding in these locations are more amenable to angiographic embolization than endoscopic therapy. Vascular lesions of the pancreatic bed or splenic artery are also identified angiographically and usually repaired surgically.

Most of the other mucosal vascular lesions and tumors of the UGI tract can be approached endoscopically and often bleeding arrested, but definitive treatment depends on the type of lesion and its location.

SUMMARY

Bleeding from the UGI tract presents a formidable clinical problem both in diagnosis and management. The high mortality reflects to a large extent the population at risk, with the elderly patient having multiple medical problems or comorbid conditions at greatest risk. Aggressive initial evaluation and resuscitation will stabilize the patient and offer an excellent opportunity for diagnostic evaluation. Endoscopy and endoscopic therapy are successful in many lesions, often at the first procedure. The risks for rebleeding and subsequent increased mortality can be evaluated and an appropriate plan for continued management determined. Surgical consultation early in the course is important to offer patients at greatest risk from persistent rebleeding and intervention an early definitive treatment for their bleeding. The success of radiographic techniques to salvage patients who fail less invasive procedures is also promising. The ultimate successful approach to managing UGI tract bleeding relies on the efforts of a skilled multidisciplinary team working in concert to effect the best outcome for the patient.

REFERENCES
Evaluation and Endoscopy

1. Gilbert DA, Silverstein FE, Tedesco FJ, et al. The national ASGE survey on upper gastrointestinal bleeding: III. endoscopy in upper gastrointestinal bleeding. *Gastrointest Endosc.* 1981;27:94–102.
2. Silverstein FE, Gilbert DA, Tedesco FJ, et al. The national ASGE survey on upper gastrointestinal bleeding:

II. clinical prognostic factors. *Gastrointest Endosc.* 1981; 27:80–93.
3. Wara P. Endoscopic prediction of major rebleeding: a prospective study of stigmata of hemorrhage in bleeding ulcer. *Gastroenterology* 1985;88:1209–1214.

These papers provide much of the data for our understanding of the clinical and endoscopic features of UGI tract bleeding. They enable a more rational approach to the problem from the time of admission through the initial endoscopy and suggest a standard treatment plan based on clinical and endoscopic criteria.

Bleeding Peptic Ulcer

1. Friedman LS, ed. Gastrointestinal bleeding I. *Gastrointest Endosc Clin.* 1993;22(4):717–911.
2. Friedman LS, ed. Gastrointestinal bleeding II. *Gastrointest Endosc Clin.* 1994;23(1):1–188.

These two issues of *Gastrointestinal Endoscopy Clinics* amplify the epidemiology, evaluation, and treatment (endoscopic, radiographic and surgical) of bleeding lesions in the GI tract. They are an excellent starting point for more in-depth review. The data on treatment of ulcer bleeding are well documented in these references, but the utility and efficacy of injection therapy is still too early to adequately evaluate.

3. Proceedings of the Consensus Conference on Therapeutic Endoscopy in Bleeding Ulcers. *Gastrointest Endosc.* 1990; 36(suppl):S1–S65.
4. Therapeutic endoscopy and bleeding ulcers: consensus conference. *JAMA.* 1989;262:1369–1372.

The first of these references provides the background information used to derive the consensus statement of the second. The conference gathered a variety of experts in the field to develop guidelines for the therapy of bleeding ulcers, and the information provided by these participants is a reasonable review of the information available at the time.

Variceal Hemorrhage

1. Henderson JM, Gilmore GT, Hooks MA, et al. Selective shunt in the management of variceal bleeding in the era of liver transplantation. *Ann Surg.* 1992;216:248–255.

This paper discusses the efficacy of shunt surgery given the increasing access to liver transplantation for patients with end-stage liver disease. The authors continue to support treatment of variceal hemorrhage with sclerotherapy as the initial treatment, selective shunt surgery for those who continue bleeding and have relatively good liver function, and transplantation for those with liver failure.

2. McCormick PA, Dick R, Burroughs AK. Review article: the transjugular intrahepatic portosystemic shunt (TIPS) in the treatment of portal hypertension. *Aliment Pharmacol Ther.* 1994;8:273–282.

This paper is a review of the most recent therapeutic option, the TIPS procedure. Although initial data was promising, more recent information on complications, encephalopathy, and shunt failure temper current enthusiasm for the TIPS. It is still useful in selected patients.

3. Orloff MJ, Orloff MS, Rambotti M, et al. Is portal-systemic shunt worthwhile in Child's class C cirrhosis? *Ann Surg.* 1992;216:256–268.

This paper is controversial but illustrates the efficacy of shunt surgery at one center. It is an uncontrolled study of 94 patients who had a nonselective shunt performed as primary therapy for variceal hemorrhage. The survival and quality of life data stand alone in the shunt literature, and most authors prefer a less invasive approach to control of hemorrhage, such as sclerotherapy, with shunt surgery as a salvage operation for those with continued bleeding.

4. Sanyal AJ, Purdum PP, Luketic VA, et al. Bleeding gastroesophageal varices. *Semin Liver Dis.* 1993;13:328–342.

These authors provide a thorough review of the current therapeutic options for the treatment of bleeding varices.

21

Acute Lower Gastrointestinal Tract Bleeding

ALAN R. BANK and STANLEY B. BENJAMIN

The management of patients with lower gastrointestinal (GI) tract bleeding remains a clinical challenge. The initial approach depends on the degree of bleeding and should be directed toward resuscitation and stabilization of the patient. A multispecialty approach involving gastroenterology, surgery, nuclear medicine, and radiology should be available to localize and treat bleeding. With judicious and timely use of nuclear scintigraphy, selective angiography, and colonoscopy, precise localization and determination of the cause of bleeding may facilitate treatment employing either angiographic vasopressin infusion, endoscopic therapy, or segmental surgical resection.

OCCULT BLEEDING

Occult bleeding is identified on routine stool examination, in screening for colorectal neoplasms, or in the evaluation of anemia. The stool is grossly normal in appearance and tests positive for blood. The evaluation of occult bleeding will not be discussed in this section.

ACUTE GI TRACT BLEEDING

Acute GI tract bleeding is manifested by the passage of melena (dark black in appearance secondary to oxidation of hematin) or hematochezia (bright red blood per rectum or maroon stool). Melena is usually a manifestation of bleeding proximal to the ligament of Treitz but can be secondary to right-sided colonic bleeding. Gross bleeding should be classified as self-limiting (80%), ongoing, or massive bleeding. Although the differential diagnosis of gross GI tract bleeding is broad (Table 21–1), three entities (angiodysplasia, diverticulosis, and upper GI tract bleeding) constitute the majority of causes.

CAUSES OF ACUTE LOWER GI TRACT BLEEDING

ANGIODYSPLASIA, ARTERIOVENOUS MALFORMATION, AND ANGIOMATA

With increasing use of angiography and colonoscopy, angiodysplasia has been recognized as a major cause of lower GI tract bleeding.[4,6,11,17] Angiodysplasia is a focal submucosal vascular ectasia that appears to be acquired with aging or associated with cardiovascular disease. These lesions are diagnosed by colonoscopy where they appear as bright red or cherry red flat lesions (Fig. 21–1), or they are diagnosed by angiography where they are identified by three major angiographic signs[4]: (1) densely opacified, dilated, tortuous, slowly emptying intramural veins reflecting ectatic changes in submucosal veins, (2) a vascular tuft, and (3) an early filling vein. These usually are right-sided lesions located in the cecum or ascending colon but can occur throughout the colon, small intestine, and upper GI tract.

Bleeding may manifest as occult bleeding, iron deficiency anemia with heme-positive stools, intermittent episodes of hematochezia or melena, or as acute massive, severe lower GI tract bleeding. Bleeding from angiodysplasia is usually not severe but has a tendency to rebleed if not treated. In persons over the age of 60

TABLE 21–1. COMMON CAUSES OF GI TRACT BLEEDING

ESOPHAGUS, STOMACH, AND DUODENUM	JEJUNUM AND ILEUM	COLON AND RECTUM
Esophagitis	Arteriovenous malformation or angiodysplagia	Arteriovenous malformation
Esophageal varices	Ulcers	Diverticula
Gastric varices	Diverticula	Colitis
Mallory-Weiss tear	Meckel's ulceration	Infective
Peptic ulcer disease	Cancer	Inflammatory bowel disease
Gastric ulcer	Crohn's disease	Ischemic
Duodenal ulcer	Polyps	Cancer
Anastomotic ulcer	Varices	Polyp
Gastritis		Hemorrhoids
Congestive gastropathy		Anal fissure
Dieulafoy's lesion		Varices
Arteriovenous malformation		Postoperative
Watermelon stomach		Polypectomy
Cancer		Anastomotic
Polyps		Ulcers
Leiomyoma		Simple
Aortoenteric fistula		Stercoral
		Infective
		Aortocolonic fistula
		Radiation colitis

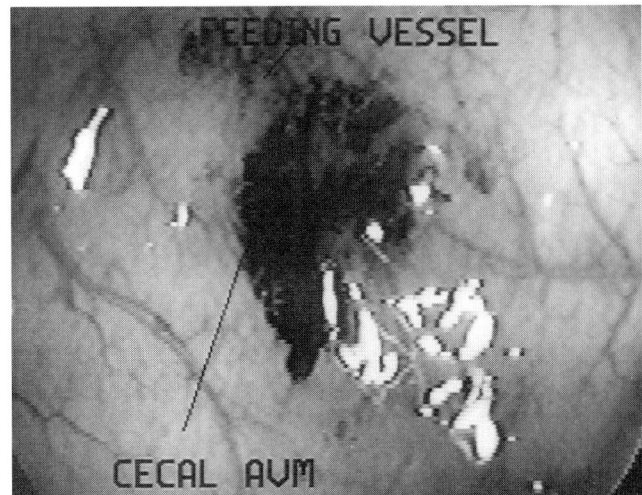

FIGURE 21–1. Colonic arteriovenous malformation with feeding vessel.

years, angiodysplasia appears to be a more frequent cause of bleeding than diverticular disease.[11,12]

DIVERTICULAR DISEASE

Diverticular disease is very prevalent in western society, especially in the elderly population, (one third to one half of persons over 60 years of age).[16] Diverticular bleeding occurs in approximately 20% of patients with diverticulosis. Diverticula are mostly left-sided lesions, but arteriographic studies have demonstrated a pattern of distribution of bleeding heavily weighted toward the right side of the colon.[8,9] These studies, however, were undertaken prior to the more aggressive use of colonoscopy and the recognition of angiodysplasia as a frequent cause of right-sided colonic hemorrhage. Recent studies using both angiography and colonoscopy in the diagnosis and treatment of acute lower GI tract bleeding have demonstrated that diverticular bleeding is a less common cause of hemorrhage than angiodysplasia.[4,11,12] Diverticular bleeding is usually arterial and, therefore, brisk, severe in nature, stopping spontaneously in 80% to 90% of patients, of which 20% to 25% rebleed.

Angiography and colonoscopy may also facilitate accurate localization and treatment of bleeding and, if bleeding is persistent or recurrent, allow the use of segmental colonic resection with an associated decrease in morbidity and mortality in comparison with subtotal colectomy.[6]

UPPER GI TRACT BLEEDING

Bleeding from an upper GI tract source should always be considered in the differential diagnosis of what appears to be acute lower GI tract bleeding. This cannot be excluded by a negative nasogastric lavage, and prior to surgical intervention esophagogastroduodenoscopy should be considered to exclude an upper GI tract lesion. As noted by Jensen et al,[11,12] an upper GI tract source for hematochezia was diagnosed in 11% of patients.

DIAGNOSTIC EVALUATION AND MANAGEMENT OF ACUTE BLEEDING

On initial presentation, patients should be assessed as to whether the rectal bleeding is moderate or severe and whether bleeding appears to be active or self-limiting. This is extremely difficult to determine clinically, and initially close monitoring and intensive care admission should be considered. The aggressiveness of the evaluation is dependent on this assessment.

Accurate localization of the site of bleeding is of paramount importance and should employ a multispecialty approach with cooperation between the internist, gastrointestinal endoscopist, radiologist, and surgeon.

Rapid bleeding is associated with acute blood loss amounting to greater than 2 U or bleeding at a rate of greater than 100 ml/h. This is characterized by tachycardia, tachypnea, and orthostatic hypotension and is indicative of at least a

TABLE 21–2. MANAGEMENT OF PATIENTS WITH ACUTE BLEEDING

1. Initial assessment
    a. History
        (1) General health status
        (2) Abdominal complaints
        (3) Bleeding history
        (4) Bleeding diathesis
        (5) Medications (i.e., NSAIDs, salicylates)
        (6) Duration of symptoms
        (7) Stool character
    b. Physical examination
        (1) Vital signs
        (2) Orthostatic measurements
        (3) Hydration status
    c. Diagnostic maneuvers
        (1) Nasogastric aspiration
        (2) Rectal examination
        (3) Anoscopy, proctosigmoidoscopy
    d. Laboratory studies
        (1) Complete blood count
        (2) Coagulation studies (PT and PTT)
        (3) Blood type and screen
2. Resuscitation
    a. Intravenous access
    b. Intensive care monitoring
    c. Transfusion of blood products
    d. Assessment of adequacy of resuscitation
        (1) Vital signs, urine output, serial blood counts and coagulation parameters
3. Definitive diagnosis
    a. Nature, location of lesions
    b. Upper endoscopy, colonoscopy, nuclear scintigraphy, angiography
4. Definitive therapy
    a. Colonoscopy (coagulation therapy)
    b. Angiography (vasopressin infusion, embolectomy)
    c. Surgical (segmental resection, subtotal colectomy)

NSAIDs = nonsteroidal antiinflammatory drugs, PT = prothrombin time, PTT = partial thromboplastin time.

15% reduction of circulating blood volume. In rapid severe bleeding, mortality may be as high as 15%.

The management of patients may be divided into four phases as outlined in Table 21–2.

COLONOSCOPY

After initial assessment and resuscitation, if bleeding appears to have stopped or slowed down, recent data suggest that the best approach is meticulous cleansing of the colon followed by urgent colonoscopy (Fig. 21–2).[11,12] Colonic preparation is undertaken with oral or nasogastric administration of a polyethylene glycol-sodium sulfate solution until rectal effluent is clear. This should take an average of 3 hours and may need 4 to 15 L (mean 5.5 L) of solution.[11,12] Data would suggest no risk of exacerbation of bleeding or of fluid retention related to this preparation.

Implicating a lesion as a cause of bleeding during colonoscopy requires (1) active bleeding, (2) adherent clot in a single diverticulum or on an ulcerated lesion resistant to washing with fresh blood nearby and no other lesions, or (3) nonbleeding visible vessel on an ulcer in the absence of other lesions.[11,12] If bleeding continues and a site is not identified with colonoscopy, then nuclear bleeding scan or angiography should be performed (Fig. 21–2). If bleeding is rapid and continuous, there is no best method of diagnosis, since evaluation depends on the availability of diagnostic tests and the rapidity with which they can be undertaken.

Emergency unprepared colonoscopy can be undertaken safely using caution and advancement of the colonoscope only under good visibility. Diagnostic findings may include (1) acutely bleeding lesions, (2) fresh blood in an area and nonbloody contents proximally, (3) fresh adherent clot, and (4) failure to localize bleeding.[10] Diffuse bleeding from colitis may also be identified.

RADIONUCLIDE SCANS

Bleeding scan uses either injection of technetium-99m (^{99m}Tc) sulfur colloid or ^{99m}Tc-labeled autologous red cells and may show extravasation into the lumen with bleeding rates of 0.1 to 0.5 ml/min. Bleeding scans are sensitive in the detection of bleeding but not specific in detecting the actual site of extravasation. With the use of autologous red blood cell labeling, sequential images may detect bleeding up to 24 hours after injection. Radiologists may prefer that a bleeding scan be obtained prior to angiography because scintigraphy provides a reliable noninvasive method of screening patients for active bleeding. However, in massive bleeding, angiography or colonoscopy should be undertaken as therapeutic intervention may be possible using vasopressin infusion,[6] embolectomy, or endoscopic coagulation.[11,12]

ANGIOGRAPHY

Selective visceral angiography may identify the site of bleeding and may facilitate therapeutic intervention. Diagnostic angiography requires active bleeding at the time of the injection, and the bleeding rate must be at least 0.5 ml/min.[20]

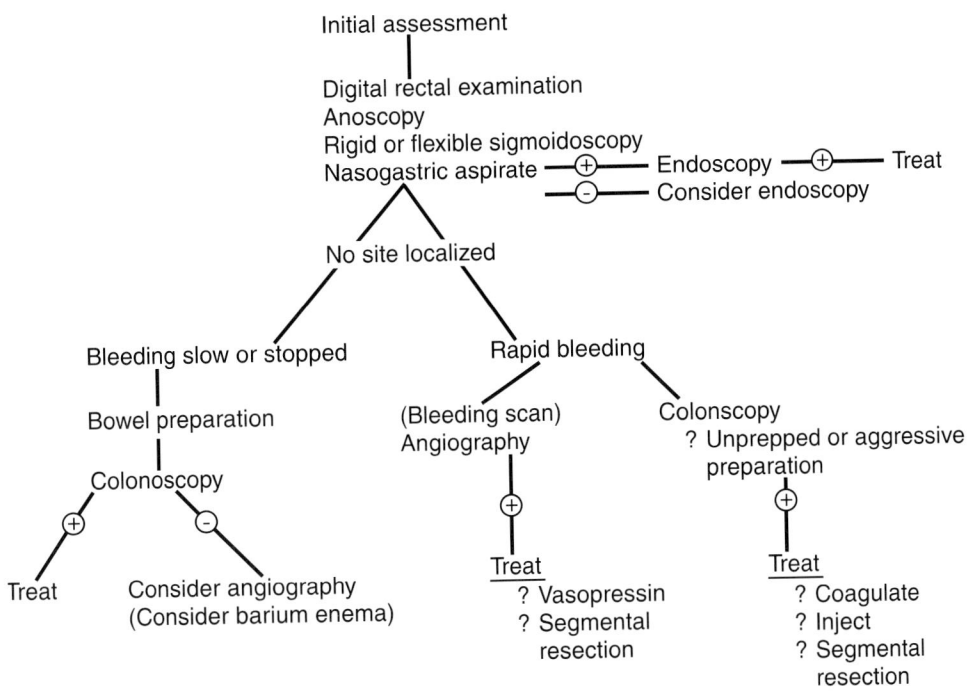

FIGURE 21–2. Algorithm for lower gastrointestinal tract bleeding.

Successful diagnosis of bleeding varies by report from 14%[11,12] to 72%,[6] and the use of vasopressin has been reported to stop bleeding in up to 92% of cases,[6] allowing stabilization of the patient in preparation for segmental colectomy. In diverticular bleeding further therapy may not be needed after vasopressin therapy. Fifty percent of patients rebleed after cessation of vasopressin.[6] If bleeding is not controlled by vasopressin, then surgery should be considered as the next step in the management. The use of embolization in the control of major bleeding should be reserved for patients in whom vasopressin has failed to stop the bleeding or vasopressin infusion is contraindicated and in whom surgery is contraindicated or considered high risk secondary to patient instability. Embolic therapy is very successful in controlling bleeding, and although its use is associated with an appreciable risk of acute colonic transmural necrosis, this risk may be less than those of emergency surgery in a hemodynamically compromised patient.[5,18] Safe embolic therapy requires accessibility of the bleeding site and subselective catheterization of the bleeding vessel.[1] Absorbable gelatin foam is most commonly used. Embolic therapy in the rectum is safer than in the proximal colon without the associated risk of transmural necrosis.

THERAPY OF ACUTE BLEEDING

Acute lower GI tract bleeding is self-limited in 75% to 90% of patients. Active bleeding identified by angiography or colonoscopy should be treated immediately. Colonoscopic methods to control bleeding include bipolar electrocoagulation (BICAP), heater probe, hot biopsy forceps, injection therapy, and laser therapy.[11,12] These modalities are mostly used in the treatment of angiodysplasia.[11,12] Angiographic methods include infusion of vasopressin and embolization.

Surgery should be performed if bleeding is continuous or not controlled by other methods.

Localization of the bleeding site by colonoscopy, angiography, or nuclear scanning should facilitate segmental colonic resection.

If surgery is necessary without preoperative localization of the site of bleeding, intraoperative panendoscopy that includes upper endoscopy, evaluation of the small intestine, and colonoscopy should be undertaken. High-flow antegrade irrigation and intraoperative colonoscopy have been used in major colonic hemorrhage.[2] It is still occasionally necessary to do a subtotal colectomy to control bleeding.

SUMMARY

Acute lower GI tract bleeding stops spontaneously in 75% to 90% of cases, allowing colonoscopy to be performed. If bleeding is continuous, diagnostic options include unprepared colonoscopy, prepared colonoscopy, red cell radionuclide scanning, and angiography. Upper GI tract causes of hematochezia occur in approximately 10% of cases and should still be considered if nasogastric aspiration shows no abnormal findings. After initial evaluation and resuscitation, patients should be managed in an intensive care unit, and localization and identification of the cause of bleeding should be aggressively undertaken.

Bleeding lesions diagnosed by angiography can be treated with vasopressin and embolotherapy, and colonoscopic treatment of bleeding sites includes BICAP, heater probe, and laser therapy. Segmental resection is preferable if surgery is necessary and the bleeding site is localized.

The mortality in severe bleeding is as high as 15% and reflects the advanced age and comorbid conditions in these patients.

REFERENCES

1. Bennett JD, Kadir S. Treatment of colorectal bleeding. In: Sadoon K, ed. *Current Practice of Interventional Radiology*. Philadelphia, Pa: BC Decker Inc; 1991:428–436.
2. Berry AR, Campbell WB, Kettlewell MGW. Management of major colonic haemorrhage. *Br J Surg.* 1988;75:637–640.
3. Birkett DH. Gastrointestinal tract bleeding. *Surg Clin North Am.* 1991;71(6):1259–1269.
4. Boley SJ, Sammariano R, Brandt LJ, Sprayregan S. Vascular ectasias of the colon. *Surg Gynecol Obstet.* 1979;149:353–359.
5. Bookstein JJ, Naderi MJ, Walter JF. Transcatheter embolization for lower gastrointestinal bleeding. *Radiology.* 1978;127:345–349.
6. Browder W, Cerise EJ, Litwin MS. Impact of emergency angiography in massive lower gastrointestinal bleeding. *Ann Surg.* 1986;204:530–536.
7. Buchman TG, Bulkley GB. Current management of patients with lower gastrointestinal bleeding. *Surg Clin North Am.* 1987;67(3):651–664.
8. Caserella WJ, Kanter IE, Seaman WB. Right-sided colonic diverticula as a cause of acute rectal hemorrhage. *N Engl J Med.* 1972;286(9):450–453.
9. Caserella WJ, Galloway SJ, Taxin RN, Follett DA, Pollack EJ, Seaman WB. Lower gastrointestinal tract hemorrhage: new concepts based on arteriography. *AJR.* 1974;121:357.
10. Forge KA, Treat MR. Colonoscopy for lower gastrointestinal bleeding. In: Dent TL, Strodel WE, Turcotte JG, et al, eds. *Surgical Endoscopy.* Chicago, Ill: Year Book Medical Publishers; 1985:261–265.
11. Jensen DM, Machicado GA. Diagnosis and treatment of severe hematochezia: the role of urgent colonoscopy after purge. *Gastroenterology.* 1988;95:1569–1574.
12. Jensen DM, Machicado GA. Endoscopic diagnosis and treatment of bleeding colonic angiomas and radiation telangiectasia. *Perspect Colon Rectal Surg.* 1989;2(1):99–113.
13. Lanthier PH, et al. Colonic angiodysplasia: followup of patients after endoscopic treatment for bleeding lesions. *Dis Col Rectum.* 1989;32(4):296–298.
14. Markisz JA, Front D, Royal HD, Sacks B, Parker JA, Kolodny GM. An evaluation of 99m Tc-labeled red blood cell scintigraphy for the detection and localization of gastrointestinal bleeding sites. *Gastroenterology.* 1982;83:394–398.
15. Nash RL, Sequeira JE, Weitzman AF, et al. Lower gastrointestinal bleeding: diagnostic approach and management conclusions. *Am J Surg.* 1981;41:478–481.
16. Painter NS, Burkitt DP. Diverticular disease of the colon, a 20th century problem. *Clin Gastroenterol.* 1975;4(1):3–21.
17. Rogers BHG, Adler F. Hemangiomas of cecum, colonoscopy diagnosis and therapy. *Gastroenterology.* 1976;71:1079–1082.
18. Rosenkrantz H, Bookstein JJ, Rosen RJ, Goff WB, Healy JF. Postembolic colonic infarction. *Radiology.* 1982;142:47–51.
19. Santos JCH, Aprilli F, Guimaraes AS, Rocha JJR. Angiodysplasia of the colon: endoscopic diagnosis and treatment. *Br J Surg.* 1988;75:256–258.
20. Schrock TR. Colonoscopic diagnosis and treatment of lower gastrointestinal bleeding. *Surg Clin North Am.* 1989;69(6):1309–1325.
21. Trudel JL, Fazio VW, Sivak MV. Colonoscopic diagnosis and treatment of arteriovenous malformations in chronic lower gastrointestinal bleeding: clinical accuracy and efficacy. *Dis Col Rectum.* 1988;31(2):107–110.

22
Gastrointestinal Tract Hemorrhage in Children

ARTHUR R. EULER and R. SCOTT SYKES

Gastrointestinal (GI) tract bleeding in infants and children is a common condition in pediatric medicine. Although typically associated with a benign prognosis, the problem can occasionally be serious and life threatening; therefore prompt assessment, diagnosis, and treatment is required. The widespread use and application of fiberoptic endoscopy, coupled with radionuclide imaging and selective angiography, have significantly improved the capability to diagnose and treat GI tract hemorrhage.[1,2]

A detailed and carefully performed history and physical examination will often provide significant clues leading to a proper diagnosis and subsequent therapy. A clear understanding of what the signs associated with GI tract hemorrhage indicate is therefore crucial. *Hematemesis* refers to the vomiting of bright red blood or "coffee-ground" material, the latter resulting from denatured blood. This presentation usually indicates bleeding from a source proximal to the ligament of Treitz. Melena refers to the passage of dark, tarry (sticky) stools and represents bleeding from the upper GI tract or proximal small bowel. Hematochezia is the passage of bright red blood per rectum and suggests a source of bleeding low in the GI tract, typically the colon. Since blood exerts a cathartic action, an upper GI tract hemorrhage of significant magnitude may also present as bright red blood per rectum. In these cases, the rectal bleeding may be massive. Perianal lesions may coat the stool with bright red blood indicating the presence of hemorrhoids or fissures. This coating of the stool with blood is an important sign of perianal disease and should be distinguished from blood mixed with the stool, indicating a more proximal source of bleeding. The presence of mucus and blood mixed with stool often indicates an inflammatory etiologic process, which could be of an infectious nature; such infections are usually invasive and should be distinguished from secretory diarrheas, which are not associated with blood loss. There are substances, often ingested by infants and children, that can cause alarm by giving the appearance of GI tract bleeding. Red food coloring as in Kool Aid, Jello, fruit juice, beets, and medications such as amoxicillin may give the appearance of blood when vomited or passed in the stool. In a child with diarrhea, these products may resemble blood per rectum. Bismuth, iron salts, spinach, dark chocolate, grape juice, and certain berries (cranberries, blueberries) may be mistaken for melena because of the dark color they impart to the stool. A number of simple chemical tests, Gastroccult and Hemoccult, performed at the bedside can confirm the presence of blood in gastric or fecal contents respectively. If epistaxis occurs, blood may be swallowed and not have originated from the patient's GI tract. In the newborn hematemesis may also result from the fetus swallowing maternal blood during delivery. The presence or absence of fetal hemoglobin can be ruled out by the Apt test.

ASSESSMENT AND DIAGNOSIS

The cause of GI tract bleeding in infants and children varies considerably from adults, therefore the diagnostic approach and subsequent therapy varies as well. The patient's age must be considered during the initial assessment and is helpful in developing a differential diagnosis.

In the newborn, for example, the most frequent sign of peptic ulcer disease is hemorrhage. These ulcers are typically related to other illnesses such as congenital heart disease, steroids, trauma (including intracranial pathology), traumatic delivery, sepsis, or asphyxia and have classically been termed secondary. Primary ulcers are those not associated with such conditions. In the newborn, whenever GI tract hemorrhage is present, it is critical to determine if vitamin K has been administered. GI tract bleeding should prompt questions to family members regarding hemophilia or other inherited coagulation factor deficits if not previously obtained during the history taking.

GI tract bleeding in the neonate may also be associated with sepsis, umbilical catheterization, or gastritis.[3] In addition, iatrogenic trauma, coagulopathy, vascular malformations, and nasopharyngeal bleeding should be considered. Similar considerations apply to the infant up to approximately 12 months of age; however, in a patient of this age the presence of esophagitis, esophageal varices, peptic ulcer, gastritis, foreign body or toxic ingestion, and various drugs including salicylates should also be considered. In the child and adolescent, signs and symptoms of portal hypertension with subsequent esophageal variceal hemorrhage, peptic ulcer disease, colonic polyps, and acquired thrombocytopenia must be considerations during history taking.

It must again be emphasized that the evaluation of an infant or child with GI tract bleeding first and foremost involves a complete history and physical examination. In the patient with acute bleeding, if hemorrhage is present, this initial assessment must be coordinated with stabilization as outlined in Table 22–1. Such early stabilization should be carefully integrated with the initial and ongoing therapeutic and diagnostic efforts. The amount of blood loss can be estimated rapidly by assessing subtle signs and symptoms such as postural hypotension, any dizziness or fainting, tachycardia, peripheral vasoconstriction, and pallor. Other factors to consider during this early diagnostic period include the nature and probable site of bleeding (upper versus lower GI tract), whether the blood is fresh or denatured, whether the blood is or is not mixed with emesis or stool, and the presence or absence of preceding signs or symptoms (i.e., pain, emesis, diarrhea).[4] The history is useful in determining if blood has actually been passed; however, biochemical analysis should always be used to confirm its presence, whether gastric or fecal.[5]

The physical examination should initially include examination of the nasopharynx to determine epistaxis as the source of bleeding. Careful dermatologic examination may reveal signs of congenital vascular or hematologic disease including the presence of petechiae, telangiectasia, ecchymoses, or purpura. Petechiae and ecchymosis may indicate a platelet defect, particularly if the lesions progress over time. Petechiae and ecchymosis of a nonprogressive nature are, however, often secondary to a traumatic delivery. Coagulopathy and fibrinolysis may manifest as diffuse bleeding or inappropriate bleeding from a phlebotomy site. Such bleeding may also be seen as a complication of septicemia, hepatic failure, or various infections. Prothrombin time, activated partial thromboplastin time, bleeding time, and platelet count should be evaluated initially in these cases. Peutz-Jeghers syndrome

TABLE 22–1. INITIAL STABILIZATION FOR ACUTE GI TRACT HEMORRHAGE IN INFANTS AND CHILDREN

1. Define need for stabilization
   a. Hct indicating >20% blood volume loss
   b. Tachycardia >150 beats/min
   c. Tachypnea >35 beats/min
   d. Dizziness or fainting
   e. Postural hypotension
   f. Peripheral vasoconstriction
   g. Decreased systolic pressure
   h. Urine output <1 ml/kg/h
2. Brief history
   a. Family history for coagulopathy
   b. Trauma
   c. Drug ingestion including caustic material, foreign body, aspirin, or NSAIDs
   d. Vitamin K prophylaxis (newborn)
   e. Character and quantity of bleeding
   f. Pain assessment
3. Brief physical examination
   a. Vital signs
   b. Skin (petechiae, telangiectasia, ecchymoses, purpura, etc.)
   c. Hepatosplenomegaly
   d. Abdominal mass or ascites
   e. Abdominal or inguinal herniation
   f. Digital rectal examination (obtain stool guaiac)
   g. Biochemical analysis of stool and blood, vomitus, aspirate
4. Procedures
   a. Protect airway for upper GI tract bleeding (if necessary, consider intubation)
   b. Two large-bore peripheral intravenous tube placements
   c. Nasogastric tube placement
   d. Foley catheter placement
   e. Laboratory: complete blood cell count, platelet count, prothrombin time, partial thromboplastin time, bleeding time, type and cross-match
   f. Central venous pressure line (only rarely required, during severe, life-threatening shock, myocardial or renal impairment, expected prolonged intravenous fluid administration, *and* the presence of a physician skilled in central venous line placement in infants and children)

NSAID = nonsteroidal antiinflammatory drug.

would be a particularly important consideration in the patient with cutaneous and oral pigmentation, although the syndrome may be present without these lesions. Coagulopathies should be considered in all infants and children with GI tract bleeding and a platelet count, prothrombin time, partial thromboplastin time, and bleeding time should be obtained. Icterus, palmar erythema, hirsutism, spider angiomata, hepatosplenomegaly, ascites, and abdominal distension with or without a prominent venous pattern may point to hepatic disease, portal hypertension, and esophageal varices. The anus should be evaluated for the presence of fissure(s) prior to digital examination, as a fissure may develop from an inappropriately performed examination.

The overall diagnostic approach for GI tract blood loss is outlined in Figure 22–1. Regardless of the presence or absence of hematemesis, a nasogastric tube should routinely be placed as one of the initial components of the diagnostic evaluation, because it can be used to differentiate upper GI tract hemorrhage (proximal to the ligament of Treitz) from lower GI tract hemorrhage (distal to the ligament of Treitz). Esophageal varices are not a contraindication to nasogastric tube placement. Once in place, the gastric contents should be gently aspirated with a syringe. The presence of blood or coffee-ground material or strongly guaiac-positive aspirate is evidence of upper GI tract bleeding. A nonbloody aspirate with a positive guaiac test may result from vigorous aspiration (a few streaks of blood may be seen in the aspirate), therefore gentle suction is important. If the aspirate is clear or bilious, the source of bleeding is usually not from the nasopharynx, esophagus, or stomach. A bleeding duodenal lesion, however, cannot be definitively ruled out by a negative aspirate, because gastroduodenal reflux of blood may not be occurring. In addition, despite the presence of a negative aspirate, esophageal, gastric, or duodenal lesion(s) may be documented at endoscopy as shown in one study of adult patients.[6]

Further diagnostic procedures for an infant or child with frank hematemesis or blood detected in the gastric aspirate or passage of large amounts of blood per rectum should usually include an esophagogastroduodenoscopy (EGD). Optimally, this procedure should be performed within the first 24 hours, after stabilization of the patient and cessation of the hemorrhage.[7] Endoscopy should rarely be performed under

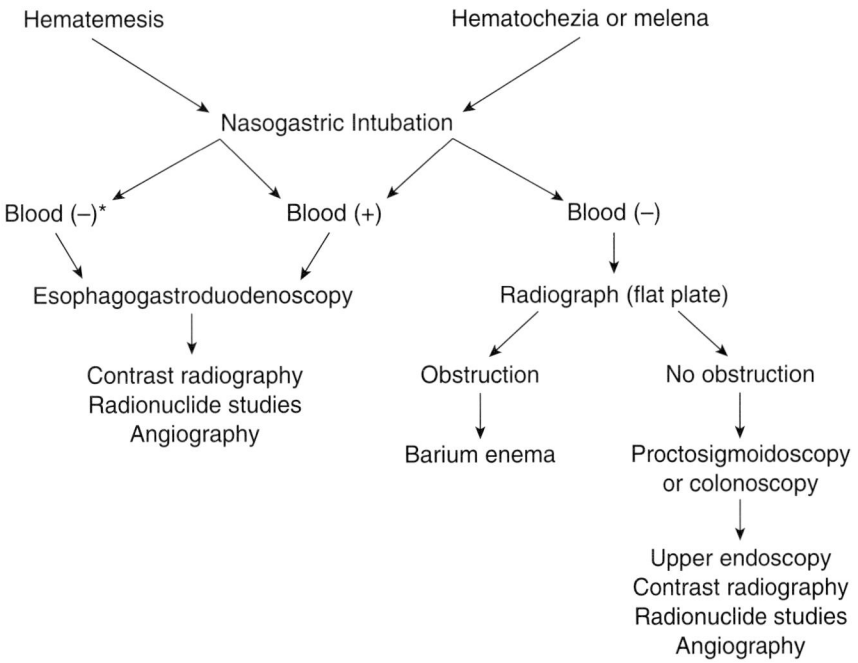

*The timing of upper endoscopy without aspirate blood depends upon the clinical presentation and physician's evaluation.

FIGURE 22–1. Diagnostic approach for GI tract blood loss.

emergent conditions, particularly if the patient has not been stabilized. Children with hematemesis and a history such as salicylate ingestion, who respond promptly to medical therapy, may have endoscopy performed during the first few days after presentation. Normally EGD is not associated with an increased risk of bleeding or rebleeding when performed under controlled conditions by an experienced endoscopist. The patient with a known coagulation disorder is, however, an exception and is at increased risk of trauma-induced bleeding during even a carefully performed endoscopic procedure; thus, endoscopy should be delayed until bleeding has abated and should be performed by an experienced gastroenterologist under optimal conditions. Infants under 12 months of age are best examined under general anesthesia with endotracheal tube placement, since tracheal compression by the endoscope is a concern in this age group. Although minimal, the risk associated with the anesthesia must be weighed against the benefit of endoscopy in a patient of this age.[8] Under most circumstances endoscopy may be performed in children and adolescents with moderate sedation only. Careful observation of vital signs is still critical in this group as in the younger patient.

Flexible fiberoptic proctosigmoidoscopy and colonoscopy are indicated in the patient with frank hematochezia, blood mixed with stool, or melena. They are also indicated in those patients without these signs when the upper GI tract endoscopy shows no abnormal findings. These procedures are well tolerated by children and provide more information than rigid instruments, which are more cumbersome and uncomfortable to the patient. With the flexible instruments, inspection of the entire rectal and colonic mucosa is also possible. Flexible sigmoidoscopy can be performed after a brief bowel cleansing and, if necessary, very mild sedation. Most bleeding lesions can be identified, including Crohn's disease involving the colon, ulcerative colitis, vascular lesions, and polyps.[9]

The indication for pancolonoscopy is the presence of blood in the stool of any kind when proctosigmoidoscopy is nondiagnostic. Smaller colonoscopes have made the examination and biopsy of the entire colon possible in a majority of infants and children. Adequate preparation of the colon is essential and requires a clear liquid diet for up to 3 days before the examination. Poorly absorbable electrolyte solutions are useful for the purpose of colonic evacuation, although their use in infants and children should be closely monitored to avoid fluid and electrolyte disturbances particularly in the smaller patient.[10] General anesthesia may occasionally be required for a complete colonic examination; however, sedation alone is preferred, allowing the patient to respond to stretching of the bowel wall, thus decreasing the risk of perforation. Appropriate precautions should be taken when obtaining biopsies or performing electrocautery or laser treatment to avoid igniting intraluminal gases. Colonoscopy can also be used to safely remove pedunculated polyps and to cauterize vascular lesions, thereby avoiding surgery.

In the preendoscopic era, in up to 50% of patients, the cause of GI tract bleeding could not be determined[11,12]; however, with modern flexible fiberoptic endoscopes, a source of bleeding can be identified in 75% to 90% of such cases.[1,3,13] Even with the modern equipment, a difficult diagnostic situation continues to exist in the patient with massive bleeding, because endoscopy may be nondiagnostic with the bleeding site being obscured by intraluminal blood. In these situations, radionuclide studies or angiography may be required. Both types of studies, particularly the former, may also be necessary if the bleeding is subacute or intermittent.

Radionuclide studies are an effective and noninvasive diagnostic approach that may involve one of several types of isotopes. The technetium-99m (^{99m}Tc)–sulfur colloid (SC) scan is sensitive, detecting bleeding rates as low as 0.1 ml/min. The half-life of this isotope is <2.5 minutes; thus after 10 minutes only 10% of the radionuclide remains in circulation. The ^{99m}Tc–SC is a tracer that is rapidly cleared from the blood and concentrated in the reticuloendothelial system. For these reasons the scan is usually best performed during the active stage of bleeding, at which time the tracer will accumulate at the bleeding site. Disadvantages include bleeding sites that would overlap the spleen or liver (which could cause misinterpretation because of the radioisotope's accumulation in these organs' reticuloendothelial systems), an intermittent bleed that is inactive at the time of injection, or a hemorrhage in which the bleeding rate has rapidly decreased.

A ^{99m}Tc-labeled red blood cell scan is another sensitive diagnostic approach to the patient with constant and intermittent bleeding. With this test, over 95% of the isotope is bound to red blood cells, thus remaining in the circulation longer than ^{99m}Tc–SC and allowing imaging for up to 24 hours following the injection. If bleeding occurs during this period, the radionuclide will accumulate at the site and may be detected during scanning. It has been estimated that a bleeding rate of >0.1 ml/min will be detected by this scan.

⁹⁹mTc-pertechnetate is another isotope used when functional gastric mucosa in an ectopic site is suspected. The isotope is useful because following intravenous injection the isotope is loosely bound to plasma proteins and selectively concentrated in areas where parietal cells are normally present, such as the stomach, but also in ectopic locations, such as a Meckel's diverticulum.[14] The diagnostic accuracy of this procedure is enhanced by the typical location of Meckel's diverticula in the right lower quadrant or midabdomen where the prominent focus of radioactivity can be easily visualized, away from the accumulation in the gastric mucosa. False-positive results can occur when ectopic gastric mucosa is present but not actively bleeding, such as with a duplication cyst. Radionuclear activity will also accumulate in other nonbleeding conditions including inflammatory bowel disease, vesicoureteral obstruction and reflux, sacral meningomyelocele, and hemangiomas, all of which therefore may also produce false-positive results. False-negative scans have occurred in the absence of or insufficient amounts of gastric mucosa within the diverticulum, massive hemorrhage (which may dilute the image), conditions impairing blood flow (torsion or intussusception), or when the ectopic mucosa's presence is overlapped by gastric mucosa.

Angiography is indicated for actively bleeding lesions or recurrent bleeding that has not been identified during other diagnostic procedures. With angiography, it is possible to detect a bleeding rate as low as 0.5 ml/min.[15] Angiography is particularly useful in detecting causes of bleeding associated with abnormal vasculature such as malformations, telangiectasias, or hemangiomas.[16,17] In many cases with chronic low-grade or intermittent GI tract bleeding, angiography will identify sites even without active bleeding.[18] Once the lesion has been located and the catheter has been placed in an afferent vessel, a therapeutic infusion of a vasoconstrictive or thrombotic agent may be performed through the catheter. Accurate localization of sites preoperatively or during surgery may also enable precise surgical excision. In children the morbidity associated with angiography must be considered. Femoral artery spasm and thrombosis may occur plus the hyperosmolarity of the contrast agent may cause fluid shifts and electrolyte imbalance, particularly in younger children.

Plain radiologic films are not of great diagnostic use in the child with GI tract bleeding but may reveal bowel obstruction and intraabdominal gas. When barium studies are used as the initial or primary diagnostic tool, incorrect diagnoses can be observed in up to 24% of patients examined for upper GI tract hemorrhage.[19] The diagnostic accuracy of the small bowel follow-through, typically difficult to evaluate, is enhanced by using enteroclysis, which provides improved filling of small bowel loops. Duodenal intubation and a constant barium infusion are required for these studies, but greater mucosal detail is obtained, thereby visualizing mucosal abnormalities with greater accuracy.[20,21] During routine small bowel barium examinations, the use of more frequent fluoroscopy and compression of all barium-filled bowel segments with an inflatable paddle will enhance the diagnostic yield. Double-contrast barium enemas are best for examining the large bowel and are highly accurate in diagnosing inflammatory bowel disease.[22] If, however, an intussusception is expected, a single-contrast barium enema should be used and may result in hydrostatic reduction. In the evaluation of lower GI tract bleeding where polyps are suspected, the only indication for obtaining contrast radiographs is failure to make a diagnosis during colonoscopy.[22] Intraluminal contrast agents will also delay or preclude the possibility of a meaningful arteriogram or isotope scan, therefore studies using them should not be undertaken if arteriograms or scans are being considered in the near future.

CONDITIONS AND TREATMENT

UPPER GI TRACT BLEEDING

As mentioned previously the cause of upper GI tract bleeding varies with the age of the patient. Regardless of age, any presentation of upper GI tract bleeding requires rapid assessment of cause (Table 22–2). For example, in the newborn period, esophageal varices are usually caused by extrahepatic portal hypertension, resulting from portal vein thrombosis. Thrombosis usually occurs following exchange transfusions, omphalitis, severe dehydration, or trauma.[23,24] Historically, this type of thrombosis was most often caused by umbilical vein catheterization where the access was used for infusion of hyperosmotic fluids and venous samples. In contrast, portal hypertension secondary to hepatic parenchymal disease such as chronic hepatitis, biliary cirrhosis associated with biliary atresia, cystic fibrosis, Wilson's disease, and a-1-antitrypsin deficiency

TABLE 22-2. CAUSES OF UPPER GI TRACT HEMORRHAGE IN INFANTS AND CHILDREN

Common	Less Common
Swallowed maternal blood	Coagulopathy
Peptic ulcer (stress ulcer)	Congenital duplication
Gastritis	Iatrogenic trauma (e.g., tube feeding)
Esophageal varices	Esophagitis
Mallory-Weiss lesion	Drug or caustic ingestion
	Foreign body
	Vascular malformation
	Nasopharyngeal bleeding

occurs in a smaller percentage of patients and manifests most often in childhood. Bleeding from extrahepatic portal hypertension usually manifests as hematemesis and melena, often being massive. Following stabilization (if necessary), management involves diagnostic esophagoscopy and therapeutic sclerotherapy on one or more occasions if hemorrhage from the varices is documented.[25] This technique does not preclude the possibility of future surgical intervention. The patient should be carefully followed to detect any evidence of rebleeding with further sclerotherapy being performed if the varices have not been obliterated during the initial session. Portal-systemic shunt surgery should be reserved for children whose variceal bleeding cannot be controlled with such intervention. Aspirin and nonsteroidal antiinflammatory drug (NSAID) use should be discouraged in these children with portal hypertension, as this may precipitate bleeding from enlarged esophageal varices.

Peptic ulcer disease in infants and children is not as frequent as in adults. The cause and clinical presentation in this patient population are also quite different. During infancy, peptic ulcer is often secondary to a stressful situation such as shock, sepsis, major surgery, burns, and respiratory insufficiency and usually presents as upper GI tract hemorrhage. In children, aspirin and NSAID use should always be sought during history taking, since they are known to cause erosions and ulcerations in the upper GI tract mucosa. Bleeding from mucosal erosions or ulcerations may also be associated with chronic renal failure. Children who develop severe medical conditions requiring admission to intensive care units (i.e., head injury, burns, etc.) have a greater risk of developing peptic ulcers (stress ulcers) similar to adult patients. Presentation of this type of peptic ulcer may also include signs of perforation or obstruction in addition to hemorrhage. Feeding difficulty and frequent vomiting may also be observed in younger children and infants. Medical management, which may include antacids or H_2 antagonists, is usually successful.[26,27] Vitamin K may be required for newborns or neonates with peptic ulcer. Antacids administered should contain both magnesium hydroxide and aluminum hydroxide to decrease the diarrhea seen with magnesium alone. Acute hemorrhage usually warrants a dose of 0.5 ml/kg of such a high-potency liquid antacid. This dose should be administered every 1 to 2 hours. Hourly measurement of gastric pH can be performed once the nasogastric tube is in place, and therapy may be adjusted to maintain an intraluminal pH ≥ 4.0. Once the acute bleeding has been controlled, the same dose can be given for maintenance; however, the frequency can be decreased to administration postprandially and at bedtime. Because of the frequency of administration required with antacids and their associated side effects, H_2 receptor antagonists are frequently used instead. The H_2 receptor antagonists, which have been evaluated most extensively in infants and children, are cimetidine and ranitidine. Both can be administered orally or intravenously. Several clinical trials, conducted in pediatric intensive care units, have been performed with the parenteral forms of these H_2 antagonists in infants and children with stress-related upper GI tract bleeding.[28-30] In these studies, intravenous cimetidine (20 to 1000 mg/kg/d) and ranitidine (6 mg/kg/d) (both administered every 6 hours) were shown to significantly increase intragastric pH, and both had acceptable safety profiles. Oral cimetidine (20 mg/kg/d; given as four doses) and ranitidine (6 mg/kg/d; given twice a day) have been proven effective for the treatment of peptic ulcer disease in children. Ranitidine, because of its documented history of fewer drug interactions may be the drug of choice in patients with both stress-related mucosal damage and peptic ulcer. Promising new drugs, including newer H_2 antagonists and proton pump inhibitors are currently being evaluated; however, there is a lack of adequate information in infants and children both in terms of efficacy and safety.

Surgery is required only for complications including continuing hemorrhage, perforation, and obstruction or in the event that medical management has been totally unsuccessful. Truncal vagotomy and pyloroplasty is the recommended surgical procedure, particularly when combined with oversewing of the ulcer in the case of hemorrhage.[27] For the rare patient with Zollinger-Ellison syndrome a total gastrectomy is required to avoid further serious complications of peptic ulcer. In the patient with hematemesis following vomiting or retching, Mallory-Weiss tears of the esophagus must be considered. This diagnosis will typically respond well to conservative medical management.

LOWER GI TRACT BLEEDING

A variety of factors may cause lower GI tract bleeding in the pediatric population as shown in Table 22–3. Lower GI tract bleeding in neonates is often secondary to anorectal disorders. Anal fissures usually involve a superficial mucosal tear, typically located posteriorly, and are associated with small amounts of bright red blood per rectum. Diarrhea with excoriation of the perineum or the passage of hard stools (more common in the older child secondary to chronic constipation) may also cause an anal fissure. Less frequently, anal trauma from a vigorous rectal examination or improper placement of a rectal thermometer may cause such a fissure. If constipation is the cause, a stool softener or a lubricant such as mineral oil may be required. Surgery is rarely required for this condition.

Necrotizing enterocolitis in the neonate is an acute fulminating conditions associated with signs of ileus such as regurgitation, vomiting, and abdominal distension plus hematochezia resulting from diffuse ulceration and necrosis of the GI tract. The ileum is most often affected; however, in approximately 75% of cases, colonic lesions are also found.[31] In the neonate, necrotizing enterocolitis can be associated with lower bowel obstruction such as with Hirschsprung's disease. In the newborn it may be associated with exchange transfusions, hyperosmolar enteric alimentation, and ischemia. There is also evidence that necrotizing enterocolitis may be infectious in origin. Diagnosis is typically confirmed on plain abdominal x-ray film, where small bowel distension, evidence of obstruction, a feathered mucosal appearance indicative of ulceration, and the presence of intramural gas may be found. With progression of this disease, gas may be found in the biliary tract, which is a particularly ominous sign, and with perforation, free air may be seen in the peritoneum. Initial treatment involves supportive care with subsequent therapy then directed at the underlying process, if any. Withholding oral feedings, nasogastric suction, and intravenous fluids should be initiated. This should be followed with definitive therapy of the primary condition such as surgical correction of a perforation or of any obstructive process. Antibiotics should be administered cautiously if at all, as morbidity from these drugs is high and the usefulness of prophylactic antibiotics is unproven; however, the acutely ill neonate with signs and symptoms of sepsis or a septic shock condition should receive appropriate antibiotic coverage.

Midgut malrotation with volvulus may present late in its course with ischemia and associated GI hemorrhage, usually melena. Often symptomatic patients present with signs of high intestinal obstruction such as bile-stained vomitus and abdominal distension. An upper GI tract series may show partial or complete obstruction manifested by dilated loops of bowel and air fluid levels on upright projections. If needed, the diagnosis may be further confirmed with a contrast study. Treatment consists of surgical correction.

Cow or soy milk protein intolerance may present with vomiting, weight loss, and GI tract bleeding, which may range from occult blood to hematochezia. The onset occurs usually between 3 to 4 months of age. Microscopic examination of the stool will reveal inflammatory and red blood cells. Sigmoidoscopy will reveal a friable, erythematous mucosa. The course may be prolonged, and treatment may require the use of elemental formulas for months. If the presentation has been severe, introduction of milk or soy protein should be delayed until after 1 year of age. Such an introduction should be made under professional supervision so that proper care can be

TABLE 22–3. CAUSES OF LOWER GI TRACT HEMORRHAGE IN INFANTS AND CHILDREN

COMMON	LESS COMMON
Upper GI tract bleeding	Coagulopathy
Milk or soy protein allergy	Vascular malformation
Necrotizing enterocolitis	Congenital duplication
Intussusception	Nodular lymphoid
Meckel's diverticulum	hyperplasia
Midgut malrotation with volvulus	Henoch-Schönlein purpura
	Hemolytic-uremic syndrome
Infectious diarrhea	Foreign body
Ulcerative colitis	
Crohn's disease	
Juvenile polyposis	
Perianal lesion or fissure	

provided in the event of a major hypersensitivity reaction when these proteins are reintroduced.

Intussusception and Meckel's diverticulum are the most common causes of lower GI tract bleeding during infancy and the preschool years. Intussusception is seen most commonly between the ages of 3 months and 3 years. Clinically, the presentation usually consists of signs and symptoms compatible with small bowel obstruction. The patient has colicky abdominal pain, vomiting, and bloody bowel movements accompanied with mucus often described as currant jelly in appearance. Prostration and fever soon appear. Auscultation of the abdomen reveals high-pitched peristaltic rushes compatible with obstruction, while on palpation an abdominal mass may be felt. The intussusception typically starts orad to the ileocecal valve, and invagination becomes ileocolic. Ileoileal and colocolic intussusceptions are also seen. Ischemia may develop with subsequent perforation and peritonitis if the circulation is significantly impaired and diagnosis delayed. Barium enema is diagnostic in the majority of children when a typical ileocolic intussusception is present. Hydrostatic reduction may be undertaken if there are no clinical signs of strangulated bowel, perforation, or severe toxicity. The overall success for such reduction is as high as 80% when performed by an experienced radiologist. The longer the diagnosis is delayed, the lower this success rate. With the presence of hematochezia, indicating that the intussusception has been long standing, the probability of therapeutic success is less. For patients not suitable for hydrostatic reduction or in whom it is unsuccessful, surgery is required.

A Meckel's diverticulum is usually located in the distal ileum and represents a remnant of the omphalomesenteric duct. The tissue often contains ectopic gastric mucosa but may also contain pancreatic tissue, jejunal, or colonic mucosa as well. Bleeding is due to peptic ulceration within the diverticulum or in the adjacent mucosa. Complications may include intestinal obstruction, secondary to a volvulus, or an intussusception with the diverticula being the invaginating segment. Clinical presentation usually consists of significant painless hematochezia unless obstruction occurs, in which case the signs and symptoms are dependent on the site. A ^{99m}Tc scan will confirm the diagnosis in the majority of cases, and treatment consists of surgical excision with a small bowel closure or segmental resection and anastomosis.[32]

Congenital duplications of the intestinal tract can occur in almost any location and may cause significant hemorrhage. The bleeding may occur from ulceration in areas of ectopic gastric mucosa and of adjacent mucosa. Intestinal obstruction occurs frequently and may develop secondary to expansion of the duplication with compression of the primary bowel lumen, a volvulus, or an intussusception. Clinical presentation usually consists primarily of the signs of such obstruction. Treatment is surgical.

The infectious diarrheas may present with blood in watery stools ranging from flecks to frank hematochezia. Invasive organisms such as *Shigella, Salmonella,* and enteroinvasive *Escherichia coli* are frequent causes with shigellosis being the most common. The sigmoidoscopic and radiologic appearances are similar to ulcerative colitis or Crohn's disease. Less frequently the presence of *Giardia, Campylobacter,* and *Yersinia* may also present with diarrhea, guaiac-positive or grossly bloody stools, fever, and ileus. This is more commonly seen with *Campylobacter* and *Yersinia* than with *Giardia*. Treatment of most infectious diarrheas is supportive, although in a minority of cases antibiotics may be required for treatment of a specific organism. Giardiasis requires antibacterial therapy for eradication, usually metronidazole.

A complication associated with the use of antibiotics for the treatment of infectious diarrhea or other infectious diseases is antibiotic-associated enterocolitis. The presentation of such antibiotic-associated enterocolitis may vary tremendously from only loose stools to hematochezia. Sigmoidoscopic findings may also range from erythema to an extremely friable mucosa with pseudomembranes. *Clostridium difficile* toxins are the usual cause. Treatment of antibiotic-associated colonic complications varies from supportive care and discontinuation of the antibiotic to the use of vancomycin or similar agents.

Juvenile polyps often cause rectal bleeding and are typically benign hamartomatous lesions. The bleeding results from the sloughing of part of the polyp surface. These polyps are usually pedunculated and located most frequently in the colon. They are often palpable during rectal examination and within reach of the sigmoidoscope. These polyps are rare in children under 1 year of age and are most common in those 3 to 5 years of age. The clinical presentation may consist of painless, episodic bright red rectal bleeding, intermittent melena with or without anemia, or prolapse of the polyp through the anal sphincter. Proctosigmoidoscopy or colonoscopy should be performed with all polyps being removed with cautery applied through a polypectomy snare. Unless signs of obstruction are present, surgery is not indicated since this endoscopic approach is usually successful. All excised polyps should be examined microscopically. Multiple juvenile polyposis is a benign condition usually presenting with intermittent mild rectal bleeding. It can be confused during endoscopy with familial adenomatous polyposis, however, so again histologic evaluation of the excised polyps is important. Familial adenomatous polyposis places the patient at risk for carcinoma development later in life, typically before 40 years of age; thus, patients with this condition should undergo colonic resection. Abdominal colectomy with ileoanal anastomosis and endorectal removal of all rectal mucosa is the procedure recommended to avoid the risk of cancer in retained bowel segments or rectal mucosa.[33,34] Other types of familial polyposis such as Peutz-Jeghers or Gardner's syndrome are rare but may also present with rectal bleeding. The initial diagnostic approach for these is similar to that described for juvenile polyps; however, once a diagnosis of either is made, all members of the affected family should be examined, as these syndromes are typically inherited.[35] This is not necessary when juvenile polyposis is diagnosed.

Although typically observed in older children and adolescents, inflammatory bowel disease can present anytime during the pediatric years. Ulcerative colitis usually presents with small amounts of blood and mucus per rectum but may be associated with hematochezia. Tenesmus, crampy abdominal pain, and extracolonic manifestations such as fever, weight loss, growth retardation, arthralgia, or arthritis may be observed. Crohn's disease may be very similar in its presentation, but usually rectal bleeding is not a predominant sign. Either disease may present as a toxic megacolon or exsanguinating hemorrhage. Histologically, ulcerative colitis reveals inflammatory cell infiltration and crypt abscesses as compared with Crohn's disease, in which a transmural process is observed with chronic granulomatous inflammatory reactions deep within the tissue. Acute management is primarily medical with frequent use of systemic steroids. Surgery must be considered when complications arise such as obstruction, perforation, fistula, abscess, or refractory hemorrhage.

Nodular lymphoid hyperplasia consists of an overgrowth of submucosal lymphoid nodules as a response to unknown stimuli, although an infectious or allergic process is frequently suspected. The condition is often detected during a barium enema or colonoscopic examination conducted for rectal bleeding. Typically patients with nodular lymphoid hyperplasia do not require specific therapy as the condition is usually self-limiting; however, patients with severe pain or bleeding may respond to antihistamines. Rarely patients require brief courses of corticosteroid therapy.

Henoch-Schönlein purpura and hemolytic-uremic syndrome may also present with lower GI tract bleeding, ranging from blood streaks to hematochezia. Henoch-Schönlein purpura usually follows a streptococcal infection with abdominal cramps, rash, nephritis, and arthritis being associated findings. Abdominal cramping and the GI tract bleeding will usually abate once corticosteroid therapy begins. Hemolytic-uremic syndrome results from a vasculitis and usually presents with hematuria, renal failure, and thrombocytopenia. Colonic ischemia is also present and often is associated with rectal bleeding as severe as hematochezia. Treatment is generally supportive with other forms of therapy such as corticosteroids, antimetabolites, exchange transfusions, and heparin having equivocal results.

Vascular lesions such as arteriovenous malformations, telangiectasias, and hemangiomas may occur in any part of the GI tract and may result in either chronic low-grade or acute, massive blood loss. GI tract hemangiomas often are associated with cutaneous hemangiomas, which represent an important diagnostic sign. A properly trained gastroenterologist may undertake endoscopic diagnosis and therapy. If such a trained gastroenterologist is not available or if lesions are not detected during endoscopy, angiography may be effective in visualizing the abnormality even if the lesion is not actively bleeding at the time.[36] In this case surgical intervention is usually necessary.

SUMMARY

GI tract bleeding in infants and children is a common problem, usually associated with benign disease but occasionally severe and life threatening. The cause is varied and age dependent. The diagnosis and management of this condition has changed considerably over the past several decades, as previously the cause and source of the bleeding usually remained unidentified. For this reason morbidity and mortality were unacceptably high. Because of the widespread and routine application of fiberoptic endoscopy, improved angiographic techniques, and imaging scans, the source of the hemorrhage is now detected in the vast majority of patients, thus decreasing morbidity and mortality. Significant therapeutic advances have also been made in the treatment of several common causes of GI tract hemorrhage in children, including acid peptic disorders, esophageal varices, and polyps. For these reasons, what was once obscure diagnostically and difficult to approach therapeutically has become manageable within a practical framework for evaluation and treatment.

REFERENCES

1. Gryboski JD. The value of upper gastrointestinal endoscopy in children. *Dig Dis Sci.* 1981;26:17–21.
2. Meyerovitz MF, Fellows KE. Angiography in gastrointestinal bleeding in children. *Am J Radiology.* 1984;143:837–840.
3. Cox K, Ament ME. Upper gastrointestinal bleeding in children and adolescents. *Pediatrics.* 1979;63:408–416.
4. Oshita Y, Okazaki Y, Takemoto T, Kawai K. What are the signs of recent hemorrhage, and what do they mean? Criteria for massive bleeding. *Endoscopy.* 1986;18(suppl 2):11–14.
5. Ahlquist DA, McGill DB, Schwartz S, et al. Fecal blood levels in health and disease: a study using Hemo Quant. *N Engl J Med.* 1985;312:1422–1428.
6. Gilbert DA, Silverstein FE, Tedesco FJ, et al. The national ASGE survey on upper gastrointestinal bleeding: III. Endoscopy in upper gastrointestinal bleeding. *Gastrointest Endosc.* 1981;27:94–102.
7. Prolla JC, Diehl AS, Benvenuti GA, et al. Upper gastrointestinal fiberoptic endoscopy in pediatric patients. *Gastrointest Endosc.* 1983;29(4):279–281.
8. Smith R. Anesthesia for infants and children. In: *Mortality in Pediatric Anesthesia.* St. Louis, Mo: The CV Mosby Co. 1980:653–661.
9. Cucchiara S, Guandalini S, Staiano A, et al. Sigmoidoscopy, colonoscopy and radiology in the evaluation of children and rectal bleeding. *J Pediatr Gastroenterol Nutr.* 1983;2:667–671.
10. Maxfield RG, Maxfield CM. Colonoscopy as a primary diagnostic procedure in chronic gastrointestinal tract bleeding. *Arch Surg.* 1986;121:401–403.
11. Caos A, Benner KG, Manier J, et al. Colonoscopy after Golytely preparation in acute rectal bleeding. *J Clin Gastroenterol.* 1986;8:46–49.
12. Spencer R. Gastrointestinal hemorrhage in infancy and childhood: 476 cases. *Surgery.* 1964;55:718–734.
13. Sherman NS, Clatworthy HW. Gastrointestinal bleeding in neonates: a study of 94 cases. *Surgery.* 1967;62:614–619.
14. Driscoll DM. The role of radionuclide imaging in the diagnosis of gastrointestinal bleeding in children. *Radiography.* 1986;52:237–239.
15. Afshani E, Berger PE. Gastrointestinal tract angiography in infants and children. *J Pediatr Gastroenterol Nutr.* 1986;5:173–186.
16. Richardson JD, Max MH, Flint LM, et al. Bleeding malformations of the intestine. *Surgery.* 1978;84:430.
17. Halpern M, Tumer AF, Citron BD. Hereditary hemorrhagic telangiectasia. *Radiology.* 1968;90:1143.
18. Meyerovitz MF, Fellows KE. Angiography in gastrointestinal bleeding in children. *AJR.* 1984;143:837–840.
19. Thoeni RF, Cello JP. A critical look at the accuracy of endoscopy and double contrast radiography of upper gastrointestinal tract in patients with substantial upper gastrointestinal hemorrhage. *Radiology.* 1980;135:305–308.
20. Maglinte DDT, Burney BT, Miller RE. Lesions missed on small bowel follow through: analysis and recommendations. *Radiology.* 1982;144:737–739.
21. Antes G, Lissner J. Double-contrast small bowel examination with barium and methylcellulose. *Radiology.* 1983;148:37–40.
22. Euler AR, Seibert JJ. The role of sigmoidoscopy radiographs and colonoscopy in the diagnostic evaluation of pediatric age patients with suspected juvenile polyps. *J Pediatr Surg.* 1981;16:500–502.
23. Altman RP, Krug J. Portal hypertension: American Academy of Pediatrics Surgical Section Survey—1981. *J Pediatr Surg.* 1982;17(5):567–570.
24. Fonkalsrud EW. Surgical management of portal hypertension in childhood. *Arch Surg.* 1980;115:1042–1045.
25. Donovan TJ, Ward M, Shepherd RW. Evaluation of endoscopic sclerotherapy of esophageal varices in children. *J Pediatr Gastroenterol Nutr.* 1986;5:696–700.
26. Johnson D, L'Hedureux P, Thompson T. Peptic ulcer disease in early infancy: clinical presentation and roentgenographic features. *Acta Paediats Scand.* 1980;69:753–760.
27. Kumar D, Spitz L. Peptic ulceration in children. *Surg Gynecol Obstet.* 1984;159:63–66.
28. Lacroix J, Infante-Rivard C, Gauthier M, et al. Upper gastrointestinal tract bleeding acquired in a pediatric intensive care unit: prophylaxis trial with cimetidine. *J Pediatr.* 1986;108:1015–1018.
29. Tam PK, Saing H. The use of H_2-receptor antagonist in the treatment of peptic ulcer disease in children. *J Pediatr Gastroenterol Nutr.* 1989;8:41–46.
30. Lopez-Herce CJ, Albajara Velasco L, Codoceo R, et al. Ranitidine prophylaxis in acute gastric mucosal damage in critically ill pediatric patients. *Crit Care Med.* 1988;16:591–593.
31. Bell MJ. Neonatal necrotizing enterocolitis: therapeutic decisions based upon clinical staging. *Ann Surg.* 1978;187:1.
32. Mackey WC, Dineen P. A fifty-year experience with Meckel's diverticulum. *Surg Gynecol Obstet.* 1983;156:56–64.
33. Martin LW, Fischer JE. Preservation of anorectal continence following total colectomy. *Ann Surg.* 1982;196(6):700–704.
34. Moertel CG, Hill JR, Adson MA. Surgical management of multiple polyposis: the problem of cancer in the retained bowel segment. *Arch Surg.* 1970;100:521–526.
35. Naylor EW, Lebenthal F. Early detection of adenomatous polyposis coli in Gardner's syndrome. *Pediatrics.* 1979;63:222–227.
36. Abrahamson J, Strandling B. Intestinal hemangianata in childhood and a syndrome for diagnosis: a collective review. *J Pediatr Surg.* 1973;8:487–495.

23
Gastrointestinal Tract Bleeding of Unknown Origin

ROME JUTABHA and DENNIS M. JENSEN

Our purpose in this chapter is to discuss *gastrointestinal (GI) tract bleeding of unknown origin*. This term refers to patients who have clinical evidence of gastrointestinal tract blood loss and who have undergone routine diagnostic tests without localization of a definitive source. Bleeding may be either overt with frank hematemesis or hematochezia, or occult with GI tract blood loss detectable only by fecal occult blood testing. Other synonyms include *occult GI tract bleeding*[21] or *obscure GI tract bleeding*.[22] We prefer the term *GI tract bleeding of unknown origin* because it is more descriptive of the diagnosis rather than the degree of bleeding, which may vary from occult to severe.

Ulcer Research and Education (CURE) data for patients with GI tract bleeding of unknown origin will be presented.

Patients with GI tract bleeding of unknown origin are typically elderly patients (mean age >60 years) with chronic iron deficiency anemia and hemoccult-positive stools.[17,24] Blood loss is usually occult in nature (detected only by fecal occult blood testing) but may manifest as hematemesis, melena, or hematochezia. Iron therapy results in a normal reticulocytosis and distinguishes anemia caused by GI tract blood loss from anemia caused by primary bone marrow dysfunction. Many patients are transfusion dependent because of chronic GI tract bleeding.[17]

CLINICAL FEATURES

Patients with GI tract bleeding of unknown origin usually have undergone extensive and often repetitive diagnostic tests including panendoscopy, colonoscopy, flexible sigmoidoscopy, air contrast barium enema, and upper GI (UGI) tract series with small bowel follow-through. In most of these cases, the localization of the bleeding site and specific diagnoses are unknown. We will review the clinical features of the various lesions responsible for GI bleeding of unknown origin and focus on the diagnostic and therapeutic endoscopic options for patients with these lesions. In addition, some of our own Center for

CLASSIFICATION

Lesions responsible for GI tract bleeding of unknown origin can be classified by their anatomic location: (1) upper gastrointestinal tract (esophagus, stomach, proximal duodenum), (2) small bowel, and (3) colon.[21] We prefer to classify patients by their clinical presentation and why the bleeding focus remains elusive despite extensive diagnostic evaluation. Our three categories are (1) lesions that are not detectable by conventional endoscopy, (2) lesions that are seen endoscopically but not recognized as a potential source of bleeding, and (3) lesions that are often missed entirely during routine endoscopic examination (see Table 23–1).

The most frequent source of GI tract bleeding of unknown origin is from the first group, lesions not detected by routine endoscopic or radiologic examination. These lesions are located in the small intestine and are not within the reach of conventional panendoscopy or colonoscopy. Thus, obscure GI tract bleeding is often

---

The CURE results and studies referred to were funded in part by an American Society of Gastrointestinal Endoscopy Career Development Grant (Dr. Jutabha), NIH Studies NIDDK R01-33273 (Dr. Jensen), and NIDDK 41301 (CURE CORE Grant).

TABLE 23–1. CAUSES OF GI TRACT BLEEDING OF UNKNOWN ORIGIN

Group 1. Lesions not detectable by conventional endoscopy, i.e., small bowel lesions
   a. Small bowel angiomas
   b. Tumors (polyps, carcinoma, lymphoma)
   c. Ulcerating lesions of the small bowel
   d. Meckel's diverticulum
Group 2. Lesions frequently unrecognized on endoscopy
   a. Gastroduodenal and rectal varices
   b. Aortoenteric fistula
   c. Watermelon stomach
   d. Angiomas of the UGI and LGI tract
   e. Submucosal masses
Group 3. Lesions often missed entirely during routine endoscopy
   a. Dieulafoy's lesion
   b. Duodenal polyp, diverticulum, duplication cyst
   c. Hemobilia and hemosuccus pancreaticus
   d. Aortoduodenal fistula
   e. Ampullary ulceration or cancer
   f. Erosions, ulcers, or Mallory-Weiss tears within a hiatal hernia
   g. Cecal lesions such as carcinoma or ulcerated lipoma

synonymous with a small bowel pathologic condition. Radiographic examination with UGI tract series and small bowel follow-through is often insensitive and nonspecific. Angiomas are the most common small bowel source of hemorrhage and are not detectable by UGI tract x-ray examination. Other less common sources of GI tract blood loss in the small bowel include tumors (polyps, carcinoma), jejunal or Meckel's diverticuli, and inflammatory bowel disease (e.g., small bowel Crohn's disease).

Lesions frequently unrecognized on endoscopy (group 2 lesions) include watermelon stomach, submucosal masses,[7] small angiomata, gastric or duodenal varices, and aortoenteric fistulas. Other lesions in this group include bleeding diverticulosis and terminal ileal lesions such as Crohn's disease.

Lesions often missed entirely during routine endoscopy (group 3 lesions) include small angiomata, ulcers, or erosions within a hiatal hernia, right-sided colon cancers, metastatic disease to the bowel, periampullary carcinoma, internal hemorrhoids, Dieulafoy's lesion, aortoenteric fistulas, hemobilia, and hemosuccus pancreaticus.

DIAGNOSTIC EVALUATION

The diagnostic approach to GI tract bleeding of unknown origin depends on the specific clinical situation. For example, one should consider the diagnosis of gastroduodenal varices in a patient with portal hypertension or right-sided colonic angiomas in an elderly patient with valvular heart disease. However, the following general principles apply to all cases of GI tract bleeding of unknown origin:

1. **Perform a careful history and physical examination.** In this age of expensive technology, one cannot overemphasize the importance of a complete history and physical examination. A detailed history provides a plethora of useful information about the location of bleeding (upper versus lower GI tract) and the frequency and degree of bleeding. This information added to physical findings may suggest a specific diagnosis. For example, a history of hematemesis, epigastric pain, and aspirin use raises suspicion of GI tract bleeding caused by peptic ulcer disease or erosions. An elderly patient with chronic renal failure or valvular heart disease who has iron deficiency anemia and hemoccult-positive stool may have GI tract angiomas or an occult malignancy. A patient with a history of severe GI tract hemorrhage any time after an abdominal aneurysm repair may have an aortoenteric fistula. Patients with mucous membrane angiomas on physical examination may have GI tract angiomas as a source of GI tract blood loss. These data will not always lead to a precise diagnosis, but can be useful in planning and guiding further diagnostic studies. Also a history and physical examination are easy and inexpensive.

2. **Obtain and review outside records.** Records include endoscopic photographs, videos and reports, biopsies, barium x-ray examinations, angiograms, and computed tomography (CT) scans. This is useful in several ways:
   a. Avoidance of unnecessary duplicate studies
   b. Recognition of lesions that may have been overlooked on initial examination
   c. Recognition of poor quality studies and repeating exams if indicated
   d. Directing further diagnostic studies if specific examinations have not been performed

3. **Repeat laboratory studies.** Studies include a complete blood and platelet count, coagulation studies including bleeding time, reticulocyte count, serial hemoccult tests, and iron studies (iron, total iron binding capacity, ferritin). The rationale for repeating these studies are:

a. To establish a baseline in the event of ongoing bleeding or rebleeding
b. To assess the chronicity and severity of bleeding, e.g., persistently hemoccult-positive stools with hypochromic, microcytic anemia and low iron studies indicative of chronic GI tract blood loss
c. To assess bone marrow function, i.e., reticulocyte count in response to iron therapy
d. To rule out a platelet dysfunction related to chronic renal failure, aspirin or nonsteroidal antiinflammatory drug (NSAID) use, or a primary platelet disorder
e. To rule out a coagulopathy especially for patients with portal hypertension

4. **Stop aspirin, aspirin-containing medications, NSAID, and anticoagulation therapy.** Aspirin or NSAIDs can cause ulceration and bleeding in all regions of the GI tract and may also inhibit platelet function. Heparin and warfarin should be stopped whenever possible in a patient with GI tract bleeding of unknown origin. The bleeding then may slow down or stop. These medications should be discontinued and the coagulopathy corrected prior to any attempts at endoscopic therapy.
5. **Consider repeating diagnostic studies.** For example, perform repeat endoscopy to exclude lesions that were either not considered or missed during the initial examination. Also consider repeat selective angiography when patients rebleed, if prior studies were incomplete or of poor quality.
6. **Perform additional endoscopic studies.** For example, consider push enteroscopy with a colonoscope or jejunoscope (with or without an overtube) to examine the distal duodenum and proximal jejunum for angiomas. With this technique one can routinely examine about 100 cm distal to the ampulla of Vater. Or consider colonoscopy with retrograde small bowel intubation to rule out Crohn's disease of the terminal ileum.
7. **Exclude small bowel pathologic conditions.** Because the major sources for GI tract bleeding of unknown origin lie within the small bowel, we will extensively discuss the various diagnostic modalities available for examining the small intestine. Additionally, some of these methods have therapeutic potential. See Table 23–2.
8. **During recurrent active bleeding consider repeating selected studies.** Studies include endoscopy such as upper panendoscopy for episodes of hematemesis or melena, and colonoscopy for hematochezia. Other tests to perform in the setting of active bleeding include angiography, or tagged red cell scan.
9. **As a last resort when bleeding persists, consider exploratory laparotomy.** Laparotomy should be combined with intraoperative enteroscopy,[4,18,24] intraoperative scintigraphy, or angiography.[13]

TABLE 23–2. METHODS OF EVALUATING THE SMALL INTESTINE

1. Radiographic and radionuclide studies
   a. UGI tract series with small bowel follow-through
   b. Enteroclysis
   c. Meckel's scan
   d. Scintigraphy
   e. Angiography
2. Enteroscopy
   a. Push enteroscopy with a colonoscope or new small bowel enteroscopes with or without overtubes
   b. Sonde enteroscopy
   c. Ropeway enteroscopy
3. Surgery or combined approaches
   a. Exploratory laparotomy
   b. Intraoperative enteroscopy
   c. Intraoperative scintigraphy
   d. Intraoperative angiography

Small intestinal lesions may be difficult to locate for a number of reasons. Barium examinations do not detect flat mucosal lesions such as angiomas and examination may be difficult because of the long and multiple loops of overlapping bowel. Nuclear medicine scans and angiograms are diagnostic only if there is active bleeding. Before the advent of small bowel enteroscopy, this region of intestine was inaccessible to the endoscopist. Because the small bowel is a free intraperitoneal structure that readily coils and loops, push enteroscopy may be difficult for the endoscopist and uncomfortable for the patient. Bleeding may be slow or intermittent making localization of the bleeding focus all the more difficult. We will briefly review the nonendoscopic methods and then focus on the various endoscopic techniques for examining the small bowel.

RADIOGRAPHIC EXAMINATION OF THE SMALL INTESTINE

Barium Studies

In a recent review of the radiographic evaluation of obscure GI tract bleeding, Rex[25] summarized various barium contrast techniques for evaluating the small bowel. UGI tract series with small bowel follow-through involves drinking barium and examining the small bowel as it moves passively through the small intestine. It is useful for detecting tumors and ulcers in the small bowel. However, this method is not sensitive, missing up to 25% of small bowel tumors eventually diagnosed by enteroclysis. This is due to poor quality x-ray images that are dependent on sufficient luminal distension with contrast to separate intestinal mucosal folds. Factors that can affect distension are the rate at which the patient drinks the contrast, the rate of gastric emptying, and small bowel motility.

Enteroclysis is performed by introducing a tube through the nose or mouth down to the ligament of Treitz and infusing barium under pressure to achieve adequate bowel distension. Glucagon or other drugs may be used to control peristalsis and examine segments of the bowel. Enteroclysis requires more time from the radiologist and more expertise than routine small bowel follow-through. Enteroclysis is superior to the traditional small bowel follow-through for detecting small bowel tumors or ulcers.[32]

It is important to remember that flat mucosal lesions such as angiomas, which account for 80% of cases of obscure GI tract bleeding from the small intestine, cannot be detected by either of these methods. In stable patients without active bleeding, we perform barium studies, preferably enteroclysis, as the initial diagnostic test for evaluating the small bowel. If this examination is nondiagnostic, then we proceed with more invasive studies such as push enteroscopy or angiography.

Angiography

Selective angiography of the celiac and mesenteric arteries is most valuable in the diagnosis and localization of vascular lesions,[13] especially if there are multiple lesions. In a series of 37 patients who underwent preoperative evaluation of obscure GI tract bleeding, emergency angiography was diagnostic in 18 of 20 examinations.[13] Selective embolization with coils or gelfoam can be performed to stop acute bleeding. Limitations include (1) requirement for active bleeding at a rate of at least 1 ml/min and (2) extravasation of contrast into the bowel lumen to make a definitive diagnosis of the lesion responsible for obscure GI tract blood loss.

RADIONUCLIDE EXAMINATION OF THE SMALL INTESTINE

A **Meckel's scan** uses technetium-99m (^{99m}Tc)-pertechnetate to image the diverticulum. This material is concentrated and secreted by gastric mucosa as well as by the ectopic gastric mucosa, which is within a diverticulum in about 80% to 90% of patients with symptomatic Meckel's diverticuli. This scan has a sensitivity of 50% to 75%. Technetium is also picked up by the reticuloendothelial system and excreted by the kidneys; thus, lesions near the spleen, liver, kidneys, and bladder may be missed. The specificity of a Meckel's scan is in the order of 80% to 90%. The specificity may even be higher in the case of a positive scan in a young patient with obscure GI tract bleeding.

Scintigraphy, like a Meckel's scan, also uses ^{99m}Tc-pertechnetate as the imaging radionuclide. This is either conjugated to red blood cells (tagged RBC scan) or to a sulphur colloid. Both scans require active bleeding to detect the responsible lesion, about 0.1 to 0.5 ml/min. The technetium colloid has a shorter half-life than the tagged RBC because it is rapidly cleared by the reticuloendothelial system. This is advantageous for detecting small bleeding sites, and it has a lower false-positive rate than the tagged RBC scan because little technetium is concentrated by the gastric mucosa. But because of the short half-life, bleeding can be detected for only a short period of time after injection.

Conversely, the long half-life of ^{99m}Tc-tagged RBC allows scanning over a 24-hour period for a lesion that may be intermittently bleeding. However, this comes at the expense of a higher background and high false-positive rate. Both the tagged RBC and sulphur colloid scans do not precisely localize the bleeding, especially in the case of rapid bleeding and increased bowel transit times.

Dynamic cine scintigraphic imaging and computer analysis is a promising new method of increasing the sensitivity and specificity for detection of bleeding in the GI tract.[20] This method also appears to be superior to traditional static scintigraphy in localizing the site of bleeding.

ENDOSCOPIC EXAMINATION OF THE SMALL INTESTINE

In a recent review of enteroscopy, Bernstein and Barkin[2] have outlined different diagnostic and therapeutic endoscopic methods available for the small bowel. We will briefly review three of these modalities.

Push Enteroscopy

Push enteroscopy is the procedure of choice for examination of the small bowel. Enteroscopy may be performed using a pediatric colonoscope or a regular adult colonoscope to inspect the small bowel up to a distance of 80 to 100 cm beyond the ligament of Treitz. With this examination, one has the ability to maneuver the endoscope, obtain biopsy specimens, perform polypectomy, and perform hemostasis with coagulation devices. Newer small bowel push enteroscopes have been developed specifically for the small bowel. Enteroscopes are longer (200 to 250 cm) and smaller in diameter (9.8 to 11.3 mm) than colonoscopes and afford a more comfortable and extensive examination to the distal jejunum or proximal ileum. These instruments have similar features as colonoscopes in terms of four-way tip deflection and biopsy channel size (2.8 mm) for therapeutic capabilities. Since these instruments are long and slender, they have a tendency to loop within the stomach, thus hindering passage of the instrument into the small bowel. A long overtube that extends from the mouth through the pylorus may be used to minimize this problem. Additionally, fluoroscopy facilitates intubation of the distal small bowel. It is important to carefully examine the mucosa as the instrument is advanced through the small bowel because scope-induced trauma may mimic angiomata.

Sonde Enteroscopy

An alternative to push enteroscopy is passive, Sonde enteroscopy.[17] This is performed using a long (279 cm) slender (5 mm diameter) small bowel enteroscope (Olympus Corp, Cherry Hill, NJ) that is fitted with an inflatable balloon at the distal tip. The enteroscope is forward viewing with a 90-degree angle of view and two internal channels (one for air insufflation and one for balloon inflation). Its capabilities are limited because it does not have tip deflection controls or suction channels for instruments to perform biopsy, snare, injection, or coagulation procedures.

The instrument is passed transnasally and carried into the duodenum with a colonoscope. The balloon is then inflated, and the colonoscope is removed. The patient is given metoclopramide to promote peristalsis and to facilitate migration of the endoscope through the small bowel. Mucosal inspection is performed during withdrawal of the instrument. In one series, the distal jejunum or beyond was reached in 57 out of 60 patients in an average of 6 hours, with a diagnostic yield for lesions beyond the ligament of Treitz of 33%.[17]

Ropeway Enteroscopy

This method involves the fluoroscopic passage of an enteroscope over a string that was previously passed perorally through the intestines and out the anus by peristalsis. This examination is both time consuming and painful to the patient, and it is not currently in clinical use.[2]

INTRAOPERATIVE ENTEROSCOPY

Despite these extensive investigations, the source of continuing GI tract blood loss may remain elusive. In these instances, intraoperative enteroscopy can be a useful tool for localizing and identifying small bowel pathologic conditions at the time of exploratory laparotomy.[4,18,24] This technique can be performed with a colonoscope or push enteroscope transorally or via a gastrotomy or duodenotomy. The colonoscope is passed beyond the duodenojejunal flexure, and then the small bowel is segmentally telescoped over the endoscope. The mucosa is carefully examined in an antegrade fashion. The endoscopist sequentially insufflates then deflates each segment of small bowel prior to advancement of the endoscope by the surgeon to avoid overdistension of the distal segments.

Although this method is effective for identifying specific mucosal abnormalities in the small intestine (diagnostic yield 70% to 83%), this technique has not been shown to decrease mortality.[4,24] Furthermore, rebleeding rates remain high (45% to 59%) despite surgical resection of the suspected bleeding source. This method is also associated with high morbidity including mucosal tears, perforation, and ischemic bowel.[24] In a series of 12 patients undergoing intraoperative enteroscopy, 10 patients had an identifiable source of bleeding.[4] Three of 10 patients had a discrete vascular lesion; however, seven of 10 patients had only "fresh blood." Operative enteroscopy was associated with a high perioperative mortality (70%) and rebleeding occurred in the three surviving patients. Therefore, intraoperative enteroscopy remains of limited clinical applicability.

GROUP 1: SMALL BOWEL SOURCES

As previously stated, the vast majority of cases of GI tract bleeding of unknown origin are due to small bowel lesions. We will discuss in detail the diagnosis and endoscopic treatment options of small bowel lesions, in particular small bowel angiomas because they are the most frequent diagnosis for obscure GI tract bleeding. Furthermore, angiomas are readily and effectively treatable by push enteroscopy and thermal coagulation.

GI TRACT ANGIOMAS

Angiomas account for 70% to 80% of cases of GI tract bleeding of unknown origin.[15] Other names that have been used synonymously with angioma are vascular ectasia, arteriovenous malformation (AVM), or angiodysplasia. We prefer the term *angioma*. Angiomas may occur as an isolated lesion within the small bowel or in conjunction with upper GI tract and colonic angiomas.[5] They may be associated with valvular heart disease,[9,27] von Willebrand's disease,[36] and with chronic renal failure.[19] They may be congenital, usually referred to as congenital arteriovenous malformations or hemangiomas, or they may be part of the Rendu-Osler-Weber syndrome (hereditary hemorrhagic telangiectasia) or CREST syndrome. However, the vascular abnormalities associated with these distinct clinical syndromes have different natural histories from typical angiomas related to aging and will not be discussed.[5]

Patients usually manifest GI tract blood loss in one of two patterns: (1) intermittent acute bleeding often requiring blood transfusions and (2) self-limited chronic occult bleeding frequently resulting in iron deficiency anemia. Rarely, patients have frank hematemesis if bleeding is from the stomach or duodenum.

Despite various diagnostic tests, angiomas of the small intestine can be very difficult to confirm because of several factors. They may be located in regions difficult to examine by standard endoscopy such as the third or fourth part of the duodenum or past the ligament of Treitz. Their small size (3 to 5 mm) often makes localization difficult. Angiomas are flat mucosal lesions and cannot be seen on barium x-ray examination. Endoscopic trauma (such as suction artifacts) resembles angiomas and therefore angiomas may be mistakenly attributed to scope trauma. The frequent use of meperidine (Demerol) for sedation prior to endoscopy can cause vasoconstriction and blanching of angiomas. Patients are often hypovolemic, thus contributing to poor mucosal blood flow. Angiomas are difficult to isolate in a surgically resected specimen unless methylene blue, fluorescein, or latex injection is performed. Endoscopic biopsy confirmation also has low diagnostic yield (<50%).

The diagnosis of angiomas may be made by endoscopy, angiography, or laparotomy with either open mucosal inspection through a jejunotomy or with intraoperative enteroscopy. The endoscopic appearance of angiomas is a tuft of dilated and engorged submucosal vessels, giving the appearance of a "cherry" red spot. The classic angiographic features of AVMs include (1) an early filling vein, (2) a vascular tuft, and (3) a slowly emptying vein. Care must be taken to exclude a primary carcinoma, which can mimic the appearance of angiomas on angiography. The distinguishing angiographic features of malignancy include a dilated intramural vein and early filling of a draining vein.

Angiomas have been classified by their anatomic location, pathologic appearance, or pattern of disease.[26] In our series of 250 patients with GI tract bleeding from GI tract angiomas, we have categorized patients into three types based on their clinical presentation and endoscopic findings:

Type 1. Isolated angioma with no other synchronous or concomitant lesion
Type 2. Multiple angiomas
Type 3. Incidental angiomas.

Each group has a distinct clinical course and more importantly, different long-term outcome following endoscopic therapy.

For 250 patients with GI tract bleeding from gut angiomata (in the UGI tract, LGI tract, or small bowel) about 10% fall into type 3. They do not have definitive hemostasis with endoscopic therapy. During further follow-up, rebleeding occurs and other (nonangioma) sources of GI tract bleeding are usually identified. For type 1 patients (about 25% of the total), the definitive hemostasis rate with endoscopic treatment is 95%. For type 2 patients, who represent 65% of the total, the definitive hemostasis rate with one or more endoscopic treatments is about 80%. Careful follow-up and reevaluation are required because new angiomata develop in the gut. We therefore consider endoscopic treatment to be palliative.

Potential treatment options for GI tract angiomas include endoscopic thermal coagulation with Gold probe, heater probe, or laser[11,30]; injection therapy; combination estrogen and progesterone therapy[34]; and surgical resection of the involved segment of bowel.[27] Most of the data regarding the treatment of GI tract hemorrhage caused by angiomas are from studies of colonic angiomas. There are no prospective randomized controlled studies comparing different treatments for bleeding small bowel angiomas. Further studies are necessary to assess the relative benefit and safety of these different treatments. We will discuss the endoscopic modalities available to treat GI tract angiomas, and then briefly discuss some of the nonendoscopic options.

Thermal Coagulation

Previous studies of thermal coagulation of colonic angiomas with argon laser, heater probe, and bipolar coagulation have shown a decrease in the rebleeding rate and transfusion requirement after treatment.[9] The goal of thermal coagulation is to achieve superficial mucosal coagulation which ablates the underlying angioma. Following is a summary of important aspects of thermal coagulation with a Gold, BICAP, or heater probe:

1. **Avoid sedation with narcotics,** e.g., meperidine, which may blanch the angioma or make it invisible from shunting of blood away from the mucosa.
2. **Localize the angioma and examine for stigmata of hemorrhage** since this will identify which angioma has bled and therefore preferentially treated.
3. **Decompress the bowel lumen** with suctioning because there is a greater risk of transmural injury with overdistension and thinning of the bowel wall.
4. **Avoid firm tamponade pressure with the probe tip** because this will increase the rate of transmural injury.
5. **Use low-power settings,** especially for right-sided colonic angiomas, because of the high rate of transmural injury, especially with heater probe at high setting.[11,30]
6. **Avoid overtreatment of an angioma;** i.e., stop once mucosal whitening is achieved. Do not attempt to stop oozing at the treatment edges by charring the lesion because this bleeding will stop spontaneously. Overaggressive treatment may increase bleeding and the risk of transmural injury and perforation.
7. **Do not use the Nd:YAG laser for colonic angiomas** because of the high risk of transmural injury and perforation.[5]
8. **Coagulate the bleeding angioma first,** i.e., the angioma with stigmata of hemorrhage. Then coagulate all the remaining angiomas. It is important to first isolate and coagulate the bleeding angioma because treatment of a nonbleeding angioma may precipitate bleeding that will confuse the endoscopist as to which angioma was responsible for the original bleeding. Also, the accumulation of blood will obscure the endoscopic view. In the case of a large angioma, we prefer to use the large bipolar probe (3.2 mm diameter) and begin treatment from the distal aspect of the angioma and work proximally.
9. **We follow up these patients at 3 months** as part of our research protocols. Annually we perform repeat endoscopy and thermal coagulation of any remaining or new angiomas.

In the event of rebleeding, angiomas are retreated with endoscopic thermal coagulation. Surgery is reserved for patients who have failed a second attempt of endoscopic therapy and continue to bleed. For colon angiomas, 18% of our patients were treated with surgery. Characteristics of these patients included multiple angiomas, severe underlying conditions (such as renal failure or valvular heart disease), and difficulty in returning for follow-up colonoscopies.

Table 23–3 lists the settings we recommend for Gold and heater probes for treatment of GI tract angiomas.

Injection Therapy

There are few clinical data of injection therapy for the treatment of bleeding UGI tract angiomas and no data for small bowel angiomas. Given the high rate of transmural injury following sclerosant injection of the canine right colon, this method should be avoided in the small bowel and colon because of the potential risk of perforation or stricture formation.[30]

TABLE 23–3. PROBE AND GENERATOR SETTINGS FOR TREATMENT OF GI TRACT ANGIOMAS

PROBE	GENERATOR TYPE AND SETTING	PULSE DURATION	TOTAL PULSES
Gold or BICAP	ACMI 50W unit at 2–3 setting (or 10–15 W)	1 s pulses	2–3 pulses per site
Heater	Olympus HPU at 10–15 J		2–3 pulses per site

BICAP = bipolar electrocoagulation, HPU = heater probe unit.

Estrogen-Progesterone Combination

Hormonal therapy has theoretic advantages for patients with extensive gut angiomas that would preclude surgical resection or endoscopic coagulation. Various combinations of estrogen and progesterone have been reported to decrease the frequency of recurrent GI tract bleeding and transfusion requirements from bleeding GI tract angiomas.[34] More recently, a large controlled trial of 64 patients with GI tract bleeding from small bowel angiodysplasia showed no significant reduction in transfusion requirement with hormonal therapy as compared with placebo.[16] Because of various side effects (gynecomastia, fluid retention) and contraindications (history of thromboembolic phenomenon, uterine or breast carcinoma), issues of compliance and risks associated with therapy are important factors limiting treatment of gut angiomas with hormonal therapy.

Surgical Resection

Surgical intervention for bleeding GI tract angiomas is not frequently required because the bleeding is usually self-limited and treatable by endoscopic modalities as described. However, surgery may be indicated if (1) bleeding is severe or recurrent requiring multiple blood transfusions, (2) the bleeding angioma is not reachable or not found endoscopically, (3) the patient has an underlying coagulopathy such as von Willebrand's disease, (4) the patient has multiple, recurrent angiomas, e.g., colonic angiomas.

In a study by Richter et al[27] 101 patients with either colonic or ileal angiomas were treated surgically (n=31), endoscopically (n=19) with thermal coagulation, or medically (n=36). They reported that the surgically treated group had less than half the rebleeding rates as compared with either the endoscopically treated patients or the medically treated patients. However, this difference was not statistically significant ($p=0.15$). The drawbacks of this study were that (1) the endoscopically treated patients had a high rate of coagulopathy and thus were at higher risk for rebleeding, (2) the patients were not randomized to different treatment groups, and (3) the small bowel was not evaluated for angiomas, therefore rebleeding may have occurred from untreated angiomas.

SMALL BOWEL TUMORS

Small bowel tumors account for 5% to 7% of cases of GI tract bleeding of unknown origin.[15] They are usually detectable by radiographic examination but can be missed by routine small bowel series or angiography. Enteroclysis is superior to UGI tract series with small bowel follow-through but requires a skilled radiologist.

In a series of 258 patients who underwent small bowel enteroscopy for evaluation of obscure GI tract bleeding, nine malignant (four lymphomas, three adenocarcinomas, one leiomyosarcoma, one carcinoid) and four benign (two lipomas, two leiomyomas) small bowel tumors were located and later surgically resected.[15] Moreover, small bowel tumors were the most common cause of obscure GI tract bleeding in patients younger than 50 years of age when a diagnosis could be made. The authors recommended surgical exploration as the treatment of choice for patients under the age of 50 with obscure GI tract bleeding, since small bowel tumors and Meckel's diverticulum were the most likely diagnoses and these lesions were readily diagnosed and treated at the time of operation. For patients over the age of 50, they recommended small bowel enteroscopy since the majority of bleeding is from small intestinal angiomas.

ULCERATING DISEASES OF THE SMALL INTESTINE

Various entities can result in small bowel ulceration and bleeding (see Table 23–4). The diag-

---

TABLE 23–4. ULCERATING DISEASES OF THE SMALL INTESTINE

1. Acid-induced
    a. Ectopic gastric mucosa
        (Meckel's diverticulum or duplication cyst)
    b. Zollinger-Ellison syndrome
2. Drug-induced
    a. Potassium
    b. Nonsteroidal antiinflammatory drugs
    c. 6-Mercaptopurine
3. Infectious
    a. Tuberculosis
    b. Syphilis
    c. Typhoid
    d. Cytomegalovirus
    e. Histoplasmosis
4. Vasculitis
    a. Polyarteritis nodosa
    b. Dermatomyositis
    c. Radiation enteritis
    d. Henoch-Schönlein purpura
5. Idiopathic
    a. Crohn's disease
    b. Ulcerative jejunitis

nostic workup is similar to that of small bowel angiomas and tumors. Treatment of the underlying disease is indicated, such as discontinuation of medication for drug-induced lesions, antibiotic therapy for infectious causes, or surgical resection for diverticuli or cysts.

GROUP 2: FREQUENTLY UNRECOGNIZED SOURCES OF GI TRACT BLEEDING

Some lesions are often misdiagnosed because they appear benign, i.e., they lack stigmata of hemorrhage (no active bleeding, visible vessel, or adherent clot). Or these lesions may be overlooked because they mimic normal structures, such as gastric varices appearing as normal gastric folds. The clinical features and endoscopic treatment options available for bleeding gastric varices will be discussed because they are relatively common, accounting for up to 20% to 30% of variceal bleeding and can lead to life-threatening hemorrhaging if they are misdiagnosed and improperly treated.

GASTRODUODENAL AND RECTAL VARICES OR ECTOPIC VARICES[14]

Gastric Varices

Gastric varices usually occur in the setting of portal hypertension, with or without esophageal varices. The incidence of gastric varices in patients with esophageal varices ranges from as low as 2% to as high as 100%.[29] However, isolated gastric varices may arise as the result of splenic vein thrombosis or following esophageal variceal obliteration by sclerotherapy. They appear as nodular or serpiginous submucosal masses, may mimic large gastric folds along the greater curvature, and can be seen on UGI tract series. In contrast to gastric folds that flatten with air insufflation during endoscopy, gastric varices do not flatten with gastric distension. They can occur in any part of the stomach, but are usually located below the gastroesophageal junction (junctional varices), in the gastric fundus, or the body of the stomach.

The optimal treatment of bleeding gastric varices remains controversial. Various endoscopic treatments for bleeding gastric varices include injection therapy with different sclerosing agents,[8,29,33] rubber band ligation,[10] and cyanoacrylate injection.[10,23]

Sclerotherapy with various sclerosants has been used successfully for initial hemostasis of bleeding gastric varices. However, this method was reported to have high complication rates of secondary ulceration and late rebleeding caused by ulceration at the injection site.[33] Unlike esophageal varices, which are situated in the superficial submucosa, gastric varices are often more deeply located. Therefore, deeper injections using higher volumes of sclerosant are often needed to arrest bleeding, thus making injections more hazardous. In spite of the possible limitations of sclerotherapy, we prefer this technique for endoscopic control of active variceal bleeding.

Cyanoacrylate, a tissue adhesive, has been used successfully in Europe for initial hemostasis and obliteration of gastric varices.[23] However, this agent has not been assessed in randomized controlled trials. Cyanoacrylate is difficult and expensive to use. Furthermore, it is not currently approved for clinical use in the United States.

Recent reports of rubber band ligation versus injection sclerotherapy for controlling active esophageal variceal bleeding have been promising.[12,31] There were fewer complications in the ligation group and fewer ligation treatments were required to achieve variceal eradication.[12] There are several technical aspects which limit the use of a rubber banding device for bleeding gastric varices as demonstrated in a canine model of bleeding gastric varices[10]:

1. The hood mechanism restricts the endoscopic view, thus making localization of the bleeding site difficult.
2. Blood tends to pool within the hood mechanism blocking the view.
3. Banding is often unsuccessful when performed with the endoscope in the retroflexed position; thus, it may be ineffective for varices located in the gastric cardia or fundus.
4. Bands often fall off with retching and require repeat banding.
5. Large gastric ulcers uniformly develop after banding of gastric varices.

There is a high risk of rebleeding from these secondary gastric ulcers. There are insufficient data on the efficacy, safety, and long-term outcome of this technique for bleeding gastric varices to recommend widespread application outside of a research protocol.

Other, nonendoscopic treatment options exist for bleeding gastric varices. These include balloon tamponade, emergency surgical portosystemic shunting, angiographic embolization, transjugular intrahepatic portosystemic shunt (TIPS),[28] and liver transplantation. These were also initially developed and assessed for esophageal variceal bleeding. The goal of these treatments is to decrease portal hypertension or to embolize the bleeding varix. However, there are no prospective randomized data comparing the effectiveness and safety of these different endoscopic and nonendoscopic hemostasis techniques for controlling gastric variceal bleeding.

Duodenal Varices

Duodenal varices may be mistaken for the normal circular folds (plicae circulares) of the second and third portion of the duodenum. Usually, duodenal varices run linearly across the plicae circulares rather than along the circular folds. Also, duodenal varices are much larger than the normal folds and may actually lead to luminal obstruction. Like gastric varices, duodenal varices do not flatten with air insufflation. Duodenal varices are much rarer than esophageal or gastric varices. Treatments of duodenal varices have been reported only as anecdotal case reports using variceal ligation, portocaval shunting, duodenal resection, and sclerotherapy.[1]

Rectal Varices

Anorectal varices develop as portosystemic collaterals in the setting of portal hypertension.[3] There have been reports of bleeding rectal varices after endoscopic sclerotherapy of esophageal varices. It is important to distinguish varices from internal hemorrhoids. This is usually easy because rectal varices are higher in the rectum and not in the rectal canal like internal hemorrhoids. Bleeding rectal varices do not respond to treatments for bleeding internal hemorrhoid such as injection, infrared cautery, or anorectal surgery.[35] Variceal ligation has been used effectively for treating anorectal varices with minimal morbidity.

WATERMELON STOMACH

Watermelon stomach (or gastric antral vascular ectasia) has a characteristic endoscopic appearance of longitudinal rows of erythematous mucosa radiating from the pylorus into the antrum.[35] These red stripes represent ectatic and sacculated mucosal vessels resembling the stripes on a watermelon, hence its name. Histologic confirmation may be achieved with endoscopic biopsy. These vessels have a propensity to bleed, and the patients most often have iron deficiency anemia. Occasionally, acute or massive UGI tract bleeding is the presentation. Endoscopic treatment consists of thermal coagulation with heater probe or laser therapy, which decreases the transfusion requirement. Antrectomy will prevent recurrent bleeding.

SUBMUCOSAL MASSES

Leiomyomas are the most common GI tract submucosal tumors and the most frequent cause of submucosal tumor bleeding.[7] Bleeding can occur from ulceration of the overlying mucosa. But these ulcers may not always be present or apparent, especially if there is delay between the bleeding episode and the diagnostic evaluation. Surgical resection is the treatment of choice for submucosal leiomyomas that have nonhealing ulcers. Injection therapy with 1:10,000 epinephrine has been used successfully for acute hemostasis of a bleeding gastric leiomyoma. Complete ulcer healing was achieved with high-dose omeprazole.

GROUP 3 LESIONS: LESIONS OFTEN MISSED BY ROUTINE ENDOSCOPY

Group 3 lesions are often overlooked or completely missed during the course of routine endoscopy because of several factors. Some are missed because of the anatomic location, rather than the lesion itself, i.e., where lesions are situated in areas that are difficult and sometimes technically impossible to examine by routine endoscopy. These "blind spots" include the gastroesophageal junction within a hiatal hernia sac, high lesser curvature of cardia, third and fourth part of the duodenum, flexures of the colon, and occasionally cecum and terminal ileum. We will divide these various lesions by their anatomic location. See Table 23–5.

Small bowel lesions have been previously discussed and are not included in this group. Likewise, angiomas were covered extensively and will not be included in this discussion. Suffice it to say, angiomas can occur in all regions of the GI tract, including these "blind spots." The diagnosis and treatment of angiomas in these areas are the same as for small bowel angiomas.

ESOPHAGOGASTRIC LESIONS

Ulcers, Erosions, or Mallory-Weiss Lesions in a Hiatal Hernia

Direct visualization of the gastroesophageal junction within a hiatal hernia can be difficult.

TABLE 23-5. LESIONS OFTEN MISSED BY ROUTINE ENDOSCOPY*

1. Esophagus and stomach
   a. Ulcers, erosions, or Mallory-Weiss lesions in a hiatal hernia
   b. Dieulafoy's lesions
2. Duodenum
   a. Small polyps
   b. Diverticuli
   c. Periampullary carcinoma
   d. Aortoduodenal fistula
   e. Hemobilia
   f. Hemosuccus pancreaticus
3. Colon
   a. Cecal carcinoma
   b. Colonic angiomata in cecum or at flexures
   c. Ulcerated lipoma such as of the ileocecal valve or fold
   d. Internal hemorrhoids
   e. Anorectal varices

*Angiomas are included in all three groups.

In the case of a sliding hiatal hernia, the gastroesophageal junction may be well above the diaphragmatic pinch within the thoracic cavity. Thus, observation must be made from a distance with the endoscope in the retroflexed position. In the setting of self-limited bleeding and absence of stigmata of ulcer hemorrhage (visible vessel, adherent clot), treatment should be conservative with antisecretory agents such as omeprazole or H_2 receptor antagonists to accelerate healing. If active arterial bleeding or stigmata of ulcer hemorrhage are present, endoscopic hemostasis may be achieved with thermal coagulation or injection therapy, similar to peptic ulcer bleeding. An exception to this recommendation is to avoid treatment with thermal coagulation in patients with esophageal varices and portal hypertension, because of the poor efficacy of this technique in these situations.

Dieulafoy's Lesions

Dieulafoy's lesion is an aneurysmal dilation of a submucosal vessel that bleeds intermittently and sometimes massively. It appears endoscopically as a raised nipple or visible vessel without an associated ulcer. This visible vessel is often overlooked if there is no active bleeding from the site. Dieulafoy's lesions are usually located in the upper stomach, primarily along the high lesser curvature and fundus. Acute hemostasis may be achieved with endoscopic thermal coagulation or injection therapy. However, there is significant risk of rebleeding following endoscopic therapy because of the persistence of the underlying artery, which may be large. Thus, surgical wedge resection may be necessary as a definitive treatment. In a recent case report, transendoscopic Doppler ultrasound was used to confirm arterial blood flow in a Dieulafoy's lesion.[6] The Doppler information guided endoscopic injection therapy and confirmed the absence of flow after treatment. The authors suggested this method may be an alternative to surgery.

DUODENAL LESIONS

The restricted endoscope tip deflection within the duodenum limits the field of view. Lesions such as angiomas may be missed if they are located on the distal or back side of a fold or at a sharp bend along the duodenal sweep. Thus, small and nonbleeding duodenal lesions may be easily overlooked unless a side-viewing endoscope (duodenoscope) is used by an experienced endoscopist. Bleeding related to an aortoenteric fistula or from the biliary or pancreatic ducts may not be readily apparent unless there is active bleeding at the time of endoscopy. Aortoenteric fistulas usually arise in the second portion of the duodenum and can be easily missed if specific attempts are not made to rule out this entity. Hemobilia or hemosuccus pancreaticus will not be diagnosed endoscopically unless there is active or recent bleeding at the time of examination.

COLONIC LESIONS

With regard to colonic lesions, the quality of the cleansing preparation prior to colonoscopy can markedly impact on the diagnostic yield of the examination. Thus, small lesions such as angiomas or polyps may be easily overlooked. Intubation of the cecum is not always successful for various reasons such as redundant colon, colonic looping, and intraabdominal adhesions. Attempts to intubate the terminal ileum in a retrograde fashion through the ileocecal valve may not have been performed but need to be considered by the skilled colonoscopist.

Internal hemorrhoids are a common clinical problem affecting 40% to 50% of the adult US population at some point during their lifetime. Bleeding internal hemorrhoids usually are evidenced by acute bleeding manifested by hematochezia. However, the hemorrhoids can bleed chronically resulting in iron deficiency anemia and thus can be a potential source of "obscure" GI tract bleeding. If they are not actively bleeding during anoscopy, internal hemorrhoids are usually a diagnosis of exclusion as the cause of hematochezia especially in elderly patients.

Other lesions such as polyps, carcinoma, colitis, and angiomas must first be excluded with either flexible sigmoidoscopy or colonoscopy.

CONCLUSION

The diagnostic evaluation of GI tract bleeding of unknown origin should be performed in a logical and orderly fashion. One should first exclude the more common causes of GI tract bleeding with routine radiologic and endoscopic tests. If the bleeding focus remains elusive, then more specialized studies to localize obscure or infrequent causes of GI tract bleeding should be used. The diagnostic and therapeutic approach to GI tract bleeding of unknown origin may require the coordinated efforts of the gastroenterologist, radiologist, and surgeon to formulate the optimal evaluation and treatment strategy.

REFERENCES

1. Barbish AW, Ehrinpreis MN. Successful endoscopic injection sclerotherapy of a bleeding duodenal varix. *Am J Gastroenterol.* 1993;88(1):90–92.
2. Bernstein D, Barkin JS. Enteroscopy. *Practical Gastroenterology.* 1993;17:12B–M.
3. Chawla Y, Dilawari JB. Anorectal varices: their frequency in cirrhotic and noncirrhotic portal hypertension. *Gut.* 1991;32:309–311.
4. Desa LA, Ohri SK, Hutton KA, Lee H, Spencer J. Role of intraoperative enteroscopy in obscure gastrointestinal bleeding of small bowel origin. *Br J Surg.* 1991;78(2):192–195.
5. Foutch PG. Angiodysplasia of the gastrointestinal tract. *Am J Gastroenterol.* 1993;88:807–818.
6. Jaspersen D. Dieulafoy's disease controlled by Doppler ultrasound endoscopic treatment. *Gut.* 1993;34:857–858.
7. Jensen DM. Benign and malignant tumors of the stomach. In: Sivak MV, ed. *Gastroenterologic Endoscopy.* Philadelphia, Pa: WB Saunders Co; 1987.
8. Jensen DM, Kovacs T, Machicado GA, CURE hemostasis research group. Sclerotherapy for actively bleeding hiatal hernia or gastric varices. *Gastrointest Endosc.* 1988;34:196–197.
9. Jensen DM, Machicado GA. Bleeding colonic angioma: endoscopic coagulation and follow-up. *Gastroenterology.* 1985;88:A1433.
10. Jutabha R, Jensen DM, Egan J, Hirabayashi K, Machicado GA. Randomized prospective study of cyanoacrylate, sclerotherapy and rubber band ligation for endoscopic hemostasis of bleeding canine gastric varices. *Gastrointest Endosc.* 1995; in press.
11. Jutabha R, Jensen DM, See J, Machicado G, Hirabayashi K. Randomized study of gold and heater probe coagulation in the canine right colon to simulate angioma therapy complications. *Gastrointest Endosc.* 1993;39(2):340(A366). Abstract.
12. Laine L, El-Newihi HM, Migikovsky B, Sloane R, Garcia F. Endoscopic ligation compared with sclerotherapy for the treatment of bleeding esophageal varices. *Ann Intern Med.* 1993;119:1–7.
13. Lau WY, Fan ST, Wong SH, et al. Preoperative and intraoperative localization of gastrointestinal bleeding of obscure origin. *Gut.* 1987;28:869–877.
14. LeBrec D, Benhamou JP. Ectopic varices in portal hypertension. *Clin Gastroenterol.* 1985;14:105–121.
15. Lewis BS, Kornbluth A, Waye JD. Small bowel tumours: yield of enteroscopy. *Gut.* 1991;32(7):763–765.
16. Lewis BS, Salomon P, Rivera-MacMurray S, Kornbluth AA, Wenger J, Waye JD. Does hormonal therapy have any benefit for bleeding angiodysplasia? *J Clin Gastroenterol.* 1992;15(2):99–103.
17. Lewis BS, Waye JD. Chronic gastrointestinal bleeding of obscure origin: role of small bowel enteroscopy. *Gastroenterology.* 1988;94:1117–1120.
18. Lewis BS, Wenger JS, Waye JD. Small bowel enteroscopy and intraoperative enteroscopy for obscure gastrointestinal bleeding. *Am J Gastroenterol.* 1991;86(2):171–174.
19. Marcuard SP, Weinstock JV. Gastrointestinal angiodysplasia in renal failure. *J Clin Gastroenterol.* 1988;10:482–484.
20. Maurer AH, Rodman MS, Vitti RA, Revez G, Krevsky B. Gastrointestinal bleeding: improved localization with cine scintigraphy. *Radiology.* 1992;185:187–192.
21. Moncure AC, Tompkins RG, Athanasoulis CA, Welch CE. Occult gastrointestinal bleeding: newer techniques and diagnosis and therapy. *Adv Surg.* 1989;22:141–177.
22. Peterson WL. Obscure gastrointestinal bleeding. *Med Clin North Am.* 1988;72(5):1169–1176.
23. Ramond MJ, Valla D, Mosnier JF, et al. Successful endoscopic obturation of gastric varices with butyl cyanoacrylate. *Hepatology.* 1989;10:488–493.
24. Ress AM, Benacci JC, Sarr MG. Efficacy of intraoperative enteroscopy in diagnosis and prevention of recurrent, occult gastrointestinal bleeding. *Am J Surg.* 1992;163:94–99.
25. Rex DK. Small intestine radiography in patients with obscure gastrointestinal bleeding. *Practical Gastroenterol.* 1993;17(1):20A–F.
26. Richardson JD. Vascular lesions of the intestines. *Am J Surg.* 1991;161:284–293.
27. Richter JM, Christensen MR, Colditz GA, Nishioka NS. Angiodysplasia: natural history and efficacy of therapeutic interventions. *Dig Dis Sci.* 1989;34(10):1542–1546.
28. Ring EJ, Lake JR, Roberts JP, et al. Using transjugular intrahepatic portosystemic shunts to control variceal bleeding before liver transplantation. *Ann Intern Med.* 1992;116:304–309.
29. Sarin SK, Lahoti D, Saxena SP, Murthy NS, Makwana UK. Prevalence, classification and natural history of gastric varices: a long-term follow-up study in 568 portal hypertension patients. *Hepatology.* 1992;16(6):1343–1349.
30. See JA, Jensen DM, Jutabha R, et al. Complications of endoscopic coagulation for bleeding colonic angiomata: post-coagulation syndrome and delayed bleeding: a 10 year prospective study. *Gastrointest Endosc.* 1993;39(2):304(A227). Abstract.
31. Stiegmann GV, Goff JS, Michaletz-Onody PA, et al. Endoscopic sclerotherapy as compared with endoscopic ligation for bleeding esophageal varices. *N Engl J Med.* 1992;326:1527–1532.
32. Taverne PP, Vander Jagt EJ. Small bowel radiography: a

prospective comparison study of three techniques in 200 patients. *Fortschr Roentgenstr.* 1985;1443:293–297.
33. Trudeau W, Prindiville T. Endoscopic injection sclerosis in bleeding gastric varices. *Gastrointest Endosc.* 1986;32:264–268.
34. Van Cutsem E, Rutgeerts P, Vantrappen G. Treatment of bleeding gastrointestinal vascular malformations with oestrogen-progesterone. *Lancet.* 1990;335:953–955.
35. Viggiano TR, Gostout CJ. Portal hypertensive intestinal vasculopathy: a review of the clinical, endoscopic, and histopathologic features. *Am J Gastroenterol.* 1992;87(8):944–954.
36. Warkentin TE, Moore JC, Morgan DG. Aortic stenosis and bleeding gastrointestinal angiodysplasia: is acquired von Willebrand's disease the link? *Lancet.* 1992;340:35–37.

SECTION II

ESOPHAGUS

24
A Gastroenterologist's View of Chest Pain

MARK H. MELLOW

The use of coronary arteriography has made it clear that there are many patients with chest pain who have normal gross coronary anatomy. Longitudinal follow-up showed that these patients had survival curves nearly identical to age-matched cohorts without chest pain. However, as late as 1980, virtually nothing was known about the cause of chest pain in these patients. In 1980, I reviewed 11 studies from the general medical and cardiologic literature, covering over 1000 patients with chest pain and normal coronary arteries. Only 200 patients had undergone any gastrointestinal (GI) tract evaluation (almost exclusively upper GI tract series and oral cholecystograms). No study mentioned upper endoscopy, acid perfusion testing, or esophageal motility testing. Thanks to the efforts of Castell, Richter, Benjamin, and many others, the ascendency of the esophagus occurred in the early 1980s, reaching its peak when it was felt that 60% to 70% of noncardiac chest pain could be ascribed to esophageal disease, especially esophageal motility disorders. The nutcracker esophagus was the esophageal motility disease of the 1980s. High-amplitude peristaltic contractions were seen with considerably greater frequency in patients with noncardiac chest pain than in controls. It was, indeed, critically important that attention was directed to the esophagus, and away from the heart, in most of these patients. However, Clouse was the first to report, in a small but startling series, that patients with "resting" esophageal motility disorders did *not* have esophageal dysmotility at the time of chest pain when studied with ambulatory motility monitoring.[1] Although further study has shown that chest pain at the time of abnormal distal esophageal motor activity does occur in some patients, they are in a minority, in the range of 20% of patients referred for studies.[2]

Gastroesophageal reflux has emerged as an important factor in the cause of noncardiac chest pain. This should not be surprising, if one considers the near ubiquitous nature of symptomatic gastroesophageal reflux. Castell, in a survey conducted in the mid-1970s, discovered that one in seven Americans had symptomatic reflux several times per week and one in 14 had daily symptoms. Patients ill with other disorders (hospitalized patients on medical service) had an even higher frequency of reflux. Thus, gastroesophageal reflux is commoner than the common cold, and it should be no surprise that it is a cause of noncardiac chest pain and, additionally, that it can be an important factor in patients with chest pain and coexistent coronary disease.

How common is gastroesophageal reflux in noncardiac chest pain? Although numerous studies have addressed the issue of the "true" incidence of symptomatic reflux as a cause of noncardiac chest pain, the numbers vary widely. Ironically, high incidence may reflect a lack of clinical acumen of the referring physician; for example, if a large number of patients with obvious reflux (classic heartburn, sour liquid regurgitation, mild nonprogressive dysphagia) are sent to a GI tract laboratory for 24-hour ambulatory pH monitoring, many patients with noncardiac chest pain will be found to have reflux disease! A more difficult statistic to determine, and really a more important one, is what percentage of patients with *none* of the typical reflux symptoms have gastroesophageal reflux as a cause of their noncardiac chest pain. Another problem is that we have tended to group all noncardiac chest pain patients together, while, in reality, there are several different categories of patients. For example, there are patients who have a single acute chest pain episode that results in their admission to the hospital and cardiac care unit,[3] patients with multiple acute episodes, patients with daily chest pain episodes, and patients with near constant chest pain. It is my feeling that daily constant chest pain is much more likely the result of anxiety or depression and that recurrent acute chest pain requiring emergency room visits is much more likely due to panic attacks than it is to either gastroesophageal reflux or esophageal motility disorders.[4] This is especially true in patients without classic reflux symptoms or dysphagia.

DIAGNOSTIC EVALUATION

I believe that most patients with serious chest pain (per categories above, either single episodes severe enough to require hospitalization or chronic repeated chest pain episodes) deserve cardiac evaluation with the gold standard testing, i.e., coronary arteriography. Although the initial cost of coronary arteriography may be considerably greater than noninvasive testing (thallium scans, treadmill testing etc.), the fact that these tests have significant false-negative rates means that everyone, both the patient and the cardiologist, cannot with certainty exclude important coronary disease as the cause of the patient's symptoms. In my experience, this has led to repeated studies, repeated hospitalizations, and the "hedging" use of coronary vasodilators, which are neither cheap nor totally harmless and can certainly aggravate gastroesophageal reflux symptoms. The risk of coronary arteriography in a patient with normal coronaries is extremely low. Thus, I believe one can make an excellent case for performing the coronary arteriogram early in the patient evaluation. An important secondary issue is whether the presence of coronary disease provides a direct link to the patient's symptoms. In certain patients, this evaluation may call for careful coordination of test results between cardiologist, gastroenterologist, psychologist, etc.

If patients with chest pain and normal coronary macroanatomy do not have gastroesophageal reflux, esophageal motility dysfunction, or gallbladder disease, what do they have? Microvascular angina is a diagnosis that has recently come to the fore. It has been shown that certain patients with chronic chest pain have abnormal myocardial metabolic responses to rapid atrial pacing.[5] Although the link between this metabolic dysfunction and clinical chest pain is far from solid, it is of great interest that many of these patients experience chest pain during routine performance of coronary arteriography itself (an event decidedly rare in patients with macrocoronary disease). Additionally, many of these patients experience chest pain with moderate atrial and right ventricular pacing, also quite uncommon in patients with macrocoronary disease. As a result of these and other observations, Cannon and Benjamin[6] have put forth the notion that many of these patients, and probably many other patients with chest pain and normal coronary macroanatomy, experience chest pain as a consequence of abnormal visceral nociception. This is an extremely important concept. Basically, it means that some people will develop discomfort as a result of a stimulus ordinarily not sufficient to cause discomfort (Benjamin's clever "The Princess and the Pea" example comes to mind). It is my belief that the vast majority of patients initially considered to have "microvascular angina" may actually be experiencing chest pain because of abnormal sensory perception of minor intracardiac events, just as it has been shown that many patients have similar pain sensations from relatively minor intraesophageal events. This has important therapeutic implications, as it takes the emphasis away from drugs such as calcium channel blockers and nitrates and focuses more on drugs that may affect sensory afferents, brainstem signal processing, or efferent responses.

Intraesophageal balloon distension was first described by Kramer in the 1950s. Recently Richter et al have refocused on it as a provocative test in noncardiac chest pain. They reported that many patients with noncardiac chest pain experienced pain at a significantly lower volume of intraesophageal balloon distension than do control subjects, another example of abnormal visceral nociception.[7,8]

ESOPHAGEAL TESTING

To my great chagrin, authors continue to recommend upper GI-tract series in the evaluation of noncardiac chest pain. In my opinion, as routinely done, the upper GI tract series is worthless in the evaluation of noncardiac chest pain. There is nothing noted on routine studies that cannot be equally or better evaluated with upper endoscopy. Clearly, upper endoscopy is a much more sensitive test for esophagitis, it is just as good for the detection of a hiatal hernia, and it is better than an upper GI tract series for evaluation of gastritis. Endoscopy, in fact, can be very helpful in evaluating the gastroesophageal valve competence mechanism as a barrier to reflux. Kozarek and Hill[9] recently presented very convincing data on this issue; easily visualized alterations of the gastroesophageal valve mechanism were closely correlated with findings on the gold standard 24-hour esophageal pH monitoring.

When endoscopy shows no positive findings (e.g., no hiatal hernia, good competent gastroesophageal valve mechanism, and grossly normal esophageal mucosa), it is my belief that the vast majority of these patients do not have symptomatic reflux. However, in a patient with frequent (i.e., more than several times per week) chest pain, a trial of intensive antireflux therapy for approximately 10 to 14 days is not unreasonable. This regimen should include proton pump blockers, avoidance of irritants, refluxogenic foods, etc. If there is not a major decrease in symptoms on this regimen, I believe one can conclude that reflux is not the issue.

ESOPHAGEAL MOTILITY DISORDERS

Standard esophageal motility testing (supine, with timed water swallows) will often reveal an abnormal pattern in patients with noncardiac chest pain. However, the link between this dysmotility and the patient's chest pain is tenuous in most instances. The worse the motility pattern, however (double- and triple-peaked waves, long duration, high-amplitude contractions, frequent nonperistaltic contractions), the more likely they are associated with symptoms. Patients with "severe" resting motility disorders deserve a therapeutic trial of "antimotility" agents (see below). Pharmacologic provocation may occasionally be of value. As pointed out by Janssens and others,[2] however, a positive provocative test (i.e., administration of edrophonium or bethanechol to cause chest pain in the motility laboratory setting) is not necessarily associated with motility-related chest pain experienced in the ambulatory setting. If a patient develops chest pain during provocative testing in conjunction with significant dysmotility, a trial of antimotility agents would be in order. If the patient develops chest pain in the absence of significant dysmotility, a trial of psychoactive medications might be in order (visceral nociceptive disorder).

Pharmacotherapy

At the standard doses, the effect of nearly all available pharmacologic agents on esophageal contractile parameters is modest at best. We found no effect on esophageal contractile parameters in normal patients and in a small group of patients with high-amplitude long-duration esophageal contractions in response to sublingual or longer acting nitroglycerin products. In fact, one patient developed esophageal spasm and chest pain under study, at a time of significant hemodynamic effect of isosorbide.[10] However, nitrates do decrease lower esophageal sphincter pressure. Whether this is a benefit in patients with painful esophageal motility disorders is unclear. Certainly we need to bear in mind that this is an undesired effect in patients with gastroesophageal reflux. Anticholinergics have a moderate effect on esophageal amplitude and duration. A decrease in lower esophageal sphincter pressure has been demonstrated, albeit the decrease is not striking. The calcium channel antagonists thus far evaluated (nifedipine, diltiazem, verapamil) have produced a modest decrease in esophageal contractile amplitude. However, the effect of these agents on chest pain frequency and severity is not striking. The one double-blind long-term study with nifedipine did not reveal an improvement in symptoms, at doses as high as 40 mg three times a day. Richter et al demonstrated a decrease in amplitude and duration of esophageal contractions in patients with nutcracker esophagus who also had decreased symptoms in an open label eight-week treatment program. Cattau demonstrated a decrease in chest pain frequency in a blind crossover study of 14 patients with nutcracker esophagus receiving diltiazem at doses between 60 and 90 mg four times daily. An arterial smooth muscle relaxant, hydralazine (Apresoline) decreased esophageal contractile amplitude and durations in five patients with painful esophageal motility disorders and blunted the "spastic" response to subsequently administered bethanechol.[10] Chest pain symptoms decreased in an open label study. I do not believe that patients with chest pain, esophageal dysmotility, but no dysphagia by history should be classified with similar patients who have concurrent dysphagia. It makes sense to me that food ingestion should be the esophageal "stress test," just as exercise is the stress test in coronary disease. Thus, I think that the case for a painful esophageal motility disorder as a cause of chest pain is much weaker in patients who never experience dysphagia.

There is a need for development of new pharmacologic agents that alter esophageal smooth muscle contractile activity, as well as development of more unique delivery systems (cutaneous administration for prolonged effects; inhalants and sublingual products for more rapid onset of action). We need to study the effect of tranquilizers on esophageal motility parameters and symptoms. In a striking double-blind crossover study, Clouse et al[11] found a decrease in chest pain severity and frequency in patients receiving low-dose trazodone, an antidepressant with no effect on esophageal contraction parameters. Future studies of psychoactive medications on symptoms and their effect on cerebral-evoked potentials to esophageal stimulation are awaited with interest.[12,13]

24-HOUR AMBULATORY ESOPHAGEAL MONITORING

Although most physicians consider 24-hour ambulatory distal esophageal pH and motility monitoring to be the gold standard test, there is considerable debate about how to interpret these studies. Since it has been observed that reflux can occur without symptoms and vice versa, a symptom index has been developed. Although it is clear that the more often symptoms and abnormal esophageal events coincide, the more certain we may be about their relevance, the converse is not necessarily true. There may be situations in which only occasional intraesophageal events are recognized by the brain. Additionally, anxiety and depression may dramatically alter one's perception of pain. A further drawback of 24-hour ambulatory monitoring is that patients often experience very few chest pain episodes during their monitoring.

Before we leave the area of esophageal testing, I feel that we have not totally excluded the possibility that lower esophageal sphincter spasm (as opposed to distal esophageal contractile abnormalities) represents an important cause of noncardiac chest pain. We currently lack the tools to monitor lower esophageal sphincter pressure in the ambulatory outpatient setting. The anatomic distribution of chest pain and its characteristics in many patients (lower chest, pressure squeezinglike) could potentially occur from an increased lower esophageal sphincter pressure (especially in patients with altered nociception). Dramatic changes in lower esophageal sphincter pressure occur frequently in the absence of distal esophageal contractile abnormalities.[14] Also, the decrease in pain frequency observed in some patients when given coronary vasodilators or calcium channel blockers, in the absence of a demonstrable distal esophageal contractile effect, might be because of the drugs' effect on lower esophageal sphincter pressure. We await the development of a comfortable catheter that straddles the lower esophageal sphincter and would, thus, be suitable for 24-hour ambulatory testing.

MANAGEMENT

We must make every effort to diagnose and treat gastroesophageal reflux in patients with noncardiac chest pain, as it is common and usually easily treatable (Fig. 24–1). The first diagnostic test is upper endoscopy, for reasons described above. If there is evidence of gastroesophageal reflux on upper endoscopy (gross esophagitis, incompetent gastroesophageal valve), a therapeutic trial of antireflux therapy is indicated. I currently use omeprazole plus standard antireflux measures. If symptoms are not improved, I then obtain a 24-hour esophageal pH study while the patient receives omeprazole. If acid reflux is demonstrable in that situation and if the patient has persistent troublesome symptoms, I recommend antireflux surgery. I generally employ a short therapeutic trial of omeprazole and antireflux measures even in patients with no obvious endoscopic correlates of reflux, but consider reflux excluded if symptoms persist after a 10- to 14-day therapeutic trial.

I encourage psychologic testing early in the negative workup of patients with noncardiac chest pain. I tell patients that it has been shown, in many patients with noncardiac chest pain, that anxiety or depression is common, that these conditions can greatly increase chest pain frequency and intensity, and that it is helpful to try medications that affect this. I also stress to patients that psychoactive medications do not work immediately. I think this is a better approach than to put patients through an exhaustive workup and then refer them, after a multitude of expensive and often unpleasant tests, to a psychiatrist. The patient then feels that "Doc feels it is all in my head."

Patients who have negative reflux workups, negative response to empiric antireflux therapy, and normal or near-normal psychologic profiles need esophageal motility testing. We presently do standard esophageal motility testing, evaluate for lower esophageal relaxation characteristics, and do motility testing during upright food ingestion. If a significant esophageal motor disorder is discovered, I initiate pharmacotherapy. As mentioned above, there is a transition zone

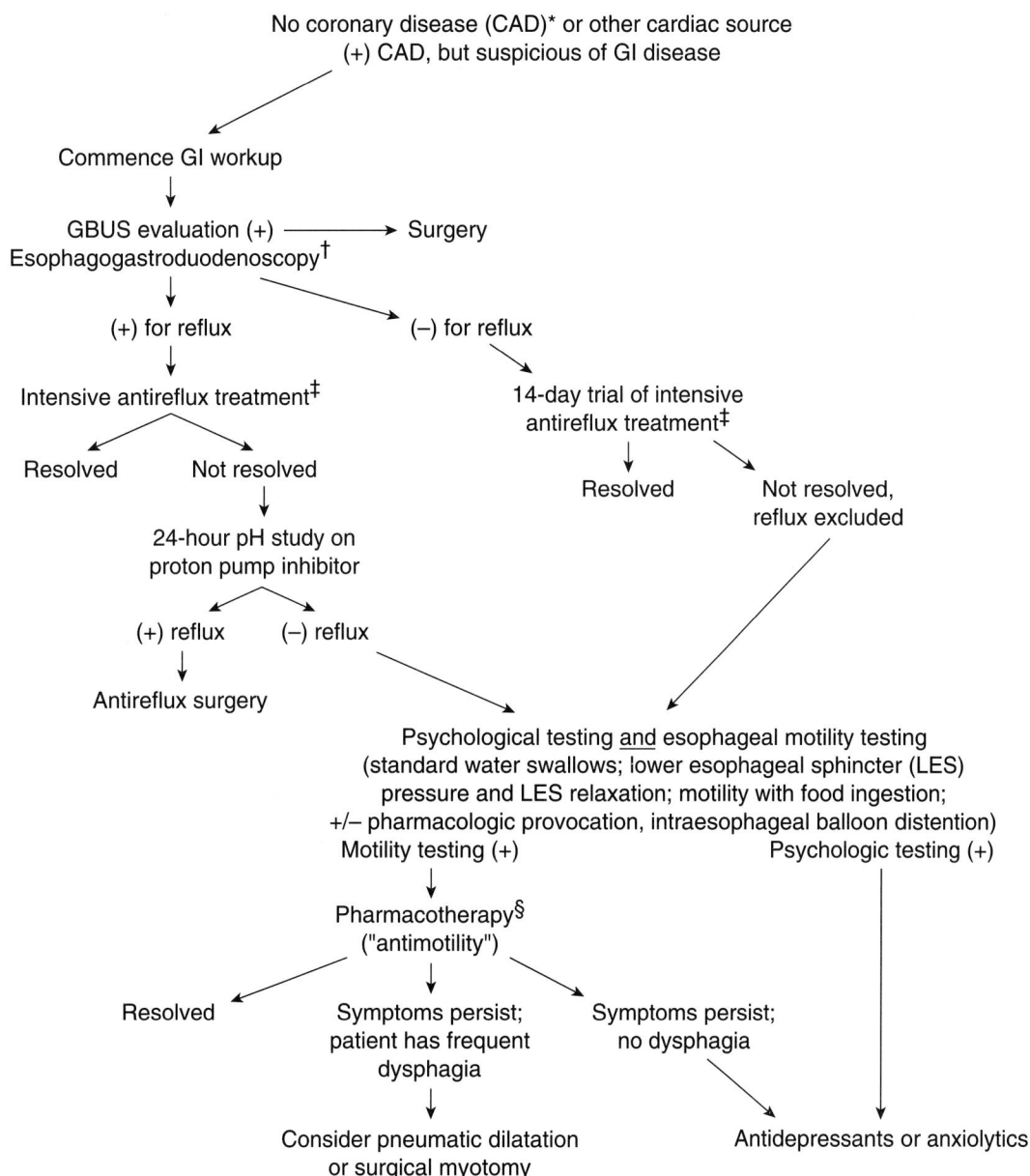

*Preferably coronary arteriogram.
†Dilate with 50 Fr mercury dilator, if dysphagia.
‡To include proton pump inhibitors.
§Calcium channel blockers; nitrates; anticholinergics; apresoline.

FIGURE 24–1. Management of noncardiac chest pain. * = preferably coronary arteriogram; ** = dilate with 50 Fr mercury dilator, if dysphagia; *** = to include proton pump inhibitors; **** = calcium channel blockers; nitrates; anticholinergics, apresoline; LES = lower esophageal sphincter.

between normal motility and markedly abnormal motility. The more abnormal the motor pattern, the more likely I am to pursue pharmacotherapy. I usually try calcium channel blockers first, consider nitrates and anticholinergics, alone or in combination. Apresoline, a smooth muscle relaxant of different type smooth muscle than nitrates, can be a potent antimotility agent, but it is more difficult to use and has more worrisome side-effects. For the relatively uncommon patient with a demonstrably severe esophageal motility disorder and persistent symptoms, pneumatic dilatation, and perhaps even a short or long esophageal myotomy, are options. I will almost always pass a large mercury dilator in patients who describe dysphagia in addition to their chest pain. I am extremely reluctant to consider "drastic" measures such as pneumatic dilatation or surgical myotomy in patients with chest pain who never have dysphagia. However, in the patient with marked esophageal motor dysfunction, significant dysphagia, and a normal or relatively normal psychological profile, who has not responded to pharmacotherapy, pneumatic dilatation or surgical myotomy can be of great benefit.

GASTROESOPHAGEAL REFLUX IN CORONARY ARTERY DISEASE

Since coronary artery disease and gastroesophageal reflux are common conditions, which therefore may coexist, we performed esophageal acid perfusion tests with concurrent blood pressure, heart rate, and 12-lead electrocardiographic monitoring in patients both with and without angiographically documented coronary disease. An index of myocardial workload was calculated. In patients with coronary disease who developed chest pain during esophageal acid perfusion, myocardial workload increased significantly in several patients, and they had concurrent electrocardiographic evidence of myocardial ischemia.[15] Additionally, over half the patients with coronary disease who developed pain during esophageal acid perfusion could not distinguish that pain from their usual angina. Furthermore, a surprising number of patients with coronary disease, whose histories did not suggest gastroesophageal reflux, had chest pain during esophageal acid perfusion in the absence of any indicators of acute myocardial ischemic changes. Therefore, esophageal acid sensitivity could not be accurately predicted by clinical history in patients with coronary disease, and misinterpretation of pain origin occurred frequently in patients with both angina and an acid-sensitive esophagus. This was best illustrated in a patient with coronary disease who underwent esophageal acid perfusion testing both with and without concurrent beta blockade. On both occasions, pain developed soon after onset of acid perfusion. Beta blockade blunted his increase in myocardial workload, and no electrocardiographic evidence of myocardial ischemia was identified. Despite this, he interpreted his pain as angina on both occasions. Because historical evidence of reflux may be lacking in patients with esophageal acid sensitivity and because major therapeutic decisions (e.g., bypass surgery) may be based on an inadequate symptomatic response to antianginal medications, it is important to seek evidence for gastroesophageal reflux disease in such patients, especially if demonstrable cardiac pathologic findings are not in keeping with the severity of the symptoms.

The rapid increase in myocardial workload that occurs in some patients with coronary disease in response to esophageal acid perfusion indicates that reflux is not merely an annoyance in these patients. Pain from an acid-sensitive esophagus may serve as a source of confusion with angina, and even if the pain is clearly recognized as heartburn, esophageal pain may induce myocardial ischemia.

Exercise has been shown to induce reflux, especially high-intensity exercise.[16] Additionally, 24-hour ambulatory esophageal pH monitoring shows reflux occurring in certain patients *only* during exercise (i.e., in patients with overall 24-hour ambulatory esophageal pH profiles within the normal range).[17] Thus, even in patients with coronary disease, "angina" may be a result of exercise-induced gastroesophageal reflux. Therefore, we must always be on guard for coexistent coronary disease and gastroesophageal reflux. Once diagnosed, aggressive antireflux therapy must be initiated.

REFERENCES

1. Clouse RE. Psychiatric disorders in patients with esophageal disease. *Med Clin North Am.* 1991;75:1081–1096.
2. Janssens J, Vantrappen G, Ghilebert G. 24 hour recording of esophageal pressure and pH in patients with noncardiac chest pain. *Gastroenterology.* 1986;90:1978–1984.
3. Lam HGT, Dekker W, Kan G, et al. Acute noncardiac chest pain in a coronary care unit: evaluation by 24 hour pressure and pH recording of the esophagus. *Gastroenterology.* 1992;102:453–460.
4. Beitman BD. Panic disorder in patients with angio-

graphically normal coronary arteries. *Am J Med.* 1992; 92(suppl 5A):33S–30S.
5. Benjamin SB. Microvascular angina and the sensitive heart: historical perspective. *Am J Med.* 1992;92(suppl 5A):53S–55S.
6. Cannon RO, Benjamin SB. Chest pain as a consequence of abnormal visceral nociception. *Dig Dis Sci.* 1993;38: 193–196.
7. Richter JE. Overview of diagnostic testing for chest pain of unknown origin. *Am J Med.* 1992;92(suppl 5A):41S–45S.
8. Deschner WK, Maher KA, Cattau EL, et al. Intraesophageal balloon distention versus drug provocation in the evaluation of noncardiac chest pain. *Am J Gastroenterol.* 1990;85:938–943.
9. Kozarek R, Hill LD. Can endoscope retroflexion at time of EGD define risk of gastroesophageal reflux? *Digestive Disease Week.* 1992;2566. Abstract.
10. Mellow MH. Effect of isosorbide and hydralazine in painful primary esophageal motility disorders. *Gastroenterology.* 1982;83:364–370.
11. Clouse RE, Lustman PJ, Eckert TC, et al. Low dose trazodone for symptomatic patients with esophageal contraction abnormalities. *Gastroenterology.* 1987;92: 1027–1036.
12. DeVault KR, Castell DO. Esophageal balloon distention and cerebral evoked potential recording in the evaluation of unexplained chest pain. *Am J Med.* 1992; 92(suppl 5A):20S–26S.
13. Smout AJPM, DeVore MS, Dalton CD, et al. Cerebral potentials evoked by esophageal distention in patients with noncardiac chest pain. *Gut.* 1992;33:298–302.
14. Freidin N, Traube M, Mittal RK, et al. Hypertensive lower esophageal sphincter: manometric and clinical aspects. *Dig Dis Sci.* 1989;34:1063–1067.
15. Mellow MH, Simpson AG, Watt L, et al. Esophageal acid perfusion in coronary artery disease: induction of myocardial ischemia. *Gastroenterology.* 1983;85:306–312.
16. Soffer EE, Merchant RK, Duethman G, et al. Effect of graded exercise on esophageal motility and gastroesophageal reflux in trained athletes. *Dig Dis Sci.* 1993;38: 220–224.
17. Schofield PM, Bennett DH, Whorwell PJ, et al. Exertional gastroesophageal reflux: a mechanism for symptoms in patients with angina pectoris and normal coronary arteriograms. *Br Med J.* 1987;294:1459–1461.

25
Disorders of the Upper Sphincter and Proximal Esophagus

REZA SHAKER

DISORDERS OF THE UPPER ESOPHAGEAL SPHINCTER

Disorders of the upper esophageal sphincter (UES) may involve its function during swallowing and, less commonly, during belching. These will be presented separately.

COMPONENTS OF UES

Although muscle fibers from the most proximal portion of the esophagus and from inferior pharyngeal constrictors contribute to the sphincter mechanism of pharyngoesophageal junction, the cricopharyngeal (CP) muscle is considered the main component of the UES. The cricopharyngeus, a striated muscle, is attached to the posterior aspect of the cricoid cartilage lamina like a C-clamp. It is innervated by branches of the vagus nerve. In the "awake" state, it maintains an active tone. This tone is augmented by reflexes originating from the lung during inspiration, esophageal body during its segmental distension, pharynx by light touch, pressure, or pharyngeal water injection, as well as from the central nervous system (CNS) during arousal and excitement. CP tone is diminished during sleep and is reduced in the elderly. It is completely abolished during swallowing, belching, vomiting, and generalized distension of the esophagus.

UES During Deglutition

During the pharyngeal phase of swallowing, the UES comprises the outlet to the pharynx, and its normal opening and closure in coordination with pharyngeal peristalsis is essential for a complete transit of the swallowed bolus out of the pharynx and into the esophagus.

For descriptive purposes, swallowing could be divided into four consecutive phases: (1) preparatory, (2) oral, (3) pharyngeal, and (4) esophageal. Dysphagia or difficulty in swallowing may involve one or more of these phases. However, disorders of the UES result in pharyngeal phase dysphagia. From a functional point of view, the pharyngeal phase of swallowing contributes to the following functions: (1) transit of the bolus through the pharynx and into the esophagus and (2) protection of the airway. The transit and protective functions are highly coordinated (Fig. 25–1). A successful pharyngeal phase swallow requires the effective and coordinated participation of the anatomic elements involved in these two functions. Pharyngeal phase dysphagia may develop when the efficacy or coordination of either transport or protective aspect of pharyngeal swallowing is compromised. Disorders of the upper sphincter, in addition to causing abnormal transit, may compromise the safety of the airway if they result in large postdeglutitive residue.

Symptoms of deglutitive UES disorders (Table 25–1) reflect the abnormalities of the two functions mentioned above. These symptoms are highly specific and should not be labeled as functional or psychogenic. Although subtle abnormalities may escape detection, every effort needs to be made to arrive at a diagnosis.

A frequently reported symptom is the sensation of inadequate clearance of the bolus from the pharynx described as "food sticks in the throat." This may be caused by the presence of large residue in the pyriform sinus or it may be a referred sensation from obstruction of the distal esophagus. Strictures of the proximal esophagus may also present themselves with cervical symptoms. For this reason, in patients with complaint of cervical symptoms, evaluation of the esophagus must be part of the dysphagia workup. Because inflammation, abrasion, or tumors of the hypopharyngeal area may produce the same sensation, a careful examination by direct visualization of this area must be included in the workup.

TABLE 25–1. SYMPTOMS OF DEGLUTITIVE UPPER ESOPHAGEAL SPHINCTER DISORDERS

Food sticking in the throat
Nasal regurgitation
Difficulty swallowing solids
Frequent repetitive swallowing
Frequent throat clearing
"Gargley" voice after meal
Hoarse voice
Swallow-related cough
Avoidance of social dining
Weight loss
Recurrent pneumonia

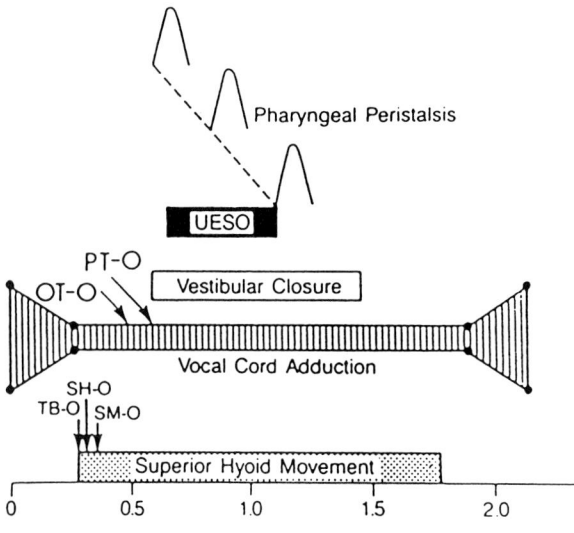

FIGURE 25–1. An example of temporal relationship between various biomechanical events of the oropharyngeal phase of swallowing during 5-ml barium swallows. Bolus transit through the pharynx and across the upper esophageal sphincter (UES) begins and ends while the vocal cords are at maximal adduction. *TB-O* = onset of tongue base movement, *SH-O* = onset of superior hyoid movement, *SM-O* = onset of submental myoelectrical activity, *UESO* = UES opening, *OT-O* = onset of bolus movement from the mouth, *PT-O* = arrival of bolus into pharynx.

Opening Mechanism of the UES During Swallowing

Normal deglutitive UES opening is determined by the following:

1. Transient UES relaxation (i.e., loss of active CP tone)
2. Persistence of minimal passive tension, namely, normal distensibility of the CP muscle
3. Active traction on the UES generated by anterior hyoid and laryngeal movement, which, in turn, is induced by contraction of the suprahyoid muscles (i.e., geniohyoid and mylohyoid)
4. Pulsion forces imparted to the relaxed UES by oncoming pharyngeal bolus

Abnormalities of any of these opening factors causes disordered UES opening, which, in turn, results in a compromised transsphincteric flow that comprises the pathophysiologic basis for the majority of disorders of the UES.

Cricopharyngeal Achalasia

Disordered deglutitive UES opening is a common clinical problem among the elderly and patients with neurologic abnormalities. It may result in incomplete pharyngeal clearance and aspiration. It is commonly referred to as cricopharyngeal (CP) achalasia. The term *cricopharyngeal achalasia* was originally used by radiologists on observation of a prominent pharyngoesophageal segment during swallowing causing inadequate opening of the pharyngoesophageal junction in patients with cervical dysphagia (Fig. 25–2). However, comparing the mechanism of closure and opening of the CP (striated) muscle

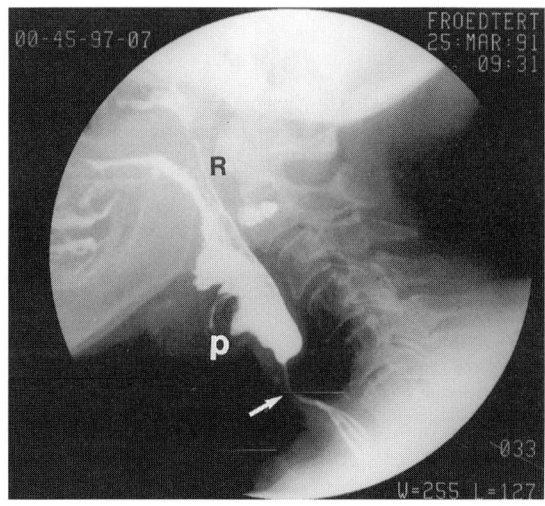
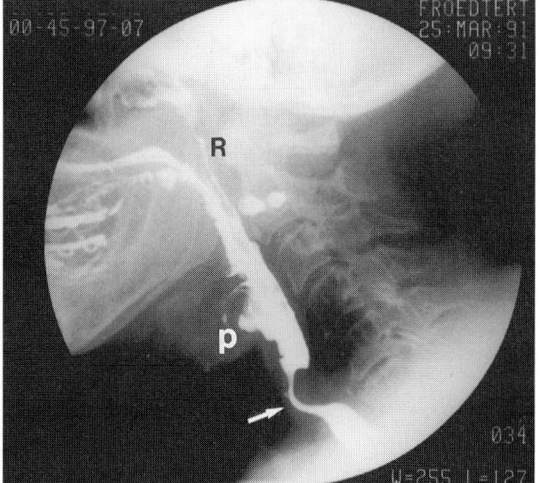
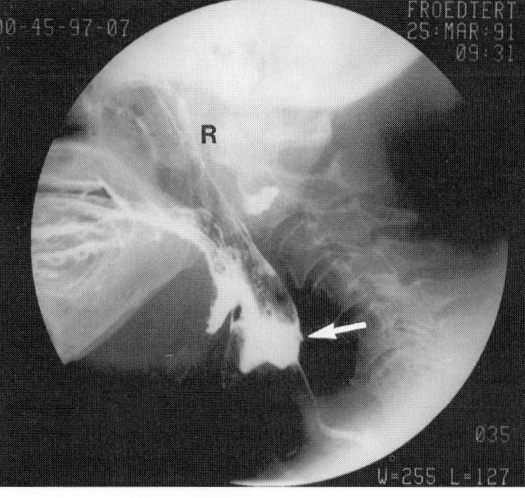

FIGURE 25–2. An example of a modified video barium swallow in a patient with cricopharyngeal (CP) achalasia resulting in a feeling of incomplete swallow, deglutitive cough, and pharyngeal residue. **A,** Barium bolus is seen in the pharynx during the pharyngeal phase of swallowing immediately before the upper esophageal sphincter (UES) opens. A trace of barium from the previous swallow is seen within the UES and proximal esophagus *(arrow)*. Vestibular penetration *(p)* and nasal regurgitation *(R)* are also seen. **B,** Barium bolus is seen traversing the UES. Prominent indentation induced by incomplete opening of the CP muscle is seen *(arrow)*. The result is severe narrowing of the UES lumen. However, barium bolus has filled the proximal esophagus. Also present is nasal regurgitation *(R)* and vestibular penetration *(p)*. **C,** Pharyngeal phase swallowing is now ended. UES has closed; however, a large amount of barium is left behind in the hypopharynx *(arrow)*. R = nasal regurgitation.

with that of the lower esophageal sphincter (smooth) muscle (to which the term *achalasia* was first applied), as well as comparing the innervation and maintenance of basal tone by the two organs, the term *cricopharyngeal achalasia* must be viewed more critically.

As discussed above, normal UES opening basically requires the existence of normal CP relaxation and distensibility, as well as normal contractile force of the suprahyoid muscles. Traditionally, UES resting tone and deglutitive relaxation have been studied by intraluminal manometry. Because of the orad displacement of the UES during swallowing and its to-and-fro movement during breathing, the use of a sleeve sensor has been advocated for this purpose. This 6 cm long sensor, which acts similar to a Starling resistor, provides continuous measurement of the UES pressure and records maximal squeeze pressure regardless of the axial sphincter movement along the length of the device. Shorter pressure sensors, either strain gauges or pneumohydraulic side holes, may remain within the sphincter at rest. However, during swallowing the sensors drop into the cervical esophagus, because of the upward movement of the sphinc-

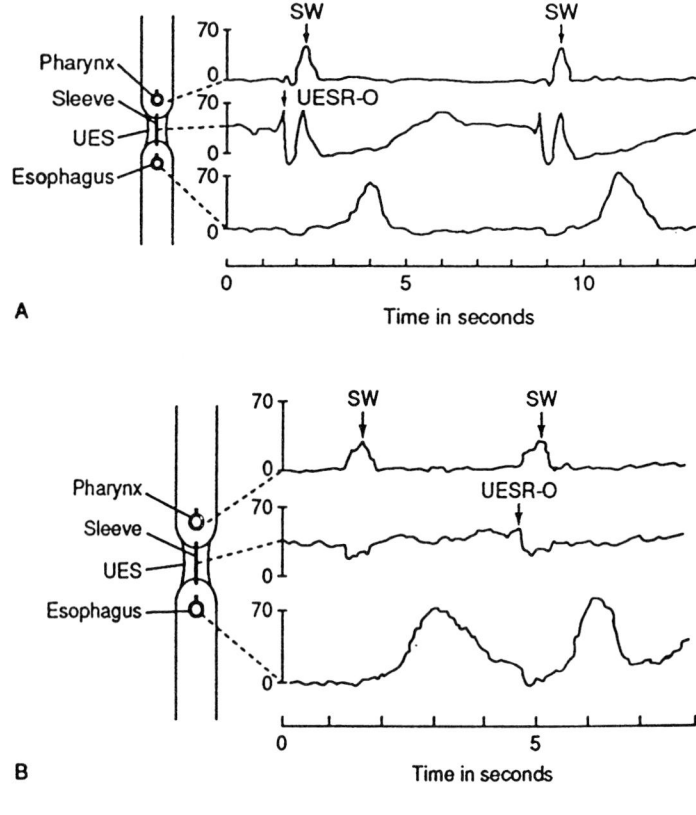

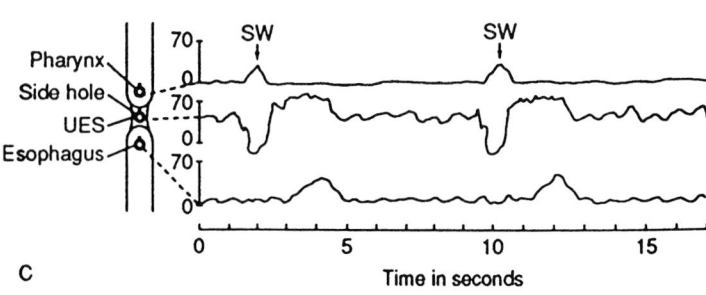

FIGURE 25–3. A, An example of complete manometric deglutitive upper esophageal sphincter (UES) relaxation in an elderly patient during UES manometry using a sleeve device. As seen, after the onset of UES relaxation *(UESR-O)*, the UES pressure sharply declines to slightly below atmospheric pressure, indicating complete UES relaxation. **B,** An example of UES manometry in a cricopharyngeal (CP) achalasia patient using a sleeve device. As seen with each swallow, contrary to the example in Figure A, although the UES pressure reduces, it does not decline to the atmospheric pressure. The reduction in UES pressure during swallowing in this patient is felt to be due to anterocephalad displacement of cricoid cartilage as a result of suprahyoid muscle contraction. **C,** An example of UES manometry using a pneumohydraulic side hole in the patient with CP achalasia. During swallowing, because of orad excursion of the UES, the side hole of the manometric catheter, which was within the UES during resting, was displaced into the proximal esophagus and recorded esophageal pressure, thus yielding a spurious UES relaxation.

ter, and yield intraesophageal pressure, which may be misinterpreted as UES relaxation (Fig. 25–3).

Differentiating between deglutitive relaxation and opening of the CP muscle by intraluminal manometry is impossible. The sudden intraluminal UES pressure decline during swallowing, commonly referred to as *UES relaxation,* reflects the effect of (1) CP relaxation and (2) UES opening of various degrees. Concurrent manometry and fluoroscopy also provide information that is the summation of the two effects of relaxation and opening. For this reason concurrent manometry, electromyography, and videofluoroscopy are essential to differentiate the effects of these phenomena.

CP muscle dysfunction is becoming an increasingly recognized cause of dysphagia. Primary neurogenic CP muscle dysfunction includes cricopharyngeal achalasia (Fig. 25–4), as well as dyscoordination of its relaxation and opening with pharyngeal peristalsis due to a variety of neurogenic causes, such as postcerebrovascular hemorrhage and Parkinson's disease. Primary myogenic CP muscle dysfunction includes loss of elasticity of the muscle and fibrotic changes that prevent its adequate opening during swallowing. A variety of causes, including gastroesophageal reflux and aging, have been suggested to be responsible for these changes. Acute CP obstruction due to dermatomyositis[1] and progressive cervical dysphagia, secondary to

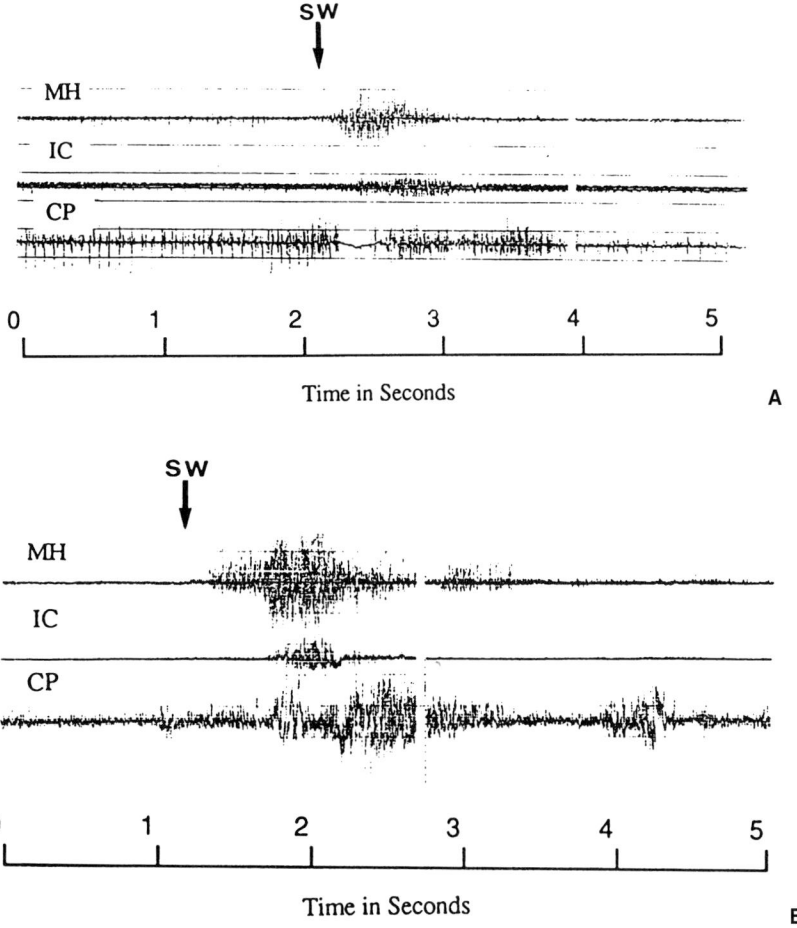

FIGURE 25–4. Examples of electromyographic recordings from the mylohyoid-geniohyoid muscle group (MH), inferior pharyngeal constrictor (IC) and cricopharyngeal (CP) muscle from a normal control **(A)** and a patient with CP achalasia **(B)** during dry swallow. As seen, the MH and IC do not exhibit any tone before swallow, whereas the CP muscle maintains a basal tone during resting. In the normal control subject, swallowing results in transient inhibition of CP tone, myoelectrical activity of the mylohyoid-geniohyoid group and the inferior constrictors. In the patient with CP achalasia, however, swallowing does not result in inhibition of the CP tone.

Crohn's disease[2] involving the CP muscle, have been reported.

In secondary CP muscle dysfunction, the relaxation and distensibility of the CP muscle is within normal limits. Whereas the suprahyoid muscles, as a result of a primary muscle disease or inflammation, are incapable of exerting adequate traction to pull open the UES. These abnormalities include inflammatory changes such as noted in myositis and inclusion body myositis. These patients may also lack normal laryngeal elevation. In this condition, excitatory impulses to the CP muscle are inhibited normally during swallowing and result in manometric relaxation of the UES. However, the UES does not open adequately because of insufficient traction. Depending on the severity of these conditions, patients may present with aspiration pneumonia, swallow-related coughing, choking, repeated swallowing, food sticking in the throat, and weight loss.

Videofluoroscopic recording of a modified barium swallow is the diagnostic modality of choice for patients with this condition. Concurrent electromyographic and manometric studies will help differentiate between neurogenic and myogenic causes of CP achalasia.

Treatment needs to be tailored to address the pathophysiology. Dilation and CP myotomy have been used to alleviate the problem with varying results. However, controlled clinical trials and outcome studies are lacking. In general, myotomy yields good results in CP achalasia due to primary CP muscle involvement. The results are less predictable for primary neurogenic causes if other parts of the swallowing apparatus are also involved (see UES and CNS disorders). The role of myotomy in secondary CP achalasia is controversial since deglutitive relaxation and abolition or resistance to flow is present in this group. Recently, endoscopic transmucosal botulinum toxin injection into the CP muscle has been tried in patients with CP achalasia. However, close proximity of the injection area and the vocal cords raises special concern about possible respiratory complications. On the other hand, because of the temporary effect of the botulinum toxin, this new technique could potentially be used to select patients who will benefit from CP myotomy.

Cricopharyngeal Bar

A relatively common change in UES structure observed during pharyngoesophageal barium studies is a prominent posterior indentation at the level of the UES (CP bar). Although rarely associated with dysphagia, its observation has been reported in 5% of patients older than 40 years who did not have symptoms.[3,4] Despite the common notion of spasm or failed relaxation, the pathogenesis of CP bar is not fully known. A recent study[5] has shown a normal resting pressure, as well as normal deglutitive relaxation, in these individuals. However, the upstream (intrabolus) pressure was found to be higher than that of normal controls. Also found was reduced dimension of the UES during passage of barium, suggestive of reduced compliance of the CP muscle. However, pharyngeal clearance is complete in individuals with CP bar.

TREATMENT. Although patients with CP bar share the feature of prominent CP muscle with patients with CP achalasia, they are generally asymptomatic and do not need intervention.

Zenker's Diverticulum

The pathophysiologic role of disordered UES opening is best defined in the pathogenesis of Zenker's diverticulum. Pharyngoesophageal diverticulum, commonly known as Zenker's diverticulum, was first described by Ludlow in the 18th century. This diverticulum (Fig. 25–5) results from herniation of the pharyngeal mucosa through a weak area of the posterior pharyngeal wall, the Killian's triangle, which is located between the lower border of oblique fibers of the inferior pharyngeal constrictor and the upper border of the transverse fibers of the CP muscle. A wide range of etiologic factors, such as incoordination between pharyngeal contraction and CP relaxation and opening, weakness of the prevertebral facial layer, and premature contraction of the CP muscle, has been proposed. However, it was only recently that concurrent manometric and radiographic studies[6] demonstrated that, in patients with Zenker's diverticulum, there was a significantly high intrabolus pressure in the hypopharynx while the pharyngeal peristaltic pressure was normal. In addition, this abnormally high intrabolus pressure was found to be accompanied by a reduced sagittal and transverse diameter of the sphincter opening. Coordination of the UES and pharynx, as well as deglutitive relaxation of the UES, was found to be normal. Interestingly, in a report of patients with Zenker's diverticulum that underwent CP myotomy, the intrabolus hypopharyngeal pressure and maximal area of deglutitive UES opening returned to normal after surgery.[7]

Patients with symptomatic Zenker's diverticulum may present with cervical dysphagia, aspiration, chronic cough, or halitosis.

TREATMENT. Transcutaneous extramucosal CP myotomy with or without diverticulectomy or diverticulopexy traditionally has been the treatment of choice depending on the size of the diverticulum and yields excellent results in over 90% of cases. However, the endoscopic transmucosal CP myotomy technique, proposed originally by Mosher and popularized by Dahlman and Mattsons, is reported to be relatively safe and yields excellent results.[8]

UES AND CNS DISORDERS

Delayed or failure of CP muscle opening has been reported in 30% to 50% of brainstem lesions,[9–11] central degenerative disorders, posterior cerebellar artery thrombosis, and bulbar paralysis. CP myotomy has been advocated for prevention of aspiration and improvement of bolus transit. The rationale for CP myotomy is to eliminate the resistance of the UES against the flow of the swallowed bolus. Under normal conditions this resistance is eliminated by timely relaxation and opening or closure of the UES. However, in a variety of conditions, because of dyscoordination of the UES and pharynx or because of ineffective pharyngeal function, the UES acts as a relative resistor to the bolus flow. It is in these conditions that CP myotomy may improve bolus transit and reduce aspiration. However, contrary to patients with Zenker's diverticulum and patients with myogenic causes of disordered UES opening such as dermatomyositis and Crohn's disease, in whom the results of myotomy are generally reported to be excellent, in these patients myotomy is reported to induce poor to satisfactory results in the majority of cases. It has been reported that the results of CP myotomy are superior when the pathophysiology is mainly limited to the UES and pharyngeal propulsive forces and patients are able to close their airways voluntarily.[12] Since the major barrier against pharyngeal regurgitation of gastric content, namely the UES, is ablated by myotomy, pulmonary complications of gastroesophageal reflux remain a major concern in patients who undergo CP myotomy.

UES DISORDERS DURING BELCHING

Recent studies have shown that the mechanism of UES opening during belching is similar to that of its opening during swallowing; i.e., initially the active tone of the CP muscle is inhibited, and then it is pulled open. However, con-

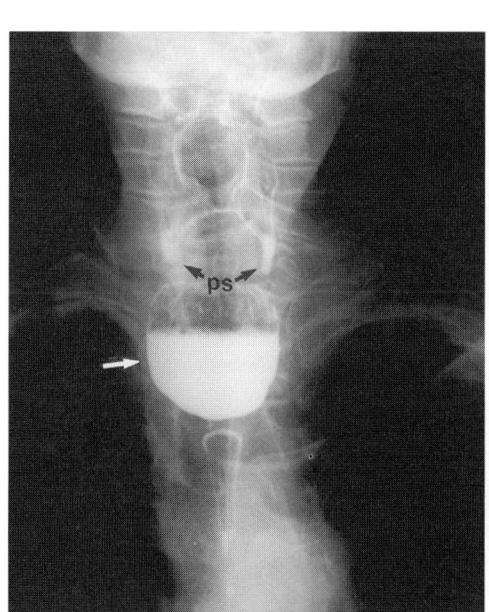
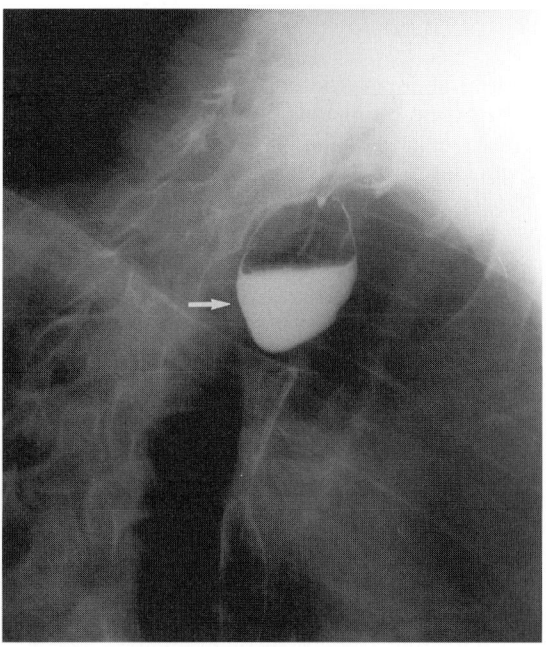

FIGURE 25–5. AP **(A)** and oblique **(B)** views of a Zenker's diverticulum. Barium bolus has been cleared from the pharynx and esophagus following swallowing. Liquid barium remains in the diverticulum *(arrow)*. Minimal residue is present in the pyriform sinuses (ps).

trary to the opening of the UES during swallowing, which involves contraction of the suprahyoid muscles that pull the UES upward and forward, during belching both supra- and infrahyoid muscles contract and pull the UES downward and forward causing it to open. These differences in the direction of traction result in differences in the shape of the UES opening during swallowing and belching (Fig. 25–6, see Color Plate II). Similar to swallowing, during belching the UES physically opens when the hyoid bone approaches the maximal distance on its orbit of movement. Disorders of UES relaxation resulting in a defective belch reflex have been reported by several investigators. These disorders may compromise the outflow of the belched gas through the UES and may result in chest pain due to severe distension of the esophagus.[13] A defective belch reflex in patients with idiopathic achalasia has also been described.[14,15] Upper esophageal sphincter pressure response to abrupt generalized distension of the esophagus is either absent or delayed in many patients with idiopathic achalasia.[16] These abnormalities may explain some of the various upper airway symptoms such as acute obstruction, acute stridor, and tracheal compression reported in achalasia patients.

DISORDERS OF THE PROXIMAL ESOPHAGUS

Structural abnormalities of the most proximal portion of the esophagus may induce obstruction and, because of the proximity to the pharynx, could present with symptoms of cervical dysphagia.

PROXIMAL ESOPHAGEAL RINGS

Proximal esophageal rings are usually reflux induced, but in rare instances they may be congenital. They may be complete or several incomplete rings arranged in a manner that results in luminal compromise (Fig. 25–7). Dysphagia is usually for solid food. Cervical symptoms and choking develop when bolus impaction occurs. Diagnosis is confirmed with an esophagram. Endoscopy and biopsy will determine the possible inflammatory nature of the ring and the status of the proximal esophagus. Reflux symptoms such as heartburn may be absent or minimal. Treatment includes dilation by either wire-guided bougienage or transendoscopic balloon dilation, followed by adequate acid suppressive therapy.

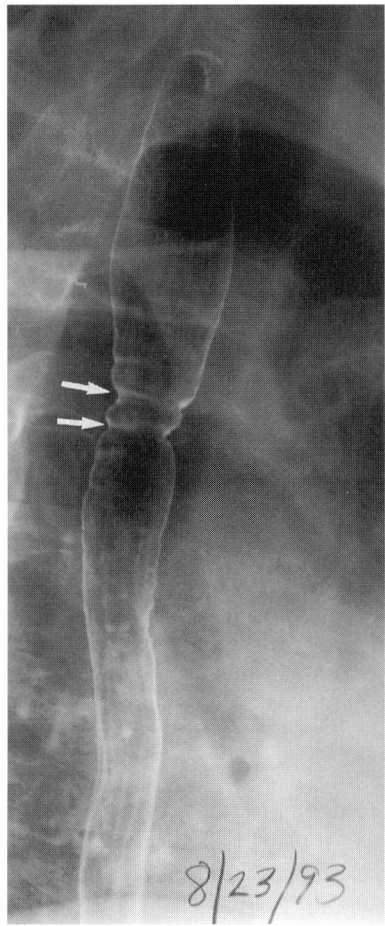

FIGURE 25–7. Proximal esophageal rings *(arrows)* acting as a series of valves causing luminal compromise, located 3 to 4 cm below the upper esophageal sphincter (UES) in a patient presenting with history of two episodes of choking on solid food requiring the Heimlich maneuver. Endoscopy in this patient revealed sequela of gastroesophageal reflux disease in the proximal esophagus. On endoscopy, however, the rings did not show signs of inflammation. Wire-guided bougienage resulted in complete alleviation of symptoms.

PLUMMER-VINSON SYNDROME

Proximal esophageal webs, as seen in Plummer-Vinson or Paterson-Brown-Kelly syndrome, occur in the upper 2 to 4 cm of the esophagus and are associated with iron deficiency anemia. Dysphagia is often associated with aspiration symptoms. There have been reports of an association between these webs and postcricoid carcinoma. Diagnosis is usually made by barium swallow study in lateral projection. Treatment is by dilation, either bougienage or transendoscopic balloon dilation. Iron stores need to be replenished to prevent recurrence. Proximal esophageal webs may be associated with Zenker's diverticulum and graft-versus-host disease following bone marrow transplantation.

PROXIMAL ESOPHAGEAL STRICTURE

These abnormalities may occur as the result of lye ingestion, nasogastric tube placement, and reflux disease. However, isolated involvement of the proximal esophagus is rare. If the proximal end of the stricture is close to the UES, patients may present with symptoms of cervical dysphagia. Reflux-induced esophageal stricture is the most common benign stricture of the esophagus. It occurs in about 10% of patients with severe reflux disease. The incidence of esophageal stricture is increased in patients with Barrett's esophagus and scleroderma esophagus. Peptic strictures commonly involve the distal esophagus and induce esophageal dysphagia. However, they may occur in the proximal esophagus and present with symptoms of cervical dysphagia such as aspiration and choking.

Malignant strictures of the proximal esophagus induced by squamous cell carcinoma or adenocarcinoma in the setting of Barrett's esophagus also present with symptoms of cervical dysphagia and must be included in the differential diagnosis of any esophageal stricture. A barium esophagram will confirm the presence of the stricture. Endoscopy and biopsy are essential to rule out malignancy. Benign strictures usually respond favorably to bougienage. Transendoscopic balloon dilation is especially effective. In case of concurrent reflux disease, adequate acid suppressive therapy usually prevents recurrence. Malignant strictures carry a poor prognosis. Surgical therapy or medical management is dictated by the extent of the tumor invasion.

COLLAGEN VASCULAR DISEASES AND THE ESOPHAGUS

Whereas a variety of collagen vascular diseases, such as progressive systemic sclerosis and mixed connective tissue disease, may involve the distal smooth muscle portion of the esophagus and the lower esophageal sphincter, dermatomyositis or polymyositis may primarily involve the proximal striated muscle portion of the esophagus and the pharynx. They may also involve the suprahyoid muscles and, by impairing their contractile function, reduce the UES opening and further increase the cervical dysphagia. If the presence of collagen vascular disease is suspected, a modified barium swallow study needs to be obtained. This may show pharyngeal or vallecular residue, nasopharyngeal reflux, and tracheal aspiration. Involvement of the swallowing apparatus is part of the general spectrum of the disease. Swallow rehabilitation techniques may be helpful for prevention of aspiration while patients are being treated for their systemic disease.

In summary, swallow-related disorders of the UES and proximal esophagus result in similar symptoms and complications. These symptoms and complications are shared by many other causes of pharyngeal phase dysphagia. For this reason, basic diagnostic studies such as barium swallow studies need to include the proximal esophagus. With the availability of newer diagnostic techniques, disorders of the UES are becoming more defined. This undoubtedly will result in a better understanding of their pathophysiology, which, in turn, will hopefully translate into more effective treatment modalities.

REFERENCES

1. Vencovsky J, Rehák F, Pafko P, et al. Acute cricopharyngeal obstruction in dermatomyositis. *J Rheumatol.* 1988;15:1016–1018.
2. Rowe PH, Taylor PR, Sladen GE, et al. Cricopharyngeal Crohn's disease. *Postgrad Med J.* 1987;63:1101–1102.
3. Seaman WB. Cineroentgenographic observations of the cricopharyngeus. *Am J Roentgenol.* 1966;96:922–931.
4. Ekberg O. Epiglottic dysfunction during deglutition in patients with dysphagia. *Arch Otolaryngol Head Neck Surg.* 1983;109:376–380.
5. Dantas RO, Cook IJ, Dodds WJ, et al. Biomechanics of cricopharyngeal bars. *Gastroenterology.* 1990;99:1269–1274.
6. Cook IJ, Gabb M, Panagopoulos V, et al. Pharyngeal (Zenker's) diverticulum is a disorder of upper esophageal sphincter opening. *Gastroenterology.* 1992;103:1229–1235.
7. Shaw DW, Cook IJ, Simula ME, et al. Restoration of normal upper esophageal sphincter compliance following cricopharyngeal myotomy in patients with Zenker's diverticulum. *Gastroenterology.* 1990;98:A122.
8. Van Overbeek JJM. Meditation on the pathogenesis of hypopharyngeal (Zenker's) diverticulum and a report of endoscopic treatment in 545 patients. *Ann Otol Rhinol Laryngol.* 1994;103(3):178–185.
9. Donner MW, Silbiger ML. Cinefluorographic analysis of pharyngeal swallowing in neuromuscular disorders. *Am J Med Sci.* 1966;251:600–616.
10. Gagic NM. Cricopharyngeal myotomy. *Can J Surg.* 1983;26:47–49.
11. Bonavena L, Khan NA, DeMeester TR. Pharyngoesophageal dysfunctions: the role of cricopharyngeal myotomy. *Arch Surg.* 1985;120:541–549.
12. Logemann JA. *Evaluation and Treatment of Swallowing Disorders.* Boston, Mass: College-Hill Press Inc; 1983.
13. Kahrilas PJ, Dodds WJ, Hogan WJ. Dysfunction of the belch reflex. A cause of incapacitating chest pain. *Gastroenterology.* 1987;92(4):818–822.

14. Holloway RH, Wyman JB, Dent J. Failure of transient lower oesophageal sphincter relaxation in response to gastric distension in patients with achalasia: evidence for neural mediation of transient lower oesophageal sphincter relaxations. *Gut.* 1989;30:762–767.
15. Waterman DC, Castell DO. Chest pain and inability to belch (letter). *Gastroenterology.* 1989;96:274–275.
16. Massey BT, Hogan WJ, Dodds WJ, et al. Alteration of the upper esophageal sphincter belch reflex in patients with achalasia. *Gastroenterology.* 1992;103:1574–1579.

26

Achalasia

HENRY P. PARKMAN and SIDNEY COHEN

Achalasia is perhaps the best understood esophageal motility disorder. Although the actual cause of idiopathic achalasia remains unknown, it is clear that whatever the underlying cause, the disease leads to damage to the innervation of the esophagus and lower esophageal sphincter (LES) producing a functional obstruction at the gastroesophageal junction. Damage to the inhibitory innervation of the LES may be the primary pathophysiologic abnormality. This chronic illness can be treated effectively in 80% to 90% of patients. Proper evaluation is necessary to ensure the diagnosis of idiopathic achalasia and exclude other esophageal motility disorders, an esophageal stricture, or secondary achalasia (a disorder usually caused by malignancy). Complications may occur in achalasia, both from the natural disease process and the treatments used for achalasia. Thus, careful patient monitoring must be performed acutely after dilation treatment for perforation and long term after treatment for gastroesophageal reflux, for the recurrence of dysphagia, or even for malignancy.

CLINICAL PRESENTATION

Achalasia can give rise to the full spectrum of esophageal symptoms: dysphagia, chest pain, regurgitation, odynophagia, and even heartburn. The chief symptom, present in virtually all patients, is dysphagia. Dysphagia for solid food is typically present from the beginning. Initially it may be intermittent but slowly worsens with time to include dysphagia for liquids. The site of obstruction is often correctly recognized by the patient as occurring at the xiphoid area. The course is an indolent one, such that at diagnosis, the symptoms of achalasia have typically been present for 6 years. Patients often develop maneuvers that enable them to finish meals, such as repeated swallowing, eating only small quantities of food, or drinking large volumes of water in an attempt to facilitate emptying of the esophagus. Dysphagia in achalasia is mainly due to a nonrelaxing LES and correlates with residual LES pressure during swallowing. Ineffective bolus transport from esophageal aperistalsis may also be contributory to dysphagia.

Regurgitation, usually of undigested food, is also a common symptom. Nocturnal regurgitation may clinically present as coughing during sleep and foodstuff on the pillow on awakening. Nocturnal regurgitation is particularly worrisome, as this may lead to aspiration pneumonia or chronic interstitial lung disease.

Chest pain is present in up to 50% of patients with achalasia. Achalasia, however, only accounts for <1% of patients presenting with noncardiac chest pain. Chest pain is rarely severe and may develop through several mechanisms. It can manifest as anginalike chest pain resulting from esophageal spasms as seen in vigorous achalasia; a variant condition is typified by high-amplitude, simultaneous, repetitive contractions. A sensation of pressure or fullness may indicate the presence of esophageal dilation from a food-filled esophagus. A burning pain localized to the epigastric area or odynophagia can be secondary to stasis esophagitis, medication-induced inflammation or *Candida* esophagitis. True heartburn related to gastroesophageal reflux is rare in untreated patients but may occur after esophagomyotomy.

Weight loss is seen in the early stages of achalasia. The weight loss is secondary to the inability to empty the esophagus adequately and poor intake from fear of pain or difficulty swallowing. As the esophagus dilates, the hydrostatic pressure of the retained food overcomes the hypertensive LES pressure, facilitating esophageal emptying and often enabling patients to regain weight. Secondary causes of achalasia, such as malignancy, must be considered if the patient's weight loss is severe, progressive, or occurs over a short time.

Secondary achalasia or pseudoachalasia refers to the development of achalasia as a result of an underlying disorder, such as malignancy (see Table 26–1). Although gastric adenocarcinoma and esophageal squamous cell carcinoma are frequently associated with secondary achalasia, malignancies distant to the esophagogastric junction have been reported to cause secondary achalasia, including lung cancer, lymphoma, hepatoma, and prostate carcinoma. Distinguishing malignancy-induced achalasia from primary achalasia on clinical grounds can be difficult.

Three clinical features suggest the possibility of malignancy as a cause of achalasia: (1) short duration of dysphagia (<1 year); (2) significant weight loss (>6.75 kg [15 lb]); and (3) age >55 years. These three clinical criteria are only guidelines, as exceptions to each have been reported.

Secondary achalasia may also develop from nonmalignant causes (see Table 26–1). Although rare in the United States, Chagas' disease should be suspected in patients who traveled or lived in Central or South America. Cases of achalasia have been reported in association with a variety of systemic disorders including amyloidosis and sarcoidosis.

DIAGNOSTIC EVALUATION

In the presence of the classic symptoms of achalasia, such as dysphagia and regurgitation of solid food hours after a meal, the diagnosis of achalasia may be self-evident. More commonly, the course of the disease is indolent and the diagnosis can remain elusive for years. Usually diagnosis of achalasia is not difficult, since nearly all patients present with dysphagia, and algorithms to investigate this symptom include the appropriate diagnostic tests: barium esophagram, upper endoscopy, and esophageal manometry.

BARIUM ESOPHAGRAM

The proper evaluation of dysphagia usually begins with roentgenographic studies: a barium esophagram and upper gastrointestinal tract series. The classic features of achalasia are esophageal dilation that tapers distally to a characteristic narrowing "bird's beak" appearance (see Fig. 26–1*B*). Often there is a midesophageal air-fluid level. These "textbook" features of achalasia on barium esophagram may not be present early in the course of the disease (see Fig. 26–1*A*). The earliest abnormalities seen by fluoroscopy are the breakdown of the normal peristaltic esophageal contractions into simultaneous contractions and a failure of the primary esophageal wave to clear the esophagus of barium. Thus, even early in the disease course, a good fluoroscopic evaluation of esophageal peristalsis by an experienced radiologist may provide the diagnosis. The radiologic evaluation should include appropriate views of the gastric cardia to exclude gastric carcinoma.

TABLE 26–1. DISORDERS ASSOCIATED WITH SECONDARY ACHALASIA (PSEUDOACHALASIA)

Malignancy-associated Causes
Gastric cancer
Esophageal cancer
Lung cancer
Pancreatic cancer
Hepatoma
Prostate cancer
Lymphoma (esophagus, gastric)
Hodgkin's disease
Mesothelioma
Reticulum cell sarcoma

Nonmalignant Causes of Achalasia
Chagas' disease
Chronic intestinal pseudoobstruction
Familial adrenal insufficiency with achalasia and alacrima
Postvagotomy
Amyloidosis
Sarcoidosis
Fabry's disease
Pancreatic pseudocyst
Diffuse esophageal leiomyomatosis
Neurofibromatosis (von Recklinghausen's disease)

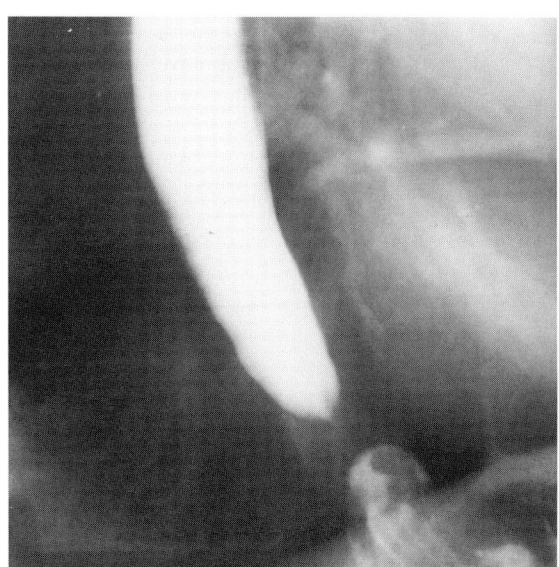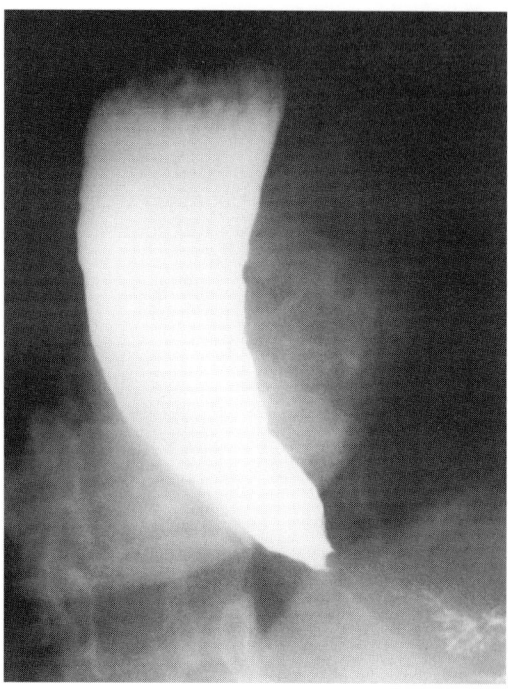

FIGURE 26-1. Radiographic progression of achalasia. Initially, this patient presented with noncardiac chest pain **(A)**. Three years later, when the predominant symptom was dysphagia, the esophagram reveals typical features of achalasia with esophageal dilation and a distal smooth tapering **(B)**.

ESOPHAGEAL MANOMETRY

Esophageal manometry is the gold standard for the diagnosis of achalasia. Usually, though, the test is confirmatory, and the diagnosis is suggested on barium studies. The three classic manometric findings for the diagnosis of achalasia are (1) aperistalsis of the esophageal body, (2) elevated LES pressure, and (3) impaired relaxation of the LES during swallowing. Depending on the duration of the disease, the classic manometric findings of achalasia may not all be present. Normal basal LES pressure is present in 10% to 30% of patients with achalasia. Several patients with radiologic manifestations of achalasia and esophageal aperistalsis have been described as having complete LES relaxation. This is believed to occur in some patients early in the course of achalasia. Subtle abnormalities of the LES may exist in these patients, such as a decreased duration of LES relaxation, making the LES relaxation functionally inadequate. Normal LES relaxation may occur after pneumatic dilation in up to 12% of patients. The presence of aperistalsis in the distal esophagus and a low LES pressure should raise the possibility of other disorders of esophageal peristalsis such as scleroderma and pseudoobstruction. Esophageal manometry does not distinguish idiopathic from malignancy-induced achalasia, as the findings on esophageal manometry are identical.

Occasionally, the manometry catheter may not pass into the stomach, preventing an assessment of the LES pressure and its response to swallowing. This may be due to coiling of the catheter in a large dilated esophagus or by the presence of a hypertensive nonrelaxing LES preventing passage. In these instances, passage of the catheter may be successful under fluoroscopy or using an endoscopically placed guide wire.

Dysphagia may also be a prominent symptom in diffuse esophageal spasm (DES). The mechanism of dysphagia in DES may be similar to achalasia. Approximately 30% of patients with DES have high pressure or impaired relaxation of the LES. Dysphagia in DES may also be due to ineffective peristalsis from the simultaneous contractions. These two syndromes are often considered different spectrums of a similar underlying disorder, since in some patients, DES may progress over time to achalasia. In both DES and achalasia, simultaneous contractions are seen; however, in DES, some normal peristalsis is retained. Absent peristalsis is a requirement for the diagnosis of achalasia, although occasional normal peristalsis may be seen after treatment with pneumatic dilation or Heller's esophagomyotomy in ~20% of patients.

UPPER ENDOSCOPY

The value of endoscopy in patients with achalasia is not to make the diagnosis of achalasia but to exclude other disease entities and to diagnose complications. In idiopathic achalasia, the mucosa is normal, and passage of the endoscope through the gastroesophageal junction is accompanied by only mild-to-moderate resistance. Residual food or fluid within the esophagus should suggest the diagnosis of achalasia even in the absence of LES resistance or dilation of the esophagus. As the disease progresses, luminal dilation and tortuosity make the diagnosis more obvious. Marked resistance or failure to pass the endoscope through the gastroesophageal junction should raise the endoscopist's suspicion of either a stricture or neoplasm as the cause of achalasia. Mass lesions of the distal esophagus and gastric cardia can produce secondary achalasia that mimics idiopathic achalasia radiologically and manometrically. Thus, a careful retroflexed view of the gastric cardia is essential. Brushings for cytologic examination and biopsy specimens for histologic examination are taken from the gastroesophageal junction whenever secondary achalasia is suspected. The concurrent development of a peptic stricture in patients with sclerodermalike smooth muscle disorder may make differentiation of these two disorders particularly difficult.

OTHER TESTS FOR EVALUATION

Depending on the suspicion of secondary achalasia, a chest x-ray examination and computed tomography (CT) of the thorax and abdomen may be appropriate when looking for a primary tumor. The thoracic CT may detect asymmetric esophageal wall thickening or nodularity, extrinsic masses, or lymphadenopathy. Endoscopic ultrasound may also be helpful when looking for submucosal tumor infiltration.

TREATMENT

The treatment of achalasia is directed toward the symptomatic relief of the functional obstruction at the LES. The aims of therapy are to reduce the LES pressure to facilitate esophageal emptying, improve symptoms, and prevent stasis-related complications. Forceful pneumatic dilation and Heller's esophagomyotomy, with the goal of partial destruction of the LES, are the two therapies currently used. Both these treatment options carry a small but appreciable morbidity. As reported recently in several small trials, endoscopic intrasphincteric injection of botulinum toxin, a potent neurotoxin, may achieve the same clinical improvement as dilation or myotomy, at least in the short term. All forms of therapy are palliative and may provide incomplete relief of symptoms and the potential for relapse. The resting LES pressure or esophageal transit after treatment is predictive of the clinical response to treatment; however, in practice, following the symptomatic outcome may be as reliable.

MEDICATION

Both long-acting nitrates (e.g., isosorbide dinitrate) and calcium channel–blocking agents (e.g., nifedipine, diltiazem) can effectively decrease LES pressure and improve symptoms of dysphagia, at least for a short time. Initial failures and further progression of disease will result in more than half failing this form of medical treatment. These agents may be useful to temporize until more permanent treatment is undertaken; they may also be used in elderly patients or patients with multiple medical problems who are at high surgical risk both for elective surgical esophagomyotomy or emergent surgery, if the need should arise, because of perforation during a pneumatic dilation.

BOUGIENAGE

Bougienage causes only passive dilation of the sphincter. This usually results in only temporary relief of dysphagia from achalasia, lasting only several days, though on occasion, it may last several months.

PNEUMATIC DILATION

Pneumatic dilation is a very effective nonsurgical treatment of achalasia. It is performed on symptomatic patients with achalasia. It is contraindicated in patients who have epiphrenic diverticula, a prior history of esophageal perforation, or adjacent aortic aneurysm. Esophagogastroduodenoscopy is performed before each dilation to rule out esophagitis or an occult neoplasm. If esophagitis is present, from *Candida* or other causes, dilation is delayed until successful treatment is accomplished.

Pneumatic dilation, performed as the initial treatment for achalasia, has a successful clinical outcome in 50% to 80% of patients. If no benefit occurs with an initial pneumatic dilation, another dilation may be performed. Although the success rate of each subsequent dilation drops off to less than 50%, the use of repeated dilations can lead to an overall successful treatment rate of 80% to 90%. If there is no response after 2 or 3 pneumatic dilations, then surgical myotomy should be undertaken. Patients with symptoms that require retreatment within several months of the initial dilation have a low likelihood of improving with a subsequent dilation. Patients who respond well to an initial dilation, but in whom symptoms recur much later, often respond in a similar manner to a repeat dilation. Of patients undergoing an initial pneumatic dilation, ~10% to 25% will eventually need esophagomyotomy for persistent or recurrent symptoms.

Pneumatic dilation is associated with a perforation rate of 2% to 8%. Other complications of this procedure include bleeding and aspiration (see Table 26–2). Careful dilation technique is important in preventing esophageal perforation. The importance of ruling out secondary achalasia, such as carcinoma or stricture, by a preceding endoscopy is generally accepted. The presence of a hiatal hernia, epiphrenic diverticulum, or fibrous stricture may increase the risk of perforation during dilation. Patients should be placed on clear liquids for 1 to 2 days and given nothing by mouth past midnight, to help ensure a clean esophagus prior to dilation. If retained food or fluid is present, the esophagus is emptied of residual content by Ewald lavage. In addition to helping with visualization during pneumatic dilation, a clean esophagus helps minimize infectious complications, such as mediastinitis, should perforation occur. The use of fluoroscopic guidance ensures proper balloon placement and helps prevent movement of the dilator during the inflation. Published dilation techniques indicate a tremendous variability in the inflation pressure, duration of inflation, and the number of inflations performed. The Rigiflex achalasia dilator is now used by many centers (see Fig. 26–2). The Rigiflex dilator is placed over a guide wire and is often preferred for patients with a markedly dilated and tortuous esophagus. In addition, the Rigiflex dilator is available with different sizes of balloons (3.0, 3.5, 4.0 cm), which may improve results in patients not responding to an initial dilation.

Following a pneumatic dilation, patients usually undergo an esophagram with water-soluble

TABLE 26–2. COMPLICATIONS OF PNEUMATIC DILATION

Esophageal perforation
Aspiration pneumonia
Gastrointestinal hemorrhage
Esophageal tear
Esophageal hematoma

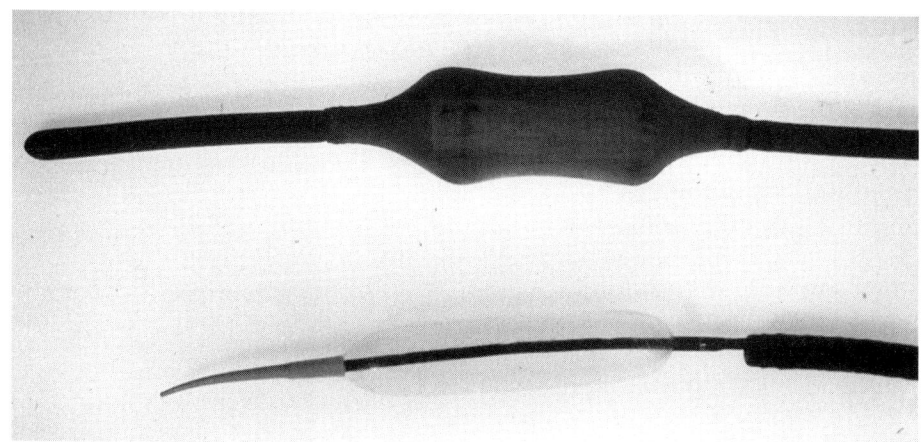

FIGURE 26–2. Pneumatic dilators used to treat achalasia. The top dilator is the old Browne-McHardy dilator, which is no longer commercially available. It consists of a graduated mercury-filled bougie with an inflatable rubber-covered radiopaque cloth bag. The bottom dilator is the newer Rigiflex achalasia dilator which is commonly used today. It consists of a polyethylene balloon and is passed over an endoscopically placed guide wire.

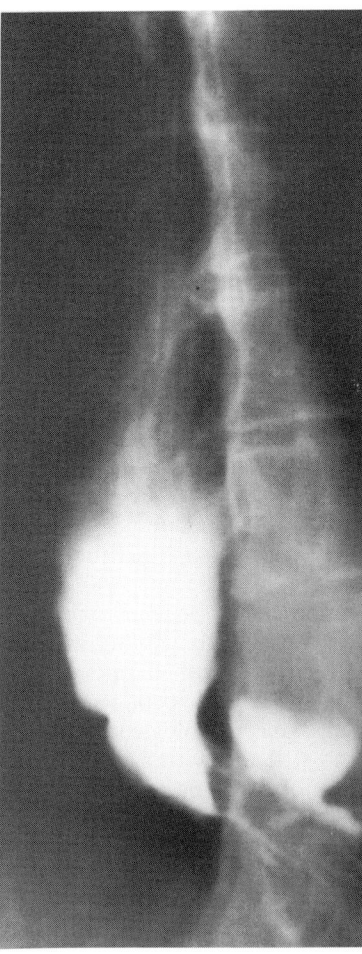

FIGURE 26-3. Perforation after pneumatic dilation. This esophagram performed after pneumatic dilation treatment of a patient with achalasia demonstrates a perforation with extravasation of contrast into the mediastinum.

contrast to detect a perforation (see Fig. 26-3). This water-soluble contrast esophagram following pneumatic dilation may not detect all perforations, so vital signs and patient symptoms are also monitored frequently for at least 6 hours after dilation. Observation of the patient is usually maintained through an overnight hospitalization. In a retrospective analysis of patients with perforation, blood on the dilator, chest pain of greater than 4 hours duration, or tachycardia were present in all patients developing a major complication after pneumatic dilation. In the appropriate setting, if there is absence of blood on the dilator, tachycardia, and prolonged chest pain, and the water-soluble contrast esophagram is normal, many patients can be safely discharged on the day of the procedure. Recently, several studies have suggested that pneumatic dilation may be performed as an outpatient procedure with postprocedure observation for 6 hours with admission reserved for those with perforation or prolonged chest pain.

The key to successful management of esophageal perforation is early recognition and treatment. Perforation is usually detected on the postdilation esophagram (see Fig. 26-3), which at our institution is performed on all patients after pneumatic dilation. Patients with a perforation of the esophagus after dilation should receive prompt surgical evaluation. Thus, pneumatic dilation should only be performed in hospitals where facilities are available for emergent surgery and where surgeons experienced in treating this complication are available. Surgical intervention usually involves a left thoracotomy, establishment of adequate drainage, closure of the laceration, and performance of a Heller's esophagomyotomy on the contralateral side. In those patients who incur a perforation requiring emergent surgical repair with the performance of an esophagomyotomy, the clinical outcome is similar to patients undergoing elective esophagomyotomy. A nonsurgical approach for treatment of perforation may be considered in clinically stable patients with minimal symptoms and signs of infection and a small perforation that is confined within the mediastinum on the initial and repeat water-soluble contrast study. This nonsurgical treatment consists of broad spectrum antibiotics, no oral intake, and parenteral hyperalimentation for 1 to 2 weeks. Occasionally esophageal drainage with a nasoesophageal tube is used.

It should be noted that only one prospective randomized study comparing pneumatic dilation with esophagomyotomy has been performed. This study, performed in Chile, showed a more favorable outcome with surgical esophagomyotomy than with a single dilation with a Mosher dilator. In the United States, pneumatic dilation is usually the initial treatment for achalasia with esophagomyotomy reserved for treatment failures. This practice is based on several points. First, a single initial pneumatic dilation will benefit a majority of patients. Second, the clinical outcome of starting treatment with initial pneumatic dilation has similar clinical benefit as starting with initial esophagomyotomy, when subsequent procedures are performed for patients remaining symptomatic. Studies have suggested that an initial treatment with pneumatic dilation, does not interfere with subsequent esophagomyotomy. Third, there are no useful predictive factors to identify before the initial treatment those patients that will require additional procedures versus those that will not. Finally, the costs to treat initially with pneumatic dilation are substantially less than performing an initial esophagomyotomy. Thus, until patients who require a Heller's esophagomyotomy can be identified at presentation, we suggest that pneumatic dilation should be the initial treatment for achalasia.

Botulinum Toxin Injection

Initial studies have suggested that intrasphincteric injection of botulinum toxin may be useful in the treatment of selected patients with achalasia. During upper endoscopy, botulinum toxin is injected directly into the LES with a sclerotherapy needle. Four injections of 1 ml of a 20 U/ml solution of botulinum toxin are delivered into each of 4 quadrants. Several studies from The Johns Hopkins Hospital have shown that this novel treatment produces clinical improvement in 70% to 80% of patients. In the patients that respond, improvement is seen within several days. This clinical improvement is associated with a decrease in LES pressure and decreased esophageal retention. At the present time, reported side effects have been minor—only a rash in several patients. By 6 months after initial injection, nearly half of the patients have had a relapse and may require repeat treatments. This relapse is similar to that seen with neurologic disorders treated with botulinum toxin. A large clinical safety and efficacy profile on the use of botulinum toxin in idiopathic achalasia will have to be developed in addition to clinical outcome studies directly comparing botulinum toxin injection to pneumatic dilation and myotomy.

Esophagomyotomy

The modified Heller's esophagomyotomy is the most common surgical procedure for achalasia. This procedure involves a single, anterior lateral myotomy. It can be performed through either a thoracic or abdominal approach. The Heller procedure yields excellent or good results in 70% to 90% of patients, with an average of 82%. Esophagomyotomy involves a thoracotomy or laparotomy which has a complication rate of 2% to 6%. Late complications such as gastroesophageal reflux, reflux esophagitis, or peptic stricture formation may occur in 11% of patients. Owing to this high incidence of reflux esophagitis after myotomy, many surgeons also perform an antireflux procedure such as partial or loose fundoplication at the time of the Heller procedure. Newer techniques for esophagomyotomy are being developed using thoracoscopic or laparoscopic esophagomyotomy.

Recurrent dysphagia following surgical treatment for achalasia may be due to several causes and patients require individualized investigation and treatment. The two most common causes of failed surgical treatment are (1) an inadequate myotomy and (2) the development of reflux esophagitis and possible stricture formation. Other reasons include excessively tight Nissen fundoplication, an incorrect preoperative diagnosis, or the subsequent development of cancer. Patients require individualized investigation, which usually includes barium esophagram, esophageal manometry, upper endoscopy, and in some cases, esophageal pH monitoring. If an incomplete myotomy was performed, a pneumatic dilation can be beneficial, in lieu of a second surgical procedure. Reflux esophagitis can often be improved with high-dose H_2 antagonists or omeprazole. A peptic stricture may respond to this pharmacologic treatment and dilation of the stricture with a TTS ("through the scope") dilator. In some patients, reoperation is needed for completion of the myotomy or addition of a fundoplication.

COMPLICATIONS OF ACHALASIA

Patients with achalasia can develop inflammatory changes of the distal esophagus by three mechanisms: infection, stasis, and medication-induced inflammation. Infectious esophagitis most frequently results from *Candida albicans*. Stasis inflammation may result from the irritant nature of foods or from the effect of bacteria that colonize the nutrient-filled esophagus. Medications or alcohol may cause a direct caustic inflammation of the esophagus. The presence of esophagitis may increase the risk of complications of pneumatic dilation, such as bleeding and perforation, and therefore should be corrected before treatment.

An association is suggested to exist between achalasia and the subsequent development of esophageal carcinoma. The average prevalence is roughly 3.5%. The duration of initial onset of symptoms typical of achalasia to the detection of cancer averages 17 to 28 years. Unfortunately, the diagnosis of carcinoma complicating achalasia is often made late, because there are no pathognomonic signs or symptoms to indicate the presence of another cause of dysphagia until the tumor is far advanced. The patients are accustomed to episodes of dysphagia and may not seek advice until the dysphagia becomes severe. Recurrence of old symptoms or the appearance of new difficulties in a patient with long-standing achalasia should suggest the possibility of a malignancy. Weight loss is often out of proportion to the dysphagia. Anemia or hemoccult-positive stool is frequent in the presence of carcinoma and cannot be explained by achalasia alone. Surveillance endoscopy is generally accepted, although when to start and how frequently to perform surveillance endoscopy are not known. Several authors suggest yearly surveillance endoscopies in patients with achalasia to detect this complication at an early treatable stage. Others suggest endoscopy with multiple random biopsies every 3 to 5 years.

REFERENCES

1. Csendes A, Braghetto I, Henriquez A, Cortes C. Late results of a prospective randomized study comparing forceful dilation and oesophagomyotomy in patients with achalasia. *Gut.* 1989;30:299–304.
2. Feldman M. Esophageal achalasia syndromes. *Am J Med Sci.* 1988;295:60–81.
3. Ferguson MK. Achalasia: current evaluation and therapy. *Ann Thorac Surg.* 1991;52:336–342.
4. Kahrilas PJ, Kishk SM, Helm JF, Dodds WJ, Harig JM, Hogan WJ. Comparison of pseudoachalasia and achalasia. *Am J Med.* 1987;82:439–446.
5. Pasricha PJ, Ravich WJ, Hendrix TR, Sostre S, Jones B, Kaloo AN. Treatment of achalasia with intrasphincteric injection of botulinum toxin—A pilot trial. *Ann Intern Med.* 1994;121:590–591.
6. Reynolds JC, Parkman HP. Achalasia. *Gastroenterol Clin North Am.* 1989;18:223–225.
7. Stark GA, Castell DO, Richter JE, Wu WC. Prospective randomized comparison of Brown-McHardy and Microvasive balloon dilators in treatment of achalasia. *Am J Gastroenterol.* 1990;85:1322–1326.
8. Tucker HJ, Snape WJ, Cohen S. Achalasia secondary to carcinoma: manometric and clinical features. *Ann Intern Med.* 1978;89:315–318.
9. Vantrappen G, Hellemans J. Treatment of achalasia and related motor disorders. *Gastroenterology.* 1980;79:144–154.
10. Vantrappen G, Jannssens J, Hellemans J, et al. Achalasia, diffuse esophageal spasm, and related motility disorders. *Gastroenterology.* 1979;76:450–457.
11. Wong RKH, Maydonovitch CL. Achalasia. In: Castell DO, ed. *The Esophagus.* Boston, Mass: Little, Brown & Co; 1992.

27

Motor Disorders of the Esophagus

RAY E. CLOUSE

Esophageal manometry is best suited for study of the distal esophagus, and the major principles of manometric interpretation have changed little over the years. A focus of attention for the past decade has been on defining and studying the seemingly minor or "nonspecific" motor abnormalities that are commonly detected in the clinical motility laboratory. The relationship of these findings to chest pain and other esophageal symptoms remains incompletely understood. The following sections highlight topics of current importance to the gastroenterologist and include discussions that are admittedly slanted toward my biases in several evolving areas.

MINIMAL MEASUREMENTS FOR INTERPRETATION OF MANOMETRIC STUDIES

The techniques employed must be capable of evaluating the esophageal body and lower esophageal sphincter (LES) region. The cervical

---

This paper was presented, in part, at a Meet-the-Professor Luncheon during the annual meeting of the American Gastroenterological Association, San Francisco, May 1992.

esophagus is better studied with videofluoroscopy and other radiologic techniques. Manometric recording methods will not be discussed here, but a high-fidelity system and attention to technical variables are essential. For example, wet swallows that employ a 3- to 5-ml swallowed water bolus produce different results from dry swallows of saliva having variable bolus volume.[1,2] Spacing the swallows by at least 20 seconds will avoid the esophageal refractory period.[3] A variety of other technical standards have been identified.[4] Some variables (such as catheter diameter) are not standardized in clinical practice, and normal values (e.g., for contraction wave parameters) are influenced by these factors.

Four types of measurements in two esophageal regions (the distal esophageal body and LES) generally are sufficient for conventional manometric interpretation today.[4] These required measurements are (1) peristaltic performance, (2) contraction wave parameters, (3) LES basal pressure, and (4) LES relaxation. Normal values have been established for each of these and are outlined below. *Peristaltic performance* refers to the percentage of swallows that are followed by normally propagating (peristaltic) waves. Correct sequencing is determined by comparing the onset of contraction at the esophageal baseline from recording ports that are spaced at approximately 5-cm intervals. For all practical purposes, this determination can be made from waves recorded in the distal 10 cm of the esophagus. Failed motor responses can also be recorded, but this measurement usually is not required for making a conventional manometric diagnosis.

Contraction wave parameters likewise are measured from the distal esophageal body. Three contraction wave parameters are most commonly calculated, reflecting the amplitude, duration, and shape of the waves in an esophageal region.[5] Although the location within the esophagus at which these measurements are taken is variably reported, it generally centers approximately 5 cm above the LES and is almost uniformly within the distal 10-cm segment. Contraction wave measurements are based on 10 or more waves recorded in that region.[4] Shape abnormalities refer to double- or triple-peaked wave forms. The percentage of waves with abnormal shapes should be recorded, although some controversy remains concerning the normal frequency of double-peaked responses.

LES basal pressure is measured using pull-through techniques or a sleeve device. The sleeve device may more accurately reflect resting pressure, but no measurement method is uniformly employed. *Relaxation of the LES* is reported as the postdeglutitive nadir in sphincter pressure over gastric baseline (residual pressure). In our laboratory, we use the lowest value observed within the first 5 seconds following the swallow, but this measurement technique is not standardized.[6] Measurements of residual pressure are more valuable than calculating a percentage of relaxation; the latter is dependent on basal resting pressure, and the range of normal values consequently is broader.

Segmental or localized abnormalities are rarely encountered. A "mapping" technique, wherein swallows are taken as the catheter is incrementally repositioned during the study, is more sensitive to these abnormalities than the stationary technique.[7] In the latter commonly used method, 10 swallows are recorded while the catheter remains in one position to sample the distal esophagus and LES. Nonstandardized, descriptive terminology is used when reporting segmental and other unusual findings.

NORMAL VALUES FOR THE PARAMETERS

Few reports of normal values wherein the studies met the above-mentioned technical standards and employed more than 30 asymptomatic subjects have been published.[2,5,8] Comprehensive sets of parameter values are available from only two of these.[2,5] Large population-based studies are unavailable because of obvious difficulties with recruiting volunteers for esophageal manometric study. Consequently, some variability related to small sample size can be expected in the reported values. Variability also relates to differences in technique and analysis methods. Richter et al[2] reported the largest series in 1987. The investigators stratified data by age group and found some age-related variation. In particular, mean distal wave amplitude of normal subjects aged >40 years was higher than that of the younger cohort. Upward adjustment in normal amplitude values derived from young subjects probably should be used for comparison with the usual population referred for clinical manometry. We have continued to use our own normal values established in 1983,[5] because other technical factors differ between our laboratory and that of Richter and colleagues. It is important for the practitioner either to establish his own normal values or to adhere to a set of values that was attained using very similar techniques as his own. The values from Richter et al[2]

TABLE 27–1. NORMAL VALUES FOR ESOPHAGEAL MANOMETRY

Parameter	Clouse and Staiano (1983)[a,b] N=40 Mean age: 40 y	Richter et al (1987)[c,d] N=95 Mean age: 43 y	Bassotti et al (1988)[c,d] N=34 Mean age: 44 y	Aliperti and Clouse (1991) N=20 Mean age: 27 y
Peristaltic performance (% of swallow)	100%	>95%	–	–
Contraction wave parameters				
Amplitude (mm Hg)	>34, <135[e,f]	<180[g]	<167[g]	–
Duration(s)	<5.6	<5.8	–	–
Double-peaked waves[g,h] (% of swallows)	<10%	<50%[i]	–	–
Triple-peaked waves (% of swallows)	0	0	–	–
LES basal pressure (mm Hg)	10–37 (RPT)	5–53 (RPT)	–	–
LES relaxation (residual pressure) (mm Hg)	–	–	–	Two of the following: 1. Mean for all leads <2.6 2. Mean for one lead <4 3. All observation <8

LES = lower esophageal sphincter, RPT = rapid pull-through technique; SPT = station pull-through technique, end-expiration.
[a]Mapping technique.
[b]Values derived from 95% confidence level.
[c]Stationary technique.
[d]Values derived from mean ± 2 SD.
[e]Contraction wave parameters taken from a zone 2–7 cm above LES.
[f]For 30 observations; normal values varied with number of waves observed.
[g]Average values from two sites, 3 and 8 cm above LES.
[h]Differences may be related to stationary versus mapping techniques.
[i]Cannot be accurately calculated from data reported in the paper.

are best suited for those using the stationary recording technique and a 5-mm diameter catheter, whereas our values[5] may be best used by those employing the "mapping" technique and a smaller catheter.

Data in Table 27–1 reflect normal values from three series; normal values for LES relaxation are also listed.[6] Most are based on 95% confidence levels; 5% of the normal subjects fall beyond the normal range. The more parameters calculated, the more likely that a normal subject will appear "abnormal." This statistical aspect of normal values also must be considered when evaluating a manometric study.

CONVENTIONAL MANOMETRIC DIAGNOSES DERIVED FROM THE MEASUREMENTS

Two disorders deviate extremely from normal and represent motor disorders with defined pathologic bases. The first is achalasia, a neural-based disorder with dyscoordination of peristalsis, unsatisfactory LES relaxation, and eventual motor failure in the esophageal body.[9] The second is the motor disorder that typifies scleroderma. The principal outcome is loss of contraction in the distal esophagus and LES region.[10] Manometric manifestations include decreased wave amplitudes in the distal body with eventual aperistalsis and hypotension of a normally relaxing LES. The manometric features of "scleroderma esophagus" likely have a pathologic basis in most if not all cases, but only 40% of patients with this manometric diagnosis have evidence of underlying connective tissue disease.[10]

A wide variety of other manometric diagnoses can be made when isolated parameter values fall outside the normal range. Only in some cases do these diagnoses represent pathologic abnormalities in the esophagus, and the term *nonspecific motor disorder* has been used as a diagnostic umbrella. I prefer to divide the nonspecific motor disorders into two groups (Table 27–2), those that fall in the direction of exaggerated contraction (group A) versus those that fall in the direction of motor failure (group B). We have shown from statistical analyses of manometric patterns that such grouping has reasonable justification.[11] Nutcracker esophagus is often singled out because of its prevalence, but the abnormality has

TABLE 27–2. NONSPECIFIC MOTILITY ABNORMALITIES

Group A: Exaggerated Contraction	*Group B: Diminished Contraction*

Vigorous contraction wave abnormalities
  Increased amplitude (the nutcracker esophagus)
  Prolonged duration
  Increased frequency of double-peaked waves
  Presence of triple-peaked waves
Hypertensive basal LES pressure
	Decreased contraction wave amplitudes
	
	Hypotensive basal LES pressure

LES = lower esophageal sphincter.

sufficient overlap with others in the group to be considered equally nonspecific.[9]

Diffuse esophageal spasm remains a dilemma in manometric diagnosis as its definition is debated. Some impairment in peristaltic performance is an important criterion to most who write on the subject, but the percentage of simultaneous responses required for diagnosis is arbitrary.[12] Patients who initially meet this criterion may have nonspecific findings (group A) on repeated manometry; the opposite is also true.[13–15] Studies that define the long-term outcome of patients with varying degrees of contraction wave abnormalities or with simultaneous contraction sequences are only beginning to appear. Thus, the set of manometric abnormalities or the severity of abnormality required for diagnosis of diffuse esophageal spasm (DES) remains poorly understood and arbitrary.

Other manometric diagnoses are infrequent compared with those discussed above, but peculiar peristaltic and wave-form abnormalities, alone or in combination, are encountered in clinical practice.[16,17] Focal or segmental abnormalities are occasionally reported and are described without consistent nosologic classification.[5,7,11]

CATEGORICAL CLASSIFICATION SCHEME TO AID WITH MANOMETRY INTERPRETATION

We first proposed the use of a categorical scheme for making manometric diagnoses in 1983.[5] A categorical scheme assumes that at each classification level (e.g., peristaltic performance, contraction wave parameters) the patient's findings can be specifically classified into one of several groupings—"pigeon-holed," if you prefer. For example, basal LES pressure could be categorized as hypotensive, normal, or hypertensive. Separation of the categories depends both on normal values and on disease-related factors. As another example, peristaltic performance is abnormal if decreased to at least 90% according to studies in volunteers; it is further abnormal if no peristaltic sequences are detected (aperistalsis). The proposed classification scheme is in an early stage of development such that most categories are defined by their deviation from normal and not because of disease-related specificity.

The categorical classification scheme modified from our initial work in 1983 is shown in Figure 27–1. Advantages to the approach include (1) its convenient use in clinical practice with improved communication between physicians who interpret tracings, (2) the ease by which it is taught to those learning manometric interpretation, and (3) its potential utility for researchers in studying and categorizing both minor and major manometric abnormalities. A computer with an appropriate algorithm could make suitable manometric diagnoses as long as each of the classification levels is categorically assigned, an additional advantage to this approach. The concept is relatively new and not yet widely accepted, but helps in organizing one's thoughts about manometric diagnosis.

The research utility is exemplified by a recent paper from my group in which manometric findings were evaluated in 1013 patients.[11] We described the prevalence of all patterns found in the subject sample and studied the statistical associations of particular manometric findings. Certain categories were highly associated with other categories. For example, strong predictive associations were found between aperistalsis and low wave amplitudes, aperistalsis and incomplete LES relaxation, low wave amplitudes and hypotensive LES, and hypertensive LES and incomplete LES relaxation. These expected associations confirm the validity of the approach. Aperistalsis and low wave amplitudes are seen both with "scleroderma esophagus" and achalasia; aperistalsis and incomplete LES relaxation

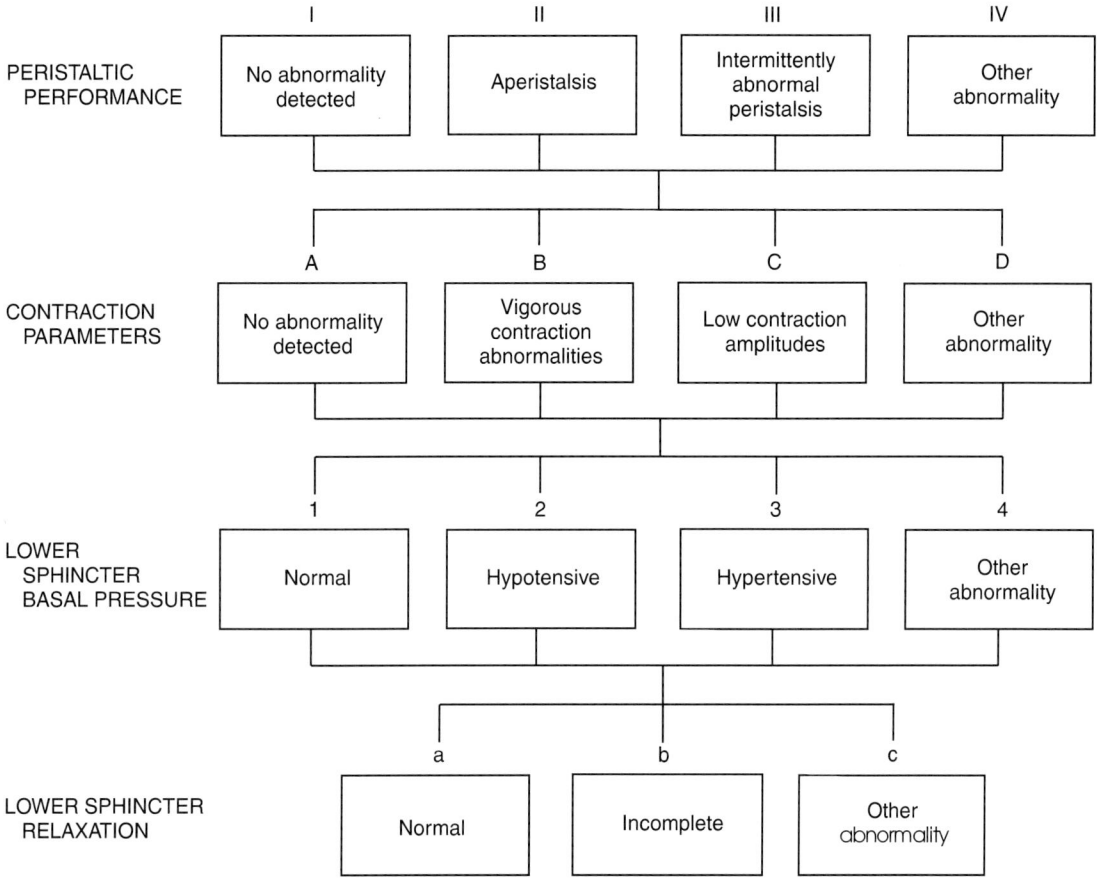

FIGURE 27–1. A recommended classification scheme for esophageal manometry. Tracings are categorized at each of the four levels, and categories within a level are mutually exclusive. Vigorous contraction abnormalities include (alone or in combination) (1) increased wave amplitude, (2) prolonged wave duration, (3) increased frequency of double-peaked waves, and (4) presence of triple-peaked waves. (Reprinted with permission from Clouse RE, Staiano A. Manometric patterns using esophageal body and lower sphincter characteristics: findings in 1013 patients. *Dig Dis Sci.* 1992;37:289–296.)

are the hallmark findings of achalasia. Low wave amplitudes and hypotensive LES are also early findings in "scleroderma esophagus"; whereas hypertensive LES and incomplete LES relaxation are commonly associated in achalasia. Thus, the pattern classification scheme statistically linked together the typical findings in patients with the pathology-based motility disorders.

Weaker associations linked some of the nonspecific motor abnormalities listed in group A in Table 27–2.[11] Features from the group A list never predicted those from the Group B list, and vice versa. Cluster analyses further distinguished these two groups of motor abnormalities.[11] Thus, the nonspecific abnormalities in each list may share common pathogenetic mechanisms, an opinion that has been suggested previously for the features of exaggerated contraction.[5] Patterns typifying DES are also associated with the nonspecific motor disorders in the group A list, but the intermittent simultaneous sequences characteristic of esophageal spasm frequently occur without any contraction wave abnormalities.[18]

INTERPRETATION OF PROVOCATIVE RESULTS IN LIGHT OF MANOMETRIC FINDINGS

Provocative testing for chest pain is often performed at the same time as manometry, but manometric findings are not required for a positive test result if typical chest pain is reproduced. Provocative tests commonly employed today include edrophonium (Tensilon) injection, intraesophageal balloon distension, and hydrochloric acid perfusion.[19,20] Each of these tests has the potential to detect unusual sensitivity of the esophagus to provocative stimulation, as normal subjects rarely develop pain or, in the case of balloon distension, respond at higher distension volumes.[21] In the absence of pathologic abnormality (such as reflux-related mucosal change) or overt motor event, a positive response assumes unusual visceral sensitivity: *sensory dysfunction* of the esophagus.

Sensory dysfunction may represent a component of neuromuscular disease that was poorly appreciated in the past.[22,23] Figure 27–2[24] highlights schematically the potential for both motor and sensory abnormalities in a variety of esophageal "motor" disorders. Provocative tests, especially balloon distension, presumably emphasize sensory over motor dysfunction.

A recent study examined both motor and sensory dysfunction in a group of symptomatic subjects referred for manometric evaluation.[25] The balloon distension test as originally described by Richter et al[21] was employed. Patients with typical esophageal chest pain and other esophageal symptoms responded to the balloon distension test even without evidence of baseline motor abnormality. Nonspecific motor disturbances, like those described in group A of Table 27–2, were common in the entire patient sample but were only partially associated with evidence of sensory dysfunction. More symptoms were reported by patients with both sensory and motor dysfunction than those with either one alone (Fig. 27–3). Thus, both types of dysfunction may contribute in some way to the symptomatic state. Richter's group had previously noted that motor dysfunction (manifested as the nutcracker esophagus) did not dependably predict the presence of sensory dysfunction as determined by balloon distension.[21]

The area needs more exploration. The balloon distension test has not been used widely, because satisfactory balloon catheters have not been marketed commercially. No diagnostic label is uniformly accepted for patients who have provocative test positivity without evidence of motor dysfunction.

CLINICAL IMPLICATIONS OF MANOMETRIC DIAGNOSES

Manometric diagnoses are valuable if they help define disease processes, if they explain symptoms, or, in particular, if they lead to specific therapy. Some diagnoses have all these desirable characteristics, whereas others may have none. No manometric diagnosis is entirely specific for an underlying disease affecting esophageal neuromuscular function. Even in the case of idiopathic achalasia, the most well-defined, pathology-based disorder, more than one process will produce the identical manometric pattern. Consequently, when the classic manomet-

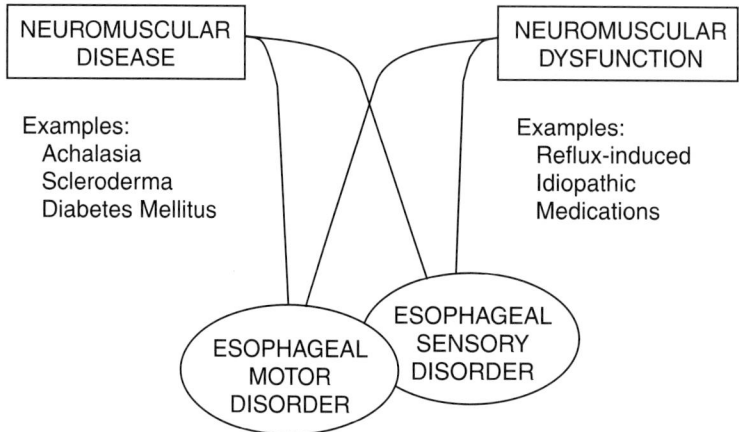

FIGURE 27–2. Esophageal motor disorders result from diseases that involve the esophageal neuromuscular apparatus or from neuromuscular dysfunction without recognized esophageal pathologic findings. In some situations, the motor disorder may be accompanied by esophageal sensory (visceral afferent) abnormalities as well. (Reprinted with permission from Clouse RE. Motor disorders of the esophagus. In: Sleisenger MH, Fordtran JS, eds. *Gastrointestinal Disease: Pathophysiology, Diagnosis, Management.* 5th ed. Philadelphia, Pa: WB Saunders Co; 1993.)

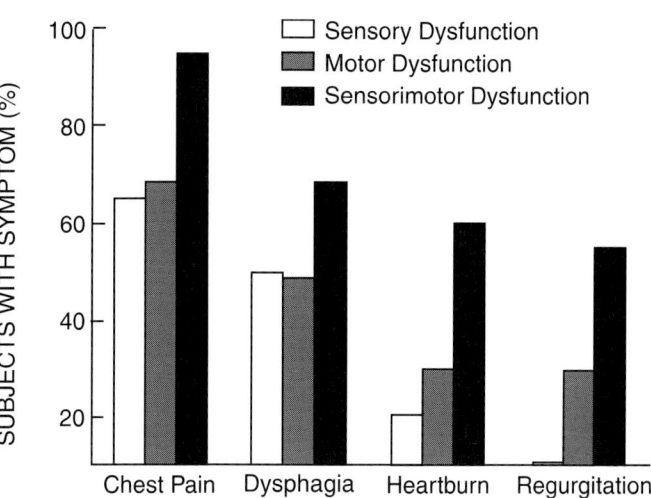

FIGURE 27-3. Prevalence of presenting symptoms in relation to findings on manometry and on the balloon distension test. Subjects with sensorimotor dysfunction (manometric abnormality and positive balloon distension test) appeared more symptomatic than the other two groups. The differences between subject groups for heartburn and regurgitation reached statistical significance ($p<0.05$ for each). (Reprinted with permission from Clouse RE, McCord GS, Lustman PJ, Edmundowicz SA. Clinical correlates of abnormal sensitivity to intraesophageal balloon distension. *Dig Dis Sci.* 1991;36:1040–1045.)

ric features are present, we make the diagnosis of "achalasia pattern" and do not commit to any specific disease—a practice that probably should be standard in manometric interpretation. Manometric findings can, however, help define the extent of a multisystem disease (e.g., amyloidosis, diabetes mellitus) or be used as contributing criteria for making diagnoses (e.g., intestinal pseudoobstruction, CREST syndrome).

A larger problem concerning the value of manometry rests with attributing symptoms to specific manometric patterns. The problem is particularly exemplified by the nonspecific motor abnormalities of exaggerated contraction (Table 27–2), the most common diagnoses made.[11] These findings are known to (1) interconvert from one pattern to another, (2) revert to normal spontaneously, and (3) correlate poorly with symptoms across patient groups and in the individual patient over time.[9] Although the evanescent nature of the findings has been used to argue against their importance, asymptomatic patient controls rarely evidence similar abnormalities on serial or prolonged monitoring studies. Thus, even intermittent demonstration of nonspecific motor abnormalities may identify an underlying symptom mechanism. Sensory dysfunction, as defined by provocative testing, may have similar interpretive value, but at least the reassurance of typical pain reproduction accompanies the positive test result.

At present it seems justified to attribute esophageal symptoms to the mechanisms underlying nonspecific motility disorders (group A, Table 27–2), most cases of DES, and provocative test positivity if (1) the symptoms have esophageal characteristics and (2) other potential esophageal and nonesophageal causes have been carefully excluded. The second unfortunate qualifier results from the poor direct association of manometric findings and symptoms and from insecurity regarding the specificity of provocative tests. Longitudinal outcome studies could help clarify the validity of the diagnoses but are only beginning to appear.[15] Outcome studies might also help in subdividing diagnostic categories to see if *degrees* of abnormality are meaningful. For example, what degree of impairment in peristaltic performance is best indicative of DES? Does the patient with 15% simultaneous sequences follow a course that differs from that of the patient with 50% simultaneous sequences? The course and prognosis of DES likely would be less ambiguous if the diagnosis were restricted, for example, to a small subset of patients with poor peristaltic performance.

Manometric patterns suggesting motor failure (e.g., "scleroderma esophagus," group B nonspecific motor abnormalities) are probably responsible for symptoms in another way. These disorders favor increased esophageal acid exposure time and could precipitate reflux-related esophageal damage. The utility of these diagnoses rests primarily in their implications for reflux disease.

Further definition of motor and sensory dysfunction hopefully will identify specific treatments. For example, low-dose antidepressant therapy for patients with DES or nonspecific motor disorders (group A) might be better suited for the subset with identified sensory dysfunction.[26] Sensory dysfunction (e.g., via the balloon distension test) was not determined in our initial report of trazodone for patients with esophageal symptoms and contraction wave abnormalities.[27] The response to the drug was heterogeneous. Possibly the subset with sensory dysfunction was responding better to this agent than the group with motor dysfunction alone. Recent work shows that nifedipine, a drug known to alter contraction wave parameters without influencing chest pain occurrence, has no sensory effect as measured by balloon distension response.[28] Such findings may help explain the unsatisfactory response to this drug by patients with chest pain of presumed esophageal origin.[29] This entire area merits further study and might have important clinical implications.

SUMMARY

Manometric interpretation is successfully performed by measuring a small number of parameters in the distal esophageal body and LES region. Attention to technical details is important for a quality study and for making comparisons with published normal values. A categoric scheme, although not yet in widespread use, is recommended for interpreting the resultant pattern because of its convenience and ability to classify the variety of manometric abnormalities encountered in practice. The clinical value of detecting and reporting common, nonspecific motor abnormalities remains unclear, and clinicians will need to persevere as research in the field continues to evolve.

REFERENCES

1. Dodds WJ, Hogan WJ, Reid DP, Stewart ET, Arndorfer RC. A comparison between primary esophageal peristalsis following wet and dry swallows. *J Appl Physiol.* 1973;35:851–857.
2. Richter JE, Wu WC, Johns DN, et al. Esophageal manometry in 95 healthy adult volunteers: variability of pressures with age and frequency of "abnormal" contractions. *Dig Dis Sci.* 1987;32:583–592.
3. Meyer GW, Gerhardt DC, Castell DO. Human esophageal response to rapid swallowing: muscle refractory period or neural inhibition? *Am J Physiol.* 1981;241: G129–G136.
4. Vantrappen G, Clouse R, Corazziari E, Janssens J, Wienbeck M. Standardisation of oesophageal manometry: an outline of required measurements and technical standards. *Gastroenterol Int.* 1989;2:150–154.
5. Clouse RE, Staiano A. Contraction abnormalities of the esophageal body in patients referred for manometry: a new approach to manometric classification. *Dig Dis Sci.* 1983;28:784–791.
6. Aliperti G, Clouse RE. Incomplete lower esophageal sphincter relaxation in subjects with peristalsis: prevalence and clinical outcome. *Am J Gastroenterol.* 1991; 86:609–614.
7. Novais L, Dalton C, Richter JE. Stationary vs. mapping manometry in evaluating dysphagia. *Dysphagia.* 1990;5: 187–191.
8. Bassoti G, Bacci G, Biagini D, et al. Manometric investigation of the entire esophagus in healthy subjects and patients with high-amplitude peristaltic contractions. *Dysphagia.* 1988;3:93–96.
9. McCord GS, Staiano A, Clouse RE. Achalasia, diffuse spasm, and non-specific motor disorders. *Baillieres Clin Gastroenterol.* 1991;5:307–335.
10. Schneider HA, Yonker RA, Longley S, Katz P, Mathias J, Panush RS. Scleroderma esophagus: a nonspecific entity. *Ann Intern Med.* 1984;100:848–849.
11. Clouse RE, Staiano A. Manometric patterns using esophageal body and lower sphincter characteristics: findings in 1013 patients. *Dig Dis Sci.* 1992;37:289–296.
12. Richter JE, Castell DO. Diffuse esophageal spasm: a reappraisal. *Ann Intern Med.* 1984;100:242–245.
13. Traube M, Aaronson RM, McCallum RW. Transition from peristaltic esophageal contractions to diffuse esophageal spasm. *Arch Intern Med.* 1986;146:1844–1846.
14. Eypasch EP, Stein HJ, DeMeester TR, Johansson KE, Barlow AP, Schneider GT. A new technique to define and clarify esophageal motor disorders. *Am J Surg.* 1990;159:144–151.
15. Rhoton AJ, Wu WC, Dalton CB, Ott DJ. The natural history of diffuse esophageal spasm (DES): a long term follow-up study. *Gastroenterology.* 1992;102:A506. Abstract.
16. Clouse RE, Ferney DM. Rhythmic spontaneous contractions in patients with esophageal symptoms. *Am J Gastroenterol.* 1986;81:666–671.
17. Traube M, Peterson J, Siskind BN, McCallum RW. "Segmental aperistalsis" of the esophagus: a cause of chest pain and dysphagia. *Am J Gastroenterol.* 1988;83: 1381–1385.
18. Dalton CB, Castell DO, Hewson EG, Wu WC, Richter JE. Diffuse esophageal spasm: a rare motility disorder not characterized by high-amplitude contractions. *Dig Dis Sci.* 1991;36:1025–1028.
19. Katz PO, Dalton CB, Richter JE, Wu WC, Castell DO. Esophageal testing of patients with noncardiac chest pain or dysphagia: results of three years' experience with 1161 patients. *Ann Intern Med.* 1987;106:593–597.
20. Barish CF, Castell DO, Richter JE. Graded esophageal balloon distension: a new provocative test for noncardiac chest pain. *Dig Dis Sci.* 1986;31:1292–1298.
21. Richter JE, Barish CF, Castell DO. Abnormal sensory perception in patients with esophageal chest pain. *Gastroenterology.* 1986;91:845–852.
22. Mayer EA, Raybould HE. Role of visceral afferent mechanisms in functional bowel disorders. *Gastroenterology* 1990;99:1688–1704.
23. Lemann M, Dederding JP, Flourie B, Franchisseur C, Rambaud JC, Jian R. Abnormal perception of visceral pain in response to gastric distension in chronic idiopathic dyspepsia: the irritable stomach syndrome. *Dig Dis Sci.* 1991;36:1249–1254.
24. Clouse RE. Motor disorders of the esophagus. In: Sleisenger MH, Fordtran JS, eds. *Gastrointestinal Disease: Pathophysiology, Diagnosis, Management.* 5th ed. Philadelphia, Pa: WB Saunders Co; 1993.
25. Clouse RE, Lustman PJ, McCord GS, Edmundowicz SA. Clinical correlates of abnormal sensitivity to intra-

esophageal balloon distention. *Dig Dis Sci.* 1991;36: 274–278.
26. Clouse RE. Chest pain of presumed esophageal origin: psychopharmacologic approaches to therapy. *Am J Med.* 1992;92(suppl):106–113.
27. Clouse RE, Lustman PJ, Eckert TC, Ferney DM, Griffith LS. Low-dose trazodone for symptomatic patients with esophageal contraction abnormalities. *Gastroenterology.* 1987;92:1027–1036.
28. Smout AJPM, Devore MS, Dalton CB, Castell DO. Effects of nifedipine on esophageal tone and perception of esophageal distension. *Dig Dis Sci.* 1992;37:598–602.
29. Richter JE, Dalton CB, Bradley LA, Castell DO. Oral nifedipine in the treatment of noncardiac chest pain in patients with the nutcracker esophagus. *Gastroenterology.* 1987;93:21–28.

28
Gastroesophageal Reflux Disease

ANDREW IPPOLITI

Gastroesophageal reflux disease, often abbreviated as GERD, is a common medical problem. Surveys estimate the prevalence of occasional symptoms of reflux at 50% to 60% of the population, whereas about 20% report frequent symptoms requiring medication. GERD is typically indicated by heartburn and regurgitation, but it can also produce chest pain, cough, or hoarseness. The disease may vary in its clinical findings from mild microscopic mucosal inflammation, to erosive esophagitis or stricture, or to Barrett's esophagus and its association with adenocarcinoma. This chapter will provide a guide to the diagnostic and therapeutic considerations in the management of patients with GERD.

DIAGNOSIS

Table 28–1 provides a list of diagnostic studies of reflux disease. The sensitivity and specificity of these tests vary widely; some are better suited to assess disease severity, whereas others are screening tests. The patient with typical reflux symptoms (Table 28–1) does not require a test to confirm the diagnosis. Objective evidence to confirm the presence of reflux disease is necessary in the patient with atypical symptoms (Table 28–1).

Reflux is often indicated by the symptoms of retrosternal burning pain and regurgitation of hot, sour contents into the throat. Symptoms are aggravated by eating or lying down, and are relieved by beverages, antacids, or sitting up. Dysphagia may occur in reflux due to dysmotility or to a stricture. Water brash, the sudden filling of the throat with a nonburning fluid, occurs infrequently but is quite specific for reflux. Reflux symptoms may be present in patients with peptic ulcers or in patients with delayed gastric emptying.

The *upper gastrointestinal (UGI) tract series* has some limited utility in the diagnosis of patients with reflux. It excludes other diseases such as peptic ulcer, gastric outlet obstruction, or carcinoma, which may cause refluxlike symptoms. The identification of a hiatal hernia is not a sole criterion for the diagnosis of reflux. Hernias are present in asymptomatic individuals, and the converse is also true, i.e., symptomatic patients without hernias. However, recent evidence suggests an association between hernias and disease pathogenesis. Patients whose hiatal hernias are fixed above the diaphragm are more likely to reflux during periods of increased intraabdominal pressure, e.g., bending over, lifting.

The UGI tract series also detects the presence of reflux of barium from stomach to esophagus. The reflux may be spontaneous, which correlates well with other evidence of reflux, or the reflux may be induced by abdominal compression. But since this is an artificial means to induce reflux, it is frequently positive in healthy subjects. In

TABLE 28–1. DIAGNOSTIC STUDIES AND SYMPTOMS OF GASTROESOPHAGEAL REFLUX

Diagnostic Studies
Upper gastrointestinal tract series
Upper gastrointestinal tract endoscopy
Esophageal motility
Bernstein or acid perfusion test
pH monitoring
Radionuclide gastric emptying

Typical Symptoms
Retrosternal burning
Regurgitation
Association of symptoms with meals and sleep
Relief with antacids
Water brash
Dysphagia

Atypical Symptoms
Anginalike chest pain
Nausea
Cough or wheezing
Throat pain, hoarseness, globus
Halitosis
Hiccups

---

summary, the UGI tract series is useful (1) to exclude other diseases or reflux complications, such as a stricture, (2) to document a hiatal hernia, and (3) to detect spontaneous reflux.

The principal use of *upper endoscopy* is to evaluate the esophageal mucosa either for the presence of acute inflammation, erosive esophagitis, ulcer, or stricture, or for the presence of a columnar epithelium, Barrett's esophagus. The prevalence of these findings in the general public is difficult to ascertain. Barrett's esophagus was found in 12% of patients selected on the basis of weekly heartburn. Some other centers have reported the prevalence of erosive esophagitis or Barrett's esophagus to be 30% to 40% of patients undergoing endoscopy. Endoscopy with biopsy is the standard for the detection of erosive esophagitis or Barrett's esophagus. Only patients with more severe reflux have these findings. Therefore, endoscopy is generally viewed as a test of disease severity. However, there is a rationale for the use of endoscopy to screen patients with chronic reflux for Barrett's esophagus. This is suggested by the association of esophageal adenocarcinoma and Barrett's epithelium.

pH monitoring has rapidly become a useful and widely available diagnostic test for reflux. The continuous recording of the esophageal pH 5 cm above the lower sphincter is the standard measure of the presence and severity of reflux disease. The advantages of this test are that it is easy to perform, the results are reproducible, and the recordings are for 24 hours under physiologic conditions, i.e., as an outpatient. The test measures the number and duration of reflux episodes, defined as a fall in pH to less than 4.0. The overall percentage of the 24-hour period that the esophageal pH was less than 4 (normally <6%) correlates well with disease severity. Patients with erosive esophagitis or Barrett's esophagus have significantly greater percentage time with acid exposure than patients with reflux symptoms without esophagitis.

The 24-hour period provides ample opportunity for symptom occurrence and the observation of associations between reflux episodes and symptoms. A positive symptom index, the number of occasions when reflux precedes a symptom divided by the total number of symptoms, is strongly supportive of the role of reflux in the causation of the complaint. This is particularly helpful for the evaluation of patients with atypical reflux symptoms. In patients with asthma, for example, the presence of reflux may represent the coexistence of two common diseases. The symptom index evaluates the likelihood of a causal relationship.

The disadvantages of pH monitoring are the inconvenience to the patient, the expense of the equipment, and the somewhat restricted nature of the test period. Patients stay home during the test and often consume a bland diet with small portions. Nonetheless, pH monitoring is the most versatile diagnostic tool. It assesses disease severity, which is especially helpful in patients with symptoms refractory to medical treatment. It is the most sensitive diagnostic test and is of most value in patients with atypical symptoms.

An *esophageal motility study* measures the resting lower esophageal sphincter pressure, the amplitude of esophageal body contractions, and the frequency of peristaltic contractions after swallows. A decrease in the resting sphincter tone is regarded as the hallmark of reflux. But this is incorrect. Only a minority of patients have sustained low pressures. In most patients with reflux the lower esophageal sphincter pressure varies greatly and often falls into the normal range. Several studies have found that reflux generally occurs during relaxation of the sphincter. The relaxation may be after swallowing or may be spontaneous, but either way it is independent of the resting sphincter tone. Similarly, changes in body contraction amplitude and the frequency of peristalsis are neither sensitive nor specific for the diagnosis of reflux. Motility is not a useful test to diagnose reflux. Its major use is to evaluate the patient with severe disease, especially one being considered for fundoplication.

The *Bernstein test,* acid perfusion of the esophagus, can be helpful in the evaluation of patients with noncardiac chest pain. It can be administered during a routine motility test and often is administered along with other provocative agents, like edrophonium (Tensilon) and balloon distension.

Radionuclide tests are of limited utility, especially to study reflux. There is value in measuring the rate of gastric emptying in certain patients with reflux, i.e., patients with symptoms of gastric stasis (such as early satiety or nausea) and patients with diseases associated with stasis (such as diabetes). These patients may be particularly benefited by the use of promotility drugs.

To summarize the diagnostic tests:

1. Screening tests
   a. UGI tract series (in patients with recent onset of symptoms, especially under 40 years)
   b. Upper endoscopy (for patients with chronic reflux symptoms to exclude erosive esophagitis or Barrett's esophagus)
2. Disease severity
   a. pH monitoring
   b. Upper endoscopy
3. Symptom-reflux association
   a. pH monitoring
   b. Bernstein test

TREATMENT

There are a variety of *supportive measures* that can lessen the frequency of reflux episodes, Table 28–2. There are several points to consider regarding these recommendations. First, their efficacy and applicability in an individual patient is variable. Second, in patients receiving medication for reflux some of these measures are superfluous. Third, most are empirical and without proven efficacy over time. Two recommendations are directed toward reducing nocturnal reflux: fasting for 2 to 3 hours before bedtime and head-of-bed elevation. Fasting before bedtime is self-taught behavior in patients with reflux. The point is to permit sufficient time for gastric emptying before lying down. The emptying half-time for a "standard" meal is 90 minutes, normally. To reduce the meal volume by 75%, two half-times (3 hours) would be required. Rich meals with high-fat content empty more slowly and

TABLE 28–2. TREATMENT OF REFLUX

Supportive Measures
Fasting before bedtime
Elevation of head of bed
Avoid tight-fitting clothing
Dietary adjustments
Weight reduction
Cessation of smoking

Medications
Histamine-2 receptor antagonists*
  Cimetidine (Tagamet) (800–1200 mg daily)
  Ranitidine (Zantac) (300 mg daily)
  Famotidine (Pepcid) (40 mg daily)
  Nizatidine (Axid) (300 mg daily)
Omeprazole (Prilosec) (20–40 mg daily)
Promotility drugs
  Metoclopramide (Reglan) (40 mg daily)
  Cisapride (Propulsid) (40–80 mg daily)
  Bethanechol (Urecholine) (100 mg daily)
Sucralfate (Carafate) (4 tablets or tablespoons daily)

*Standard starting doses; higher doses may be required.

could take 4 to 5 hours. Unfortunately, these are the type of meals generally eaten late at night. Sleeping on a bed that has been elevated 6 inches has been shown to reduce nocturnal reflux. The bed itself must be raised; sleeping on several pillows is not effective. Patients on acid-suppressing medications for reflux usually will not need to sleep in this position. Activities that increase intraabdominal pressure, such as lifting or bending, may result in excess reflux. However, if the activity is important to the patient's state of mind, such as exercising or gardening, it is more appropriate to prescribe medication than restrict the practice.

There are a number of specific food items that can be associated with heartburn and reflux. These include onions, garlic, spicy foods, coffee, and peppermint. However, the degree of postprandial reflux has never been shown to be substantially modified by diet adjustment. Thus, it is best to recommend that patients refrain only from specific foods that they associate with symptoms. Coffee, even without caffeine, is a potent stimulant of acid secretion. Its use particularly between meals should be minimized.

Cessation of smoking and weight loss may be helpful in reducing reflux but the evidence for this is empirical. Smoking delays acid clearance, lowers sphincter pressure, and slows gastric emptying. Reflux is another good reason not to smoke. Weight reduction in selected patients may be very important. Specifically, patients whose symptoms began in association with some weight gain may obtain sustained relief of reflux with dieting.

Antacids are extensively used by patients with reflux on an as-needed basis. There is no evidence that antacids promote healing or sustained symptom relief with prolonged therapy. But the acute relief of pain with antacids is generally accepted. There are no specific antacid formulations that are more or less effective. Virtually all antacids have been enhanced to increase their buffering capacity. Most antacids are either aluminum-magnesium combinations, which can cause altered bowel function with regular use, or calcium antacids, with less bowel effect but more potential problems with absorption of the calcium. The use of an antacid-alginate combination (Gaviscon) may be preferable to some patients, and a few limited studies support its efficacy. Antacids have a longer duration of action when given after meals at 1 and 3 hours.

The *histamine-2 (H_2) receptor antagonists* are widely prescribed for the treatment of reflux and are very effective in symptom relief. They are more convenient than antacids, are usually free of side effects, and take the place of many of the supportive measures. The disadvantages are their expense, the need for dosage adjustment, low healing rates for esophagitis, and the failure to achieve a sustained remission. Table 28–2 lists the currently available H_2 blockers and their initial doses. These doses have been shown to heal peptic ulcers over 4 to 8 weeks' treatment. However, symptom relief or healing of erosive esophagitis may require two to four times the initial dose. There is a direct correlation between dosage, reduction in acid secretion, and reduction in gastroesophageal reflux. Some patients require near achlorhydria to be symptom free. Fortunately, even at four times the usual dose H_2 blockers are not associated with increased side effects.

The *proton-pump antagonists* such as omeprazole (Prilosec) are a major advance in the treatment of reflux. These are the most potent antisecretory drugs and reduce acid secretion by 80% to 90% with one or two pills daily. As with the H_2 antagonists, side effects are uncommon. However, safety considerations for long-term use have resulted in an FDA recommendation that continuous treatment with omeprazole be limited to 8- to 12-week periods. To date, there has been no evidence of tumor formation in general in patients receiving omeprazole at variable doses for an average of 5 years. The healing rates for esophagitis are significantly higher in patients treated with omeprazole than for those treated with H_2 blockers at standard doses. Omeprazole is generally indicated for complicated reflux disease, esophagitis or Barrett's esophagus, or for patients poorly responsive to H_2 blockers. In these settings it may be difficult to wean the patient from omeprazole. It may be necessary to taper the use of omeprazole or switch from omeprazole to a high-dose H_2 blocker and then taper. Omeprazole is more expensive than standard doses of H_2 blockers, and it may not confer any sustained symptom relief when treatment is stopped.

There are three types of *promotility drugs* that have reported efficacy in the treatment of reflux (Table 28–2). The first was bethanechol (Urecholine), a choline esterase inhibitor. Metoclopramide (Reglan) has been widely used for this purpose for 20 years. Its mode of action is complex, but it stimulates smooth muscle directly by enhancing acetylcholine release and indirectly by antagonizing dopamine, a smooth muscle inhibitor. The most recent agent is cisapride (Propulsid). It also enhances acetylcholine release, but is a serotonin agonist without effect on dopamine. Bethanechol often produces typical cholinergic side effects (cramping, sweating, tearing) at conventional doses. Because of its antidopamine effects metoclopramide can cause Parkinson-like reactions. These are fortunately rare, but agitation or sedation may be found in elderly patients. Cisapride's principal advantage is that there are fewer side effects. The most common of these are diarrhea and abdominal cramps. Although it is clear that reflux symptoms and even esophagitis are improved during treatment with promotility drugs, the mechanism is uncertain. The agents stimulate smooth muscle contraction and potentially shorten acid clearance time and raise sphincter pressure, all of which would reduce esophageal acid exposure. However, in patients with severe reflux and marked loss of motor function it is unlikely that the drugs provide much esophageal stimulation. Here their principal effect may be to stimulate gastric emptying.

The final drug to consider is *sucralfate (Carafate)*. This agent has no antisecretory activity. Its main use in reflux is for its potential to bind bile acids. Occasionally patients have nonacid reflux of small bowel contents. This would generally be patients who have had a gastric resection or an antrectomy. Carafate on empiric grounds is possibly helpful.

In summary, the approach to the treatment of GERD may be viewed as three levels of therapy.

Level 1 is antacids and supportive measures. This level of treatment may be put into effect by the patient long before a physician is seen. Even if the treatment is physician initiated, patient compliance can be difficult to achieve. Some patients even at the initial evaluation will be clearly unsuited to this approach. Level 2 is the use of H_2 receptor antagonists. Patients with uncomplicated reflux should receive H_2 blockers. There is no particular advantage for one agent over the other. H_2 blockers should be prescribed at regular intervals, e.g., at bedtime or two to four times daily, as indicated. Antacids may be used on an as-needed basis. Supportive measures are recommended as necessary. Fasting before bedtime is always advisable, but elevating the head of the bed may not be needed when an H_2 blocker is taken at bedtime. Most patients with reflux will respond substantially to these treatments. Level 3 is for those patients with complex reflux, erosive esophagitis, stricture, or Barrett's esophagus and those refractory to H_2 blockers. There are three ways to treat the level 3 patient: (1) increase the H_2 blocker dosage, (2) discontinue the H_2 blocker and start omeprazole, and (3) add a promotility drug to the antisecretory regimen. At this level omeprazole alone is the most cost effective. H_2 blockers will require two or three times the usual dose and expense. Promotility drugs alone are not effective for a level 3 patient. It is a waste of money to prescribe combinations of H_2 blockers or omeprazole plus an H_2 blocker.

The acute phase of treatment at any level will require about 4 weeks. But acute treatment may last 12 or 16 weeks in some patients. Once symptoms have been substantially reduced and esophagitis, if present, has healed, maintenance therapy can be considered. Patients, responding to H_2 blockers alone, may not require a regular program of maintenance treatment. This is particularly true if some lifestyle adjustment was made, such as weight loss or cessation of smoking. However, most level 3 patients require maintenance because symptom recurrence within the next year is practically universal in this group. Maintenance is often achieved with a lower dosage of the antisecretory drug alone on a daily or every other day basis. Unfortunately, many level 3 patients require on-going active treatment with higher doses and multiple drugs. This is particularly true for the patients with frequent symptoms but without esophagitis. They never experience the benefit of "healing" a mucosal inflammation. Their symptoms are correlated with their acid exposure times, and regular full-dose treatment is needed to reduce the time. These patients may be good candidates for antireflux surgery (see below).

Finally, it is important to remember that some medications can directly irritate esophageal mucosa causing erosions or ulcers even without much reflux. Other drugs may interfere with intrinsic antireflux properties such as sphincter pressure and increase the frequency of reflux. Both types of drugs are delineated in Table 28–3.

TABLE 28–3. DRUGS TO AVOID IN REFLUX

Mucosal Irritants
Antibiotics (doxycycline)
Potassium (Slow-K)
Iron
Quinidine
Nonsteroidal antiinflammatory agents (aspirin)

Smooth Muscle Inhibitors
Anticholinergics
Calcium channel blockers
b-Adrenergic agonists
Nitrates
Theophylline

ANTIREFLUX SURGERY

Fundoplication is gaining greater acceptance in the management of reflux disease. The operation may be performed by a thoracic approach (Belsey procedure) or an abdominal approach (Nissen procedure). The essential features are to increase pressure across the lower esophageal sphincter by wrapping the stomach around all or a portion of the distal esophagus. Any herniation is corrected by restoring the intraabdominal portion of the esophagus. Two large US studies have documented the effectiveness of antireflux surgery when compared with medical treatment for reflux. Medical treatment has included supportive measures, antacids, H_2 antagonists, and promotility drugs. Comparative trials with omeprazole have not been done as yet. Fundoplication should be considered when there is objective evidence of reflux disease by endoscopy, erosive esophagitis, Barrett's esophagus, or pH monitoring and when the patient has not responded to adequate medical treatment. One would also consider patients who are unwilling or unable to continue chronic medical treatment. Preoperative assessment should include endoscopy, motility, pH monitoring if endoscopy results are negative, and gastric emptying. Laparoscopic antireflux surgery has been developed, and its efficacy is being evaluated.

SPECIAL CONSIDERATIONS IN REFLUX DISEASE

REFLUX AND LUNG AND LARYNGEAL DISEASES

Cough, wheezing, throat pain, and hoarseness are listed as atypical symptoms of reflux. Although the exact mechanisms whereby gastroesophageal reflux leads to laryngeal inflammation or bronchospastic diseases are not known, there is mounting evidence of such relationships. Reflux can be detected by pH monitoring in many patients with adult-onset, nonallergic asthma. In fact some surveys have noted an 80% prevalence of abnormal monitoring in patients with asthma. Such a high association is not surprising when one considers that reflux and asthma are common diseases, smoking adversely affects both, and many bronchodilators increase reflux. Several studies have documented improvement in pulmonary function and symptoms after medical and surgical treatment of reflux. Nocturnal wheezing may be an important clue to the coexistence of the two conditions as many of these patients have frequent reflux when lying down. However, not all patients will have typical reflux symptoms. Reflux should be considered in any patient with adult-onset asthma, patients with idiopathic pulmonary fibrosis, and patients with chronic cough. pH monitoring will be the single best test for this possible disease association. Treatment should follow the above guidelines, and a reduction in number and doses of the pulmonary medications is excellent evidence of a favorable effect.

As with pulmonary diseases laryngeal inflammation may be a result of reflux. Vocal lesions such as ulceration, granuloma, or intraarytenoid erythema are signs of reflux-induced irritation and are termed *acid posterior laryngitis*. Patients typically complain of hoarseness, excessive expectoration, thick saliva, throat pain, or a lump in the throat. A few studies have documented an excessive reflux of acid into the proximal esophagus in these patients. Standard acid reflux measures plus H_2 blockers benefit many patients. Best results are found with omeprazole 20 to 40 mg daily for 2 to 3 months.

BARRETT'S ESOPHAGUS

Barrett's esophagus is defined as the presence of columnar epithelium in the esophagus and is a consequence of chronic gastroesophageal reflux. The columnar change begins in the distal esophagus and extends proximally for variable distances. Columnar epithelium may also be occasionally found just below the upper esophageal sphincter, but this is a developmental abnormality, unrelated to reflux, and is not Barrett's esophagus. Barrett's esophagus has been reported to occur in 12% of patients with weekly symptoms of heartburn. It is more common in patients with complicated reflux disease, e.g., 35% of patients with erosive esophagitis and 44% with strictures have Barrett's esophagus. Barrett's esophagus occurs predominantly in white men, but neither age nor duration of symptoms is predictive of its presence.

The pathophysiology of Barrett's esophagus is not certain. When it is present, other associated features include decreased lower esophageal sphincter pressure, decreased body amplitude and peristalsis, and high rates of reflux, i.e., percent time esophageal pH is less than 4. Thus, patients with Barrett's esophagus are at the severe end of the spectrum of reflux disease. Additional findings include a lack of sensitivity to acid infusion, a negative Bernstein test, and an increased basal acid output. The symptomatic response to H_2 blockers or omeprazole is comparable to that of patients with reflux but without Barrett's esophagus. Ulcers and strictures respond well to medical treatment. To date, there is no evidence that medical treatment results in a regression of the columnar change. However, this is a subject of intense investigation at present.

Barrett's esophagus is an important consequence of reflux because of its potential to lead to adenocarcinoma. The prevalence of adenocarcinoma in patients with Barrett's esophagus is 10% to 15%. Recent prospective studies report an incidence of 1/50 to 100 patient-years. Adenocarcinoma of the esophagus, esophagogastric junction, or gastric cardia is the fastest rising cancer in the last 20 years. A recent study comparing the incidence before 1971 and after 1974 described a fivefold increase. Adenocarcinoma from this region is, like Barrett's esophagus, predominantly a disease of white men. Its frequency in white men is 5.1/100,000, which is the 15th most common cancer in this country. Based on incidence figures the rate of adenocarcinoma in patients with Barrett's esophagus is 1000/

100,000, which is twice the lung cancer rate for white men of similar age. Unlike squamous esophageal cancer, alcohol and tobacco use are less frequent in adenocarcinoma. In light of an almost epidemic incidence of adenocarcinoma of the esophagus and cardia, surveillance of patients with Barrett's esophagus has become quite important. It is well-documented that dysplastic changes in the columnar epithelium precede the development of cancer. Regular examinations at yearly intervals to diagnose dysplasia are recommended. Further, routine screening of patients with chronic heartburn to detect Barrett's esophagus is also advised.

REFERENCES

1. Bell NJV, Hunt RH. Role of gastric acid suppression in the treatment of gastro-esophageal reflux disease. *Gut.* 1992;33:118–124.
2. Dodds WJ, Dent J, Hogan WJ, et al. Mechanisms of gastroesophageal reflux in patients with reflux esophagitis. *N Engl J Med.* 1982;307:1547–1552.
3. Hameeteman W, Tytgat GNJ, Houthoff HJ, van den Tweel JG. Barrett's esophagus: development of dysplasia and adenocarcinoma. *Gastroenterology.* 1989;96:1249–1256.
4. Jacob P, Kahrilas PJ, Herzon G. Proximal esophageal pH-metry in patients with 'reflux laryngitis'. *Gastroenterology.* 1991;100:305–310.
5. Johnson LF, DeMeester TR. Twenty-four hour monitoring of the distal esophagus: a quantitative measure of gastroesophageal reflux. *Am J Gastroenterol.* 1974;62:325–332.
6. Pera M, Cameron AJ, Trastek VF, et al. Increasing incidence of adenocarcinoma of the esophagus and esophagogastric junction. *Gastroenterology.* 1993;104:510–513.
7. Spechler SJ, and the Dept. of Veterans Affairs Gastroesophageal Reflux Disease Study Group. Comparison of medical and surgical therapy for complicated gastroesophageal reflux disease in veterans. *N Engl J Med.* 1992;326:786–792.
8. Toussaint J, Gossuin A, Deruyttere M, et al. Healing and prevention of reflux oesophagitis by cisapride. *Gut.* 1991;32:1280–1285.
9. Wiener GJ, Richter JE, Copper JB, et al. The symptom index: a clinically important parameter of ambulatory 24-hour esophageal pH monitoring. *Am J Gastroenterol.* 1988;83:358–361.
10. Winters C, Spurling TJ, Chobanian SJ, et al. Barrett's esophagus: a prevalent, occult complication of gastroesophageal reflux disease. *Gastroenterology.* 1987;92:118–124.

29
Gastroesophageal Reflux During Infancy and Childhood

CRAIG HILLEMEIER

Gastroesophageal reflux, or the reflux of gastric contents into the body of the esophagus, occurs in both children and adults and is an example of a motility disorder that has markedly different clinical symptoms in the two age groups. Although virtually all infants have some degree of gastroesophageal reflux, the severity of the symptoms may vary from an occasional wet burp to persistent emesis and may occasionally have associated failure to thrive or respiratory symptoms. The adult with gastroesophageal reflux will often complain of heartburn and will rarely have emesis.

It must be remembered that the infant who is suffering from significant regurgitation or vomiting may be responding to disease outside the gastrointestinal tract. However, evaluations of most infants who have persistent symptoms of vomiting reveal no easily definable, anatomic, metabolic, infectious, or neurologic cause, and they are often labeled with the descriptive term *gastroesophageal reflux* (GER). Although there are a large number of tests available to detect and quantitate the amount of GER that occurs during infancy, the precise cause often remains unclear. It is important to remember that, since most infants have some degree of GER, one should not fall into the trap of assuming a cause-and-effect relationship between GER and other health-related problems such as growth failure, respiratory disease, apnea, or behavioral problems. The clinical determination of the relationship between these conditions and GER is often difficult and must be approached with a degree of skepticism.

CLINICAL PRESENTATION

The majority of infants with GER become symptomatic during the first few months of life, and usually the overt symptoms resolve by 1 to 2 years of age. Most infants who have clinically significant problems with GER are thriving and healthy and therefore require little in the way of diagnostic or therapeutic maneuvers. However, an infant who suffers health problems such as failure to thrive, recurrent pneumonia, hematemesis, or episodes of apnea and who also has GER requires thoughtful consideration as to the relationship between the two.

It should also be noted that infants and older children who have significant neurologic deficits or psychomotor retardation often have significant GER and may suffer from serious complications. Recurrent pneumonia or blood loss from erosive esophagitis in these children is not uncommon. These patients are likely to have hiatal hernias, and they are more likely to require aggressive or definitive therapy such as surgical fundoplication to reduce the likelihood of esophagitis with bleeding or pneumonia.

The other significant group of children who are likely to present with symptoms of GER are school-aged children and adolescents who have significant amounts of heartburn. These patients often have worsening symptoms associated with exercise or periods of stress. It is likely these children represent a variant of the way GER often presents in adults.

DIAGNOSTIC EVALUATION

Immunologic, neurologic, metabolic, or renal disease may not be obvious in an infant with significant clinical symptoms suggestive of GER, but an appreciation of the diseases' symptoms may save the infant needless diagnostic procedures and result in more appropriate and timely therapy. If there is any sign of neurologic impairment a serum ammonia level should be obtained to rule out a urea cycle enzyme deficit, and electrolytes with anion gap should be calculated to rule out a metabolic acidemia. Careful physical examination including measurement of head circumference and an examination of fundi may lean to a diagnosis of increased intracranial pressure. Blood urea nitrogen, creatinine, urinalysis, urine culture, and attempts to show if the infant can concentrate his urine will help to rule out renal disease, hydronephrosis, or urinary tract infection that may present with persistent vomiting. The presence of projectile vomiting should alert the health care provider to the possibility of an anatomic problem such as pyloric stenosis or a malrotation.

An infant who has significant symptoms of GER but who is thriving and growing well and has no other health problems does not require or benefit from extensive diagnostic evaluations. Often these children will have a history of vomiting for several hours after a feeding and usually will not vomit much during the night. If pH probes are performed on many of these healthy children, they are found to show significant reflux that diminishes with increasing age. A careful history and physical examination should be sufficient to confirm the fact that the child merely suffers from a moderately severe variant of GER during infancy and is suffering no associated sequelae.

If a child has symptoms of GER that are extremely severe or thought to be associated with other health problems such as failure to thrive or recurrent pneumonia, the child should undergo a contrast study of the upper gastrointestinal tract to rule out an anatomic obstruction. During the swallowing phase of the examination the hypopharynx should be carefully evaluated for signs of aspiration or an anatomic abnormality such as a web or stricture. This is particularly important if there is a history of pneumonia, which aspiration during swallowing can promote as readily as aspiration during an episode of reflux. The body of the esophagus should be carefully evaluated to look for signs of stricture or ulceration. The stomach and duodenum must be examined to detect signs of pyloric stenosis, gastric outlet obstruction secondary to ulcerations, or other anatomic obstruction such as mucosal web. In general, most physicians do not find quantitation of the amount of GER on a radiologic contrast study of the upper gastrointestinal tract to be very helpful.

pH probes in these children are very accurate ways in terms of quantitating the amount of acid reflux that occurs during GER. However, this test in and of itself does nothing other than quantitate the amount of reflux and does little to allow correlation between reflux and symptoms such as recurrent pneumonia. It may be helpful if a specific therapeutic maneuver is to be evaluated and a pH probe is performed both before and after to determine the effectiveness of therapy.

The performance of upper gastrointestinal tract endoscopy and esophageal biopsy in an infant who is otherwise thriving probably has little role. Nuclear scintigraphy to evaluate gastric emptying may be appropriate in a child who has severe reflux or who is being considered for surgical fundoplication. Children who have delayed gastric emptying associated with GER may well benefit from a procedure to facilitate gastric emptying at the time of their fundoplication.

Many children with severe neurologic impairment often benefit from a feeding gastrostomy because of inability to swallow adequate nutrients. In these children it is often helpful to quantitate the amount of reflux with a pH probe plot prior to placement in gastrostomy so that fundoplication can be used when appropriate.

THERAPY

The infant who has significant reflux who seems to be growing well and has no other significant health problems benefits most from little or no therapy. A careful history and physical examination with appropriate reassurance to the child's caregiver is the most appropriate course. Small or frequent feedings are probably the most effective way to reduce the amounts of reflux. Sitting a child up in the infant seat after feeding has not been shown to reduce the amount of reflux that occurs. In the past it had been suggested to place the child on his stomach with the head elevated to reduce the amount of reflux. However, recent concerns over the possible relationship of sudden infant death syndrome associated with this position have reduced reliance on this therapy.

It is often suggested that thickened feedings may be helpful in children who have GER. However, most studies that have examined this issue in a quantitative fashion have not been able to reveal a reduced amount of reflux time associated with thickened feedings. It is possible, however, that early satiety associated with thickened feedings may make the infant more comfortable, reduce the amount of crying, and result in better weight gain because of increased calories.

Probably the most effective medical therapy for infants who have severe problems with GER is small, frequent feedings. This presumably reduces the amount of formula in the stomach that is available for reflux. I commonly will suggest that a child who is taking 8 oz of formula every 4 to 5 hours might benefit from a reduction to perhaps 4 to 6 oz of feeding every 3 to 4 hours.

For those infants who have more severe reflux and who are being considered for surgery, it is often helpful to consider continuous nasal gastric feedings or postpyloric feedings. This is often important prior to surgery because one wants to make sure that the intestinal tract is capable of handling adequate amounts of enteral feeding. If a fundoplication is performed in a child whose intestinal tract is unable to handle adequate calories, the child may still have significant vomiting after surgery but will be unable to relieve the pressure in the stomach because of the fundoplication. A child who chronically vomits from postpyloric feeding may benefit from antroduodenal motility in both the pre- and postprandial periods to evaluate the possibility of intestinal pseudoobstruction.

PHARMACOTHERAPY

Despite the fact that most children with GER symptoms during infancy tend to thrive and do quite well, much research has been done on pharmacologic therapy to suppress the symptoms of what appears to be an almost physiologic process. However, in large part these efforts to find an agent to reduce GER during infancy have been unsuccessful.

Since many infants who have significant amounts of reflux will have esophagitis, there have been many attempts to treat them with gastric acid–neutralizing techniques. Although it certainly can be shown that acid suppression reduces the amount of acid present in the gastric contents and therefore in the amount of acid that is refluxed into the esophagus, beneficial effects of these regimens have rarely been shown. Although it may seem intuitively obvious that the infant with GER has discomfort, the infant who has excessive crying or colicky behavior rarely, if ever, benefits from a trial of these gastric acid–neutralizing agents. One also must be careful in the use of traditional antacids in infants and older children because of the potential for aluminum toxicity with such agents.

Other pharmacologic agents such as bethanechol, a muscarinic agonist, have been shown to markedly increase lower esophageal sphincter pressure in infants who have GER. However, since the majority of these infants do not have decreased lower gastroesophageal sphincter pressure, the rationale for using bethanechol is somewhat shaky. It has been shown to somewhat reduce the amount of reflux as quantitated by pH probes if one uses a high dose; however, these high doses are often associated with side effects such as cramping and diarrhea, and bethanechol is rarely used to treat GER during infancy.

Metoclopramide, a dopamine antagonist that seems to sensitize tissues to acetylcholine, is commonly used to treat GER in adults. It has been used somewhat in children, but it has been difficult to show effectiveness in terms of reducing the amount of GER during infancy. It probably has some effect on increasing lower gastroesophageal sphincter pressure, and it may have a mild effect on speeding up the gastric emptying of ingested foodstuffs. However, the fact the drug has been widely used is somewhat unfortunate since it seems to have a high degree of side effects in children and very little documented success in treating GER. It has been estimated that up to a third of children who take metoclopramide with have increased drowsiness or restlessness, and not an insignificant number will have a dystonic reaction that manifests as neck pain rigidity, dizziness, and an oculogyric crisis.

A newer gastric prokinetic agent, cisapride, has recently been introduced in this country and approved for use in adults. There has been limited use with this noncholinergic nonantidopaminergic agent, which appears to work through enhancing the postganglionic release of acetylcholine.

SURGERY

Surgical procedures to increase the competence of the lower esophageal sphincter area and thereby prevent the reflux of the gastric contents have been widely used in children. In many pediatric centers fundoplication is indeed one of the common forms of surgical procedure. This is a procedure that should not commonly be performed on infants who have a normal central nervous system. However, for an infant or child who has GER that seems to be associated with unacceptable symptoms, there is little doubt that a surgical fundoplication is the most effective way to deal with the problem of GER.

Often a child who has severe neurologic impairment does not respond to conservative medical therapy and may require a fundoplication. However, it is important that the child's ability for gastric emptying be measured prior to the fundoplication. If one performs a fundoplication on a child who has markedly delayed gastric emptying, he may end up with significant retching against the fundoplication. The child with delayed gastric emptying who undergoes a fundoplication will benefit from a surgical procedure to increase the gastric emptying rate. A child who has had a fundoplication, especially a child with severe neurologic impairment, is especially at risk from surgical complications of this procedure. The incidence of small intestine obstruction secondary to adhesions is not small in series of pediatric patients who have had fundoplications. It is important to realize that those children who have severe neurologic impairment and who undergo fundoplication are most likely to have a delayed diagnosis of intestinal obstruction because their caregivers do not understand that the children are having symptoms of intestinal obstruction.

SUMMARY

Most infants with symptoms of GER benefit from no invasive diagnostic or therapeutic maneuvers. Infants and older children with profound central nervous system dysfunction are likely to have severe GER, which requires more aggressive or possibly surgical management.

REFERENCES

1. Cucchiara S, Bortolotti M, Raffaele M, Auricchio S. Fasting and postprandial mechanisms of gastroesophageal reflux in children with gastroesophageal reflux disease. *Dig Dis Sci.* 1993;38:86–92.
2. Cucciara S, Staiano A, Romaniello G, Capobianco S, Auricchio S. Antacids and cimetidine treatment for gastroesophageal reflux and peptic esophagitis. *Arch Dis Child.* 1984;59:842–847.
3. Euler AR, Ament ME. Detection of gastroesophageal reflux in the pediatric age patient by esophageal intraluminal pH probe measurement (Tuttle test). *Pediatrics.* 1977;60:65–68.
4. Fonkalsrud EW, Foglia RD, Ament ME, et al. Operative treatment for the gastroesophageal reflux symptom in children. *J Pediatr Surg.* 1989;24:525–529.
5. Hillemeier AC, Lange R, McCallum R, Seashore J, Gryboski JD. Delayed gastric emptying in infants with gastroesophageal reflux. *J Pediatr.* 1981;98:190–193.

6. Kurlandsky LE, Vaandrager V, Davy CL, Stockinger FS. Lipoid pneumonia in association with gastroesophageal reflux. *Pediatr Pulmonol.* 1992;13:184–188.
7. Orenstein SR. Effects on behavior state of prone versus seated positioning for infants with gastroesophageal reflux. *Pediatrics.* 1990;1985:764–767.
8. Orenstein SR, Whitington PF. Positioning for prevention of infant gastroesophageal reflux. *J Pediatr.* 1983; 103:534–537.
9. Orenstein SR, Magill LH, Brooks P. Thickening of infant feedings for therapy of GER. *J Pediatr.* 1987;110: 181–186.
10. Vandenplas Y, deRoy C, Sacre L. Cisapride decreases prolonged episodes of reflux in infants. *J Pediatr Gastro Nutr.* 1991;12:44–47.

30
Hiatal Hernia

JEFFREY H. PETERS and TOM R. DeMEESTER

With the advent of clinical roentgenology, it became evident that a hiatal hernia was a relatively common abnormality and was not always accompanied by symptoms. Three types of esophageal hiatal hernias were identified:

1. The sliding hernia (type I), characterized by an upward dislocation of the cardia in the posterior mediastinum (Fig. 30–1A)
2. The rolling or paraesophageal hernia (type II), characterized by an upward dislocation of the gastric fundus alongside a normally positioned cardia (Fig. 30–1B)
3. The combined sliding-rolling or mixed hernia (type III), characterized by an upward dislocation of both the cardia and the gastric fundus (Fig. 30–2A)

The end stage of a type I or II hernia occurs when the whole stomach migrates up into the chest by rotating 180 degrees around its longitudinal axis with the cardia and pylorus as fixed points. In this situation the abnormality is usually referred to as an intrathoracic stomach (Fig. 30–2B).

INCIDENCE AND ETIOLOGY

The true incidence of a hiatal hernia in the overall population is difficult to determine because of the absence of symptoms in a large number of patients. When roentgenographic examinations were done in response to gastrointestinal symptoms, the incidence of a sliding hiatal hernia was seven times more frequent than a paraesophageal hernia. The age distribution of patients with paraesophageal hernias is significantly different from that observed in sliding hiatal hernias. The former has a median age of 61 years, whereas the latter is 48 years. Paraesophageal hernias are more likely to occur in women by a ratio of four to one.

Structural deterioration of the phrenicoesophageal membrane over time may explain the higher incidence of hiatal hernias in the older age group (Fig. 30–3).[1] These changes involve thinning of the upper fascial layer of the membrane (supradiaphragmatic-continuation of the endothoracic fascia) and loss of elasticity in the lower fascial layer (infradiaphragmatic-continuation of the transversalis fascia). Consequently, the membrane yields to stretching in the cranial direction because of persistent intraabdominal pressure. The upper fascial layer is formed only by loose connective tissue and is of little importance. The lower fascial layer is thick and stronger and of more importance. It divides into an upper and lower leaf about 1 cm before attaching intimately with the esophageal adventitia. Because of stretching in the cranial direction from intraabdominal pressure, the attachment of the lower leaf protrudes upward and can frequently be identified in the thoracic cavity. These observations suggest that the development of a

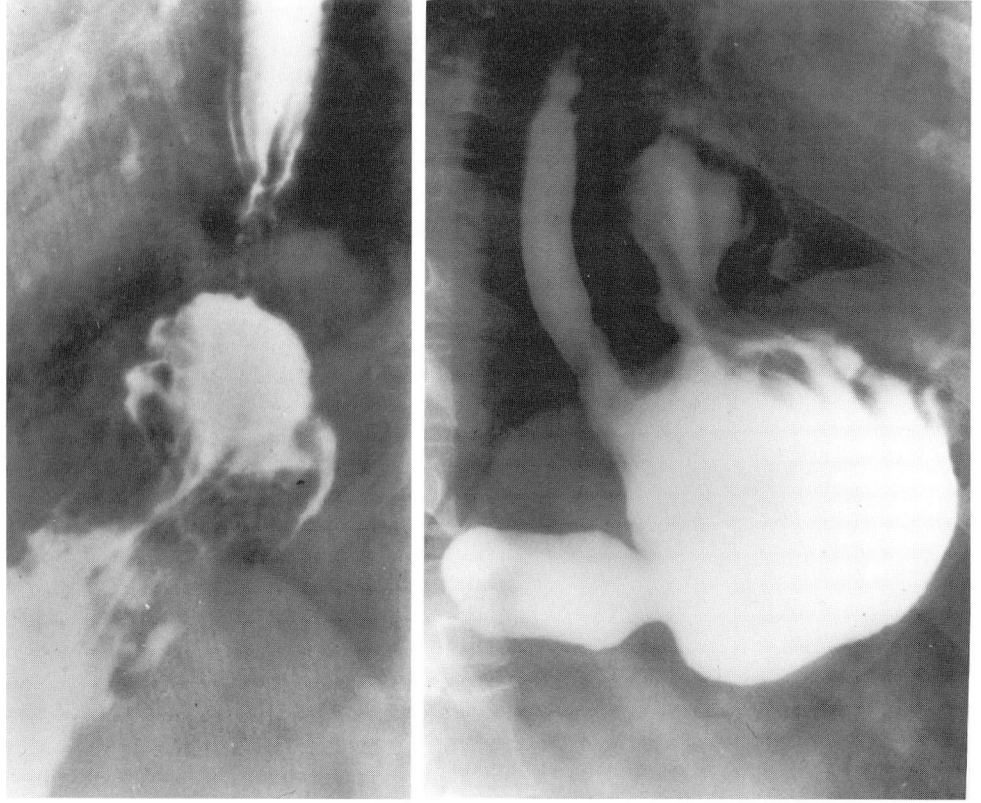

FIGURE 30–1. A, Roentgenogram of a type I sliding hiatal hernia. **B,** Roentgenogram of a type II rolling or paraesophageal hernia. (From DeMeester TR, Bonavina L. Paraesophageal hiatal hernia. In: Nyhus LM, Condon RE, eds. *Hernia.* 3rd ed. Philadelphia, Pa: JB Lippincott Co; 1989:684, 685, with permission.)

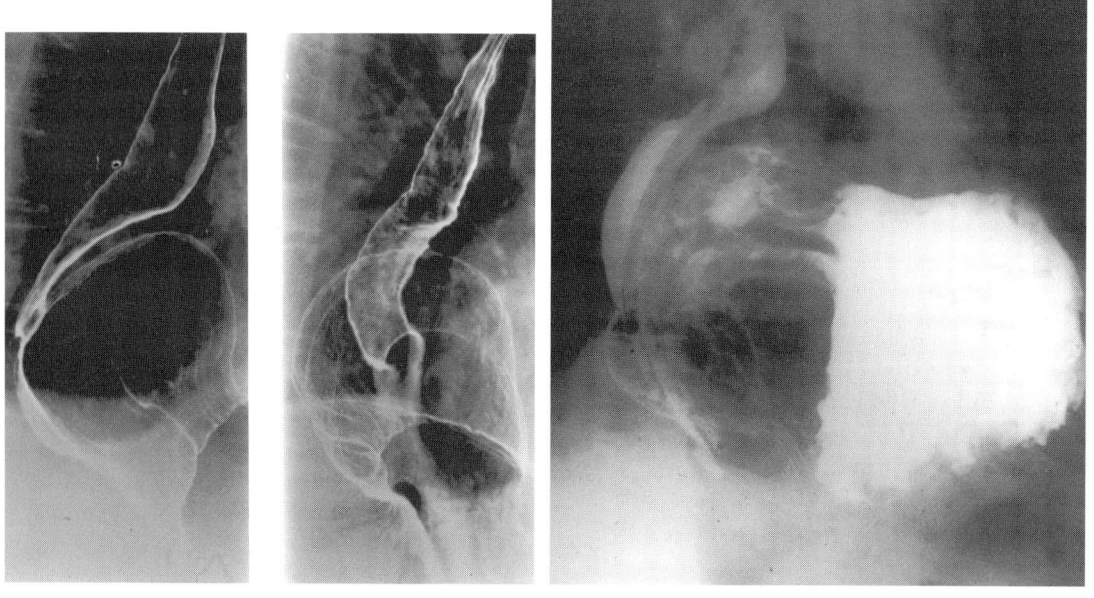

FIGURE 30–2. A, Roentgenogram of a type III combined sliding-rolling or mixed hernia. **B,** Roentgenogram of an intrathoracic stomach. This is the end stage of a large hiatal hernia regardless of its initial classification. Note that the stomach has rotated 180 degrees around its longitudinal axis with the cardia and pylorus as fixed points. (From DeMeester TR, Bonavina L. Paraesophageal hiatal hernia. In: Nyhus LM, Condon RE, eds. *Hernia.* 3rd ed. Philadelphia, Pa: JB Lippincott Co; 1989:685, 686, with permission.)

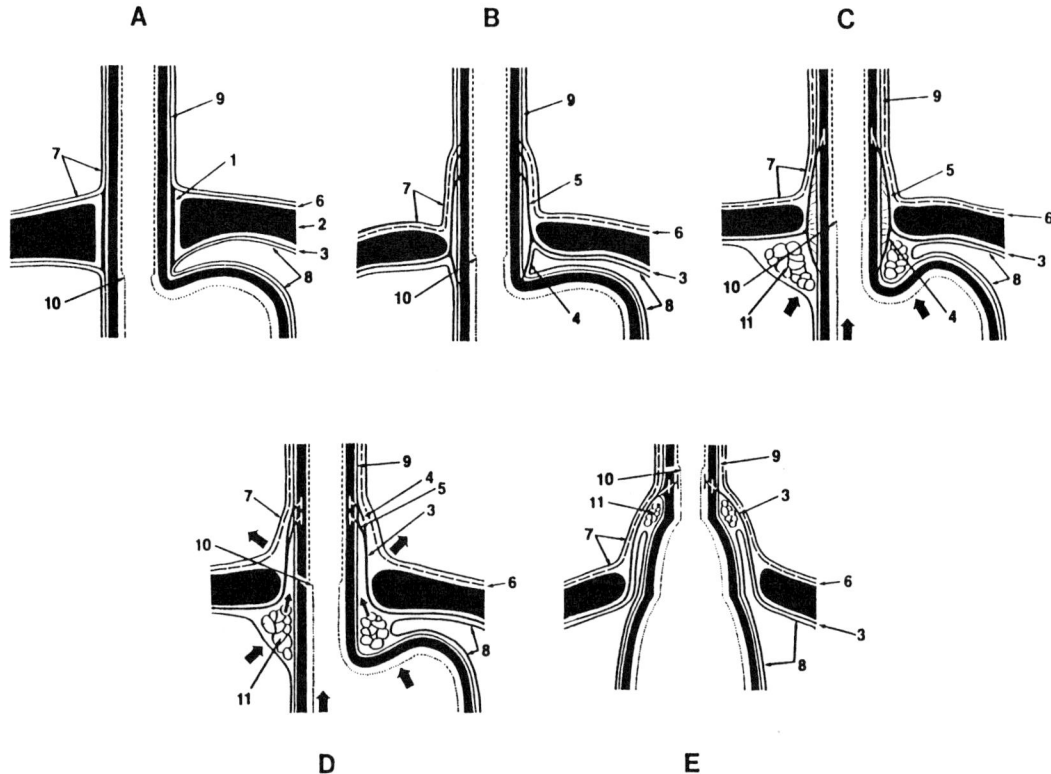

FIGURE 30–3. Changes in the anatomy of the phrenoesophageal membrane over time based on the dissection of 163 human cadavers from the fetal period to age 75 years. **A,** Fetus. **B,** Newborn and small infants and young adults 20 to 30 years of age. **C,** Old adults 55 to 70 years of age. **D,** Old adults in transition to a hiatal hernia. **E,** Old adults with hiatal hernia. In the fetus the membrane is closely attached to the adventitia of the esophagus. In neonates, children, and young adults the membrane is slightly stretched. In old adults, loose connective tissue develops in the lower fascial layer. In old adults in transition to hiatal hernia, the lower fascial tissue is pushed cranially to form the developed hernia shown in **E.** *Broad arrows* indicate direction of stretch owing to intraabdominal pressure and movement of the esophagus during swallowing. *1,* phrenoesophageal membrane; *2,* diaphragmatic crus; *3,* lower fascial tissue; *4,* lower leaf of lower fascial layer; *5,* upper leaf of lower fascial layer; *6,* upper fascial layer; *7,* pleura; *8,* peritoneum; *9,* esophageal adventitia; *10,* gastroesophageal epithelial junction; *11,* subperitoneal fat. (From DeMeester TR, Bonavina L. Paraesophageal hiatal hernia. In: Nyhus LM, Condon RE, eds. *Hernia.* 3rd ed. Philadelphia, Pa: JB Lippincott Co; 1989:687, with permission.)

hiatal hernia appears to be a phenomenon related to age and is secondary to repetitive upward stretching of the phrenicoesophageal membrane owing to up-and-down movements of the esophagus during swallowing and the upward pushing of the membrane by intraabdominal pressure. A paraesophageal hernia rather than a sliding hernia develops when there is a defect, perhaps congenital, in the esophageal hiatus anterior to the esophagus.[2] The persistent posterior fixation of the cardia to the preaortic fascia and the median arcuate ligament is the only essential difference between a sliding and paraesophageal hernia. When an anterior defect in the hiatus occurs in association with a loss of fixation of the cardia, a mixed or type III hernia develops.

SYMPTOMS

The clinical presentation of a paraesophageal hiatal hernia differs from that of a sliding hernia.[3] There is usually a higher prevalence of symptoms of dysphagia and postprandial fullness with paraesophageal hernias, but the typical symptoms of heartburn and regurgitation present in sliding hiatal hernias can also be present. Both are caused by gastroesophageal reflux secondary to an underlying mechanical deficiency of the cardia. The symptoms of dysphagia and postprandial fullness in patients with a paraesophageal hernia are explained by the compression of the adjacent esophagus by a distended cardia or twisting of the gastroesophageal junction by the torsion of the stomach that occurs as it becomes progressively displaced in the chest.[4]

About one third of patients with a paraesophageal hernia complain of hematemesis due to recurrent bleeding from ulceration of the gastric mucosa.[3] Respiratory complications are frequently associated with a paraesophageal hernia and consist of dyspnea from mechanical compression and recurrent pneumonia from aspiration. Intermittent esophageal obstruction can develop in patients with an intrathoracic stomach because of the rotation that has occurred as the organ migrates into the chest. Conversely, many patients with paraesophageal hiatal hernia are asymptomatic or complain of very minor symptoms.

The condition is life threatening in one fifth of patients in that the hernia can lead to sudden catastrophic events, such as excessive bleeding or volvulus with acute gastric obstruction or infarction. With mild dilation of the stomach, the gastric blood supply can be markedly reduced causing gastric ischemia, ulceration, perforation, and sepsis.

The symptoms of sliding hiatal hernias are usually due to functional abnormalities associated with gastroesophageal reflux and include heartburn, regurgitation, and dysphagia. These patients have a mechanically defective lower esophageal sphincter giving rise to reflux of gastric juice and to the symptoms of heartburn and regurgitation. The symptom of dysphagia occurs from the presence of mucosal edema, Schatzki's ring, stricture, or the inability to organize peristaltic activity in the body of the esophagus as a consequence of the disease. There are a group of patients with hiatal hernias unassociated with reflux disease who have dysphagia without any obvious endoscopic or manometric explanation. Video barium roentgenograms have shown the cause of dysphagia in these patients to be an obstruction to the passage of the swallowed bolus by diaphragmatic impingement on the herniated stomach. Manometrically, this is reflected by a double-humped, high-pressure zone at the gastroesophageal junction caused by diaphragmatic impingement of the herniated stomach and the true distal esophageal sphincter. These patients usually have a mechanically competent sphincter, but the impingement of the diaphragm on the stomach can result in propelling the contents of the supradiaphragmatic portion of the stomach up the esophagus and into the pharynx, resulting in patient complaints of regurgitation and aspiration, often confused with typical gastroesophageal reflux disease. Surgical reduction of the hernia results in relief of the dysphagia in 91% of patients.

DIAGNOSIS

A roentgenogram of the chest with the patient in the upright position can diagnose a hiatal hernia if it shows an air fluid level behind the cardiac shadow (Fig. 30–4). This is usually caused by a paraesophageal hernia or an intrathoracic stomach. The accuracy of the upper gastrointestinal barium study in detecting a paraesophageal hiatal hernia is greater than for a sliding hernia, since the latter can often spontaneously reduce. The paraesophageal hiatal hernia is a permanent herniation of the stomach into the thoracic cavity, so that a barium swallow provides the diagnosis in virtually every case. When seen, attention should be focused on the position of the gastroesophageal junction to differentiate it from a type II hernia (Figs. 30–1B and 30–2A).

Fiberoptic esophagoscopy is very useful in the diagnosis and classification of a hiatal hernia be-

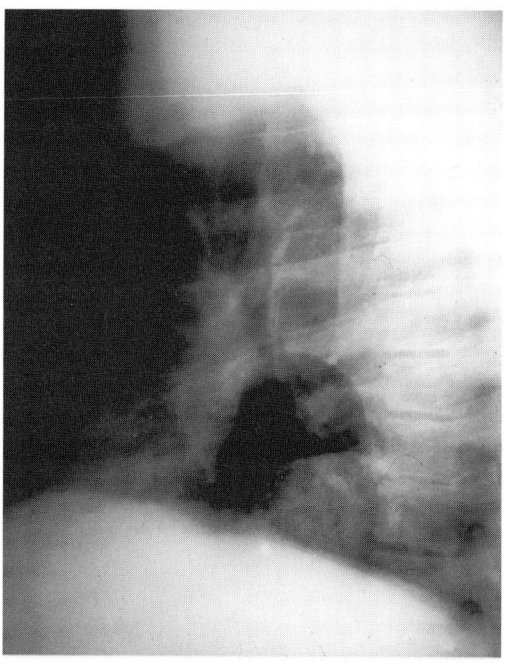

FIGURE 30–4. Lateral chest roentgenogram showing a posterior mediastinal air-fluid level in a gas bubble, indicating the presence of a paraesophageal hernia. (From DeMeester TR, Bonavina L. Paraesophageal hiatal hernia. In: Nyhus LM, Condon RE, eds. *Hernia.* 3rd ed. Philadelphia, Pa: JB Lippincott Co; 1989:688, with permission.)

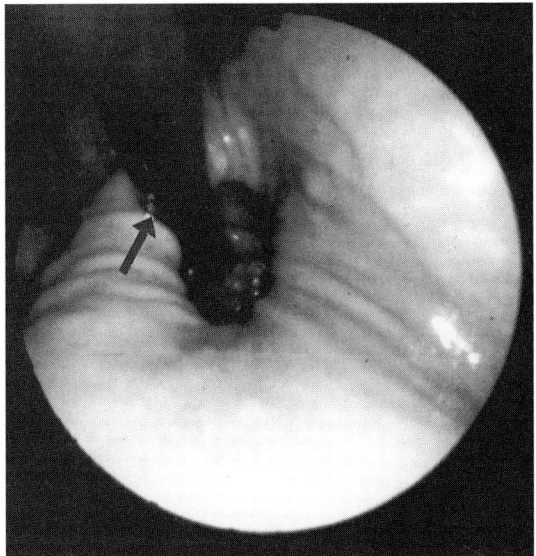
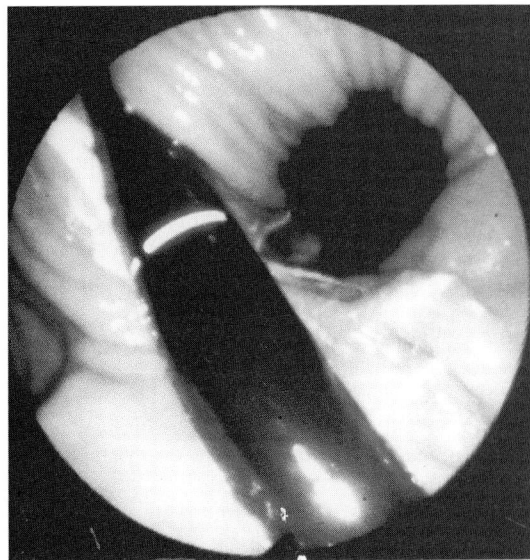
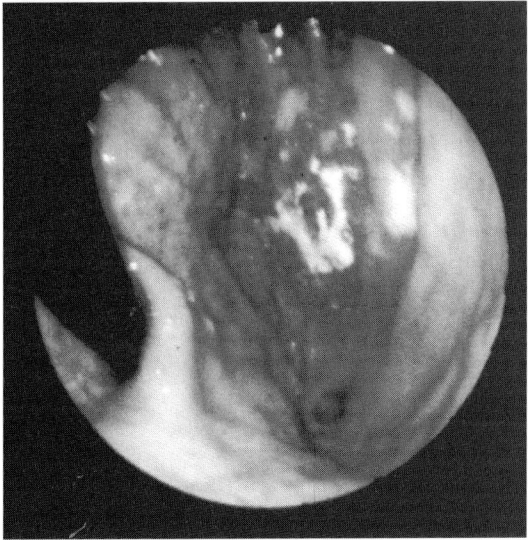

FIGURE 30-5. **A,** Endoscopic view through a retroflexed fiberoptic gastroscope showing the shaft of the scope *(arrow)* coming down through a sliding hernia. Note the gastric rugae extending above the impression caused by the crura of the diaphragm. **B,** Endoscopic view through a retroflexed fiberoptic gastroscope showing the shaft of the scope coming down through the gastroesophageal junction adjacent to a separate orifice of the paraesophageal hernia into which the gastric rugae ascend. **C,** Endoscopic view through a retroflexed fiberoptic gastroscope showing the shaft of the scope entering a hernia about midway up the side of a mixed hiatal hernial pouch that extends high into the thorax. (From DeMeester TR, Bonavina L. Paraesophageal hiatal hernia. In: Nyhus LM, Condon RE, eds. *Hernia.* 3rd ed. Philadelphia, Pa: JB Lippincott Co; 1989: 689, with permission.)

cause of the ability to retroflex the scope. In this position, a sliding hiatal hernia can be identified by noting a gastric pouch lined with rugae extending above the impression caused by the crura of the diaphragm (Fig. 30–5A) or measuring at least 2 cm between the crura (identified by having the patient sniff) and the squamous columnar junction on withdrawal of the scope.[4] A paraesophageal hernia is identified on retroversion of the scope by noting a separate orifice adjacent to the gastroesophageal junction into which gastric rugae ascend (Fig. 30–5B). A sliding-rolling or mixed hernia can be identified by noting a gastric pouch lined with rugae above the diaphragm with the gastroesophageal junction entering about midway up the side of the pouch (Fig. 30–5C).

PATHOPHYSIOLOGY

It has been assumed for a long time that a sliding hiatal hernia is associated with an incompetent distal esophageal sphincter, whereas a paraesophageal hiatal hernia constitutes a pure anatomic entity and is not associated with an incompetent cardia. Accordingly, surgical therapy has been directed toward making the cardia functional in patients with a sliding hernia and simply reducing the stomach into the abdominal cavity and closing the crura for a paraesophageal hernia.

Over the past three decades there has been an increased interest in the physiology of the gastroesophageal junction and its relationship to the various types of hiatal hernias. Physiologic testing with 24-hour esophageal pH monitoring has shown increased esophageal exposure to acid gastric juice in 60% of the patients with a paraesophageal hiatal hernia compared with the observed 71% incidence in patients with a sliding hiatal hernia. No relation was found between the symptoms experienced by the patient with a paraesophageal hernia and the competency of the cardia (Table 30–1). Thus, it is now recognized that paraesophageal hiatal hernia can be associated with pathologic gastroesophageal reflux.

Physiologic studies have shown that the competency of the cardia depends on an interrelationship of distal esophageal sphincter pressure, its length exposed to the positive pressure environment of the abdomen, and its overall length. A deficiency in any one of these manometric characteristics of the sphincter is associated with incompetency of the cardia regardless if a hernia is present.[4,5] Patients with a paraesophageal hernia who have incompetent cardias have been shown to have a distal esophageal sphincter with normal pressure but a shortened overall sphincter length that is displaced outside the positive pressure environment of the abdomen (Fig. 30–6A). In a sliding hernia, even though the sphincter appears to be within the chest on a roentgenographic barium study, it still can be exposed to abdominal pressure because of the surrounding hernia sac that functions as an extension of the abdominal cavity (Fig. 30–6B).[7] A high insertion of the phrenoesophageal membrane into the esophagus gives adequate length of the distal esophageal sphincter exposed to abdominal pressure. A low insertion gives inadequate length. The importance of the anatomic length of esophagus within the hernia sac has been emphasized by Bombeck, Dillard, and Nyhus[6] in their careful dissections of the hiatus. They showed that in 55 patients who underwent postmortem dissection, there were eight who had a hiatal hernia, five of whom had no evidence of esophagitis and therefore a competent cardia. In these five patients the phrenoesophageal membrane inserted 2 to 5 cm with a mean of 3.6 cm above the gastroesophageal junction. The other three patients had evidence of esophagitis and therefore an incompetent cardia. In these patients the membrane inserted 0 to 1 cm with a mean of 0.5 cm above the gastroesophageal junction. This difference was significant and emphasized the importance of an adequate length of intraabdominal esophagus in maintaining competency of the cardia even in the presence of a hiatal hernia.

In contrast to a paraesophageal hernia where the sphincter remains fixed in the abdomen, in a mixed type III hernia the sphincter moves extraperitoneally into the thorax through the widened hiatus along with a portion of the lesser curvature of the stomach and cardia and forms part of the wall of the hernia sac. Consequently, the lower esophageal sphincter lies outside the abdominal cavity and is unaffected by its environmental pressures. The loss of normal esophageal fixation that occurs in a type I sliding hernia or a type III mixed hernia results in the body of the esophagus being less able to carry out its propulsive function. This contributes to a greater exposure of the distal esophagus to refluxed gastric juice when components of an incompetent cardia are present.

In summary, the cause for a mechanical incompetency of the cardia is similar regardless of the type of hernia and is identical in patients who have an incompetent cardia and no hiatal hernia.

THERAPY

The presence of a paraesophageal hiatal hernia is an indication for surgical repair. The catastrophic, life-threatening complications of bleeding, infarction, and perforation that are part of the natural history of the hernia in about 25% of patients drive its surgical correction even in the elderly with a shorter life expectancy.

TABLE 30–1. SYMPTOMS IN 15 PATIENTS WITH A PARAESOPHAGEAL HERNIA COMPARED WITH RESULTS OF 24-HOUR ESOPHAGEAL pH MONITORING

Status	Positive	Negative
Heartburn	6 of 9	4 of 6
Regurgitation	6 of 9	3 of 6
Dysphagia	6 of 9	4 of 6
Postprandial fullness	8 of 9	3 of 6
Bleeding	4 of 9	1 of 6

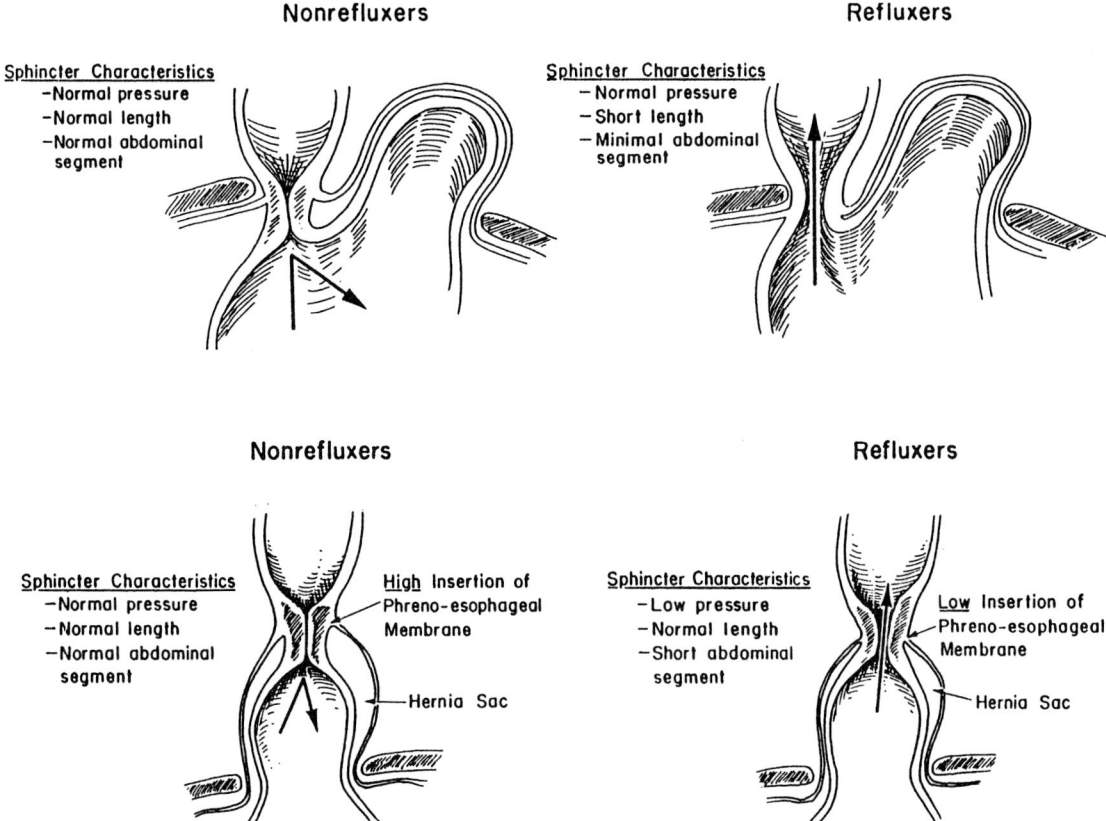

FIGURE 30-6. **A,** Anatomic and manometric difference between patients with a **paraesophageal hiatal hernia** with reflux and those without it, based on 24-hour esophageal pH monitoring. **B,** Anatomic and manometric difference between patients with a **sliding hiatal hernia** with reflux and those without it, based on 24-hour esophageal pH monitoring. (From DeMeester TR, Bonavina L. Paraesophageal hiatal hernia. In: Nyhus LM, Condon RE, eds. *Hernia*. 3rd ed. Philadelphia, Pa: JB Lippincott Co; 1989:690, 691, with permission.)

In the classic report of Skinner and Belsey,[7] 6 of 21 patients with a paraesophageal hernia treated medically because of minimal symptoms died from the complications of strangulation, perforation, exsanguinating hemorrhage, or acute dilation of the herniated intrathoracic stomach. These catastrophes occurred for the most part without warning. With this in mind, patients with a paraesophageal hernia are counseled to have elective repair of their hernia regardless of the severity of their symptoms or the size of the hernia. If surgery is delayed and repair is done on an emergency basis, there is a 19% operative mortality,[8] compared with less than 1% for an elective repair.[9]

Based on pathophysiologic studies on patients with a paraesophageal hiatal hernia, the repair of a paraesophageal hernia should include an antireflux procedure to correct the sphincter characteristics associated with a mechanically incompetent cardia. This is particularly necessary when the operation is performed on an urgent basis without preoperative studies. If time permits, preoperative evaluation with 24-hour esophageal pH monitoring and esophageal manometry allows the identification of patients with competent cardias. Such patients are candidates for a simple anatomic repair provided it can be done without surgical dissection of the cardia. If dissection of the cardia is necessary, an antireflux procedure should be added to the repair. Operative repair of sliding hiatal hernias are driven by symptoms of or complications of gastroesophageal reflux disease unless the patient is determined to have impingement of the stomach by the diaphragm as a cause of symptoms as discussed above.

REFERENCES

1. Eliska O. Phreno-oesophageal membrane and its role in the development of hiatal hernia. *Acta Anat.* 1973;86:137–150.
2. Kleitsch WP. Embryology of congenital diaphragmatic hernia. I. Esophageal hiatus hernia. *Arch Surg.* 1958;76:868–873.
3. Walther B, DeMeester TR, Lafontaine E, Courtney JV, Little AG, Skinner DB. Effect of paraesophageal hernia on sphincter function and its implication on surgical therapy. *Am J Surg.* 1984;147:111–116.
4. DeMeester TR, Lafontaine E, Joelsson BE, et al. Relationship of a hiatal hernia to the function of the body of the esophagus and the gastroesophageal junction. *J Thorac Cardiovasc Surg.* 1981;82:547–558.
5. Bonavina L, Evander A, DeMeester TR. Length of the distal esophageal sphincter and competency of the cardia. *Am J Surg.* 1986;151:25–34.
6. Bombeck TC, Dillard DH, Nyhus LM. Muscular anatomy of the gastroesophageal junction and role of the phrenoesophageal ligament. *Ann Surg.* 1966;164:643.
7. Skinner DB, Belsey RHR. Surgical management of esophageal reflux and hiatus hernia: long-term results with 1030 patients. *J Thorac Cardiovasc Surg.* 1967;53:33–54.
8. Postlethwait RW. *Surgery of the Esophagus.* New York, NY: Appleton-Century-Crofts; 1979:195–255.
9. DeMeester TR, Bonavina L, Albertucci M. Nissen fundoplication for gastroesophageal reflux disease: evaluation of primary repair in 100 consecutive patients. *Ann Surg.* 1986;204:9–20.

31

Esophageal Tumors

BRIAN SPIVACK and SAMUEL ERIC WILSON

Tumors of the esophagus are known to present late in their clinical course. Symptoms may be absent until the lumen is more than two thirds obstructed. The presenting symptom in most cases is dysphagia. Progressive dysphagia (from solids to liquids) should always be investigated with barium esophagogram or esophagoscopy or both. Odynophagia, pain, and hematemesis are late findings. Weight loss (often as much as 9 kg [20 lb]) in conjunction with esophageal carcinoma carries a worsened prognosis for survival.

BENIGN TUMORS

Benign tumors are rare and account for approximately 1% of neoplasms of the esophagus in most series. The actual incidence is no doubt higher since most are small and asymptomatic and are never discovered.

The most common benign esophageal tumor is the leiomyoma, most often seen in the 20- to 60-year age group. In autopsy series, leiomyomas are encountered on average in 1 in 1100 patients. Most (80% to 90%) are found in the middle or distal third of the esophagus. They are intramural lesions with typically intact overlying mucosa, although pressure ulceration with disruption of the mucosa can occur.

Barium swallow demonstrates a characteristically smooth outline, which is different from malignant tumors. Other benign lesions such as myoblastomas, congenital cysts or duplications, and neurofibromas can present with similar findings. Extrinsic lesions like mediastinal tumors, lymph nodes, bronchogenic cancers, and saccular aneurysms of the thoracic aorta can also mimic the leiomyoma. Aortogram is indicated if aneurysm is suspected.

The treatment for benign leiomyomas is excision by shelling out the lesion. No attempt at endoscopic biopsy should be made because scarring at the biopsy site may make extramucosal excision more difficult. In the case of giant leiomyoma or multiple tumors, esophageal resection may be necessary.

ESOPHAGEAL CARCINOMA

EPIDEMIOLOGY

Esophageal carcinoma represents 1% of all malignancies and 4% of gastrointestinal (GI) tract malignancies. The two most common histologic types are squamous cell carcinoma and adenocarcinoma. Historically, squamous cell carcinoma represented 90% to 95% of all tumors, but adenocarcinoma has been increasing rapidly over the past decade. By the mid-1980s, adenocarcinoma accounted for one third of all esophageal cancers, representing an increase of 4% to 10% per year, the most rapid increase in incidence of any malignancy. This increase in adenocarcinoma may be the result of more aggressive surveillance in patients with Barrett's esophagus (a premalignant lesion). There are 10,000 new cases of esophageal cancer each year and 9800 deaths per year. The male-to-female ratio is 2:1 and the peak age is 50 to 60 years. Traditionally, 20% of tumors occurred in the upper third of the esophagus, 35% in the middle third, and 45% in the lower third. This distribution is changing though because of the increase in adenocarcinoma which is almost exclusively found at or near the esophagogastric junction.

Like all upper aerodigestive carcinomas, tobacco and alcohol are causative factors. Certain diets, especially those high in nitrosamines and food contaminants like silica, have also been implicated. The incidence of esophageal cancer in the United States is between 1 and 2.6/100,000. In some endemic areas such as Iran, parts of Russia, South Africa, and Northern China, the incidence may reach as high as 100/100,000.

Barrett's esophagus is associated with a 10% incidence of adenocarcinoma. The rise in adenocarcinoma has paralleled a noted rise in recognition of Barrett's esophagus. Between 8% and 11% of patients with gastroesophageal reflux who have symptoms warranting biopsy are found to exhibit histologic evidence of Barrett's esophagus.

Other risk factors for the development of carcinomas include achalasia, reflux esophagitis, caustic burns (e.g., lye or acid ingestion), Plummer-Vinson syndrome, leukoplakia, esophageal diverticula, and tylosis.

Most patients present with advanced disease. Thus, the overall 5-year survival averages 5% to 10%. Prognosis is improved in early tumors; the 5-year survival for stage I disease may be as high as 55% to 85% and for stage II, approximately 30%.

CELL BIOLOGY AND PROGNOSIS

The recent growth in the field of oncogenes has taken on clinical significance. The gene product p53 or "tumor suppressor gene" has been found in 50% of Barrett's esophageal specimens but in fewer than 10% of Barrett's esophagus with adenocarcinoma. The loss of expression of this gene may be a marker for malignant potential. High levels of the ras p21 protein have been reported in some esophageal squamous cell specimens, as well as in other GI tract malignancies. The amplification of the int2 and hst1 genes has been reported in multiple malignancies. Their coamplification has been reported in 30% of esophageal tumors and is associated with a significantly higher metastasis rate and lower survival rate.

The evaluation of DNA ploidy in esophageal squamous cell carcinoma shows that aneuploidy is related to a worse prognosis, although the validity of ploidy as an independent factor is still under consideration.

The degree of differentiation and stage at diagnosis remain the most important prognostic indicators. If the tumor is confined to the mucosa without nodal metastases, and 80% 5-year survival has been reported.

MECHANISM OF SPREAD

The absence of a serosal barrier and the presence of a complex network of submucosal lymphatics that extends the length of the esophagus promote rapid local extension. Spread can then take place by a combination of (1) local mediastinal invasion, (2) dissemination by bloodstream, and (3) by lymphatics. The lymphatic and venous flow make spread from distal to proximal the most problematic. Adequate margins of 10 cm proximally are recommended. The tumor will have spread 3 cm in 65% of cases, 6 cm in 20%, and 9 cm in 10%. Skip lesions are common, and 15% of cases have malignant cells 5 cm from the primary. Lymph node metastases are present in 80% of cases; 50% in primary tumors smaller than 5 cm and 90% for primary tumors larger than 5 cm.

Pathologists have identified two types of tumor growth. The more common "vertical growth" type penetrates the submucosa early and is prone to metastasize via the bloodstream and lymphatics. The "superficial spreading" form of carcinoma is confined to the mucosa, and 80% 5-year survival rates have been reported.

Symptoms and Complications

The most common symptom of esophageal malignancy is dysphagia, often with the patient experiencing progression of dysphagia from solids to liquids before seeking help. Approximately 30% of patients will complain of pain and as many as a third of patients admitted to a cardiac unit for chest pain will be found to have pain of esophageal origin (most often, reflux esophagitis). Hoarseness as a result of recurrent laryngeal nerve compression, obstruction, weight loss, anemia, shortness of breath, and cardiac arrhythmias are late signs.

Complications of larger lesions include compression and invasion into surrounding structures. Aortoenteric fistula is lethal. Approximately 10% of patients develop a tracheal fistula and constant aspiration pneumonias. Median survival for patients with malignant tracheoesophageal fistulae is measured in weeks and palliation with radiotherapy or surgical bypass, while superior to esophageal intubation, provides limited relief.

TABLE 31–1. ESOPHAGEAL CANCER DEFINITION OF TNM*

Primary Tumor (T)
TX	Primary tumor cannot be assessed
T0	No evidence of primary tumor
Tis	Carcinoma in situ
T1	Tumor invades lamina propria or submucosa
T2	Tumor invades muscularis propria
T3	Tumor invades adventitia
T4	Tumor invades adjacent structures

Regional Lymph Nodes (N)
NX	Regional lymph nodes cannot be assessed
N0	No regional lymph node metastasis
N1	Regional lymph node metastasis

Distant Metastasis (M)
MX	Presence of distant metastasis cannot be assessed
M0	No distant metastasis
M1	Distant metastasis

Staging Grouping
Stage 0	Tis	N0	M0
Stage I	T1	N0	M0
Stage IIA	T2	N0	M0
	T3	N0	M0
Stage IIB	T1	N1	M0
	T2	N1	M0
Stage III	T3	N1	M0
	T4	Any N	M0
Stage IV	Any T	Any N	M1

*From American Joint Committee on Cancer. *Handbook for Staging of Cancer*, 4th ed. Philadelphia, Pa: J.B. Lippincott Co.; 1993:78.

Staging and Diagnosis

Accurate staging for esophageal cancer allows planning of an appropriate treatment strategy. Staging is dependent on the evaluation of intramural spread and nodal involvement. Prior to computed tomography (CT) scanning, only 28% of tumors were accurately staged using endoscopy and barium studies. The advent of CT allowed clinicians to increase the accuracy of staging to between 50% and 90%. Limitations of CT include the inability to evaluate depth of wall invasion and the reliance on size of lymph nodes as the sole indication of nodal metastases. CT remains the most accurate method of detecting distant metastases.

A recent advance in preoperative staging uses an endoscopically placed ultrasound probe (EUS) to detect depth of invasion and lymph node involvement. EUS is more sensitive to nodal metastases because it detects heterogenous areas within nodes, whether or not they are enlarged. The use of EUS to evaluate tumor size and nodal involvement, coupled with the use of CT for distant metastases has resulted in an 86% accuracy in preoperative staging according to a group from Memorial Sloan-Kettering Hospital.

Staging of esophageal carcinoma relies on the TNM system, see Table 31–1 for details.

Screening

Esophageal carcinoma is relatively rare in North America and Europe, making screening tests impractical for the general population. In endemic areas, however, simple screening tests are used to great advantage in discovering early tumors. In China, "Lawang" (literally, pulling in a net) employs a swallowed balloon covered by silk or nylon mesh with subsequent cytologic analysis of cells. Both early gastric and esophageal tumors are discovered in this way.

To improve the yield on standard tests for the evaluation of dysphagia or other complaints, experts suggest a number of improvements. Use of double contrast (barium and air) in esophagography improves the sensitivity of this examination. Endoscopy is likewise enhanced when Lugol spray is used for the evaluation of small, difficult-to-see lesions.

Preoperative Management

In addition to having a debilitating GI tract malignancy, patients with esophageal cancer often have multiple other health problems, making them poor treatment candidates. Respiratory status must be optimized by the cessation of tobacco smoking and the institution of bronchodilators as necessary. Nutritional status should be improved in cachectic patients for 1 to 2 weeks before operation but should not interfere with timely treatment. The use of total parenteral nutrition (TPN) and enteral feedings per se have not been shown to improve survival but are invaluable in maintaining constitutional status during radiation therapy. Bronchoscopy for upper lesions and in any patient with a history of pneumonia or hoarseness should be performed. Perioperative antibiotics should begin a few hours before operation.

Surgery

Operative treatment remains the mainstay of therapy. Lesions amenable to surgery include those without evidence of local or distant spread. Approximately 50% of patients have a resectable lesion, although some surgeons believe that preoperative radiotherapy increases this number. Lesions larger than 10 cm are usually not resectable. Even if cure is not possible in the fit patient, many would agree that surgery offers the best palliation. The fact that operative mortality remains 6% to 10%, however, should be considered in the incurable, debilitated patient.

The choice of operation varies somewhat ac-

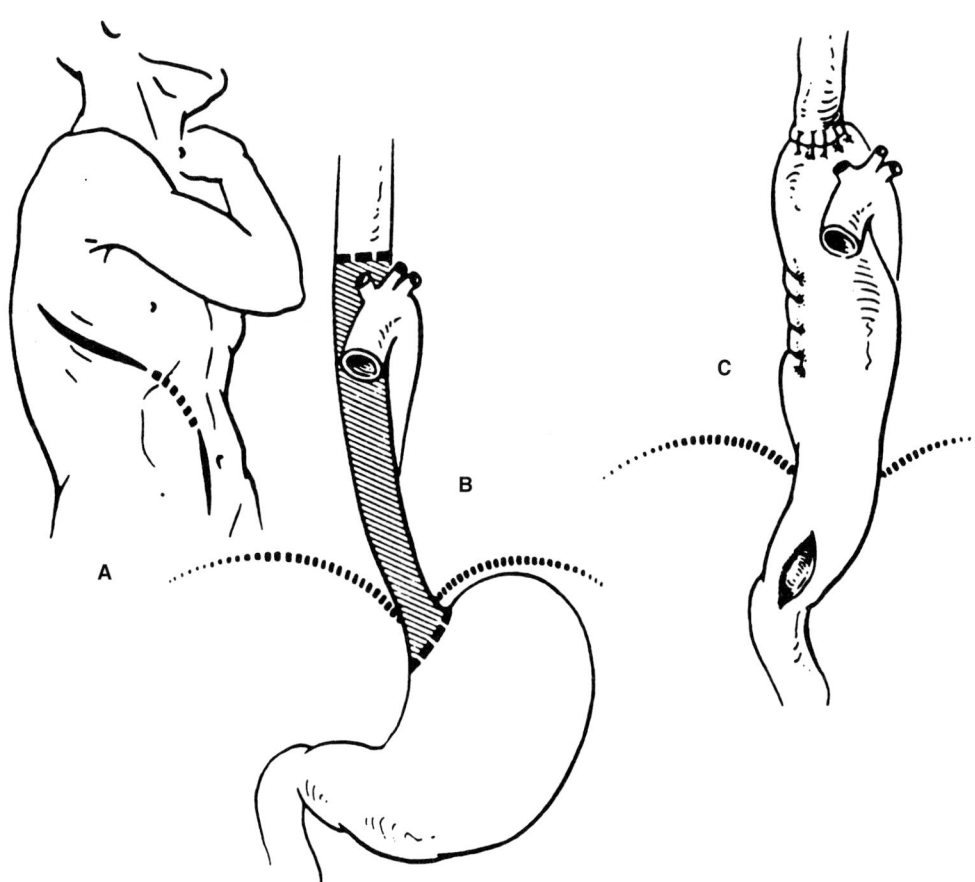

FIGURE 31–1. Standard thoracoabdominal Ivor-Lewis esophagogastrectomy for lesions of the lower and middle third of the thoracic esophagus. **A,** The continuous thoracoabdominal incision and the separate thoracic or abdominal incisions that may be used. **B,** Portion of the esophagus to be resected *(shaded area)*. **C,** Completed reconstruction with high intrathoracic esophagogastric anastomosis and gastric drainage procedure. (From Ellis FH Jr. Treatment of carcinoma of the esophagus and cardia. *Mayo Clin Proc.* 1960; 35:653.)

cording to the experience of the individual surgeon, no one procedure having been shown superior. For lower third lesions the left thoracoabdominal incision is commonly used. The most frequently used operation for any tumor, however, remains the Ivor-Lewis approach, which employs a laparotomy and right thoracotomy (Fig. 31–1). The stomach is mobilized on the right gastroepiploic vessels so that it may be pulled up into the chest for anastomosis with the proximal esophagus. The esophagus and gastric cardia are resected en bloc with a 10 cm proximal margin. The spleen is not removed. Pyloroplasty (since the vagus nerves are transected) and feeding jejunostomy are preformed. Wide chest tube drainage is employed, and an intact anastomosis is demonstrated by Hypaque swallow before beginning feeding.

Orringer et al have recently popularized the transhiatal esophagectomy without thoracotomy or "blunt esophagectomy," (Fig. 31–2). The entire procedure is carried out through a laparotomy and a cervical incision with the anastomosis performed in the neck. This operation may be used for any tumor not adherent to the tracheobronchial tree. Critics of this procedure cite the greater risk of bleeding, tracheal or thoracic duct tear, injury to the recurrent laryngeal nerve, and the failure to remove lymph nodes en bloc with the surgical specimen. Orringer and others, however, have reported no increased morbidity or mortality with similar survival rates. The need for thoracotomy and anastomosis in the chest is obviated, which is advantageous in these debilitated patients. Approximately 10% of esophageal anastomoses leak and an intrathoracic leak carries a 50% mortality. An anastomotic leak in the neck is much easier to treat than an intrathoracic leak (usually with local drainage only).

Some authors support the use of alternative bowel grafts (like colon) in patients with expected long-term survival. Patients with colonic interposition have superior functional results with better long-term swallowing and less reflux. This procedure is most often reserved for benign processes.

High cervicothoracic lesions present special problems in surgical management. It is often impossible to attain a full 10-cm margin. If these tumors are very high, a laryngopharyngoesophagectomy with or without neck dissection may be necessary. Adherence to the trachea might require resection and mediastinal tracheostomy. Reconstruction of the esophagus and pharynx with skin and muscle flaps or a free transfer of jejunum are complicated procedures and often need to be multistaged. Many clinicians treat these types of lesions with radiation and chemotherapy only with 5-year survival as high as 30%.

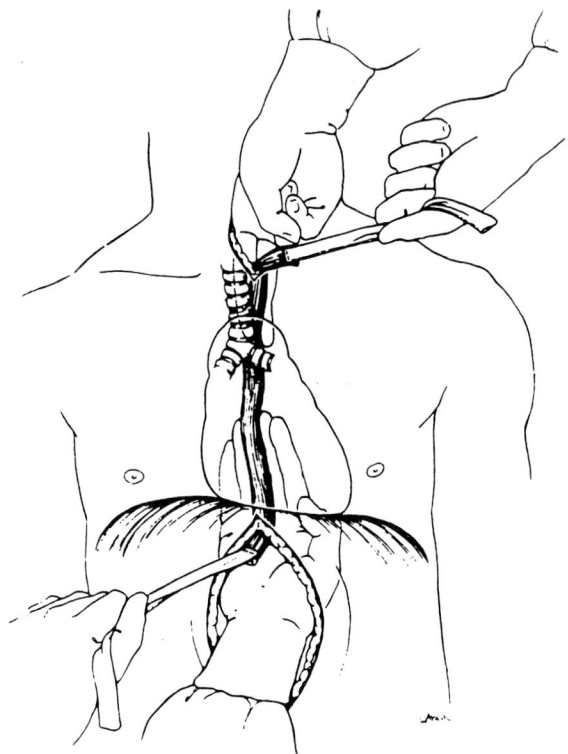

FIGURE 31–2. Transhiatal dissection of the lower esophagus through the diaphragmatic hiatus is achieved through an upper midline abdominal incision. Penrose drains around either end of the esophagus are used for traction during the dissection. The upper thoracic esophagus is mobilized through a limited cervical incision. (Modified from Orringer MB, Sloan H. Esophagectomy without thoracotomy. *J Thorac Cardiovasc Surg.* 1978;76:643.)

ADJUVANT MANAGEMENT

Treatment failures are characterized by both local recurrence and distant metastasis. Radiation therapy, chemotherapy, or both, used in conjunction with surgery, have been gaining favor in the management of this frequently systemic disease.

Investigators at Wayne State University (1983–1985) tested a nonsurgical treatment regimen including cisplatin, 5-FU, and 3000 cGy radiotherapy followed by bleomycin and mitomycin with 2000 cGy. Good control of disease was obtained, but toxicity was felt to be prohibitive. Enthusiasm over the results of the Wayne

State group led others to search for a more tolerable regimen to be used in conjunction with surgical extirpation.

In three early studies, regimens employing preoperative radiotherapy and a combination of chemotherapeutic drugs including cisplatin and infusional 5-FU have yielded an approximately 25% pathologic complete response with apparent improved survival in all resectable cases. Very little, if any, difference between adenocarcinoma and squamous cell carcinoma is shown in these studies. Further prospective, randomized trials to elucidate the appropriate dose of chemotherapeutic agents and radiotherapy are currently ongoing.

PALLIATION

The best form of palliation remains surgery with placement of a nonanatomic jejunal or colonic segment for bypass if the tumor-bearing esophagus cannot be removed. Radiotherapy can effectively treat dysphagia in about 50% of patients who are too ill to undergo surgery.

Intubation of the esophagus can be performed by esophagoscopy or laparotomy (e.g., Celestin's, Souttar, or Mousseau-Barbin tubes). Use of such tubes is fraught with complications including bleeding, blockage, perforation, and slippage either up into the pharynx or down into the stomach. These tubes have become unpopular and are generally reserved for high-risk patients with a 1- to 2-month survival expectancy who are in danger of obstruction.

Recently, enthusiasm over endoscopic laser therapy (ELT) has been gaining. Either the Nd:YAG or the argon laser has been used to recanalize the esophagus in patients with obstruction who are unresectable. Good palliation has been reported with frequent treatments of 6 to 8 weeks. Use of hematoporphyrin derivatives to enhance the argon dye method has been reported and may even be used for cure in some instances. Lasers have been used most successfully in short lesions such as those found in anastomotic recurrences.

OTHER MALIGNANT TUMORS

Other malignant tumors of the esophagus, besides squamous cell carcinoma and adenocarcinoma, are uncommon. Series of esophageal neoplasms report a 1.2% to 7.2% incidence of other histologic findings. Presenting symptoms of progressive dysphagia, pain, and weight loss are the same as in the other malignancies.

Rare case reports of carcinoid tumor, various sarcomas, and lymphomas are found in the literature. The three most common "other tumors" include leiomyosarcoma, melanoma, and oat cell carcinoma. All are treated in similar fashion: resection with or without chemotherapy and radiation. Leiomyosarcoma tends not to spread as rapidly as the others and 5-year survival rates have been reported at 25%. Melanoma is widely resistant to all therapies but surgical resection and lymphadenectomy. Nodal metastases are frequent, resulting in a poor 5-year survival rate. Small cell carcinoma of the esophagus has the worst survival rate and is treated by chemotherapy with surgery reserved for palliation. Small cell carcinoma may present with a paraneoplastic syndrome as occasionally occurs in lung cancer of this cell type.

REFERENCES

1. Botet JF, Lightdale CJ, Zauber AG, et al. Preoperative staging of esophageal cancer: comparison of endoscopic US and dynamic CT. *Radiology.* 1991;181(2):419–425.
2. Caldwell CB, Bains MS, Burt M. Unusual malignant neoplasms of the esophagus. *J Thorac Cardiovasc Surg.* 1991;101(1):100–107.
3. Duhaylongsod FG, Wolfe WG. Barrett's esophagus and adenocarcinoma of the esophagus and gastroesophageal junction. *J Thorac Cardiovasc Surg.* 1991;102(1):36–42.
4. Kelsen D, Atiz OT. Therapy of upper gastrointestinal tract cancers. *Curr Probl Cancer.* 1991;15(5):239–284.
5. Ohno S, Mori M, Tsutsui S, et al. Growth patterns and prognosis of submucosal carcinoma of the esophagus. *Cancer.* 1991;68(2):335–340.
6. Postlethwait RW. Benign tumors and cysts of the esophagus. *Surg Clin North Am.* 1983;63(4):925–931.

32
Obstructing Esophageal Disease

DAVID G. RIMER

This chapter addresses the techniques and treatments currently available to deal with a problem common to almost all esophageal diseases, benign and malignant, a problem that may often be the presenting symptom and is sometimes the only disability—esophageal obstruction. In benign esophageal stricture proper dilation technique is easy, safe, and very rewarding. The technique of esophageal dilation is similar for both benign and malignant lesions, but special problems and special applications of dilation to benign and malignant lesions are reviewed in this chapter. The poor prognosis and the limitations of therapy in the treatment of malignant lesions forces us to focus primarily on palliation. Surgery, radiation, chemotherapy, and mechanical interventions for palliation of malignant esophageal obstruction are reviewed.

BENIGN STRICTURE

The great majority of benign strictures are the result of peptic esophagitis. This can occur at any age, even during childhood, but is more common after age 40. The fundamental abnormality is that of excessive acid reflux resulting in an inflammatory reaction in the distal esophagus, which leads to scarring after repeated injury and healing. There may or may not be ulceration, which would influence the nature of the stricture. Benign strictures are often concentric but may be "valvular" or eccentric (semilunar). Whatever scar occurs will contract with healing, which narrows the lumen. A hiatus hernia may often be present. Whether this contributes to the acid reflux is still a matter of controversy, but when a hiatus hernia is present, blind bougienage may be more hazardous (see below).

There are many other causes of benign stricture. The older literature reports strictures secondary to infectious diseases, such as tuberculosis, which are rare in today's practice. Currently the differential diagnosis includes: achalasia, corrosive injury, scleroderma with associated reflux esophagitis, radiation injury, postsurgery stricture, congenital webs, and Schatzki's ring. Treatment of the stricture may be modified depending on its origin.

Congenital malformations may occur in the form of a membranous diaphragm or web. These may occur in the distal esophagus, but most are in the proximal esophagus at the level of the cricopharyngeus. Most are quite fragile. Since the flexible endoscope is introduced essentially "blind" to a point just beyond the cricopharyngeus, a congenital web may not be visualized prior to being ruptured. With careful observation as the scope is withdrawn, the operator may only see a fragment of the web or a raw area of bleeding. If the web is not dilated by the scope, it will usually respond to a single passage of a 48F or 50F Maloney bougie. Occasionally, thicker, tougher, semilunar webs require serial dilations.

The lower esophageal ring, or Schatzki's ring, occurs at the squamocolumnar junction. It is fibrous, but it is a static process; it does not ordinarily close down as does a cicatricial stricture. When a ring is discovered, one can assume it has been there for years. Rings rarely cause dysphagia or symptomatic obstruction. It is not proper to blame new onset dysphagia on an old ring. If a ring does require dilation, the passage of a single 54F Maloney bougie will often be sufficient.

MALIGNANT OBSTRUCTION: POOR PROGNOSIS, LIMITED GOALS

There are 11,000 new cases of cancer of the esophagus per year, or 10 per 100,000 men in the United States. Cancer of the esophagus is more common among blacks (6:1), more in men (10:1), and strongly correlated with smoking and excessive alcohol ingestion, especially during young adulthood. In the United States the incidence of squamous cell carcinoma has remained constant, but the incidence of adenocarcinoma has risen 100% in the last 15 years and now exceeds the rate of squamous cell carcinoma in white men below 55 years of age. Barrett's esophagus (metaplastic gastric mucosa in the lower esophagus) is much more common in men than women and more common in whites. The incidence of Barrett's esophagus is rising; when these lesions show dysphagia, there is a risk for adenocarcinoma. This may account for the observed increase in adenocarcinoma.

The treatments available for carcinoma of the esophagus have been disappointing. There are differences between adenocarcinoma, arising from gastric mucosa, and squamous cell carcinoma, but surgical resection gives a 15% 5-year survival at best and recurrence after radiation, chemotherapy, and laser therapy is inevitable.

Several factors, which encourage spread, including the rich lymphatic network and the lack of a serosal barrier, make for late discovery and poor prognosis. Only in the rare serendipitous finding of an early lesion confined to the mucosa, without node involvement, can one consider resection for cure. Alternatively, palliation may be achieved through surgery, chemotherapy, radiation, stent placement, laser, tumor probe, injection, or a combination of modalities.

Earlam and Cunha-Melo reviewed outcome in patients with squamous cell carcinoma of the esophagus. Surgery was considered in 58%, and 39% had the tumor resected. The overall operative mortality was 13%. The survival rates for 1, 2, and 5 years were 18%, 9%, and 4%, respectively. This dismal outlook may be improved for highly selected cases, but the 5-year survival rate is 15% to 18% at best. In view of this, it is most helpful, early on, to define treatment goals that are appropriate to the clinical state. Aggressive, invasive, hazardous therapy cannot be justified if the patient spends his remaining weeks disproportionately the captive of a futile medical effort.

Failing surgical resection for cure, we try to extend life, and, most importantly, palliate the dysphagia, pain, or fistula that the cancer may cause.

Dysphagia is often the presenting symptom and is by far the most common problem early in the disease. Other than surgery, a variety of treatments are available to reduce tumor bulk or keep the esophageal lumen open.

Dilation is often sufficient to keep the esophageal lumen open. It should be done slowly, with gentle progression every 2 to 3 days until an adequate caliber is reached. Periodic reinforcement is necessary, but as long as the patient can go at least 2 weeks between sessions, this usually is very acceptable treatment. This is particularly true if the lesion is suitable for dilation with Maloney bougies. Wire-guided dilators are more often necessary for malignant lesions, but episodic dilation with either technique is still often the safest and most convenient method of therapy.

Surgical palliation is effective for many patients with carcinoma of the esophagus; however, surgical mortality is still 5% to 10%, and the attendant morbidity and recovery time may occupy a considerable percentage of the patient's remaining life. With the alternatives now available, surgical palliation is often inappropriate and less often necessary than it used to be.

The decision for palliative treatment should be driven by symptoms, not by laboratory data or imaging. It is rare that treating an asymptomatic metastatic lesion will be rewarding; save your ammunition.

Muller et al surveyed 1201 papers on surgery in esophageal cancer during the decade ending 1990. Postoperative mortality was reduced from 18% during the 24-year period prior to 1978 to 11% during the period 1980 to 1988. In contrast, long-term survival has not improved in spite of extensive excision procedures and adjuvant chemotherapy and radiation therapy. They found that 56% of patients presenting to surgeons had resectable disease. Of these, 80% left the hospital, 27% survived 1 year, and 10 % survived 5 years. Even with localized disease they found no difference in 5-year survival between surgery and radiotherapy.

Radiation therapy alone does not extend survival, but may offer temporary tumor shrinkage relieving dysphagia for many weeks. Preoperative therapy with radiation or chemotherapy alone has not proven effective in improving objective response, surgical outcome, or recurrence rate. However, low-dose radiation in combination with agents such as cis-platinum, 5-FU, mitomycin-C, and vincristine has been used as preoperative adjuvant therapy, and between 10% to 36% of such patients enjoy a complete remission. Patients who have a good preoperative response have a better survival rate than those who do not respond. Thus, a preoperative trial of therapy may provide a prognostic indicator for postoperative long-term survival. Radiation and chemotherapy are more effective in squamous cell carcinoma than in adenocarcinoma.

Whereas surgery may provide good palliation for some patients with cancer of the lower two thirds of the esophagus, radiation provides good palliation in about 50% of patients and is preferred to surgery for lesions of the upper third.

Other innovations in treatment such as injection with ethanol or 5-FU plus sodium morrhuate, or intraluminal radiation, are of interest but remain unproven. At best, however, we can expect only alternative palliative treatments.

TECHNIQUES OF ESOPHAGEAL DILATION

The initial endoscopic examination of a patient with symptomatic obstructing esophageal disease may not only reveal the diagnosis but presents an opportunity for initiating treatment in both benign and malignant obstruction. The initial dilation may often be accomplished by passage of the endoscope through the lesion under direct visual control. The initial endoscopy also delineates the characteristics of the lesion, which will determine how subsequent dilations should be done. If the endoscope cannot be passed initially, a subsequent endoscopy after appropriate dilation must be planned to completely visualize the lesion and obtain biopsy specimens. Always obtain a turnaround view of a lower esophageal stricture to check for adenocarcinoma of the stomach invading the esophagus.

WIRE-GUIDED DILATION

If a stricture is narrow (<12 mm/36 F), very long, tortuous, or angulated or has a shelf or diverticulum, use a guide wire. The guide wire is usually placed endoscopically, but in the case of a very tight stricture, it may be placed (with great care) under fluoroscopic guidance. Watch that the spring tip of the wire seeks the lumen easily, without undue pressure, and remains straight. Stop and withdraw if the tip begins to curl. The spring tip is easy to see fluoroscopically.

The Savary guide wire is better than the Puestow, because the spring tip is graduated and is less likely to bend or break at the junction with the wire and cause injury to the gastric wall. The Microvasive wire (#5174) is also useful. It has a long and very flexible tip, but the wire itself is quite stiff (Fig. 32–1). In any case, use a wire with indelible markers to indicate the depth of insertion.

Endoscopic placement of the wire is appropriate if the scope can traverse the lesion or if the distal lumen and gastric cavity can be seen well enough to allow safe passage under direct vision in advance of the scope. Lay the wire on the greater curve, in the antrum. The assistant then pulls the scope out in 5-cm increments as the operator feeds the wire at the same rate. The assistant grabs the wire at the teeth as the scope is being removed, and secures the position of the wire at this point. With the scope completely removed

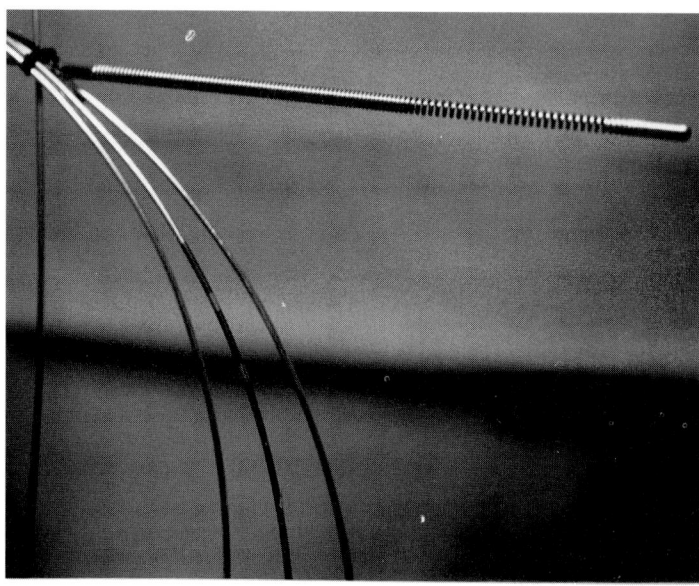

FIGURE 32–1. Insertion guide wire with markers.

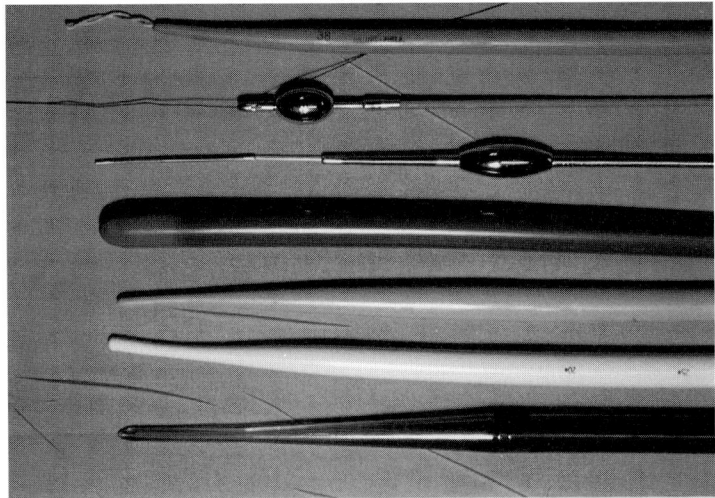

FIGURE 32–2. Various dilators: Tucker (pull through), Pilling (silk thread guided), Puestow, Hurst, Maloney, American Endoscopy (wire guided), Savary-Guillard (wire guided).

and set aside, the operator then advances the dilator over the wire. When the tip of the dilator reaches the teeth, the assistant shifts position to hold the wire beyond the butt of the dilator firmly in place to maintain position. The wire should not advance as the dilator is passed into the esophagus and the lesion dilated. Be careful not to impact the dilator on the spring tip. The operator then withdraws the dilator by holding the wire rigidly in place a short distance from the butt end of the dilator and sliding the dilator to that fixed point, repeating the process so that the dilator, but *not* the wire, moves, until the assistant can grasp the wire at the teeth again and maintain the position of the wire, while dilators are changed and the process repeated. With this technique the wire should not move once it has been positioned, and fluoroscopy is not necessary. Check the markers on the wire each time to make sure the position is maintained. Fluoroscopy is only necessary (except for initial passage of the wire through a tight stricture as mentioned above) if the physician needs to check the position of the spring tip in the stomach as the dilators are changed.

Both American Endoscopy and Savary-Guillard dilators (Wilson-Cook) work well. However, American Endoscopy wire-guided dilators have a shorter taper (Fig. 32–2); this is helpful when there is limited space distal to the stricture. The Savary-Guillard dilator has a 20-cm taper, which may require a loop of guide wire in the stomach. This gentle taper makes the dilation easier, sometimes deceptively so, and one may be tempted to overdilate. It is helpful to have markers on the dilator indicating the distance from the tip and from the shoulder of the dilator. Always note the point where the shoulder of the dilator enters the stricture and note any resistance or pain at that point. Using American Endoscopy dilators, when the first dilator is passed, with the shoulder 5 to 10 cm beyond the stricture, the wire may be repositioned and excess wire withdrawn. This prevents angulation of the wire distally, which can injure the stomach and ruin the wire.

BALLOON DILATION

Balloon dilators can be passed either through the scope or over a wire, and the dilation is either under direct vision or fluoroscopic control. The plastic balloons have a low compliance and will not expand beyond a fixed diameter (but may burst with excessive force). The advantages claimed for balloon dilation are several: The force is applied radially only, whereas bougies transmit axial longitudinal force as well. The greatest force is applied to the narrowest point, and all of the force is directed to the stricture. Balloons do not require as much room distal to the stricture as the taper of a Savary-type dilator, and they can be used even with a narrow esophageal inlet, which would limit the size of a bougie.

Balloons are usually inflated with water. For fluoroscopy, use 60% Hypaque diluted 1:3 with water. Always use an "inflation gun" to control the pressure and keep it constant. Test the balloon first, deflate it, then lubricate it with silicone before sliding it through the biopsy channel. The response to dilation may be monitored in several ways. Most important is to abort immediately if the patient experiences undue pain. Under direct vision, test for the ability of the balloon to slide easily to and fro through the previously strictured area. With fluoroscopic monitoring, position the partially filled balloon, and watch the waist gradually efface as you increase the pressure. After the dilation be sure to deflate completely before pulling the balloon back through the channel of the scope.

Blind dilation (without fluoroscopy) may be done with a balloon over a guide wire. Test the balloon as usual, then insert over the wire *past* the stricture. Inflate fully and pull back snugly against the stricture. Deflate, withdraw 2 to 3 cm, and reinflate. This may need to be repeated several times. Finally, pull the inflated balloon through the strictured area, thus documenting and calibrating a successful dilation.

Balloon dilators are useful as an initial treatment on first encounter with a tight stricture. After dilation under direct vision the scope may then be advanced and the lesion thoroughly examined along with the rest of the upper gastrointestinal tract. Balloons may also be useful in larger (>12 mm) but asymmetric strictures. Some authorities also recommend balloon dilation for very fibrotic, lengthy, or irregular strictures.

Balloons continue to be useful, but our initial enthusiasm for balloons has waned. Balloon dilators are not safer than Maloney or Savary-type dilators. There is no tactile sensation, and one may lack assurance that the dilation was achieved without fluoroscopy. Very fibrotic strictures may not respond to the pressures obtainable. Fibrotic strictures require finely controlled serial dilations, and they often crack rather than stretch. There is the risk of excessive dilation and rupture, especially if a large diameter balloon is used. Lastly, the balloons are relatively fragile and are much more expensive and labor intensive for the assistant than bougies.

MALONEY MERCURY-FILLED BOUGIES

Rubber mercury-filled bougies have been used for generations to dilate esophageal lesions, and they remain the cheapest and simplest of dilators. Hurst dilators, originally used, have a blunt end and have been supplanted by Maloney dilators, which are tapered (Fig. 32-2). The taper makes the Maloney dilator easier and more comfortable to pass, and acts as a seeker to guide the dilator into the esophagus and through the lesion.

When the channel through the lesion is relatively straight, at 10 to 12 mm (30 to 36 F) or more in diameter, not too long, and without hazards such as a diverticulum or blind pouch, then "blind" dilation with Maloney dilators is safe, quicker, easier, and far less expensive than other techniques. In practice, Maloney dilators are used most often for benign lesions, but many malignant lesions will meet the above criteria.

Intravenous premedication is not necessary unless the patient is unduly anxious. We anesthetize the back of the throat prior to the procedure. Dilation may be done with the patient sitting, but most prefer lying on the left side. The dilator should be wet and lubricated with K-Y jelly. Hold the dilator with the right hand and guide the tapered end along the base of the tongue with the left index finger. This projects the force of the dilation downward, in the axis of the esophagus, rather than allowing the dilator to push against the posterior pharynx. The left index finger also can help to keep the tip in the midline as it passes the hypopharynx, may help to push the dilator through a lesion, and provides greater sensitivity to the feel of the dilator as it traverses the lesion. Keep the patient's head flexed forward, chin down, then pass the dilator as the patient swallows or just after a cough. When the tip nears the distal esophagus, have the patient take a deep breath. This lowers the diaphragm and straightens the esophagus, and the dilator will slip through. Do not forget to allow for esophageal stretching; be sure the shoulder of the dilator actually passes beyond the stricture.

It is very important to know when the shoulder of the dilator enters the lesion and to know where the tip and the shoulder of the dilator are relative to important landmarks: the top of the lesion, bottom of the lesion, and lower esophageal sphincter or diaphragmatic hiatus. The measurements of these landmarks (distance from the teeth) made during the preliminary endoscopy should be clearly in mind before starting any blind dilation, and the bougie must be marked so you know, from the outside, where the tip and the shoulder are relative to the lesion. (American Endoscopy dilators have two scales, measuring the distance from the tip and the distance from the shoulder of the dilator.) A ballpoint pen makes a convenient temporary marker; (it wipes off with an alcohol sponge). If the dilator meets an obstruction *where it should not,* stop and pull back.

Dilate frequently, every 2 to 3 days, and start each dilation at least two sizes below the previous maximum. Limit dilation at one session to three sizes that actually stretch (meet resistance). With a stricture that is very tight, long, or due to scarring postradiation therapy, dilate slowly and gently, limiting increments to one or two sizes that meet resistance per session. At 13 mm (40 F) the patient will still have dysphagia for solids. The goal would be at least 15 mm (45 F); at this level symptoms are still present but acceptable (see Table 32–1). Reflux peptic strictures are mucosal, therefore can be dilated to a larger size more easily. Some authorities dilate these abruptly with the passage of a single 50-F Maloney dilator, but I do not recommend it. A tough fibrous stricture such as a congenital web may respond better if you first take bites with a biopsy forceps. A fibrous stricture will crack, not stretch, and must be kept open with repeat dilations during healing. Look for blood on the dilator. Radiation strictures and carcinoma are transmural with greater risk of disruption, so dilate slowly and more cautiously with less stretching per session.

Even with a malignant lesion dilation alone is often sufficient treatment. If a lesion can be kept open with dilation no more often than every 2 weeks, it may not be necessary to resort to more invasive or expensive therapy.

CONTRAINDICATIONS AND HAZARDS TO DILATION

The various problems leading to esophageal obstruction are more common with advancing age, and age may be accompanied by other problems as well. Poor dentition often leads to poorly masticated food, which is more likely to plug a narrowed segment. Cervical arthritis becomes more common, and osteophytes protruding from the bodies of the cervical vertebrae may interfere with endoscopy and make dilation more hazardous. It would be quite rare for deformity of the cervical spine to make endoscopy and dilation impossible, but be alert to coexisting problems such as narrowed esophageal inlet or Zenker's diverticulum. I recently encountered a patient with all these problems, a very narrowed inlet, cervical osteophytes, and a hypopharyngeal diverticulum, who required very careful passage of a 6-mm bronchoscope into the distal esophagus so that a wire could be introduced for wire-guided bougienage.

Zenker's diverticulum is the most common esophageal diverticulum. It results from herniation of the esophageal mucosa posteriorly through the space between the inferior pharyngeal constrictor (above) and the cricopharyngeus (below). The orifice of the diverticulum is directly posterior, opposite the cricoid cartilage, at the junction of the hypopharynx and esophagus. The pouch swings caudad as it enlarges, putting it in the same axis as the esophagus. Thus, there is great risk that any per oral intubation may seek the wrong orifice and perforate the sac of the diverticulum if forced. If a patient has cervical dysphagia, obtain a barium swallow before endoscopy. Midesophageal and epiphrenic diverticuli are less common and pose less risk because the opening is at right angles to the esophageal lumen.

A hiatus hernia may present a problem because of slackness of the esophagus and the herniated stomach. The axis of the esophagus, stricture, and herniated stomach may be curved so that the bougie will point toward the gastric wall lying on the surface of the diaphragm medial to the hiatus. The danger from blind bougienage in this instance is that the resistance of the hernia wall and diaphragm may easily be confused with the resistance of the stricture itself. A wire guide should be used to minimize risk in all these instances.

When an upper respiratory infection occurs during a course of dilations, one should start the session two to three sizes below usual. Certain particularly dangerous coexisting problems, such as thoracic aortic aneurysm, severe chronic pulmonary disease, recent esophageal surgery or perforation, bleeding disorders, or recent myocardial infarction, require careful thought before embarking on a series of dilations. Coexistent esophageal varices and stricture (or postsclerotherapy stricture) present a serious dilemma. There is no reliable rule, even though experienced endoscopists allege that varices rarely bleed with dilation for peptic stricture, and each case must be individually judged.

TABLE 32–1. MAXIMUM SIZES FOR DILATION OF VARIOUS STRICTURES

Benign short distal stricture due to reflux	50 F–56 F
Radiation stricture	50 F
Carcinoma	50 F
Lye stricture	45 F
Stricture longer than 8–10 cm	40 F

The principal complications of esophageal dilation are perforation, bleeding, and pulmonary aspiration. The overall risk is about 0.3%, and is higher in complex strictures (longer, narrower, more angulated, and lye induced). The risk of perforation in esophageal stent placement is about 10%. Bacteremia is more common after esophageal dilation than most other gastroenterologic procedures. Prophylactic antibiotics may be indicated in selected cases.

ESOPHAGEAL STENTS

The concept of stenting the obstructing malignant lesion to maintain a patent lumen is an old one, but it fell into disrepute because the surgical placement of Celestin tubes in the esophagus caused excessive morbidity and mortality. More recently, Boyce in the United States and Tytgat in Holland have proposed a relatively simple method of stent manufacture and placement, which has led to their widespread use. Several commercial stents and placement systems are now available, and newer expandable stents promise an even greater range of usefulness.

SELECTION OF PATIENTS FOR STENT PLACEMENT

When the stent is used for the palliation of dysphagia, it will usually be a secondary maneuver in patients who have failed other cancer therapy. Do not use a stent before radiation therapy or chemotherapy. When the lesion shrinks, the stent will slip out.

On the other hand, a patient with a fistula should be stented immediately; there is no other satisfactory treatment of tracheoesophageal fistula (glues and tissue injections are yet to be proven), and symptomatic palliation of this miserable complication deserves top priority.

CONTRAINDICATIONS TO STENT PLACEMENT

There are four main contraindications to the use of a stent. With a high lesion, less than 1 to 2 cm below the cricopharyngeus, the top funnel of the stent may cause unacceptable discomfort. A custom-made stent with a very short funnel may overcome this objection. The uncooperative patient or the patient "in extremis" may not benefit, although any patient with a fistula should be considered for stenting; even a few days of respite are worth it. A lesion that can be kept open with periodic dilation should not be stented unless the frequency of dilation becomes a burden.

PRELIMINARY EVALUATION FOR STENT PLACEMENT

Preliminary evaluation of the patient should include a chest x-ray, barium swallow, and computed tomography of the chest. Note the location of the lesion, its length and overall characteristics, and the axis of the lumen in relation to the stomach. Is the lumen straight? Check for anterior cervical spurs that will interfere with placement, and rule out Zenker's diverticulum. If the patient has had previous manipulation, look for mediastinal paraesophageal abscess. Bronchoscopy may be useful, especially when a fistula is present.

At the time of endoscopic evaluation, certain observations are important. What is the overall configuration? Is the channel straight? Is there a shoulder to hold the stent from slipping down? Is the lesion concentric? Will it be safe to dilate blind with Maloney bougies? Accurate measurements must be made from the teeth to (1) the upper esophageal sphincter, (2) the top of lesion, (3) the bottom of lesion, and (4) the lower esophageal sphincter or esophagogastric junction. The lesion is then dilated, as described above, and made ready for stent insertion.

A very firm lesion may squeeze a mercury-filled bougie, and one may falsely assume more dilation than has actually occurred. In preparation for stent placement, the Savary-type dilators are preferable.

CHOOSE THE RIGHT STENT

Choose the right stent for the lesion. The top funnel and the distal flange need to "straddle" the lesion to prevent movement, and the stent diameter must be small enough to be passed without undue trauma but big enough so the lesion squeezes the stent. Either the top funnel or the distal end may need to extend farther beyond the main growth to prevent satellite lesions from growing into the lumen. With a fistula, the top funnel may need to be larger to block the fistula opening. Anticipate how the stent will lie; do not let the distal end impact on the diaphragmatic curve of the esophagus. Lesions near the cricopharyngeus (upper esophageal sphincter) need a short funnel as mentioned above. The minimum clearance is about 1 cm. If the top of the stent protrudes into the area of the upper esophageal sphincter or above, it is poorly tolerated. In this case, make a trial placement of a stent without the distal flange (retaining ring). If it is tolerated, replace with a permanent stent.

STENT PLACEMENT

Stent insertion is traumatic. The patient should have prophylactic antibiotics, if indicated, and should be generously premedicated with meperidine (Demerol) and midazolam (Versed). Fluoroscopy may be helpful, but is usually not necessary; the procedure is akin to esophageal dilation, with or without a wire guide. The stent may be inserted with the endoscope, a rubber bougie, a microvasive balloon, or with a commercial introducer such as the one by Wilson-Cook (Fig. 32–3*A*). The steps for stent placement follow:

1. Assemble *everything* before starting the procedure: wire guide, pusher tube, stent, retrieval line (11.25 kg [25-lb] test monofilament nylon fishing line) (Fig. 32–3*B*).
2. Mark the pusher tube with the distances from the teeth so the position of the stent relative to the lesion is known during insertion (Fig. 32–3*C*): (1) the tip of the stent is entering the tumor constriction, (2) the distal flange is entering the tumor constriction, (3) the top funnel of the stent lies just above the shoulder of the lesion, and the stent is in proper position.
3. Execute a "dry run," without inserting the stent into the patient, reviewing each step in the process of introducing the stent and then removing the apparatus leaving the stent in place. Reassemble the stent placement apparatus.
4. Start the procedure by dilating the lesion using a wire guide and Savary-Guillard type dilators, not balloon dilators. The most common custom-made (see below) or commercial stents would require dilation to either 45 F or 54 F depending on the size stent selected. Leave the wire in and go directly to step 5.
5. Slide the introducer (with pusher tube, stent, and retrieval line in place) over the wire and place the stent.
6. Remove the introducing apparatus in the following sequence. (1) Deflate the balloon and remove the introducer and the wire guide. (2) Slide the scope through the pusher tube and check the position of the stent. Be sure to note the position of the distal end, and verify that there is no obstruction to outflow. (3) Remove the retrieval line. It is better to pull the end coming back through the pusher tube, so the force of the pull does not cut the tongue. (4) Disengage the pusher tube under direct vision with the scope in place, and remove it, leaving the stent in place.

FOLLOW-UP

After placement of a stent order a barium swallow and a routine chest x-ray. Assume that there will be gastroesophageal reflux. Even if the stent does not traverse the lower esophageal sphincter, the esophageal clearing mechanism will be impaired; order routine antireflux measures and an appropriate diet. Further follow-up depends on the individual clinical situation.

PROBLEMS, HAZARDS, AND COMPLICATIONS

Perforation of the esophagus may occur for various reasons (excessive force, too rapid dilation, too large a stent, bad angle, no clearance at distal end of lesion, etc.) and is seen about 10% of the time. Stent migration is more common. The patient can usually tell if the stent has migrated upward, with the sensation of a foreign body, blockage, and increased salivation. In this case remove the stent and make the appropriate modifications. Migration downward occurs if the stent was placed early and the lesion shrinks with therapy. It may pass spontaneously or may be left safely in the stomach, and further manipulation should be performed only if required. More rarely a stent may erode into the esophageal wall and surrounding structures. This is usually a terminal event. Stent blockage is usually due to poorly chewed meat. Have the patient swallow a slurry of meat tenderizer (1 teaspoon in small amount of water). Gently pass a small dilator to unplug, and perform endoscopy to check for tumor overgrowth.

In the cervical esophagus, the funnel of the stent may press on the posterior tracheal wall and cause pressure necrosis. Anterior lipping of the cervical spine can interfere with placement, cause pressure necrosis, and interfere with removal of the stent (see below).

Extrinsic lesions causing esophageal obstruction such as bronchogenic carcinoma are problematic. If the stent is not anchored by a constricting *circumferential* mucosal lesion, it will slip out. This may be remedied by anchoring the stent from above with an infant feeding tube placed through the nose and secured externally.

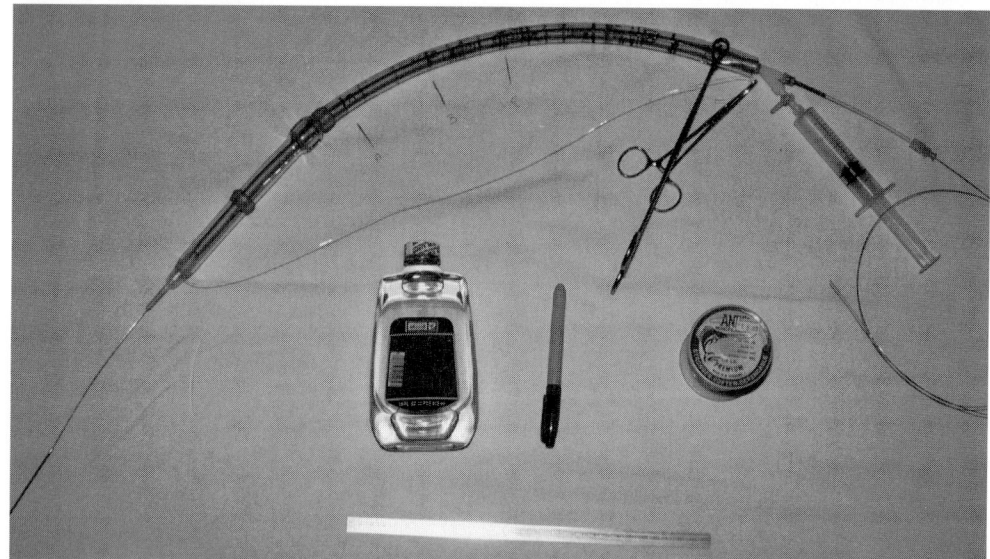
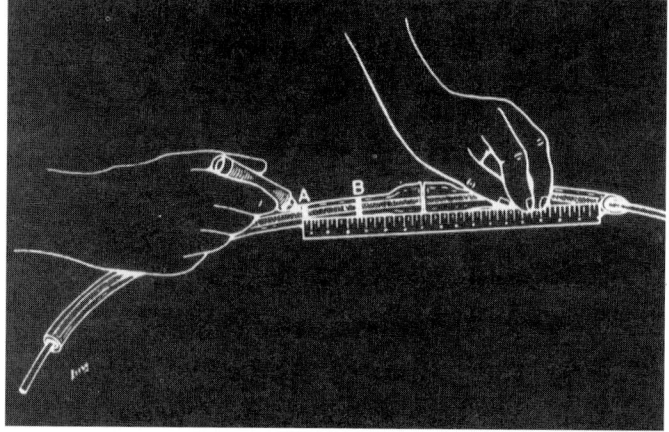

FIGURE 32–3. A, Various insertion guides. **B,** Apparatus assembled, ready for insertion. Stent and pusher tube over a Wilson-Cook insertion guide with balloon inflated, large sponge forceps holding the pusher, and small clamp holding the retrieval line; all placed on a Puestow wire (which would have already been positioned in the patient). **C,** Marking the pusher tube. (*C* from Peura DA, Heit HA, Boyce HW, Johnson LF. Esophageal prosthesis in cancer. Washington, DC: Walter Reed Army Medical Center, 1976.)

Very rarely, one may elect to use an extra long stent and anchor the distal end surgically.

TECHNIQUES OF STENT REMOVAL

It is tempting to try to pass the scope through the stent and hook the scope to remove it. This is not recommended. It does not work well, is more traumatic for the patient, and may damage the scope. The proper technique is to use a balloon catheter. Always use a "pusher tube" or overtube to couple with the funnel of the stent so the rim will not catch. If the stent is in the upper esophagus, pass a Foley catheter with a 30-cc balloon and inflate with 10 ml of water. Passage may be facilitated by stiffening the catheter with a biopsy forceps (Fig. 32–4). For more distal stent retrieval, position the pusher tube with the scope, then withdraw the scope and pass an appropriate-sized balloon dilator through the pusher tube and the stent. Then inflate and withdraw. A single balloon may not be big enough, but two small balloons in tandem work well.

TREATMENT OF FISTULAE

Fistulae, a dreadful complication of esophageal malignancy, present a difficult treatment challenge. Noninvasive therapies, chemotherapy, and radiation therapy are not effective. Surgical treatment causes excessive postoperative morbidity, and the complication rate and treatment failure rate are high. The most direct, practical, and effective therapy is to plug the hole, and this is done with a stent. A stent designed simply to maintain the lumen may also close a fistula, but it often fails. The funnel may be adequate to engage the shoulder of the lesion and prevent downward displacement, but not nearly fill the proximal normal esophagus, and food and fluid can seek the space outside the stent. A fistula more likely occurs in an area of extensive necrosis and disease with an irregular lumen, and a good tight fit to seal the fistula is difficult.

There are several innovative techniques to overcome these difficulties. The Wilson-Cook balloon cuff prosthesis is the most useful, commercially available stent designed to treat fistulae. As illustrated (Fig. 32–5), the cuff of latex foam is naturally expanded, but it is collapsed with suction during insertion. It will reexpand passively to fill the lesion and seal off the hole. A custom-made stent (see below) can be tailored to the patient, for example, by making the top funnel extra large (provided cervical osteophytes will not impede placement). A number of innovative injection techniques have been reported using tissue glue, cyanoacrylate, or dermal collagen tissue expanders.

The most intriguing new development is a self-expanding stent—the Gianturco Z-stent. These are currently marketed for biliary strictures, and larger versions are being tested for esophageal lesions. The Z-stent looks like tubular chain-link fencing with silicone webbing. It is

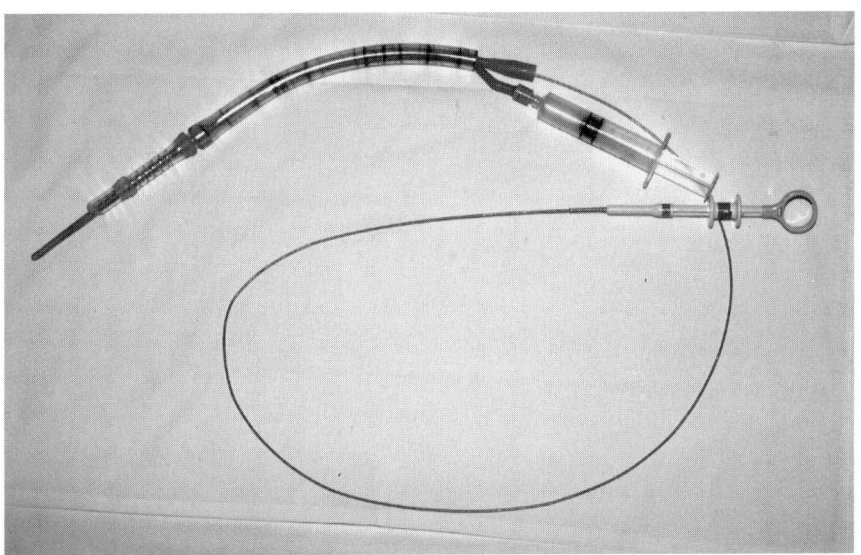

FIGURE 32–4. Retrieval technique. Foley catheter with 30-cc balloon, biopsy forceps used as stiffener, and a short pusher tube to ease withdrawal.

234 ESOPHAGUS

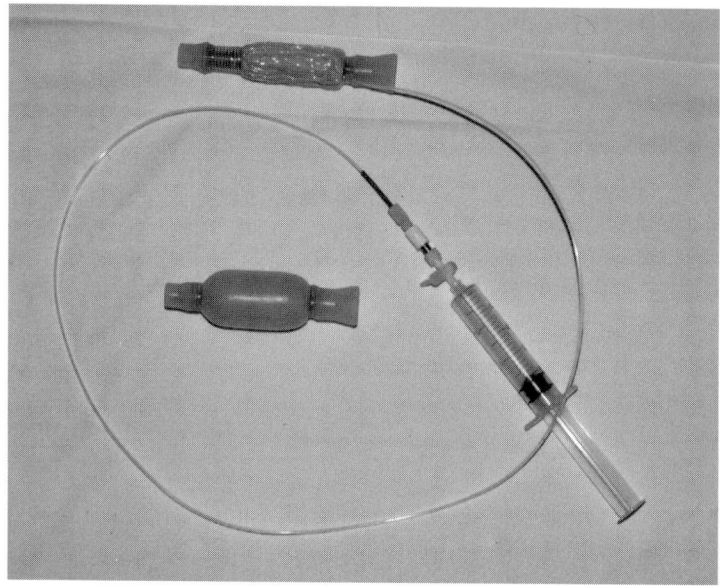

FIGURE 32–5. Wilson-Cook balloon cuff prosthesis.

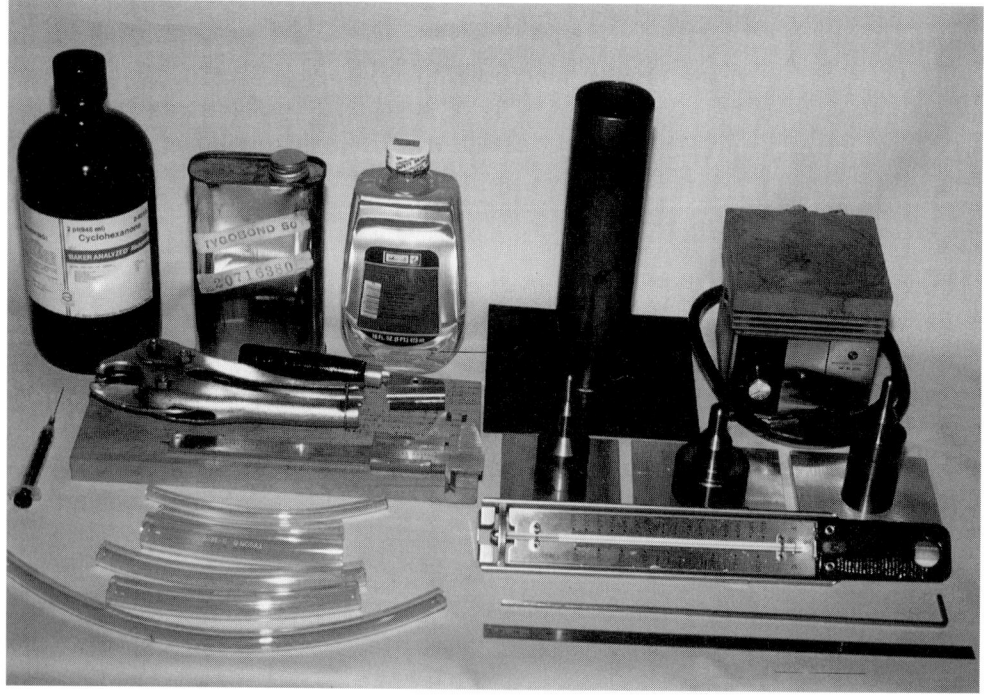

FIGURE 32–6. Supplies and equipment necessary to make stents. Solvent, mineral oil, cylinder to heat oil, hot plate, cutting board and cutting apparatus, forms to shape funnel, thermometer, holder, ruler, and assorted pieces of tubing.

placed while collapsed, then expands in place, opening up the lumen, and sealing off the fistula. The ease of placement, the way it may conform to the lesion, and the integral tendency to dilate the lesion all make this a most attractive new technique. Preliminary evaluation indicates excellent technical and functional success. It is preloaded in a 29-F delivery catheter. The length varies from 8 to 14 cm, with an internal expanded diameter of 18 mm, a 22-mm diameter flanged proximal end, rounded wires, a silicone bumper at the distal end, and hooks to anchor the stent within the tumor. The silicone coating provides a barrier to tumor growth through the mesh into the lumen and prevents perforation by the exposed wire expanding into the tumor, as well as sealing off the fistula.

The silicone self-expanding Z-stents are currently undergoing clinical testing. They appear to be appropriate for any situation where a conventional stent would be used and especially for patients with a tracheoesophageal fistula. Complications are similar but less frequent than with rigid stents. Correct placement technique is essential, because repositioning or removal is problematic; but compared with conventional rigid endoprostheses, they are easier to insert and less traumatic.

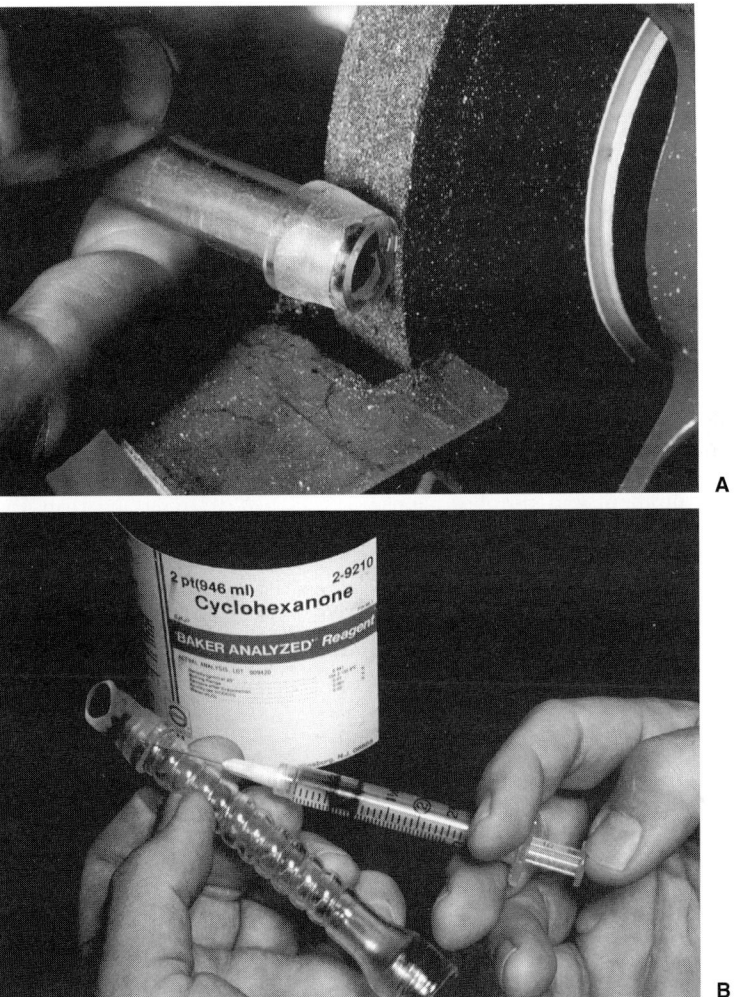

FIGURE 32–7. A, Tapering a 1-cm length of the next larger size tubing to make the distal retaining ring. **B,** The distal ring is glued in place with solvent (the ridges on the shaft of the stent illustrated are not necessary and are no longer made).

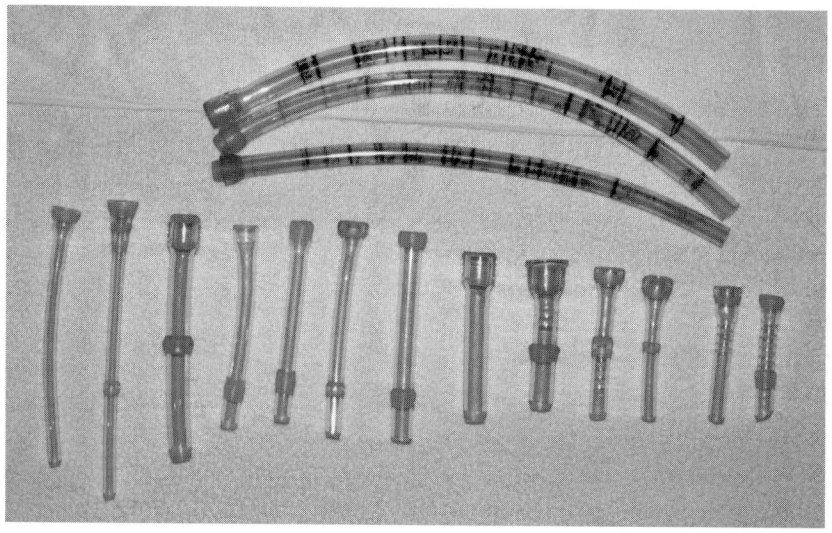

FIGURE 32–8. An assortment of stents and pusher tubes.

STENT MANUFACTURE

I began the manufacture of custom-made stents, at the instigation of a patient with obstructing carcinoma of the esophagus who also happened to be an expert in plastic design and manufacture, and with the guidance and inspiration of Boyce and Tytgat, at a time before commercial stents were available. There continues to be the occasional patient whose lesion requires a special shape or design. The technique of stent manufacture presented here is inexpensive, simple, and can be adapted to a wide variety of patient needs. The equipment and supplies we use are illustrated in Figure 32–6.

The basic material is inexpensive surgical grade Tygon plastic tubing (5-50-HL) (Norton Plastics and Synthetics Division, PO Box 350, Akron, Ohio 44309). The most commonly used tube diameter is ⅝-inch (16mm) OD (52 F). The steps in making a stent follow:

1. Select tubing size based on the appearance of the lumen and the results of preliminary dilation. Calculate the length from measurements made at endoscopy rather than on x-ray examination. Allow an extra 3 cm each for the top funnel and the distal end; cut the tubing to the length of the lesion plus 6 cm.
2. Heat mineral oil (or glycerin) to 200°F (94°C) minimum, 280°F (135°C) maximum. Immerse the cut length for 2 to 3 minutes to straighten it (if desired). Form the funnel-shaped top of the stent by pressing the hot tubing onto the proper-sized mandrel. Originally, a large Hurst bougie was used for this purpose. The funnel should be straight, as illustrated, not flanged, so the edge will not erode into the wall.
3. Make a distal flange from a ring of the next larger-sized tubing. Shape it with a standard high-speed fine grit grinder (Fig. 32–7A); slide it on the stent and cement it in place by injecting a bonding agent with syringe and 23-gauge needle (Fig. 32–7B). Use either cyclohexanone, Tygobond-50 (#20716380 Norton Plastics Division) or tetrahydropurane for bonding.
4. Smooth and taper the edges with a high-speed grinder (or freeze, and smooth with fine grit abrasive paper).
5. Make a pusher tube to fit the stent. This should be a length of the ⅝-in or ¹¹⁄₁₆-in tubing with a distal cuff, which couples with the stent so as to disengage easily with stent placement, and serve as an overtube if necessary for stent removal. The length is limited by the length of the insertion guide but must be long enough to allow a hand's breadth for grasping the external end in addition to the depth of insertion (Fig. 32–8).

REFERENCES

1. Anderson JR. Oesophageal injury Part 1. The changing face of the management of instrumental perforations. *Gullet.* 1990;1:10–15.

2. Barkin JS, Taub S, Rogers AI. The safety of combined endoscopy, biopsy and dilatation in esophageal strictures. *Am J Gastroenterol.* 1981;76:23–26.
3. Boyce HW, Palmer ED. *Techniques of Clinical Gastroenterology.* Springfield, Ill: Charles C Thomas Publisher; 1975:sect III.
4. Buset M, Des Marez B, Cremer M. Endoscopic palliative intubation of the esophagus invaded by lung cancer. *Gastrointest Endosc.* 1990;36:357–359.
5. Cox J, Bennett JR. Light at the end of the tunnel? Palliation for esophageal cancer. *Gut.* 1987;28:781–785.
6. Earlam R, Cunha-Melo JR. Oesophageal squamous cell carcinoma. I. A critical review of surgery. *Br J Surg.* 1980;67:381–390.
7. Earlam R, Cunha-Melo JR. Oesophageal squamous cell carcinoma. II. Critical review of radiotherapy. *Br J Surg.* 1980;67:457–461.
8. Graham DY. Dilatation for the management of benign and malignant strictures of the esophagus. In: Silvis SE, ed. *Therapeutic Gastrointestinal Endoscopy.* New York, NY: Igaku-Shoin; 1985, chap I.
9. Graham DY, Smith JI. Balloon dilatation of benign and malignant strictures. *Gastrointest Endosc.* 1985;31:171–174.
10. Grobe JL, Kozarek RA, Sanowski RA. Self-bougienage in the treatment of benign esophageal stricture. *J Clin Gastroenterol.* 1984;6:109–112.
11. Herskovic A, Martz K, Al-Sarraf M, et al. Combined chemotherapy and radiotherapy compared with radiotherapy alone in patients with cancer of the esophagus. *N Engl J Med.* 1992;236:1593–1598.
12. Kelsen DP, Minsky B, Smith M, et al. Preoperative therapy for esophageal cancer: a randomized comparison of chemotherapy vs. radiation therapy. *J Clin Oncology.* 1990;8:1352–1361.
13. Kozarek RA, Ball TJ, Patterson DJ. Metallic self-expanding stent application in the upper gastrointestinal tract: caveats and concerns. *Gastrointest Endosc.* 1992; 38:1–6.
14. Kozaric RA. Hydrostatic balloon dilatation of gastrointestinal stenoses: a national survey. *Gastrointest Endosc.* 1986;32:15–19.
15. Lightdale CJ. Self-expanding stents for esophageal and gastric cancer. *Gastrointest Endosc.* 1992;38:86–88.
16. Muller JM, Erasmi H, Stelzner M, et al. Surgical therapy of esophageal carcinoma. *Br J Surg.* 1990;77:845–857.
17. Palmer ED. Peroral prosthesis for the management of incurable esophageal carcinoma. *Am J Gastroenterol.* 1973;59:487–498.
18. Patterson DJ, Graham DY, Smith JL, et al. Natural history of benign esophageal strictures treated by dilatation. *Gastroenterology.* 1983;85:346–350.
19. Pera M, Cameron AJ, Trastec VF, Carpenter HA, Zinsmeister AR. Increasing incidence of adenocarcinoma of the esophagus and esophagogastric junction. *Gastroenterol.* 1993;104:510–513.
20. Peura DA, Heit HA, Boyce HW, Johnson LF. Esophageal prosthesis in cancer. Washington, DC: Walter Reed Army Medical Center; 1976.
21. Puestow KL. Conservative treatment of stenosing diseases of the esophagus. *Postgrad Med.* 1955;18:6–14.
22. Tulman AB, Boyce HW. Complications of esophageal dilatation and guidelines for their prevention. *Gastrointest Endosc.* 1981;27:229–234.
23. Tytgat GNJ. Esophageal perforation: diagnosis, prevention and therapy. *Eur J Gastroenterol and Hepatol.* 1990; 2:193–202.
24. Webb WA. Esophageal dilatation: personal experience with current instruments and techniques. *Am J Gastroenterol.* 1988;83:471–475.
25. Webb WA. Management of foreign bodies of the upper gastrointestinal tract. *Gastroenterol.* 1988;94:204–216.
26. Webb WA. Balloon dilatation of esophageal strictures. *Gastrointest Endosc.* 1985;31:224–225.
27. Webb WA, McDaniel L, Jones L. Endoscopic evaluation of dysphagia in 293 patients with benign disease. *Surg Gynecol Obstet.* 1984;158:152–156.

33

Esophageal Infections

DONALD P. BRANNAN and EUGENE MICHAEL BOZYMSKI

Many infectious agents may cause esophagitis (Table 33–1). Most often the clinical setting is that of an immunocompromised patient, but normal individuals may develop fungal or viral esophagitis, particularly if they are receiving antibiotics or corticosteroids. Infectious esophagitis was previously regarded to be rather uncommon; however, the acquired immunodeficiency syndrome (AIDS) epidemic has dramatically changed this perception and is probably the single most important factor accounting for the increasing incidence of infectious esophagitis. Growing numbers of immunosuppressed organ transplant patients also provide an at-risk popu-

TABLE 33–1. COMMON CAUSES OF INFECTIOUS ESOPHAGITIS

Organism	Typical Symptoms	Endoscopic Findings	Histologic Features
Candida albicans	Dysphagia or odynophagia	Raised white plaques without ulceration; confluent exudate with ulceration	Hyphae admixed with squamous cells or invading hyphal forms on biopsy
Herpes simplex virus	Sudden odynophagia	"Punched-out" ulcers with raised yellow borders (volcano ulcers)	Multinucleate squamous cells with intranuclear inclusion bodies
Cytomegalovirus	Odynophagia or chest pain	Usually small 3- to 5-mm ulcers; at times giant >1-cm longitudinal ulcers usually in distal third of esophagus	Epithelial or endothelial cytoplasmic inclusions

lation that contributes to the upsurge. These infections are responsible for serious morbidity and mortality in compromised patients.

Most patients with esophageal infections present with odynophagia or dysphagia. Although reflux esophagitis is generally not a predisposing factor, other causes of esophagitis such as radiation therapy or cytotoxic chemotherapy may be responsible for symptoms in this group of patients or may provide a portal of entry for infection to occur. Still, gastroesophageal reflux disease, pill-induced esophageal injury, pericardial disease, and myocardial ischemia must be considered in the differential diagnosis of acute odynophagia and dysphagia.

Candida albicans and herpes simplex virus (HSV) are the most commonly encountered pathogens, although a number of other agents including cytomegalovirus (CMV), *Aspergillus*, and tuberculosis and a variety of bacteria may infect the esophagus. In this section we will discuss the infections by cause—fungi, viruses, and bacteria—and review the clinical presentation, diagnosis, and therapeutic options.

CANDIDA ESOPHAGITIS

Candida albicans has been reported to cause esophagitis in immunocompetent patients and to be the most common cause of esophagitis in AIDS.[1-3] Oral thrush is often present concurrently with esophageal candidiasis, but it is an *insensitive* predictor of esophageal involvement. However, in patients with AIDS presenting with oral thrush and odynophagia, candidal esophagitis is so likely as to make empiric therapy without further diagnostic testing reasonable in this setting.[4] Individuals with severe neutropenia are at risk for dissemination of infection from *Candida* mucositis.[5] As noted, infections with *Candida* may occur in other clinical settings such as the immunocompetent patient receiving antibiotics or corticosteroids.

DIAGNOSIS

The diagnosis of *Candida* esophagitis is best made by upper endoscopy. Classically, patients will display small, raised white plaques that adhere to the mucosa despite washing (Fig. 33–1, see Color Plate II). Some patients with severe immunodeficiency may have a very large fungal burden with endoscopy revealing an extensive white-yellow pseudomembrane covering a diffusely erythematous and friable mucosa. Brushings for cytologic examination and KOH preparation should be obtained along with mucosal biopsy. Since *Candida* may colonize without causing disease, one would ideally like to see squamous cells admixed with hyphae or invading hyphae forms on biopsy. Obtaining brush cytologic specimens via a small bore nasogastric tube (without endoscopy) in patients with AIDS and patients with odynophagia or dysphagia has been demonstrated to be a rapid, safe, and economic means of diagnosing *Candida* esophagitis in this population.[6]

Barium esophagography may be a useful initial step and will typically reveal an irregular, shaggy mucosa suggestive of mucosal inflammation and ulceration. Other abnormalities seen include plaques, cobblestoning, nodularity, strictures, and even fistulae. Single contrast studies are fairly insensitive for detecting early mucosal changes, and double contrast studies are, therefore, preferred.

Complications of *Candida* esophagitis may include stricture formation, fistulae, perforation, dissemination of infection, and secondary bacterial infection. Fatal gastrointestinal bleeding from *Candida* esophagitis in a patient with AIDS has been reported recently.[7]

TREATMENT

A number of effective antifungal compounds are available (Table 33–2). The appropriate choice depends on the clinical situation and the patient's immunologic status. Oral nonabsorbable agents such as nystatin (Mycostatin, Nilstat) suspension or clotrimazole (Mycelex) may be appropriate for the basically immunocompetent, clinically stable patient who develops *Candida* esophagitis while receiving corticosteroids or antibiotics. A typical dose of 400,000 to 600,000 U of nystatin suspension is given as a "swish and swallow" six times daily. If possible, antibiotics or corticosteroids should be reduced or eliminated. Nystatin is not adequate therapy for esophageal candidiasis in AIDS or other compromised patients. Clotrimazole vaginal tablets 100 mg orally three times a day have been reported to be effective in esophageal candidiasis in AIDS patients. The tablet is allowed to slowly dissolve in the mouth. This therapy has the advantage of reduced cost when compared with newer agents such as fluconazole.[8] Similarly, one study reported that oral miconazole given as a gel, 50 mg four times daily, was effective in the treatment of *Candida* esophagitis in patients with AIDS.[9] However, since the advent of oral, systemically absorbed agents (discussed below), many physicians no longer use these nonabsorbable agents as primary therapy for any patients with esophageal candidiasis.

Oral systemically absorbed drugs such as ketoconazole (Nizoral) and fluconazole (Diflucan) have become the drugs of choice for ambulatory, clinically stable patients with AIDS, neoplastic abnormalities, or other disease who develop esophageal candidiasis. Ketoconazole was the first orally administered systemic antifungal medication available. Ketoconazole, like other imidazole derivatives, alters fungal cell permeability by interfering with the biosynthesis of sterols, chiefly ergosterol. Optimal absorption requires an acid milieu. Many AIDS patients have gastric hypochlorhydria and thus may have less than optimal absorption of this drug.[10] Taking the drug with an acidic vehicle such as a cola drink may help. In immunocompetent patients a dosage of 200 mg/d is sufficient. In patients with AIDS an initial dose of 400 mg/d is commonly used and this may be increased to 800 mg/d. Candidal resistance to ketoconazole does occur and may require changing to another agent.[11]

The major toxicity of ketoconazole is nausea and vomiting, which is dose dependent and occurs in about 3% of patients. Ketoconazole causes asymptomatic elevations of liver function tests in 2% to 5% of patients and may rarely (1:10,000) cause progressive hepatic toxicity, which may be fatal if not recognized and the drug is continued. Toxicity usually becomes evident during the first 4 weeks of therapy. Liver function tests should be checked prior to beginning administration of the drug and every 1 to 2 weeks during the initial month of therapy and less frequently thereafter. Chronic administration of ketoconazole may impair the biosynthesis of steroids and thereby affect adrenal and testicular function. Ketoconazole may increase the blood levels of warfarin, phenytoin, cisapride, and cyclosporin A by its effect on the hepatic mi-

TABLE 33–2. THERAPEUTIC OPTIONS FOR *CANDIDA* ESOPHAGITIS

DRUG	DOSAGE	ADVANTAGES OR DISADVANTAGES	COST PER TREATMENT*
Nystatin suspension	500,000 U q.i.d.	Least cost; frequent dosing; unsuitable for immunocompromised patients	$16.50 for 10 d
Clotrimazole tablets	100 mg t.i.d.	Low cost; appears effective in AIDS patients; nonsystemic therapy; requires allowing tablets to dissolve in mouth three times per day	$22.50 for 10 d
Ketoconazole	200 mg b.i.d.	Least costly oral systemic antifungal agent; side effects include nausea, vomiting (3%), hepatotoxicity (2-5%); requires checking liver function tests; needs acidic environment for good absorption	$54.50 for 10 d
Fluconazole	100 mg b.i.d.	Lacks many side effects seen with ketoconazole and may effectively treat ketoconazole-resistant *Candida* species; very high cost	$137.50 for 10 d

*Based on average wholesale price.

crosomal cytochrome P-450 mixed function oxidase system.

Fluconazole (Diflucan) is a newer imidazole derivative that has some advantages over ketoconazole. This agent does not require an acidic environment for absorption, appears to lack the hepatotoxic potential of ketoconazole, and does not appear to affect adrenal or testicular function. However, like ketoconazole, fluconazole increases the blood levels of warfarin, phenytoin, and cyclosporin A. Candidal resistance has not yet been reported. The usual dosage for fluconazole is 100 to 200 mg/d.

Patients with neutropenia, receiving aggressive immunosuppressive therapy or who are otherwise at high risk for disseminated candidiasis, are candidates for intravenous amphotericin B (Fungizone) therapy. Febrile neutropenic patients with esophageal candidiasis may have occult diffuse gastrointestinal or systemic candidiasis. Amphotericin B should be administered at a dose of 0.5 to 0.6 mg/kg/d. A 1-mg test dose is usually administered first to observe for serious systemic reactions (e.g., hypotension, bronchospasm). Premedication with acetaminophen, meperidine, or hydrocortisone may ameliorate the frequent febrile reactions.

Of note, imidazole agents (ketoconazole, fluconazole) may antagonize the antifungal activity of amphotericin B. Ergosterol is the primary sterol-binding site for amphotericin B in fungal cell membranes. Imidazole agents inhibit a cytochrome P-450 enzyme important in the synthesis of ergosterol, thus reducing this binding site for amphotericin B. Therefore, these agents should not be used concurrently. Selection of either agent should be guided by clinical criteria discussed above.

Flucytosine (Ancobon) is an oral antifungal agent with a narrow spectrum of activity and should not be used alone as drug resistance will rapidly develop. In patients with disseminated candidiasis, flucytosine used in conjunction with amphotericin B may allow for greater efficacy with less toxicity. Flucytosine does have significant potential for adverse effects with rash, diarrhea, and hepatic and bone marrow toxicity the most commonly reported.

Patients who are not at high risk for disseminated candidiasis but who are unable to swallow medications are also candidates for amphotericin B. Such nonneutropenic patients may be treated with lower doses of amphotericin (0.1 to 0.3 mg/kg/d). After resolution of symptoms a switch to an oral agent for the duration of therapy may be made.

Neutropenic patients who are not candidates for endoscopic evaluation are often treated empirically with an oral systemic antifungal agent or amphotericin B. Esophageal candidiasis is so common in patients with AIDS as to make empiric therapy reasonable in those with odynophagia or dysphagia and oral thrush. If symptoms do not significantly improve after 3 to 4 days, endoscopy can be performed.

DURATION OF ANTIFUNGAL THERAPY

The appropriate duration of therapy in patients with esophageal or disseminated candidiasis is uncertain.[12] Neutropenic patients should certainly receive therapy until signs and symptoms of esophagitis and neutropenia have resolved. Neutropenic patients with evidence of dissemination such as candidemia, endophthalmitis, or cutaneous lesions require longer courses of amphotericin (i.e., >15 mg/kg total dose). However, patients who are not neutropenic or otherwise profoundly immunocompromised may do quite well with a 1- to 2-week course of treatment with a total dose of 3 to 5 mg/kg. Esophageal candidiasis in patients with AIDS is a chronic recurrent problem. Chronic suppressive therapy may be appropriate in this group. When used as a lozenge, clotrimazole (Mycelex) troches, from which the drug is slowly released, are useful at a 10-mg dose four times daily for this purpose. Nystatin suspension 500,000 to 1.5 million U every 6 hours or ketoconazole 100 to 200 mg every 12 hours may be effective in reducing recurrence. Relapse while receiving oral therapy should prompt one to consider other causes of infective esophagitis (i.e., herpes simplex virus or CMV), although recurrent resistant *Candida* is still more likely.[13]

OTHER FUNGI

Esophageal infection with other fungi is rare. Esophagitis due to *Aspergillus* may be grossly and microscopically indistinguishable from that caused by *Candida*. Next to *Candida*, *Aspergillus* species is the most common mycotic cause of infectious esophagitis in patients with cancer. Mixed infection with *Aspergillus* and *Candida* has been reported as a cause of tracheoesophageal fistula.[14] In general, aspergillosis should be considered in apparent candidal esophagitis resistant to usual therapy. Invasive aspergillosis should be treated with amphotericin B.

Histoplasmosis and blastomycosis may also involve the esophagus. Histoplasmosis should be considered in endemic areas (midwestern United States) particularly if pulmonary or splenic calcifications are present along with hilar adenopathy. Blastomycosis should be considered in patients with typical skin lesions and dysphagia. Diagnosis can be confirmed by examination of smears and cultures. Histoplasmosis frequently resolves without treatment. If required, amphotericin B and ketoconazole or fluconazole should be effective against both histoplasmosis and blastomycosis. Itraconazole, an oral, triazole-derivative antifungal agent, can be used to treat systemic fungal infections in immunocompromised and nonimmunocompromised patients. It has been used to treat pulmonary and extrapulmonary blastomycosis and histoplasmosis. Rare cases of idiosyncratic hepatitis have been reported.

VIRAL ESOPHAGITIS

HSV and CMV are the most common viral pathogens that infect the esophagus. Varicellazoster virus may infect the esophagus as well, whereas other agents are much less common. HSV, like *Candida,* may occur in immunocompetent individuals, whereas CMV is more common in patients who are immunosuppressed because of transplantation or AIDS.

HERPES SIMPLEX VIRUS

HSV type 1 (HSV-1) is the most common virus to infect the esophagus and is second only to *Candida* as a cause of infectious esophagitis. Although HSV esophagitis is most commonly associated with immunocompromised hosts, it can occur in healthy individuals without apparent risk factors.[15,16]

HSV esophagitis most often presents with severe, sudden-onset odynophagia. Herpes labialis or other upper respiratory tract viral infection may precede the onset of esophagitis. In immunocompetent patients resolution of esophageal infection occurs in 1 to 2 weeks. In immunocompromised patients such as those with AIDS, HSV esophagitis may cause deep ulceration with hemorrhage, perforation, and dissemination.

Endoscopic examination is the best way to make the diagnosis. If it is performed early after symptom onset, one may observe vesicular lesions that are ephemeral. More often the gastroenterologist will find multiple discrete ulcers in the distal esophagus with raised yellow borders (volcano ulcers); however, the ulcers may become confluent. At the time of endoscopy a biopsy specimen of the involved mucosa may be obtained for histologic examination and culture. The classic histologic finding is that of multinucleated giant cells with eosinophilic intranuclear (Cowdry type A) inclusions within epithelial cells. Cultures are only likely to be positive if obtained during the vesicular phase of the disease. *Candida* is commonly described in association with HSV esophagitis and in most cases is a likely colonizer of ulcer bases.[15] Barium esophagography generally reveals focal "stellate" ulcers in the distal esophagus. Severe herpetic esophagitis may yield the nonspecific findings of diffuse ulceration, cobblestoning, or a "shaggy" mucosal appearance.

Acyclovir (Zovirax) has been demonstrated to shorten the duration of viral shedding and speed healing of lesions in immunocompromised patients with oral and genital herpes. Intravenous acyclovir at a dosage of 250 mg/m^2 every 8 hours for 7 to 10 days in HSV esophagitis in patients with AIDS reduces viral shedding and promotes the healing of lesions.[17] Side effects are few and include local phlebitis and rash. Immunocompetent patients may only require analgesia in the form of viscous 2% xylocaine or other systemic analgesia to treat the odynophagia. However, oral acyclovir is frequently prescribed for these patients because of its perceived safety and efficacy. Nausea and vomiting are the most frequent adverse effects associated with acyclovir, occurring in 2.7% of patients. Local phlebitis and rash may also occur. Resistance of herpes simplex to acyclovir may occur during chronic administration.[18]

CYTOMEGALOVIRUS

Unlike HSV-1, CMV esophagitis does not occur in immunocompetent people. CMV esophagitis, therefore, strikes those patients with AIDS or other immunodeficiency states such as organ transplant recipients. More than 90% of homosexual men infected with human immunodeficiency virus (HIV) have serologic evidence of CMV infection. Thus, CMV esophagitis is likely a consequence of systemic infection.

Patients typically complain of odynophagia with or without dysphagia.[19] Endoscopic findings typically reveal multiple small ulcers in the distal esophagus. Occasionally one finds "giant ulcers," 2 to 3 cm in length in the distal esophagus (Fig. 33-2, see Color Plate II). Radiographically the changes resemble those seen with HSV-1 esophagitis; however, "giant ulcers" seem more common with CMV. Cytologic and biopsy specimens reveal epithelial or endothelial cytoplasmic inclusions. CMV can be grown in culture if the specimen is placed in an appropriate viral transport media. CMV ulcerations may heal with stricture formation requiring dilation.[20]

Ganciclovir (Cytovene), an acyclovir derivative, has been demonstrated to be useful in treating CMV infections in patients with AIDS; however, at present it is only approved for use in CMV retinitis. A recent report in which this agent was used at a dosage of 2.5 mg/kg every 8 hours to 5 mg/kg every 12 hours for 10 days led to complete symptom resolution in 50% and partial response in 30% of patients.[19] Because of frequent relapse after successful therapy, many physicians continue maintenance therapy indefinitely. The major route of excretion is renal, and therefore, the dosage must be decreased in accordance with the creatinine clearance. The most frequent toxicity associated with ganciclovir is leukopenia, which occurs in about 40%, and thrombocytopenia, which occurs in about 20% of patients. In most cases the cytopenias are reversible with discontinuation of the drug. Patients should have frequent hematologic monitoring throughout treatment, and the drug should not be administered if the neutrophil count falls below 500/mm^3 or the platelet count below 25,000/mm^3.

Foscarnet (trisodium phophonoformate hexahydrate), a pyrophosphate analog that inhibits viral DNA polymerase and reverse transcriptase, is under investigation for the treatment of CMV gastrointestinal disease. A recent trial reported that 15 of 18 patients with CMV esophagitis treated with foscarnet had a complete response and only three had relapse of their disease after 1, 4, and 7 months, respectively.[21] This agent may cause renal dysfunction and anemia.

Varicella-Zoster Virus

The frequency of esophageal infection in conjunction with chicken pox or zoster infection is unknown. Lesions seen mimic those found in infection with HSV-1. Esophagitis in association with herpes zoster involving thoracic dermatomes has been reported in two patients.[22] Esophageal stricture has been a complication of esophagitis associated with herpes zoster.[23] Acyclovir is effective against the varicella virus; however, no controlled trials for this indication have been reported.

MYCOBACTERIAL INFECTION

Although tuberculous involvement of the esophagus is quite rare, the marked increase in systemic tuberculosis associated with AIDS may result in clinicians encountering this entity. Most commonly, esophageal ulceration results from fistulae from involved mediastinal lymph nodes. Structural abnormalities of the esophagus such as benign or malignant strictures may provide a suitable environment for the growth of ingested organisms. Esophageal involvement due to hematogenous spread with a miliary pattern can occur but is rare. Primary esophageal tuberculosis without pulmonary disease has been reported but likewise is extremely rare.[24]

Patients may present with odynophagia caused by ulceration or primarily dysphagia due to fibrotic stricture. Esophageal tuberculosis should be considered in patients with known pulmonary or extrapulmonary tuberculosis who develop odynophagia or dysphagia. Barium studies are nonspecific and may show ulceration or stricture. An ulcerated tuberculous mass may resemble primary squamous cell carcinoma of the esophagus. Upper endoscopy is the best way to make the diagnosis as biopsy specimens from the edge of the lesions may contain granulomas or acid-fast bacilli. Biopsy material should always be cultured if mycobacterial infection is a consideration.

Serious complications of esophageal tuberculosis include esophagotracheal or esophagopleural fistulae. Coughing after ingestion of food or liquid should prompt one to consider this entity. Serious hemorrhage from esophageal ulcers and esophagoarterial fistulae have been reported.[25]

Multidrug therapy is required for treatment. Fistulae may not close with medical therapy and may require surgery. Esophageal strictures can be managed by dilation or endoscopic methods depending on the nature and severity of the stricture.

BACTERIAL INFECTION

Bacterial esophagitis may be much more common than generally appreciated. Most have regarded bacterial infection to be a secondary event following infection with a more common agent, such as *Candida,* or damage following injury with a caustic. However, primary bacterial esophagitis does occur. In one series of immunocompromised patients, 11% of endoscopic biopsy specimens obtained showed purely bacterial esophagitis.[26] Bacterial pathogens are usually oral flora such as *Streptococcus viridans,* staphylococci, and *Bacillus* species. *Pseudomonas aeruginosa* usually infects the esophagus in patients with acute leukemia. Bacterial infection probably follows some disruption in the squamous epithelium caused by trauma, i.e., nasogastric tubes, acid reflux, or cytotoxic therapy.

The typical patient who develops bacterial esophagitis with odynophagia or dysphagia and fever is neutropenic and receiving chemotherapy for leukemia. Bacterial esophagitis may provide a source for bacteremia and sepsis. Endoscopy should be performed and biopsy specimens obtained for Gram stain and culture. Broad spectrum coverage should be initiated to cover likely pathogens pending the culture and sensitivity results.

REFERENCES

1. Matheison R, Dutta S. *Candida* esophagitis. *Dig Dis Sci.* 1983;28:365–370.
2. Andersen L, Freeriksen H-J, Appleyard M. Prevalence of esophageal candida colonization in a Danish population: special reference to esophageal symptoms, benign esophageal disorders, and pulmonary disease. *J Infect Dis.* 1992;165:389–392.
3. Bonacini M, Young T, Laine L. The causes of esophageal symptoms in human immunodeficiency virus infection. *Arch Intern Med.* 1991;151:1567–1572.
4. Raufman J-P. Odynophagia/dysphagia in AIDS. *Gastroenterol Clin North Am.* 1988;17:599–614.
5. DeGregorio M, Lee W, Ries C. *Candida* infections in patients with acute leukemia: Ineffectiveness of nystatin prophylaxis and relationship between oropharyngeal and systemic candidiasis. *Cancer.* 1982;50:2780–2784.
6. Bonacini M, Laine L, Gal A, et al. Prospective evaluation of blind brushings of the esophagus for *Candida* esophagitis in patients with the human immunodeficiency virus infection. *Am J Gastroenterol.* 1990;85:385–389.
7. Cappell M, Gupta A. Gastrointestinal hemorrhage due to gastrointestinal Mycobacterium avium intracellulare or esophageal candidiasis in patients with the acquired immunodeficiency syndrome. *Am J Gastroenterol.* 1992; 87:224–229.
8. Lalor E, Rabeneck L. Esophageal candidiasis in AIDS: successful therapy with clotrimazole vaginal tablets taken by mouth. *Dig Dis Sci.* 1991;36:279–281.
9. Deschamps M-M, Pape J, DeHovitz J, et al. Treatment of candida esophagitis in AIDS. *Am J Gastroenterol.* 1988;83:20–21.
10. Lake-Bakaar G, Quadros E, Beidas S, et al. Gastric secretory failure in patients with the acquired immunodeficiency syndrome (AIDS). *Ann Intern Med.* 1988;109: 502–504.
11. Tavitian A, Raufman J-P, Rosenthal L, et al. Ketoconazole-resistant candida esophagitis in patients with acquired immunodeficiency syndrome. *Gastroenterology.* 1986;90:443–445.
12. Medoff G. Controversial areas in antifungal chemotherapy: short-course and combination therapy with amphotericin B. *Rev Infect Dis.* 1987;9:403–407.
13. Parente F, Cernuschi M, Rizzardini G, et al. Opportunistic infections of the esophagus not responding to oral systemic antifungals in patients with AIDS: their frequency and treatment. *Am J Gastroenterol.* 1991;86: 1729–1734.
14. Obrecht W, Richter J, Olympio G, Gelfland D. Tracheoesophageal fistula: a serious complication of infectious esophagitis. *Gastroenterology.* 1984;87:1174–1179.
15. Yacono J. Type I herpes simplex esophagitis with candidal esophagitis in an immunocompetent host. *N Y State J Med.* 1985;656–658.
16. Shortsleeve M, Levine M. Herpes esophagitis in otherwise healthy patients: clinical and radiographic findings. *Radiology.* 1992;182:859–861.
17. Kadakia S, Oliver G, Peura D. Acyclovir in endoscopically presumed viral esophagitis. *Gastrointest Endosc.* 1987;33:33–35.
18. Sacks S, Wanklin R, Reece D, et al. Progressive esophagitis from acyclovir-resistant herpes simplex. *Ann Intern Med.* 1989;111:893–899.
19. Wilcox C, Diehl D, Cello J. Cytomegalovirus esophagitis in patients with AIDS: a clinical, endoscopic and pathologic correlation. *Ann Intern Med.* 1990;113:589–593.
20. Goodgame R, Ross P, Kim H-S, et al. Esophageal stricture after cytomegalovirus ulcer treated with ganciclovir. *J Clin Gastroenterol.* 1991;13:678–681.
21. Nelson M, Connolly G, Hawkins D, Gazzard B. Foscarnet in the treatment of cytomegalovirus infection of the esophagus and colon in patients with the acquired immunodeficiency syndrome. *Am J Gastroenterol.* 1991;86: 876–881.
22. Gill R, Gebhard R, Dozeman R, Sumner H. Shingles esophagitis: endoscopic diagnosis in two patients. *Gastrointest Endosc.* 1984;30:26–27.
23. Kroneke K, Cuadrado R. Esophageal stricture following esophagitis in a patient with herpes zoster: case report. *Mil Med.* 1984;149:479–481.
24. Seivewright N, Feehally J, Wicks A. Primary tuberculosis of the esophagus. *Am J Gastroenterol.* 1984;79:842–843.
25. Chase R, Haber M, Pootage J, et al. Tuberculous esophagitis with erosion into aortic aneurysm. *Arch Pathol Lab Med.* 1986;110:965–966.
26. Walsh T, Belitsos N, Hamilton S. Bacterial esophagitis in immunocompromised patients. *Arch Intern Med.* 1986; 146:1345–1348.

SECTION III

STOMACH

34
Gastric Motor Disorders

FREDERICK H. WEBER and RICHARD W. McCALLUM

Motor disorders of the stomach are common, varied in their clinical presentation, and may present with symptoms suggestive of impaired storage or impaired emptying of chyme. Although impaired storage leads to accelerated gastric emptying and has been described in selected patients with hyperthyroidism (nonnutrient liquids only) and Zollinger-Ellison syndrome, it usually occurs as a postoperative sequelae when the antropyloric apparatus is either surgically eliminated or bypassed. In contrast, impaired gastric emptying is much more commonly encountered by the clinician and may result from a wide array of underlying disorders. Remarkable technologic advances over the past decade have provided an expanding number of diagnostic and therapeutic modalities, which warrant a systematic approach in their use. Therapy is symptomatic and should be directed at the underlying pathologic process whenever possible. In addition to addressing nutritional and antiemetic needs, therapy frequently includes use of one or more of an expanding number of prokinetic drugs to enhance and coordinate gastroduodenal motility. This chapter reviews the disorders associated with delayed gastric emptying and treatment approach in such patients with a focus on established and putative prokinetic agents.

DISORDERS ASSOCIATED WITH DELAYED GASTRIC EMPTYING
(Table 34–1)

Clinical manifestations of delayed gastric emptying are nonspecific but frequently include nausea, vomiting (particularly of food ingested many hours previously), early satiety, postprandial bloating, and abdominal pain. Motor disorders of the antrum characteristically manifest delayed solid emptying due to inadequate trituration of digestible solids but preserved liquid emptying through a maintained ability to generate an adequate gastroduodenal pressure gradient. In contrast, motor disorders of the body and fundus of the stomach may delay both solid and liquid emptying as even adequately triturated chyme cannot empty properly in the setting of an inadequate gastroduodenal pressure gradient.[1] When clinical evaluation has excluded regurgitation, rumination, pregnancy, and offending medications and reveals objective impairment of gastric emptying, a wide range of potential underlying disorders require consideration.

MECHANICAL OBSTRUCTION

Obstruction of either the antropyloric junction or immediate postbulbar area results in gastric retention. Initially this involves indigestible solids but later includes digestible solids and liquids. Causes are numerous (see Table 34–1). Esophagogastroduodenoscopy and small bowel barium radiographic examination will adequately exclude obstruction, and endoscopic advances now permit dilation and even stenting of obstructive gastroduodenal lesions in poor operative candidates.

DIABETES MELLITUS

Symptoms of chronic nausea and vomiting are common in diabetes mellitus, being described in 29% of unselected diabetic outpatients.[2] Objective evidence of delayed solid or liquid gastric emptying is much more common, however, occurring in 58% of a group of randomly selected type I diabetic patients[3] and suggesting that many patients can remain asymptomatic or have fluctuating symptoms. Conversely, many patients with symptoms suggestive of gastroparesis have repeatedly normal solid and liquid gastric emptying studies. Here fluctuations of blood sugar (>200 mg/dl), electrolyte changes, infec-

TABLE 34–1. CLINICAL SITUATIONS ASSOCIATED WITH DELAYED GASTRIC EMPTYING

- **Mechanical obstruction**, i.e., duodenal ulcer, prepyloric ulcer, pyloric channel ulcer, idiopathic hypertrophic pyloric stenosis, gastric carcinoma, duodenal carcinoma, pancreatic carcinoma or pseudocyst, duodenal Crohn's disease, superior mesenteric artery syndrome
- **Acid-peptic diseases**, i.e., gastric ulcer, gastroesophageal reflux disease
- **Diabetes mellitus**
- **Gastric surgery sequelae**, i.e., vagotomy, gastric resection, Roux-en-Y gastrojejunostomy, fundoplication
- **Psychogenic disorders**, i.e., anorexia nervosa, bulimia, depression
- **Disorders of gastric smooth muscle**, i.e., hollow viscus myopathy, scleroderma, polymyositis, dermatomyositis, muscular dystrophy, amyloidosis, systemic mastocytosis
- **Neuropathic disorders**, i.e., hollow viscus neuropathy, Shy-Drager syndrome, Parkinson's disease, paraneoplastic syndrome, CNS or labyrinthine disorders, scleroderma, abdominal epilepsy, abdominal migraine, high cervical cord lesions
- **Gastritis**, i.e., atrophic gastritis, viral gastroenteritis
- **Metabolic endocrine disorders**, i.e., hypothyroidism, hyperthyroidism, adrenal insufficiency, hyperparathyroidism
- **Medications**, i.e., anticholinergics, narcotic analgesics, L-dopa, tricyclic antidepressants, aluminum-containing antacids, sucralfate, alcohol, beta-agonists, progesterone, calcium channel blockers
- **Ischemia**
- **Idiopathic disorders**, i.e., nonulcer dyspepsia, gastric dysrhythmias, gastroduodenal dissynchrony, idiopathic pseudo-obstruction, irritable bowel syndrome

tions, and acidosis contribute to the temporal course of symptoms. It seems likely that diabetic gastropathy is a heterogeneous disorder variably involving gastric emptying dysfunction of digestible solids, an isolated abnormality of nondigestible solid emptying,[4] antral dysrhythmias,[5] pyloric dysmotility,[6] or abnormal postprandial bursts of the duodenum and jejunum that have a braking effect on the transit of chyme. These abnormalities are usually but not invariably associated with concomitant diabetic end-organ damage, autonomic dysfunction, and peripheral neuropathy and most closely accompany type I disease. The acute effects of hyperglycemia and acidosis on gastric emptying function in the diabetic patient and on the relationship between gastroparesis and poor diabetic control must be appreciated.

POSTOPERATIVE GASTRIC STASIS

Although the pathogenesis remains poorly understood, a range of 1% to 9% of patients who undergo gastric surgery develop gastric atony (vagotomy with pyloroplasty, 1.25%; vagotomy with antrectomy, 2.4%; subtotal gastrectomy, 3%; vagotomy with subtotal gastrectomy, 9%).[7] The incidence approaches 50% in patients with preoperative gastric outlet obstruction probably due to irreversible antral decompensation from prolonged preoperative distension. Postsurgical patients frequently demonstrate a shortened half-emptying time for liquids (due to loss of fundic receptive relaxation) with a possible "dumping syndrome" and diarrhea, concomitant with markedly delayed solid gastric emptying (due to diminished antral peristalsis, possible associated changes in the gastric electrical control, and abnormal migrating motor complex activity) and vomiting. Diminished migrating motor complex activity, combined with hypochlorhydria, accounts for frequent bezoar formation.

The pathogenesis of delayed gastric emptying in such patients remains poorly understood. Its occurrence after complete antral resection suggests that abnormal antral motility is not the only mechanism. Postoperative maldigestion has been well described[8]; exposure of the distal small intestine to fatty acids and partially digested carbohydrates may contribute directly to postprandial symptoms or indirectly through an "ileal brake" mechanism.[8]

EATING DISORDERS

Anorexia nervosa is a highly prevalent neuropsychiatric disorder that may be associated with signs and symptoms of delayed gastric emptying. Objective evidence of impaired gastric emptying may be found in 80% of such patients but is more variable in those with bulimia.[9] Diminished antral contraction amplitude and both fasting and postprandial gastric dysrhythmias are common.[10] As malnutrition alone may cause impaired gastric emptying, and weight gain can often improve the gastric emptying and gastric rhythm,[11] it seems likely that in many of these patients delayed gastric emptying is not a primary abnormality. Whether pharmacologic improvement of gastric emptying improves symptoms remains unclear.

DISORDERS OF GASTRIC SMOOTH MUSCLE

Delayed gastric emptying frequently occurs in familial or nonfamilial hollow viscus myopathy as part of the spectrum of chronic idiopathic intestinal pseudoobstruction. These primary disorders of gut smooth muscle may affect gut function ranging from the esophagus to the colon and may also involve other hollow organs lined by smooth muscle such as the urinary bladder. Secondary gastric muscle involvement occurs in scleroderma (late phase), polymyositis, dermatomyositis, amyloidosis, muscular dystrophies, and systemic mastocytosis.

NEUROPATHIC DISORDERS

These may include primary disorders such as familial or nonfamilial hollow viscus neuropathy (another form of chronic intestinal pseudoobstruction). Such disorders often present in childhood and have clinical characteristics similar to those of myopathic pseudoobstruction. They can be distinguished from a myopathy manometrically and histopathologically. Disorders that may secondarily affect gastric emptying include diabetes mellitus, Riley-Day syndrome, paraneoplastic syndromes, central nervous system (CNS) or labyrinthine disorders, scleroderma (early phase), abdominal epilepsy, migraine, and high cervical cord lesions.

GASTRITIS OR GASTROENTERITIS

Atrophic gastritis and achlorhydria are associated with impaired solid (but not liquid) emptying, although patients may remain relatively asymptomatic. Adequate trituration of solid food requires a prolonged time in patients with diminished gastric acid, and this prolonged contact time may even play a role in carcinogenesis. Postviral gastroparesis has been described with associated antral hypomotility[12]; many recover completely, but some patients with a less apparent acute phase may present with chronic "idiopathic gastroparesis." Chronic type B gastritis due to *Helicobacter pylori* does not delay gastric emptying; *H. pylori*–positive patients with non-ulcer dyspepsia empty faster than *H. pylori*–negative patients. *H. pylori* is not more common in gastroparetic patients than controls.[13] *H. pylori* colonization of the stomach, however, may present as severe nausea in some patients.

METABOLIC OR ENDOCRINE DISORDERS

Hyperthyroidism, either overt or occult, may cause gastric and small bowel myoelectrical abnormalities and symptoms that resolve entirely with restoration of the euthyroid state. Hyperparathyroidism should always be excluded as well. The acute effects of hyperglycemic hyperosmolar states and acidosis on gastric emptying have been described previously with respect to diabetes mellitus and may also play a role in delays in gastric emptying related to total parenteral nutrition (TPN).

MEDICATIONS (Table 34–2)

Commonly implicated agents include anticholinergics, narcotic analgesics, L-dopa, tricyclic antidepressants, and phenothiazines. More subtle effects may be seen with aluminum-containing antacids, sucralfate, beta agonists, progesterone, potassium salts, alcohol (high concentrations), nicotine, and octreotide. Calcium channel blockers do not seem to have much impact on gastric emptying, although they do alter antral and colonic motility.[14] Urine toxic screens to exclude the possibility of surreptitious ipecac use also must be considered.

ISCHEMIA

Ischemic gastroparesis has been reported in a few patients with gastroparesis and gastric dysrhythmias and should be considered in older patients with unexplained gastroparesis and risk factors for vascular disease; often there is some accompanying abdominal pain. Symptoms and dysrhythmias normalize after mesenteric revascularization.[15] It is conceivable that smaller vessel disease due to vasculitis (i.e., systemic lupus erythematosus or polyarteritis nodosa) could play a role in some patients as well.

IDIOPATHIC

This heterogeneous group remains as a substantial (approximately 25%) subset of the gastroparetic population. The demographics are characterized by 90% being women and 90% being under 45 years of age. Some of these patients have an associated impairment of small bowel or colonic motility and overlap either a pseudoobstruction picture or irritable bowel syndrome.

Primary antral dysrhythmias such as sustained bradygastrias (1 to 2 cpm) and tachygas-

TABLE 34–2. AGENTS THAT DELAY GASTRIC EMPTYING

Alcohol (high concentration)	Octreotide
Aluminum antacids	Opiates
Anticholinergics	Phenothiazines
Beta agonists	Potassium salts
Calcium channel blockers (?)	Progesterone
L-Dopa	Sucralfate
Nicotine	Tricyclic antidepressants

trias (4 to 9 cpm) have been noted in the fed and fasted state of some patients with idiopathic gastroparesis,[16] although to date research continues in order to sort out cause from effect because similar dysrhythmias may be spontaneously seen in normal subjects for very brief periods. The effects of prokinetic agents on dysrhythmias and symptoms in such patients are incompletely studied. Subgroups with clinical suggestions of a postviral cause or variation of symptoms with the menstrual cycle appear to be emerging; an additional subgroup includes those with significant abdominal pain located in the epigastrium or right upper quadrant. Frequently such patients have had prior abdominal surgeries (i.e., cholecystectomy), and abdominal pain may be disproportionately greater than any objective findings. The role of isolated pyloric dysfunction has not been well addressed. Psychologic factors (personality type, depression, history of physical or sexual abuse) require further investigation as a risk factor or a vulnerability factor for manifesting stress in the form of abdominal pain and gastrointestinal motility symptoms often out of proportion to objective demonstration of dysmotility.

GASTROESOPHAGEAL REFLUX, NONULCER DYSPEPSIA, AND PEPTIC ULCER DISEASE

Delayed gastric emptying plays a role in a subgroup of gastroesophageal reflux disease patients.[17] This is specific for solids; it generally does not result in actual vomiting but rather profound postprandial distress. It has been suggested that patients with refractory symptoms and failed fundoplication may have a high incidence of an underlying delay in gastric emptying.

Although delayed gastric emptying may be identifiable in approximately 50% of patients with nonulcer dyspepsia,[18] it has not yet been demonstrated that there is a relationship between symptom categories, objective abnormalities, or response to therapy. However, a gastric motor disorder must be considered in patients who are considered to have an ulcer or "acid-peptic problem" and in turn fail therapy on H_2 receptor blockers. Duodenal ulcer patients may have accelerated gastric emptying, whereas chronic gastric ulcer patients (non-NSAID related) generally have delayed gastric emptying, and a number of "nonulcer dyspepsia" patients may be underappreciated gastroesophageal reflux patients in whom results of endoscopy generally are negative.

THERAPEUTIC APPROACH TO PATIENTS WITH DELAYED GASTRIC EMPTYING

After identifiable gastroduodenal disease, systemic disease, and offending drugs have been excluded and a primary or secondary disorder of gastric emptying defined, management centers on hydration, dietary manipulation, nutritional supplementation, and pharmacologic therapy. When possible, therapy should be directed at the underlying disease process as this may obviate the need for long-term pharmacologic therapy directed specifically at gastric emptying dysfunction. Surgery may include placement of a feeding jejunostomy or even gastric resection as a last resort. Bezoars should always be identified and eliminated.

HYDRATION

Hydration and dietary plans should capitalize on the ability of these patients to empty liquids better than solids. One or more liters per day should be ingested in the form of water, fruit juices, or other low-fat drinks. During periods of acute decompensation, intravenous hydration is often necessary. At such times even fasting salivary and gastric secretions may be retained; nasogastric decompression along with antisecretory therapy may be necessary to reduce gastric volume.

NUTRITION

Liquids and mechanical soft solids should be emphasized. Frequent (i.e., six per day) small, low-fat, low-fiber meals that emphasize complex carbohydrates and avoid bulky nondigestible solids are administered. Maintaining an erect posture may assist gastric emptying. Multivitamin supplements and liquid caloric supplements are often useful, and any identified nutritional abnormalities should be addressed. Jejunal feedings may be necessary in more severe cases; rarely will home TPN be necessary.

ANTIEMETICS

Phenothiazine derivatives prove to be very useful. Promethazine (Phenergan) can be administered in a dose of 12.5 mg to 25 mg every 4 to 6 hours as needed. Parenteral, oral, and rectal preparations are available. A dose of 10 mg of prochlorperazine (Compazine) may be administered orally or parenterally twice daily as required. These drugs have sedative properties that may enhance the effects of concomitant low-dose narcotic administration if the latter is required for control of pain. Extrapyramidal symptoms including tardive dyskinesia may occur with this family of medications.

Trimethobenzamide (Tigan) can be administered orally (250 mg three times a day), rectally (200 mg three times a day), or intramuscularly (200 mg three times a day). It is not recommended for intravenous administration. Efficacy is similar to the phenothiazines, drowsiness may occur, and extrapyramidal symptoms have been reported.

Scopolamine (Transderm Scop) patches should also be tried. Their sustained release is a positive factor, although the anticholinergic component may prove detrimental.

Ondansetron (Zofran), a serotonin receptor antagonist (specifically a $5-HT_3$ antagonist), has been found more effective than metoclopramide in chemotherapy-related nausea and vomiting[19]; there may be a role for its parenteral use in the hospitalized gastroparetic patient despite its lack of a gastrokinetic effect. It is currently available in a parenteral form and may be administered at 0.15 mg/kg every 6 hours. The oral formulation is now available, and doses of 8 mg two or three times daily are recommended. Because it is so expensive, it can be recommended only sparingly when long-term use is anticipated.

PROKINETICS

The place of prokinetic drugs in the overall approach to the therapy of delayed gastric emptying is indicated in Table 34–3.

Agents that accelerate gastric emptying are the mainstay of chronic therapy. Such "prokinetic" agents enhance gut contractility and transit of chyme from the stomach into the duodenum and through the small bowel by coordination of regional motor activity. Selecting a particular prokinetic agent involves characterizing the risk-benefit ratio for an individual patient. Proper selection incorporates drug characteristics with clinical parameters such as age, underlying diseases, appropriate route for administration, need for concomitant antiemetic activity, and market availability (although several investigational agents may also be obtained through compassionate clearance). In general, the efficacy of these agents is better in neuropathic rather than myopathic disorders.

Metoclopramide

Metoclopramide (methoxychloroprocainamide [Reglan]) was first developed in the 1960s, and although a procainamide derivative, it lacks the anesthetic and antiarrhythmic properties of procainamide. Through both dopamine-antagonistic,[20] $5-HT_3$ antagonistic, cholinergic-enhancing,[21] and $5-HT_4$ agonistic effects, it can coordinate antral, duodenal, and pyloric muscle function. Its ability to increase lower esophageal sphincter pressure[22] and accelerate gastric emptying[23] has made it efficacious in the treatment of gastroesophageal reflux. Metoclopramide has also been shown to increase jejunal peristalsis and accelerate intestinal transit time from the proximal small bowel to the ileocecal valve.[24]

Since its approval in 1981, metoclopramide has been used via the oral, subcutaneous, and intravenous routes for a variety of diseases. It is efficacious in the treatment of gastroparesis, gastroesophageal reflux, and drug-induced nausea and vomiting. Patients with delayed gastric emptying due to weakened antral contractions or poorly coordinated antroduodenal activity may benefit particularly from metoclopramide. It is especially useful in patients with severe symptoms who cannot take oral medication as it can be administered in a parenteral form.

In gastroesophageal reflux disease, metoclopramide has been shown to increase lower esophageal sphincter pressure,[22] enhance gastric emptying,[23] and significantly improve symptoms.[25–28] Since it does not reliably heal macroscopic esophagitis,[28] it has primarily been used as an adjunct to H_2 blockers for long-term maintenance in chronic gastroesophageal reflux disease (GERD).

Controlled trials have suggested that metoclopramide provides symptomatic relief of diabetic gastroparesis.[29,30] Gastric emptying of both solids and liquids is enhanced acutely, but a prokinetic effect has been less consistently observed after chronic oral administration. Nausea may be improved significantly by the centrally acting antiemetic properties of the drug. Gastric emp-

---

TABLE 34–3. PROKINETIC AGENTS IN 1992

Established
Metoclopramide (Reglan)
Domperidone (Motilium)
Cisapride (Propulsid)
Erythromycin

Putative
$5-HT_3$ receptor antagonists and $5-HT_4$ receptor agonists
Opiate antagonists
Gonadotropin-releasing hormone agonists
Cholecystokinin receptor antagonists

tying improvement often correlates poorly with symptomatic response, suggesting that the antiemetic effect may be as important as its prokinetic effect. Similar gastrokinetic effectiveness has been reported in idiopathic gastric stasis and anorexia nervosa.[9] In other settings, such as chronic idiopathic intestinal pseudoobstruction, metoclopramide may be less effective and may require much higher doses to achieve any clinical response. Its potent and central antiemetic effect accounts for its wide use in the treatment of nausea and vomiting associated with chemotherapy. Appetite improvement and improved sense of well-being may precede any demonstrable change in gastric emptying.

Following oral dosing, peak plasma drug levels are reached in 60 to 120 minutes, although there may be further delay in patients with abnormal gastric emptying. Onset of its prokinetic effect occurs 60 minutes after an oral dose and within 3 minutes after intravenous administration. The drug is available in tablet, liquid, and parenteral forms. The latter is particularly useful in the hospitalized patient (e.g., decompensated diabetic gastroparetics) in whom intravenous metoclopramide can be administered every 2 to 3 hours. Intravenous loading of the drug for several days to stabilize the patient and improve symptoms may be needed prior to conversion to subcutaneous or oral administration. Initial oral dose of the drug is 10 mg given 15 to 30 minutes before meals and at bedtime but may be increased as necessary and tolerated. In older patients or those with renal impairment, the initial dose should be 5 mg and slowly increased as tolerated to a clinically effective level. A syrup preparation is available for children or patients with dysphagia. The intravenous dosage for most patients is 10 mg every 4 to 6 hours; however, these authors have given up to 240 mg/d as a 20 mg every 2 hour bolus or as a continuous infusion. These very high doses may occasionally be required in the severely ill patient to control intractable nausea and vomiting. In such patients with coexisting renal failure, increased dosing requirements after dialysis sessions can be anticipated since metoclopramide is completely dialyzed.

Considerable experience in the use of subcutaneous metoclopramide is accumulating.[31] It provides an effective alternate route of administration for patients who have unpredictable absorption of oral medication because of intractable vomiting. Local side effects at the injection site are rare. Using this method, 5 mg (1 ml) three or four times daily may be initially tried in managing many severely affected patients. The dose may be increased to 10 mg (2 ml) three or four times daily depending on CNS side effects. Such a regimen may be supplemented with concomitant oral medication until the patient can be maintained solely via the oral route. Subcutaneous administration may decrease the need for intravenous therapy to maintain hydration status and avoid emergency room visits and hospital admissions. Subcutaneous injection provides serum concentrations that peak at 30 minutes and are sustained for 4 hours. Self-administration is easy to teach and well tolerated at these dosages. Once symptomatic relief is achieved, attempts should always be made to reduce or discontinue the drug; the chronic relapsing course of many gastroparetic patients, however, frequently requires indefinite therapy. In diabetics the use of subcutaneous metoclopramide (Reglan) to address morning nausea, typically with a blood glucose greater than 200 mg/dl, can be beneficial.

Potent CNS action contributes both to the drug's efficacy and side effect profile. Its antidopaminergic properties remain the major obstacle to the drug's more widespread use. Side effects may occur in up to 20% to 30% of patients, but the incidence of side effects has exceeded 30% in some studies.[32] Symptoms due to CNS dopamine inhibition include restlessness, anxiety, drowsiness, tremor and muscle rigidity; the addition of diphenhydramine (Benadryl) or benztropine (Cogentin) may be helpful and allow drug continuation. Acute dystonic reactions such as torticollis, trismus, facial spasms, and opisthotonos are more common in younger patients, whereas parkinsonian reactions and irreversible tardive dyskinesia are more common in the elderly. Dopamine receptor inhibition may lead to hyperprolactinemia and subsequent impotence, gynecomastia, amenorrhea, or galactorrhea. Cholinergic side effects such as abdominal cramps or diarrhea are rare. Dosing, particularly in children, the elderly, and those with renal impairment, should begin with low doses and gradually be increased to achieve a therapeutic response. Concurrent sedatives such as alcohol, barbiturates, and benzodiazepines should be avoided, as should anticholinergic drugs and narcotics, which may antagonize the drug's prokinetic action.

Domperidone

Domperidone (Motilium), a benzimidazole derivative, was first synthesized in 1974. It is a dopamine antagonist that blocks DA_2 receptors in the central and peripheral nervous systems. It is structurally related to the butyrophenones and has been shown to antagonize the inhibition of gastric motility caused by dopamine. In contrast to metoclopramide, domperidone is active in the peripheral circulation only; it has rare (if any) CNS side effects because it poorly crosses the blood-brain barrier. A potent central antiemetic effect is present, however, since its site of action on the chemoreceptor trigger zone lies outside the blood-brain barrier. Domperidone is currently available in 58 countries primarily for the indication of nonspecific dyspepsia. Approval in the United States is pending further clinical evaluation and is expected in 1995.

Like metoclopramide, the effects of domperidone are mainly on the proximal gastrointestinal tract. It enhances gastric and duodenal contractions, improves gastroduodenal coordination, and has a potent antiemetic effect.[33] It increases lower esophageal sphincter pressure and enhances gastric emptying, with the latter effect occurring through inhibition of receptive fundic relaxation and improvement of antroduodenal coordination. Unlike metoclopramide, this motor effect is not cholinergically mediated since it is not blocked by atropine.

Lower esophageal sphincter pressure increases after intravenous administration of domperidone.[34] In contrast, effects of oral administration of the drug on lower esophageal sphincter pressure are less consistent. Domperidone's clinical efficacy in the treatment of gastroesophageal reflux has been more variable than that of prokinetic agents, which have cholinergic effects.

Although single oral doses of 20, 30, or 40 mg of domperidone significantly increase gastric emptying, double-blind placebo controlled trials using 20 or 30 mg four times daily have shown variable effects on gastric emptying despite significant improvement in symptoms of gastric retention.[35,36] Koch et al[37] suggested that resolution of gastric dysrhythmias by domperidone, not normalization of emptying rates, correlates best with symptomatic improvement in diabetic gastroparesis and that this may explain such discrepancies between symptomatic responses and "prokinetic" effects. The long-term prokinetic effect may disappear with chronic administration[36]; however, one study suggested that the drug's favorable effect on symptoms and gastric emptying is sustained for at least 12 months.

Domperidone has a unique pharmacologic niche in patients with Parkinson's disease in whom gastrointestinal symptoms such as nausea, bloating, vomiting, and pyrosis frequently are side effects of dopamine agonist therapy. As a peripheral dopamine antagonist, domperidone has been studied at our center to evaluate its improvement in these symptoms. In a small group of patients with a mean age of 68 years, a baseline gastric emptying test was compared with posttherapy measurements. The mean rate of gastric emptying was significantly accelerated in each of the studied patients. Symptom scores also significantly improved in comparison with baseline evaluation, and this improvement exceeded all other groups of gastroparetic patients. No adverse effects were reported; we concluded that in a small group of Parkinson's patients, long-term oral domperidone therapy significantly reduces gastrointestinal symptoms without adverse effects on the underlying disease.

Direct comparative studies of domperidone versus metoclopramide are not available. Dosage of domperidone can be titrated upward to larger doses than are possible for metoclopramide without bothersome side effects because of its lack of blood-brain barrier penetration. Suppository forms of the drug are valuable in patients with nausea and vomiting who do not need hospital admission but cannot tolerate oral therapy. Peak plasma levels are achieved in 30 to 120 minutes after oral administration. The usual dose is 20 mg taken 15 to 30 minutes before meals and at bedtime. The dose may be increased to 30 mg four times daily as needed. An oral suspension (1 mg/ml) may be used in a dose of 0.3 mg/kg of body weight three times a day and at bedtime for children. Bioavailability of oral domperidone is decreased by alkalinization of the stomach with H_2 blockers or sodium bicarbonate; antacids should be avoided within 30 minutes of a dose. Side effects with oral administration occur in less than 7% of patients and include headaches, dry mouth, diarrhea, and anxiety. Dystonic and extrapyramidal side effects are rare. Hyperprolactinemia may occur with resultant breast enlargement, nipple tenderness, galactorrhea, and amenorrhea. Gynecomastia in males is rarely seen. Often these side effects are more inconvenient than serious, and patients who benefit from the drug are generally willing to accept some of these side effects.

Cisapride

Cisapride (Propulsid) is a substituted piperidinyl benzamide chemically related to metoclopramide. It is currently undergoing clinical trials as a prokinetic agent for the treatment of gastrointestinal motility disorders extending from the esophagus to the colon. Unlike metoclopramide and domperidone, cisapride is not antidopaminergic[38] and has no antiemetic effect. It increases the release of acetylcholine from postganglionic nerve endings of the myenteric plexus and leads to improved proximal, mid, and distal gut propulsion. 5-HT_3 receptor antagonism and 5-HT_4 receptor agonism may also play a major role in its mode of action,[39] and the drug may influence transmission of intrinsic gut chemical messengers.

Experimentally, cisapride increases lower esophageal sphincter pressure, increases antral motility, decreases duodenogastric reflux, increases jejunal propulsive activity, and accelerates colonic transit.[40-44] Two large multicenter trials have evaluated cisapride in the treatment of gastroesophageal reflux disease. Cisapride at a dose of 10 mg or 20 mg four times daily reduced symptoms and antacid consumption, healed macroscopic esophagitis better than placebo, and seemed more effective in those patients with severe disease. Experimentally, increases in lower esophageal sphincter pressure are most consistently demonstrated with the 20-mg dose. In the United States in August 1993, cisapride was approved for treatment of nocturnal symptoms of gastroesophageal reflux disease.

Cisapride significantly increases gastric emptying of solids in normal subjects and dyspeptic patients.[45,46,47] Preliminary short-term studies mainly evaluating small numbers of patients have investigated the effect of cisapride in patients with delayed gastric emptying. In diabetic gastroparesis, dose-ranging studies have suggested that 2.5, 5, and 10 mg given intravenously restore gastric emptying to normal.[46] A study evaluating 20 diabetic gastroparetic patients using a 4-week trial of cisapride (20 mg orally four times daily) versus placebo found a significant improvement in gastric emptying but not symptoms.[48] A similar trial of 18 patients found significant improvement in solid phase gastric emptying and total symptom score in patients treated with cisapride (10 mg four times daily) when compared with those treated with placebo.[49]

Cisapride has been found effective in the acute management of gastroparesis due to progressive systemic sclerosis, anorexia nervosa,[50] dystrophia myotonica, and idiopathic gastroparesis.[51] Studies evaluating 2- to 6-week treatment durations have shown significant improvement in gastric emptying but inconsistent symptom improvement, perhaps reflecting the refractory nature of gastroparetic patients who are enrolled in such trials.[52] Three long-term studies involving follow-up of up to 1 year in a total of 33 patients have demonstrated sustained improvement in gastric emptying rates but variable improvement in symptoms.[53] Several direct comparison studies with metoclopramide in gastroparesis suggest at least equal efficacy of cisapride and a more favorable safety profile.[54]

Combination therapy with dopamine receptor antagonists or motilin receptor agonists may capitalize on synergistic prokinetic mechanisms of action. Tatsuta et al[55] have reported in a controlled trial of eight dyspeptic patients that cisapride (2.5 mg) plus domperidone (10 mg three times daily) improved gastric emptying and symptoms significantly better than cisapride plus placebo. Clearly combination therapy in gastroparetic patients requires further investigation.[55] Cisapride should be combined with an antiemetic for the first few weeks of treatment until gastric motility has been accelerated adequately.

Cisapride is 98% protein bound in plasma and extensively metabolized with metabolites being excreted equally in urine and feces. After oral administration, peak plasma levels are achieved within 2 hours. Elimination is somewhat delayed in the elderly and those with hepatic or renal failure.

Cisapride has been well tolerated in clinical studies and has very few side effects. The most commonly reported side effects include abdominal cramping, diarrhea, and headache; they lead to drug discontinuation in 2% to 3% of patients. CNS effects are much less frequent when compared with metoclopramide, likely reflecting the absence of a central mechanism of action. Bioavailability of cisapride may be increased by cimetidine or ranitidine administration, possibly because of inhibition of oxidative metabolism of cisapride by these drugs.[46]

Cisapride is available throughout the world as an oral tablet and suspension, but no intravenous form is currently marketed. In the United States it was approved in July 1993 for the treatment of nighttime heartburn in patients with gastroesophageal reflux disease. Further indications for cisapride's efficacy in other areas of gastrointestinal motility disorders await the results of clinical trials. The recommended dose is 10 mg orally 15 to 30 minutes before each meal, with an additional 10-mg dose taken at bedtime as needed. This dose can be increased as necessary to 20 mg given three or four times daily. Lower doses (e.g., 5 mg three or four times daily) can be considered initially for patients with hepatic insufficiency or those receiving CNS depressants such as diazepam or alcohol, as cisapride may enhance their clinical effect.

Bethanechol

Bethanechol is a cholinomimetic agent that increases gastric acid and salivary secretion. It is *not* a prokinetic agent despite its ability to increase gastric contractions[27] since it does not coordinate upper gastrointestinal motility and does not accelerate gastric emptying. Other limitations include the development of cholinergic side effects in 15% to 20% of patients, stimulation of gastric acid secretion, and lack of an antiemetic effect. There may, however, be some conceivable role for bethanechol in augmenting metoclopramide's therapeutic effect in patients who fail to respond to metoclopramide alone. The usual oral dose is 25 mg four times daily; peak levels are obtained in 30 to 90 minutes, and there is a 1- to 2-hour duration of action. Cholinergic effects may include abdominal cramps, loose stools, salivation, bradycardia, flushing, sweating, lacrimation, nausea, bronchoconstriction, and urinary urgency.

Erythromycin

Erythromycin, a commonly used macrolide antibiotic, has emerged as a potential prokinetic agent through investigations into the mechanism of the well-recognized gastrointestinal side effects of the drug. Observations in both animals and humans suggest that erythromycin acts as a motilin receptor agonist and serves to stimulate fasting and fed state antral contractions.[56] This effect is specific for erythromycin and related 14-membered macrolides, as macrolides with similar antibiotic spectrums do not stimulate similar contractile activity in vivo or in vitro.[56] Radionuclide-labeled gastric emptying studies in patients with diabetic gastroparesis given 200 mg intravenously or 1 g intravenously have revealed dramatically increased solid and liquid emptying that approached or exceeded values for normal controls. Significant but less dramatic effects occur with oral dosing. The minimum erythromycin dose required to induce proximal gut motor activity is 40 mg intravenously, a dose much lower than the drug's antimicrobial dose.

Janssens et al[57] studied 10 patients with diabetic gastroparesis who were treated with 250 mg oral erythromycin ethylsuccinate three times daily, given 30 minutes before meals. After 4 weeks, gastric emptying of both solids and liquids remained significantly improved; symptomatic changes were not quantitated. We performed a similar study in 14 patients with idiopathic or diabetic gastroparesis.[58] Gastric emptying of solids remained significantly improved after 4 weeks of oral treatment with 500 mg of erythromycin base 30 minutes before meals and at bedtime. Although global assessment scores improved, however, individual symptom scores of nausea, bloating, pain, anorexia, early satiety, heartburn, and vomiting were unchanged.

Further studies are necessary to determine optimal dosing; it appears that low doses (i.e., 250 mg once or twice daily) are appropriate for initiation of therapy and may prove as effective as higher doses. In the absence of controlled double-blind studies, erythromycin should be used as an adjunct to the well-established and proven prokinetic agents—cisapride, metoclopramide, or domperidone—to enhance treatment responses. The initial starting dose of erythromycin in this setting should be 250 mg once a day to reduce the possibility of dose tolerance, with options to increase to 2 or 3 times daily during symptom exacerbations. (Liquid preparations are also available if necessary.) Remaining questions include the effect of motilin agonists on chronic symptoms, whether tachyphylaxis will occur, whether postsurgical or antrectomized patients will respond, and whether such agents will play a role in combination therapy. Preliminary evidence suggests that erythromycin accelerates gastric emptying in postsurgical gastroparesis patients[59,60]; there may therefore be prokinetic effects of the drug that do not require the presence of antral motilin receptors. Several 14-membered macrolides that have much greater motilinlike activity and no antibiotic component are the subject of active clinical investigation.[61]

Leuprolide Acetate

Progesterone or relaxins are known to alter the function of the gastrointestinal tract in women during their menstrual cycle.[62] Prolonged orocecal transit has been found in the luteal phase, and some patients with gastroparesis link worsening of symptoms with the luteal phase. Leuprolide acetate is a gonadotropin-releasing hormone (Gn-RH) agonist that inhibits ovulatory cycle fluctuations in gonadal hormones. A single small uncontrolled report has described dramatic improvement in abdominal pain, nausea, and vomiting in four female patients with debilitating "functional" disease when leuprolide was administered at a dose of 0.5 mg subcutaneously daily for up to 15 months.[63] A challenge with progesterone or withdrawal of leuprolide was associated with a return of baseline symptoms within 3 to 5 days. Symptomatic improvement and improvement of disturbed duodenal motility has been reported in seven diabetic patients with neuromuscular gastrointestinal tract involvement after 4 months of leuprolide. A depot form of the drug is currently being investigated on a research basis. The potential long-term risk of accelerated osteoporosis remains a concern, although intermittent therapy or concomitant estrogen replacement may prove helpful in this regard. This therapeutic area is obviously interesting given the female dominance in gastroparesis. However, rigorous and controlled studies are needed to advance this treatment approach. Leuprolide should be considered when there is clearly a cyclical correlation with symptom relapse or there are unexplained peaks and valleys in the patient's course.

5-Hydroxytryptamine (5-HT$_3$) receptor antagonists and 5-HT$_4$ receptor agonists

Since metoclopramide and cisapride are 5-HT$_3$ receptor antagonists and 5-HT$_4$ receptor agonists, some of their prokinetic effect has been proposed to relate to action on these 5-HT receptors.[39,64] This concept has led to investigation of other 5-HT$_3$ receptor antagonists, which, devoid of dopamine receptor antagonism, may prove preferable to metoclopramide. Preliminary evidence has suggested that other agents with combined 5-HT$_3$ antagonism and 5-HT$_4$ agonism (e.g., ICS/205-930) accelerate gastric emptying in normal humans.[65] Ondansetron, a 5-HT$_3$ antagonist with potent antiemetic properties exceeding those of metoclopramide, does not modify gastric emptying in normal subjects suggesting that 5-HT$_3$ receptor antagonism alone does not accelerate gastric emptying. Selective 5-HT$_4$ agonists (SC-49518) have been shown to increase gastric emptying of solids and liquids in dogs. The relative contributions that 5-HT$_3$ receptor antagonism and 5-HT$_4$ receptor agonism have on the mechanisms of action of existing prokinetic agents remain to be determined, but evidence has accumulated to suggest that neuronal 5-HT may normally regulate gastrointestinal motor activity. Another area of excitement regarding 5-HT receptors is their potential role as part of the afferent arc of the enteric reflex. Through relationships with the gut peptide substance P some of the pain component of the gastrointestinal tract could be related to luminal events stimulating 5-HT related reflexes. This adds further interest to exploring 5-HT neurons as part of the spectrum of irritable bowel syndrome, and further development of specific agonists and antagonists may play an important role in future drug therapy.

Opiate Receptor Antagonists

Enkephalins have been demonstrated in the myenteric plexus, and it appears that both mu and kappa opiate receptors are important in the regulation of gastric emptying. Mu opiate receptor agonists such as morphine inhibit gastric emptying of solids, but kappa receptor agonists appear to increase solid gastric emptying. Naloxone has no effect on solid and liquid gastric emptying in normal volunteers, but it accelerates gastric emptying in patients with chronic idiopathic intestinal pseudoobstruction.[66] A paucity of adverse effects of the opiate antagonists and the recent availability of a new oral opiate antagonist (naltrexone) may lead to a future therapeutic role for such agents as prokinetic drugs.

Cholecystokinin Receptor Antagonists

Cholecystokinin (CCK) receptor antagonists accelerate gastric emptying in experimental animals and humans, possibly through interfering with the feedback regulation that CCK has on gastric emptying.[67] Whether interrupting such feedback is useful in gastroparetic patients (who may already have diminished feedback because of delayed duodenal filling) requires further investigation. The possibility remains that such patients may have an underlying sensitivity to the gastric inhibitory effect of CCK.

NUTRITION SUPPORT AND SURGERY

Nasojejunal, endoscopically placed, or surgically placed jejunostomy tubes are important in the management of some refractory patients. Cessation of oral intake generally improves nausea and vomiting, and nocturnal tube feedings can then meet caloric requirements. Medications (including prokinetics) may be administered via the tube. In this manner, weight may be stabilized, and the need for recurrent hospitalization may be reduced. At the time of jejunostomy tube placement, which now can be successfully performed by a laparoscopic technique, a full-thickness small bowel or gastric biopsy specimen can be obtained for diagnostic purposes. Patients with chronic intestinal pseudoobstruction may also benefit from periodic "venting" to relieve distension. Venting is best done by placing a gastrostomy tube endoscopically.

In patients with prior gastric surgery who present with vomiting, once anastomotic obstruction is excluded, a gastric emptying study must be performed. Refractory gastric stasis following vagotomy and pyloroplasty may occasionally be improved with partial gastrectomy and gastroenterostomy. Total gastric resection may be used as a last resort in patients with gastric stasis following partial gastrectomy. Our successful experience with completion gastrectomy in eight patients with refractory gastroparesis following surgery for peptic ulcer disease has been recently reported.[68] The procedure entailed a 95% or complete resection of the remaining stomach, construction of an esophagojejunal anastomosis, and lengthening of a preexisting Roux-en-Y limb to greater than 45 cm if necessary. Further stomal revisions or de novo Roux-en-Y constructions do not resolve the symptoms of chronic gastric atony in such patients and may even worsen gastrointestinal transit. Completion gastrectomy, although seemingly radical, is usually successful in improving quality of life.

We do not recommend pyloroplasties or antrectomies in the treatment of refractory gastroparesis. In our experience patients may become up to 50% better with an antrectomy but still require medical therapy and may have symptoms secondary to their surgery. Rather, the feeding jejunostomy concept provides clinical stability while development of better pharmacologic agents is awaited. Therapy is better with an anatomically intact stomach (including vagus nerve), and no other complications will have been induced by the surgery. We do not recommend TPN. This method of nutrition support is fraught with potentially life-threatening complications. Also, the economics of TPN are not defendable when an intact small bowel is available.

In summary, a wide array of underlying disorders may be responsible for delayed gastric emptying. In most cases this is a chronic condition that requires a thorough initial search for treatable underlying disease followed by individualized therapy that focuses on hydration, dietary manipulation, nutritional supplementation, and pharmacologic therapy. An expanding group of prokinetic agents with better side effect profiles has emerged. Future approaches will include combination therapy focusing on correction of specific receptor abnormalities in this heterogeneous group of patients with different pathophysiologic mechanisms responsible for delayed gastric emptying.

REFERENCES

1. Minami H, McCallum RW. The physiology and pathophysiology of gastric emptying in humans. *Gastroenterology.* 1984;86:1592–1610.
2. Feldman M, Schiller LR. Disorders of gastrointestinal motility associated with diabetes mellitus. *Ann Intern Med.* 1983;98:378–384.
3. Horowitz M, Harding PE, Maddox A, et al. Gastric and esophageal emptying in insulin-dependent diabetes mellitus. *J Gastroenterol Hepatol.* 1986;1:97.
4. Feldman M, Smith HJ, Simon TR. Gastric emptying of solid radiopaque markers: studies in healthy subjects and diabetic patients. *Gastroenterology.* 1984;87:895–902.
5. Koch KL, Stern RM, Stewart WR, et al. Gastric emptying and gastric myoelectrical activity in patients with diabetic gastroparesis: effect of long-term domperidone treatment. *Am J Gastroenterol.* 1989;84:1069–1075.
6. Mearin F, Camilleri M, Malagelada JR. Pyloric dysfunction in diabetes with recurrent nausea and vomiting. *Gastroenterology.* 1986;90:1919–1925.
7. Herman G, Johnson V. Management of prolonged gastric retention after vagotomy and drainage. *Surg Gynecol Obstet.* 1970;130:1044–1048.
8. Spiller RC, Trotman IF, Adrian TE, et al. Further characterization of the "ileal brake" reflex in man: effect of ileal infusion of partial digests of fat, protein and starch on jejunal motility and release of neurotensin, enteroglucagon and peptide YY. *Gut.* 1988;29:1042–1051.
9. McCallum RW, Grill BB, Lange R, et al. Definition of a gastric emptying abnormality in patients with anorexia nervosa. *Dig Dis Sci.* 1985;30:713–722.
10. Abell TL, Malagelada JR, Lucas AR, et al. Gastric electromechanical and neurohumoral function in anorexia nervosa. *Gastroenterology.* 1987;93:958–965.
11. Rigaud D, Bedig G, Merrouche M, et al. Delayed gastric emptying in anorexia nervosa is improved by completion of a renutrition program. *Dig Dis Sci.* 1988;33:919–925.
12. Oh JJ, Kim CH. Post-viral gastroparesis: clinical features and prognosis. *Gastroenterology.* 1989;96:A373. Abstract.
13. Wegener M, Borsch G, Schaffstein J, et al. Are dyspeptic symptoms in patients with *Campylobacter pylori*-associated type B gastritis linked to delayed gastric emptying? *Am J Gastroenterol.* 1988;83:737–740.
14. Santander R, Mena I, Gramisu M, et al. Effect of nifedipine on gastric emptying and gastrointestinal motility in man. *Dig Dis Sci.* 1988;33:535–539.
15. Liberski SM, Koch KL, Atnip RG, et al. Ischemic gastroparesis: resolution after revascularization. *Gastroenterology.* 1990;99:252–257.
16. You CH, Lee KY, Chey WJ, et al. Electrogastrographic study of patients with unexplained nausea, bloating and vomiting. *Gastroenterology.* 1980;79:311–314.
17. McCallum RW, Mensh R, Lange R. Definition of the gastric emptying abnormality in gastroesophageal reflux patients. In: Weinbeck M, ed. *Motility of the Digestive Tract.* New York, NY: Raven Press; 1982:355–362.
18. Jian R, Ducrot F, Ruskoff A, et al. Symptomatic radionuclide and therapeutic assessment of chronic idiopathic dyspepsia. *Dig Dis Sci.* 1989;34:657–664.
19. Pieter HM, DeMulder MD, Seynaeve C, et al. Ondansetron compared with high-dose metoclopramide in prophylaxis of acute and delayed cisplatin-induced nausea and vomiting. *Ann Intern Med.* 1990;113:834–840.
20. Valenzuela JE. Dopamine as a possible neurotransmitter in gastric relaxation. *Gastroenterology.* 1971;71:1019–1022.
21. Stadaas J, Aune S. Clinical trial of metoclopramide on postvagotomy gastric stasis. *Arch Surg.* 1972;104:684–686.
22. Heitman P, Moler N. The effect of metoclopramide on the gastroesophageal junctional zone and distal esophagus in man. *Scand J Gastroenterol.* 1970;5:620–626.
23. Fink SM, Lange RC, McCallum RW. Effect of metoclopramide on normal and delayed gastric emptying in gastroesophageal reflux patients. *Dig Dis Sci.* 1983;28:1057–1061.

24. Johnson AG. Gastroduodenal motility and synchronization. *Postgrad Med J.* 1973;49(suppl 4):29–33.
25. Bright-Asare P, El Bassoussi M. Cimetidine, metoclopramide or placebo in the treatment of symptomatic gastroesophageal reflux. *J Clin Gastroenterol.* 1980;25:750–755.
26. McCallum RW, Ippoliti AF, Coon C, et al. A controlled trial of metoclopramide in symptomatic gastroesophageal reflux. *N Engl J Med.* 1977;296:354–357.
27. McCallum RW, Fink SM, Lerner E, et al. Effects of metoclopramide and bethanechol on delayed gastric emptying present in gastroesophageal reflux patients. *Gastroenterology.* 1983;84:1573–1577.
28. McCallum RW, Fink SM, Einnan GR, et al. Metoclopramide in gastroesophageal reflux disease: rationale for its use and results of a double-blind trial. *Am J Gastroenterol.* 1984;79:165–172.
29. Loo FD, Palmer DW, Soergel KH, et al. Gastric emptying in patients with diabetes mellitus. *Gastroenterology.* 1983;86:485–494.
30. Schade RR, Duas MC, Lhotsky DM, et al. Effect of metoclopramide on gastric liquid emptying in patients with diabetic gastroparesis. *Dig Dis Sci.* 1985;30:10–15.
31. McCallum RW, Valenzuela G, Polepalle S, et al. Subcutaneous metoclopramide in the treatment of symptomatic gastroparesis: clinical efficacy and pharmacokinetics. *J Pharmacol Exp Ther.* 1991;258:136–142.
32. Albibi R, McCallum RW. Metoclopramide: pharmacology and clinical application. *Ann Intern Med.* 1983;98:86–95.
33. Brogden RN, Carmine AA, Heel RC, et al. Domperidone: a review of its pharmacological activity, pharmacokinetic and therapeutic efficacy in the symptomatic treatment of chronic dyspepsia and as an anti-emetic. *Drugs.* 1982;24:360–400.
34. Bron B, Massih L. Domperidone: a drug with powerful action on the lower esophageal sphincter pressure. *Digestion.* 1980;20:375–378.
35. Albibi R, DuBovic S, Lange RC, et al. A dose response study of the effects of domperidone on gastric retention states in man. *Am J Gastroenterol.* 1982;77:679.
36. Horowitz M, Harding PE, Chatterton BE, et al. Acute and chronic effects of domperidone on gastric emptying in diabetic autonomic neuropathy. *Dig Dis Sci.* 1985;30:1–9.
37. Koch KL, Stern RM, Stewart WR, et al. Gastric emptying and gastric myoelectrical activity in patients with diabetic gastroparesis: effect of long-term domperidone treatment. *Am J Gastroenterol.* 1989;84:1069–1075.
38. VanNeuten JM, Schuurkes JAJ. Pharmacodynamics of cisapride, a prokinetic agent with indirect cholinergic properties. *Digestion.* 1986;34:137.
39. Cooke HJ, Carey HV. The effects of cisapride on serotonin-evoked mucosal response in guinea pig ileum. *Eur J Pharmacol.* 1984;98:147–148.
40. Wallin L, Kruse-Anderson S, Madsen T, et al. Effect of cisapride on the gastro-oesophageal function in normal human subjects. *Digestion.* 1987;37:160–165.
41. McCallum RW, Prakash C, Campoli-Richards DM, et al. Cisapride: a preliminary review of its pharmacodynamic and pharmacokinetic properties, and the therapeutic use as a prokinetic agent in gastrointestinal motility disorders. *Drugs.* 1988;36:652–681.
42. Coremans G, Janssens J, Vantrappen G, et al. Cisapride stimulates propulsive motility patterns in human jejunum. *Dig Dis Sci.* 1988;33:1512–1519.
43. Lee KY, Chey WY, You CH, et al. Effect of cisapride on the motility of gut in dogs and colonic transit time in dogs and humans. *Gastroenterology.* 1984;86:1157.
44. Krevsky B, Maurer AH, Malmud LS, et al. Cisapride accelerates colonic transit in patients with colonic inertia. *Am J Gastroenterol.* 1989;84:822–887.
45. Jian R, Ducrot F, Piedeloup C, et al. Measurement of gastric emptying in dyspeptic patients: effects of a new gastrokinetic agent (cisapride). *Gut.* 1985;26:352–358.
46. McCallum RW. Cisapride: a new class of prokinetic agent. *Am J Gastroenterol.* 1991;86:135–152.
47. Muller-Lissner SA, Fraas C, Hartl A. Cisapride offsets dopamine-induced slowing of fasting gastric emptying. *Dig Dis Sci.* 1986;31:807–810.
48. Horowitz M, Maddox A, Harding PE, et al. Acute and chronic effects of cisapride on gastric esophageal emptying in insulin-dependent diabetes mellitus. *Gastroenterology.* 1987;92:1899–1907.
49. Champion MC, Gulenchyn K, Braaten J, et al. Cisapride improves symptoms and solid phase gastric emptying in diabetic gastroparesis (DGP). *Diabetes.* 1988;37(suppl 1);84:37.
50. Stacher G, Bergmann H, Wiesnagrotzki S, et al. Intravenous cisapride accelerates delayed gastric emptying and increases antral contraction amplitude in patients with primary anorexia nervosa. *Gastroenterology.* 1987;92:1000–1006.
51. Corinaldesi R, Stanghellini V, Raiti C, et al. Effect of chronic administration of cisapride on gastric emptying of a solid meal and on dyspeptic symptoms in patients with idiopathic gastroparesis. *Gut.* 1987;28:300–305.
52. Richards RD, Valenzuela GA, Davenport KG, et al. Objective and subjective results of a randomized, double-blind, placebo controlled trial using cisapride to treat gastroparesis. *Dig Dis Sci.* (In press.)
53. Abell TL, Camilleri M, DiMagno EP, et al. Cisapride is effective in the long-term treatment of gastric motor disorders. *Gastroenterology.* 1987;92:A1287.
54. DeCastecker JS, Ewing DJ, Clarke BF, et al. Double-blind placebo-controlled trial comparing cisapride and metoclopramide in diabetes with autonomic neuropathy. *Digestion.* 1986;34:148–149.
55. Tatsuta M, Iishi H, Nakaizumi A, et al. Effect of treatment with cisapride alone or in combination with domperidone on gastric emptying and gastrointestinal symptoms in dyspeptic patients. *Alim Pharmacol Ther.* 1992;6:221–228.
56. Peeters T, Matthijs G, Depoortere I, et al. Erythromycin is a motilin receptor agonist. *Am J Physiol.* 1989;257:G470–G474.
57. Janssens J, Peeters TL, Vantrappen G, et al. Improvement of gastric emptying in diabetic gastroparesis by erythromycin. *N Engl J Med.* 1990;322:1028–1031.
58. Richards RD, Davenport K, McCallum RW. The treatment of idiopathic and diabetic gastroparesis with acute intravenous and chronic oral erythromycin. *Am J Gastroenterol.* 1993;88:203–207.
59. Kendall BJ, Weber FH, Samy NH, et al. Effect of a single dose of IV erythromycin on gastric emptying in chronic postsurgical gastroparesis. (Submitted.)
60. Mozwecz H, Pavel D, Pitrak D, et al. Erythromycin stearate as prokinetic agent in postvagotomy gastroparesis. *Dig Dis Sci.* 1990;35:902–905.
61. Itoh Z, Omura S. Motilide, a new family of macrolide compounds mimicking motilin. *Dig Dis Sci.* 1987;32:915.
62. Wald A, Van Thiel DH, Hoechstetter L, et al. Gastrointestinal transit: the effect of the menstrual cycle. *Gastroenterology.* 1981;80:1497–1500.

63. Mathias JR, Ferguson KL, Clench MH. Debilitating "functional" bowel disease controlled by leuprolide acetate, gonadotropin-releasing hormone (GnRH) analog. *Dig Dis Sci.* 1989;34:761–766.
64. Costall B, Naylor RJ. 5-Hydroxytryptamine: new receptors and novel drugs for gastrointestinal motor disorders. *Scand J Gastroenterol.* 1990;25:769–787.
65. Akkermans LMA, Vos A, Hoekstra A, et al. Effect of ICS 205–930 (a specific 5-HT$_3$ receptor antagonist) on gastric emptying of solid meal in normal subjects. *Gut.* 1988;29:1249–1252.
66. Schang JC, Devroede G, Perrault R. Naloxone therapy in small intestinal obstruction: preliminary results about two cases. *Am J Gastroenterol.* 1984;79:828.
67. Shillabeer G, Davison JS. Proglumide, a cholecystokinin antagonist, increases gastric emptying in rats. *Am J Physiol.* 1987;252:R353–R360.
68. McCallum RW, Polepalle SC, Schirmer B. Completion gastrectomy for refractory gastroparesis following surgery for peptic ulcer disease. *Dig Dis Sci.* 1991;36:1556–1561.

35
Rapid Gastric Emptying
ROBIN D. ROTHSTEIN and WILLIAM B. LONG

Rapid gastric emptying has been demonstrated in a myriad of medical conditions, and has been a well-recognized problem following gastric surgery. A subset of patients with rapid gastric emptying have associated symptoms, which may be severe and difficult to control.

POSTGASTRECTOMY DUMPING

Rapid gastric emptying has been implicated as the cause of the "dumping syndrome." This syndrome has been divided into early and late stages. Early symptoms are those that typically occur within 30 to 60 minutes of food ingestion and are thought to occur because of the rapid exit of fluid from the stomach into the small bowel. The fluid discharged from the stomach is relatively hypertonic and is thought to stimulate influx of extracellular fluid into the small bowel to establish osmotic equilibrium.

However, the development of an isosmotic state occurs at the expense of decreased plasma fluid and proximal small bowel distension and may be the main factor in early dumping. Support for this theory includes the observation that the rate of gastric emptying does correlate with a decrease in plasma volume and the development of symptoms of dumping.[1] In addition, instillation of hypertonic fluid, including amino acids and glucose solution, into the jejunum or balloon distension of the jejunum causes similar symptoms.[2]

Clinically, rapid gastric emptying does appear to be a prime factor in the cause of symptoms. Patients with dumping usually have the most rapid phase of gastric emptying within the first 15 to 30 minutes after food ingestion, and this time course correlates to symptom development. There is often a worsening of symptoms with large volume liquid consumption or ingestion of hypertonic fluids, both of which can cause greater jejunal distension. Liquids consumed with solids accelerate the emptying of the solids in postgastrectomy patients, in contrast to no effect on solid emptying in normal individuals.[3]

Therefore, it is not surprising that the typical symptoms of early dumping are often vasomotor and include lightheadedness, flushing, sweats, tachycardia, and orthostatic hypotension. In addition, patients may experience abdominal distension and cramps, which may be attributable to autonomic reflexes from small bowel distension and possible serotonin release. Other symptoms include nausea, vomiting, and early satiety.

However, additional factors must be important in the etiology of the early dumping syndrome. The degree of hypovolemia does not correlate well with symptoms and peripheral infusion of fluid does not thwart the development of early dumping.[4]

Alterations in peptides have been noted and provide some insight into the mechanism for the pathophysiology of dumping. Vasoactive intestinal peptide (VIP) has been noted to be increased in gastrectomy patients following glucose ingestion but not in normal subjects. In addition, VIP levels correlate with both packed cell volume and blood glucose level. In symptomatic patients following gastrectomy, the rise in VIP levels is greater than in patients without symptoms.[5] Neurotensinlike immunoreactivity was demonstrated to be elevated in patients with postoperative dumping syndrome. As neurotensin does delay gastric emptying in physiologic doses, the postprandial elevation seen in patients with dumping symptoms may potentially be an attempt to slow emptying.[6] Other peptides or hormones may also play a role, including serotonin and bradykinin.[7]

Some patients may develop late postcibal symptoms. These late dumping symptoms occur 90 and 180 minutes after a meal and are thought to be induced by hypoglycemia. Glucose tolerance has been documented to be abnormal following gastric surgery. In the immediate postprandial state, hyperglycemia occurs, followed by elevated insulin levels and a subsequent period of reactive hypoglycemia.[8] Initially, these changes were thought to be secondary to rapid gastric emptying with rapid glucose absorption.[9] However, in a study examining glucose tolerance following vagotomy and pyloroplasty, nearly one third of ingested glucose did not reach the systemic circulation. Therefore, although there is rapid emptying of glucose from the stomach, there appears to be diminished absorption possibly due to glucose malabsorption and an abbreviated absorption period.[10]

A role for glucagonlike peptide-1 (GLP-1) in late dumping has also been implicated. The peak concentration of GLP-1 in patients with late dumping following total gastrectomy is 10-fold greater than in normal controls. GLP-1 induces insulin release and may be important in reactive hypoglycemia. Alternatively, stimulation of the pancreas may also trigger reactive hypoglycemia.[11]

There also appears to be a link between cholecystokinin and postprandial insulin release. Loxiglumide (a specific cholecystokinin receptor antagonist) increases gastric emptying of a mixed meal and a pure glucose meal. In addition, it causes a rapid increase in early postprandial insulin levels, which closely correlates to meal emptying.[12]

In addition to the aforementioned symptoms that occur with early and late dumping, some postgastric surgery patients develop diarrhea. Rapid gastric emptying, especially in the first 15 minutes following ingestion, has been noted to occur more often in patients with diarrhea.[13] Potentially the cause for the diarrhea is the rapid transit of chyme to the colon.

OTHER CAUSES OF RAPID GASTRIC EMPTYING

Multiple medical problems have been associated with rapid gastric emptying. Although the relationship between rapid gastric emptying and duodenal ulcer disease remains controversial, there is evidence to suggest that some patients with duodenal ulcers have more rapid gastric emptying. Gastric scintigraphy has demonstrated that the overall rate of gastric emptying is increased in patients with duodenal ulcers.[14-16] Other studies have not confirmed this finding but suggest that the initial phase of emptying is more rapid.[17]

Rapid gastric emptying has been implicated to be important in the pathophysiology of duodenal ulcer development as there is increased emptying of an acid load into the duodenum, promoting ulceration of the first portion of the duodenum. This theory is relatively simplistic as abnormal gastric emptying is not uniformly observed in all patients with duodenal ulcer nor does it normalize after treatment and resolution of the duodenal ulcer.[18]

Some patients with gastric ulcers have also been noted to have rapid gastric emptying. These are primarily patients with ulcers in the proximal portion of the stomach, in contrast to distal gastric ulcers that tend to be associated with delayed gastric emptying. Potentially, patients with proximal gastric ulcers have altered receptive relaxation of the proximal stomach.[19]

Associated gastric motor abnormalities have been implicated in patients with achalasia. The half-time for gastric liquid emptying is significantly accelerated in patients with achalasia (10 minutes) compared with normal controls (19 minutes).[20] However, symptoms of dumping in patients with achalasia are uncommon, possibly because of the impairment of esophageal emptying. Potentially, patients with achalasia have vagal impairment that results in alteration of fundic relaxation. However, the vagal neuropathy must be specific to the nonadrenergic noncholinergic pathway as the cholinergically mediated gastric acid secretion pathway remains intact.[20]

There is some evidence that rapid gastric emptying is part of the cause of obesity. Rats with iatrogenic lesions of the ventromedial aspect of the hypothalamus overeat and rapidly become obese. Rapid gastric emptying is felt to be the primary abnormality in these rats.[21] In human subjects, in a comparative study of lean compared with obese adults, gastric emptying was more rapid in the latter group. In a follow-up study of four patients with near-normalization of their weight, the gastric emptying rate for solids and liquids was unchanged, which may explain the high rate of repeat weight gain in obese patients.[22] However, the cause for obesity appears to be more complex. The administration of secretin, which delays gastric emptying, does not cause a significant decrease in food consumption. Cholecystokinin-8 inhibits feeding and gastric emptying when given immediately before a meal. Thus, although cholecystokinin-8 decreases food consumption, its mechanism does not appear to be mediated via altered gastric emptying.[23]

Patients with pancreatic insufficiency have accelerated gastric emptying of liquid fatty meals. This defect is corrected by treatment with pancreatic enzymes or by replacing the triglycerides with fatty acids, indicating that the control mechanism of gastric emptying is still intact once the luminal defect is corrected. Such rapid emptying has been speculated to contribute to the maldigestion by overwhelming limited digestive function.[24]

Studies evaluating patients with bulimia have demonstrated two subsets of patients: those with delayed gastric emptying and subjects with more rapid emptying. In one study, approximately 40% of patients had accelerated emptying.[25] Patients with anorexia nervosa also demonstrate a spectrum of gastric dysmotility. Approximately 50% of patients have scintigraphic evidence of rapid gastric emptying.[26]

Gastric dysmotility has also been demonstrated in rats with experimentally induced portal hypertension. Emptying for both solids and liquids was more rapid than in controls. Reduced compliance of the stomach wall may play a role in altered emptying rates as rats with portal hypertension have histologic evidence of submucosal edema.[27] Although these data are of interest, the clinical significance remains unclear.

Rapid gastric emptying has also been encountered in some patients with insulin-dependent diabetes mellitus, especially early on in their disease. In this setting, the most commonly observed disturbance is rapid early liquid emptying.[28]

Dumping syndrome in a child can be potentially life threatening and may result in severe symptoms of anorexia, irritability, weight loss, abdominal distension, diaphoresis, and failure to thrive. Symptomatic rapid gastric emptying has been documented to occur in a patient who inadvertently received duodenal feeds via an antrally placed gastrostomy tube and in a patient with a colonic interposition for esophageal atresia.[29] Scintigraphically measured rapid gastric emptying has also been documented in an 11-month-old infant after a Nissen fundoplication and pyloroplasty.[30] Some children with intestinal malrotation, including omphalocele, gastroschisis, and Ladd's bands have persistent gastrointestinal symptoms, including diarrhea and bloating, despite corrective surgery. These patients have been noted to have rapid gastric emptying.[31]

A majority of patients following severe head trauma have documented alterations of gastric emptying in the early phases of their recovery. Overall, patients with rapid gastric emptying tolerated enteral feeds sooner than patients with delayed gastric emptying.[32] It remains unclear what the pathophysiology is for the altered gastric emptying in head trauma patients.

Thyroid disease has a controversial effect on gastric emptying. In rats with chemically produced thyrotoxicosis, gastric emptying rates were faster than in controls.[33] In a study of four hyperthyroid subjects, gastric emptying was unchanged in both the hyperthyroid and subsequently treated euthyroid state.[34]

In an initial study of patients with Zollinger-Ellison syndrome, rapid gastric emptying was demonstrated compared with normal subjects. Normal subjects who received pentagastrin had either no change or a reduction in their gastric emptying, implicating that hypergastrinemia and gastric hypersecretion do not play a role in rapid gastric emptying.[35] In a follow-up study, patients with Zollinger-Ellison syndrome had decreased $t_{1/2}$ of gastric emptying compared with both normal subjects and patients with duodenal ulcer disease. The $t_{1/2}$ remained unchanged in patients with Zollinger-Ellison syndrome despite pretreatment with high-dose cimetidine. Additionally, although fatty meal ingestion severely inhibited normal gastric emptying, there was no delay in gastric emptying in patients with Zollinger-Ellison syndrome.[36]

TREATMENT

Treatment of symptomatic rapid gastric emptying remains less than satisfactory. Diet is important. Small, frequent meals, without accompanying liquids, and decreased simple carbohydrate ingestion are the building blocks of therapy directed at diminishing dumping symptoms. Liquids not only empty more rapidly than solids, but they also accelerate the emptying of solids in postgastrectomy patients. Food items containing lactose are best avoided, as a relative intolerance may occur because of the rapid transit of hypertonic fluid in the small intestine.[3] Patients with dumping syndrome frequently find that lying down after eating helps with reducing their symptomatology, possibly by reducing gravitational forces that may facilitate gastric emptying. Both glucose and starch are emptied more slowly from the stomach in the supine rather than the erect position.[37]

High-viscosity meals may benefit some patients with dumping. After distal gastrectomy dogs have a very rapid initial rate of emptying low-viscosity meals compared with animals with intact stomachs. In contrast, medium-viscosity meals empty from the stomach at the same rate in both operated and nonoperated animals. This effect was felt to be related to the viscosity of the meal and not related to its nutrient value.[38] The authors used cellulose to add viscosity to the meal, suggesting that the addition of fiber to meals may delay gastric emptying in human beings with dumping syndrome.

Pectin has been demonstrated to help relieve symptoms of dumping. Patients with dumping syndrome were given oral glucose solutions with and without the addition of pectin. Patients who ingested the pectin-supplemented glucose had few or no symptoms of dumping, did not experience hypoglycemia, and had less significant plasma volume changes. Pectin also led to prolongation of gastric emptying and reduced postprandial insulin levels.[39] Therefore, the addition of pectin before or during meals may decrease symptoms. Alternatively, the use of a disaccharidase inhibitor, e.g., acarbose, may provide some relief.[40]

Alteration of gastrointestinal peptides may provide some benefit to patients with dumping. Fat, in the form of soya bean oil, stimulates the release of neurotensin, enteroglucagon, and gastric inhibitory polypeptide. Patients ingesting soya oil within 20 minutes of a meal have less rapid early emptying of a meal.[41]

Medications, including opiates and anticholinergic medications, have been used with mixed success in treatment of dumping syndrome.

Octreotide acetate has been used as a relatively effective agent in the treatment of early dumping syndrome, potentially by decreasing both gastric and intestinal motility or by inhibiting peptide release of neurotensin, insulin, glucagon, or pancreatic polypeptide. Octreotide reduces the symptoms of dumping, decreases the length and amplitude of the fed pattern, and induces migrating myoelectrical complexes.[42] Acute administration of this medication has been documented to delay gastric emptying, and long-term use does ameliorate symptoms.[43]

As a last resort in selected patients, surgical intervention may be appropriate, especially those patients who developed dumping syndrome as a postsurgical complication. Surgical alteration to a Roux-en-Y loop may provide relief for some patients. Alternatively, a jejunal loop with an intussusceptive valve can be interposed between the stomach remnant and the duodenum. A decrease in the degree of dumping has been noted in these patients.[44] Interposition of an antiperistaltic loop of bowel may also increase transit time.[45] However, with reoperation there is the risk of substituting symptoms of rapid gastric emptying for those associated with gastroparesis. Electrical pacing of the small bowel requires further study, but it is a possible exciting future alternative.[46]

REFERENCES

1. Ralphs DNL, Thomson JPS, Haynes S, Lawson-Smith C, Hobsley M, LeQuesne LP. The relationship between the rate of gastric emptying and the dumping syndrome. *Br J Surg.* 1978;65:637–641.
2. Machella TE. Mechanism of post-gastrectomy dumping syndrome. *Gastroenterology.* 1950;14:237.
3. Kroop HS, Long WB, Alavi A, Hansell JR. Effect of water and fat on gastric emptying of solid meals. *Gastroenterology.* 1979;77:997–1000.
4. LeQuesne LP, Hobsley M, Hand BH. The dumping syndrome. I. Factors responsible for symptoms. *Br Med J.* 1960;1:141.
5. Sager GR, Bryant MG, Ghatei MA, Kirk RM, Bloom SR. Release of vasoactive intestinal peptide in the dumping syndrome. *Br Med J.* 1981;282:507–514.
6. Blackburn AM, Lawaetz O, Bloom SR. Plasma neurotensin release and gastric emptying in the dumping syndrome. *Life Sci.* 1983;32:833–837.
7. Editorial. Dumping syndrome and gut peptides. *Lancet.* 1980;2:1173.
8. Breuer RS, Moses H III, Hagen TC, et al. Gastric operations and glucose homeostasis. *Gastroenterology.* 1972;62:1109–1119.
9. Leichter SB, Arnold AC, Lewis SB. Glucose tolerance insulin secretion and glucose utilization in subjects after gastric surgery. *Am J Clin Nutr.* 1977;30:2053–2060.
10. Radziuk J, Bondy DC. Abnormal oral glucose tolerance and glucose malabsorption after vagotomy and pyloroplasty. *Gastroenterology.* 1982;83:1017–1025.
11. Miholic J, Orskov C, Holst JJ, Kotzerke J, Meyer HJ. Emptying of the gastric substitute, glucagon-like pep-

tide-1 (GLP-1) and reactive hypoglycemia after total gastrectomy. *Dig Dis Sci.* 1991;36:1361–1370.
12. Fried M, Schwizer W, Beglinger C, Keller U, Jansen JB, Lamers CB. Physiological role of cholecystokinin on postprandial insulin cholecystokinin receptor antagonist loxiglumide. *Diabetologia.* 1991;34:721–726.
13. Parr NJ, Grime S, Brownless S, Critchley M, Baxter JN, Mackie CR. Relationship between gastric emptying of liquid and postvagotomy diarrhoea. *Br J Surg.* 1988;75:279–282.
14. Lam SK, Isenberg JI. Grossman MI, Lane WH, Hogan DL. Rapid gastric emptying in duodenal ulcer patients. *Dig Dis Sci.* 1982;27:598–604.
15. Maddern GJ, Horowitz M, Hetzel DJ, Jamieson GG. Altered solid and liquid gastric emptying in patients with duodenal ulcer disease. *Gut.* 1985;26:689–693.
16. Harasawa S, Tani N, Suzuki S, et al. Gastric emptying in normal subjects and patients with peptic ulcer: a study using the acetaminophen method. *Gastroenterol Jpn.* 1979;14:1–10.
17. Parr NJ, Grime S, Critchley M, Baxter JN, Mackie CR. Abnormal pattern of gastric emptying of liquid in chronic duodenal ulcer. *Digestion.* 1988;40:237–243.
18. Holt S, Heading RC, Taylor TV, Forrest JA, Tothill P. Is gastric emptying abnormal in duodenal ulcer? *Dig Dis Sci.* 1986;37:685–692.
19. Kanaizumi T, Nakano H, Matsui T, et al. Gastric emptying in patients with gastric and duodenal ulcer. *Tohoko J Exp Med.* 1989;158:133–140.
20. Eckardt VF, Krause J, Bolle D. Gastrointestinal transit and gastric acid secretion in patients with achalasia. *Dig Dis Sci.* 1989;34:665–671.
21. Duggan JP, Booth DA. Obesity, overeating, and rapid gastric emptying in rats with ventromedial hypothalamic lesions. *Science.* 1986;231:609–611.
22. Wright RA, Krinsky S, Fleeman C, Trujillo J, Teague E. Gastric emptying and obesity. *Gastroenterology.* 1983;84:747–751.
23. Conover KL, Collins SM, Weingarten HP. Gastric emptying changes are neither necessary nor sufficient for CCK-induced satiety. *Am J Physiol.* 1989;256:R56–R62.
24. Long WB, Weiss JB. Rapid gastric emptying of fatty meals in pancreatic insufficiency. *Gastroenterology.* 1974;67:920–925.
25. Shih WJ, Humphries L, Digenis GA, Castellanos FX, Domstad PA, Deland FH. Tc-99m labeled triethylene tetraamine polystyrene resin gastric emptying studies in bulimia patients. *Eur J Nucl Med.* 1987;13:192–196.
26. Domstad PA, Shih WJ, Humphries L, DeLand FH, Digenis GA. Radionuclide gastric emptying studies in patients with anorexia nervosa. *J Nucl Med.* 1987;28:816–819.
27. Reilly JA, Forst CF, Quigley EM, Rikkers LF. Gastric emptying of liquids and solids in the portal hypertensive rat. *Dig Dis Sci.* 1990;35:781–786.
28. Oliveira RB, Troncon LE, Meneghelli UG, Dantas RO, Godoy RA. Gastric accommodation to distention and early gastric emptying in diabetics with neuropathy. *Braz J Med Biol Res.* 1984;17:49–53.
29. Lavind JE, Hattner RS, Heyman MB. Dumping in infancy diagnosed by radionuclide gastric emptying technique. *J Pediatr Gastroenterol Nutr.* 1988;7:614–618.
30. Pittschieler K. Dumping syndrome after combined pyloroplasty and fundoplication. *Eur J Pediatr.* 1991;150:410–412.
31. Jolley SG, Tunell WP, Thomas S, Young J, Smith EI. The significance of gastric emptying in children with intestinal malrotation. *J Pediatr Surg.* 1985;20:627–631.
32. Tibbs P, Ryo UY. Altered gastric emptying in the head-injured patient: relationship to feeding intolerance. *J Neurosurg.* 1991;74:738–742.
33. Ikeda T, Fujiyama K, Hoshino T, Takeuchi T, Tominaga M, Mashiba H. Glucose intolerance and gastric emptying in thyrotoxic rats. *Metabolism.* 1989;38:874–877.
34. Wiley ZD, Lavigne ME, Liu KM, MacGregor IL. The effect of hyperthyroidism on gastric emptying rates and pancreatic exocrine and biliary secretion in man. *Am J Dig Dis.* 1978;23:1003–1008.
35. Dubois A, Van Eeerdewegh P, Gardner JD. Gastric emptying and secretion in Zollinger-Ellison syndrome. *J Clin Invest.* 1977;59:255–263.
36. Hawsa A, Ippoliti A, Cullin R. Rapid gastric emptying in Zollinger-Ellison syndrome (ZE). *Gastroenterology.* 1980;78:1180.
37. Gulsrud PO, Taylor IL, Watts HD, Cohen MB, Elashoff J, Meyer JH. How gastric emptying of carbohydrate affects glucose tolerance and symptoms after truncal vagotomy with pyloroplasty. *Gastroenterology.* 1980;78:1463–1471.
38. Ehrlein HJ, Thomas G, Keinke O, Tsiamitas C, Schumpelick V. Effects of nutrients on gastrointestinal motility and gastric emptying after distal gastrectomy with Roux-Y gastrojejunostomy in dogs. *Dig Dis Sci.* 1987;32:538–546.
39. Leeds AR, Ralphs DN, Ebied F, Metz G, Dilawari JB. Pectin in the dumping syndrome: reduction of symptoms and plasma volume changes. *Lancet.* 1981;1:1075–1078.
40. McLoughlin JC, Buchanan KD, Alam MJ. A glycoside-hydrolase inhibitor in treatment of dumping syndrome. *Lancet.* 1979;2:603.
41. Lawaetz O, Bloom SR, Stimpel H, Siemssen OJ. Effect of soya bean oil on symptoms, gastric emptying and gut hormone release in patients with postvagotomy symptoms. *Annal Chir Gynaecol.* 1986;75:308–313.
42. Richards WO, Geer R, O'Dorisio TM, et al. Octreotide acetate induces fasting small bowel motility in patients with dumping syndrome. *J Surg Res.* 1990;19(6):103–107.
43. Geer RJ, Richards WO, O'Dorisio TM, et al. Efficacy of octreotide acetate in treatment of severe postgastrectomy dumping syndrome. *Ann Surg.* 1990;212:678–687.
44. Svensson JO, Olbe L. Intestinal intussusception valve for postgastrectomy bile reflux and/or dumping. *Acta Chir Scand.* 1985;151:355–360.
45. Sawyers JL, Herrington JL Jr. Superiority of antiperistaltic jejunal segments in management of severe dumping syndrome. *Ann Surg.* 1973;178:311.
46. Bjork S, Phillips SF, Kelly KA. Mechanisms of enhanced intestinal absorption with electrical pacing. *Gastroenterology.* 1984;86:1029.

36
Gastric Outlet Obstruction

MILES AUSLANDER

Gastric outlet obstruction is the mechanical cause of gastric retention. Failure of the stomach to empty may result from organic narrowing or blockage of the exit of the stomach, from abnormalities of the motility of the upper intestinal tract, or from a combination of factors. Abnormalities of motility are considered in more detail, elsewhere in this volume.

GASTRIC EMPTYING

The stomach empties liquids, digestible solids, and nondigestible solids by different mechanisms.[1] Liquids empty from the stomach in a linear relationship to the pressure within the gastric body. If 500 ml of isotonic neutral liquid is placed in the normal stomach, it will be half emptied in about 12 minutes. Hypertonic or strongly acidic liquids empty more slowly (Table 36–1).

· Solid particles larger than 2 mm in diameter cannot exit the normal stomach during the digestive phase of gastric motility. From a pacemaker located high on the greater curvature, a propagated slow wave of electrical activity cycles at three to four per minute.[2] Some of these waves have spike potentials and associated muscular contractions. This peristaltic ring moves to the pylorus, which closes as the electrical wave reaches it. Pressures up to 60 cm H_2O pulverize the food. The strong peristaltic contractions against the antral muscular blockade reduce particle size below the critical 2 mm to allow exit from the stomach.

The rate of emptying depends on hormonal and neural control. Pain, emotional upset, and nausea slow gastric emptying through central mechanisms. Adrenergic tone slows emptying, while parasympathetic fibers may have a stimulatory or inhibitory effect on the muscle. Cholecystokinin and gastrin both delay emptying. Receptors for acid, amino acids, or fatty acids in the small bowel finely regulate the emptying of solids during the digestive phase of motility. One hundred kilocalories of fat empties at about the same rate as 100 kcal of carbohydrate or protein.

Nondigestible material that cannot be crushed by the antral pump must await the interdigestive period during fasting to exit the stomach. This migrating motor complex or housekeeper wave is phase 3 and lasts 5 to 15 minutes, emptying the stomach of nondigestible solids.

Gastric emptying is complex, affected by central neural output, local neural reflexes, and hormonal influence. Although the character of the gastric contents is the most important determinant of gastric emptying, other factors have influence. Mild activity speeds emptying, whereas maximal exercise impedes it[3]; alcohol use slows emptying[4]; and emptying is slower in the postmenopausal state, even in women who experience menopause prematurely.[5]

SYMPTOMS

The symptoms of gastric retention depend on the extent and duration of delay and the underlying disease. Vomiting is the most common symptom and is usually the presenting complaint. Associated nausea, anorexia, upper abdominal fullness, and bloating are common. Diminished intake leads to weight loss in some two thirds of patients. Constipation is also common, leading to the mistaken assumption that impaction has led to the vomiting rather than decreased intake. Pain will be reported more often with acute and complete obstruction, often mechanical in cause, and especially if peptic ulcer is the cause (Table 36–2).

Prolonged outlet obstruction will lead to dehydration and electrolyte and acid-base imbalance. The gastric distension may result in aspiration. Nocturnal vomiting strongly supports gastric retention over functional dyspepsia or other

TABLE 36–1. MECHANISMS OF GASTRIC EMPTYING	
Liquids	Continuous emptying (linear to gastric pressure)
Digestible solids	Acid-pepsin digestion
	Digestive motility pulverizes to less than 2 mm
	Peristalsis empties
Nondigestible solids	Interdigestive houskeeper wave

TABLE 36–2. SYMPTOMS OF GASTRIC OUTLET OBSTRUCTION	
ACUTE	CHRONIC
Vomiting	Weight loss
Pain	Hypochloremic alkalosis
Abdominal distension	Dehydration
Early satiety	Aspiration pneumonia
Anorexia	Constipation
Nausea	

causes of vomiting. Although other conditions may result in forceful, repetitive, or projectile vomiting, gastric retention is an important factor.

SIGNS

Physical examination may be useful in the diagnosis of gastric outlet obstruction. Obvious evidence of malnutrition, dehydration and abdominal distension may wrongly suggest disseminated abdominal cancer or chronic liver disease. The typical succussion splash should correctly distinguish the pathophysiology. In a patient who has not eaten for 4 hours, gentle rocking of the abdomen should not produce the sloshing sound of free liquid within the stomach heard with the stethoscope. This positive splash is evidence for retention. In the very thin patient, vigorous gastric peristalsis may be visible through the abdominal wall, especially in acute and complete obstruction.

ETIOLOGY (Table 36–3)

PEPTIC ULCER DISEASE

Peptic ulcer disease is the most frequent cause of gastric outlet obstruction. Although only 2% of ulcer patients have the complication of obstruction, 80% of obstructions occur in patients with acute or chronic ulcer disease.[6] The most common presentation is a middle-aged patient with a longer than 10-year history of peptic ulcer. Prior complications of bleeding, perforation, or obstruction are frequent. The expected epigastric burning pain is gradually replaced by fullness, early satiety, and vomiting. Gastric ulcer in the body of the stomach impairs gastric emptying by interfering with normal peristaltic contractions. Ulcer in the prepyloric antrum, channel, or duodenal bulb is more likely to physically obstruct the exit and is responsible for 90% of ulcer obstruction. Three quarters of patients with ulcer causing retention have active ulcer at the time of diagnosis, often with associated penetration. Acute ulcer disease related to nonsteroidal anti-inflammatory drugs can rapidly progress to pyloric obstruction.

Some changes in the physiology of emptying in patients with peptic ulcer disease may be caused by the ulcer or may actually play a part in causing the ulcer.[7] Acidic gastric juice entering the duodenum usually slows emptying by a local vagal reflex. Patients with duodenal ulcer disease, even without active ulcer, empty acidic liquid more rapidly than normal. Gastroesophageal reflux disease is associated with delayed emptying of liquids and solids. Patients with gastric ulcer have abnormal pyloric function. There is some delay of emptying solids, which may be caused by fibrosis of the antrum. There is also increased reflux of duodenal bile back to the stomach, perhaps playing a part in damage of the gastric mucosal barrier.

The onset of partial obstruction can also cause intractability of previously manageable disease. The partial obstruction leads to gastric retention. The distended antrum is stimulated to release gastrin, which causes acid hypersecretion. The gastrin drive may exceed the inhibition of H_2-blocking agents, perpetuating the ulcer and increasing the obstruction.

INFLAMMATION

Inflammation not related to peptic ulcer disease may also detain gastric contents. Crohn's disease of the upper intestinal tract will more likely inflame and scar the antrum, but the duodenum can also be involved. Transient motility disturbances, as well as inflammatory edema, may delay emptying of the stomach in patients with acute cholecystitis or pancreatitis.

TABLE 36-3. CAUSES OF MECHANICAL OBSTRUCTION

Peptic Ulcer Disease
Gastric ulcer
Pyloric channel ulcer
Duodenal ulcer

Inflammatory
Crohn's disease
Cholecystitis
Pancreatitis

Neoplasm
Gastric cancer
Gastric polyps
Duodenal polyps
Ampullary carcinoma
Pancreatic carcinoma
Metastatic carcinoma

Postoperative Stenosis
Stricture
Gastroenterostomy intussusception
Gastroenterostomy edema
Transverse mesocolon obstruction of Billroth II
Complications of obesity surgery

Other
Annular pancreas
Bezoar
Caustic stricture
Duodenal webs
Hypertrophic pyloric stenosis
Superior mesenteric artery syndrome

NEOPLASM

Neoplasm may obstruct the stomach. Gastric or duodenal polyps can prolapse and block the pylorus. Gastric, duodenal, ampullary, and pancreatic cancers are responsible for closure of the exit. Malignant obstruction of the gastric outlet usually leads to slowly progressive retention. The systemic findings of weight loss and pain may overshadow the gastric symptoms. In some indolent tumors, particularly pancreatic, gastric retention may be the presenting feature.

Neoplasia of the colon, retroperitoneum, or cancers metastatic to the abdomen may also lead to obstruction of the gastric outlet. Breast and lung cancer may invade the gastric wall. Ovarian tumors disseminate intraperitoneally, and melanoma may metastasize to the small bowel. It is sometimes difficult to distinguish clinically, whether nausea, anorexia, and weight loss are caused by obstruction or centrally mediated systemic symptoms of carcinomatosis.

GASTRIC SURGERY

Surgery is both a treatment of retention and an important cause of mechanical and motility disturbances of gastric emptying. Transient ileus and delayed gastric emptying is the rule after abdominal and many other major surgical procedures. Surgery directed at esophageal reflux, peptic ulcer disease, and gastric neoplasia all have major effects on gut motility.

Vagotomy affects emptying, whether the vagotomy is performed specifically to reduce gastric acidity or incidentally during fundoplication or esophageal transection for varices. Vagotomy eliminates the normal receptive relaxation reflex. This leads to increased pressure in the gastric body and speeds the emptying of liquids.[8] Superselective or parietal cell vagotomy spares the antral-pyloric vagal fibers and, other than a brief and mild decrease of solid emptying, plays little role in gastric retention. Truncal or selective vagotomy, however, significantly deters the emptying of solids from the stomach.

Because of the delay of emptying after vagotomy (other than superselective vagotomy), drainage procedures must be done. Pyloroplasty normalizes both liquid and solid emptying. After a period of adjustment, patients with antrectomy and gastroenterostomy empty more rapidly than normal and may produce dumping, not retention, as the primary complication.

Mechanical outlet obstruction occurs following gastric surgery in 1% to 3% of patients.[9] The most common cause is a transient edema of the stoma of the gastroenterostomy. Blockage can also be due to intussusception of the small bowel into the stoma, to torsion of the efferent limb by the transverse mesocolon (especially in the obese patient), or to stricture. Stenosis of the stoma may occur rapidly after surgery and is often due to technical problems such as a leak at the anastomosis. Obstructing stenosis that occurs months or years after surgery is usually due to recurrent peptic disease with marginal ulceration. Although edema will subside within a few days of nasogastric drainage, many of the mechanical postoperative obstructions require repeat surgery for correction.

Gastric outlet obstruction can be a complication of surgery for obesity, though currently it is not commonly performed. A variety of techniques have been used to limit dietary intake, and many suffer from being too loose, and therefore ineffective, or too tight, causing degrees of obstruction. The various gastroplasty procedures, including staples or bands, may occlude excessively. Surgery is usually required in these cases, although endoscopic balloon dilation has successfully decreased symptoms.

OTHER

Other, less common causes of mechanical occlusion include hypertrophic pyloric stenosis of the infant or adult, duodenal webs, annular pancreas, and superior mesenteric artery syndrome. Caustic ingestion, especially strong acids, may cause stricture and obstruction of the distal antrum. Patients with gastric retention from any cause may collect nondigestible solids, which form a bezoar, making retention more severe.

DIAGNOSIS

As in any illness, the history and physical examination direct the clinician toward the correct diagnosis. Laboratory tests are useful only to document the degree of chronic malnutrition or dehydration resulting from decreased dietary intake (Table 36–4).

Contrast radiographs are often the first test ordered when disorders of emptying are suspected. A liquid contrast medium is sometimes used, especially if perforation or penetration is suspected. Thin barium gives a better demonstration of the mucosal detail but may be difficult to remove if the obstruction is high grade. Upper gastrointestinal tract radiographs demonstrate both retention and often the cause of the obstruction. In many cases, it is difficult to distinguish gastric retention caused by motility disorders from retention caused by obstruction. The deformity of surgery may make postoperative radiographs difficult to interpret.

Upper gastrointestinal endoscopy is used to delineate the cause of gastric retention. Aspiration is a risk in the patient with significant retention of gastric contents. The stomach may need to be lavaged for safety and to allow observation of the mucosa. In some cases, computed tomography aids in assessing possible tumor, abscess, or other extraintestinal cause of obstruction.

Quantitative tests of gastric emptying are very important both in diagnosis, in evaluating the response to therapy, and in deciding if surgery is necessary. A gastric residual, measured by nasogastric suction, of over 300 ml obtained more than 4 hours after eating or 200 ml overnight suggests retention. For a rapid but quite useful guide to emptying, the saline load test may be done. After a 16-F sump tube has been placed and its location in the distal antrum confirmed by radiography, the stomach is lavaged until empty. Then 750 ml of normal saline is infused rapidly into the stomach. The fluid remaining after 30 minutes is withdrawn and measured. If less than 300 ml remains, emptying is normal. Between 300 and 400 ml is borderline, and over 400 ml is clearly retention. This test can be repeated after 3 days of nasogastric suction. If the study is still abnormal, nonsurgical improvement is unlikely.

The saline load test only measures liquid emptying and, if abnormal, usually indicates significant obstruction. More detailed information about gastric function is obtained with nuclear medicine gastric emptying studies. Liquids tagged with nuclear agents may be tested simultaneously with solids labeled differently to allow solid and liquid emptying rates. The normal emptying curves are determined for each laboratory, but about 10% per minute for liquids and 5% per minute for solids are reasonable.

TABLE 36–4. DIAGNOSIS OF GASTRIC OUTLET OBSTRUCTION

Tests for Emptying
Saline load test
  750 ml normal saline
  Aspirate after 30 min:
    Less than 300 ml: normal
    300–400 ml: borderline
    More than 400 ml: retention
Nuclear medicine gastric emptying
  Liquid: 10%/min
  Solid: 5%/min

Tests for Etiology
Upper gastrointestinal radiography
  Liquid contrast
  Thin barium
Upper gastrointestinal endoscopy
Computed tomography

THERAPY

The therapy for high-grade, chronic gastric outlet obstruction is usually surgical. In cases where there is a mixed picture of motility disturbance and partial obstruction, prokinetic agents may allow nutritional balance. Endoscopic dilation can occasionally obviate the need for surgery.

Acute peptic ulcer disease with complicating obstruction is diagnosed by endoscopy or upper gastrointestinal radiography. The initial therapy includes nasogastric suction and intravenous H_2-blocking agents. The degree of obstruction can be determined with the saline load test. It is essential that good evacuation of the stomach be maintained. Continued gastric distension leads to gastrin hypersecretion, the risk of aspiration pneumonia, and the serious problem of gastric atony even if the obstruction is eventually relieved surgically. Other causes of gastric retention should be investigated during this period of suction. Diabetes, electrolyte disturbances, and neurologic disorders are evaluated and corrected. Computed tomography of the abdomen is useful to detect neoplasm or contained perforation and abscess which may perpetuate the obstruction.

Even if medical management succeeds, the nasogastric tube is removed, feedings are begun, continued close observation is necessary. The use of aspirin or other nonsteroidal antiinflammatory drugs must be avoided. Even with continued maintenance with H_2-blocking drugs or sucralfate, recurrent obstruction requiring eventual surgery is not unusual.

Patients failing medical care require surgery. Ulcer surgery in the setting of obstruction requires more aggressive technique. The risk of postoperative gastric atony is up to 27% in these patients, over five times that in routine ulcer surgery. The gastric retention following surgery is related to poor emptying of solids and, interestingly, to loss of the phase 3 interdigestive period or housekeeper wave. Studies have recommended that if vagotomy was accompanied by pyloroplasty or Billroth I anastomosis, it be revised to an antrectomy and Billroth II. Billroth II drainage may be converted to Roux-en-Y drainage. Investigators have suggested that in view of the high incidence of postoperative atony, the first surgery should be at least a hemigastrectomy with gastroenterostomy. The Roux-en-Y drainage may also lead to symptomatic retention. In one study,[10] the slow wave electrical activity of the proximal small bowel was reversed in those patients who were symptomatic after this surgery.

Some patients continue to have symptoms of retention even after several surgical procedures. Recurrent mechanical obstruction, often due to marginal peptic ulcer, must be treated. Two studies have suggested total[11] or near total[12] gastrectomy for continued retention postoperatively. The results are improvement of overall satisfaction; however, these patients have considerable debility from these major surgeries.

Fundoplication may enhance the emptying of liquids and solids from the stomach, perhaps by its effect on the size of the gastric reservoir.[13,14] Gastric retention may, however, follow surgery for esophageal reflux, esophageal variceal bleeding, esophageal cancer, and obesity.[8,15,16] Enhanced surgical drainage may be required if vagotomy has been performed or emptying otherwise disturbed.

Nonsurgical treatment of gastric retention, either postoperative or not, includes the use of dietary manipulation and drugs. In some cases, patients tolerate easily digestible solid foods better than liquids. After vagotomy, however, gastric retention is worst for nondigestible solids, better for digestible solids, and best for liquids. In these patients the use of complete liquid nutrition may sustain the patient until motility improves, usually 3 to 6 months at most.

Prokinetic medication is designed to enhance gastric emptying. Bethanechol and other cholinergic acting drugs actually have little benefit in most cases. Better experience has been noted with metoclopramide. This chemical has both strong cholinergic effects and antidopaminergic action. It is the central antidopaminergic activity that suppresses the vomiting center of the brain and provides the antiemetic function. In the stomach the effects are to enhance antral contractions, reduce receptive relaxation, and coordinate antral-pyloric-duodenal motility.

Newer agents include cisapride, a prokinetic agent that facilitates the release of acetylcholine in the myenteric plexus postganglionic synapse[17–19]; domperidone, similar to metoclopramide but without central nervous system effects or side effects,[20] which is still under evaluation; and the recently described use of erythromycin for this purpose.[21,22]

CONCLUSION

Mechanical obstruction of the stomach leads to gastric retention and the symptoms of vomiting, abdominal fullness, early satiety, and nausea. Peptic ulcer disease is the most common cause, both acutely and in chronic cases. Obstruction can also develop because of inflammatory disease, tumor, or prior gastric surgery. Although medical decompression and therapy of the underlying cause of obstruction should be attempted and prokinetic agents may facilitate emptying, therapy is often surgical.

REFERENCES

1. McCallum R. Motility. In: Sleisenger M, Fordtran J, eds. *Gastrointestinal Disease*. Philadelphia, Pa: WB Saunders Co; 1989:675–712.
2. Davenport H. *Physiology of the Digestive Tract*. Chicago, Ill: Year Book Medical Publishers Inc; 1977.
3. Marzio L, Formica P, Fabiani F, et al. Influence of physical activity on gastric emptying of liquids in normal human subjects. *Am J Gastroenterol*. 1991;86:1433–1436.
4. Wegener M, Schaffstein J, Dilger U, et al. Gastrointestinal transit of solid-liquid meal in chronic alcoholics. *Dig Dis Sci*. 1991;36:917–923.
5. Wedmann B, Schmidt G, Wegener M, et al. Effects of age and gender on fat-induced gallbladder contraction and gastric emptying of a caloric liquid meal: a sonographic study. *Am J Gastroenterol*. 1991;86:1765–1770.
6. Jordan P Jr. Gastric Surgery. In: Sleisenger M, Fordtran J, eds. *Gastrointestinal Disease*. Philadelphia, Pa: WB Saunders Co; 1989:939–951.
7. Taylor IL. Gastrointestinal hormones in the pathogenesis of peptic ulcer disease. In: Isenberg J, Johansson C, eds. *Clinics in Gastroenterology*. 1984;13:376–377.
8. Koelz H, Gewertz B. The stomach. In: Blum A, Siewert J, eds. *Clinics in Gastroenterology*. 1979;8:310–312.
9. Moody F, McGreevy J, Miller T. Gastric surgery. In: Schwartz S, Shires GT, Spencer FS, eds. *Principles of Surgery*. New York, NY: McGraw-Hill Book Co; 1989:1157–1188.
10. VanTrappen G, Coremans G, Janssens J, et al. Inversion of the slow-wave frequency gradient in symptomatic patients with Roux-en-Y anastomoses. *Gastroenterology*. 1991;101:1282–1288.
11. Karlstrom L, Keely KA. Surgical treatment of chronic gastric atony. *Am J Surg*. 1987;157:44–49.
12. McCallum R, Polepalle SC, Schirmer B. Completion gastrectomy for refractory gastroparesis following surgery for peptic ulcer disease: long-term follow up with subjective and objective parameters. *Dig Dis Sci*. 1991;39:1556–1561.
13. Maddern GJ, Jamieson GG. Fundoplication enhances gastric emptying. *Ann Surg*. 1985;201:296–299.
14. Jamieson GG, Maddern GJ, Myers JC. Gastric emptying after fundoplication with and without proximal gastric vagotomy. *Arch Surg*. 1991;126:1414–1417.
15. Maddern GJ, Myers JC, McIntosh N, et al. The effect of the Angelchik prosthesis on esophageal and gastric function. *Arch Surg*. 1991;126:1418–1422.
16. Fok M, Cheng SW, Wong J. Pyloroplasty versus no drainage in gastric replacement of the esophagus. *Am J Surg*. 1991;162:447–452.
17. Carnilleri M, Malagelada JR, Abell TL, et al. Effect of six weeks of treatment with cisapride in gastroparesis and intestinal pseudo-obstruction. *Gastroenterology*. 1988;96:704–712.
18. Stacher G, Granser GV, Bergmann H, et al. Slow gastric emptying induced by high fat content of meal accelerated by cisapride administered rectally. *Dig Dis Sci*. 1991;39:1259–1265.
19. Madsen JL. Effects of cisapride on gastrointestinal transit in healthy humans. *Dig Dis Sci*. 1990;35:1500–1504.
20. Wengrower D, Zaltzman S, Karmeli F, Goldin E. Idiopathic gastroparesis in patients with unexplained nausea and vomiting. *Dig Dis Sci*. 1991;36:1255–1258.
21. Sarna SK, Soergel KM, Koch TR, et al. Gastrointestinal motor effects of erythromycin in humans. *Gastroenterology*. 1991;101:1488–1496.
22. Janssens J, Peters TL, VanTrappen G, et al. Improvement of gastric emptying in diabetic gastroparesis by erythromycin: preliminary study. *N Engl J Med*. 1990;322:1028–1031.

37

Gastroparesis

HENRY P. PARKMAN and ROBERT S. FISHER

DEFINITION AND SYMPTOMS OF GASTROPARESIS

Gastroparesis is a chronic motility disorder of the stomach caused by delayed transit of intraluminal contents from the stomach into the duodenum in the absence of mechanical obstruction.

Symptoms of gastric stasis (gastroparesis) include early satiety, postprandial abdominal bloating or distension, nausea often accompanied by vomiting, and abdominal pain. Patients with gastroparesis may vomit food that has been eaten hours previously. Abdominal discomfort is often a part of the clinical picture of gastroparesis, but pain is usually not prominent or severe. Symptoms of gastroparesis are nonspecific and are similar to those associated with mechanical obstruction. The severity of symptoms does not necessarily correlate with the degree of gastric stasis; the clinical features of gastroparesis may be variable. Other disorders such as small intestinal dysmotility, nonulcer dyspepsia, irritable bowel syndrome, and gastritis from *Helicobacter pylori* may be associated with similar symptoms.

CLINICAL DISORDERS OF GASTRIC STASIS

Impaired or altered motility in different anatomic regions of the stomach may result in delayed gastric emptying. For example, decreased fundic tone, decreased antral peristalsis, dysrhythmias of the gastric pacemaker, incoordination between the antral peristaltic wave–pyloric sphincter relaxation-proximal duodenal contractions, pylorospasm, and even intestinal dysmotility have all been reported to delay gastric emptying.

The cause of gastroparesis is multifactorial (see Table 37–1). The three most common causes of gastroparesis are diabetes mellitus, prior surgery for peptic ulcer disease, and idiopathic (i.e., gastroparesis with no obvious cause).

TABLE 37–1. CAUSES OF GASTROPARESIS (NONOBSTRUCTIVE DELAYED GASTRIC EMPTYING)

1. Idiopathic
2. Metabolic
    a. Diabetes
    b. Thyroid disease
    c. Renal insufficiency
3. Postgastric surgery
4. Neuromuscular disorders
    a. Polymyositis or dermatomyositis
5. Connective tissue diseases
    a. Scleroderma
6. Infiltrative disorders
    a. Lymphoma
    b. Amyloidosis
7. Diffuse gastrointestinal motility disorder
    a. Intestinal pseudoobstruction
8. Medication-induced
    a. Narcotic analgesics
    b. Antidepressants
    c. Anticholinergics
    d. Calcium channel blockers
9. Electrolyte imbalance
    a. Potassium
    b. Calcium
    c. Magnesium

POSTGASTRIC SURGERY

The vagus nerve is particularly important to the neural control of gastric emptying. Vagal stimulation induces fundic relaxation and antral contractions. Thus, truncal vagotomy may be associated with delayed emptying of solids and accelerated emptying of liquids. In theory, parietal cell vagotomy should not alter gastric motor function. Surgically induced gastroparesis is usually from peptic ulcer disease surgery. Any procedure involving a vagotomy, especially Roux-en-Y diversion of the biliary system, may produce a wide array of upper gastrointestinal tract symptoms in up to as many as 50%. A subset of patients with preoperative symptoms of gastric outlet obstruction may develop a particularly severe chronic nonmechanical gastric stasis after surgery. One wonders about the role of dysmotility in the original presentation of these patients.

DIABETIC GASTROPARESIS

Diabetic gastroparesis is a well-recognized complication of long-standing diabetes mellitus. Delayed gastric emptying is present in up to 50% of patients with insulin-dependent diabetes mellitus (IDDM) and is usually associated with other diabetic complications such as retinopathy, neuropathy, and nephropathy. Frequently, these patients have other signs of autonomic neuropathy such as orthostatic hypotension and signs of peripheral neuropathy. Diabetic gastroparesis should be suspected in patients with long-standing insulin-dependent diabetes and postprandial upper abdominal complaints such as nausea, vomiting, early satiety, and belching.

In some diabetic patients, delayed gastric emptying may contribute to poor glucose control (hypoglycemia or hyperglycemia) because of unpredictable delivery of food into the duodenum. Impaired gastric emptying may lead to hypoglycemia. Conversely, improved emptying (for example, during treatment of gastroparesis) may lead to hyperglycemia.

Hyperglycemia, of itself, may delay gastric emptying in normal subjects and patients with diabetes. Intraluminal manometric recordings have shown that hyperglycemia-induced delayed gastric emptying is associated with a decrease in antral contractility, a decrease in antral phase 3 migrating motor complex (MMC) activity, and an increase in pyloric contractions. Normalization of serum glucose in hyperglycemic diabetics can restore antral phase 3 activity in some patients.

IDIOPATHIC GASTROPARESIS

Overall, idiopathic gastroparesis is the most common form of gastroparesis, accounting for nearly half of all cases. This disorder is most frequently seen in women.

GASTROESOPHAGEAL REFLUX DISEASE

Although some investigators have claimed that gastric retention with accumulation of acid and gastric contents may be a contributory factor in up to 40% of patients with gastroesophageal reflux disease (GERD), other studies have been conflicting.

GASTRIC ULCER

Delayed gastric emptying has been reported in some patients with gastric ulcers. Of interest, gastroparesis has resolved in some patients after ulcer healing. It is not clear whether gastroparesis is a result or a cause of the ulcer.

MEDICATION-INDUCED GASTROPARESIS

Many drugs including anticholinergics, narcotic analgesics, antidepressants, and possibly calcium channel blockers are known to delay gastric emptying. Drug-induced gastroparesis may be asymptomatic but must be considered when interpreting gastric emptying scans.

METHODS OF MEASURING GASTRIC EMPTYING AND MOTILITY

Four diagnostic modalities are used to measure gastric motility: (1) roentgenographic examinations, (2) intraluminal manometry, (3) radionuclide scintigraphy, and (4) electrogastrography.

UPPER GASTROINTESTINAL TRACT RADIOGRAPHIC SERIES

A diagnosis of gastric retention is supported by poor emptying of barium from the stomach, gastric dilation, or the presence of retained food or a gastric bezoar. Roentgenographic studies, however, are nonphysiologic, nonquantitative, associated with significant radiation exposure, and do not adequately assess total gastric emptying time. The upper gastrointestinal tract radiographic series (upper GI) is primarily useful to rule out mechanical obstruction or gross mucosal abnormalities such as peptic ulcer disease.

INTRALUMINAL GASTROPYLORODUODENAL MANOMETRY

Intubation of the gastric-antral-duodenal area with perfused catheters or solid-state pressure probes may be used to measure intraluminal contractile activity. These studies may show decreased motor activity in the fundus and antrum or phase 3 migrating motor activity originating in the small intestine rather than the stomach in patients with gastroparesis. Occasionally, pylorospasms or irregular bursts of small intestinal contractions, which increase outflow resistance, can be recorded. Manometric tests may be uncomfortable and prolonged in that at least 5 hours' recording time is required to assess the fasting- and fed-state motility patterns.

RADIONUCLIDE GASTRIC EMPTYING SCINTIGRAPHY

Gastric scintigraphy is currently the gold standard test to quantitate gastric emptying. Gastric scintigraphic studies can be performed on an outpatient basis without intubation and are readily accepted by the patient. In this test, the patient ingests small amounts of a gamma-emitting radiopharmaceutical, and the aboral movement of the radiolabel is measured using a gamma counter (see Figs. 37–1A and 37–2A). Initially solid-phase gastric emptying tests were performed using chicken liver after injection of the wing vein with ^{99m}technetium (Tc)-sulfur colloid. Today, most tests are performed using ^{99m}Tc-sulfur colloid–labeled eggs. Measuring gastric emptying of liquids is of little clinical use since it does not become abnormal until gastroparesis is far advanced.

The simplest approach to interpreting gastric emptying data for solids is to report the percentage of emptying at some specific time after ingestion (usually 1 hour) or the time to 50% emptying ($t_{1/2}$) (see Figs. 37–1B and 37–2B). Other parameters of potential use are the lag phase for solids and the slopes of the emptying curves. The lag phase most likely represents the time required for trituration of solid food before emptying from the stomach occurs. A prolonged lag phase suggests antral hypomotility. The slope (rate at which solids leave the stomach once emptying begins) may be prolonged by antral hypomotility or by intestinal dysmotility.

ELECTROGASTROGRAM

Measurements of gastric myoelectric activity can be obtained with cutaneous electrodes. The

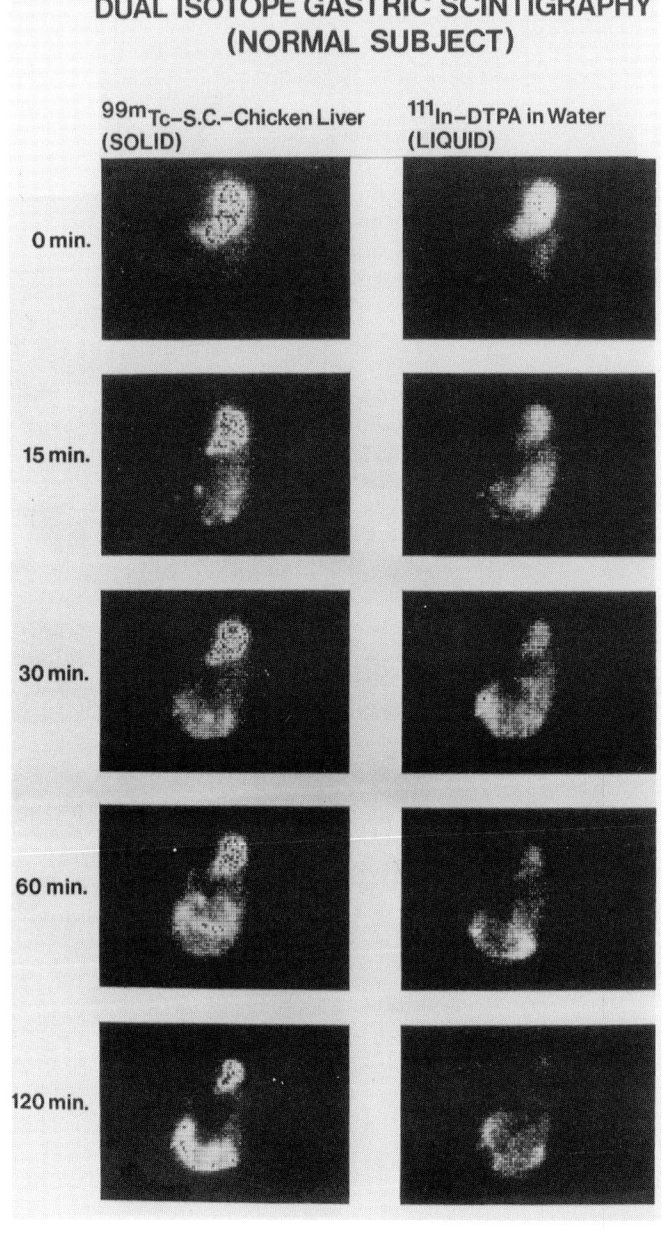

FIGURE 37–1. Normal scintigraphic gastric emptying test. **A,** Serial scans of a gastric emptying test in a normal subject using two radioisotopes to simultaneously measure solid and liquid gastric emptying. The solid marker is ^{99m}technetium-sulfur colloid in chicken liver, and the liquid marker is ^{111}indium in water. Scintigraphic scans at 0, 15, 30, 60, and 120 minutes after ingestion of the radioisotopes are shown. At 0 minutes, the outline of the stomach is shown and emptying from the stomach is seen in the subsequent scans. Note that the liquid empties from the stomach faster than the solid marker. **B,** Average values for gastric emptying of solids and liquids in normal patients as a function of time. Note that the $t_{1/2}$ (time for 50% gastric emptying) for liquids is ~30 minutes, whereas the $t_{1/2}$ for solids is ~90 minutes.

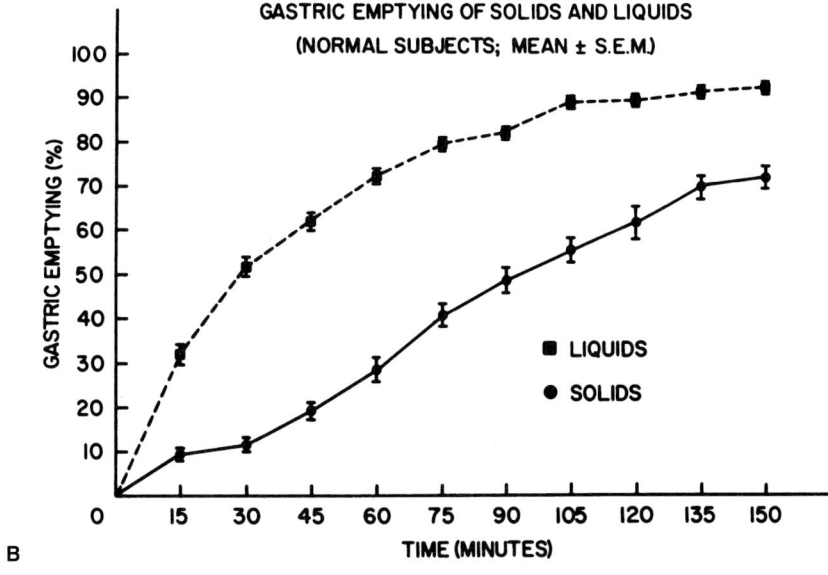

FIGURE 37–1 Continued

electrogastrogram (EGG) is analogous to an electrocardiogram (ECG) and provides an analysis of gastric rhythm but not gastric emptying. Electrogastrography enables detection of gastric dysrhythmias. The normal gastric rhythm is 3 cpm. Gastric dysrhythmias such as tachygastria, bradygastria, and flat line patterns have been described in idiopathic and diabetic gastroparesis. In addition, gastric dysrhythmias may produce symptoms such as nausea and vomiting without a change in gastric emptying.

EVALUATION OF SUSPECTED GASTROPARESIS

The first step in diagnosing gastroparesis is to have a high index of clinical suspicion (see Table 37–2). Signs of a severe gastric emptying disorder, such as presence of bezoars and old food particles in the stomach, may be detected when an upper GI tract series or endoscopy is performed. Systemic causes including diabetes, hypothyroidism, hypercalcemia, and pregnancy are usually considered at the initial visit.

The second step in diagnosing gastroparesis is to exclude other abnormalities by performing barium roentgenography or upper endoscopy. Mechanical gastric outlet obstruction can be caused by pyloric stenosis secondary to an acute duodenal, pyloric channel, or prepyloric ulcer, scarring from prior ulcers, chronic ulcer disease, or neoplasia. In all cases of presumed gastroparesis, mechanical obstruction of the stomach, duodenum, or small bowel must be excluded. Often, the stomach is decompressed for several days using a nasogastric tube before testing for mechanical obstruction.

The third step is to obtain a solid-phase gastric emptying scintigraphic test. Patients are instructed to discontinue medications that may affect gastric emptying for approximately 48 hours prior to gastric scintigraphy. An abnormal gastric emptying test suggests, but does not prove, that the symptoms are caused by gastroparesis. If the gastric emptying test is normal, a careful reevaluation of the patient is needed. Although abdominal pain may be caused by gastroparesis, this is usually evaluated separately.

TREATMENT OF SYMPTOMATIC GASTROPARESIS

The treatment of gastroparesis varies depending on the setting in which a patient is initially seen (see Table 37–3). In an ambulatory outpatient complaining of early satiety and abdominal distension, treatment may merely consist of pre-

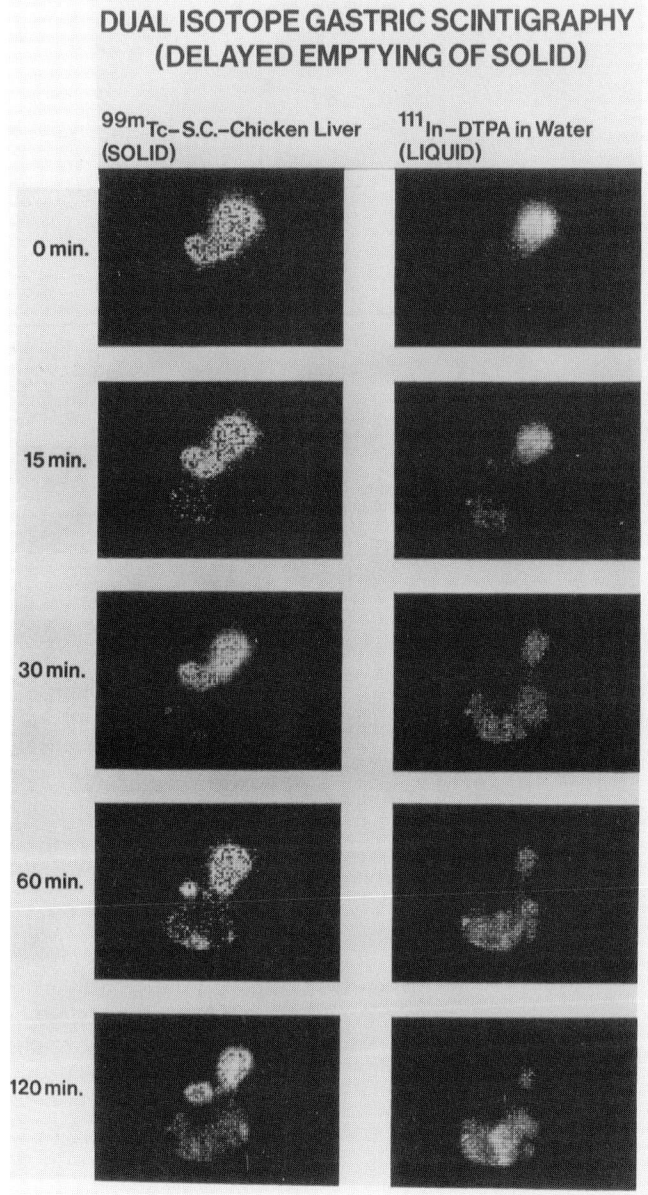

FIGURE 37–2. A, Scintigraphic gastric emptying in a patient with gastroparesis. Serial scans at 0, 15, 30, 60, and 120 minutes after ingestion of a meal with two radioisotopes: ^{99m}Tc-sulfur colloid in chicken liver for solid emptying and ^{111}indium in water for liquid emptying. Note that there is retention of the radiolabel in the stomach for solids but not for liquids (compare with Figure 37–1*A*).

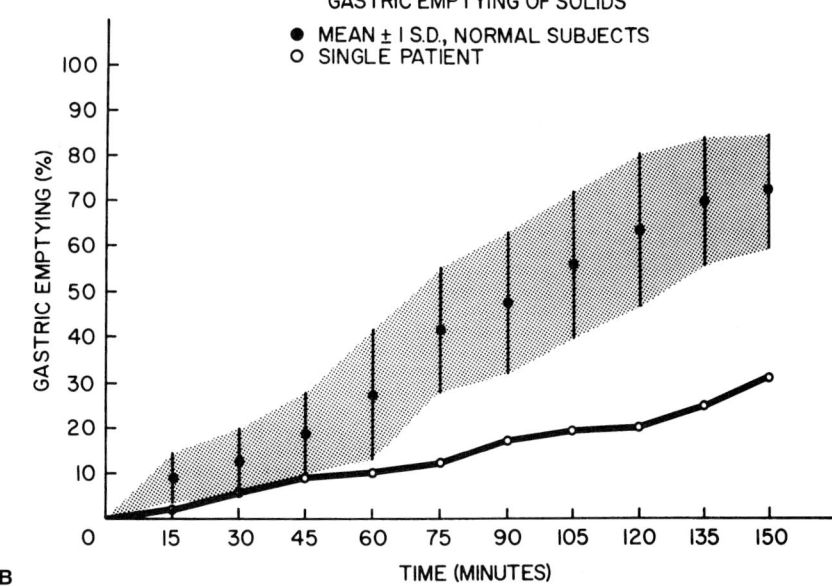

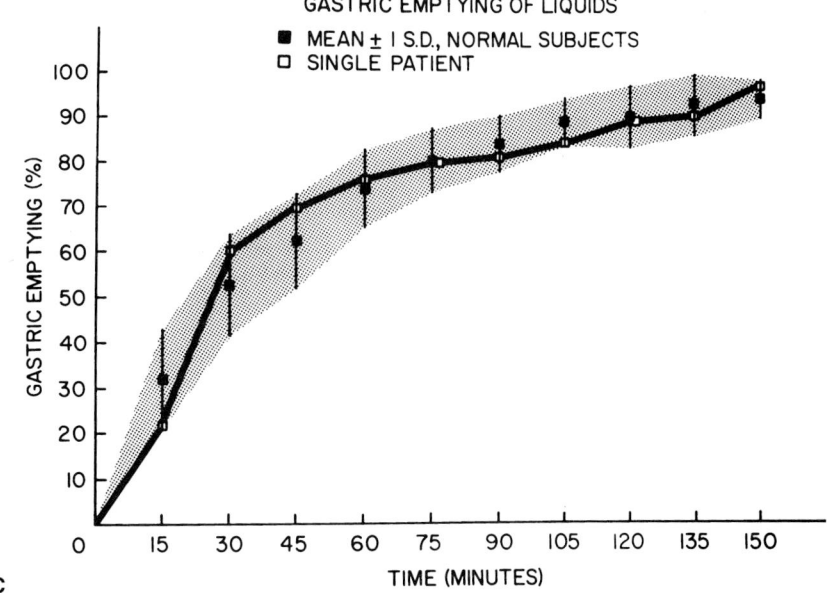

B, Gastric emptying curves for solids in a patient with gastroparesis compared with the normal values from Figure 37–1B. At 120 minutes, normal subjects have 65% emptying, whereas this patient had only 20% emptying. **C,** Gastric emptying curves for liquids in a patient with gastroparesis compared with the normal values from Figure 37–1B. Note that the gastric emptying of liquids is normal in this patient with gastroparesis.

TABLE 37–2. EVALUATION OF PATIENTS WITH SUSPECTED GASTROPARESIS

1. Consider the diagnosis of gastroparesis
2. Evaluate for mechanical obstruction
    a. Upper gastrointestinal tract series
    b. Upper endoscopy
3. Document gastroparesis
    a. Solid phase gastric emptying test
4. Evaluate for secondary causes
    a. Check glucose, potassium, creatinine, calcium, magnesium, thyroid tests

TABLE 37–3. TREATMENT OF GASTROPARESIS

1. Treat underlying disease process, if possible
2. Dietary
    a. Hydration
    b. Small, frequent meals
    c. Liquid feedings often better tolerated
    d. Avoid fatty foods, fiber, indigestible solids
3. Pharmacologic therapy
    a. Antiemetics
    b. Prokinetic agents
        (1) Metoclopramide
        (2) Domperidone
        (3) Cisapride
        (4) Erythromycin
        (5) Bethanechol

scribing an oral prokinetic agent. In severe cases with nausea, vomiting, and signs of dehydration and poor glucose control, however, treatment may require hospital admission, intravenous hydration, careful regulation of blood glucose, nasogastric decompression, and intravenous administration of prokinetic agents.

The goals of treatment are to reduce symptoms and maintain hydration and nutrition. This may be accomplished in several ways. First, underlying medical illnesses and causes for symptomatic gastroparesis (electrolyte imbalance, renal insufficiency, thyroid dysfunction, mucosal disease, etc.) must be sought and treated appropriately. This includes eliminating causative drugs such as narcotic analgesics. Second, the general medical condition of the patient should be assessed and addressed. This includes hydration, correction of electrolyte disturbances, and, if appropriate, controlling blood glucose concentrations.

Nausea and vomiting may be treated directly with antinauseants or antiemetics including prochlorperazine (Compazine) or trimethobenzamide (Tigan). Conventional antiemetic drugs, such as phenothiazines, act centrally. Some antiemetics may have adverse effects on gastric motility because of their anticholinergic properties. Ondansetron, a serotonin (5-HT$_3$) receptor antagonist available only in an intravenous form, has been shown to be helpful in chemotherapy-induced nausea and vomiting.

Third, the nutritional status of the patient should be addressed. This often involves increasing liquid nutrients in the diet because emptying of liquids may be less affected than the emptying of solids; eliminating bulky, indigestible solids from diet; and introducing small frequent feedings of easily digestible foods low in fat. Indigestible food (fiber) should be avoided. Fat and lactose in the diet should be decreased. Alcohol should be avoided, since even low doses of alcohol can decrease antral contractility and impair gastric emptying. Commercial formula diets or self-prepared liquid homogenized meals may be well tolerated. Sometimes enteral alimentation (if the small intestine works) may be needed. For severe cases of gastroparesis, parenteral nutrition may be needed, although this is not an ideal long-term solution because of the high incidence of catheter-induced bacteremia.

Fourth, pharmacologic therapy with prokinetics may be needed for symptomatic control. Several prokinetic agents enhance the motility of the upper gastrointestinal tract and accelerate the aboral movement of the intraluminal contents. In general, prokinetic agents increase gastric contractions, improve antral contractility and antroduodenal coordination, resolve gastric dysrhythmias, and may also act centrally to decrease symptoms (see Table 37–4). Usually prokinetic agents are given 30 minutes preprandially to maximize the gastric prokinetic effect at the time of the meal. In addition, an evening dose is often important to empty the stomach of indigestible solids. Since gastrointestinal symptoms may correlate poorly with objective measurements of gastric emptying, the response to treatment is judged by clinical symptoms and not by gastric emptying tests. The reason that some patients respond to one of these prokinetic agents, whereas others do not, is uncertain. Limited data suggest that the prokinetic efficacy of metoclopramide, domperidone, and erythromycin may diminish during prolonged administration. A wide variety of side effects may be observed with some prokinetic agents. Usually side effects are seen at the higher doses; however, some patients, especially elderly patients, may display side effects at the normal dosage.

TABLE 37–4. MECHANISMS OF ACTION FOR PROKINETIC AGENTS IN TREATMENT OF GASTROPARESIS

1. Normalization of gastric emptying
   a. Increase antral contractility
   b. Improve antroduodenal coordination
2. Resolution of gastric dysrhythmias
3. Central antiemetic effect

In contrast to published studies on prokinetic agents suggesting that they are very effective, the experience of individual clinicians has not been nearly that good. Factors that may explain this discrepancy include the duration of treatment (acute versus chronic), the route of administration (intravenous versus oral), medication side effects preventing appropriate prokinetic doses, wrong diagnosis with symptoms of the patient from another disorder, and different patient populations with different severity of gastroparesis.

METOCLOPRAMIDE

Metoclopramide has three major effects on the gastrointestinal tract: release of acetylcholine from intrinsic cholinergic neurons, peripheral dopamine receptor antagonism on gastrointestinal smooth muscle, and an antiemetic action due to central dopamine receptor antagonism in the chemoreceptor zone for vomiting. Gastrointestinal actions of metoclopramide include increased amplitude of gastric contractions in the fundus, antrum, and duodenum with an increased coordination between antral contractions and pyloric relaxation. There is also an increased amplitude of esophageal contractions and resting lower esophageal sphincter (LES) pressure. Controlled trials have shown that metoclopramide may provide symptomatic relief while accelerating gastric emptying of solids and liquids in patients with idiopathic, diabetic, and postvagotomy gastroparesis and in patients with gastroesophageal reflux disease. Metoclopramide may also improve symptoms with a minimal effect on gastric emptying because of its central antiemetic effects. The usual dose of metoclopramide in adults is 10 mg, 30 minutes before each meal and at bedtime; but this dose often must be increased in patients who do not respond clinically. In patients with severe gastroparesis, oral metoclopramide might not be adequately absorbed because of nausea and vomiting or delayed gastric emptying. In these patients, it must be given intravenously to improve gastric emptying. Although metoclopramide is an effective drug in the acute treatment of gastroparesis, there is evidence that metoclopramide's therapeutic effect disappears at least partly during long-term treatment.

Side effects due to the antidopaminergic properties of metoclopramide are the major factor restricting its use and may occur in up to 30% of patients. Side effects are more frequent with higher doses and occur more commonly in young children and the aged. Side effects associated with metoclopramide include agitation, irritability, drowsiness, lethargy, akathisia, and increased prolactin release resulting in breast engorgement, lactation, and menstrual irregularity. In addition, extrapyramidal effects including facial spasm, oculogyric crisis, trismus, and torticollis may occur.

CISAPRIDE

Cisapride acts to facilitate release of acetylcholine from cholinergic nerves in the myenteric plexus. It may also function as a serotonin (5-HT_4) agonist. Cisapride increases antral and duodenal contractions, improves antroduodenal coordination, and increases gastric emptying. Cisapride also increases esophageal contractions and resting LES pressure and thus is beneficial for some patients with gastroesophageal reflux disease. At the present time, cisapride is approved for use in gastroesophageal reflux disease. Studies also suggest that cisapride improves gastric emptying and symptoms in patients with gastroparesis. Its beneficial results may last for at least 1 year. Cisapride has no antidopaminergic effects and thus does not cause extrapyramidal side effects or prolactin secretion. Side effects of cisapride are few, less severe than with metoclopramide, and include diarrhea, light-headedness, and abdominal cramps. In patients with a seizure focus, cisapride may rarely result in an increase in seizure activity.

ERYTHROMYCIN

Erythromycin, which mimics the effect of the gastrointestinal peptide, motilin, on gastrointestinal motility, may have therapeutic value in patients with gastroparesis. Erythromycin accelerates gastric emptying by increasing the amplitude and frequency of antral contractions and improving gastroduodenal coordination. In addition, erythromycin causes an early reappearance of propagative phase 3 motor activity in the stomach. The motor response to erythromycin is less during the fed state than during the fasted state. In the fed state, erythromycin significantly shortens the duration of time in which the migrating motor complex is disrupted by a meal. The gastrointestinal prokinetic effects of erythromycin may occur at dosages lower than that required for antibacterial effects. Intravenous infusion of erythromycin lactobionate (200 mg) accelerates the slow emptying of solids in patients with diabetic gastroparesis. In these same patients, 4 weeks of oral erythromycin ethylsuccinate (250 mg orally three times a day, 30 minutes before meals) accelerated the delayed emptying of solids and liquids but not as much as was observed in response to the single intravenous dose. A stimulatory effect of erythromycin has also been reported in postvagotomy gastroparesis and gastroparesis associated with progressive systemic sclerosis. Studies of longer duration are needed to assess whether tachyphylaxis may develop with high doses or frequent administration. In addition, side effect profiles associated with erythromycin must be established. Some side effects include nausea, bloating, and upper abdominal cramping pain. Analogs of erythromycin are being designed that have more potent motilin agonist activity and little antibiotic action.

BETHANECHOL

Bethanechol is a nonspecific cholinergic muscarinic agonist. It enhances the amplitudes of contractions throughout the gastrointestinal tract. Unfortunately, bethanechol does not coordinate contractions; therefore, gastric emptying and small bowel transit are not necessarily accelerated. Some gastroenterologists do not consider bethanechol to be a true prokinetic agent. Occasionally, it may be helpful as adjuvant treatment to be used with prokinetic agents. Specific effects of bethanechol include increased amplitude of contractions of the esophagus, LES, gastric antrum, small bowel, colon, and gallbladder. The direct cholinergic action of bethanechol may also stimulate the secretion of gastric acid and saliva. Potential side effects of bethanechol include increased salivation, blurring of vision, abdominal cramps, and bladder spasm.

DOMPERIDONE

Although domperidone is an investigational agent in the United States, it is widely available in Europe, Canada, Mexico, and Japan. Domperidone is a specific peripheral dopamine antagonist, with no cholinergic activity. Domperidone stimulates upper gastrointestinal tract motility by enhancing gastroduodenal contraction and coordination and can improve gastric emptying in some patients with gastroparesis. Domperidone does not readily cross the blood-brain barrier; therefore, it rarely causes extrapyramidal side effects. The side effects of domperidone are less than metoclopramide and are usually secondary to increased prolactin release (e.g., breast engorgement and galactorrhea). Central nervous system side effects are minimal.

SURGICAL TREATMENT

Surgery for gastroparesis is performed rarely, with great caution, and only as a last resort. Surgery may be performed to provide a feeding route or to decompress the stomach. A surgical jejunostomy may be placed for enteral alimentation with or without a gastrostomy tube to serve as a decompressive outlet. Surgical jejunostomies are very effective in providing nutrition and often function better than percutaneously placed gastrostomies of jejunostomies.

In patients with postsurgical gastric atony, patients may require even more radical surgery to eliminate hold-up in the atonic stomach and prevent enterogastric reflux. Extensive subtotal or near total gastrectomy and Roux-en-Y gastrojejunostomy may lead to improvement in some patients with chronic gastric atony. Unfortunately, many patients have no benefit even after extensive surgery. Thus, at the current time, present surgical treatments are usually unsatisfactory and, not infrequently, the patient is not improved.

On rare occasion, a total gastrectomy may be performed in patients with gastroparesis to remove the offending organ. Caution is advised, since symptoms may be transient and the motility problem may extend into the small bowel.

Gastric pacing with surgically implanted electrodes provides an exciting future therapeutic possibility for augmenting gastric electromechanical activity.

CLINICAL OUTCOME OF GASTROPARESIS

Few studies have provided long-term follow-up of patients with gastroparesis. Thus, it is difficult to prognosticate for an individual patient with gastroparesis on the course of his illness. Patients with postviral gastroparesis often improve and do well in the long term without recurrence of symptoms. Patients with diabetic gastroparesis often have recurrent or persistent symptoms.

A recent study evaluated the clinical outcome of 60 patients with gastroparesis failing to improve symptomatically or experiencing unacceptable side effects with metoclopramide. Over a follow-up of 16 months, 58% responded to initial therapy with another single prokinetic agent; 32% required switching from one prokinetic to another; 7% underwent surgical jejunostomy; and one patient underwent gastric resection with Roux-en-Y anastomosis.

CONCLUSION

In the last several years, advances have been made in several areas related to gastroparesis. Electrogastrography has been used to help understand that symptoms may be related not only to delayed gastric emptying but also to an abnormal gastric myoelectrical rhythm (either bradygastria or tachygastria). Treatment with prokinetic agents may improve the symptoms and gastric rhythm to the normal 3 cpm without necessarily a change in the gastric emptying rate. Side effects of the prokinetic agents may limit their efficacy. Currently, prokinetic agents with a selective action on the gastrointestinal tract with few side effects are being sought. Over the next few years, several new prokinetic agents will become available for use in patients with gastroparesis. The goal of drug development is to develop agents with prokinetic actions that persist during long-term treatment and have few side effects. Which prokinetic agents should be employed for initial treatment and which categories of gastroparesis respond to specific prokinetic agents will be determined with future studies. The application of surgical treatment with gastric pacing or gastric resection to improve symptoms is starting to be developed.

REFERENCES

1. Annese V, Janssens J, Vantrappen G, et al. Erythromycin accelerates gastric emptying by inducing antral contractions and improved gastroduodenal coordination. *Gastroenterology.* 1992;102:823–828.
2. Fraser RJ, Horowitz M, Maddox AF, Harding PE, Chatterton BE, Dent J. Hyperglycaemia slows gastric emptying in type I (insulin-dependent) diabetes mellitus. *Diabetologia.* 1990;33:675–680.
3. Horowitz M, Edelbroek M, Fraser R, Maddox A, Wishart J. Disordered gastric motor function in diabetes mellitus: recent insights into the prevalence, pathophysiology, clinical relevance, and treatment. *Scand J Gastroenterol.* 1991;26:673–684.
4. Horowitz M, Harding PE, Chatterton BE, Collins PJ, Shearman DJC. Acute and chronic effects of domperidone on gastric emptying in diabetic autonomic neuropathy. *Dig Dis Sci.* 1985;30:1–9.
5. Janssens J, Peeters TL, Vantrappen G, et al. Improvement of gastric emptying in diabetic gastroparesis by erythromycin: preliminary studies. *N Engl J Med.* 1990; 322:1028–1031.
6. Koch KL, Stern RM, Stewart WR, Vasey MW. Gastric emptying and gastric myoelectric activity in patients with diabetic gastroparesis: effect of long-term domperidone treatment. *Am J Gastroenterol.* 1989;84:1069–1074.
7. Menomi H, McCallum RW. The physiology and pathophysiology of gastric emptying in humans. *Gastroenterology.* 1984;85:1592–1610.
8. Oster-Jorgense E, Gerner T, Pederson SA. The determination of gastric emptying rate. *Eur J Surg.* 1991; 564(suppl):31–43.
9. Parkman HP, Schwartz SS. Esophagitis and gastroduodenal disorders associated with diabetic gastroparesis. *Arch Intern Med.* 1987;147:1477–1480.
10. Read NW, Houghton LA. Physiology of gastric emptying and pathophysiology of gastroparesis. *Gastroenterol Clin North Am.* 1989;18:359–373.
11. Reynolds JC. Prokinetic agents: a key in the future of gastroenterology. *Gastroenterol Clin North Am.* 1989;18: 437–457.
12. Rock E, Malmud L, Fisher RS. Motor disorders of the stomach. *Med Clin North Am.* 1981;65:1269–1289.
13. Sarna SK, Soergel KH, Koch TR, et al. Gastrointestinal motor effects of erythromycin in humans. *Gastroenterology.* 1991;101:1488–1496.
14. Snape WJ, Battle WM, Schwartz SS, Braunstein SN, Goldstein HA, Alavi A. Metoclopramide to treat gastroparesis due to diabetes mellitus. *Ann Intern Med.* 1982;96:444.
15. Varis K. Diabetic gastroparesis. *Scand J Gastroenterol.* 1989;24:897–903.

38
Bezoars
THOMAS J. DEVERS

Bezoars are a fascinating topic of medical history and present many challenging treatment options. Bezoars result from the accumulation of foreign ingested material and have been reported to occur in any area of the intestinal tract from the esophagus to the rectum. The most common site of bezoar formation is in the stomach, and the most common type of patient is one who has had previous gastric surgery. A patient with a vagotomy and Billroth II gastrectomy who ingests unpeeled persimmon fruit has a calculated risk 56 times greater than that of age- and sex-matched controls.[1] Persimmon bezoars are one of the few types that can occur in patients with normal gastric motility.

In addition to gastric surgery, diseases associated with delayed gastric emptying such as diabetic gastroparesis, certain neuromuscular disorders, and intestinal pseudoobstruction increase the risk of gastric bezoars. There are several reported cases of gastric carcinoma presenting with bezoars, so mechanical obstruction may be a predisposing cause. Health faddism is a risk factor for bezoars. Lupini beans are used by unorthodox healers for arthritic pain and are an increasing cause of bezoars. Lecithin ingested in bulk form by people believing it will improve memory and lower cholesterol has been a cause of the gastric bezoar. Per diem bulk type psyllium may cause an esophageal or gastric bezoar. Medication bezoars are increasingly being reported with long-acting theophylline, and nifedipine preparations, and enteric coated aspirin are known to produce bezoars composed mostly of their insoluble residues. There is a reported case of fatal theophylline overdose secondary to a medication bezoar that weighed 318.8 g and contained 29 g of theophylline in a white waxy mass found in the stomach at autopsy.[2] Sucralfate has been reported on multiple occasions to produce bezoars and should not be used in patients with delayed gastric emptying.

Trichobezoars are usually found in young women or girls in association with psychiatric disorders or mental retardation. These cases commonly present with a mobile abdominal mass, and trichophagia (hair eating) is usually preceded by trichotillomania (hair pulling). These types of bezoars are notoriously difficult to treat. A trichobezoar may have hair extending throughout the intestinal tract to the cecum, a condition given the fairy-tale designation, Rapunzel syndrome.[3] Polystyrene cups may produce bezoars through ingestion of material. Primary colonic bezoars are rare, but there is a report of a lecithin vitamin B_{12} bezoar in an 81-year-old man. Sunflower seeds and popcorn can produce a rectal bezoar. There is a single case report of a child ingesting a large amount of gummi bear candy which produced a rectal bezoar (Table 38–1).

CLINICAL MANIFESTATION OF BEZOARS

The most frequent clinical manifestation of bezoars is intestinal obstruction secondary to migration of the entire bezoar or a substantial portion of the bezoar. Any patient with previous gastric surgery for peptic ulcer disease who presents with intestinal obstruction should be considered a likely candidate for a bezoar causing the obstruction. In a series of 56 patients with bezoars following gastric surgery, 80% presented with intestinal obstruction (Fig. 38–1, see Color Plate III).[4] Ulceration of the stomach from mechanical pressures of the bezoar is well recognized. Perforation and peritonitis especially as a consequence of intestinal obstruction is a very serious complication. Mortality associated with complications of bezoars such as obstruction or perforation ranges from 30% to 47%. Bezoars may occur in patients with life-threatening acute

TABLE 38-1. CLASSIFICATION OF BEZOARS

1. Phytobezoar
   a. Persimmon
   b. Psyllium
   c. Fruit: raisins, oranges, coconuts, figs, apples
   d. Vegetable: green beans, brussel sprouts, sauerkraut, potato peels, lupini beans
2. Trichobezoar
   a. Gastric
   b. Rapunzel syndrome
3. Medication Bezoar
   a. Enteric coated aspirin
   b. Sustained release capsules, theophylline, nifedipine
   c. Lecithin
   d. Sucralfate
4. Others
   a. Polystyrene, styrofoam cup, exchange resins
   b. Lactobezoar
   c. *Candida*

TABLE 38-2. BEZOAR THERAPY

1. Dissolution
   a. Cellulase
   b. Acetylcysteine
   c. Adolph's Meat Tenderizer
2. Mechanical disruption
   a. Endoscopic snare or biopsy
   b. Endoscopic or nasogastric tube water jet fragmentation
3. Laser or lithotripsy
   a. Electrohydraulic
   b. ND:YAG laser
   c. Extracorporeal lithotripsy
   d. Pulse dye laser
4. Surgery
5. Prevention
   a. Diet
   b. Gastric prokinetic agents
     (1) Metoclopramide
     (2) Cisapride

medical problems such as bone marrow and liver transplants and may greatly increase their morbidity. Bezoars may complicate endoscopic sclerotherapy for bleeding esophageal varices presumably secondary to damage of the vagus nerve from the injection of the sclerosing agent.

BEZOAR THERAPY

The type of bezoar and the presence or absence of complications largely determine the therapeutic options (Table 38-2). An uncomplicated phytobezoar has many possible effective forms of therapy. On the other hand, a trichobezoar with or without complications has limited effective therapeutic options. There are only two reported cases of successful endoscopic removal of a trichobezoar. The most important principle in dealing with bezoars is to use the most conservative effective form of therapy first and to reserve the "high-tech" invasive procedures for failures. The following compounds have been used successfully to dissolve phytobezoars.

CELLULASE

Cellulase has been used to dissolve phytobezoars since 1968. A review by Walker-Renard[5] examined a total of 19 patients receiving cellulase with a 100% dissolution rate with no adverse effects (Table 38-3). The length of therapy ranged from 2 to 7 days. Various cellulase preparations have been used. Gastroenterase tablets, which contain pepsin, pancreatic enzymes, dehydrocholic acid, and cellulase, were a common choice, but they are no longer available in the United States. Pure cellulase has been used dissolved in water, given over 3 to 5 days with a 100% success rate. Cellulase can be obtained from Valley Research (South Bend, Indiana; phone [219]232-5000). Cellulase is clearly the drug of choice for medical dissolution therapy for phytobezoars.[5]

ACETYLCYSTEINE

There is one reported case of acetylcysteine oral mucomist instilled by nasogastric tube; 15 ml of acetylcysteine was diluted in 50 ml of NaCl 0.9%. The tube was clamped for 3 hours, and the procedure was repeated three more times over the next 24 hours. The bezoar was dissolved, and no side effects were reported.

PAPAIN

Papain is a protease that has been used successfully in the treatment of phytobezoars. A total of 15 patients have been reported, and papain was effective in treating 13 of the 15 patients (87%). The length of therapy ranged from 1.5 to 180 days. The source of papain used most commonly today is Adolph's Meat Tenderizer. This is usually mixed with water and administered by nasogastric tube or consumed orally. The use of Adolph's Meat Tenderizer in the esophagus has

TABLE 38-3. CELLULASE TREATMENT OF PHYTOBEZOARS

Patients (N)	Treatment Regimen	Length of Therapy (Days)	Success Rate	Adverse Effects
1	Gastroenterase 3 tablets after each meal	3	100%	NR
1	Gastroenterase 3 tablets after each meal	3	100%	NR
4	Gastroenterase 2 tablets t.i.d. with meals	3–7	100%	NR
1	Gastroenterase	3	100%	NR
1	Gastroenterase 3 tablets after each meal	5	100%	NR
1	Cellulase 0.5% solution in 300 ml water every 4 h	5	100%	NR
4	Cellulase 5 g in 300–500 ml water daily	2–3	100%	NR
5	Cellulase 0.5% solution in 300 ml water every 4 h	3	100%	NR
1	Cellulase 4 g in 300 ml water daily	5	100%	NR

NR = none reported.
From Walker-Renard P. Update on the medicinal management of phytobezoars. 1993;88(10):1663–1666.

been associated with esophageal perforation in two cases. Hypernatremia is also a risk since each 20 cc of Adolph's Meat Tenderizer contains over 7 g of NaCl.

Endoscopic Bezoar Therapy

Endoscopic disruption and removal of phytobezoars has been well described. Disruption or destruction of the bezoar can be accomplished by using a polypectomy snare or biopsy forceps. The bezoar can be fragmented into small particles and can either pass or be removed by the endoscope. Another successful endoscopic method is water jet fragmentation, available in most endoscopic units. Nasogastric tubes with vigorous lavage or Ewald tubes have been used successfully to disrupt phytobezoars.

Endoscopic therapy of trichobezoars is risky and is based on little published experience. There are only two reported cases of successful removal of trichobezoars by endoscopy. The first case required over 100 passages of the endoscope over a 3-hour period. In the second case an overtube was used and the trichobezoar was removed with the patient receiving endotracheal general anesthesia. The main danger of endoscopic removal of a trichobezoar is airway obstruction, and no attempts may be made to remove this type of bezoar without endotracheal intubation for airway protection.

Laser Therapy or Lithotripsy

A variety of endoscopically assisted devices have been used to disrupt large or hard phytobezoars not amenable to mechanical disruption as described above. These devices include the electrohydraulic lithotripter, the ND:YAG laser, and the pulse dye laser. All these devices can be used with an endoscope and an overtube in place to facilitate fragment removal.[6] Extracorporeal lithotripsy has also been used successfully to disrupt phytobezoars allowing endoscopic removal. Although these devices have been successful, they are not the first line of therapy for bezoars.

Surgery

Surgery is the treatment of choice for bezoars associated with intestinal obstruction or perforation. Patients who are found to have bezoar obstruction of the small intestine should have the foreign material milked through the ileocecal valve to relieve the obstruction. Prior to making the surgical skin incision, the possibility of a bezoar should be considered in patients who have had previous gastric surgery and who present with intestinal obstruction. There is a high risk of postoperative infection in bezoars removed by small bowel enterotomy. Surgery is the treatment of choice for trichobezoars. These bezoars are frequently found in patients with major psychiatric illness and may contain foreign bodies such as pins or razor blades. This should be considered before attempting endoscopic removal.

PREVENTION

Once a bezoar has been treated by many of the above methods, it is important to initiate a program to prevent recurrence. Bezoar removal has done nothing to correct gastric motility or gastric outlet obstruction. The most important factor in the formation of a phytobezoar is diet. The patient should be given explicit instructions to avoid eating oranges, persimmons, coconuts, berries, green beans, figs, apples, sauerkraut, brussel sprouts, and potato peels. No patient who has had gastric surgery for peptic ulcer disease or who has delayed gastric emptying for any reason should ever eat a peeled or even unpeeled persimmon.

Once the diet has been addressed, the next consideration is gastric emptying. If there is a delay in gastric emptying, consideration for using metoclopramide, 10 mg before meals, or cisapride, 10 to 20 mg before meals, should be considered. This may prevent bezoar reformation when delayed gastric emptying is the primary disorder.

SUMMARY

The treatment of bezoars affords the clinician many options. Some of these are high tech, high cost, and risky, and some such as surgery are obviously necessary in certain cases. The therapy of phytobezoars with cellulase is safe, effective, and inexpensive and should be considered the treatment of choice whenever possible.

REFERENCES

1. Benharroch D, Krugliak P, Porath A, Zurgil E, Niv Y. Pathogenetic aspects of persimmon bezoars. A case-control retrospective study. *J Clin Gastroenterol.* 1993;17(2):149–152.
2. Bernstein G, Jehle D, Bernaski E, Braen GR. Failure of gastric emptying and charcoal administration in fatal sustained-release theophylline overdose: pharmacobezoar formation. *Ann Emerg Med.* 1992;21(11):1388–1390.
3. Balik E, Ulman I, Taneli C, Demircan M. The Rapunzel syndrome: a case report and review of the literature. *Eur J Pediatr Surg.* 1993;3(3):171–173.
4. Cifuentes Tebar J, Robles Campos R, Parrilla Paricio P, Lujan Mompean JA, et al. Gastric surgery and bezoars. *Dig Dis Sci.* 1992;37(11):1694–1696.
5. Walker-Renard P. Update on the medicinal management of phytobezoars. *Am J Gastroenterol.* 1993;88(10):1663–1666.
6. Lubke HJ, Winkelmann RS, Berges WM, Necklenbeck W, Wienbeck M. Gastric phytobezoar: endoscopic removal using the gallstone lithotripter. *Z Gastroenterol.* 1988;26(8):393–396.

39

Gastric Volvulus

RAFAEL A. AMARAL and KENNETH L. KOCH

Volvulus is derived from the Latin word *volvere*, which means "to twist around." Gastric volvulus is defined as a rotation of the stomach exceeding 180 degrees, a rotation that may cause a closed loop obstruction and possible strangulation and necrosis of the stomach.

Gastric volvulus is an uncommon clinical condition discovered by Berti[1] in 1866 during an autopsy of a 60-year-old woman. In 1896 Berg[2] was the first to correct gastric volvulus at a surgical operation. Rosselet[3] reported the first case of chronic gastric volvulus detected by radiologic studies.

Acute gastric volvulus is a surgical emergency. The mortality for acute gastric volvulus is 30% to 50%,[4] but if the condition is recognized early, the mortality can be reduced to 0% to 13%.[5,6] More than 350 cases of gastric volvulus have been reported in the medical literature.[6–9]

ANATOMY

The stomach is fixed in the abdomen by the gastrophrenic ligament and by the peritoneum covering the second portion of the duodenum; it is limited in mobility between these two points by the lesser curvature of the stomach and the gastrohepatic omentum (Fig. 39–1). The gastrosplenic ligament in the upper part of the gastric cardia and the gastrocolic ligament on the greater curvature help to anchor the other re-

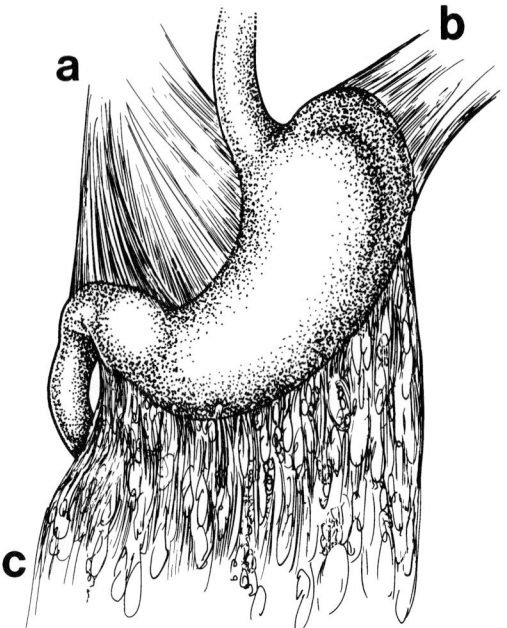

FIGURE 39–1. Main ligamentous attachments of the stomach: hepatogastric and hepatoduodenal ligaments (a); gastrosplenic ligament (b); gastrocolic ligament (c).

gions of the stomach (Fig. 39–1). Dalgaard[9] showed in cadavers that the normal stomach cannot be rotated 180 degrees unless the gastrosplenic and gastrocolic ligaments are cut. He also showed that a fluid-filled stomach rotated more easily than an empty stomach. Rotation in the postprandial state is easier because the ligaments are relaxed and the weight of the stomach brings the pylorus and the cardia closer together, setting the stage for a volvulus to occur.

Despite the various ligamentous attachments, the stomach is a very mobile intraabdominal organ. Intermittent episodes of gastric rotation without symptoms occur more often than appreciated.[8,9] The stomach may rotate in several directions, using itself, its ligaments, or gastric adhesions as an axis of rotation. A 180-degree rotation in a specific axis is needed for a complete volvulus.[10] A partial volvulus involves rotation of less than 180 degrees. For complete or partial volvulus to occur the peritoneal-gastric ligamentous support must relax or be absent altogether.

PREDISPOSING FACTORS

Congenital Factors

Certain conditions promote or are associated with the formation of a gastric volvulus (Table 39–1). Adhesions, either congenital or acquired, can form an axis for gastric rotation. The greater omentum, gastrocolic ligament, and the gastrosplenic ligament were absent in a patient with gastric volvulus.[11] Additional important promoting factors for gastric volvulus are diaphragmatic defects such as eventration or paraesophageal hernias. During eventration, when there is a raised diaphragm, the increased subphrenic potential space is filled with abdominal viscera. The most mobile viscera of the upper part of the abdomen, the greater curve of the stomach, fills this potential space first. The upward stomach movement draws up the transverse colon and may lead to organoaxial volvulus of the stomach.[12] The negative intrathoracic pressure and paradoxic movements of the diaphragm increase the eventration, and the degree of torsion in the gastric volvulus tends to increase with time.

Acquired Factors

Other factors that can precipitate volvulus are intractable vomiting, abdominal trauma, rapid increase in intraabdominal pressure, hiatal hernia, elevation of the left diaphragm secondary to phrenic nerve paralysis, and left lung resection or intrapleural adhesions (Table 39–1). Aerophagia presumably contributed to the formation of gastric volvulus in two mentally retarded patients.[13] Volvulus may also be initiated by gastric ulcers or neoplasms that cause obstruction or distension of the stomach,[6,11,14] by enlarged organs (like the spleen), overfilling of the stomach and vigorous gastric peristalsis.

Azmy and Morey[15] also consider colonic distension secondary to mechanical obstruction as an etiologic factor for gastric volvulus. Stremple[12] described a patient in whom colonic disten-

TABLE 39–1. PREDISPOSING FACTORS FOR GASTRIC VOLVULUS

Congenital	Acquired
Adhesions	Adhesions
Absence of ligaments	Hiatal hernia
Diaphragmatic defects	Phrenic nerve paralysis
Paraesophageal hernias	Lung resection
	Aerophagia
	Intractable vomiting
	Abdominal trauma
	Peptic ulcer disease
	Gastric neoplasm
	Enlarged organ (splenomegaly)
	Colonic distension

sion contributed to chronic intermittent gastric volvulus by pulling the greater curvature of the stomach upward and to the right. Llaneza et al[16] reported a patient who presented with jaundice secondary to a gastric volvulus. The stomach had assumed an inverted and displaced position in the thorax; the common bile duct was pulled cephalad and across the diaphragmatic hiatus and became obstructed. Yin and Nowak[14] reported the possibility of familial occurrence of intrathoracic gastric volvulus, although all cases previously reported were sporadic in occurrence. One third of patients with gastric volvulus have no predisposing abnormalities and are termed *idiopathic* or *primary gastric volvulus*.

CLASSIFICATION

Three types of gastric volvulus are described: (1) organoaxial volvulus, (2) mesenteroaxial volvulus, and (3) combined volvulus. This classification provides no prognostic value. The acuteness of clinical presentation, the cause of the volvulus and the degree of vascular occlusion are the most important factors in predicting which patients will require immediate surgical intervention. A gastric volvulus classification based on anatomic rotations is shown in Table 39–2.

ORGANOAXIAL ROTATION AND GASTRIC VOLVULUS

Organoaxial rotation is the most common form of gastric volvulus in the adult and pediatric population. Most cases in childhood are secondary to deficient gastric fixation with ligaments and increased gastric mobility at the diaphragmatic hiatus. Acute gastric volvulus in childhood may present as an early complication of these diaphragmatic defects. In organoaxial volvulus the stomach rotates around its longitudinal axis defined by a line extending from the esophagocardiac junction to the pylorus (Fig. 39–2a).

Partial gastric volvulus occurs more often in patients with acute presentations. In one series 9 of 11 patients had partial organoaxial volvulus. Even in partial gastric volvulus, necrosis of the stomach wall may occur. The anterior rotation of the stomach is more common than posterior rotation. In the posterior organoaxial rotation the transverse colon must pass behind the stomach. In one series 8 of 93 patients had organoaxial volvulus of the posterior type.[8] As the stomach rotates, elongating or tearing the mesocolon, the vascular supply of the stomach is jeopardized.

TABLE 39–2. CLASSIFICATION OF GASTRIC VOLVULUS

1. Type of stomach rotation
   a. Organoaxial rotation
   b. Mesenteroaxial rotation
   c. Combined
2. Extent of rotation
   a. Total: entire stomach involved in the rotation
   b. Partial: a portion of stomach is involved in the rotation
3. Direction of gastric rotation
   a. Anterior: rotating part moves anteriorly over the stomach
   b. Posterior: rotating part moves posteriorly (very rare)
4. Etiology (see Table 39–1)
   a. Congenital
   b. Acquired
5. Onset or severity
   a. Acute: emergent
   b. Chronic: recurrent with range of symptoms

When organoaxial gastric volvulus is complete, the entire organ is involved, and occlusion at the pylorus and the esophagus occurs (Fig. 39–2b). The pylorus is occluded first through twisting and kinking of the distal stomach. Gastric distension rapidly ensues. As air and fluid are swallowed, gastric distension is exacerbated, accentuating the degree of torsion at the esophagogastric junction and increasing the patient's difficulty in eructing or vomiting. At this point saliva cannot enter the stomach, and any effort to eruct air in the stomach is futile. The marked distension of the stomach produces bluish discoloration and thinning of the wall. Edema of the duodenum and esophagus develops.

Severe impairment of gastric blood flow during gastric volvulus is not the rule, however. Timely restoration of gastric position prevents ischemic necrosis. Most series estimate a 5% prevalence of gastric strangulation, although Carter et al[17] reported a 28% prevalence. If gastric strangulation is not corrected, the patient may develop hypovolemic shock from third space fluid accumulation in the stomach. In addition, the distended stomach may become ischemic and progress to gastric perforation, peritonitis, and septic shock. The volvulus may also cause secondary distension of the right transverse colon as the colon is pulled up by the omentum and interposed between the dilated stomach and the anterior abdominal wall. Rupture of the splenic vessels and fat necrosis near

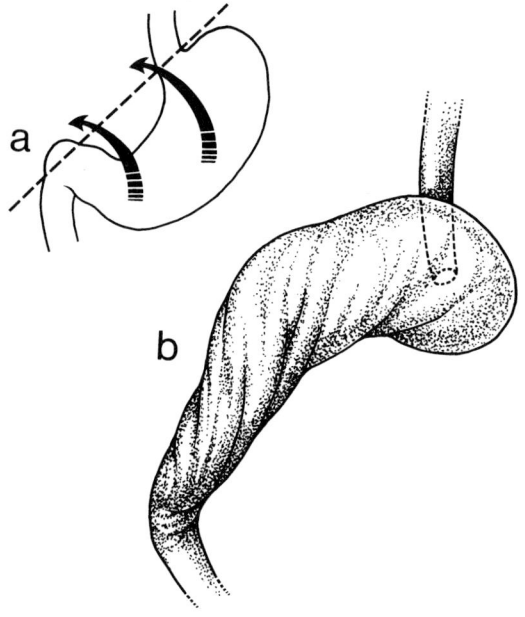

FIGURE 39–2. Schematic representation of organoaxial gastric volvulus. Cardiopyloric axis of rotation in organoaxial gastric volvulus (a). As anterior rotation occurs cardia and pyloric obstruction will develop (b).

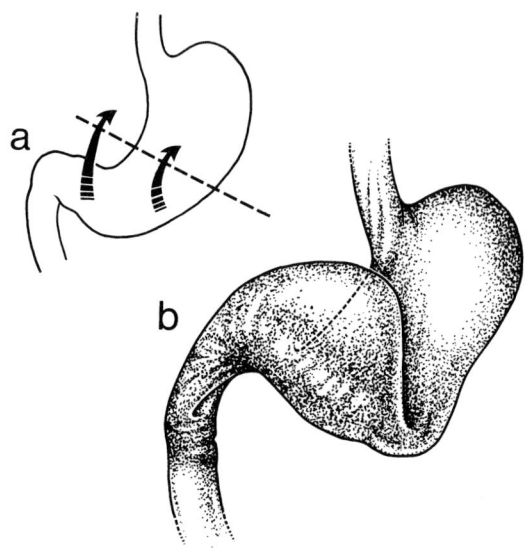

FIGURE 39–3. Schematic representation of mesenteroaxial gastric volvulus. Transverse axis of rotation in mesenteroaxial gastric volvulus (a). As the anterior wall moves upward and folds on itself, pyloroantral obstruction develops (b).

the tail of the pancreas have been associated with organoaxial gastric volvulus,[6] secondary to displacement of the spleen and pancreas.

Mesenteroaxial Rotation and Gastric Volvulus

In mesenteroaxial volvulus the stomach rotates in a cephalad or vertical plane in an axis perpendicular to the lesser curvature (Fig. 39–3a). The rotation is limited by the mobility of the pylorus where the obstruction actually occurs. Strangulation is less likely in mesenteroaxial volvulus compared with organoaxial rotations. In mesenteroaxial volvulus the anterior gastric wall folds on itself and separates the cardia from the pylorus. The antropyloric region rotates upward from right to left and the posterior surface of the antrum becomes an anterior surface (Fig. 39–3b).

Combined Volvulus

If the fundus undergoes secondary organoaxial rotation, a combined gastric volvulus is produced. A combined volvulus is rare.

CLINICAL PRESENTATION

Volvulus occurs in men and women with approximately the same frequency. Peak incidence occurs during the fifth and sixth decades. Gastric volvulus is rare, however, in the pediatric population where only 51 cases have been reported[18]; most children were less than 1 year of age. In a combined series of 206 adult cases, 122 patients (59%) had organoaxial rotations, 60 patients (29%) had mesenteroaxial rotation, 5 patients (2%) had combined rotations, and 19 patients (10%) were not classified.[6]

Acute gastric volvulus presents with a striking clinical picture and usually requires an emergency operation. However, early on in the development of the volvulus the patient's history usually reveals few upper gastrointestinal tract complaints. The symptoms usually start shortly after meals. Patients may complain of nonspecific symptoms suggestive of peptic ulcer disease, gallbladder disease, or gastritis, especially in the patients with chronic and intermittent gastric volvulus. Patients may complain of bloating, nausea, vomiting, belching, early satiety, abdominal distension, postprandial pain, and lower thoracic pain that may radiate to the back, neck, or the interscapular region. Vomiting during a partial volvulus is usually replaced by unproductive retching as the volvulus becomes complete.

The lower abdomen remains relatively soft on examination. As the volvulus becomes complete, abdominal pain exacerbates, the pulse increases, and low-grade fever may develop. Respiratory rate increases and epigastric pain becomes generalized.[5] Septic shock from perforation and peritonitis may develop if the condition is not corrected.

In 1904 Borchardt[18] described a diagnostic triad for acute gastric volvulus: (1) retching and inability to vomit, (2) severe epigastric pain and abdominal distension, and (3) inability to pass a nasogastric tube. The Borchardt triad reflects an initial blockage at the pylorus followed by occlusion at the cardia, i.e., an organoaxial rotation. This classic volvulus causes a closed loop obstruction of the stomach, resulting in the patient's inability to vomit and the physician's inability to pass a nasogastric tube.

Carter et al[17] referred to three other findings that help in the diagnosis of gastric volvulus: (1) minimal abdominal findings when the stomach is in the thorax; (2) a gas-filled viscus in the lower chest or upper abdomen as shown by plain x-ray films of the chest and abdomen, especially when associated with a paraesophageal hernia; and (3) obstruction at the site of volvulus as demonstrated by emergency upper gastrointestinal tract barium series. Vomitus may or may not contain bile depending on the degree of pyloric obstruction.

DIFFERENTIAL DIAGNOSIS

The differential diagnosis of acute gastric volvulus includes acute myocardial infarction, acute pancreatitis, peptic perforation of the stomach or other viscus, mesenteric embolus, strangulated ovarian cyst, ruptured gallbladder, and cholecystitis. Hematemesis secondary to necrosis from vascular strangulation may occur acutely. The physical examination may reveal frank or borderline shock with a silent or slightly tender abdomen, a large tympanitic area in the left epigastrium, and a relatively benign lower abdomen. The complete blood count may show leukocytosis and hemoconcentration as the process progresses.

The patient with chronic or recurrent gastric volvulus may remain asymptomatic for many years or may present with postprandial discomfort, belching, vomiting, bloating, early satiety, or weight loss. In the differential diagnosis of chronic gastric volvulus, peptic ulcer disease, gastritis, gallbladder and biliary disease, gastric atony, and pyloric obstruction must also be considered.

DIAGNOSTIC TESTS

Abdominal radiography is essential for diagnosis of gastric volvulus. A plain scout film of the abdomen will show a large air-filled viscus in the upper abdomen in organoaxial gastric rotations. The greater curvature of the stomach will be located higher than the lesser curvature. Identification of the greater curvature adjacent to the diaphragm is also characteristic of organoaxial gastric volvulus. If a hiatal hernia or a diaphragmatic defect is present, then an upright film will reveal a grossly distended viscus or a large air-fluid level in the lower chest area.

Barium studies are very helpful depending on the degree of esophageal obstruction created by the volvulus. Barium will outline the site of the proximal twist and the relative inability of the barium to enter the stomach.[19] The stomach will be in the highest position and the duodenal bulb will be pointing downward and to the right. In addition the stomach has a cascade appearance, with a spiral appearance of the rugae demonstrated by the barium.[19]

In the mesenteroaxial rotation a plain film of the abdomen will show a double fluid level with the antrum representing the upper fluid level and the fundus the lower fluid level. In the partial or chronic mesenteroaxial volvulus the upper gastrointestinal tract series will reveal the abnormal position of the stomach.

THERAPY

Acute gastric volvulus requires immediate surgical intervention. Intravenous fluids must be administered; shock must be immediately corrected. A nasogastric tube should be introduced into the stomach if possible for immediate decompression. An abdominal surgical approach is recommended, even when the stomach lies in the chest, to identify any associated gastrointestinal anomalies and to facilitate accurate crural repair. Placement of a gastrostomy tube is recommended, especially in infants, for both stomach fixation and postoperative enteral feeding.[20] In general, surgical intervention involves decom-

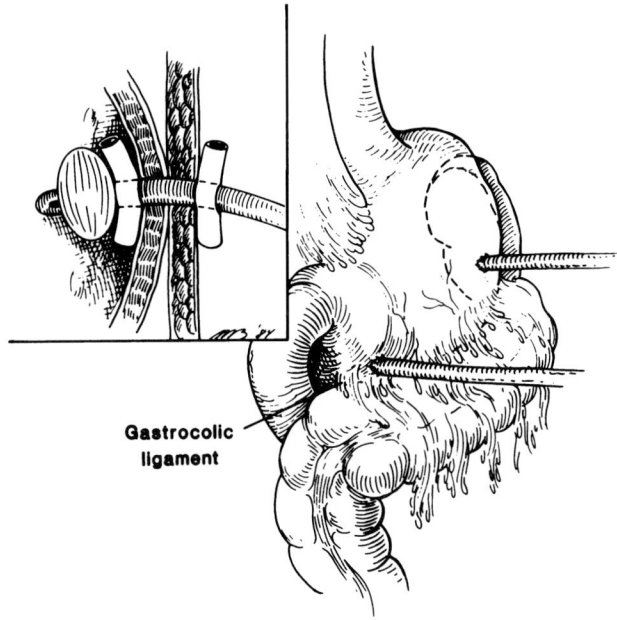

FIGURE 39–4. Insertion of two tubes for correction of gastric volvulus with percutaneous endoscopic gastrostomies.

pression of the stomach, detorsion of the stomach, and fixation of the stomach to prevent recurrence. Fixation has been achieved by different means: plication of the stomach ligaments and suture of the greater curvature to the transverse colon. In cases with gastric neoplasm or ulcer (or if gastric necrosis has occurred), partial gastrectomy with anterior gastropexy and anterior or posterior gastroenterostomy may be performed.

Endoscopy has also been used to diagnose and treat gastric volvulus. Patel[21] described a simple endoscopic technique to correct gastric volvulus. With minimal air-insufflation the endoscope was introduced into the stomach, a loop was allowed to form in the stomach, and counterclockwise or clockwise rotation of the stomach was accomplished by rotating the endoscope 180 degrees. The result was a sudden "jar" which indicated the completed rotation of the stomach. This maneuver was helpful in patients with either organoaxial or mesenteroaxial rotation.[21] In patients with combined volvulus, surgery is necessary. Such endoscopic maneuvers resolve the episode of gastric volvulus but do not prevent future recurrences.

More recently dual percutaneous endoscopic gastrostomy (PEG) tubes were inserted to prevent recurrent chronic gastric volvulus.[22] In this endoscopic technique, two PEG tubes were inserted into the stomach to anchor the stomach to the abdominal wall (Fig. 39–4). The first PEG tube was inserted in the antrum and the second was placed anterolaterally in the body of the stomach. These tubes were drained by gravity for 24 hours; thereafter the patient was allowed to eat. Two weeks later the PEG tubes were removed. Follow-up at 1 year showed that all patients were asymptomatic and had normal stomach position documented by x-ray studies.

REFERENCES

1. Berti L. Singolare attortigliamento dell'esofagacol duodeno sequito da rapida morte. *Gazz Med Ital.* 1866;9:139–141.
2. Berg J. *Zwei Falle On des Magens.* 1897;19:1.
3. Rosselet A, Gilbert R. Observation radiologique d'un volvulus de l'estomac. *J Radiol Electrol.* 1922;6:76.
4. Smith RJ. Volvulus of the stomach. *J Natl Med Assoc.* 1983;75:393.
5. Pillay SP, Angorn IB, Baker LW. Gastric volvulus unassociated with hiatal hernia. *S Afr Med J.* 1977;52:880.
6. Wastell C, Ellis H. Volvulus of the stomach. *Br J Surg.* 1971;58:39.
7. Gurnsey JM, Connolly JE. Acute complete gastric volvulus. *Arch Surg.* 1963;86:423.
8. Buchanan J. Volvulus of the stomach. *Br J Surg.* 1930;18:99.
9. Dalgaard JB. Volvulus of the stomach. *Acta Chir Scand.* 1952;103:131.
10. Sawyer KC, Hammer RW, Fenton WC. Gastric volvulus as a cause of obstruction. *AMA Arch Surg.* 1956;72:764.
11. Stremple JF. A new operation for the anatomic correction of chronic intermittent gastric volvulus. *Am J Surg.* 1973;125:360.

12. Tanner NC. Chronic and recurrent volvulus of the stomach. *Am J Surg.* 1968;115:505–515.
13. Ziprokowski MN, Teele RL. Gastric volvulus in childhood. *AJR.* 1979;132:921–925.
14. Yin RL, Nowak TV. Familial occurrence of intrathoracic gastric volvulus. *Dig Dis Sci.* 1988;33(11):1483–1487.
15. Azmy S, Morey A. Volvulus of the stomach. *Am J Roentgenol.* 1932;27:420.
16. Llaneza PP, Salt WB, Partyka EK. Extrahepatic biliary obstruction complicating a diaphragmatic hiatal hernia with intrathoracic gastric volvulus. *Am J Gastroenterol.* 1986;81(4):292–294.
17. Carter R, Brewer LA, Hinshow DB. Acute gastric volvulus. *Am J Surg.* 1980;140:99–105.
18. Borchardt M. Zur Pathologie und Therapie des Magenvolvulus. *Arch Klin Chir.* 1904;74:243.
19. Cantor MO, Reynolds RP. Obstruction of the stomach and sphincters. In: Cantor MO, Reynolds RP eds. *Gastrointestinal Obstruction.* 1st ed. Baltimore, Md: Williams & Wilkins; 1957:67.
20. Idowu J, Aitken DR, Georgeson KE. Gastric volvulus in the newborn. *Arch Surg.* 1980;115:1046–1049.
21. Patel NM. Chronic gastric volvulus: report of a case and review of literature. *Am J Gastroenterol.* 1985;80(3):171.
22. Eckhauser ML, Ferron JP. The use of dual percutaneous endoscopic gastrostomy (DPEG) in the management of chronic intermittent gastric volvulus. *Gastrointest Endosc.* 1985;31(5):340–342.

Acknowledgments

We wish to acknowledge and thank Mary Maiolo for her excellent secretarial support in completing this chapter.

40
Gastric Adenocarcinoma

JOSEPH R. MURPHY

Despite a continual decrease in its incidence over the last 50 years, gastric carcinoma remains a significant cause of death in the United States. There are approximately 23,200 new cases annually and more than 13,000 deaths.[1] Carcinoma of the stomach is the most common cancer in the world, accounting for approximately 10.5% of cancers worldwide.[2] There is great variation by region with a 6.5 times higher death rate in Japan than in the United States.[3]

The overall cure rate for gastric cancer has changed little over the last 30 years. The cumulative 5-year survival rates have remained bleak at less than 20%.[1] Patients continue to present for treatment with advanced disease in which 40% of patients have either local lymph node involvement or metastatic carcinoma. Often by the time endoscopy is performed, there is a significant mass lesion such as that shown in Figure 40–1 (see Color Plate III). The median survival of patients with metastatic carcinoma is less than 6 months.

PATHOPHYSIOLOGY

Epidemiology studies have shown a strong association between atrophic gastritis with achlorhydria and stomach cancer. The pathologic sequence appears to involve an agent or organism in which the gastric epithelium is damaged with a reduced secretion of acid that permits the generation of potential carcinogens. The gastric epithelium appears to undergo intestinal metaplasia. Neoplasia then develops within the metaplastic tissue.

Recent interest has focused on *Helicobacter pylori* as an organism whose infection results in mucosal atrophy and achlorhydria. A significant correlation between areas with a high prevalence of *H. pylori* and the incidence of gastric cancer in regions of Columbia have been found.[4] Several recent reports have also implicated *H. pylori*

The opinions and assertions contained herein are the private views of the author and are not to be construed as official or as reflecting the views of the Department of the Army or the Department of Defense.

with progressive gastric pathology that predisposes to cancer.[5-8] However, data on *H. pylori* infection in Africa are at odds with the notion that this infection is the inciting agent leading to cancer.[9] Pernicious anemia is another disorder in which atrophy and achlorhydria may predispose a patient to gastric cancer,[8] although the risk appears to be low.[10]

The natural history of gastric epithelial dysplasia and its relation to gastric cancer is ill defined. In one study of 13 patients with high-grade dysplasia, 11 (85%) were found to have gastric cancer within 15 months.[11] Another series found that moderate and severe gastric dysplasias are preneoplastic lesions and a valuable marker of gastric cancer risk.[12] Moreover, the cancers associated with high-grade dysplasia are usually pathologically favorable and curable.

The most recent commonly used histologic classification was described by Lauren in 1965.[13] He reported two types of gastric cancer, intestinal and diffuse. The intestinal type is a well differentiated lesion that tends to form glands and is associated with chronic gastritis, atrophy, metaplasia, and dysplasia. Spread is most often by blood-borne pathogens to distant organs. In contrast, the diffuse form of gastric cancer is typified pathologically by a lack of gland formation and cell adhesion. There is no antecedent history of gastritis but there is a possible association with blood group A.[13,14] This form of gastric cancer tends to spread by transmural extension into the peritoneal cavity and through lymphatic invasion.[13]

SCREENING AND DIAGNOSIS

Mass screening by photofluorography has been effective in Japan, where in 1985 over 5 million people were screened and 6240 (0.12%) cases of gastric cancer were detected. Approximately half of these were early stage cancers.[3] From these studies it is believed that mass screening for gastric cancer has been effective in reducing the death rate.

Without a mass screening program like that in Japan, Western clinicians must maintain a high index of suspicion for the diagnosis of gastric cancer. Since the symptoms of gastric cancer are nonspecific, the endoscopist must be able to recognize early gastric cancer whenever examining the stomach. Groups in which the clinician should be especially vigilant are those patients with intestinal metaplasia, pernicious anemia, gastric polyps, prior gastric surgery, or immunodeficiency.

When performed by an experienced endoscopist, upper endoscopy with biopsy has a high level of accuracy. The need for multiple biopsy specimens over endoscopic appearance alone was confirmed by Dekkar and Tytgat.[15] Biopsy specimens from both the base and rim of an ulcer should be obtained for the best accuracy.[16] Graham et al[17] have shown that seven biopsy specimens per patient yielded the correct diagnosis in 98% of carcinomas. Early gastric cancer may be especially difficult to diagnose, and staining the mucosa with Congo red-methylene blue to perform a biopsy on the blue intestinal metaplasia has demonstrated improvement in diagnostic accuracy.[18]

STAGING

Currently, most staging systems for gastric cancer use the American Joint Commission version of the TNM staging system as is shown in Table 40–1.[19,20] The staging system is largely pathologic in orientation but can accurately predict 5-year survival rates. The major disadvantage is that in the majority of patients, the stage cannot be accurately assessed prior to surgery.

A number of classification systems have attempted to examine prognostic factors that

TABLE 40–1. THE AMERICAN JOINT COMMISSION TNM STAGING SYSTEM FOR GASTRIC CANCER

Stage	Description
T	Primary tumor
T_1	Confined to the mucosa
T_2	Extends through muscularis propria but not through mucosa
T_3	Penetrates through serosa without involving contiguous organs
T_4	Involves entire thickness of stomach wall (includes linitis plastica)
N	Regional lymph nodes
N_0	No lymph nodes involved
N_1	Perigastric lymph nodes in close proximity
N_2	Perigastric lymph nodes distant or on both curvatures
M	Distant metastasis
M_0	No distant metastasis
M_1	Distant metastasis including nodes beyond regional lymph nodes but excluding contiguo penetration

might be used in alternative staging systems. Schmitz-Moorman et al[21] found tumor size, Lauren type, number of infiltrating lymphocytes, tumor fibrosis, and nodal status as important prognostic factors, while Hemanek[22] found Lauren type and depth of tumor invasion as the most important factors. Shennib et al[23] also showed that the presence of intestinal metaplasia had higher survival rates.

Endoscopic appearance also appears to have prognostic implications. Sakita et al[24] characterized three types of gastric cancer by their endoscopic appearance: type I (protruded), type II (superficial, including IIa elevated, IIb flat, IIc depressed), and type III (excavated). Correlation of the endoscopic and histologic types of gastric cancer has been found.[25] These findings show that type I and II lesions are predominantly intestinal, whereas a significant portion of type III lesions are diffuse and have a poorer prognosis.

The introduction of endoscopic ultrasound has made it possible to assess the depth and pattern of stomach wall penetration.[26,27] In the hands of an experienced operator, the accuracy of assessing depth of invasion is 85%.[26] As shown in Figure 40–2, endoscopic ultrasound (EUS) may confirm infiltration of gastric carcinoma into the esophagus. EUS also appears superior to computed tomography (CT) and magnetic resonance imaging (MRI) for detecting lymph node involvement. Lightdale and colleagues[28] performed a prospective evaluation of 50 patients with gastric cancer in which all were evaluated via CT scan, MRI scan of the chest and abdomen, and EUS. Surgery on all patients permitted pathologic staging. EUS was found superior to CT and MRI for assessing T and N stage.

With both the Lauren classification (which gives histologic prognostic factors on endoscopic biopsy tissue) and endoscopic ultrasound (which gives morphovolumetric prognostic factors), there now appears to be a basis for a preoperative gastric staging system.[29] Factors to be considered in such a system are summarized in Table 40–2.

Gastric cancer can spread either locally by direct extension or distally via lymphatic, hematogenous, or peritoneal routes. Lymph nodes and organs most commonly involved are summarized in Table 40–3. The use of CT evaluation instead of laparotomy to detect spread has not borne out. Cook et al[30] found 51% of patients had more extensive disease than predicted by CT, whereas 18% had less extensive disease. More recently, laparoscopy is being investigated as a potential staging procedure to determine if surgical resection with a clear margin is possible and to rule out metastatic disease in the liver and peritoneum.

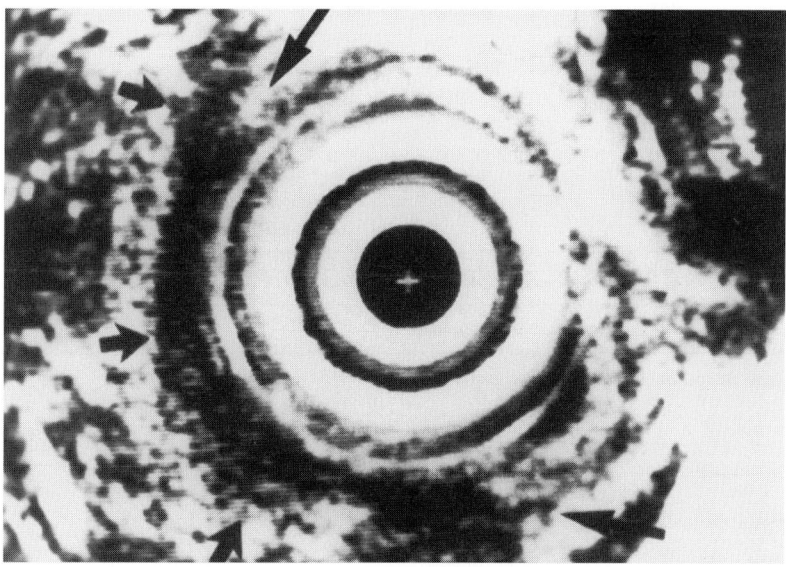

FIGURE 40–2. Submucosal tumor infiltration arising from the stomach with the second and third hypoechoic layers *(large and small arrows)* at the gastroesophageal junction.

TABLE 40-2. PROGNOSTIC PREOPERATIVE FACTORS

Histologic	Lauren type (intestinal versus diffuse)
	Tumor size
	Lymphocyte infiltration
	Tumor fibrosis
	Intestinal metaplasia
Endoscopic appearance	Type I (protrudes)
	Type II (superficial)
	a (elevated)
	b (flat)
	c (depressed)
	Type III (excavated)
Endoscopic ultrasound	Depth of invasion
	Extension into adjacent organs
	Lymph node involvement

TREATMENT

SURGERY

Surgery is the only curative treatment for gastric carcinoma, although overall survival rates are still quite low. Table 40-4 summarizes the operative mortality and 5-year survival rates for curative resection of gastric carcinoma. Surgery is still the major approach for palliation. Gradual progress for surgical therapies has been seen with operative mortalities as high as 20% 15 years ago down to 6% now.[31] In fact operative mortality of less than 1% has been reported from some centers in both Japan and the United States.

The extent of gastric resection does not appear to influence 5-year survival rates independent of pathologic staging. A recent study showed no significant difference in either operative mortality or overall 5-year survival rates (48%) in patients undergoing total versus subtotal gastrectomy.[32] Several studies have reported recurrent carcinoma in the gastric remnant of long-term survivors of subtotal gastrectomies.[33,34] Total gastrectomy in theory would carry a lower risk of late recurrences in long-term survivors.

Much controversy has been raised over the role of radical lymphadenectomy in the operative treatment of gastric adenocarcinoma. Several studies from Japan have shown a markedly increased survival rate with low operative morbidity and mortality.[35,36] However, most Western countries have not been able to demonstrate a similar improvement in survival.[37,38] A recent report evaluating the morbidity of radical lymphadenectomy by Smith et al[39] from Memorial Sloan Kettering found no difference in the morbidity and mortality or in the length of stay in patients who recently (1985 to 1989) underwent extensive lymph node resection.

The increased survival rate in Japan may be related to several factors. First, mass screening has led to a finding of gastric cancer at an earlier stage with a younger patient population without other major medical problems. Second, the Japanese use a meticulous nodal staging system with all relevant nodal systems removed, whereas many Western series understage patients with removal of only perigastric nodes. Finally, the prevalence of disease is greater in Japan making surgeons more technically adept because they perform the operation more frequently.

The Japanese Research Society for gastric cancer defines an absolute curative resection as one in which patients without serosal involvement or peritoneal or liver metastases have had

TABLE 40-3. SPREAD OF GASTRIC CANCER

	NODES	ORGANS
Local extension	Perigastric	Omentum
		Esophagus
		Liver
		Pancreas
		Spleen
		Colon
Distant metastases	Celiac	Liver
	Common hepatic	Lungs
	Left gastric	Bone
	Supraclavicular (Virchow)	Central nervous system
	Left axillary (Irish)	Ovarian (Krukenberg)
	Umbilical (Sr. Mary Joseph)	Rectal shelf (Blumer)

TABLE 40–4. CURATIVE RESECTION OF GASTRIC CARCINOMA

OPERATION	OPERATIVE MORTALITY	5-YEAR SURVIVAL
Gastric resection		
Subtotal gastrectomy	3.2%	48%
Total gastrectomy	1.3%	48%
Lymph node resection		
Perigastric (R_1)	1.1%	26%
Regional (R_2)	1.6%	63%

gastric resection with a lymph node dissection that extends one level beyond the pathologic level of lymph node involvement. A relative curative resection is one in which there is no serosal, peritoneal, or hepatic metastases and in which the level of pathologic lymph node involvement is equal to the level of lymph node dissection.[40] In this system, the extent of gastric resection in R_1 is removal of all or part of the stomach, omentum, and N_1 (perigastric lymph nodes), and in R_2 is removal of the stomach en bloc with greater and lesser omenta, the superior leaf of the transverse mesocolon, and the pancreatic capsule and an extensive lymphadenectomy in the infraduodenal and supraduodenal areas and along the common hepatic, celiac, and splenic arteries with ligation of the left gastric artery at its origin.[41]

A recent report reveals the difficulty that Western centers have in implementing radical gastrectomy. Of 122 consecutive patients undergoing operative exploration, only 6% had early gastric cancer, and only 12% of potentially curative patients had N_1 involvement.[42] These results suggest that accurate intraoperative staging and proper selection of patients will be required to obtain dividends with an aggressive approach to surgical resection.

CHEMOTHERAPY

Gastric carcinoma is only potentially curable with surgical resection. Most patients die either because they are unresectable or after a curable resection, which occurs in a majority of patients with gastric carcinoma, there is relapse at either locoregional or distant (including intraperitoneal) sites. The median survival duration ranges between 12 and 25 months for patients undergoing curative resection[43,44] and is less than 6 months for patients undergoing incomplete or no resection.[44,45]

The strategy of adjuvant chemotherapy for patients undergoing curative resections to potentially eliminate relapses resulting in higher cure rates appears to be justified. Adjuvant chemotherapy in breast, head, and neck cancers has met with some success. However, adjuvant chemotherapy in gastric cancer has not been as successful. Initially encouraging results for adjuvant 5-FU and MeCCNU[46] have not been confirmed.[47,48] The lack of survival benefit may be from either ineffective chemotherapy combinations or the lapse of time between the curative resection and the initiation of chemotherapy. Recent trials have begun to investigate combination chemotherapy begun prior to operation and continued in the postoperative period in resectable patients.[49] Currently, adjuvant chemotherapy should be restricted to clinical trials until a survival benefit can be demonstrated.

Metastatic gastric cancer is still an incurable disease. New therapeutic strategies continue to evolve. Much of the difficulty in interpreting most trials is the use of response rate (tumor reduction of 50%) rather than effect on survival. Single agent response rates are summarized in Table 40–5. Most response rates are less than 30% with infrequent complete response (CR).

The existence of modestly active single agents provided the impetus to combine these agents. Table 40–5 also summarizes the response rates found by combining various chemotherapeutic agents. Drug combinations with 5-FU and mitomycin C were the standard, with response rates of 30% to 45%. However, these responses were of short duration (<6 months) with no prolonged survival benefit noted and very low (<5%) complete response.

More recently combinations of etoposide and cisplatin often in combination with 5-FU, doxorubicin, leucovorin, or methotrexate have been reported to have response rates as high as 57% with 15% complete response.[50] Median survival for patients with locally advanced carcinoma was 17 months. However, toxicities to these regimens include myelosuppression, nausea, vomiting, alopecia, weight loss, and mucositis. Several investigations with etoposide and cisplatin in the United States are ongoing.

RADIATION

Radiation therapy either alone or in combination with chemotherapy appears to have little role in the treatment of gastric cancer. The dose and area of interest restriction to spare adjacent radiosensitive organs precludes the delivery of

TABLE 40-5. SINGLE AGENT AND COMBINATION THERAPY RESPONSE RATES

	NUMBER OF PATIENTS	RESPONSE (%)
Single Agent Regimen		
Mitomycin	221	30
Doxorubicin	68	27
5-Fluorouracil	392	21
Etoposide	14	21
Cisplatin	115	20
Methotrexate	28	11
Combination Regimen		
EAP	145	57
FAMTX	187	43
FAP	187	36
FAM	656	30
AMF	36	22

EAP: etoposide, doxorubicin, cisplatin; FAMTX: 5-FU, doxorubicin, methotrexate; FAP: 5-FU, doxorubicin, cisplatin; FAM: 5-FU, doxorubicin, mitomycin C; AMF: endoxorubicin, methotrexate, 5-FU.

adequate therapy. The combined toxicity of radiation and chemotherapy is greater than chemotherapy alone in locally advanced gastric cancer and offers no survival advantage.[51]

FUTURE THERAPIES

Efforts to improve therapy for locoregional and metastatic gastric cancers will most likely involve multiple modalities. Extensive surgery with radical lymphadenectomy in selected patients may permit increased cure rates. Also, newer active chemotherapy agents need to be incorporated into regimens. Approaches using autologous bone marrow transplants and colony-stimulating factor to permit higher dose chemotherapy are likely strategies to pursue. Preoperative chemotherapy in patients with resectable cancer may permit higher cure rates.

Intraperitoneal strategies for gastric cancer are theoretically enticing in view of the failure pattern of the disease. Local recurrence in the tumor bed and peritoneal or hepatic failure are exceedingly common with gastric malignancies. Several trials are now in progress using intraperitoneal chemotherapy in the immediate postoperative period.

Endoscopic treatment of gastric tumors has mainly been palliative with relief of obstruction or hemostasis. In addition to endoscopic monotherapy, new trials in therapeutic endoscopy include combining endoscopy with laser therapy and other treatment modalities for massive tumor destruction in multimodal protocols for advanced cancer.

Prospective randomized treatment trials that demonstrate not only short-term response rates but also long-term survival benefits are needed. Research should continue to develop tumor markers that will adequately screen at-risk populations, resulting in more patients presenting with early stage gastric cancer.

REFERENCES

1. Silverberg E, Boring CC, Sauives TS. Cancer statistics 1990. *CA.* 1990;40:9.
2. Parkin DM, Laara E, Muir CS. Estimates of the worldwide frequency of sixteen major cancers in 1980. *Int J Cancer.* 1988;41:184.
3. Hisamichi S. Screening for gastric cancer. *World J Surg.* 1989;13:31.
4. Correa P, Haenszel W, Carlos C, et al. Gastric precancerous process in a high risk population: cross sectional studies. *Cancer Res.* 1990;50:4731.
5. Nomura A, Stemmerman GN, Chyou P, et al. *Helicobacter pylori* infection and gastric carcinoma among Japanese Americans in Hawaii. *N Engl J Med.* 1991;325:1132.
6. Parsonnet J, Friedman GD, Vandersteen DP, et al. *Helicobacter pylori* infection and the risk of gastric carcinoma. *N Engl J Med.* 1991;325:1127.
7. Recavarren S, Leon-Barue R, Cok J, et al. *Helicobacter pylori* and progressive gastric pathology that predisposes to gastric cancer. *Scand J Gastroenterol.* 1991;26(suppl 181):51.
8. Brinton LA, Gridley G, Hrubec Z, et al. Cancer risk following pernicious anemia. *Br J Cancer.* 1989;59:810.
9. Holcombe C. *Helicobacter pylori:* the African enigma. *Gut.* 1992;33:429.
10. Schafer L, Larson DE, Melton LJ, et al. Risk of development of gastric carcinoma in patients with pernicious anemia: a population based study in Rochester, Minnesota. *Mayo Clin Proc.* 1985;60:444.
11. Lansdown M, Quirke P, Dixon MF, et al. High grade dysplasia of the gastric mucosa: a marker for gastric carcinoma. *Gut.* 1990;31:977.
12. Coma del Corral M, Pardo Minden FJ, Razquin S, et al. Risk of cancer in patients with gastric dysplasia. *Cancer.* 1990;65:2078.
13. Lauren P. The two main types of gastric carcinoma: diffuse and so-called intestinal type carcinoma. *Acta Pathol Microbiol Immunol Scand.* 1965;64:31.
14. Viste A, Erde GE, Halvorsen K, et al. The prognostic value of Lauren's histopathological classification system and ABO blood groups in patients with stomach carcinoma. *Eur J Surg Oncol.* 1986;12:135.
15. Dekkar W, Tytgat GN. Diagnostic accuracy of fiberendoscopy in the detection of upper intestinal malignancy: a follow-up analysis. *Gastroenterology.* 1977;73:710.
16. Hatfield ARW, Slavin G, Segal AW, et al. Importance of the site of endoscopic gastric biopsy in ulcerating lesions of the stomach. *Gut.* 1975;16:884.
17. Graham DY, Schwartz JJ, Cain GD, et al. Prospective evaluation of biopsy number in the diagnosis of esopha-

geal and gastric carcinoma. *Gastroenterology.* 1982;82:228.
18. Tatsuta M, Tishi H, Okuda S, et al. Diagnosis of early gastric cancers in the upper part of the stomach by the endoscopic Congo-red methylene blue test. *Endoscopy.* 1984;82:379.
19. Fielding JWL, Roginski G, Ellis DJ, et al. Clinicopathological staging of gastric cancer. *Br J Surg.* 1984;74:877.
20. Kennedy BJ. Staging of gastric cancer. *Semin Oncol.* 1985;12:19.
21. Schmitz-Moorman P, Pohl C, Himmelman GW, et al. Morphological predictors of survival in advanced gastric carcinoma: univariate and multivariate analysis. *J Cancer Res Clin Oncol.* 1980;112:156.
22. Hermanek P. Prognostic factors in stomach cancer surgery. *Eur J Surg Oncol.* 1986;12:241.
23. Shennib H, Lough J, Klein HW, et al. Gastric carcinoma: intestinal metaplasia and tumor growth patterns as indicators of prognosis. *Surgery.* 1986;100:774.
24. Sakita T, Ogura Y, Takasu S, et al. The development of endoscopic diagnosis of early carcinoma of the stomach. *Jpn J Clin Oncol.* 1971;1:113.
25. Bearzi I, Ranaldi R. Early gastric cancer: a morphological study of 41 cases. *Tumori.* 1982;68:223.
26. Yamanaka T, Kimura K. The use of ultrasonographic endoscopy in the assessment of depth of invasion of gastric cancer. In: Maruyama M, Kimura K, eds. *Review of Clinical Research in Gastroenterology.* Tokyo: Igaku Shein; 1988:93.
27. Tio TL, Schouwink MH, Cikot RJL, et al. Preoperative TNM classification of gastric endosonography in comparison with pathological TNM system: a prospective study of 72 cases. *Hepatogastroenterology.* 1989;36:51.
28. Lightdale C, Botet J, Brennan M, et al. Endoscopic ultrasonography compared to computerized tomography for preoperative staging of gastric cancer. *Gastrointest Endosc.* 1989;35:154.
29. Tio TL, der Hertog J, Tytgat GN. The role of endoscopic ultrasound in assessing local resectability of esophagogastric malignancies: accuracy, pitfalls, and predictability. *Scand J Gastroenterol.* 1986;123:78.
30. Cook AO, Levine BA, Sirenek KR, et al. Evaluation of gastric adenocarcinoma: abdominal CT does not replace celiotomy. *Arch Surg.* 1986;121:603.
31. Boddie AW, McMurtey MJ, Giacco GG, et al. Palliative total gastrectomy and esophagogastrectomy: a reevaluation. *Cancer.* 1983;51:1195.
32. Gouzi JL, Hugier M, Fagniez PL, et al. Total vs subtotal gastrectomy for adenocarcinoma of the gastric antrum. *Ann Surg.* 1989;209:162.
33. Hoerr SO. Long term results in patients who survive five or more years after gastric resection for primary carcinoma. *Surg Gyn Obstet.* 1981;153:820.
34. Saario I, Schroder T, Lempinen M, et al. Analysis of 58 patients surviving more than 10 years after operative treatment of gastric cancer. *Arch Surg.* 1987;122:1052.
35. Kadama Y, Sugimachi K, Soejma K, et al. Evaluation of extensive lymph node resection for carcinoma of the stomach. *World J Surg.* 1981;5:241.
36. Marwyama K, Gunrin P, Okabayashi K, et al. Lymph node metastases of gastric cancer: general pattern in 1931 patients. *Ann Surg.* 1989;210:596.
37. Gilbertsen VA. Results of treatment of stomach cancer: an appraisal of efforts for more extensive surgery and a report of 1983 cases. *Cancer.* 1969;23:305.
38. Dent DM, Madden MV, Price SK. Randomized comparison of R_1 and R_2 gastrectomy for gastric carcinoma. *Br J Surg.* 1988; 75:110.
39. Smith JW, Shiu MH, Kelsey L, et al. Morbidity of radical lymphadenectomy in the curative resection of gastric carcinoma. *Arch Surg.* 1991;126:1469.
40. Japanese Research Society. The general rules for the gastric cancer study in surgery and pathology. *Jpn J Surg.* 1981;11:127.
41. Nakijima T, Kajitani T. Surgical treatment of gastric cancer with special reference to lymph node resection in diagnosis and treatment of upper gastrointestinal tumors. In: Friedman M, Ogawa M, Kisner D, eds. *Diagnosis and Treatment of Upper Gastrointestinal Tract Tumors.* Amsterdam: Exerpta Medica; 1981.
42. Irvin TT, Bridges JE. Gastric cancer: an audit of 122 consecutive cases and the results of R_1 gastrectomy. *Br J Surg.* 1988;75:106.
43. Diehl JT, Hermann RE, Coopererman AM, et al. Gastric carcinoma: a ten year review. *Ann Surg.* 1983;198:9.
44. Dupont JB, Lee JR, Burton GR, et al. Adenocarcinoma of the stomach: review of 1497 cases. *Cancer.* 1978;41:941.
45. McBride CM, Broddie AW. Adenocarcinoma of the stomach: are we making any progress? *South Med J.* 1987;80:283.
46. Gastrointestinal Tumor Study Group. Controlled trial of adjuvant chemotherapy following curative resection for gastric cancer. *Cancer.* 1982;49:116.
47. Engstrom PF, Lavin PT, Douglas HO, et al. Postoperative adjuvant 5FU plus MeCCNU therapy for gastric cancer patients. *Cancer.* 1985;55:1868.
48. Higgins GA, Amadeo JH, Smith DE, et al. Efficacy of prolonged intermittent therapy with combined 5FU and MeCCNU following resection for gastric carcinoma: a Veterans Administration surgical oncology report. *Cancer.* 1983;52:1105.
49. Ajani JA, Ota DM, Jackson DE. Current strategies in the management of locoregional and metastatic gastric carcinoma. *Cancer.* 1991;67:260.
50. Preusser P, Wilke H, Achterrath W, et al. Phase II study with the combination of etoposide, doxorubicin, and cisplatin in advanced measurable gastric cancer. *J Clin Oncol.* 1989;7:1310.
51. Gastrointestinal Tumor Study Group. A comparison of combination chemotherapy and combine modality therapy for locally advanced gastric carcinoma. *Cancer.* 1982;49:1771.

41

Gastric Lymphoma*

HERMAN KATTLOVE

Although the incidence of gastric non-Hodgkin's lymphoma is increasing, it still remains an uncommon malignancy and accounts for only about 5% of all gastric neoplasms. This increase in incidence probably results from (1) early detection by endoscopy (2) reclassification of pseudolymphomas into true malignancies, and (3) an overall unexplained increase in the incidence of all lymphomas. Gastric lymphoma occurs equally in men and women and increases in frequency with age.[1] Most patients present after 60 years of age. Because this disease is uncommon, almost all discussions of its therapy have been derived from retrospective analyses. Although recent advances in understanding the etiology and pathogenesis of gastric lymphoma, as well as the recent maturation of modern lymphoma therapy, have left us without a standard treatment for this disease, this new information has allowed oncologists to formulate an intelligent approach that can provide both good long-term survival and quality of life.

ETIOLOGY AND PATHOGENESIS

The stomach can be involved in approximately 10% of patients with nodal lymphomas. Gastric lymphomas, where the stomach constitutes the primary disease site, are considered a separate disease since these latter neoplasms probably arise from a different source than nodal lymphomas. This source, mucosa-associated lymphoid tissue (MALT),[2] may account for most, if not all, gastric lymphomas and may have a different natural history. Most investigators feel these lymphomas have a better prognosis, grade for grade, than their nodal counterparts.

In over 90% of patients with gastric lymphoma, investigators have found the stomach infected with *Helicobacter pylori,* which has led them to ascribe the cause of this lymphoma to an excessive immune response to gastric infection with this organism.[3] This immune response is thought to lead to the formation of what was formerly called *pseudolymphoma,* but which has been shown by molecular-genetic studies to represent an early form of a low-grade MALT lymphoma.[4] It has been postulated that the high-grade lymphomas may develop from these low-grade lymphomas.[5]

Lymphomas have been classified in numerous ways, but I find most useful that of the World Health Organization, which classifies them into low-, intermediate-, and high-grade according to their growth rates. Surprisingly, the low-grade lymphomas tend to be more widespread at presentation and, although associated with a good long-term prognosis, are rarely curable. Conversely, the high-grade lymphomas, which are more likely to be localized at presentation, can be cured by chemotherapy but, when not cured, usually lead to the patient's death in 1 to 2 years. Most recent studies of gastric lymphoma have combined the intermediate- into the high-grade category, and I will continue that practice in this discussion.

CLINICAL PICTURE

PRESENTING SYMPTOMS

Pain predominates as the major symptom of this disease and was present in 70% of patients in a British series of 153 patients[6] and a German series of 145 patients.[7] Anorexia, nausea, and weight loss occur less often (20% to 50%), whereas bleeding is found in 10% to 40%. A gastric mass may be palpable in the more advanced lesions, but peripheral adenopathy and hepatosplenomegaly are uncommon.

---

*Lymphoma refers to non-Hodgkin's lymphoma, since gastric Hodgkin's lymphoma is rare.

Diagnosis

The diagnosis is usually made through endoscopic biopsy. Low-grade lymphomas may present as (1) large ulcers with raised edges, (2) gastritis, (3) erosions, or (4) thickening of gastric folds.[8] Since they often grow submucosally, they may be difficult to diagnose, and multiple biopsy specimens should be taken. Gastric endoscopic ultrasound may help by localizing the preponderant area of involvement. High-grade lymphomas often appear as a mass indistinguishable from carcinoma. The incidence of high-grade and low-grade lesions is approximately equal.

Prognosis

The prognosis of patients with gastric lymphoma reflects the stage and histology of their disease. Most patients present with either stage IE or IIE (E represents *extranodal*) disease. That is, the disease is either confined to the stomach (IE) or includes possible extension to regional lymph nodes (IIE). Occasionally, patients also present with abdominal lymph node involvement (stage III) or bone marrow or other organ involvement (stage IV). Therefore, once the diagnosis of gastric lymphoma is made, patients should undergo an abdominal computerized tomographic scanning. Bone marrow evaluation rarely proves fruitful and should be reserved for patients who exhibit extensive disease or hematologic compromise.

Low-Grade Gastric Lymphomas

The prognosis of patients with low-grade gastric lymphomas is excellent. Several recent series[7–9] have reported very few deaths in treated patients with low-grade gastric lymphomas followed 5 to 13 years. One reason for this good prognosis of low-grade lymphomas has been the inclusion in these studies of lesions previously called pseudolymphoma. These, of course, present as stage IE lesions. Patients with stage IIE low-grade lymphomas suffer a higher mortality, perhaps 25% at 10 years.[7]

High-Grade Gastric Lymphomas

Patients with high-grade lymphomas experience a higher mortality. Several early series report only a 30% to 50% 5-year survival rate for these patients.[10–12] The stage of the disease also predicts prognosis with increased mortality found in patients whose disease presents in higher stages.

TREATMENT OF GASTRIC LYMPHOMAS

Treatment of gastric lymphoma has evolved considerably since gastric endoscopy has been widely used for its diagnosis. When, in preendoscopic times, the diagnosis required laparotomy, most patients underwent either partial or total gastric resection. Indeed, most early series were reported from surgical departments. Many of these studies reported improved survival in those patients who were viable candidates for gastric resection. However, the role of surgery has become less clear now that we have endoscopy available to make the diagnosis and chemotherapy and radiotherapy available for treatment and can avoid some of the disabling effects of extensive gastric resections. Unfortunately, no randomized clinical trials to define the roles of these treatment modalities have been performed.

Principles of Lymphoma Therapy

Low-Grade Lymphomas

To understand the treatment of patients with gastric lymphomas, one must understand how patients with typical nodal lymphomas are treated. As I stated earlier, low-grade lymphomas are rarely curable but in general progress slowly with patient survival measured in decades. Unfortunately, they can transform into higher grade lymphomas, which are more virulent and often fatal. When we treat these low-grade diseases, we tend to use single agent therapy such as the alkylating agents chlorambucil or cyclophosphamide and reserve polychemotherapy for more aggressive disease. Patients are usually treated until they achieve a significant regression of their disease; the treatment is then stopped and the patient observed. Our hand is somewhat stayed by the tendency of these drugs to cause bone marrow transformation into myelodysplasia and myelocytic leukemia. Thus, we try to avoid their excessive use, particularly in these patients with good long-term prognoses.

High-Grade Lymphomas

Because patients with intermediate- or high-grade lymphomas will die of their disease within 2 years if treatment is unsuccessful, we treat them aggressively with polychemotherapy. Most polychemotherapy combinations used to treat these lymphomas achieve similar success rates of about 50% long-term survival.[13] The combination of cyclophosphamide, doxorubicin, vincristine, and prednisone (CHOP) is most often used because it is well tolerated and easy to administer. Radiotherapy may also be administered to sites of bulky disease since these will be the most likely sites of recurrence. This is usually delayed until chemotherapy has been completed to take advantage of the reduced size of the tumor and avoid distant progression of the lymphoma that might occur during radiotherapy. For a more thorough review of lymphoma therapy, see the recent article by Armitage.[14]

GASTRIC LYMPHOMAS

Treatment of gastric lymphoma reflects the above principles modified by this lymphoma's specific location. I will limit this discussion to patients in which the lymphoma is confined to the stomach and its draining nodes (IE, IIE). Once there is extensive abdominal lymph node involvement or extraabdominal disease, the treatment is that of systemic nodal lymphomas.

Low-Grade Lymphomas

Since low-grade lymphomas have such good prognoses, aggressive therapy has little to offer. A unique approach to these early low-grade lymphomas has been proposed by Wotherspoon et al.[15] These investigators found *H. pylori* in 92% of gastric lymphomas and, reasoning that this antigenic stimulus led to lymphomatous growth, treated this infection. They reported that in 5 of 6 patients the lymphoma, which was a low-grade early lesion, completely regressed, whereas in the remaining patient it mostly regressed. This response of early low-grade gastric lymphomas to antibiotic therapy of *H. pylori* has also been reported by other investigators. Thus, in early low-grade lymphomas, I would look for *H. pylori* infection and, if found, treat this before administering chemotherapy. I would follow two parameters: the patient's symptoms and the size of the lymphoma, which is evaluated by endoscopy every 3 to 6 months.

If this fails I would treat these patients with single agent alkylating therapy, either chlorambucil or cyclophosphamide. Therapy is continued until there is a major remission of disease but for no longer than 1 year. If the disease has regressed, I then recommend endoscopy every 6 to 12 months and reinstitute therapy if it recurs.

If the disease proves refractory to this approach, I then recommend radiation therapy. Since the low-grade lesions often involve a significant portion of the stomach, radiation therapy provides better quality of life than does an extensive gastric resection, and retrospective reviews by Castrillo et al,[9] Blazquez et al,[8] and Gobbi et al[16] confirm that surgery does not provide better survival.

If the disease does present with a large tumor mass, I would treat it like the high-grade disease since its behavior better reflects its propensity to grow than does its histology.

High-Grade Lymphomas

High-grade lymphomas or extensive low-grade lymphomas (bulky mass or extensive nodal involvement) require a more aggressive approach. These traditionally have been treated by surgical resection, and most series have reported poor outcomes in those who were unresectable and good outcomes in those who could be resected. This may reflect the aggressiveness of the disease rather than the benefit of surgical intervention. The single factor that has changed our approach to high-grade gastric lymphomas has been the introduction of effective chemotherapy. Two recent studies[17,18] have used this modality after resection and found that the most important prognostic factor for long-term survival was whether the patients responded to chemotherapy.

The relative unimportance of surgery was emphasized in a recent[16] retrospective review of a large group of patients who were treated in a nonrandomized fashion with either surgery and radiation therapy or chemotherapy or, if resection was not possible, with radiation and chemotherapy. These investigators found no benefit for the patients who underwent surgery in spite of their less extensive disease. This benefit for chemotherapy and radiotherapy without surgery was championed by recent studies,[19,20] which found that surgery was not needed to provide a good long-term survival for gastric high-grade lymphoma patients.

It has become clear that chemotherapy is the primary life-saving modality in high-grade gastric lymphoma. The major question has now become when to administer it and whether it needs to be combined with surgery or radiation therapy. I do not see any advantage in using both radiotherapy and surgery since both are intended to treat the primary lesion. Many have argued that surgery is needed to prevent either perforation or bleeding that might accompany successful chemotherapy or radiotherapy. However, Gobbi et al[16] have shown that the complications of surgery far exceed those of nonsurgical treatment.

RECOMMENDATIONS

My primary approach to these lesions, therefore, would begin with accurate staging including, if possible, gastric endoscopic sonography. If the lesion is early low grade with no bulky component, I would first treat any *Helicobacter* infection. If this is absent or the lymphoma does not respond, then I would administer single-agent chemotherapy with either cyclophosphamide or chlorambucil. Therapy would be administered for 6 to 12 months and monitored every 6 months by endoscopy. If the lesion does not respond or if the patient responds only partially and remains symptomatic after that period, I would consider radiation therapy to the stomach.

High-grade lesions as well as bulky low-grade ones should be treated with intravenous chemotherapy. My regimen of choice would be CHOP, although one might eliminate the doxorubicin for low-grade lesions. I would treat *first* with chemotherapy and carefully observe the patient both clinically and endoscopically for evidence of impending perforation or bleeding. Treatment would continue for 4 to 6 months depending on the response. In the absence of any good clinical trial to the contrary, I feel obliged at this point to add local treatment. In almost all cancers, recurrence is most likely at the site of bulky disease, usually the primary lesion, and these are then often incurable. Therefore, I would want to sterilize the area of the primary lesion with radiation therapy.

Is there any role for primary surgery? Clearly for bleeding or obstructing lesions, surgery may be the best approach prior to chemotherapy. Sometimes surgery is needed to make a diagnosis; if the lesion is small, a small partial gastrectomy would not add that much morbidity to that of the laparotomy and would be worthwhile. However, I would not recommend it otherwise although no clinical trial has tested the role of elective surgery in this disease. Indeed, although it might be tempting to resect small lesions, these are just the malignancies that respond best to chemotherapy.

REFERENCES

1. Severson RK, Davis S. Increasing incidence of primary gastric lymphoma. *Cancer.* 1990;66:1283–1287.
2. Isaacson PG, Spencer J, Finn T. Primary B-cell gastric lymphoma. *Hum Pathol.* 1986;17:72–82.
3. Wotherspoon AC, Ortiz-Hildago C, Falzon MR, Isaacson PG. *Helicobacter pylori*–associated gastritis and primary B-cell gastric lymphoma. *Lancet.* 1991;338:1175–1176.
4. Sanchez L, Algara P, Villuendas R, Martinez P, et al. B-cell clonal detection in gastric low-grade lymphomas and regional lymph nodes: an immunohistologic and molecular study. *Am J Gastroenterol.* 1993;88:413–419.
5. Chan JKC, Ng CS, Isaacson PG. Relationship between high-grade lymphoma and low-grade B-cell mucosa-associated lymphoid tissue lymphoma (MALToma) of the stomach. *Am J Pathol.* 1990;136:1153–1164.
6. Hockey MS, Powell J, Crocker J, Fielding JWL. Primary gastric lymphoma. *Br J Surg.* 1987;74:483–487.
7. Cogliatti SB, Schmid U, Schumacher U, et al. Primary B-cell gastric lymphoma: a clinicopathological study of 145 patients. *Gastroenterology.* 1991;101:1159–1170.
8. Blazquez M, Haioun C, Chaumette M-T, et al. Low grade B cell mucosa associated lymphoid tissue lymphoma of the stomach: clinical and endoscopic features, treatment, and outcome. *Gut.* 1992;33:1621–1625.
9. Castrillo JM, Montalban C, Obeso G, et al. Gastric B-cell mucosa associated lymphoid tissue lymphoma: a clinicopathological study in 56 patients. *Gut.* 1992;33:1307–1311.
10. Brooks JJ, Enterline HT. Primary gastric lymphomas. *Cancer.* 1983;51:701–711.
11. Azab MB, Henry-Amar M, Rougier P, et al. Prognostic factors in primary gastrointestinal non-Hodgkin's lymphoma. *Cancer.* 1989;64:1208–1217.
12. Dragosics B, Bauer P, Radaszkiewicz T. Primary gastrointestinal non-Hodgkin's lymphomas. *Cancer.* 1985;55:1060–1073.
13. Fisher RI, Gaynor ER, Dahlberg S, et al. Comparison of CHOP vs m-BACOD vs ProMACE-CytaBOM vs MACOP-B in patients with intermediate or high-grade lymphoma. *N Engl J Med.* 1993;328:1002–1006.
14. Armitage JO. Treatment of non-Hodgkin's lymphoma. *N Engl J Med.* 1993;328:1023–1030.
15. Wotherspoon AC, Doglioni C, Diss DC, et al. Regression of primary low-grade B-cell gastric lymphoma of mucosa-associated tissue type after eradication of *Helicobacter pylori*. *Lancet.* 1993;342:575–577.
16. Gobbi PG, Dionigi P, Barbieri F, et al. The role of surgery in the multimodal treatment of primary gastric non-Hodgkin's lymphomas. *Cancer.* 1990;65:2528–2536.
17. Bellesi G, Alterini R, Messori A, et al. Combined surgery and chemotherapy for the treatment of primary gastrointestinal intermediate- or high-grade non-Hodgkin's lymphomas. *Br J Cancer.* 1989;60:244–248.
18. Sheridan WP, Medley G, Brodie GN. Non-Hodgkin's lymphoma of the stomach: a prospective pilot study of surgery plus chemotherapy in early and advanced disease. *J Clin Oncol.* 1985;3:495–500.
19. Maor MH, Velasquez WS, Fuller LM, Silvermintz KB. Stomach conservation in stages IE and IIE gastric non-Hodgkin's lymphoma. *J Clin Oncol.* 1990;8:266–271.
20. Salles G, Herbrecht R, Tilly H, et al. Aggressive primary gastrointestinal lymphomas: review of 91 patients treated with the LNH-84 regimen. *Am J Med.* 1991;90:77–84.

42
Gastric Polyps
MONROE H. SPECTOR

A gastric polyp(s) may be discovered as a result of clinical presentation or radiographic or endoscopic evaluations. The lesion may represent a normal variant of mucosa, i.e., exaggerated gastric tissue, or represent a true polypoid projection. Its exact nature should be analyzed to determine the correct clinical approach. True gastric polypoid structures are derived from either gastric epithelium or mesenchymal tissue. This chapter confines its remarks to polyps of epithelial origin, i.e., hyperplastic and adenomatous polyps.

INCIDENCE

Gastric epithelial polyps were initially felt to be rare lesions. First discovered by Morgagni at autopsy, then radiographically by Heinz and finally endoscopically by Schendler.[1] The incidence varies from 0.4% to 0.7%.

Hyperplastic polyps constitute a much more frequent subgroup (7% to 91%),[2,3] and are not felt, in general, to be precursors of carcinoma. Adenomatous polyps, on the other hand, are premalignant and much less frequent. The incidence of adenomatous polyps appears to be somewhat higher in familial polyposis coli and Gardner's syndrome.[4]

PATHOLOGY

Hyperplastic Polyps

Hyperplastic polyps (also referred to as *regenerative polyps*)[5] are generally small (less than 2 cm), sessile or pedunculated, solitary, usually occurring in the fundus or gastric body areas of the stomach. Histologically, they consist of numerous dilated, cystic, branching glandular structures surrounded by a fibrous muscular stroma with infiltration by chronic inflammatory cells such as lymphocytes and are not true neoplastic polyps. Hyperplastic polyps, however, are associated with gastric dysplasia, intestinal metaplasia, pernicious anemia, atrophic gastritis, Ménétrier's disease and familial polyposis coli, which in turn are associated with an increased incidence of carcinoma of the stomach and small intestine. In some instances, hypergastrinemia has been noted, which may be an etiologic factor in the genesis of hyperplastic polyps.[6]

Adenomatous Polyps

Adenomatous polyps are true neoplastic lesions and, like hyperplastic polyps, can be sessile or pedunculated, more commonly confined to the gastric antrum, but can occur anywhere in the stomach and are frequently solitary. There is a much higher incidence of these polyps in patients with gastric cancer. Histologically, they are similar to adenomatous polyps of the colon. Transition from polyp to normal mucosa is usually abrupt; nuclei may be mildly to severely dysplastic and may be part of a frankly invasive adenocarcinoma, which is uncommonly seen in these polyps.[2,5] Additionally, intestinal metaplasia (also associated with an increased incidence of adenocarcinoma of the stomach) has been associated with adenomatous polyps.[6]

CLINICAL PRESENTATION

Most polyps, either hyperplastic or adenomatous, are asymptomatic. They are frequently discovered radiographically or endoscopically. Infrequently, symptoms occur, usually vague and nonspecific, consisting of abdominal discomfort, pain, anemia, occult or frank gastrointestinal tract bleeding, fatigue, or nausea, all of which may be unrelated to the presence of a polyp(s).

Antral pedunculated lesions may prolapse through the pylorus and cause symptoms of intermittent gastric outlet obstruction. Bleeding from polyps presents as melena and anemia and less frequently, hematemesis. Additionally, gastric polyps are associated with atrophic gastritis and pernicious anemia.[7]

Gastric polyps can occur in all age groups, but the peak incidence is the fifth to seventh decades of life.

RELATION TO CARCINOMA

Ming and Goldman[5] and Tomasulo[2] clearly demonstrated the association of gastric polyps with carcinoma of the stomach. Hyperplastic polyps rarely undergo malignant transformation, although as previously discussed, these polyps are associated with carcinoma developing in gastric mucosa.[5] Adenomatous polyps, on the other hand, albeit infrequently, can clearly undergo malignant transformation within the polyp itself and are also associated with cancer occurring elsewhere within the stomach.

Polyp size is of great importance with regard to malignant potential. A 24% incidence of malignancy was noted in Tomasulo's study[2] in polyps greater than 2 cm, whereas polyps less than 2 cm, had a 4% chance of harboring carcinoma. As demonstrated by Ming and Goldman,[5] hyperplastic polyps greater than 2 cm had no increased incidence of carcinoma.

An additional factor of importance with regard to malignancy is polyp morphology as noted by Yamada.[8] In addition to confirming Tomasulo's and Ming's observations that size is of great importance, Yamada noted that sessile polyps had the highest incidence of malignancy, even if the polyp was less than 2 cm.

Tomasulo and others have shown no association with multiple polyps and carcinoma (i.e., solitary versus multiple).

DIAGNOSIS

Diagnosis of gastric polyps is usually fortuitous. They are found less commonly because of specific symptoms than by chance. More often today, with frequent use of endoscopy, polyps are discovered coincidentally. Less commonly, but with greater frequency than clinical presentation, radiographic discovery may lead to specific endoscopic evaluation of the polyp. Clinical presentation may result from occult or frank gastrointestinal tract bleeding or intermittent gastric outlet obstruction by a pedunculated polyp prolapsing back and forth through the pyloric channel.

MANAGEMENT OF GASTRIC POLYPS

Once discovered, either radiographically or endoscopically, the exact nature of a gastric polyp must be elucidated. With the advent of improved fiberoptic techniques and more recently, video endoscopy, the physician has the ability to determine whether polyps are of epithelial or mesenchymal origin. Additionally, the investigator must determine the gastric mucosal background in patients with gastric polyps. In case of solitary larger polyps, the entire lesion must be removed to determine its histologic factors and potential to progress to carcinoma.

Seifert and Elster[9] reviewed their experience of gastric polypectomy and found that discrepancies frequently occurred between the histologic findings of superficial biopsies and whole polyp mounts. They were required to change the histologic diagnosis in 75% of cases. Exfoliative cytologic examination via saline lavage may be helpful, but resulted in a large number of false-negative results in another study (20% to 40%).[10]

Additionally, Seifert and Elster[9] found that polyps that seemed hyperplastic on superficial biopsy contained adenomatous features after the entire polyp was removed and were frequently of mixed variety, i.e., hyperplastic-adenomatous.

Hyperplastic Polyps

As previously discussed, hyperplastic polyps are the most frequently encountered gastric neoplasm. They are most often solitary, but occasionally multiple and numerous, can be limited to the gastric body, but may also be predominantly fundic. Fundic polyps are more commonly seen in women and the familial polyposis syndromes. Additionally, fundic polyps frequently do not occur in the background of abnormal mucosa elsewhere in the stomach.[4,11–13] Hence, the approach to fundic polyps need not be as rigorous as to polyps located elsewhere in the stomach.

The approach to hyperplastic polyps involving the gastric body and antrum should be much more cautious. Two issues are of importance: (1) the exact histologic type of polyp and (2) the background of surrounding mucosa. With regards to the latter problem, because many hyperplastic polyps are associated with chronic active gastritis, hypergastrinemic states or pernicious anemia, and a tendency to form dysplastic mucosa distant to the polyp, not only should large polyps be removed, but background mucosa should be carefully examined by biopsy and analyzed histologically for dysplastic changes.[5] In fact, Tomasulo[2] and Ming and Goldman[5] noted the presence of coexisting carcinoma in patients with hyperplastic polyps.

ADENOMATOUS POLYPS

Although much less common than hyperplastic polyps,[2,5,9] adenomatous polyps present a risk to patients. Frequently solitary and antral, they may occur in the gastric body and rarely in the gastric fundus. Frequently they are radiographically and endoscopically indistinguishable from larger hyperplastic polyps and must be completely removed. Polyps that are greater than 2 cm and sessile have a great propensity to malignant transformation. Therefore, when one approaches these polyps, careful consideration is required as to the most expeditious way to manage them, i.e., endoscopic versus surgical removal.

THERAPEUTIC APPROACH TO GASTRIC POLYPS

ENDOSCOPIC POLYPECTOMY

With improved endoscopic techniques, it is now possible to remove large gastric polyps, up to 5 cm. The decision concerning endoscopic removal must be based on the risk-benefit ratio, i.e., benefit versus risk of hemorrhage, perforation, and incomplete removal of a malignant lesion.

Seifert and Elster[9] and ReMine and colleagues[14] have provided the largest experience to date of endoscopic polypectomies. Seifert and Elster evaluated 138 patients for a total of 244 polyps removed by electroresection. Hyperplastic polyps (47.7%) and focal areas of hyperplasia (14.8%) were the most common lesions removed. Adenomatous polyps occurred much less frequently (7.4%). Other lesions included in his series were inflammatory pseudopolyps (6.3%), chronic erosions (9.7%), xanthoma (2.3%), neurinomas (2.8%), "mesenchymal" tumors or fibromatous polyps (2.8%), lipomas (0.6%), pancreatic heterotopy (1.7%), eosinophilic granulomas (1.1%), and early gastric cancer (1.1%).

Based on their findings, the following classification of polyps was proposed:

1. Focal hyperplasia
2. Hyperplastic polyps
3. Adenoma
4. Proliferation of glandular neck with epithelial atypia (borderline lesion, protruded type)
5. Early gastric cancer.

In these groups, transition from a reactive regenerative process to frank carcinoma was noted. While lesions in groups 1 and 2 were benign, without tendency to malignant degeneration, Seifert and Elster felt that groups 3 and 4 were precancerous. Additionally, discrepancies occurred between superficial biopsy material and whole mount preparations.

ReMine and colleagues[14] reviewed 48 consecutive gastric polypectomies in 43 patients who ranged in age from 43 to 86 years, mean of 66 years. The most common symptoms were epigastric discomfort or indigestion (44%) and anemia (21%). The most common anatomic location of lesions included the antrum (67%) and fundus (30%). Pedunculated polyps occurred in 77% of cases and sessile polyps in 22%. Polyp size ranged from 0.5 to 3.5 cm. Multiple polyps occurred in 5% of patients. Histologic types included: hyperplastic (58%), adenomatous (25%), carcinoid (6%), mesenchymal (13%), aberrant pancreas, inflammatory pseudotumors, hamartomas, and Peutz-Jeghers polyps occurring in the remainder. In addition, 2 of 12 adenomatous polyps showed foci of in situ carcinoma, and one was noted to have marked dysplasia. Seventy-five percent of adenomatous polyps were antral and 67% were pedunculated. ReMine and colleagues found a ratio of hyperplastic to adenomatous polyps of 2.3:1, similar to Tomasulo's experience[2] but lower than noted by Ming and Goldman.[5] Additionally, ReMine and colleagues felt that the lower incidence of malignant change in their experience correlated with a smaller size of polyps compared with other reviewers.

Safety of Endoscopic Polypectomy

The experience concerning the safety of endoscopic polypectomy has been reassuring. Seifert and Elster[9] noted complications in 3 of 244 cases. Complications included bleeding (two patients), controlled by electrocoagulation in one case and by surgery in the second. One patient developed severe abdominal pain, was taken to surgery, and found to have a large ulcer at the polypectomy site; perforation was not reported by Seifert and Elster.

ReMine and colleagues[14] reported a 6% complication rate, i.e., three complications and no deaths. However, two of the patients required laparotomy for uncontrolled bleeding. A third case was complicated by poor patient compliance; no sequela was reported in this case.

SURGERY

In most cases, endoscopic polypectomy suffices as definitive intervention. Surgery is indicated for the following reasons:

1. *In situ malignant degeneration noted in the polyp after endoscopic removal:* One cannot assume the entire lesion has been resected. Further experience from large series is needed to determine whether endoscopic polypectomy with no tumor invasion beyond the muscularis mucosa can be managed in a similar manner as colon polyps, i.e., no surgical resection. If surgical intervention is not chosen, careful endoscopic follow-up with multiple additional biopsies is advisable. If invasive carcinoma is found, surgical intervention is warranted.
2. *Incomplete removal of a large (greater than 2-cm) polyp, either pedunculated or sessile:* As previously discussed, these polyps have a greater potential for malignant transformation. Additionally, they may be of a mixed variety, i.e., hyperplastic-adenomatous.
3. Very large, nonremovable polyps.

THE DECISION-MAKING PROCESS: WHICH POLYPS SHOULD BE REMOVED?

Because endoscopic polypectomy and surgical intervention are not without morbidity, possibly even mortality, discussion with the patient should occur concerning indications for polyp removal. After careful review of the literature, the following recommendations can be made with regard to complete excision:

1. Polyps greater than 2 cm
2. Sessile polyps
3. Polyps that present with symptoms: bleeding, gastric outlet obstruction
4. Evidence for malignancy
5. True adenomas
6. Age greater than 50 years in patients with adenomatous and hyperplastic polyps, with abnormal background mucosa

Multiple polyps do not require gastrectomy. The major problem in this group, however, is sampling. In most cases, multiplicity is due to hyperplastic polyps. Caveats do occur, however: Huppler et al[15] reported in a surgical series from the Mayo Clinic that when multiple polyps occurred, the incidence of cancer was 14%, in contrast to 9% when a single polyp was present. This series was preendoscopic and does not conform to endoscopic literature. A more disturbing report from Japan[16] reviewed 470 hyperplastic polyps removed by endoscopic polypectomy, where the authors studied polyp dysplastic changes and malignant transformation. Focal carcinoma was noted in 2.1% of hyperplastic polyps (10 polyps). Location of cancer was in the polyp head or at the polyp surface. Dysplasia was also found in the polyp and near foci of carcinoma in 10 polyps. Additionally, dysplastic foci were found in 4% of hyperplastic polyps (19 polyps). All 10 polyps with foci of cancer were larger than 2 cm. The authors concluded that cancer develops from dysplastic foci as the polyp grows larger. Furthermore, they suggested that as the polyp enlarges and becomes semipedunculated or pedunculated, dysplastic foci appear first followed by carcinoma.

HELICOBACTER PYLORI

Although a body of literature has developed associating *Helicobacter pylori* with gastric carcinoma,[17,18] little information is available at this time to relate the organism to gastric polyps.

FOLLOW-UP OF GASTRIC POLYPS

STOMACH FREE OF POLYPS AFTER POLYPECTOMY

Insufficient data regarding follow-up after polypectomy exist to draw conclusions. ReMine and colleagues[14] and Hughes[19] noted in follow-up examinations in over 50% of their patients that no new adenomatous polyps formed. However, one patient had a recurrent hyperplastic polyp that was removed twice over a 2-year period. Long-term follow-up studies, however, are not available. Seifert[9] reported follow-up examinations 1 year after polypectomy in 64 patients. In six, a polypoid remnant was noted: three had recurrence at the same site indicating incomplete removal of the polyp(s), and three were at sites elsewhere in the stomach.

FOLLOW-UP OF GASTRIC POLYPS NOT REMOVED

Hyperplastic Polyps

Kamiya et al[20] evaluated 93 hyperplastic polyps in 56 patients followed endoscopically and microscopically for 5 to 12 years. Thirty patients (54%) showed changes in the number, size, or shape of polyps during the follow-up period. Three lesions showed transformation from hyperplastic to adenomas associated with polyp enlargement, severe atypia, and finally progression to frank carcinoma. Others in the Japanese literature have demonstrated similar results. It is not clear, however, that the Japanese experience is analogous to the experience seen in the West.

Adenomas

Kamiya et al[21] evaluated 85 adenomatous polyps in 74 patients observed from 6 months to 12 years. As age increased, so did the incidence of adenomas (0.1% in the third decade; 3.7% in the ninth). Gastric cancers that coexist with gastric adenomas were noted in 14 patients (8%). Moderate-to-severe dysplasia in polyps was noted as a transition to cancer. The authors suggest that as lesions enlarge, the degree of dysplasia increases, which leads to subsequent carcinomas.

CONCLUSIONS

Gastric epithelial polyps present a therapeutic challenge to the practicing physician. Concurrent management and follow-up must be guided by several important factors:

1. Large polyps (greater than 2 cm) are at risk for development of gastric carcinoma.
2. The larger the polyp, the greater the risk of dysplasia, a precancerous state.
3. Although hyperplastic polyps carry a very low risk for cancer, malignancy can occur in a polyp as it enlarges and transforms to an adenoma. Additionally, cancer may also occur in abnormal background gastric tissue, i.e., atrophic and dysplastic mucosa.
4. Adenomatous polyps are premalignant and tend to increase in size, which carries an increased risk of cancer. Additionally, cancer may also develop in nonadenomatous gastric tissue.
5. Endoscopic follow-up of both hyperplastic and adenomatous polyps is important. There are no data, however, as to how often to perform endoscopic evaluation, although the literature seems to support frequent endoscopic evaluation for both adenomatous and large hyperplastic polyps.
6. Sessile polyps appear to increase the risk of the dysplasia to carcinoma sequence.
7. Age greater than 50 years appears to be a risk factor for development of dysplasia and carcinoma in polyps.

REFERENCES

1. Monaco A, Roth S, Castleman B, et al. Adenomatous polyps of the stomach. *Cancer.* 1962;15:456–466.
2. Tomasulo J. Gastric polyps: histologic types and their relationship to gastric carcinoma. *Cancer.* 1971;27:1346–1355.
3. Deppisch LM, Vigil VT. Epithelial polyps: a ten-year study. *J Clin Gastroenterol.* 1989;11:110–115.
4. Watanabe H, Enjoji M, Yao T, et al. Gastric lesions in familial adenomatous coli. *Hum Pathol.* 1978;9:269–283.
5. Ming SC, Goldman H. Gastric polyps: a histologic classification and its relation to carcinoma. *Cancer.* 1965;18:721–726.
6. Nakano H, Person B, Slezak P. Study of gastric mucosal background in patients with gastric polyps. *Gastrointest Endosc.* 1990;36:39–42.
7. Neimark S, Rogers A. Gastric polyps: a review. *Am J Gastroenterol.* 1989;77:585–587.
8. Yamada T, Ichikawa H. X-ray diagnosis of elevated gastric lesions of the stomach. *Radiology.* 1974;110:79–83.
9. Seifert E, Elster K. Gastric polypectomy. *Am J Gastroenterol.* 1975;63:451–456.
10. Carney JA. Gastric exfoliative cytology. *Surg Clin North Am.* 1971;51:979.
11. Haruma K, Sumii K, Yoshihara M, et al. Gastric mucosa in female patients with fundic glandular polyps. *Clin Gastroenterol.* 1991;13:565–569.
12. Kinosita Y, Tojo M, Yano T, et al. Incidence of fundic gland polyps in patients without familial adenomatous polyposis. *Gastrointest Endosc.* 1993;39:161–163.
13. Marcial MA, Villafa M, Hernandez-Denton J, et al. Fundic gland polyps: prevalence and clinical pathologic features. *Am J Gastroenterol.* 1993;88:1711–1713.
14. ReMine SG, Hughes RW Jr, Weiland LH. Endoscopic gastric polypectomies. *Mayo Clin Proc.* 1981;56:371–375.
15. Huppler EG, Priestly JT, Morlock CG, et al. Diagnosis and results of treatment of gastric polyps. *Surg Gynecol Obstet.* 1960;110:309–313.
16. Daibo M, Itabashi M, Hirota T. Malignant transformation of gastric hyperplastic polyps. *Am J Gastroenterol.* 1987;82:1016–1025.
17. Nomura A, Stemmermann GN, Chyou PH, et al. Helicobacter pylori infection and gastric carcinoma among Japanese Americans in Hawaii. *N Engl J Med.* 1991;325:1132–1136.
18. Parsonnet J, Friedman GF, Van Der Steen DP, et al. Helicobacter pylori infection and the risk of gastric carcinoma. *N Engl J Med.* 1991;325:1127–1131.
19. Hughes RW. Gastric polyps and polypectomy: rationale, technique and complications. *Gastrointest Endosc.* 1984;30:101–102.
20. Kamiya T, Hitoshi A, Yoshio M, et al. Histoclinical long-standing follow-up study of hyperplastic polyps in the stomach. *Am J Gastroenterol.* 1981;75:275–281.
21. Kamiya T, Tetsuo M, Hitoshi A, et al. Long-term follow-up study of gastric adenoma and its relation to gastric protruded carcinoma. *Cancer.* 1982;50:2496–2503.

43
Carcinoid Tumors and Carcinoid Syndrome

RALPH R. HALL and KARL H. HANSON

Carcinoid tumors are ubiquitous tumors found primarily in the gastrointestinal tract but have been described in most organ systems. They represent a spectrum from benign, highly curable tumors, which produce symptoms because of inflammation or perforation, to a group of long-surviving patients with bizarre and fascinating clinical presentations. There are those with 99% cure rates from initial surgical procedures such as the appendiceal carcinoid. In one series of patients with 820 appendiceal carcinoids, there was only one patient who died during a 5-year follow-up period.[1] Finally, there is a small number of patients with undifferentiated tumors that are associated with an aggressive course with rare patients living 6 months after the initial diagnosis.

The term *carcinoid syndrome* identifies a group of patients who manifest symptoms of flushing, diarrhea, hypotension, and bronchial constriction due to the neurohumoral hormones secreted by this small proportion of patients with carcinoid tumors. The name was given to these interesting slow-growing tumors because they have an appearance of carcinoma but they follow a clinical course that is much less aggressive than other malignancies. The widespread origin of carcinoid tumors is a result of the extensive distribution of the Kulschitsky's cells, which are found in virtually all body organs. The cells are thought to arise from the neural crest as described by Bolande.[2] These are the same cells Pearce[3] has dubbed APUDomas (alanine precursor uptake and decarboxylation). For the most part, carcinoid tumors consist of benign-appearing cells with only rare mitotic figures.

The histologic findings from metastatic sites, such as the liver and biopsy specimens, cannot be relied on to differentiate between gastrointestinal tumors and those tumors that do not originate from gastrointestinal sites. The immunohistologic findings of these tumors have been helpful in identifying which tumors were multihormonal. The production of hormones from these tumors is complicated. There are now more than 80 peptides that are secreted by at least 20 different types of neuroendocrine cells.[4] As many as six different active hormones have been identified as being secreted by a single carcinoid tumor. These findings probably underlie the various presentations and varied responses of the carcinoid syndrome to treatment. It is of interest that carcinoid tumors at different sites in the gastrointestinal tract produce different and somewhat specific hormonal peptides. For instance, gastrin tends to be produced by the stomach and duodenal tumors, whereas serotonin and substance P are produced by ileal tumors. Rectal carcinoids produce glucagon, b-endorphins, enkephalin, and insulin.

Carcinoid tumors have been found in the esophagus, bile ducts, Meckel's diverticulum, throughout the small and large intestines, the lung, and even, in a small group, in the ear. There is a high frequency of abdominal noncarcinoid tumors found concurrently with the carcinoids. In one large series, 8% of the appendiceal carcinoids, 10% of colon carcinoids, and 13% of large intestinal carcinoids had other tumors concurrently identified at the time the initial tumor was found.[5]

INITIAL PRESENTATION

There is an amazing variation in the reasons why patients with carcinoid tumors seek help from their physicians. In the series reported by Moertel (Table 43–1) in which the findings from 91 patients with carcinoid syndrome were described, diarrhea and flushing was the most frequent pre-

TABLE 43-1. PRESENTING CLINICAL MANIFESTATIONS IN 91 PATIENTS WITH THE MALIGNANT CARCINOID SYNDROME

Clinical Signs and Symptoms	Percentage of 91 Patients
Diarrhea	73
Flushing	65
Asthma	8
Pellagra	2
None*	12

From Moertel, CG. Gastrointestinal tumors and the malignant carcinoid syndrome. In: Sleisenger MH, Fordtran JS, eds. *Gastrointestinal Disease.* 5th ed. Philadelphia: WB Saunders Co; 1993:1363-1378.
*Elevated 5-hydroxyindoleacetic acid (5-HIAA) only.

sentation. This is consistent with other reported studies.

In another series, flushing and diarrhea were present in only 35% of patients with carcinoid metastases to the liver when the original tumor site was unknown. It was present in 18% of the patients with metastases known to be from the ileum.[1]

One of our patients presented with a purple pigmentation over his entire body. His presentation was initiated because he was disturbed by his appearance. His previous physicians had been unable to explain his skin changes. Because his appearance resembled that of a patient with the carcinoid syndrome who had a purplish patch over his face and neck pictured in another text, a 5-hydroxyindoleacetic acid (5-HIAA) test was ordered and found to be elevated. He gave a history of mild diarrhea and flushing in the past but had managed to control this by eliminating alcohol and caffeine from his diet. He had a palpable liver and a barely detectable heart murmur, which was thought to represent a right-sided valvular defect.

Another young patient has been described with similar skin findings, which were thought to be cyanosis due to valvular heart disease.[6] At autopsy the patient had subendocardial valvular heart disease due to a metastatic carcinoid tumor. The histologic findings of profound dermal capillary dilation were identical to those of our patient and to those lesions described on the head and neck of other patients with carcinoid tumors.

The severity of the syndrome by all accounts is directly related to the tumor size and its metastasis to the liver. Symptoms are usually not present until the tumor reaches the liver where it can secrete biologically active amines directly into the circulation. This circumvents inactivation of the amines by the enzymatic processes in the liver. Carcinoid tumors from the ovaries and testes may secrete their active amines directly to the circulation and thus produce symptoms without liver metastasis.

The cutaneous flushing is usually easily distinguished from the flushing of other causes, i.e., menopause, since there is a distinct red color appearing with the feeling of heat during the flush by the patient. The diarrhea occurring with the carcinoid syndrome is not easily distinguished from other causes of diarrhea. It has been attributed to mechanical factors and hypermotility. In some instances it may resemble a secretory diarrhea with large volumes associated with steatorrhea. In rare instances it may become profuse and life threatening with an accompanying hypokalemia and metabolic acidosis.

The frequency of valvular heart disease in reported series varies from 10% to 69%. Pulmonary disease and tricuspid valvular heart disease usually appear late in the course of the disease and are due to subendocardial fibrosis. Cardiac symptoms in a few instances have been the presenting complaint.

Abdominal pain is often an initial presenting symptom. This can be due to a large tumor mass with or without obstructive symptoms or possibly due to gastrointestinal cramping. Widespread retroperitoneal fibrosis resulting from serotonin or other active amine secreted by the tumor is usually a late development in the course of the disease.

BIOLOGIC MARKERS FOR CARCINOID TUMORS

In the patient with "typical" carcinoid syndrome 5-HIAA is excreted in excess. Various studies have shown that 5-HIAA was elevated in urine specimens from 87% to 99% of the time. Feldman[7] found that the sensitivity of the urine 5-HIAA test to be 73% and the specificity to be 100%.

Many other markers have been used but have not been found to be as useful as the urine 5-HIAA level. In Feldman's studies serum tryptophan levels were normal in most patients. In rare patients the conversion of serotonin to 5-HIAA is so rapid that the level of tryptophan is low and the patient develops pellagra because of tryptophan deficiency.

The usual metabolism of serotonin involves the conversion of tryptophan to 5-hydroxytryptophan (5-HTP). 5-HTP is then converted to 5-hydroxytryptamine (5-HT = serotonin) by dopa decarboxylase in the tumor. The 5-HT that is formed is then either stored in neurosecretory granules, which under the influence of stress or other factors release the serotonin. A portion of the serotonin remains in the plasma where it is converted into 5-HIAA. The 5-HIAA is then excreted by the kidney and appears in the urine. Urinary 5-HIAA levels correlate well with the extent and size of the tumor, as well as the propensity for the rare carcinoid crisis.

Many neurohumoral hormones, i.e., tachykinins, gastrointestinal peptides, prostaglandins, have been studied and evaluated for their diagnostic applications and their influence on the patients' symptoms. The subunits of human chorionic gonadotropin have been evaluated and are present in as many as 28% of patients with carcinoid syndrome. The measurement of carcinoembryonic antigen (CEA) has not been useful in distinguishing carcinoid tumors from other endocrine tumors. The concentration of CEA may be very high in other tumors such as neuroblastoma and medullary carcinoma of the thyroid. If the CEA antigen is markedly elevated in patients with carcinoid syndrome, concomitant tumors should be suspected.

A number of unusual endocrine and metabolic disturbances have been associated with carcinoid tumors. These include acromegaly, ectopic adrenocorticotropic hormone (ACTH) syndrome, hyperparathyroidism, and diabetes. All these disturbances have been improved with the removal of the tumor. These findings have led to the association of carcinoid syndrome with multiple endocrine neoplasia. Hypercalcemia may occur because of bone metastases although a high percentage of patients with bone metastases do not have hypercalcemia. The origin of the tumor is of little help in arriving at the cause of the hypercalcemia. It is therefore necessary to determine the cause of the hypercalcemia by the usual methods.

PHARMACOLOGIC TREATMENT

A number of pharmacologic agents have been used to treat patients with carcinoid syndrome. When using these agents, it is best to remember that the majority of these patients remain active and are only intermittently disturbed by the flushing and diarrhea. In our experience a number of medications can produce such severe drowsiness or other side effects that the disease was less disturbing than the side effects of the treatment.

Most of the agents used in the past only controlled one symptom of the disease such as either the diarrhea or the flushing. Simple agents such as the antidiarrheal drugs, loperamide and diphenoxylate, often are effective in controlling the diarrhea. Paracholoro-phenylalanine has been used with some success. Despite varying and titrating the dose, many patients are unable to drive or carry out other activities because of problems with memory and somnolence.

α-Methyldopa has limited effectiveness in blocking the conversion of 5-HTP to serotonin. It is somewhat helpful for the flushing but does not usually improve the diarrhea. Phenoxybenzamine and phenothiazine have been useful for the flushing. In the few patients with gastric carcinoids the pruritic flush is thought to be due to histamine and possibly other associated peptides. H_1 and H_2 antagonists have been helpful in preventing these symptoms in patients with gastric carcinoids.

More recently interferon[8] and octreotide[9] have been found to inhibit both the flushing and the diarrhea. These agents are expensive and have to be given subcutaneously or intravenously. The interferons have been associated with fever and malaise and again in our experience have been more difficult for patients to tolerate than is generally reported. Interferon and octreotide decrease the excretion of 5-HIAA and have been reported to be associated with regression of the tumor or at least responsible for its lack of progression in 10% to 15% of the patients. Octreotide has been associated with fat malabsorption and gallstones due to an alteration in gallbladder and gastrointestinal tract motility.

It has been suggested that there may be a difference in response to interferon produced by different pharmaceutical firms.[7] As pointed out by Feldman, the results reported by Moertel were in studies using interferon alfa-2a (Roferon-A) made by Roche rather than the preparation produced by Schering. The results reported from the Roche preparation were more favorable. The chemical structures of these two interferons are not identical.

The exact cause of carcinoid syndrome, i.e., flushing, diarrhea, lacrimation, bronchoconstriction, and variation in blood pressure, is poorly understood. Serotonin has been documented to cause diarrhea in some patients. Serotonin levels in the plasma are certainly correlated with the severity of diarrhea. It is to be noted, however, that not all patients with elevations of their serum serotonin have diarrhea. The diarrhea has been described as due to decreased transit time, as well as a secretory type of diarrhea. A recent study in a small number of patients documented a decrease in transit time.[10] These patients did not have evidence of a secretory type of diarrhea. More patients must be studied to rule out the possibility that some patients do have the secretory type of diarrhea determined by the humoral peptides produced by the tumor.

OCTREOTIDE ACETATE (SANDOSTATIN)

Clinical Pharmacology

The use of octreotide represents a significant advance in the management of the carcinoid syndrome. Octreotide exerts pharmacologic actions similar to the natural hormone somatostatin. In normal subjects, it has the ability to suppress secretion of serotonin, gastroenteropancreatic peptides such as gastrin, vasoactive intestinal peptide, insulin, glucagon, secretin, motilin, and pancreatic polypeptide. In addition, octreotide acetate suppresses growth hormone release. After subcutaneous injection, octreotide is absorbed rapidly and completely from the injection site. Intravenous and subcutaneous doses have been found to be bioequivalent. The duration of action of octreotide is reported to be variable but extends up to 12 hours when given in doses of 100 µg or more.

Therapy with octreotide is associated with cholelithiasis, presumably by altering fat absorption and possibly by decreasing the motility of the gallbladder. Data from controlled studies suggest an incident of between 15% to 20% of the development of gallstones or sludge. It is therefore recommended that patients undergoing prolonged therapy with octreotide be monitored for gallbladder disease with the use of ultrasound of the gallbladder and bile ducts.

It has been found that in carcinoid syndrome gradual increases in the dose may be needed to maintain symptomatic control. The precipitation of hypothyroidism and reduction in insulin requirements have occurred during the initiation or long-term use of octreotide. Octreotide has been administered concomitantly with H_2 antagonists, antimotility agents, and diuretics without apparent serious drug interactions. When the drug is administered with other agents, however, it is recommended that patients be monitored closely for adjustment in the other therapies. Imbalances in fluid and electrolytes may be the result of correction of preexisting abnormalities and not directly to octreotide. Octreotide has also been found to give prompt and complete relief of the joint pain in patients with the arthropody that sometimes accompanies the carcinoid syndrome.[11] It is also of great interest that insulinlike growth factor 1 (IGF-1) has been found to stimulate the growth of carcinoid tumor culture cells and that octreotide inhibits the production of IGF-1 in vivo and in carcinoid cell cultures.[12]

Although it is expensive, octreotide appears to be one of the most useful agents for the treatment of carcinoid syndrome, as well as for the prevention and treatment of carcinoid crises.

HEPATIC ARTERY EMBOLIZATION

Hepatic artery embolization with and without chemoembolization has now been carried out in several centers with some success.[13] Ruszniewske and others[13] treated 18 patients with carcinoid tumors with chemoembolization. Eleven of these patients exhibited the carcinoid syndrome. The diarrhea and flushing improved after the first treatment in all patients and had disappeared in eight patients at the end of treatment regimens. 5-HIAA levels improved in eight patients by greater than 50% and were completely normalized in three patients. At follow-up (median 20.5 months) (range 4 to 48 months), a decrease in tumor volume occurred in 6 of 18 patients and there were two complete regressions at 20 and 36 months.

Wangberg and others[14] used simple embolization therapy in 48 patients with midgut carcinoids with disseminated disease. The patients first underwent surgical procedures, and subsequently 27 patients with liver metastases had hepatic embolization. Thirteen patients had a greater than 50% reduction in liver metastasis size. Of specific interest, in three patients with bilobar disease who underwent unilobar embolization, their 5-HIAA level normalized and the bilateral lobar tumor regressed. Wangberg and others interpreted these results to indicate that there was a systemic effect from the ischemia produced by the embolization. The unexplained regression in some tumors after all forms of therapy and the slow progression of these tumors in general cause some to speculate that a few of these tumors regress without treatment, perhaps because of the ischemia produced by the tumor because of blockage of the venous vascular structure. There were no deaths related to treatment in either of these series.

Hepatic embolization remains one consideration for those with advanced tumors. To prevent carcinoid crises, patients are usually given octreotide in a dose of 200 µg subcutaneously beginning 24 hours prior to the scheduled embolization procedure and administered at least every 8 to 12 hours following the procedure. In most reported cases, the patients with carcinoid syndrome are treated for 10 days postoperatively with octreotide. The complications from this procedure are related to abdominal pain, fever, and an increase in the symptoms of the carcinoid syndrome in some of the patients. The symptoms of the carcinoid syndrome are controllable with octreotide administration.

Recently Moertel and others[15] have reviewed the Mayo Clinic experience with hepatic artery embolization and follow-up chemotherapy. In their series, there were four deaths associated with the hepatic artery occlusion procedure.

SURGERY

Reviews of the surgical treatment of advanced carcinoid tumors indicate that the evaluation of all various treatments of carcinoid tumors are difficult because of the heterogeneity of these tumors. Surgery for advanced carcinoid tumors has been successful in resolving symptoms associated with the size of the tumor and in giving relief of diarrhea and flushing of the carcinoid syndrome.

Soreide et al[16] have reviewed their experience with 75 patients with advanced disease. Thirty-three percent of these patients had abdominal debulking procedures. Debulking was defined as attempts at removing extraintestinal tumor growth. The survival rates reported by Soreide and colleagues in patients with midgut tumors who underwent debulking were significantly better than those with similar disease who did not undergo debulking procedures.

There was no significant difference in the survival of those with midgut tumors and tumors originating elsewhere. Patients who had carcinoid syndrome had more advanced disease, i.e., liver metastasis, lymph node involvement, and weight loss. The presence of carcinoid syndrome did not affect survival. Of the 48 patients with liver metastasis from midgut tumors, 23 (48%) had surgical debulking treatment directed at the liver. The median survival rate for those with intervention procedures was 216 months versus 48 months for those not receiving this treatment. The survival rate of patients with liver metastasis who underwent intervention directed at the liver, i.e., resection, hepatic artery ligation, or embolization, was significantly better ($p<0.001$) than those who received no treatment.

In this series, only 15% of the patients had midgut tumors without lymph node metastases and 80% of the patients had distant metastases. This series, as the authors point out, is representative of patients who present with symptoms from far more advanced disease than those carcinoid tumors that are discovered incidentally at the time of surgery.

Symptoms compatible with intestinal obstruction are present in 30% to 50% of the patients in different series. The likelihood of intestinal obstruction, infarction, and perforation are decreased in all large series in which surgical intervention is reported. The presence of abdominal pain, however, is not necessarily due to obstructive disease and is well documented in patients who did not have obstruction. The pain is often permanently relieved by debulking procedures even though no obstruction was found at the time of the procedures.

The surgical treatment of patients with carcinoid syndrome is clearly effective in reducing the flushing, diarrhea, lacrimation, and bronchoconstriction that are part of the syndrome. One might speculate that the reduction of these symptoms suggests that the humors or hormone secreted by these tumors is markedly reduced and that therefore the retroperitoneal or subendocardial fibrosis is likely to be arrested or at least its progression decelerated.

CHEMOTHERAPY

Chemotherapy in patients with carcinoid syndrome has not been shown to increase life span in patients with carcinoid syndrome or with large carcinoid tumors. Some tumors occasionally do respond to chemotherapy with shrinkage or more often fail to show evidence of progression. Some tumors have a mixed response to chemotherapy where a portion of the tumor shrinks and other portions do not. Streptozocin, 5-fluorouracil, cyclophosphamide, doxorubicin, etoposide, and dacarbazine have all been used individually and in combination. Reduction in tumor size and lack of progression of the tumor have occurred in 11% to 40% of these patients. The usual side effects of these drugs are nausea, vomiting, lowering of the white blood cell count and platelets, as well as renal damage from streptozocin and cardiac toxicity from doxorubicin.

When combined with hepatic artery occlusion, however, higher rates of tumor shrinkage and symptomatic improvement have been reported. Moertel et al[15] reported that with single hepatic artery ligation and embolization combined with chemotherapy there was a 12% incidence of complete hormonal regression. This was compared with a 50% incidence of complete hormonal regression in pancreatic islet cell tumors.

Since the national history of the disease often includes long asymptomatic periods and long intervals without evidence of tumor growth, the lack of progression following any therapy is difficult to evaluate.

Interferon alfa has been used in multiple trials. In general, 15% of these patients have had an objective reduction in size, and again 43% of the patients seem to have stabilized. As with other treatment modalities, therapy with interferon has not been shown to prolong life.

CARCINOID CRISIS

Carcinoid crisis is mentioned frequently in reviews of the treatment of these interesting tumors. However, the incidence of crisis appears to be rare. Bissonnette et al[17] reported a fatality following fine needle aspiration of hepatic metastases. They reviewed their experience and other experiences with hepatic biopsy of carcinoid tumors. The most frequent complication was intrahepatic hematomas. This complication was found only in patients in which a 14-gauge cutting needle was used. It was also noted that a mild flushing and an elevated blood pressure occurred transiently with transbronchial forceps biopsy of a carcinoid tumor.

Soreide et al,[16] in reporting surgery in 75 patients with advanced carcinoid tumors, did not have any patients who exhibited carcinoid crisis. However, only 18 of these patients reported symptoms of carcinoid flush, diarrhea, etc., prior to the procedure. Others have reported a worsening of symptoms during the preparation and induction of anesthesia and during the surgical manipulation of the tumor.

Kvols and others[18] first reported the successful treatment of carcinoid crisis. The patient was known to have carcinoid syndrome and was being prepared for surgery to relieve small bowel obstruction. She had been flushing 8 to 9 times per day and had 24-hour urine 5-HIAA levels of 417 mg/24 h. When anesthesia was induced, the blood pressure became unobtainable, and the patient was deeply flushed. She failed to respond to intravenous calcium, phenylephrine (Neo-Synephrine), and epinephrine. A dose of 50 µg of somatostatin analog was given intravenously followed by a second dose of 50 mg 15 seconds later. Within 30 to 40 seconds, the pulses returned and the blood pressure rose to 130/80 mm Hg. The planned surgical procedure was then carried out without recurrence.

Since carcinoid crisis has been reported to occur spontaneously during induction of anesthesia and from minor invasive procedures associated with chemotherapy, it is recommended that octreotide be available during any invasive procedure in patients with carcinoid syndrome. In those patients in whom the symptoms are frequent and severe, it may be given prophylactically prior to the procedure of surgery. An appropriate approach would be to give 100 µg subcutaneously 1 hour prior to the procedure. Others have recommended slightly higher dosages beginning 24 hours prior to surgery.

In the event of an abrupt crisis, 200 to 500 µg may be given intravenously and repeated if there is no response or if the response is inadequate. Since there is not a large number of patients who have been treated by any one physician or any one group of physicians, one must rely on the published reports cited by this review to gauge the treatment of carcinoid crisis.

CARCINOID HEART DISEASE

It is not unusual for patients with carcinoid tumors to present as a direct result of carcinoid heart disease. There are now a number of patients who have undergone either valve replacement or percutaneous balloon valvuloplasty successfully.[19] The proper selection of patients may result in 1 or more years of productive lifestyle. As we learn to control the symptoms and progression of the carcinoid tumors, the need for definitive therapy of the carcinoid complications becomes more important. The decision on whether to perform cardiac surgery or balloon valvuloplasty will obviously depend on the ability of the patient and physicians to deal successfully with complications of this complex disorder.

The patients with carcinoid heart disease characteristically have levels of 5-HIAA that are higher than those without heart disease. The levels of 5-HIAA, however, are not a factor in the selection of patients who should be referred for echocardiography. The history, physical findings, and other complications will influence the need for ultrasound evaluation of patients with cardiac valvular disease.

Recently there have been patients reported who have high-output cardiac failure due to the tumor's secretion of substance P. These patients did not have accompanying valvular heart disease. Since there are several substance P antagonists, there may be specific therapies for this disorder.[20]

SUMMARY

At the current time, the decisions to treat the carcinoid tumor or the syndrome need to be approached conservatively when the use of pharmacologic agents is considered. The simpler the therapy, the less likely one is to interfere with what may be many years of mild discomfort and perhaps minor alterations in lifestyle. Cytotoxic reductive therapy of carcinoid tumors may prolong patients' lives. A surgical approach or hepatic embolization is a more effective approach than medically managing the patients who have severe symptoms and a large tumor mass.

When patients are no longer amenable to physical debulking treatment, interferon or octreotide may be preferable. The side effects of octreotide tend to be less than those from the interferons. The side effects from both of these modalities are reversible when the treatment is stopped. There is a need for a large control trial of all treatment modalities in carcinoid syndrome. Because of the slow growth of what occasionally appears to be spontaneous tumor shrinkage, a control group receiving only symptomatic treatment should be included in these trials. The rarity of these tumors makes it difficult to implement such trials. It will also be important to measure the quality-of-life issues related to each type of therapy for metastatic carcinoid tumors.

REFERENCES

1. Godwin JD. Carcinoid tumors: an analysis of 2837 cases. *Cancer.* 1975;36:560.
2. Bolande RP. The neurocrestopathies: a unifying concept of disease arising in neural crest maldevelopment. *Hum Pathol.* 1974;5:409–429.
3. Pearce ACE. The APUD concept and hormone production. *Clin Endocrinol Metab.* 1980;9:211–222.
4. Modlin IM, Basson MD. Clinical applications of gastrointestinal hormones. *Endocrinol Metab Clin North Am.* 1993;22:4, 823–844.
5. Moertel, CG. Gastrointestinal carcinoid tumors and the malignant carcinoid syndrome. In: *Gastrointestinal Disease,* 5th ed. Philadelphia, Pa: WB Saunders Co; 1993: 1363–1378.
6. Biorck G, Axen O, Thorson A. Unusual cyanosis in a boy with congenital pulmonary stenosis and tricuspid insufficiency: fatal outcome after angiocardiography. *Am Heart J.* 1952;44:143–148.
7. Feldman JM. Carcinoid tumors and the carcinoid syndrome. *Curr Probl Surg.* 1989;24(12):831–885.
8. Oberg K, Eriksson B. The role of interferons in the management of carcinoid tumors. *Acta Oncol.* 1991;30:519–523.
9. Kvols LK, Moertel CG, O'Connell M, et al. Treatment of the malignant carcinoid syndrome: evaluation of a long acting somatostatin analogue. *N Engl J Med.* 1987; 317:162–168.
10. von der Ode MR, Camilleri M, Kvols LK, Thomforde GM. Motor dysfunction of the small bowel and colon in patients with the carcinoid syndrome and diarrhea. *N Engl J Med.* 1993;329(15):1073–1078.
11. Smith S, Anthony L, Roberts LJ, Oats JA, Pincus T. Resolution of musculoskeletal symptoms in the carcinoid syndrome after treatment with the somatostatin analog octreotide. *Ann Intern Med.* 1990;112:66–68.
12. Ahlman H, Wangberg B, Nilsson O. Growth regulation in carcinoid tumors. *Endocrinol Metab Clin North Am.* 1993;22:889–915.
13. Ruszniewski P, Rougier P, Roche A, et al. Hepatic arterial chemoembolization in patients with liver metastases and endocrine tumors: a prospective phase II study in 24 patients. *Cancer.* 1993;71(8):2624–2630.
14. Wangberg B, Gerterul K, Nilsson O, et al. Embolization therapy in the midgut carcinoid syndrome: just tumor ischemic? *Acta Oncol.* 1993;32(2):251–256.
15. Moertel CG, Johnson CM, McKusick MA, et al. The management of patients with advanced carcinoid tumors and islet cell carcinomas. *Ann Intern Med.* 1994; 120:302–309.
16. Soreide O, Berstad T, Bakka A, et al. Surgical treatment as a principle in patients with advanced abdominal carcinoid tumors. *Surgery.* 1992;111(1):48–54.
17. Bissonnette RT, Gibney RG, Berry BR, Buckley AR. Fatal carcinoid crisis after percutaneous fine-needle biopsy of hepatic metastasis: case report and literature review (review). *Radiology.* 1990;174(suppl 3, pt 1):751–752.
18. Kvols LK, Martin JK, Marsh HM, Moertel CG. Rapid reversal of carcinoid crisis with a somatostatin analogue. *N Engl J Med.* 1985;313:1229–1230.
19. Yun D, Heywood JT. Metastatic carcinoid disease presenting solely as high-output heart failure. *Ann Intern Med.* 1994;120:45–46.
20. Morimoto H, Murai M, Maeda Y, Hagiwara D, Miyake H, Metusuo M. FR11360: a novel tripeptide substance P antagonist with NK1 receptor selectivity. *Br J Pharmacol.* 1992;106:123–126.

44
Gastric Ulcers

GARY R. ZUCKERMAN and GIUSEPPE ALIPERTI

The anatomic location of a gastric ulcer is bounded by the gastric cardia on the proximal side and the pylorus on the distal aspect. Gastric ulcers represent mucosal defects that extend into the muscularis mucosae, as opposed to erosions that only involve the mucosa and heal without a fibrous scar or deformity. Although acute stress ulcers or erosions are also located primarily in the stomach, they have a different pathophysiology than peptic ulcers, and the best approach to their management is directed at prevention; therefore this chapter addresses only the therapy of established gastric peptic ulcer. It is important at this point to emphasize that although duodenal ulcers are characteristically benign, gastric ulcers on occasion may represent an ulcerated malignancy. Also, gastric ulcers typically take longer to heal than duodenal ulcers. Thus, because of these two characteristics, the follow-up for a gastric ulcer will differ from duodenal ulcer. Gastric ulcers have been categorized by some authors according to their location in the stomach, but the significance of these associations has decreased with time. The prediction of malignancy based on ulcer location has also not been helpful. Ulcers in the pyloric channel and prepyloric antrum were thought to have common pathophysiology to duodenal ulcers, but more recent evidence does not show a similarity in acid secretory profiles.[1] Ulcers that occur within a large hiatal hernia may represent a diagnostic and therapeutic subset.

ETIOLOGY AND ASSOCIATED PATHOLOGY

An understanding of the different causes and associated pathology of gastric ulcer is important in developing an overall management plan for therapy. As with duodenal ulcer there appear to be three primary associations or causes for gastric ulcer: nonsteroidal antiinflammatory drugs (NSAIDs), *Helicobacter pylori* and acid hypersecretory states as in Zollinger-Ellison syndrome (ZES). ZES is classically associated with duodenal ulcers; isolated gastric ulcers are uncommon, if not rare, in this condition. Duodenal reflux of bile salts into the stomach and antral hypomotility with resultant gastric stasis of acid have both been implicated in contributing to gastric mucosal injury. Other uncommon associations with gastric ulcer include infections such as cytomegalovirus (CMV), syphilis, and radiation-induced ulcers.

H. pylori is a microaerophilic bacterium that has been found to be responsible for antral chronic active gastritis and its attendant polymorphonuclear infiltration. This form of gastritis is found in the majority of patients with peptic ulcer disease. Koch's postulates have been fulfilled for the casual relationship between *H. pylori* and gastritis; however, the etiologic association of *H. pylori* with peptic ulcer disease is not as conclusive, although the circumstantial evidence is impressive.[2] Although the majority of *H. pylori*–infected subjects do not develop peptic ulcer disease, 70% to 80% of patients with gastric ulcers (not associated with NSAID use) are infected with *H. pylori*. The most impressive evidence for a causal relationship is found in the marked decrease in recurrence rates of peptic ulcer when the organism is eradicated. This decrease in ulcer recurrence rate is greater for duodenal ulcer than gastric ulcer. Both recurrence rates are less than 10% in 1 year.

Aspirin and NSAIDs are a common source of gastric mucosal damage as only about one third of chronic users have normal findings on endoscopic examination and ulcers are found in 5% to 30% of subjects.[3,4] Although NSAID-associated ulcers are found in both the stomach and duodenum, gastric ulcers appear to be the more common presentation. Regular daily use of aspirin has been shown to increase the risk of hospitalization for gastric ulcer.[5] Aspirin and other NSAIDs have also been implicated in increasing the risk for ulcer complications (bleeding and perforation) and ulcer-related mortality. This risk has ranged from a 1- to 10-fold increase for NSAID users.[4]

The pathophysiology of NSAID-induced ulcers can, in part, be accounted for by local or topical action in which weak acids such as aspirin are unionized in the acidic environment of the stomach and thus can penetrate the gastric mucosa. There is also evidence for a systemic action as shown by the development of ulcers after parenteral administration of NSAIDs. The proposed explanation for this systemic action is that NSAIDs reduce gastroduodenal mucosal prostaglandin production.

There is no evidence that NSAIDs cause diffuse gastritis, whereas the majority of gastric ulcers found in patients that do not have a history of NSAID ingestion, are associated with both gastritis and *H. pylori* infection. When gastric ulcers are found in patients with a history of NSAID ingestion, only about 50% of cases are associated with gastritis and *H. pylori* infection.[6] These data support both the separate association of *H. pylori* and NSAIDs in the pathogenesis of gastric ulcer and the overlap of *H. pylori* with the ubiquitous use of NSAIDs.

The greatest risk for NSAID complications appears to occur within the first month of ingestion.[5] Other risk factors for ulcer development include advanced age, in particular patients over 65 years of age, and smoking.[7,8] The combination of steroids and NSAIDs appears to be a greater risk for ulcer development than either agent alone, and the risk of gastrointestinal tract hemorrhage from ulcer is 10-fold greater with the combination compared with NSAIDs alone.[9] Alcohol does not appear to be a risk factor. Gastric ulcers also appear to be more prevalent in patients with underlying chronic pulmonary disease, and the frequency of both gastric and duodenal ulcers appear to be increased in patients with cirrhosis.[10]

SYMPTOMS AND NATURAL HISTORY

Although the classic symptom pattern of abdominal pain-food-relief of pain has been described in patients with peptic ulcer disease, it will not discriminate between gastric and duodenal ulcer, and it is absent in many patients. Ulcer patients first presenting with bleeding or perforation without preceding pain are frequently encountered in the hospital situation. These "silent" ulcers tend to occur more commonly in elderly patients and in those patients taking NSAIDs. The gastrointestinal tract bleeding can present as acute hemorrhage or as iron deficiency anemia. In a study of patients with rheumatoid arthritis receiving long-term NSAID therapy who presented with iron deficiency anemia, one fourth were found to have a gastric ulcer.[11] Pyloric channel and prepyloric antral ulcers may present more commonly with nausea and vomiting than other peptic ulcer locations, but again, symptoms alone may be misleading.

The natural history of uncomplicated gastric ulcers can be extrapolated from the placebo arms of ulcer treatment trials. About 30% of gastric ulcers showed spontaneous healing at the end of 4 weeks, but healing rates continued to increase over 12 weeks in the remaining patients.[12] Gastric ulcers can recur in 40% to 80% of patients within 12 months.[13]

EVALUATING GASTRIC ULCERS FOR MALIGNANCY

The overwhelming majority of gastric ulcers are benign, although they rarely may represent an ulcerated malignancy. For this reason, and differently than for duodenal ulcers, gastric ulcers will necessitate radiographic or endoscopic evaluation for malignancy. Cost considerations prevent the use of endoscopy for all patients with ulcer symptoms, thus the initial diagnosis is often made by radiographic means. Endoscopy with tissue sampling will be necessary for all radiographically equivocal (benign versus malignant) ulcers, and an index endoscopy with biopsies may be warranted for many other gastric ulcers detected radiographically.[14,15] A prospective study would be needed to determine which patients with gastric ulcers detected radiographically need endoscopy, but such a study was thought not to be feasible by a subcommittee of the American Society for Gastrointestinal Endoscopy.[16] Such a study, because of the low incidence of malignant ulcers, would require a very large number of ulcer patients to reach statistic significance.[17] Endoscopy for biopsy and cytologic examination can be performed immediately after radiographic diagnosis of a benign gastric ulcer or after a period of adequate therapy, so that a persistent ulcer can be sampled for histologic examination.[14] Endoscopy is more sensitive than x-ray examination in both detecting ulcers and in determining their likelihood of being malignant.[18,19] Endoscopy additionally allows tissue sampling for histologic examination in the same setting. The combination of endoscopic visual impression and endoscopic biopsy and cytologic examination, results in a diagnostic accuracy of 98% to 99% for distinguishing malignant from benign ulcer.[20,21] For satisfactory sampling, 6 to 10 specimens should be obtained from the ulcer base and margins.[18,20,21] Exudative and necrotic material should be avoided for more reliable areas of tissue sampling.

A relatively small risk of missing malignancy persists despite good initial biopsies. This risk, less than 2%,[22-24] has perpetuated a tradition of endoscopic and histologic follow-up of gastric ulcers until complete healing. Lack of prospective studies in support of or against this practice has generated considerable controversy in the current era of cost containment. In a Danish study reporting endoscopic follow-up in 760 patients with gastric ulcers, a total of 1269 follow-up endoscopies yielded 10 malignancies, only five of which were curable.[25] Each curable malignancy was found at the expense of approximately 250 endoscopies.[25] Another study from Italy reported on the routine follow-up of 144 patients at 3, 6, and 12 months, and confirmed that delays in the diagnosis of malignancy are not unusual.[26] Of 10 patients with malignancies, six were found at 3 months, three at more than 6 months, and one at 41 months. Dysplasia at the edge of the ulcer was documented in 6 of the 10 patients, and was considered an indication for closer follow-up.[26] A study on endoscopic follow-up of gastric ulcers in 597 patients from Germany noted that the 5-year survival rate for the eight patients with a malignancy was not different in patients who kept their appointments for endoscopic follow-up, compared with patients who did not.[22] A recent Japanese study followed 2529 patients with medially treated gastric ulcers for a period of 9 to 23 years to ascertain whether benign gastric ulcers could antedate gastric malignancy.[27] Patients who developed cancer within 1 year were excluded. Only nine patients developed gastric cancer in the same site as the initial ulcer, and in seven of these review of the initial specimens could not exclude malignancy.[27]

The major question is whether all gastric ulcers need endoscopic follow-up. The lack of prospective studies leaves many important issues unresolved, making the establishment of firm guidelines very difficult. It will be easier to identify those patients that will require endoscopy: (1) patients with a malignant or indeterminant (equivocal)-appearing gastric ulcer on upper gastrointestinal tract series and (2) follow-up of an indeterminant (equivocal) gastric ulcer ascertained by endoscopic appearance or by endoscopic biopsy or cytologic examination. Endoscopic follow-up should also be obtained if the quality of the initial examination is questionable or if doubt exists about the adequacy of histologic interpretation. If the ulcer has not healed, biopsies and brushings for cytologic examination should be repeated. Since gastric ulcers usually require longer healing times than duodenal ulcers (related to the larger size of gastric ulcers) endoscopy follow-up is usually performed 8 to 12 weeks after the index endoscopy. A recent study would imply that follow-up endoscopy may not be necessary for the great majority of ulcers and that repeat endoscopy could be reserved for persistent symptoms or when the endoscopic appearance or biopsies were suggestive of cancer.[28] It has recently been recommended that if a gastric ulcer lacking the endoscopic criteria for malignancy has an adequate histology specimen interpreted as negative, follow-up endoscopy is not cost effective, given the very low incidence of malignancies disclosed on subsequent studies.[29] The follow-up of patients with gastric ulcers is changing, but the approach should still be individualized, taking into account the various clinical and histologic parameters.

THERAPEUTIC APPROACH

The treatment plan for gastric ulcer will be based on the previously reviewed causes, which in most cases will involve therapy aimed at NSAID- or *H. pylori*–induced ulcers. Patients with NSAID-induced ulcers should not only be admonished to avoid the known offending agent, but they should also be informed of the various over-the-counter aspirin and nonaspirin NSAIDs that need to be avoided. They should also be told that prescription drugs for pain and arthritis frequently contain NSAIDs and that they will need to mention their ulcer history during any future physician encounters. It may be helpful to detail these admonitions in writing to further emphasize their importance. Obviously, in some patients an NSAID may need to be continued for various therapeutic reasons, and in these cases, an antisecretory agent or prostaglandin analog administered concomitantly may reduce ulcer risk. Since there is some evidence that NSAID ulcers may be dose dependent, it may be helpful to decrease the dose to the lowest level necessary to still obtain a clinical benefit.[30] Aspirin appears to be more damaging to the gastric mucosa than nonaspirin NSAIDs, whereas the use of enteric-coated agents does not seem to confer any added protection. There is also evidence that nonacetylated salicylates may be less ulcerogenic than other NSAIDs, but in our experience rheumatologists are very reluctant to switch to these agents because of their apparent decreased anti-inflammatory activity. Although there may be differences in the relative risk of gastric mucosal injury produced by various NSAIDs, it has not been shown that switching from one NSAID to another will improve the clinical course. It should be emphasized that ulcer healing is delayed with continued NSAID use, even in the face of concomitant H_2-receptor antagonist (H_2-RA) administration.[31] Thus, whenever possible, discontinuation of NSAIDs will be the optimal approach for healing NSAID-induced ulcers.

Most, if not all gastric ulcers require some form of gastric antisecretory therapy. For patients that have a gastric ulcer and *H. pylori* infection, an antisecretory drug and therapy for *H. pylori* will be needed. If aspirin or nonaspirin NSAIDs are felt to be the only cause for gastric ulcer, then H_2-RA should be sufficient therapy. H_2-RA has been shown, in placebo controlled studies, to result in faster healing of a gastric ulcer. The standard doses of H_2-RA used for treating duodenal ulcer have been applied to gastric ulcer. Healing takes longer (8 to 12 weeks), and is likely related to the larger size of most gastric ulcers compared with duodenal ulcers. At present, only cimetidine, ranitidine, and famotidine have Food and Drug Administration (FDA) approval for treatment of gastric ulcers. Sucralfate has also been shown to be superior to placebo for gastric ulcer healing. Parietal cell proton pump inhibition with omeprazole at doses of 20 to 40 mg daily will also induce more rapid healing of gastric ulcer than placebo or even H_2-RA. We reserve the use of omeprazole for special situations such as the need for more rapid healing in patients with a complicated gastric ulcer, rather than frontline therapy.[32] The effectiveness of antacids for gastric ulcer healing has not been extensively evaluated. Because symptom relief will frequently precede ulcer healing, patients should understand the need to continue therapy for the full 8 to 12 weeks. Gastric ulcers should not be considered refractory to healing until a 12-week course of treatment has been completed. Although stopping the patients' NSAID ingestion may be all that is necessary to accomplish ulcer healing, it would seem reasonable to coadminister an antisecretory agent.

The National Institutes of Health (NIH) consensus conference on *H. pylori* and peptic ulcer disease has now given us the guideline to treat all *H. pylori*–infected patients with an ulcer with therapy that will eradicate the infection.[2] Even patients without a complicated gastric ulcer should benefit from *H. pylori* eradication. Eradication is defined as the absence of *H. pylori* 4 weeks after discontinuation of therapy. Because of the potential for resistant organisms, combination therapy or "triple therapy" is used. The most common oral regimens used in the United States combine two antibiotics with bismuth. The regimen of metronidazole (Flagyl 250 mg three times daily), combined with tetracycline (500 mg four times daily) and bismuth (two Pepto-Bismol tablets four times a day) for a 14-day course has achieved 90% eradication of *H. pylori*.[33] Patient compliance would appear to be an important factor in reaching this high eradication rate. Other antibiotic regimens have used amoxicillin (500 mg four times a day) in combination with metronidazole and bismuth. Omeprazole in combination with amoxicillin has also been an effective therapy against *H. pylori*.[34] Antisecretory therapy with an H_2-RA is frequently started simultaneously with "triple therapy," but with evolving information from ongoing research studies it may be that only eradication of the organism will be necessary, without the need for simultaneous antisecretory therapy. On the other hand, our experience suggests that when patients have symptoms of partial gastric outlet obstruction, triple therapy for *H. pylori* usually must be deferred until symptoms have improved with antisecretory drugs.

The outcomes of therapy can be determined two ways, ulcer healing and eradication of *H. pylori*. It follows that ulcer healing should occur with eradication of the organism, but the reverse is not necessarily true. If complete healing does not occur with elimination of *H. pylori* from the stomach, superimposed NSAID ingestion may be a factor. Once *H. pylori* has been eradicated, recurrence of the infection appears to be very uncommon, less than 1% per year.[35] *H. pylori*–associated ulcers can of course heal without

TABLE 44–1. KEY ELEMENTS IN GASTRIC ULCER THERAPY

- Determine etiology
  Malignant versus benign
  Helicobacter pylori
  NSAIDs
  Combination *H. pylori* and NSAID
- Stop NSAID use
- Inform patient of other NSAIDs
- Treat with H$_2$-receptor antagonists (H$_2$-RA)
- Treat *H. pylori* with antibiotic regimen

NSAID = nonsteroidal antiinflammatory drug.

eliminating the organism, but ulcer recurrences are more frequent. If the patient will require a follow-up endoscopy, which is frequently done for gastric ulcers, gastric mucosal biopsies can detect the organism either by histologic demonstration or with detection of urease activity in the tissue specimen. A 20% reduction of *H. pylori* immunoglobulin G antibody serum concentration at 6 months after treatment has also been associated with successful elimination of the organism.[36] In summary, the key element in gastric ulcer management involves the determination of cause, which should in turn direct therapy (Table 44–1).

REFERENCES

1. Collen M, Sheridan M. Gastric ulcers differ from duodenal ulcers: evaluation of basal acid output. *Dig Dis Sci.* 1993;38:2281–2286.
2. NIH Consensus Development Conference. *Helicobacter pylori* in peptic ulcer disease. Feb 7–9, 1994.
3. Silveso G, Ivey K, Butt J, et al. Incidence of gastric lesions in patients with rheumatic disease on chronic aspirin therapy. *Ann Intern Med.* 1979;91:517.
4. Kurata J. Assessment of nonsteroidal anti-inflammatory drugs as a risk factor in ulcer disease. *Ann Intern Med.* 1991;114:311.
5. Kurata J, Abbey D. The effect of chronic aspirin use on duodenal and gastric ulcer hospitalizations. *J Clin Gastroenterol.* 1990;12:260.
6. Laine L, Marin-Sorensen M, Weinstein W. *Helicobacter pylori* prevalence and mucosal injury in gastric ulcers: relationship to chronic NSAID ingestion. *Gastroenterology.* 1991;100:A103. Abstract.
7. Fries J, Williams C, Bloch D, Michel B. Nonsteroidal anti-inflammatory drug-associated gastropathy: incidence and risk factor model. *Am J Med.* 1991;91:213.
8. McCarthy D. Smoking and ulcers: time to quit (editorial). *N Engl J Med.* 1984;311:726.
9. Piper J, Ray W, Daugherty J, Griffin M. Corticosteroid use and peptic ulcer disease: role of nonsteroidal anti-inflammatory drugs. *Ann Int Med.* 1991;114:735.
10. Sonnenberg A. Factors which influence the incidence and course of peptic ulcer. *Scand J Gastroenterol.* 1988;155:119.
11. Upedhyay R, Torley H, McKinlay A, Sturrock R, Russell R. Iron deficiency anemia in patients with rheumatic disease receiving non-steroidal anti-inflammatory drugs: the role of upper gastrointestinal lesions. *Ann Rheum Dis.* 1990;49:359.
12. Howden C, Hunt R. The relationship between suppression of acidity and gastric ulcer healing rates. *Aliment Pharmacol Ther.* 1990;4:25.
13. Berlin R, Root J, Cook T. Nocturnal therapy with famotidine for one year is effective in preventing relapse of gastric ulcer. *Aliment Pharmacol Ther.* 1991;2:161.
14. Richardson CT. Gastric ulcer. In: Sleisenger MH, Fordtran JS, eds. *Gastrointestinal Disease.* 4th ed. Philadelphia, Pa: WB Saunders Co; 1989.
15. Appropriate use of gastrointestinal endoscopy. A consensus statement from the American Society for Gastrointestinal Endoscopy. Prepared by the Committee on Endoscopic Utilization. Reviewed and approved by the Standards of Training and Practice Committee and by the Governing Board, June 1986.
16. Tedesco FJ, Best WR, Littman A, et al. Role of gastroscopy in gastric ulcer patients. *Gastroenterology.* 1977;73:170–177.
17. Weinstein WM, et al. Gastroscopy for gastric ulcer. *Gastroenterology.* 1977;73:1160.
18. Dekker W, Tytgat GN. Diagnostic accuracy of fiber-endoscopy in the detection of upper intestinal malignancy: a follow-up analysis. *Gastroenterology.* 1977;73:710.
19. Kiil J, Anderson D. X-ray examination and/or endoscopy in the diagnosis of gastroduodenal ulcer and crater. *Scan J Gastroenterol.* 1980;15:39.
20. Rowland R, Durbridge T, Hecker R, et al. How many endoscopic biopsy specimens? *Med J Aust.* 1976;2:172.
21. Graham DY. Prospective evaluation of biopsy number in the diagnosis of esophageal and gastric carcinoma. *Gastroenterology.* 1982;82:228.
22. Eckardt VF, Giebler W, Kanzler G, et al. Does endoscopic follow-up improve outcome of patients with benign gastric ulcers and gastric cancer? *Cancer.* 1992;69:301–305.
23. Teagardh B, Haglund U. Endoscopic diagnosis of gastric ulcer. *Acta Chir Scand.* 1985;151:37–41.
24. Llanos O, Guzman S, Duarte I. Accuracy of first endoscopic procedure in the differential diagnosis of gastric lesions. *Ann Surg.* 1982;195:224–226.
25. Bytzer P. Endoscopic follow-up study of gastric ulcer to detect malignancy: is it worthwhile? *Scand J Gastroenterol.* 1991;26:1193–1199.
26. Farinati F, Cardin F, DiMario F, et al. Early and advanced gastric cancer during follow-up of apparently benign gastric ulcer: significance of the presence of epithelial dysplasia. *J Surg Oncol.* 1987;36:263–267.
27. Lee S, Mitsuo I, Tsuneyoshi Y, et al. Long term follow-up of 2,529 patients reveals gastric ulcers rarely become malignant. *Dig Dis Sci.* 1990;35:763–768.
28. Pruitt RE, Truss CD. Endoscopy, gastric ulcer, and gastric cancer: Follow-up endoscopy for all gastric ulcers? *Dig Dis Sci.* 1993;38:284–288.
29. Kochman ML, Elta GH. Gastric ulcers: when is enough, enough? *Gastroenterology.* 1993;105:1582–1584.
30. Griffin M, Piper J, Daugherty J, Snowden M, Ray W. Nonsteroidal anti-inflammatory drug use and increased risk for peptic ulcer disease in elderly persons. *Ann Intern Med.* 1991;114:257.

31. Lancaster-Smith M, Jaderberg M, Jackson D. Ranitidine in the treatment of non-steroidal anti-inflammatory drug associated gastric and duodenal ulcers. *Gut.* 1991; 32:252–255.
32. Maton PN. Omeprazole. *N Engl J Med.* 1991;324:965–975.
33. Graham DY, Lew GM, Malaty HM, et al. Factors influencing the eradication of *Helicobacter pylori* with triple therapy. *Gastroenterology.* 1992;102:493–496.
34. Labenz J, Gyenes E, Ruhl GH, Borsch G. Two weeks treatment with amoxicillin/omeprazole for eradication of *Helicobacter pylori. Gastroenterology.* 1992;30:776–778.
35. Graham DY, Lew GM, Klein PD, et al. Effect of treatment of *Helicobacter pylori* infection on long-term recurrence of gastric and duodenal ulcer. *Ann Intern Med.* 1992;116:705–708.
36. Cutler A, Shubert A, Shubert T. Role of *Helicobacter pylori* serology in evaluating treatment success. *Dig Dis Sci.* 1993;38:2262–2266.

45

Gastritis

FELIX W. LEUNG

Gastritis is a group of disorders that involves varying degrees of alterations of the normal gross or histologic appearance of the gastric mucosa. It is not a single disease. Patients with gastritis can be asymptomatic or have a constellation of symptoms including abdominal discomfort, anorexia, heartburn, indigestion, bloating, nausea, and vomiting. Signs of weight loss, abdominal tenderness, hematemesis, coffee ground emesis, frank or occult blood in the stool, and anemia or even diarrhea can accompany these symptoms. Because many of these symptoms are nonspecific, it is essential to obtain a thorough history initially, and to request tests to rule out problems associated with the gallbladder, pancreas, liver, or kidney.

Gastritis is usually composed of localized or diffuse lesions of variable sizes confined to the mucosa (erosions), edema, and subepithelial hemorrhage with or without inflammation in the adjacent mucosa. The lesions arise as a result of an imbalance between aggressive and defensive factors. Examples of aggressive factors include alcohol, aspirin, nonsteroidal antiinflammatory drugs (NSAIDs), local trauma, irradiation, bile reflux, uremia, ischemia, caustics, and drugs. Examples of defensive factors include mucus bicarbonate secretion, gastric mucosal barrier, endogenous prostaglandins, and mucosal blood flow.

The most common forms of acute gastritis are induced by drugs, e.g., aspirin, NSAIDs, or alcohol. Withdrawal of the causative agent is the mainstay of treatment of drug-induced gastritis. Spontaneous resolution is common, and long-term sequelae are unusual. Acute infectious gastritis in healthy individuals is often due to viral organisms and is self-limiting. Treatment is limited to supportive care. *Helicobacter pylori* infection of the gastric mucosa has been recognized as a unique condition that can give rise to both an acute and a chronic form of inflammation of the mucosa. The association of the chronic form of gastritis with ulcer disease makes it particularly interesting. Recent reports have suggested that eradication of the *H. pylori* leads to a significant reduction in the recurrence rate of duodenal ulcer disease in these patients. The most well-known form of chronic gastritis is the atrophic type associated with pernicious anemia. Of note in the therapy is the need to replace vitamin B_{12} to prevent neurologic and hematologic complications.

Supported in part by Veterans Administration Medical Research Funds and by the California Tobacco Related Disease Research Program Grant 1RT 80.

In the assessment of patients with gastritis, the upper gastrointestinal tract radiologic examination may be entirely normal. Together with a history of recent ethanol, aspirin, or NSAID ingestion and self-limited upper gastrointestinal tract bleeding, the normal radiologic examination will be most consistent with a diagnosis of alcoholic or drug-induced gastritis. The radiographs may reveal varying degrees of thickening of the gastric folds or multiple small but persistent filling defects, suggestive of acute infectious gastritis. At endoscopy, varying degrees of redness, breaks in the mucosa with or without overlying exudates, friability, and evidence of recent bleeding such as fresh blood or blood clots may be recognized. An associated gastric or duodenal ulcer may be present in gastritis because of *H. pylori* infection. Alternatively, thinning of the gastric mucosa with prominence of the underlying blood vessels may be present in atrophic gastritis. Gastric biopsy is indicated when specific types of gastritis are suspected. Other forms of gastritis are less common. Characteristic features in the history and gastric biopsy results usually point to a specific diagnosis.

If the patient has significant vomiting, food should be withheld, nasogastric suction instituted, and parenteral fluid and electrolyte supplements administered. If there is evidence of gastrointestinal tract bleeding and endoscopic examination is contemplated, antisecretory treatment may be started. The treatment does not alter the outcome of the bleeding but is started on the assumption that there is either an ulcer or gastritis present. Antacids and sucralfate ingestion make endoscopic examination harder to carry out because parts of the mucosa are obscured by the adherent antacid or sucralfate. Once gastritis is diagnosed by endoscopic examination and if there is no active ulcer disease present, the less expensive treatment with antacid should be substituted as needed for symptom relief.

ALCOHOLIC GASTRITIS OR GASTROPATHY

Patients with alcoholic gastritis usually present during a binge drinking episode. Abdominal pain, nausea, vomiting, hematemesis, and melena are major presenting symptoms. In assessing these patients, a history of recent aspirin or NSAID ingestion must be ruled out. A history of bringing up normal gastric content followed by hematemesis should indicate Mallory-Weiss lesion in the differential diagnosis. If there are stigmata of portal hypertension, variceal bleeding should be kept in mind. Bleeding from peptic ulcer disease can be ruled out by upper gastrointestinal tract series or endoscopic evaluation. In managing these patients, prompt assessment of hemodynamic status and resuscitative measures with intravenous fluids and blood products are indicated. Assessment of gastric contents either by inspection of the vomitus or passage of a nasogastric tube to lavage the gastric contests establishes whether continued bleeding is present. If the patient has evidence of continued bleeding, endoscopic examination with possible therapeutic interventions, e.g., epinephrine injection, bipolar electrocoagulation, or heat probe treatment, may be indicated as soon as the patient's condition can be stabilized with intravenous fluids and blood products. The gastritis itself is not amenable to endoscopic interventions because of the diffuse nature of the mucosal involvement. The associated variceal bleeding, solitary bleeding source such as in an ulcer, can be treated endoscopically with reductions of transfusion requirement and need for urgent operative intervention. Additionally, the alcohol-induced gastric lesions have been more precisely defined as alcoholic gastropathy recently based on the histologic finding that there are minimal inflammatory changes but very prominent subepithelial hemorrhages in the gastric mucosa of patients with recent alcohol ingestion. Symptoms resolve rapidly, and in the absence of coagulopathy the bleeding associated with the alcohol-induced gastric lesions ceases quickly after withdrawal of the alcohol. Unless endoscopic examination reveals ulcer disease, H_2 blockers and other antiulcer drugs need not be administered. Although some authors recommend the use of H_2 blockers for pain in these patients, antacids may be a less expensive mode of therapy after endoscopic examination has ruled out treatable bleeding lesions. Replacement of clotting factors is the treatment of choice in the presence of coagulopathy and continued bleeding. Gastric biopsy may provide an opportunity to rule out *H. pylori* infection. If the patient's symptoms completely resolve after withdrawal of the alcohol, it is debatable whether the patient will need therapy for the *H. pylori* infection even if confirmed. Unless the long-term effects of treating a large number of asymptomatic subjects with *H. pylori* infection is known, treatment of *H. pylori* infection in a patient symptomatic from alcoholic gastritis is difficult to justify at this time.

ASPIRIN- OR NSAID-INDUCED GASTRITIS

Acute exposure to aspirin or NSAIDs produces spotty red lesions in the gastric mucosa. These can be associated with occult blood in the stool but usually not profound hemorrhage. On the other hand, older patients not infrequently present with bleeding ulcers and recent ingestion of aspirin or NSAIDs as a prominent part of the history. Unless the patients develop symptoms while on the drug, it is impractical to initiate diagnostic studies on all patients taking aspirin or NSAIDs. For patients who have complications such as bleeding associated with these drugs, endoscopic examination usually reveals the source of bleeding. Ulcers with active bleeding or stigmata of recent hemorrhage can be treated endoscopically. Withdrawal of the offending agent is the most logical and effective way in preventing further progression of the mucosal lesions. Ulcers discovered at the time of endoscopy can be treated with antiulcer therapy: antacids, H_2 blockers, sucralfate, or omeprazole. Efficacy is comparable. History of drug reaction and cost are the determining factors in the choice of medication. Patients with arthritis frequently require long-term treatment with aspirin or NSAIDs for pain control. Misoprostol 100 to 200 g four times a day prevents NSAID-induced mucosal lesions. Although the effect of misoprostol on ulcers associated with NSAID use is less well studied, misoprostol is often administered with the goal of preventing aspirin- or NSAID-induced complications. Misoprostol has the major undesirable side effects of inducing diarrhea and abortions. In patients with occult blood in the stool and anemia, a diagnosis of gastric lesions induced by aspirin or NSAIDs should be accompanied by withdrawal of the offending agent. If the anemia and the occult blood in the stool do not resolve, a workup to rule out colonic lesions is appropriate. Whether an incidental finding of *H. pylori* infection in a patient symptomatic from aspirin- or NSAID-induced gastritis requires treatment is debatable. Again, in the absence of long-term follow-up data, empiric treatment is probably not justified.

H. PYLORI–ASSOCIATED GASTRITIS

Most patients with *H. pylori* infection are asymptomatic and have normal-appearing gastric mucosa. Symptomatic patients may have swollen gastric folds. *H. pylori* infection is the major cause of nonerosive chronic active gastritis. Histologic examination of gastric biopsy specimens is the most useful method of diagnosis because both the presence of gastritis and *H. pylori* can be determined. The antral mucosa within 1 to 2 cm of the pylorus is the best location for sampling biopsy specimens. Serology is useful in epidemiologic studies. After eradication both immunoglobulin G and immunoglobulin A levels fall. The rapid urease and urea carbon breath test are based on the ability of *H. pylori* to split urea into ammonia and carbon dioxide by its urease. In the urease test (probably less expensive than histologic examination), a gastric biopsy specimen is placed in contact with urea and a pH indicator. The ammonia raises the pH leading to a change in the color of the indicator. In the breath test, urea labeled with carbon 13 or carbon 14 is fed to the patient. The carbon dioxide in the expired air is analyzed for the labeled carbon. The evidence that *H. pylori* causes gastritis includes the development of gastritis after ingestion of the organisms, attenuation of the gastritis with eradication of the organisms, and transmission of the infection by contaminated nasogastric tubes or endoscopic equipment. Whether *H. pylori*–associated ulcer disease or gastritis should be treated or not is controversial. In favor of treatment is the evidence that eradication of *H. pylori* reduces ulcer recurrence rate and significantly attenuates the severity of the gastritis. Confirmation of *H. pylori* infection is recommended prior to treatment. A combination of bismuth (Pepto-Bismol, 30 ml or 2 tablets four times daily on an empty stomach; De-Nol, currently not available in the United States) and antibiotics for 2 weeks has been suggested. Amoxicillin, erythromycin, or tetracycline (each 2 g/d) or metronidazole (1 to 1.5 g/d) has been used with reports of eradication of *H. pylori*. On the other hand, *H. pylori* gastritis is frequently asymptomatic, most ulcers heal with antisecretory therapy, recurrence is reduced by maintenance treatment, and the long-term effects of treating a large number of patients with bismuth and antibiotics are not known. At present it would appear to be prudent to limit the treatment of *H. pylori* to symptomatic patients with gastritis for which other causes are absent and *H. pylori* infection is confirmed and to patients with ulcers that are frequently recurring and responding poorly to antisecretory treatment.

STRESS-INDUCED GASTRITIS

In patients with multiorgan failure, diffuse gastritis can develop with gastrointestinal tract bleeding as a major mode of presentation. The approach to management is the same as for other causes of upper gastrointestinal tract bleeding: supportive measures to stabilize the vital signs, followed by endoscopic examination to establish the diagnosis. This condition is rather uncommon. Although there is very little dispute that patients with multiorgan failure require acid antisecretory prophylaxis, the routine use of such treatments in all patients monitored for single problems in the intensive care unit is unnecessary. In patients in whom prophylaxis is indicated, supportive measures to optimize cardiac, respiratory, acid-base, and electrolyte balance is indicated. Intravenous cimetidine, 300 mg every 8 hours or 300 mg priming dose followed by 37.5 mg/h continuous infusion, or ranitidine, 50 mg every 12 hours, has been used with adequate elevation of intragastric pH to above 3.5. Endoscopic examination after ingestion of sucralfate is usually suboptimal because of adherence of the sucralfate to the mucosa. Its use should be avoided if endoscopic examination is contemplated.

CAUSTIC GASTRITIS

Patients with caustic gastritis present after ingestion of caustic substances. In addition to gastric injury the esophagus usually sustains damage. Treatment is supportive, including analgesics, intravenous fluids, and sedatives. If the patient can swallow, a large quantity of orally administered water dilutes the ingested caustic substance. Antacids to neutralize ingested acid and dilute vinegar or lemon juice to neutralize alkali may also be indicated. Gastric lavage or emetics should be avoided to minimize the risk of perforation and aspiration. Endoscopic examination determines the extent of damage. Surgery is necessary if there is evidence of gangrene or perforation. After the acute stage, if pyloric stenosis develops, surgery is also indicated.

ATROPHIC GASTRITIS

Atrophic gastritis is found in patients with achlorhydria, vitamin B_{12} malabsorption, and pernicious anemia. There is severe atrophic fundic gland gastritis. There is reduced secretion of intrinsic factor. Antibodies to intrinsic factor and parietal cells are present. In severe cases endoscopic examination reveals thin gastric folds and prominent vessels. Some patients retain the ability to secrete intrinsic factor and do not develop pernicious anemia despite the presence of atrophic gastritis. Midbody along the greater curvature is the best location for sampling biopsy specimens. There is no specific treatment for the gastritis, but vitamin B_{12} replacement is indicated, e.g., 1000 g intramuscular or deep subcutaneous injection on a monthly basis. Periodic endoscopic examination may be indicated to rule out dysplasia or malignancy.

HYPERTROPHIC GASTRITIS

Hypertrophic gastritis, also known as Ménétrier's disease is a rare condition in which patients present with diarrhea, hypoalbuminemia, significant protein loss from the gastric lumen, and dramatic thickening of the gastric folds. Full thickness gastric biopsy may be necessary to rule out lymphoma or carcinoma. Treatment is supportive. Documented ulcerations can be treated with usual antiulcer therapy.

POSTGASTRECTOMY GASTRITIS

After ulcer surgery some patients present with abdominal discomfort associated with the endoscopic finding of diffuse gastritis and bile in the stomach. The condition is called *bile reflux gastritis, alkaline reflux gastritis,* or *duodenal gastric reflux.* Ingestion of aspirin, NSAIDs, or alcohol must be excluded by taking a careful history. Endoscopic examination and biopsy may assist in excluding *H. pylori* infection. Medical management is of limited success. A Roux-en-Y anastomosis has relieved symptoms in patients with incapacitating symptoms.

ISCHEMIC GASTRITIS

Gastric ischemia can develop acutely as a result of atheromatous embolization to the stomach. Emphysematous gastritis with air in the portal tract has been reported as a preterminal event in gastric ischemia. Chronic gastric ischemia has also been described. These patients present with symptoms not unlike those of abdominal angina. There is chronic postprandial abdominal pain, fear of eating, weight loss, and evidence of vascular disease. Endoscopic examination reveals gastroduodenal mucosal lesions and ulcers. These are resistant to conventional ulcer therapy. Angiography usually reveals obstruction or stenosis of two of the three mesenteric arteries. If the correct diagnosis is made in a timely fashion, repair of the obstructed or stenotic vessels leads to resolution of the gastroduodenitis and ulcerations. Ischemic gastritis can arise as a result of vasculitis. Treatment of the underlying disease is indicated. Surgery may be necessary if findings consistent with an acute abdomen develop.

EOSINOPHILIC GASTRITIS

Patients with eosinophilic gastritis present with eosinophilia and vomiting due to gastric outlet obstruction. There is thickening of the gastric folds, particularly involving the antrum as a result of infiltration of the mucosa and the muscular layer by eosinophils. Differential diagnosis includes milk allergy, connective tissue disorder, and parasitic infestation. Operative intervention may be necessary when corticosteroid treatment fails. Specific diagnosis associated with eosinophilic gastritis includes Churg-Strauss syndrome.

GRANULOMATOUS GASTRITIS

Granulomas in the gastric mucosa occur in sarcoidosis, Crohn's disease, or infections such as tuberculosis, histoplasmosis, syphilis, and Whipple's disease. Rigidity of the gastric wall, thickened folds, and ulcerations are the usual radiographic or endoscopic findings, making the exclusion of malignancy a priority in the workup of these patients. If a specific diagnosis can be made, the treatment is directed toward the underlying systemic illness.

RADIATION-INDUCED GASTRITIS

Gastric mucosal damage as a result of radiation exposure can be treated with antacids or antisecretory drugs. If gastric outlet obstruction has developed, surgical intervention may be indicated.

WATERMELON STOMACH

Patients with watermelon stomach present with gastrointestinal bleeding or iron deficiency anemia. Endoscopic examination reveals erythematous folds in the antrum converging at the pylorus, giving the appearance of a watermelon. Biopsy results reveal dilated vasculature. If a discrete bleeding site is identified, conventional endoscopic therapeutic interventions are indicated. Corticosteroids have been tried with some success, but uncontrolled persistent bleeding may necessitate treatment with antrectomy.

PHLEGMONOUS GASTRITIS

Phlegmonous gastritis is an uncommon but fulminant infection of the gastric wall due to streptococci, staphylococci, *Escherichia coli,* or *Proteus.* Surgical intervention is the therapy of choice, although initial management with antibiotics is also indicated.

GRAFT-VERSUS-HOST GASTRITIS

Gastric lesions are encountered in bone marrow transplant patients with abdominal pain or gastrointestinal tract bleeding. Gastric biopsy to rule out opportunistic, treatable infections is indicated. Otherwise care is supportive.

GASTRITIS IN THE IMMUNOCOMPROMISED HOST

A variety of viral, bacterial, fungal, and parasitic infestations can affect the gastric mucosa of the immunocompromised host. Examples include cytomegalovirus, herpesvirus, tuberculosis, syphilis, candidiasis, histoplasmosis, mucormycosis, cryptococcosis, aspergillosis, *Cryptosporidium,* anisakiasis, *Strongyloides stercoralis,* schistosomiasis, hookworm, toxoplasmosis, amebiasis, leishmaniasis, and *Pneumocystis carinii.* Gastric biopsy or positive culture of the organism is necessary for diagnosis. Treatment is directed toward the specific infection, although the degree of underlying immunodeficiency will be the more important determinant of the outcome of therapy.

REFERENCES

1. Blaser MJ. Hypotheses on the pathogenesis and natural history of *Helicobacter pylori*–induced inflammation. *Gastroenterology.* 1992;102:720–727.
2. Marshall BJ. Treatment strategies for *Helicobacter pylori* infection. *Gastroenterol Clin North Am.* 1993;22:183–198.
3. Soll AH. Gastritis. In: Wyngaarden JB, Smith LH, Bennett JC, eds. *Cecil Textbook of Medicine.* 19th ed. Philadelphia, Pa: WB Saunders Co; 1992:648–652.
4. Van Damme H, Jacquet N, Belaiche J, Creemers E, Limet R. Chronic ischemic gastritis: an unusual form of splanchnic vascular insufficiency. *J Cardiovasc Surgery.* 1992;33:451–453.
5. Weinstein WM. Gastritis and gastropathies. In: Sleisenger MH, Fordtran JS, eds. *Gastrointestinal Disease: Pathophysiology, Diagnosis, Management.* 5th ed. Philadelphia, Pa: WB Saunders Co; 1993:545–570.

46

Zollinger-Ellison Syndrome

DAVID C. METZ and ROBERT T. JENSEN

Gastrinomas are gastrin-secreting endocrine tumors that generally originate in the pancreas or proximal duodenum. Because of gastrin's abilities to induce gastric parietal cell hypertrophy and stimulate gastric acid secretion, gastrinomas give rise to the Zollinger-Ellison syndrome, which is characterized by a non-beta islet cell tumor, gastric acid hypersecretion, and severe, often fulminant, peptic ulcer disease.[1-4]

Only a small fraction of all patients with acid-peptic disease are ultimately proven to have the Zollinger-Ellison syndrome. Therefore, it is inappropriate to screen all patients with acid-peptic symptoms or even all patients with documented peptic ulcer disease for the Zollinger-Ellison syndrome. However, it is important to consider the possibility of Zollinger-Ellison syndrome in certain subsets of patients with acid-peptic disease and to establish the diagnosis when it is present because the natural history and therefore the approach to management as well differ significantly in patients with Zollinger-Ellison syndrome as opposed to patients with idiopathic peptic ulcer disease. The only problem requiring management in patients with idiopathic peptic ulcer disease is the peptic ulcer disease itself. In Zollinger-Ellison syndrome, the clinician is confronted by two separate processes, gastric acid hypersecretion and a malignant tumor of endocrine origin. Each of these processes require adequate therapy.[1,2]

Many studies have demonstrated that there generally is a long delay between the onset of symptoms and the diagnosis of Zollinger-Ellison syndrome so that a high index of suspicion is required if the diagnosis is to be made early on in the course of the disease process. Because of the severe risks of uncontrolled gastric acid hypersecretion, adequate antisecretory therapy should be started as soon as the possible diagnosis of Zollinger-Ellison syndrome has been raised. The consequences of short-term overtreatment of a patient with idiopathic peptic ulcer disease during the period when the diagnosis is being established are minimal in comparison with the risks of uncontrolled acid hypersecretion in a patient who has Zollinger-Ellison syndrome.[1,5]

Once acid hypersecretion has been safely controlled and the patient has been placed on an effective long-term antisecretory regimen, attention can then be turned to the management of the tumor itself. The first important variable on which the approach to the tumor itself depends is the extent of disease. Adequate staging is essential to establish the likelihood of surgical resectability since complete removal of the gastrinoma will cure both the gastric acid hypersecretion as well as the potentially malignant process.[1,4]

A second, equally important, variable on which the approach to the tumor depends is the presence or absence of multiple endocrine neoplasia type 1 (MEN-1). MEN-1 is an autosomal dominant syndrome characterized by multiple tumors in endocrine glands. Its major manifestations include primary hyperparathyroidism (in over 95% of cases), pituitary tumors (in up to 60% of cases), and pancreatic tumors (in up to 75% of cases).[4] Twenty-five percent of cases of Zollinger-Ellison syndrome occurs in the setting of MEN-1, whereas 75% is noninherited (sporadic). These two forms of the disease differ in that whereas the sporadic form of Zollinger-Ellison syndrome is characterized by a single tumor, which is potentially surgically resectable, the inherited form of Zollinger-Ellison syndrome is characterized by multiple tumors, and it is not clearly established that these patients are able to be cured by simple enucleation of the tumor.

The following chapter describes the general approach to patients suspected of having Zollinger-Ellison syndrome and highlights when to suspect the disease, how to establish the diagnosis, treatment of the gastric acid hypersecretion, determination of disease extent, and management of the tumor dependent on disease extent and the presence or absence of MEN-1 syndrome.

WHEN TO SUSPECT ZOLLINGER-ELLISON SYNDROME (Table 46–1)

Gastrinomas generally present during adulthood, the male-to-female ratio is approximately 3:2 and most cases are diagnosed in persons over 40 years of age.[1] The mean time to diagnosis after the development of initial symptoms is 6.4 years. All the manifestations of the Zollinger-Ellison syndrome can be explained on the basis of gastrin's ability to stimulate gastric acid hypersecretion and induce parietal cell hypertrophy.[1]

Abdominal pain is the major presenting symptom in up to 93% of patients. Generally, the pain is associated with diarrhea (up to 55% of patients). Occasionally diarrhea occurs in the absence of abdominal pain (7% to 35% of patients). In recent years, it has become clear that gastroesophageal reflux symptoms (heartburn, dysphagia, pyrosis) are far more common than was initially believed, occurring in up to two thirds of patients. Consequently, patients with peptic ulcers who also complain of diarrhea or severe esophageal symptoms should be suspected of having Zollinger-Ellison syndrome.[1]

TABLE 46–1. WHEN TO SUSPECT ZOLLINGER-ELLISON SYNDROME

1. Duodenal ulcers coexisting with diarrhea or severe esophageal disease
2. Multiple duodenal ulcers in unusual locations
3. Complicated duodenal ulcers (perforation, bleeding, obstruction)
4. Failure to relieve acid-peptic symptoms with standard doses of antisecretory medication
5. Duodenal ulcers that do not heal or that recur after medical therapy
6. Duodenal ulcers that are severe enough to require surgery or that recur after surgery
7. Duodenal ulcers with a family history suggestive of MEN-1
8. Chronic diarrhea of undefined origin
9. Gastric rugal hypertrophy on endoscopy or upper gastrointestinal tract series
10. Duodenal ulcers with no *Helicobacter pylori* present

Most patients with Zollinger-Ellison syndrome have ulcers that are clinically indistinguishable from those occurring in idiopathic peptic ulcer disease. However, peptic ulcer patients who present in an atypical manner should be suspected of having an underlying gastrinoma since atypical presentations do occur more commonly in patients with Zollinger-Ellison syndrome. These atypical presentations include multiple ulcers in unusual locations, ulcers that present with complications such as bleeding, perforation, or gastric outlet obstruction, ulcers that do not respond to standard medical therapy, and any ulcers that are severe enough to warrant surgery or that recur after apparently appropriate surgery. In addition, patients with peptic ulcers who also have hyperparathyroidism or a family history suggestive of MEN-1 syndrome should be suspected of having Zollinger-Ellison syndrome as opposed to idiopathic peptic ulcer disease. Patients with Zollinger-Ellison syndrome occasionally come to the attention of the physician following the recognition of gastric rugal hypertrophy on upper gastrointestinal (GI) tract series or endoscopy or as part of the workup for chronic diarrhea of unclear origin. Lastly, more than 90% of duodenal ulcers are associated with *H. pylori,* whereas it is found in less than 50% of patients with Zollinger-Ellison syndrome. Therefore, in a patient with duodenal ulcer with *H. pylori* present, Zollinger-Ellison syndrome should be suspected.[6]

ESTABLISHING THE DIAGNOSIS OF ZOLLINGER-ELLISON SYNDROME

Other than by definitive histologic examination, the diagnosis of Zollinger-Ellison syndrome depends on a combination of criteria including fasting serum hypergastrinemia (Table 46–2), elevated acid output measurements (Table 46–3), and positive provocative testing with secretin stimulation (Table 46–3, Fig. 46–1) or calcium infusion (Fig. 46–1). The initial screening test in all patients should be a fasting serum gastrin determination during a period when the patient is thought to be producing gastric acid (i.e., ingesting no antisecretory medications, at least briefly). However, the ultimate diagnosis requires proof of autonomous secretion of gastrin by the tumor that does not respond to physiologic feedback control mechanisms (i.e., hypergastrinemia in the presence of increased gastric acid production or inappropriate hypergastrinemia).[1]

Table 46–2 lists the causes of hypergastrinemia and divides them into those causes that are appropriate or physiologic and those that are inappropriate such as occurs in Zollinger-Ellison syndrome. The causes of physiologic hypergastrinemia (Table 46–2) can be excluded by demonstrating that the hypergastrinemia has resulted from achlorhydria or hypochlorhydria causing a feedback increase in serum gastrin in an attempt to restore acid output. To this end, a fasting gastric juice pH of >2.5 in a patient who is not taking any antisecretory medications rules out the possibility of Zollinger-Ellison syndrome regardless of the magnitude of the elevation of serum gastrin levels. With respect to the causes of inappropriate hypergastrinemia (Table 46–2), a fasting serum gastrin concentration of >1000

TABLE 46–2. DIFFERENTIAL DIAGNOSIS OF FASTING HYPERGASTRINEMIA

1. Physiologic hypergastrinemia (achlorhydria or hypochlorhydria)
   a. Atrophic gastritis
   b. Pernicious anemia
   c. Postvagotomy or gastric resection
   d. Gastric acid antisecretory medications (H_2-receptor antagonists, H^+-K^+ATPase inhibitors (omeprazole, lansoprazole)
   e. *Helicobacter pylori*
2. Inappropriate hypergastrinemia (with gastric acid present)
   a. Retained gastric antrum
   b. Massive small bowel resection
   c. Chronic gastric outlet obstruction
   d. Chronic renal failure (rarely)
   e. Antral G-cell hyperfunction or hyperplasia
   f. Zollinger-Ellison syndrome
   g. *Helicobacter pylori*

H_2 = histamine-2.

TABLE 46–3. DIAGNOSTIC PROCEDURES IN ZOLLINGER-ELLISON SYNDROME

1. BAO-MAO
   a. Patients taking H^+-K^+ ATPase inhibitors (omeprazole, etc.) should be switched to high-dose oral H_2-receptor antagonists (at least 300 mg ranitidine q 6 h) 2 weeks before the test.
   b. Discontinue the oral H_2-receptor antagonist 30 h before the test (12 h for intravenous drug).
   c. Insert a nasogastric tube after an overnight fast.
   d. Confirm tube placement (aspiration or fluoroscopy) on the morning of the test.
   e. Discard overnight residual secretions and ensure the patient is well hydrated (i.e., urine specific gravity <1.020).
   f. Collect acid output in four 15-min aliquots and measure the volume of each sample in milliliters (S_1–S_4).
   g. Dilute 1 ml from each sample in 20 ml of distilled water; titrate each specimen to pH 7.0 with 0.01 N NaOH, and measure the volume of base required in milliliters (B_1–B_4).
   h. $[(S_1 \times B_1)+(S_2 \times B_2)+(S_3 \times B_3)+(S_4 \times B_4)]/100$ = basal acid output (BAO) in milliequivalents of H^+ per hour.
   i. Inject pentagastrin subcutaneously (6 μ/kg).
   j. Repeat steps d to f above = maximal acid output (MAO).
   k. Inject 150 mg of cimetidine intravenously at completion of test.
2. Secretin stimulation test
   a. Do this test on the same day as the BAO-MAO (just before administering the intravenous cimetidine) to ensure the presence of gastric acid since achlorhydria-induced false-positive tests have been described.
   b. Draw two baseline blood samples (serum separator tubes) for fasting serum gastrin determination 15 min apart.
   c. Administer Kabi secretin intravenously (2 U/kg) by bolus injection.
   d. Draw blood samples at 2, 5, 10, and 20 min to measure the gastrin response to secretin stimulation.
   e. Positive results are defined as an increase in the serum gastrin of >200 pg/ml above the average of the two baseline values and occur in 87% of patients with Zollinger-Ellison syndrome.

H_2 = histamine-2.

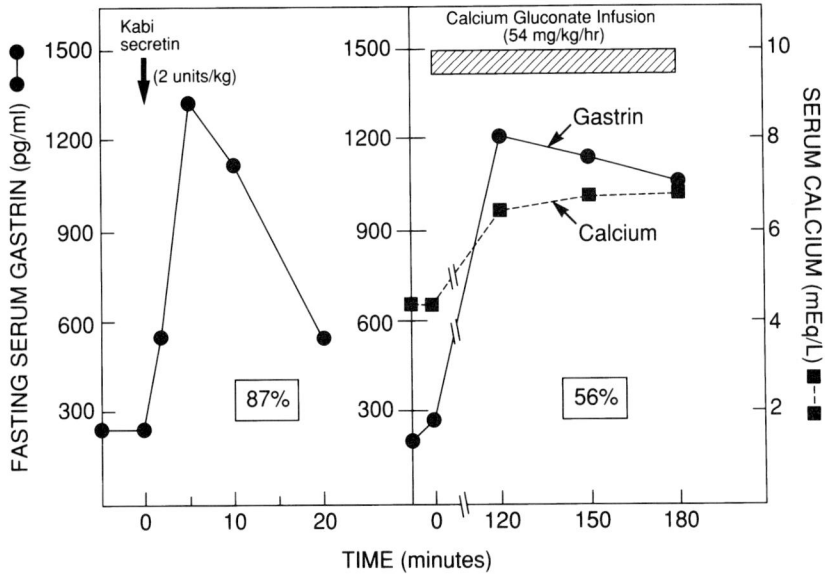

FIGURE 46–1. Provocative diagnostic tests in Zollinger-Ellison syndrome. Positive results from a secretin stimulation test are illustrated on the left, and positive results from a calcium infusion test are illustrated on the right. Positive secretin stimulation test results (seen in 87% of patients with Zollinger-Ellison syndrome) require an increase in serum gastrin of greater than 200 pg/ml over pretreatment values following intravenous stimulation with 2 U/kg of Kabi secretin. Positive calcium infusion test results (seen in 56% of patients with Zollinger-Ellison syndrome) require an increase in serum gastrin of greater than 395 pg/ml over pretreatment values following continuous infusion of 54 mg/kg/h of calcium gluconate. The serum calcium must increase by >1.5 mEq/L over pretreatment values for the test to be interpretable. Calcium infusion test results are positive in one third of patients with Zollinger-Ellison syndrome who have negative results on a secretin provocative test.

pg/ml in the presence of a gastric juice pH of <2.5 in a patient who has not undergone previous gastric surgery is diagnostic of Zollinger-Ellison syndrome and no further testing is required. The retained antrum syndrome must be considered in patients who have undergone previous gastric surgery.[1] In this rare condition, following a Billroth II gastrectomy, a piece of antrum is left behind and excluded from the flow of gastric juice so that inappropriate hypergastrinemia as high as >1000 pg/ml can result. The retained antrum syndrome can be diagnosed by technetium-99m (^{99m}Tc)-pertechnetate scan, and Zollinger-Ellison syndrome can be excluded by negative provocative testing (see below). Approximately one third of patients with Zollinger-Ellison syndrome will have fasting serum gastrin levels >1000 pg/ml and will be diagnosed this way.[1] The remaining two thirds of patients who have moderate inappropriate hypergastrinemia (100 to 1000 pg/ml) require provocative testing and formal acid secretory studies to firmly establish the diagnosis.[1]

The generally used acid secretory criterion for Zollinger-Ellison syndrome is a basal acid output (BAO) of >15 mEq/h in the absence of previous gastric acid-reducing surgery (>5 mEq/h following acid-reducing surgery).[1] However, an elevated BAO measurement alone (Table 46–3) can only be considered suggestive of Zollinger-Ellison syndrome because idiopathic hypersecretion, another hypersecretory syndrome characterized by gastric acid hypersecretion in the absence of hypergastrinemia, limits the accuracy of BAO measurement alone in the diagnosis of Zollinger-Ellison syndrome. To make acid secretory data more discriminating, many investigators have attempted to expand the definition to include assessment of the maximal acid output (MAO) (Table 46–3) and the BAO-MAO ratio (>0.6 being suggestive of the disease), but these modifications have not resulted in an improved accuracy of acid secretory criteria alone. Despite this limitation, the combination of an elevated BAO together with serum hypergastrinemia is highly suggestive of Zollinger-Ellison syndrome.[1]

The two provocative tests for the diagnosis of Zollinger-Ellison syndrome that have stood the test of time are the secretin stimulation test and the calcium infusion test. The secretin stimulation test is easy to perform (Table 46–3), is easy to interpret (Fig. 46–1, Table 46–3), and has only one known cause for a false-positive result (i.e., achlorhydria), which is easily excluded by performing the test on the same day as the BAO-MAO evaluation. Therefore, it is the initial diagnostic provocative test of choice. Unfortunately, the secretin test results are only positive in 87% of cases. The calcium infusion test (Fig. 46–1) is more cumbersome to perform, is more difficult to interpret, and has significant side effects in certain patients so that its use should be reserved for patients who are strongly suspected of having Zollinger-Ellison syndrome but in whom the secretin test results are negative.[1] The calcium infusion test results are positive in a third of patients with Zollinger-Ellison syndrome who have a negative secretin test so that <10% of patients with Zollinger-Ellison syndrome test negative with both provocative tests. In these cases (see Table 46–2), the diagnosis is usually confirmed by the absence of associated features suggestive of the other causes of moderate hypergastrinemia (e.g., renal insufficiency, bowel obstruction, previous abdominal surgery). There is much controversy regarding the diagnosis, incidence, and even existence of the antral G-cell hyperplasia or hyperfunction syndromes (Table 46–2). In these conditions, the inappropriate hypergastrinemia is said to be of antral origin. The standard meal test, in which the serum gastrin response to a standard meal is measured, has been claimed to be helpful in the diagnosis of these syndromes. However, the standard meal test is positive in up to 30% of patients with Zollinger-Ellison syndrome so that we do not believe that a positive meal test should prevent a patient with Zollinger-Ellison syndrome from benefitting from surgery, if indicated, even if the other provocative test results are negative.[1]

MANAGEMENT OF GASTRIC ACID HYPERSECRETION

In recent years, it has become clear that gastric acid hypersecretion can be controlled medically in all cases of Zollinger-Ellison syndrome provided sufficient medication is administered.[1,5,7] As a result, total gastrectomy, which previously was the mainstay of therapy, should now be reserved for the occasional patient who is unable or unwilling to take medication. The shift toward medical therapy has come about as a result of a number of factors including the development of safe and effective oral and intravenous antisecretory medications, the realization that the efficacy of therapy cannot be guided by the control of symptoms alone, and the establishment of reliable acid secretory criteria with which therapy can be safely instituted and effectively monitored.

In most patients with Zollinger-Ellison syndrome, if gastric acid output is reduced to less than 10 mEq/h in the last hour before the next dose of medication, symptoms will be controlled, peptic ulcers will heal, and recurrent acid-peptic disease will be prevented.[1,5,7] However, certain subgroups of patients with complicated forms of disease require more aggressive therapy with reduction of acid output to even lower levels. Patients with previous partial gastrectomies require reduction of acid output to <5 mEq/h to heal all mucosal disease and prevent recurrence. Patients with severe gastroesophageal reflux disease require reduction of acid output to <1 mEq/h to control symptoms of heartburn and heal reflux-induced strictures in all cases although most reflux patients only require reduction to <5 mEq/h.[8] Finally, patients with MEN-1 syndrome who often have associated hyperparathyroidism, which can cause fluctuations in serum calcium levels and therefore acid output as well, generally require more medication than patients who have sporadic Zollinger-Ellison syndrome.[1,5]

Medical management of gastric acid hypersecretion in patients with Zollinger-Ellison syndrome can be divided into two phases because the approach differs in the acute setting as opposed to the long term (Table 46–4). In most cases, treatment can be started with oral antisecretory agents (i.e., long-term management from the start); however, in certain situations, patients initially require parenteral therapy. Some patients initially present with severe vomiting, electrolyte disturbances, and dehydration prior to diagnosis. Other patients initially present with a complication of peptic ulcer disease requiring emergency surgery. In both these groups of patients, once the possible diagnosis has been considered, acid output must be controlled rapidly to prevent the development of severe, often life-threatening, complications such as perforation or gastrointestinal tract hemorrhage, and parenteral therapy is required (Table 46–4). Because intravenous H^+-K^+ ATPase inhibitors are unavailable in the United States, histamine-2 (H_2)-receptor antagonists are required for the management of acid output in the acute setting or when patients cannot take oral med-

TABLE 46–4. HOW TO CONTROL GASTRIC ACID HYPERSECRETION IN PATIENTS WITH ZOLLINGER-ELLISON SYNDROME

1. Acute management
   a. Continuous IV ranitidine or cimetidine infusions have been studied the best.
   b. For ranitidine, give an IV bolus injection of 100–150 mg of ranitidine at the start of treatment.
   c. If the effective oral ranitidine dose is known, start the IV at 100% of the daily oral dose (effective in 95% of patients).
   d. If the effective oral ranitidine dose is not known, start the IV at 1 mg/kg/h (effective in >36% of patients).
   e. Measure acid output 4 h later.
   f. Titrate the IV rate upward in 0.5 mg/kg/h increments and repeat acid output measurements q 4 h until it has been reduced to <10 mEq/h (1.5 mg/kg/h effectively controls acid output in 84% of patients and 2.5 mg/kg/h in 100%).
   g. Begin oral drug when the patient has resumed eating.
   h. For cimetidine, proceed as above but remember that cimetidine is three to fourfold less potent than ranitidine so that three to four times larger doses will be required.
2. Long-term management
   a. Omeprazole is now the oral drug of choice. Administer the first dose 1 to 2 h after an IV bolus of ranitidine (omeprazole is acid-labile).
   b. Start with 60 mg/d in patients with uncomplicated disease.
   c. Patients with severe reflux esophagitis, previous partial gastrectomy, or MEN-1 with hyperparathyroidism should start with 40 mg twice daily.
   d. Measure acid output the next day in the last hour before the next dose of drug.
   e. Titrate the dose upward by 20 mg per dose interval and repeat acid output measurements daily until it has been reduced to <10 mEq/h (<5 mEq/h in patients with previous gastric resections and <1 mEq/h in certain patients with severe gastroesophageal reflux disease).
   f. Patients who are not controlled with 120 mg once daily should be switched to 60 mg twice daily (about 25% of patients need twice daily dosing).
   g. Omeprazole will control acid secretion in all patients with Zollinger-Ellison syndrome (median daily dose requirements are 60–100 mg/d).
   h. Acid control in MEN-1 patients with hyperparathyroidism may be facilitated by parathyroidectomy.
   i. Once acid output is effectively controlled, long-term maintenance dose requirements can be safely reduced with appropriate monitoring in most patients with uncomplicated disease.
   j. Reinforce the need for continual lifelong therapy and warn patients that they may require intermittent IV medication during periods when they are unable to take it orally (e.g., surgery, vomiting).

ications for any other reason (e.g., perioperatively or during an episode of gastroenteritis). In the short term, there is little difference between equipotent doses of these agents, although famotidine is eight times more potent than ranitidine, which is four times more potent than cimetidine. It must be stressed that relatively high doses of medication are required for effective control of acid output in patients with Zollinger-Ellison syndrome as opposed to patients with idiopathic peptic ulcer disease and that the physician should not become concerned even if extremely high doses of medication are required.[1,5] Table 46–4 outlines an effective approach for rapid control of gastric acid output in the acute setting in patients with suspected Zollinger-Ellison syndrome. In addition, simple gastric decompression using a nasogastric tube placed to low intermittent suction often affords patients significant relief in the acute setting, but this maneuver must be combined with careful attention to overall fluid balance so that patients are not rendered profoundly dehydrated by ongoing nasogastric losses, which can be massive.

The H^+-K^+ ATPase inhibitors such as omeprazole or lansoprazole are currently the agents of choice for the long-term management of gastric acid hypersecretion in patients with Zollinger-Ellison syndrome because of their safety, efficacy, and ease of administration (Table 46–4).[1,5,7] Omeprazole will control acid output effectively in all patients with Zollinger-Ellison syndrome. Tachyphylaxis is not a problem, the drug is well tolerated, and recent studies in Zollinger-Ellison syndrome patients, treated for up to 7 years, show no evidence of drug-induced carcinoid tumors.[1,7] Patients with Zollinger-Ellison syndrome, especially those with MEN-1 syndrome as well, have a predisposition to carcinoid tumors of the stomach anyway presumably because of their chronic hypergastrinemia. Table 46–4 provides an effective approach for the long-term management of gastric acid output in patients with Zollinger-Ellison syndrome using omeprazole.

Other agents that can be used for long-term management of gastric acid hypersecretion in patients with Zollinger-Ellison syndrome include H$_2$-receptor antagonists, anticholinergic agents, prostaglandins, and octreotide. H$_2$-receptor antagonists are effective in most cases of Zollinger-Ellison syndrome, although extremely high doses are required; at least one dose increase per year is usually required, and the drug must be taken as often as every three to four hours in some cases.[1,5] In addition, long-term use of cimetidine in men is associated with gynecomastia and impotence. Despite known antisecretory activity, anticholinergic agents (e.g., propantheline [Pro-Banthine]) and prostaglandin analogs (e.g., misoprostol [Cytotec]) have significant side effects and limited efficacy so that they no longer have a role in the medical therapy of gastric acid hypersecretion in patients with Zollinger-Ellison syndrome. The synthetic somatostatin analog, octreotide, has a potential role in the medical management of gastric acid hypersecretion in these patients. Octreotide inhibits gastric acid secretion both by a direct effect on the parietal cell and by lowering serum gastrin levels by acting on the gastrinoma cells. As a result it potentially has the additional theoretical benefits of reversal of the trophic effect of gastrin on the stomach and other tissues, as well as a possible direct antitumor effect. However, the need for subcutaneous administration two or three times daily and the potential side effects of long-term therapy (gallstones, steatorrhea, abdominal cramps) make its use for long-term control of gastric acid hypersecretion in patients with Zollinger-Ellison syndrome questionable and experimental at present.

The role for surgery in the long-term management of gastric acid hypersecretion in patients with Zollinger-Ellison is limited.[1-3] Parathyroidectomy in patients with MEN-1 who have documented hyperparathyroidism may prevent fluctuations of acid output making it easier to manage acid output medically. Parietal cell vagotomy may have a role in women of childbearing age who undergo surgery for attempted cure because this may allow some patients to stop all antisecretory medications during a future pregnancy when these medications may be harmful. As mentioned above, total gastrectomy should be reserved for patients who are unwilling or unable to take oral medications.[1]

DETERMINATION OF DISEASE EXTENT AND MEN-1 STATUS

Once the gastric acid hypersecretion has been brought under control medically, consideration can be given to surgical removal of the gastrinoma. This is the only form of therapy that is able to definitively cure the endocrine syndrome. In addition, 60% to 90% of gastrinomas are malignant so that early surgery is indicated to remove tumors prior to the development of metastatic disease.[1-3] However, the likelihood of achieving a successful response with surgery depends on the extent of disease at presentation and the patient's MEN-1 status.

EXTENT OF DISEASE

Surgical extirpation of the gastrinoma can only be successful in the setting of localized (resectable) disease. One of the major roles of imaging studies is therefore to exclude the presence of unresectable metastases thereby preventing the performance of unnecessary surgery in patients who are unlikely to benefit from the procedure. In this regard, ultrasound, computed tomography (CT) scan, magnetic resonance imaging (MRI) scan, and angiography have very high specificity for the detection of liver metastases (Table 46–5). As a result, if any findings from these studies are positive for unresectable metastatic disease, a biopsy of the metastasis should be performed to confirm its nature histologi-

TABLE 46–5. UTILITY OF VARIOUS LOCALIZING MODALITIES IN PATIENTS WITH ZOLLINGER-ELLISON SYNDROME

	SENSITIVITY (%)	SPECIFICITY (%)
Liver Metastases		
1. Ultrasound	63	100
2. CT scan	72	98
3. MRI scan	83	88
4. Angiography	86	100
Primary Tumor Detection		
1. Imaging modalities		
a. Ultrasound	30	94
b. CT scan	59	95
c. MRI scan	21	33
d. Angiography	68	94
2. Hormonal techniques		
a. Portal venous sampling (PVS)	73	33
b. Secretin angiography	78	100
3. Intraoperative methods		
a. Intraoperative ultrasound	83	Not done
b. Duodenal transillumination*	83	88

*For duodenal tumors only.

cally, and surgery can be avoided. The combination of CT scan with selective abdominal angiography has been shown to detect >95% of liver metastases in some studies. We therefore advise a stepwise approach beginning with CT scanning (noncontrast scans are better than contrast-enhanced scans of the liver) and ultrasound followed by MRI scan if results from both initial studies are negative. If observations from the MRI scan are also negative for metastatic disease, selective hepatic artery angiography should be done before any patient is taken to surgery since this is the procedure that is most likely to identify liver metastases that may have been missed prior to surgery. Using this approach, we have found that almost all patients with unresectable disease can be identified without having to subject them to unnecessary surgery.[1]

Patients without evidence of unresectable liver metastases are potential surgical candidates. A second important role for localization studies is to aid the surgeon by identifying the primary gastrinoma preoperatively. Gastrinomas are commonly small and multiple and may be located in a variety of sites including the duodenum or pancreas (most commonly), although primary tumors originating in lymph nodes, the hepatic hilus, the ovary, and even the heart have been described.[1,3] As a result, most early surgical series of gastrinomas revealed a significant percentage of patients in whom no tumors were found at surgery. With regard to the identification of primary tumors, routine imaging modalities such as ultrasound, CT scan (contrast-enhanced scans are better than noncontrast scans of the pancreas), MRI scan, and angiography have a low sensitivity (Table 46–5), although angiography is clearly the best modality for this purpose. The major limiting factor in the ability of routine imaging modalities to localize gastrinomas is tumor size. Routine imaging studies will identify less than 10% of tumors smaller than 1 cm, 30% to 40% of tumors 1 to 3 cm in diameter, and 70% to 80% of tumors larger than 3 cm.[1,3] Furthermore, routine imaging modalities are much more likely to identify pancreatic gastrinomas preoperatively than duodenal gastrinomas.[1,3] With the recent advent of endoscopic ultrasonography, dynamic bolus-enhanced CT scanning, and of [^{111}Im-DTPA-DPhe^1] octreotide scanning, this may change in the future.

In recent years, with improvements in both localization techniques and the surgical approach, tumors are now being found in over 90% of patients.[1,3] Tumors are now frequently found in patients with negative results from preoperative localization studies. These improvements have resulted from the use of improved localization techniques such as intraoperative ultrasound, duodenal endoscopic transillumination, and routine duodenotomy (Table 46–5). We therefore believe that negative imaging should not preclude a patient from being offered surgery. It is unclear whether all patients should undergo either portal venous sampling or secretin angiography preoperatively (Table 46–5); however, all patients should have intraoperative ultrasound and duodenal transillumination performed during the operation (Table 46–5) and possibly a duodenotomy as well.

MEN-1 STATUS

Previous studies have demonstrated that the natural history of gastrinoma differs between patients with or without MEN-1 syndrome. The likelihood of achieving cure with exploratory laparotomy in patients with MEN-1 syndrome has previously been shown to be low so that many authorities do not believe in subjecting MEN-1 patients with gastrinoma to surgery with intent to cure.[1] This viewpoint has been supported in the past by the contention that gastrinomas in MEN-1 patients are less aggressive than those that occur in patients with the sporadic form of the disease.[1]

MEN-1 syndrome is diagnosed by demonstrating two or more of the endocrinopathies that are typical phenotypic manifestations of the disease in the same patient (about two thirds of cases) or by the appearance of one typical endocrinopathy in a patient with a strong family history (about one third of cases). Thus, patients who already have gastrinoma can be diagnosed as having MEN-1 syndrome either if they have a strong family history of MEN-1 syndrome (e.g., a first-degree relative with the syndrome) or if they manifest a second endocrinopathy. In over 95% of cases, gastrinoma is not the first manifestation of MEN-1 syndrome. Gastrinomas usually develop in the fourth decade of life and are almost invariably preceded by hyperparathyroidism (which may be asymptomatic) in the third decade.[4] We therefore screen all patients with Zollinger-Ellison syndrome with simultaneous serum calcium and serum parathyroid hormone levels (using a sensitive IRMA assay from Nichols Institute, San Juan Capistrano, Calif.). If hyperparathyroidism is not present, MEN-1 syndrome is unlikely. In addition, it may also be necessary to measure a serum prolactin level and a 24-hour urinary free cortisol level in equivocal cases. Although the vast majority of MEN-1 syndrome patients are identified using this approach, it is becoming clear that occasionally patients do present with Zollinger-Ellison syndrome as the first manifestation of their disease, and the underlying MEN-1 syndrome only becomes apparent years later with the development of a second endocrinopathy.

THERAPY FOR NONMETASTATIC, NON-MEN-1 DISEASE

As alluded to above, negative imaging should not be a reason to avoid surgical exploration. Current statistics from the National Institutes of Health (NIH) indicate that tumor is found in over 90% of sporadic Zollinger-Ellison syndrome patients without evidence of metastases preoperatively regardless of preoperative imaging results.[3] Furthermore, almost two thirds of these patients are rendered disease-free immediately postoperatively, and about 30% of patients are cured long-term.[3] To date, because of the slow-growing nature of gastrinomas in general, there are no data available regarding any potential long-term survival benefit from early surgical intervention. However, it has been estimated that 50% to 70% of deaths in patients with metastatic disease are due to tumor progression.[1]

The preoperative workup should include a bowel preparation in anticipation of a duodenotomy and administration of pneumococcal vaccine in the event that splenectomy is required. Since the patient will be unable to take oral medication for some time, it is essential to determine the effective intravenous antisecretory drug requirement in the individual patient (Table 46–4) and to start this therapy preoperatively. It is essential that the exploration be done by an experienced surgeon.

At exploration, the liver should be carefully examined for evidence of metastatic disease. In the event that extensive metastases not previously visualized are found, the surgery should be modified to avoid subsequent performance of any morbidity-associated procedures (e.g., partial pancreatectomy or duodenotomy). If there is no evidence of unresectable liver disease, the primary tumor should then be sought. The entire abdomen should be explored with special attention being paid to the so-called *gastrinoma triangle* (the area contained by the junction of the cystic and common bile ducts superiorly, the junction of the neck and body of the pancreas medially, and the junction of the second and third portions of the duodenum inferiorly). This procedure requires an extended Kocker maneuver.[3]

Most often, primary tumors are found in the pancreatic head or duodenal wall. These gastrinomas should be carefully enucleated only. More aggressive resections (e.g., pancreaticoduodenectomy) have not been shown to provide a benefit that outweighs the increased morbidity associated with aggressive surgery despite the fact that these tumors are commonly malignant. Even if one tumor is found, the entire abdomen still must be explored carefully because there may be more than one tumor causing the disease. With the addition of routine duodenal transillumination and duodenotomy to the NIH protocol, it has recently become clear that duodenal gastrinomas are as common as pancreatic gastrinomas despite previous assertions to the contrary. We therefore believe that all patients undergoing exploration with intent to cure require a duodenotomy as a routine part of the procedure.[3]

If an isolated, resectable liver metastasis is found, it should be removed with the primary tumor. If no tumor is found, blind pancreatic resections are not recommended since extrapancreatic gastrinomas are common and total pancreatectomy is contraindicated.

The routine use of parietal cell vagotomy at the time of surgery is controversial. Following gastrinoma resection, parietal cell vagotomy reduces antisecretory drug requirements; however, unless they are cured surgically, no patients can stop antisecretory therapy completely.[1]

THERAPY FOR MEN-1 DISEASE

Therapy for gastrinoma patients who also have MEN-1 syndrome can be divided into three major areas: treatment of the gastrinoma, treatment of the MEN-1 syndrome, and treatment of the patient's family. With regard to the gastrinoma itself, the primary aim is to control the gastric acid hypersecretion with an effective antisecretory regimen coupled with consideration for parathyroidectomy in patients who have documented hyperparathyroidism. Successful parathyroidectomy reduces the subsequent antisecretory drug requirements significantly in all patients and in up to 10% of patients even seems to result in a complete disappearance of the Zollinger-Ellison syndrome with normalization of serum gastrin levels and reduction of acid output to within normal limits.[9] The mechanism for this response is unknown. We recommend twice-daily omeprazole therapy in all MEN-1 patients since these patients appear to require more medication than patients with sporadic Zollinger-Ellison syndrome, and even after successful parathyroidectomy, these patients are at risk for recurrent hyperparathyroidism and recurrent fluctuations of acid secretion with changes in serum calcium levels.[7] The role of exploratory surgery in MEN-1 syndrome patients, even with localized disease, is controversial at present, and we do not recommend routine exploration in MEN-1 syndrome patients.[1] However, in recent years it is becoming clear that gastrinomas in the setting of MEN-1 syndrome are more likely to metastasize than previously thought and that the primary gastrinomas are commonly located in the proximal duodenal submucosa. Therefore, with recent improvements in the ability to detect and resect duodenal tumors it may become possible to surgically cure certain MEN-1 patients with gastrinomas. However, multiple other nongastrinoma pancreatic endocrine tumors, which also have malignant potential, will remain behind.

With regard to the MEN-1 syndrome itself, it is essential to evaluate all MEN-1 syndrome patients fully for associated endocrinopathies and to tailor therapy as indicated in the individual patient. As mentioned earlier, MEN-1 syndrome is primarily characterized by hyperplasia of the parathyroid glands and tumors of the pituitary gland and pancreas. Other less common manifestations effect a variety of other tissues. The approach to hyperparathyroidism in the absence of Zollinger-Ellison syndrome depends on the degree of bone mineral loss (best assessed by bone densitometry), underlying renal function, and the history of renal stones. All patients require imaging of the sella turcica (MRI scan is better than CT scan for this purpose) since pituitary tumors are common.[4] If a pituitary tumor is found, long-term oral bromocriptine to shrink prolactinomas with intermittent repeat imaging is necessary. About one fifth of MEN-1 patients also develop mild Cushing's disease (pituitary Cushing's syndrome), which must be distinguished from Cushing's syndrome secondary to ectopic adrenocorticotropic hormone (ACTH) production that occasionally occurs in patients with widespread sporadic Zollinger-Ellison syndrome and is usually severe.[4] Other endocrinopathies that must be considered in MEN-1 patients are pheochromocytomas, other pancreatic islet cell tumors (especially nonfunctional tumors and insulinomas), thyroid tumors, carcinoid tumors of the lung and gastrointestinal tract, and lipomas.

MEN-1 syndrome is an autosomal dominant condition with high penetrance. The genetic defect has recently been localized to the long arm of chromosome 11 in a region close to the centromere (11q13).[4] At present, there is no genetic marker with which to screen family members of patients with MEN-1 syndrome to identify heterozygotes prior to the development of clinical disease. Because most cases present with hyperparathyroidism as their first manifestation and because this usually occurs in the third decade of life, we believe that all family members of patients with MEN-1 syndrome should have intermittent serum calcium determinations done in early adulthood. Screening for other endocrinopathies should only be performed if family members develop symptoms attributable to the development of a specific endocrinopathy.[4]

THERAPY FOR METASTATIC DISEASE

Patients with widespread metastatic gastrinoma require lifelong therapy with omeprazole to control gastric acid hypersecretion. There is general agreement that therapy directed against the metastatic disease is also indicated because the overall 5-year survival in patients with widespread metastatic disease is as low as 20% and up to 70% of deaths in patients with metastatic disease are due to tumor progression.[1,4] However, controversy exists regarding when to start therapy and about which modalities to use. The reasons for the lack of agreement are that patients with widespread metastatic disease often feel well once their acid output has been controlled and that the available therapeutic modalities for metastatic disease are both toxic and of limited efficacy.[1,4]

With regard to the decision of when to start therapy, we believe that all patients should have clear evidence of active tumor growth or symptoms of metastatic disease that may respond to direct antitumor therapy before therapy is instituted.[1,4] In addition, no patient should be subjected to potentially toxic therapeutic regimens without histologic confirmation of metastatic disease.

Chemotherapy, interferon, and chemoembolization have been used therapeutically for gastrinoma metastatic to the liver.[4] However, bone metastases develop in up to one fourth of patients with advanced metastatic disease so that therapy such as hepatic artery chemoembolization, which is directed only at the liver, is unlikely to be helpful and systemic chemotherapy or interferon with or without local radiotherapy is indicated in patients with documented bony metastases. Once widespread symptomatic metastatic disease has developed, much of the therapy is palliative in nature, and therapy should be directed against specific symptoms of the disease. To this end, local radiation therapy can be extremely helpful. It must also be stressed that gastrinomas are generally slow-growing tumors and that, even with massive tumor loads, careful attention to the palliative control of symptomatic metastases can provide the patient with many years of quality life.

Chemotherapy using streptozocin appears to be the best single agent in the treatment of metastatic gastrinomas.[1,4] The combination of streptozocin plus 5-fluorouracil has been shown to be more effective than streptozocin alone. Streptozocin with doxorubicin is more effective than streptozocin and 5-fluorouracil, and therefore this regimen, with or without 5-fluorouracil, is the current therapy of choice for metastatic gastrinoma.[1,4,10,11] The NIH protocol (Table 46–6) employs all three agents. Unfortunately, the response rate using this three-drug regimen is only 40%, and in no cases does tumor disappear completely.[10] The recent addition of ondansetron, a $5-HT_3$-inhibitor, to control chemotherapy-induced vomiting has significantly reduced

TABLE 46–6. REGIMENS FOR METASTATIC ZOLLINGER-ELLISON SYNDROME

Combination Chemotherapy (NIH Protocol)[9]
1. Obtain pretreatment parameters (ejection fraction, blood count, renal function, pregnancy test).
2. Antisecretory medication should be taken at least 4 hours before chemotherapy is administered.
3. On day 1 (of a 30-day cycle):
   a. Ondansetron 0.15 mg/kg in 50 ml 5% dextrose over 15 min for three doses
   b. Streptozocin 1.5 g/m^2 in 150 ml 5% dextrose over 10–20 min
   c. Doxorubicin (Adriamycin) 40 mg/m^2 over 3–5 min into a rapidly flowing intravenous infusion
   d. 5-Fluorouracil 600 mg/m^2 in 100 ml 5% dextrose over 10–15 min.
4. Repeat drug administration as above on day 8 except do not give doxorubicin.
5. Monitor response to therapy every 3 mo (imaging including bone scan)
6. Monitor for side effects of therapy:
   a. Blood count and renal function (creatinine clearance, 24-h protein) before each cycle
   b. Ejection fraction every 3–6 months
7. Duration of treatment:
   a. For as long as an objective response occurs (seen in 40% of patients)
   b. Discontinue Adriamycin treatment once the cumulative Adriamycin dose reaches 550 mg/m^2
   c. A complete response (disappearance of tumor) is rare
   d. Stop whenever tumor growth occurs or new lesions appear
8. Dose modifications:
   a. Renal dysfunction (streptozocin)
   b. Cardiac dysfunction (doxorubicin [Adriamycin])
   c. Hematologic dysfunction (5-fluorouracil)
9. Side effects:
   a. Vomiting unusual since addition of ondansetron to the regimen (previously 100%)
   b. Alopecia in most patients (80%)
   c. Transient proteinuria (40%)
   d. Leukopenia requiring dose modification (20%)
   e. Mucositis (common)

Interferon (NIH Protocol)
1. Less toxic to the patient
2. Requires patient cooperation and training for self-administration of drug
3. Human recombinant interferon alfa, available as a lyophilized powder, requires reconstitution with bacteriostatic water for injection and remains stable at 2–8°C for 1 mo
4. Dose: 5 million units by daily subcutaneous injection
5. Duration of therapy: indefinitely provided the tumor does not grow
6. Tumor growth is arrested in about one third of patients; objective tumor regressions are rare
7. Monitor response to therapy every 3 mo (imaging including bone scan)
8. Dose modifications:
   a. Marrow suppression (responds to dose reduction)
   b. Psychiatric disturbances (requires discontinuation)
   c. Rash or pruritus (usually responds to dose reduction)
   d. Other side effects rarely requiring dose modification include fatigue, flulike symptoms, pain and erythema at the injection site, reversible alopecia, laboratory abnormalities of thyroid function, liver function, and lipids

the morbidity associated with this regimen, but renal dysfunction and leukopenia are still major problems that often require dose modification. Cardiotoxicity with the current regimen is not commonly encountered. In another recent study,[11] the combination of streptozocin and doxorubicin was reported to provide a 69% response rate in patients with metastatic islet cell tumors.

Because of the toxicity and generally poor response rates to chemotherapy, other agents have recently been investigated in an attempt to develop better therapeutic approaches to metastatic gastrinoma. Another agent that has shown some promise in some studies is interferon (Table 46–6).[1,4] Interferon has been well studied in carcinoid tumors that histologically resemble gastrinomas and has been found to exert a tumoristic effect that can be prolonged.[4] Studies thus far at the NIH suggest that an objective response with interferon alfa (Table 46–6) occurs in about one third of patients with metastatic gastrinoma such that tumor growth is halted for at least 3 months although tumor regression has not been seen in any cases. Our present policy is to treat most patients with interferon initially because it is well tolerated. Those patients who later demonstrate failure of a continued response with interferon (i.e., the tumor starts growing again) are switched to combination chemotherapy.

Octreotide may also be useful for controlling tumor growth in some patients with metastatic gastrinomas.[4] All tumors appear to have somatostatin receptors, and octreotide definitely inhibits the secretion of gastrin from gastrinomas. Preliminary results suggest that octreotide may have a tumoristic effect as well in some patients.[4]

SUMMARY

Figure 46–2 provides a flow diagram summarizing the approach to patients suspected of having Zollinger-Ellison syndrome. The first thing to be done as soon as the possibility of Zollinger-Ellison syndrome has been raised is to control acid

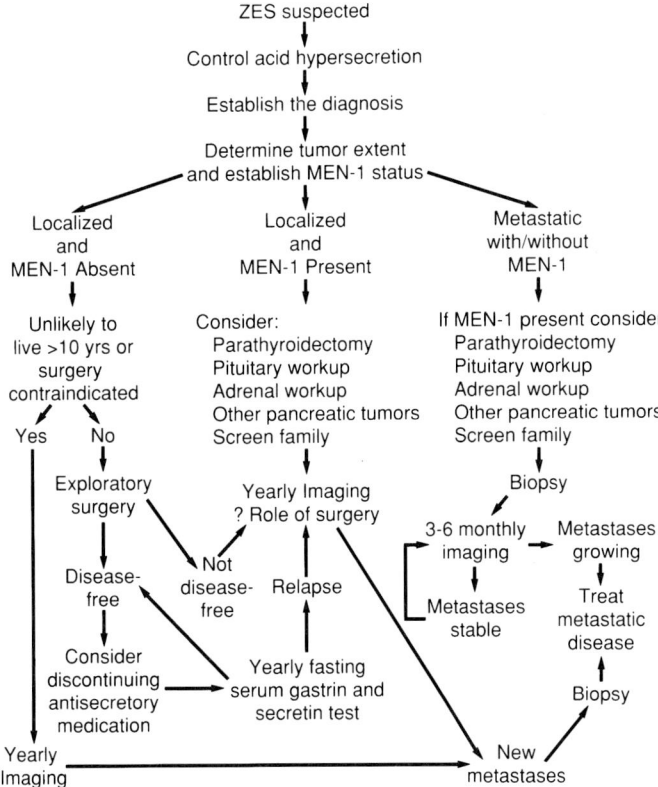

FIGURE 46–2. Flow diagram summarizing the general approach to patients suspected of having Zollinger-Ellison syndrome. For details, see text. *MEN-1* = multiple endocrine neoplasia type 1, *ZES* = Zollinger-Ellison syndrome.

output to prevent the development of complications (which can develop rapidly) and to provide time to establish the diagnosis, define the extent of disease, and establish whether the patient also has MEN-1 syndrome. Thereafter, the therapeutic approach depends on the extent of disease and the presence or absence of associated MEN-1 syndrome.

Patients who have sporadic Zollinger-Ellison syndrome and no evidence of metastases should undergo early surgical exploration with intent to cure unless surgery is contraindicated or they are unlikely to outlive the natural history of their disease. Patients who are rendered disease-free should be followed yearly with fasting serum gastrin determinations and secretin stimulation tests. If these patients continue to appear cured, it may be possible to discontinue their antisecretory therapy. Patients who are not rendered disease-free after exploratory laparotomy should be followed yearly with imaging studies since, if metastatic disease develops, decisions must be made regarding chemotherapy or interferon therapy. The role of repeated surgery in patients who relapse or who are not initially rendered disease-free is controversial.

The role of surgery in patients who have MEN-1 syndrome and potentially resectable disease is also controversial. The treatment approach in this group of patients involves controlling acid output medically with consideration for parathyroidectomy. Yearly imaging studies are important since, if metastatic disease develops, these patients must also be considered candidates for chemotherapy or interferon. In addition, a full endocrine workup to detect and treat other manifestations of the MEN-1 syndrome and family counseling are required.

Patients with metastatic disease require regular imaging studies including a bone scan. Those in whom the metastases appear to be stable can be monitored without subjecting them to toxic therapy with a limited benefit. However, if the tumor is growing, systemic therapy with interferon or combination chemotherapy is indicated once a histologic diagnosis has been obtained. There also is a role for regional therapies in patients with metastatic disease primarily for control of symptoms.

REFERENCES

1. Jensen RT, Gardner JD. Zollinger-Ellison syndrome: clinical presentation, pathology, diagnosis and treatment. In: Dannenberg A, Zakim D, eds. *Peptic Ulcer and Other Acid-Related Diseases.* New York, NY: Spectrum Publishing Co; 1991:117.
2. Andersen DK. Current diagnosis and management of Zollinger-Ellison syndrome. *Ann Surg.* 1989;210:685.
3. Norton JA, Doppman JL, Jensen RT. Curative resection in Zollinger-Ellison syndrome: results of a ten year prospective study. *Ann Surg.* 1992;215:8.
4. Norton JA, Jensen RT. Cancer of the endocrine syndrome. In: DeVita VT, Hellman S, Rosenberg SA, eds. *Principles and Practice of Oncology.* 4th ed. Philadelphia, Pa: JB Lippincott; 1993:1333–1435.
5. Metz DC, Pisegna JR, Fishbeyn VA, Benya RV, Jensen RT. The control of gastric acid hypersecretion in the management of patients with Zollinger-Ellison syndrome. In: Norton JA, ed. Progress Symposium on the Treatment of Islet Cell Tumors. *World J Surg.* 1993;17:468–480.
6. Metz DC, Weber C, Orbuch M, Strader DB, Lubensky IA, Jensen RT. *Helicobacter pylori* infection: a reversible cause of hypergastrinemia and hyperchlorhydria which can mimic Zollinger-Ellison syndrome. *Dig Dis Sci.* 1995;40:153–159.
7. Frucht H, Maton PN, Jensen RT. The use of omeprazole in patients with Zollinger-Ellison syndrome. *Dig Dis Sci.* 1991;36:394.
8. Miller LS, Vinayek R, Frucht H, Gardner JD, Jensen RT, Maton PN. Reflux esophagitis in patients with Zollinger-Ellison syndrome. *Gastroenterology.* 1990;98:341.
9. Norton JA, Cornelius MJ, Doppman JL, Maton PN, Gardner JD, Jensen RT. Effect of parathyroidectomy in patients with hyperparathyroidism and Zollinger-Ellison syndrome and multiple endocrine neoplasia type I: a prospective study. *Surgery.* 1987;102:958.
10. von Schrenck T, Howard JM, Doppman JL, et al. Prospective study of chemotherapy in patients with metastatic gastrinoma. *Gastroenterology.* 1988;94:1326.
11. Moertel CG, Lefkopoulo M, Lipsitz S, Hahn RG, Klaassen D. Streptozotocin-doxorubicin, streptozotocin-fluorouracil or chlorozotocin in the treatment of advanced islet-cell carcinoma. *N Engl J Med.* 1992;326:519.

47

Complications of Peptic Ulcer Disease

DOUGLAS A. HALE and ANDRE DUBOIS

Great strides have been made over the past two decades regarding the pathophysiology and therapy of peptic ulcer disease. The addition of histamine-2 H_2-receptor antagonists to the clinicians armamentarium has improved healing rates of ulcers while causing fewer side effects than anticholinergic agents and antacids. The more recent clarification of the role of *Helicobacter pylori* in peptic ulcer disease has helped reduce the rate of recurrence through appropriate antibiotic therapy. Despite these gains however, complications of peptic ulcer disease continue to plague clinicians due to the fact that they now tend to occur in older and sicker patients. These complications include bleeding, perforation, obstruction, and intractability. The purpose of this chapter is to review the currently accepted means of evaluating and treating these complications and to explore options that may be available in the near future.

HEMORRHAGE

Hemorrhage remains the most common serious complication of peptic ulcer disease, occurring in 15% to 20% of all patients.[1] The average mortality from this complication is 4% to 8%.[2] Predictors of poor outcome include hematemesis, blood-tainted nasogastric aspirate that fails to clear after 6 L of lavage, presence of shock on presentation, age greater than 60 years, and presence of four or more preexisting medical illnesses.[3] These clinical factors are useful for stratifying patients into appropriate risk categories and in guiding the appropriate level of aggressiveness of management (see Fig. 47–1).

The opinions and assertions contained herein are the private ones of the authors and are not to be construed as official or reflecting the views of the Department of Defense or the Uniformed Services University of the Health Sciences.

INITIAL MANAGEMENT AND ASSESSMENT

Initial attention is focused on the assessment and resuscitation of the patient with upper gastrointestinal tract hemorrhage. Assessment of the magnitude of hemorrhage is initially based on the patient's vital signs on presentation and the response of the vital signs to resuscitation over time. Resuscitation is initiated with a balanced crystalloid solution via large bore intravenous access. A baseline hematocrit and type and cross-match are drawn and supplemental oxygen administered. A Foley urinary catheter is inserted to aid in the assessment of the patient's response to ongoing resuscitative measures.

Once these emergency measures have been taken, an oral gastric tube is placed, the gastric contents are aspirated, and the stomach is lavaged with normal saline. It is now recognized that the role of gastric lavage is mainly diagnostic in nature, and information provided is helpful in determining the severity and activity of hemorrhage. The presence of a coffee-ground type material in an otherwise clear aspirate indicates that hemorrhage is most likely not active and that the process of definitive evaluation and therapy can proceed at a semielective pace. The presence of bright red blood that fails to clear after 6 L of irrigation indicates that hemorrhage is active and further evaluation and therapy should be pursued with a sense of urgency. A non-blood-tinged aspirate devoid of coffee-ground material indicates that the source of hemorrhage is likely to be distal to the ligament of Treitz. This finding is only reliable if bile is present in the aspirate, demonstrating that there is mixture of fluids from the duodenum and stomach.

Following the confirmation of an upper gastrointestinal tract source of hemorrhage via the oral gastric tube, the next step in the evaluation is esophagogastroduodenoscopy (EGD). Thorough irrigation prior to EGD is essential for an accurate appraisal of the esophagus, stomach, and duodenum. If a lesion is identified, several

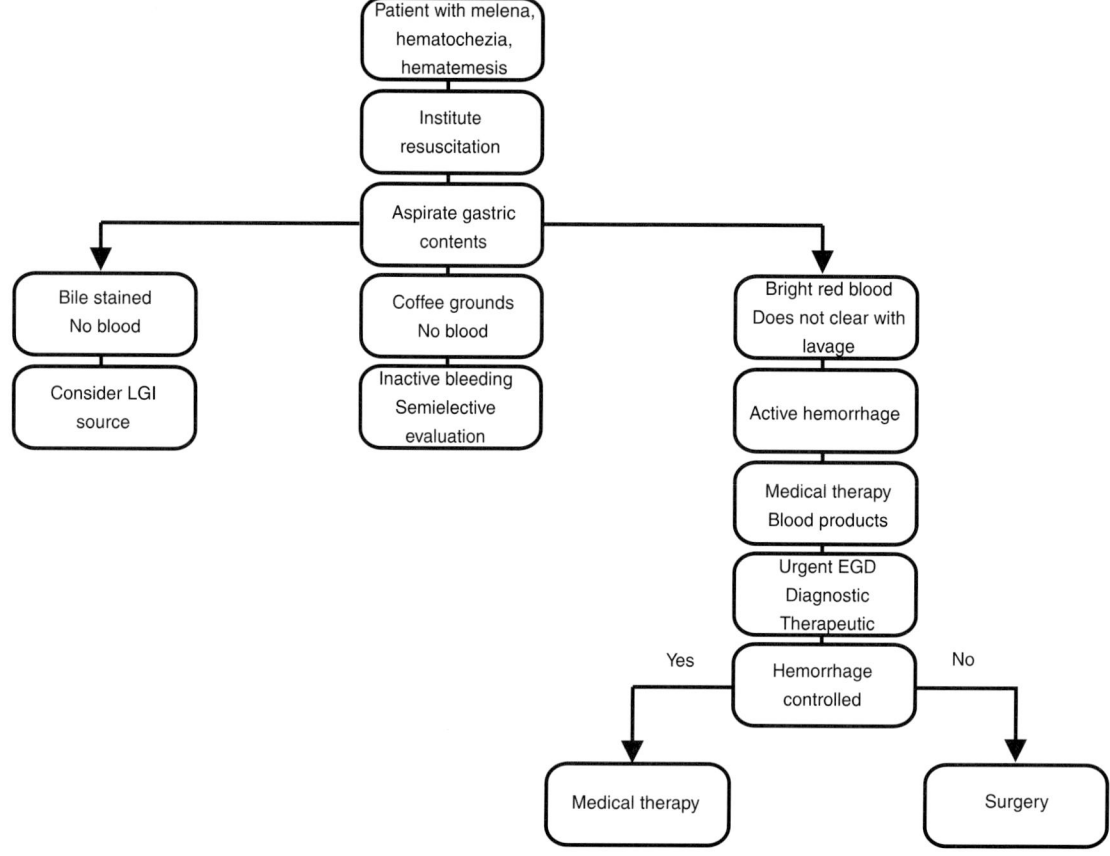

FIGURE 47–1. Management of bleeding with peptic ulcer disease.

characteristics allow the endoscopist to predict the likelihood of recurrent hemorrhage and need for intervention (see Table 47–1). If an actively bleeding ulcer is present on examination, spontaneous cessation of hemorrhage occurs in only 20% to 30% of cases. The presence of a nonbleeding visible vessel in an ulcer base indicates a rebleeding rate of 40% to 50%. The use of a Doppler probe allows for stratification of visible vessels into high and low risk based on the presence or absence of pulsatile flow.[4] The presence of adhering clot predicts a 20% chance of rebleeding, whereas a clear ulcer base is indicative of a rebleeding rate of less than 5%.[5]

MEDICAL MANAGEMENT

The tradition of using iced saline lavage as a means to control upper gastrointestinal tract hemorrhage is without scientific foundation. As mentioned previously, gastric lavage serves two primary functions; it allows the evaluation of the severity and activity of hemorrhage, and it permits cleansing of the stomach to facilitate an unobscured endoscopic evaluation. The use of lavage, iced or otherwise, in an attempt to stem active hemorrhage serves only to delay the institution of more effective therapeutic modalities.

Pharmacologic therapy of upper gastrointestinal tract hemorrhage attempts to control bleeding by either preventing dissolution of existing clot or by decreasing blood flow to the stomach and duodenum. Decreasing proteolytic activity in the stomach by decreasing acid secretion, increasing pH and thereby reducing the activity of pepsin remains the most common pharmacologic intervention used in the therapy of bleeding ulcers. H_2-receptor antagonists have traditionally filled this role and some experimental data support this practice.[6] The H^+-K^+ ATPase (proton pump) inhibitor omeprazole has also been used with impressive results.[7] In this study, 19 patients with upper gastrointestinal tract hemorrhage were treated with omeprazole, 20 were treated with ranitidine. Only three patients in the omeprazole group experienced recurrent hemor-

TABLE 47–1. ENDOSCOPIC FINDINGS AND ASSOCIATED RISK OF RECURRENT HEMORRHAGE

Endoscopic Characteristic	Risk of Continued/ Recurrent Hemorrhage
Active bleeding	80%
No bleeding vessel visible	40%–50%
Adhering clot	20%
Clear ulcer base	<5%

rhage compared with 17 in the ranitidine group. Unfortunately, a more recent and much larger double-blind, placebo-controlled trial failed to document any improvement in mortality, recurrent hemorrhage, and rates of emergent operation with omeprazole therapy.[8]

Tranexamic acid is an antifibrinolytic agent that has been studied in the setting of upper gastrointestinal tract hemorrhage. Two controlled, randomized studies failed to document any significant decrease in rates of recurrent hemorrhage between treatment and control groups.[9,10]

Decreasing splanchnic blood flow through the use of vasopressin or somatostatin in the setting of bleeding peptic ulcer has not been shown to significantly decrease rebleeding rates or otherwise significantly affect the clinical course of these patients.[11,12]

ENDOSCOPIC MANAGEMENT

The selective application of endoscopic hemostatic techniques has made a significant contribution to the management of patients with upper gastrointestinal tract hemorrhage. Whether it is performed as definitive therapy or as a temporizing measure allowing for adequate preoperative resuscitation, these methods have demonstrated potential for reducing morbidity and mortality. This form of therapy, however, should be reserved for those individuals who are either actively bleeding at the time of endoscopy or at high risk of recurrent hemorrhage based on clinical and endoscopic factors. A National Institutes of Health Consensus Conference held in 1989 confirmed this sentiment.[13] Currently accepted indications for therapeutic endoscopy are active bleeding on endoscopic evaluation, continuing rapid hemorrhage (clinically demonstrated by hematochezia, shock, or continuing transfusion requirement), recurrent hemorrhage in the hospital, and presence of a visible vessel or sentinel clot. Individuals over the age of 60 years and those with serious associated medical illnesses should be considered candidates for early intervention because of their higher risk status.

There are two primary forms of endoscopic hemostatic therapy available today: (1) thermal coagulation techniques and (2) injection techniques. Thermal techniques include monopolar and bipolar electrocautery, heater probes, and laser photocoagulation and are the most widely used methods in the United States. Injection therapy, which was developed to treat variceal hemorrhage, is now being applied to nonvariceal upper gastrointestinal tract hemorrhage with similar success.

Thermal techniques use a variety of heat sources to effect hemostasis by shrinkage and contraction of blood vessels, tissue desiccation, protein denaturation, and tissue edema. Conversion of electrical energy of varying frequencies provides the heat source for all these modalities.

Earliest attempts at hemostasis using thermal energy were made with monopolar cautery devices. These devices convert radio frequency electrical energy (1 million Hz) into heat by causing the current to flow from the electrode to a ground plate applied to the patient. The heat produced at the electrode contact site coagulates tissue, thereby effecting contraction and shrinkage of the responsible vessel wall. Energy is generally applied at multiple sites in a circumferential pattern to produce hemostasis. Controlled and uncontrolled studies of monopolar therapy for upper gastrointestinal tract hemorrhage have demonstrated successful initial hemostasis rates of approximately 80%.[14] Although effective, this technique is hampered by its rather imprecise application of thermal energy and the concomitant difficulty in predicting the depth of tissue injury.

Bipolar and multipolar electrocautery devices contain multiple electrodes at the tip of the instrument that serve as both energy source and ground. This arrangement allows for tangential application of heat energy around the bleeding site and a more shallow depth of tissue injury than that caused by monopolar devices. This device, like the heater probe, allows for application of direct pressure to the vessel thereby tamponading the hemorrhage and coapting the vessel walls. This allows for very efficient application of thermal energy while causing minimal injury to the immediately surrounding tissue. Studies evaluating this therapeutic modality in patients with active hemorrhage or a nonbleeding visible vessel in an ulcer indicate shorter hospitalizations, less frequent need for emergency surgery, and lower transfusion requirements compared with controls.[15]

Another method of endoscopic intervention is the use of a heater probe. With this instrument, no electrical energy is transferred directly to the target area. A low-frequency electrical current increases the temperature of a heating element contained within the probe itself. This heat energy is transferred to the target tissue through the probe covering to cause tissue coagulation. A benefit of this method of endoscopic hemostasis is that the probes are designed with a rounded tip, which allows for coaptation of the vessel prior to coagulation of vessel wall proteins. The heater probe can also be applied in a circumferential manner for larger lesions. Studies of the effectiveness of heater probe therapy in arresting upper gastrointestinal tract hemorrhage have demonstrated initial hemostasis rates of approximately 80% or greater.[16]

Laser photocoagulation is another endoscopic method of hemostasis which involves the transfer of heat energy. The efficacy of argon and Nd:YAG (neodymium:yttrium-aluminum-garnet) crystal lasers has been studied. The argon laser light has a wavelength of 500 nm. This energy is then absorbed primarily by red pigments, thus producing 1-mm depth of coagulation. The Nd:YAG laser emits light with a wavelength of 1060 nm, which is rather poorly absorbed by red pigments. The result is a greater depth of coagulation necrosis that can extend below the mucosa. Technical considerations dictate that the bleeding lesion must be addressed head on by the laser energy as tangential application can be dangerous, as well as ineffective. Therefore, this technique is somewhat limited when dealing with duodenal ulcers where the capability of maneuvering the scope is reduced. Nevertheless, recent evaluations of laser photocoagulation as a means of upper gastrointestinal tract hemostasis have demonstrated reduced rebleeding rates and mortality.[17]

The final endoscopic hemostatic modality to be discussed is injection therapy. Depending on the type and volume of solution used, the hemostatic effect arises from vasoconstriction, tissue sclerosis, or vessel tamponade. The various sclerosants include dehydrated alcohol, hypertonic saline, and polidocanol. The most commonly used vasoconstrictive agent is epinephrine. The various solutions are generally injected in three or four locations surrounding the bleeding lesion using a catheter or retractable needle. Because of the great variety of solutions used and injection schedules followed, comparison of many reported trials of sclerotherapy is difficult. The initial hemostasis rates reported using these techniques are generally in the 90% range with rebleeding rates comparable with those reported with thermal hemostatic methods (approximately 5% to 15%).[18]

SURGICAL MANAGEMENT

Although there has been a marked decline in the number of operations performed for peptic ulcer disease over the last decade, the number of emergent operations performed appears to have decreased only slightly.[19] This has been brought about through more effective medical therapy and the use of endoscopic hemostatic techniques which obviate the need for surgery in some patients and allow definitive resuscitation and semielective operative intervention in others.

As one might imagine, the indications for operative intervention vary based on available local resources. The time-honored criteria of operating when 6 U of packed cells have been transfused, continuous blood loss exceeding 1000 ml/d following stabilization, and rebleeding episode during the hospitalization period still apply when competent therapeutic endoscopy is unavailable. Patients with multiple medical problems and those greater than 60 years of age tolerate the stress of upper gastrointestinal tract hemorrhage poorly and operative intervention should be considered sooner rather than later. A more expeditious operation should also be considered in those patients who have had previous complications from peptic ulcer disease and in those patients with a rare blood type or antibodies that make cross-matching difficult.

When therapeutic endoscopy is available, active hemorrhage or stigmata indicative of a high risk of recurrence should be treated in an attempt to stabilize the patient. Once the patient is stabilized, a semielective surgical procedure should be considered. Should endoscopic methods fail to stop active hemorrhage or prevent recurrent hemorrhage, urgent operative intervention is indicated.

The operation performed for hemorrhage secondary to peptic ulcer disease depends primarily on the location of the ulcer and the clinical stability of the patient prior to, and during, surgery. The standard operative approach for a reasonably stable patient with a bleeding duodenal ulcer is to perform a longitudinal gastroduodenotomy over the ulcer site and oversew the ulcer. The incision is then closed transversely, effecting a pyloroplasty. A truncal or proximal gastric vagotomy is then typically performed prior to closure. An alternative operation is truncal vagotomy and antrectomy. Although associated with a slightly lower risk of recurrence, this procedure is also associated with a small increase in perioperative morbidity.

The treatment of choice for bleeding gastric ulcers is gastric resection, which includes the ulcer in the specimen. For ulcers located high in the stomach, local excision should be incorporated along with gastric resection, and an appropriate reconstruction should be performed. In cases where the ulcer cannot be excised, a thorough biopsy specimen should be taken from the ulcer bed and the margins prior to oversewing. Vagotomy is generally not performed if a sufficient portion of the stomach is resected.

PERFORATION

Although the incidence of peptic ulcer perforation appears to be decreasing, it remains a major cause of peptic ulcer disease morbidity and mortality. Most perforations occur in duodenal ulcers, although gastric ulcer perforations do occur and are generally associated with a higher mortality.

INITIAL MANAGEMENT AND ASSESSMENT

The diagnosis of perforated peptic ulcer is generally apparent based on the history and physical examination. A history consistent with chronic peptic ulcer disease can be elicited in approximately two thirds of patients with a perforated ulcer.[20] The patient will lie still on the gurney in a vain attempt to minimize what is typically described as an excruciating, stabbing abdominal pain. The patient can usually be quite specific regarding the time of onset and location of what is usually described as a sharp, piercing, or burning epigastric pain that can be localized with the tip of one finger. As peritonitis becomes more generalized, the patient will describe a more diffuse abdominal pain and demonstrate its location with his entire hand. On physical examination, the patient appears anxious, pale, and diaphoretic. Vital signs demonstrate tachycardia, and the patient may be hypotensive. The abdomen is rigid, and bowel sounds are usually absent. An upright chest x-ray examination will demonstrate free air under the diaphragm only 65% of the time, therefore lack of free air does not exclude this diagnosis.[21]

MEDICAL MANAGEMENT

While the medical management of patients with a perforated peptic ulcer usually consists of resuscitative measures taken in preparation for surgery, there does appear to be a limited role for the nonoperative therapy of this disease process. The traditional role of surgical intervention in perforated peptic ulcer disease was called into question in 1957 when 256 patients with perforated peptic ulcers were treated with nasogastric suction and fluid hydration. Of these patients, 80% sealed their perforations spontaneously and were spared laparotomy.[22] The mortality rate of 11% compared favorably with that of surgical closure at that time. More recently, a prospective randomized study comparing nonoperative management to immediate surgery and closure was performed.[23] Again, 70% of patients treated nonoperatively with antibiotics, H_2-receptor antagonists, nasogastric decompression, and intravenous fluid hydration were spared a laparotomy. Morbidity and mortality were equivalent for both groups, but the nonoperative patients required intensive observation by experienced surgeons and were hospitalized 1.5 times as long as the operative group. Criteria followed included pulse, temperature, abdominal examination, and the advance in general well-being of the patient. An upper gastrointestinal tract series using gastrografin was performed in 38 of 40 patients followed nonoperatively, and, interestingly enough, a demonstrated leak was not an absolute indication to take patients to the operating room provided their clinical status continued to improve. Elderly patients, in whom operative intervention is least desired, actually faired more poorly with nonoperative management.

These studies demonstrate just how resilient the human body can be in the face of caustic peritoneal soilage and that peritoneal cells may be effective in eliminating these toxins. It should be noted that the price paid for nonoperative management is a prolongation of the injury and rehabilitation phases of this disease process. It seems clear that going to this length to avoid operative intervention in anyone other than an individual who presents a prohibitive anesthetic risk is unwarranted given the recent availability of laparoscopic surgery (see below).

SURGICAL MANAGEMENT

The surgical evaluation and management of a patient with a perforated peptic ulcer revolves around three central issues. First to be considered is the overall clinical stability of the patient preoperatively and intraoperatively. The patient's capacity to tolerate an anesthetic and operation influences the surgeon's choice of procedure. Second to be considered is whether or not the patient has a history of chronic peptic ulcer disease for which a definitive procedure should be done in addition to closure of the perforation. The final issue to be considered is the level of experience of the surgeon and the ability of the surgeon to perform a safe, expeditious, definitive ulcer operation.

Patients who are in shock, have severe associated medical problems, or severe peritoneal sepsis should undergo as expeditious a procedure as possible. This would most typically consist of an omental patch and copious irrigation of the peritoneal cavity. These patients should then receive intravenous H_2-receptor antagonist in the immediate postoperative period to effect ulcer healing. If the presence of *H. pylori* in gastric biopsies is demonstrated, this infection should be cured. Alternatively, the patients should receive long-term oral prophylaxis with an H_2-receptor antagonist, as three quarters of these ulcers recur after discontinuation of this therapy.[24] Verification of the efficacy of this treatment in suppressing intragastric acid can then be done. These recommendations may have to be reconsidered in view of recent studies demonstrating that eradication of *H. pylori* appears effective in preventing ulcer relapse. The patient in good clinical condition, without a history of peptic ulcer disease should also undergo ulcer closure with the possible addition of a definitive ulcer-treating procedure. Most commonly, this would involve either an omental patch with proximal gastric vagotomy or vagotomy and pyloroplasty with excision of the ulcer incorporated into the pyloroplasty. Performed by competent surgeons in properly selected patients, these procedures add minimal morbidity to the operation and reduce the risks of recurrence from approximately 35% to 5%.[24]

There is little controversy that a definitive acid-reducing operation should be performed at the time of perforation closure in patients with a history consistent with chronic peptic ulcer disease. This assumes the patient is an appropriate anesthetic risk. Again omental patch and proximal gastric vagotomy is the most commonly favored procedure, other options include vagotomy and pyloroplasty or vagotomy and antrectomy, both of which would include excision of the ulcer if at all possible.

More recently, a laparoscopic approach has been described for the management of perforated peptic ulcer. The procedure includes an omental patch, anterior proximal gastric vagotomy, posterior truncal vagotomy, and copious peritoneal lavage.[25] As more surgeons become facile with laparoscopic techniques, this procedure will undoubtedly be applied more often.

PYLORIC STENOSIS

Pyloric stenosis remains a significant source of morbidity in patients with chronic peptic ulcer disease and occasionally occurs in patients with an acute ulcer. In the acute setting, the obstruction to gastric outflow is due to edema from the inflammatory processes surrounding the ulcer bed. In the chronic setting, the obstruction is usually due to a constricting scar and ongoing inflammation secondary to long-term injury.

INITIAL MANAGEMENT AND ASSESSMENT

Patients present with a well-defined history of symptoms consistent with acute or chronic peptic ulcer disease and progressively worsening symptoms of gastric outlet obstruction (i.e., satiety, nausea, bloating, vomiting, reflux). The findings on physical examination are generally nonspecific although in severe cases a markedly distended stomach can be delineated through percussion.

An easy way to confirm the diagnosis is with a saline loading test. The test is performed by instilling 750 ml of 0.9% saline into an empty stomach. After 30 minutes with the patient in an upright position, the patient's stomach is aspirated. Aspiration of greater than 400 ml of saline at this time is consistent with a diagnosis of gastric outlet obstruction. Specific diagnosis of gastric retention can be provided by intragastric or intraduodenal marker dilution techniques. A fractional emptying rate of less than 10%/min (= half-life of 6 minutes) after water or saline meals strongly suggests gastric retention.[26]

In advanced cases, laboratory evaluation may reveal a hypokalemic, hypochloremic metabolic alkalosis typically associated with repeated loss of gastric secretions. If the loss is prolonged and associated with hypovolemia, paradoxic aciduria may result.

Radiologic evaluation can be significant for a dilated gastric air bubble shown on upright films. An upper gastrointestinal tract series can accurately delineate the anatomic characteristics of the stenosis (i.e., degree of narrowing, length of stenosis, location of stenosis) although it does not necessarily correlate well with the functional degree of obstruction. This can best be evaluated by observing clearance of a solid nuclear meal over time with a gamma camera. A fractional emptying rate of less than 0.5%/min after a chicken liver meal is diagnostic of gastric retention.

Symptoms of gastric distension without retention of food may be observed in the presences of normal gastric emptying if there is gastric hypersecretion. This association was observed in atypical cases of the Zollinger-Ellison syndrome, in which symptoms of gastric distension completely disappeared after treatment with cimetidine.

Esophagogastroduodenoscopy is helpful in excluding a cancer as the cause of the obstruction and can allow for the placement of a guide wire through the area of stenosis. This wire can then be used for guiding a feeding tube or dilator through the lesion.

Medical Management

The medical therapy of pyloric stenosis secondary to peptic ulcer disease has two primary components. The first goal is to stop the continuing injury to the area of stenosis. This is usually accomplished with long-term administration of H_2-receptor antagonists, which is periodically punctuated by short-term omeprazole therapy for flaring episodes of peptic ulcer disease. The second goal is to promote gastric emptying. This can occasionally be accomplished through the addition of a prokinetic agent (i.e., metoclopramide or cisapride) but more commonly requires dilation of the stricture.

Dilation of esophageal strictures with metal olives or weighted bougie catheters has been practiced for several decades. These techniques, due to technical limitations, could not be successfully applied to strictures of the pylorus or gastroenterostomies on a wide-scale basis. Over the past 10 years, the availability of balloon dilation catheters that can be introduced through an endoscope has led to more widespread application of dilation to other areas of the intestinal tract (e.g., the pylorus, gastroenterostomies, enterocolostomies, and colonic strictures).

There is abundant evidence that through-the-scope balloon dilation of pyloric stenosis is safe and efficacious over a short period of time. Despite the fact that balloon dilation has been practiced for a decade, it is only very recently that intermediate or long-term assessment of its efficacy was evaluated. A recent retrospective review undertaken to determine long-term results of balloon dilation in patients with gastric outlet obstruction included 23 patients who were followed a mean of 31 months.[27] At completion of this study, 14 of 23 patients remained asymptomatic, although two of these patients required a second dilation at a subsequent nonspecified time interval. Four patients required surgical relief of their obstruction at a mean of 15 months; one patient required an emergency operation for perforation secondary to the dilation. No prospective, randomized trial comparing balloon dilation and acid suppression therapy with conventional surgical management has been reported.

The role of *H. pylori* in this complication of peptic ulcer is at present unknown.

Surgical Management

Patients unresponsive to medical therapy are referred for surgical intervention. Again, the aim of therapy is twofold: relieve the obstruction and treat the ulcer diathesis. Multiple factors are considered when determining the correct operation to perform. These factors include the length of the stricture, the amount of locoregional scarring and distortion of tissue planes, and the patient's general clinical status. Vagotomy with antrectomy remains the commonly accepted procedure of choice. It is recognized, however, that the amount of scarring may be so limited that a pyloroplasty can be performed without undue risk of breakdown. In these cases, vagotomy with pyloroplasty is a viable option. If the patient's clinical status precludes antrectomy and if a pyloroplasty is not possible, vagotomy and gastrojejunostomy should be performed. Recently, reports of a small number of patients managed with proximal gastric vagotomy and dilation have been published. As in the case of medical therapy and balloon dilation, no prospective evaluation of this technique has been performed, although short-term results in these small series are encouraging. This technique has the added attraction of being amenable to a laparoscopic approach, and this will no doubt be sufficient reason for some to adopt it as their standard approach. Until prospective randomized studies compare the various medical and surgical approaches for ulcer recurrence and reobstruction rates, the most cost-effective and efficacious means of treating this problem will remain unknown.

INTRACTABILITY AND RECURRENCE

Intractability of peptic ulcer disease is the most common reason for elective acid-reducing surgery. For purposes of this discussion, intractability is defined as incomplete healing of an ulcer in response to adequate medical or surgical therapy. It also includes those individuals who might initially have a complete response to therapy but who subsequently relapse following discontinuation of the medical regimen or after a surgical procedure.

INITIAL EVALUATION

After the diagnosis of peptic ulcer has been made and appropriate therapy instituted, approximately 90% of patients have a complete clinical response based on symptomatic improvement and documentation of ulcer healing. Those few patients who remain symptomatic or who have documented persistence of an ulcer after 2 to 3 months of medical therapy require further evaluation. Reasons for treatment failure are numerous and include patient noncompliance with prescribed treatment, cigarette smoking, basal acid hypersecretion, Zollinger-Ellison syndrome, *H. pylori* infection, use of nonsteroidal antiinflammatory drugs (NSAIDs), and malignancy. A combination of directed history, secretin-stimulated serum gastrin levels, gastric acid secretion studies, and multiple biopsies for culture, histologic examination, and urease testing is usually sufficient to eliminate these possibilities.

Recurrence of peptic ulcer disease after successful initial management is extremely frequent. Patients who receive no therapy after initial healing have a 70% to 80% chance of recurrence over 1 year. Initiation of a maintenance regimen after healing decreases relapse rates to the 20% range. No specific evaluation is required for a routine recurrent duodenal ulcer since this phenomenon is fairly commonplace. It is now believed that most of these recurrences are due to *H. pylori* infection,[24] as eradication of the bacterium reduces the relapse rate to less than 10% per year. Patients with exceptionally rapid or persistent relapse should be evaluated in a similar fashion as those patients with primary failure of therapy.

The recurrence rate of peptic ulcer disease following surgery varies based on the procedure performed. The currently popular proximal gastric vagotomy is associated with a recurrence rate of 10% to 15%. Recurrence following a vagotomy and antrectomy by comparison, is only about 1%.

The most common causes of recurrence following surgical therapy are incomplete vagotomy, insufficient resection of parietal cell mass, retained antrum, and gastrinoma. Depending on the initial operation performed, these possibilities can be evaluated with acid secretion studies, serum gastrin levels, upper gastrointestinal tract series, and endoscopy.

MEDICAL THERAPY

The medical therapy of patients who have an incomplete response to initial therapy should be tailored to the individual patient based on the results of the evaluation outlined above. If this evaluation suggests that acid suppression is incomplete, the type or dose of H_2-receptor antagonist can be increased or the patient can receive a more potent inhibitor of acid secretion (e.g., omeprazole). If cultures, histologic examination, or urease testing suggests *H. pylori* colonization, appropriate antibiotic therapy should be instituted.

A great deal at attention has been paid to the role of *H. pylori* in the pathogenesis of peptic ulcer disease, especially that of the duodenum. This is somewhat of a paradox since it is well recognized that this organism typically colonizes gastric-type epithelium preferentially. Recently it has become apparent that patients with duodenal ulcers have patches of gastric metaplasia in the duodenum. It seems that this gastric metaplasia is present in more than 90% of patients with duodenal ulcers and that in 50% of cases these patches are colonized with *H. pylori*.[28] Gastric metaplasia of the duodenum has been induced in animals by chronic stimulation of gastric acid secretion and has been noted to be associated with acid hypersecretion in humans.[29] Once present, the *H. pylori* may aggravate injury through local inflammatory effects or toxins, which serve to decrease mucosal defenses. Whatever the mechanism involved, it has been clearly demonstrated that eradication of *H. pylori* with standard triple therapy (bismuth, tetracycline, metronidazole) or amoxicillin and metronidazole can markedly improve healing rates and decrease relapse rates in patients with refractory peptic ulcer disease.[24,30]

SURGICAL THERAPY

There may be as many opinions regarding the actual time at which medical therapy has failed as there are gastroenterologists and patients. This would seem to be appropriate in light of the fact that intensive medical regimens affect varying lifestyles differently. This determination is also influenced by the quantity and quality of surgical support available. Surgery becomes a viable option when, at some point in time, the gastroenterologist has exhausted available therapies and either the patient's symptoms or the medical regimen is perceived as interfering sufficiently with his lifestyle.

The goal of surgical intervention in intractable peptic ulcer disease is to eliminate the ulcer diathesis, minimize the mortality associated with the procedure, and minimize the alterations in gastrointestinal tract function that can sometimes result from these procedures. No one procedure satisfies all these criteria, and hence the surgeon must have a repertoire of several procedures from which to choose the one most applicable to each patient.

The most popular procedure done currently is the proximal gastric vagotomy. The reasons for its popularity include a near-zero mortality and minimal effects on postoperative gastric emptying. Its shortcoming is a 10% to 15% incidence of ulcer recurrence.

Truncal vagotomy with pyloroplasty also is associated with a 10% to 15% incidence of ulcer recurrence. Other shortcomings included unregulated gastric emptying predisposing to dumping syndrome, loss of pyloric function resulting in duodenogastric reflux, and denervation of the hepatobiliary tract, pancreas, and small intestine. Mortality is usually quoted as 0.5% to 1.0%.

Vagotomy with antrectomy is associated with the lowest rate of recurrence of any of the more commonly performed antiulcer procedures. This risk is usually described as being in the 1% range. Unfortunately, this procedure is associated with a close to 30% incidence of significant postoperative side effects, which may be as capable of detracting from the patient's quality of life as the original peptic ulcer disease.

Recent advances in laparoscopic techniques have made minimally invasive antiulcer surgery a reality. The best-known technique involves performing an anterior proximal gastric vagotomy or seromyotomy in combination with a posterior truncal vagotomy. Preliminary results are encouraging in terms of reduction in gastric acid output. Further study is necessary before these laparoscopic procedures become a standard of care.

Peptic ulcer disease that recurs following surgery is sometime amenable to medical management, but more often than not, a second procedure is required. The procedure should be selected on the basis of the patient's evaluation and the nature of the primary procedure. In general, operative recurrences are treated by the next highest effective procedure. For instance, recurrence following proximal gastric vagotomy should be treated with truncal vagotomy and a drainage procedure (either pyloroplasty or antrectomy); recurrence following a vagotomy and antrectomy should be treated with a subtotal gastrectomy. This reasoning assumes that the original procedures were correctly performed. If gastric acid secretion tests indicate that an incomplete vagotomy is the source of the recurrence, a completion vagotomy is an acceptable second procedure. This can be done through either an abdominal or thoracic approach.

The role of *H. pylori* in postoperative recurrence of peptic ulcer is currently unclear.

GENERAL CONCLUSIONS

The introduction of new medical and surgical therapies for the treatment of peptic ulcer disease has revolutionized its treatment during the past 15 years. In addition, it is now generally agreed that the vast majority of peptic ulcers are associated with, and probably caused by, *H. pylori*. The novel therapeutic approaches that are currently being developed are likely to provide safer and more effective treatment for this condition. However, eradication of this bacterium remains difficult in some patients, and resistant strains have recently emerged. This concern may be tempered somewhat by the knowledge that multiple antibiotic regimens of equivalent efficacy have been reported in the literature. Finally, the role of NSAIDs in the production of these complications remains unclear, although it is probably important. Therefore, it will take some time before one can determine whether there will be a significant decrease in the complications of peptic ulcer disease that have been described in this chapter. Only well-controlled, double-blind studies will permit a definition of the best treatment(s) for this important cause of morbidity, mortality, and economic losses to our nation.

REFERENCES

1. Graham DY. Complications of peptic ulcer disease and indications for surgery. In: Sleisenger MH, Fordtran JS, eds. *Gastrointestinal Disease: Pathophysiology, Diagnosis, Management.* 4th ed. Philadelphia, Pa: WB Saunders Co; 1989:925–938.
2. Silverstein FE, Gilbert DA, Tedesco FJ, et al. The national ASGE survey on upper gastrointestinal bleeding,

II: clinical prognostic factors. *Gastrointest Endosc.* 1981; 27:80–93.
3. Larson G, Schmidt T, Gott J, et al. Upper gastrointestinal bleeding: predictors of outcome. *Surgery.* 1986;100: 765–773.
4. Fullarton GM, Murray WR. Prediction of rebleeding in peptic ulcers by visual stigmata and endoscopic Doppler criteria. *Endoscopy.* 1990;22:68–71.
5. Chojkier M, Laine L, Conn HO, et al. Predictors of outcome in massive upper gastrointestinal hemorrhage. *J Clin Gastroenterol.* 1986;8:16–22.
6. Collins R, Langman M. Treatment with histamine H_2 antagonists in acute upper gastrointestinal hemorrhage: implications of randomized trials. *N Engl J Med.* 1985; 313:660–666.
7. Brunner G, Chang J. Intravenous therapy with high doses of ranitidine and omeprazole in critically ill patients with bleeding peptic ulcerations of the upper intestinal tract: an open randomized trial. *Digestion.* 1990; 45:217–225.
8. Daneshmend TK, Hawkey CJ, Langman MJ, et al. Omeprazole versus placebo for acute upper gastrointestinal bleeding: randomised double blind control trial. *Br Med J.* 1992;304:143–147.
9. Barer D, Ogilvie A, Henry D, et al. Cimetidine and tranexamic acid in the treatment of acute upper gastrointestinal tract bleeding. *N Engl J Med.* 1983;308:1571–1575.
10. Holstein CCS, Eriksson SBS, Kallen R. Tranexamic acid as an aid to reducing blood transfusion requirements in gastric and duodenal bleeding. *Br Med J.* 1987;294: 44–50.
11. Magnusson I, Ihre T, Johansson C, et al. Randomized double blind trial of somatostatin in the treatment of massive upper gastrointestinal haemorrhage. *Gut.* 1985; 26:221–226.
12. Stump DL, Hardin TC. The use of vasopressin in the treatment of upper gastrointestinal haemorrhage. *Drugs.* 1990;39:38–53.
13. Consensus Conference: Therapeutic endoscopy and bleeding ulcers. *JAMA.* 1989;262:1369–1372.
14. Papp JP. Monopolar and electrohydrothermal treatment of upper gastrointestinal bleeding. *Gastrointest Endosc.* 1990;36:S34–S37.
15. Laine L. Multipolar electrocoagulation in the treatment of peptic ulcers with nonbleeding visible vessels: a prospective controlled trial. *Ann Intern Med.* 1989;110:510–514.
16. Fullarton GM, Birnie GG, Macdonald A, et al. Controlled trial of heater probe treatment in bleeding peptic ulcers. *Br J Surg.* 1989;76:541–544.
17. Matthewson K, Swain CP, Bland M, et al. Randomized comparison of Nd:YAG laser, heater probe, and no endoscopic therapy for bleeding peptic ulcers. *Gastroenterology.* 1990;98:1239–1244.
18. Chen PC, Wu CS, Leaw YF. Hemostatic effect of endoscopic local injection with hypertonic saline-epinephrine solution and pure ethanol for digestive tract bleeding. *Gastrointest Endosc.* 1986;32:319–323.
19. Gustavsson S, Kelly KA, Melton LJ, et al. Trends in peptic ulcer surgery. *Gastroenterology.* 1988;94:688–694.
20. Friedman F. Peptic ulcer disease. *Clin Symp.* 1988;40(5): 1–32.
21. Gunshefski L, Flancbaum L, Brolin RE, et al. Changing patterns in perforated peptic ulcer disease. *Am Surg.* 1990;56:270–274.
22. Taylor H. The nonsurgical treatment of perforated peptic ulcer. *Gastroenterology.* 1957;33:353–368.
23. Crofts TJ, Park KGM, Steele RJC, et al. A randomized trial of nonoperative treatment for perforated peptic ulcer. *N Engl J Med.* 1989;320:970–973.
24. Jordan PH Jr. Surgery for peptic ulcer disease. *Curr Probl Surg.* 1991;28(4):267–322.
25. Tate JJ, Dawson JW, Lay WY, Li AK. Sutureless laparoscopic treatment of perforated duodenal ulcer. *Br J Surg.* 1993;80:235.
26. Dubois A, Price SF, Castell DO. Gastric retention in duodenal ulcer disease, a reappraisal. *Am J Dig Dis.* 1978;23:993–997.
27. Kozarek RA, Botoman VA, Patterson DJ. Long-term follow-up in patients who have undergone balloon dilation for gastric outlet obstruction. *Gastrointest Endosc.* 1990;36:558–561.
28. Fitzgibbons PL, Dooley CP, Cohen H, Appleman MD. Prevalence of gastric metaplasia, inflammation and *Campylobacter pylori* in the duodenum of members of a normal population. *Am J Clin Pathol.* 1988;90:711–714.
29. Rhodes J. Experimental production of gastric epithelium in the duodenum. *Gut.* 1964;5:454–458.
30. Rauws EA, Tytgat GNJ. Cure of duodenal ulcer associated with eradication of *Helicobacter pylori*. *Lancet.* 1990;335:1233–1235.

48

Surgery for Peptic Ulcer Disease: For Whom and When

DANNY O. JACOBS and JAMES M. BECKER

Peptic ulceration is thought to occur when the complex balance between ulcerogenic and protective factors is disturbed. Examples of protective factors include mucous secretions, blood flow, bicarbonate production, and various prostaglandins. Recognized aggressive factors are, for example, smoking, alcohol, stress, family history, nonsteroidal antiinflammatory drugs, and most recently the presence of *Helicobacter pylori*.

Current treatment modalities emphasize the restoration of the balance between these naturally occurring forces. Both duodenal and gastric ulcers have a cyclical natural history with spontaneous healing and recurrence rates that may be highly variable. At least half the recurrences are symptomatic. However, introduction of new medications to decrease intragastric acidity, neutralize or suppress acid production, and enhance the protective and restorative properties of the gastric and duodenal mucosa, as well as apparent changes in disease incidence, have altered the profile of patients who require surgical intervention. Nevertheless, the **basic indications for surgery** are unchanged and fall under four broad headings:

1. Intractability or failure of medical therapy
2. Uncontrollable, unrelenting hemorrhage
3. Perforation
4. Obstruction

After a brief consideration of pertinent surgical anatomy and physiology, this chapter reviews the indications for and timing of operative intervention in patients who have peptic ulcer disease. In addition, recent recommendations regarding the types of operation that should be performed for patients with ulcer disease are reviewed.

SURGICAL ANATOMY

The stomach has a very generous blood supply. The right gastric artery, which is usually a branch of the hepatic artery and the left gastric artery, which is typically a direct branch off the celiac axis, form a vascular arcade along the lesser curvature of the stomach. Other branches of the celiac axis include the splenic and common hepatic arteries. The right gastroepiploic artery, arising from the gastroduodenal artery, and the left gastroepiploic artery, which is a branch of the splenic artery, form a second vascular arcade along the distal two thirds of the greater curvature of the stomach. The proximal portion of the greater curvature receives its blood supply from short gastric vessels which originate from the left gastroepiploic and splenic arteries. The blood supply of the duodenum is derived in large part from the anterior and posterior pancreaticoduodenal arteries. The anterior pancreaticoduodenal artery usually branches from the gastroduodenal artery, whereas the posterior pancreaticoduodenal artery most typically originates from the superior mesenteric artery.

Any one of the four major vessels feeding the stomach, either the left or right gastric arteries or the left or right gastroepiploic arteries, is capable of maintaining the viability of the organ. However, in extensive gastric resection where all four major vessels are ligated, necrosis of the gastric remnant is possible. The blood supply of the duodenum is far more tenuous. Injury to the main branch of the gastroduodenal artery, for example, may put this portion of the intestine at risk for loss of viability (Fig. 48–1*A*).

Both parasympathetic and sympathetic nerves innervate the stomach. The vagus nerves moderate acid secretion and gastric motility through

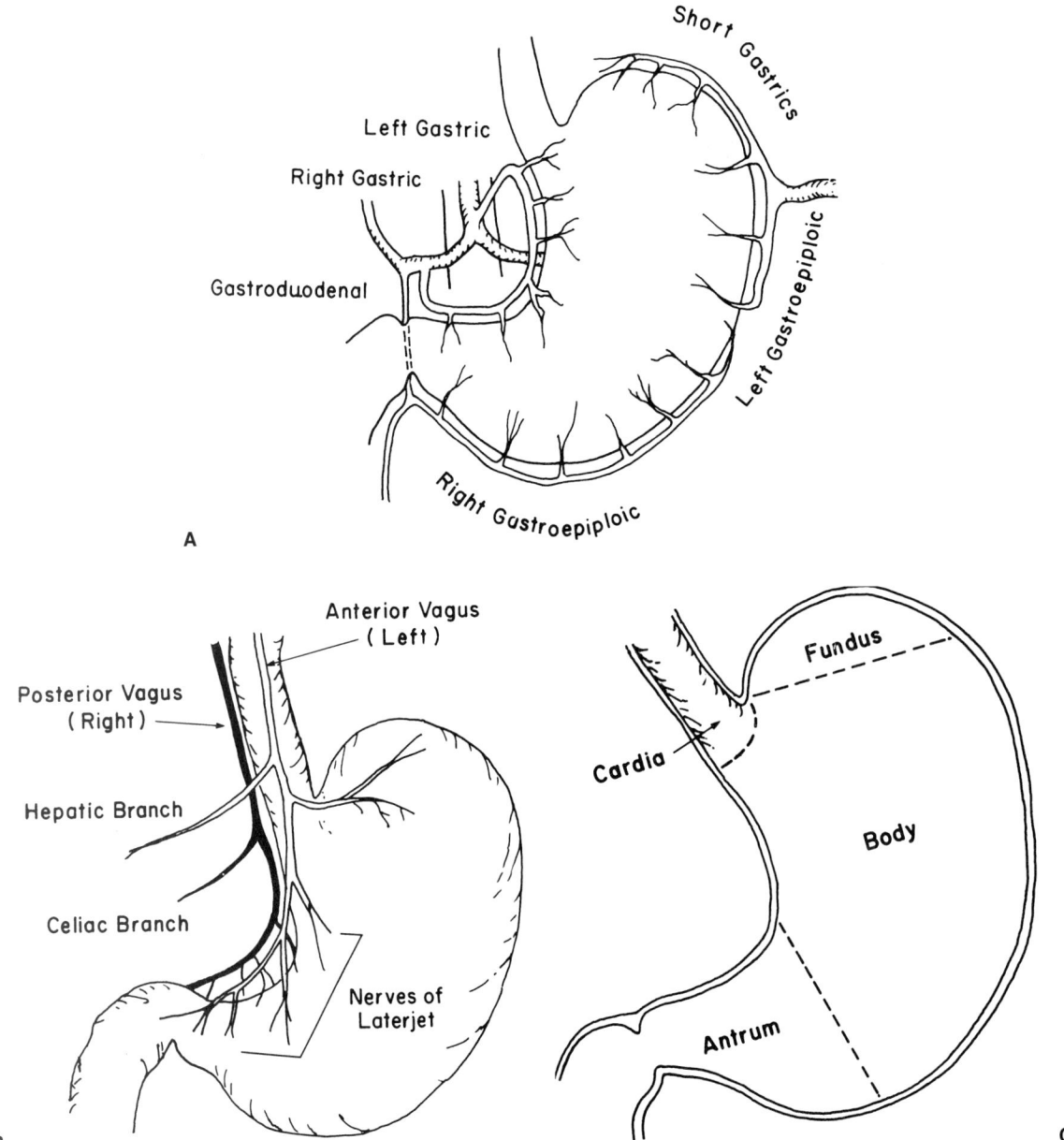

FIGURE 48–1. A, Vessels that maintain blood supply to the stomach. B, Nerves that innervate the stomach. C, Divisions of the stomach.

the actions of their efferent fibers. The anterior or left vagus nerve passes through the esophageal hiatus anterior to the esophagus and subsequently divides into hepatic and gastric branches. Some of the gastric efferents innervate the anterior aspect of the lesser curvature of the stomach. These nerves are known as the anterior nerves of Laterjet. The posterior or right vagus nerve runs posterior to the esophagus in the adventitial space near the aorta. This vagal trunk divides into a celiac branch, which ultimately supplies the small bowel and the pancreas. However, branches of this nerve also supply the posterior aspect of the lesser curve of the stomach as the posterior nerves of Laterjet. The anterior and posterior nerves of Laterjet give off branches in the fundus and body of the stomach before they terminate in the antrum (Fig. 48–1B).

The stomach is typically divided into the cardia, fundus, body, and the antrum (Fig. 48–1C). The pylorus identifies the junction between the stomach and the duodenum. The proximal two thirds of the stomach contains the fundic glands, which secrete acid and pepsin in response to ingested food. The distal third of the stomach, represented by the antrum, is responsible for food mixing and propulsion, and it contains the mucosal G cells, which produce gastrin.

INCIDENCE

Peptic ulcer disease affects between 5% and 10% of Americans during their lifetime.[1] The annual incidence is about 1.6%, i.e., 4 million ulcers per year. Important risk factors include cigarette smoking, which is especially implicated in ulcer recurrences and retardation of ulcer healing, and the use of salicylates, steroids, and nonsteroidal antiinflammatory agents.

The number of elective surgical operations performed for peptic ulcer disease worldwide has decreased from a rate of 72.1 per 100,000 citizens in 1956 to a low of 10.7 elective cases per 100,000 in 1986.[2] Whereas, previously, ulcer disease was approximately four times more common in men than in women, recently the ratio has approached equality for the two sexes (being approximately 1.5:1). However, the ratio of duodenal to gastric ulcer disease has not changed. The rate of operation for complications is also smaller. In Sweden, the frequency of operation for perforation has decreased by approximately 50%, from 12.8 to 6.4 operations for each 100,000 inhabitants. The dramatic decline in elective operations for peptic ulcer began long before the introduction of modern fiberoptic endoscopy or H_2-receptor antagonists. This reduction in the number of elective and emergency procedures suggests that the incidence and/or the severity of peptic ulcer disease has truly changed.

Nevertheless, other data suggest that the decline in elective surgery for peptic ulcer disease can be at least partially attributed to the use of H_2-receptor antagonists. In Helsinki, during the last decade,[3] the introduction of these drugs was associated with a fall in the annual incidence of elective duodenal ulcer operations from 15.5 to 6.7 per 100,000 and a fall in the annual incidence of elective gastric ulcer operations from 9.4 to 3.1 per 100,000 subjects. The decrease was greatest among men with duodenal ulcers. In contrast, the incidence of emergency surgical operations for hemorrhage or perforation complicating ulcer disease remained relatively stable, between 7.2 and 10.2 per 100,000 patients.

A similar pattern has been observed in the United States where the number of admissions for peptic ulcer disease decreased by 39.3% after the introduction of H_2 blockers.[4] The number of operations performed has decreased by approximately 20% with the greatest decline being in the number of operations performed for duodenal ulcer. The number of emergency operations performed for massive unrelenting hemorrhage or acute perforation and the number of deaths from operation have remained essentially constant. The mean age of patients undergoing elective operation has not changed, but the age of patients undergoing emergency operation has increased.

Another factor that likely has contributed to the decreased overall incidence of peptic ulcer disease is the decreased prevalence of smoking. In contrast, increased use of nonsteroidal antiinflammatory drugs has increased the incidence of ulceration in the older population. Serious complications from the use of these drugs, such as perforation and bleeding, have been observed, especially in older women.[5]

GASTRIC ULCERS

Gastric ulcers are a heterogeneous group of disorders that appear to have a variety of pathophysiologic associations. They are usually divided into three categories for convenience and to facilitate decision making as regards surgical correction. Type I ulcers are the most common, accounting for 60% of all cases. They can occur anywhere in the stomach proximal to the antrum. However, they are most commonly located along the lesser curvature and, as demonstrated by immunohistochemical mapping, are identified most frequently at the interface between antral and corporal mucosa. Type II gastric ulcers are associated with concomitant duodenal ulcers, which occur in about 40% of patients, especially when the gastric ulcer occurs in close proximity to the pylorus. The associated duodenal ulcer usually points to the benign nature of the gastric ulcer and does not appear to affect its rate of healing. Patients with pyloric channel ulcers usually do poorly while receiving medical therapy; most will require surgical correction. Type III ulcers are the so-called *prepyloric ulcers*. Like duodenal ulcers, they may be associated with extremely high levels of gastric acid output as a primary etiologic factor.

The pathogenesis of gastric ulcers is unclear and somewhat arbitrary except perhaps for type II ulcerations where it is clearer. Type II ulcers are closely related to duodenal ulcers clinically in the sense that they respond to surgical treatment much like duodenal ulcers and should be approached similarly. This similarity in pathophysiology is borne out by studies which have shown that patients with pyloric or prepyloric ulcers treated by antrectomy and Billroth I gastroduodenostomy without vagotomy have a 30% chance of recurrence, whereas the inclusion of truncal vagotomy with antrectomy significantly reduces the recurrence rate for this particular disease entity.

Because roentgenographic findings are often incorrect, endoscopy has become the mainstay in the diagnosis of gastric ulcers. Ulcers larger than 2 cm in diameter have a greater chance of being malignant. In a series of 153,000 endoscopies, only 37 (0.024%) revealed carcinoma within the ulcer when the study was performed for duodenal ulcer disease.[6] However, because 5% to 10% of gastric ulcers are malignant, every gastric ulcer should be subjected to endoscopic biopsy. Lastly, many gastric ulcers that harbor a malignant lesion may heal, emphasizing the point that, even after gastric ulcers heal, they should be subjected to routine follow-up endoscopy and biopsy.

The selection of patients for therapy is based on three factors:

1. The natural history of the disease
2. The effectiveness of therapy
3. The cost

The goals of therapy are control of symptoms, healing of the ulcer, and prevention of recurrence and complications. Spontaneous healing may occur in 50% of patients with gastric ulcers, but ulceration may recur in the other 50% within the first year; 80% may recur on a long-term basis. Ten percent of patients with gastric ulcers have complications largely consisting of bleeding, perforation, or stenosis. Whereas it is widely accepted that medical therapy is effective, especially in terms of relieving symptoms, the natural history, in fact, may not be affected at all. Recurrences may be prevented by continuous prophylaxis, but no reduction in the rate of complications has been achieved by this modality.

Nevertheless, the initial management of a gastric ulcer, once a malignant lesion is definitively excluded, is medical. Treatment should consist of an appropriate H_2-receptor antagonist such as ranitidine for at least 6 to 8 weeks of therapy. Antacids and sucralfate are typically not combined, because such therapy is more expensive and is not more efficacious than either agent used alone if they are taken properly. Although medical therapy is likely to be more successful when the patient is hospitalized, in-hospital treatment is largely impractical. The patient should be encouraged to stop smoking and to omit salicylates and nonsteroidal antiinflammatory drugs. Once the ulcer has healed, and repeat endoscopy has confirmed this finding in the absence of malignant change, H_2-receptor blockers may be used prophylactically to prevent ulcer recurrence.

However, as mentioned previously, gastric ulcers recur almost 50% of the time, usually within the first 6 months of treatment. They recur in older patients with chronic medical illnesses or because of the continuing use of antiinflammatory agents. Age, in particular, appears to affect recurrence; the patient's sex and the size or position of the ulcer do not. Gastric acid output or hemorrhage similarly do not appear to affect the rate of ulcer recurrence. When carefully managed, recurrent ulcers heal at the same rate as the initial ulcer on appropriate medical therapy. Coexisting duodenal ulcers may occur in up to 40% of patients, especially when the ulcer is distal to the incisura. An associated duodenal ulcer usually points to the benign nature of the gastric ulcer, but it does not appear to affect healing when managed appropriately.

Thus, for medical therapy to be an adequate alternative to surgical treatment of recurrent ulcers, the drug used for treatment must be effective, safe, and inexpensive, and patient compliance must be good. There are **five indications for surgical therapy for gastric ulcer:**

1. Failure of the ulcer to heal after 3 months of effective H_2-receptor antagonist therapy
2. Poor long-term control, especially of recurrent ulcers, many of which may be asymptomatic
3. Poor compliance with medical therapy or significant side effects from the drugs
4. Complications such as perforation, hemorrhage, or fibrosis
5. Dysplasia or carcinoma within the ulcer

The Billroth I operation (gastric resection with direct anastomosis to the duodenum) is curative in more than 95% of gastric ulcers, with minimal major morbidity. Furthermore, this form of reconstruction has late metabolic advantages (better fat, iron, and calcium absorption) as compared with the Billroth II reconstruction where the duodenum is closed and the stomach is anastomosed to the jejunum. For these reasons, the Billroth I reconstruction should be preferentially used following gastric resection if the duodenum is usable, which it usually is in type I gastric ulcers. For type II ulcers, vagotomy may be required to decrease acid production satisfactorily. Type III, prepyloric ulcers are often treated like duodenal ulcers, largely because of the extremely high acid production occurring in such instances and because these ulcers often extend into the duodenal mucosa.

The management of high-lying gastric ulcers poses a particular challenge for surgical management. When assessing operations for high-lying gastric ulcers close to the gastroesophageal junction, the morbidity and mortality, recurrence rate, and side effects of the operation are especially pertinent. In this situation, a generous distal gastrectomy is performed in combination with a freehand excision along the lesser curvature to incorporate the ulcer at the juxtaesophageal position. Closure is then accomplished as a standard Billroth I operation. This procedure can be used to successfully manage patients with this difficult problem with minimal postoperative morbidity and mortality and a low recurrence rate.[7]

BLEEDING

The initial management of patients with active gastrointestinal tract hemorrhage should include both diagnostic and therapeutic maneuvers. On presentation, the primary goals are to diagnose, to localize the site of bleeding, and to determine the extent and activity of hemorrhage. Volume resuscitation should occur concomitantly as the patient undergoes various diagnostic and therapeutic maneuvers. In the event of massive life-threatening bleeding, prompt operative intervention is needed. If urgent operative intervention is not required, then upper gastrointestinal tract endoscopy can be performed. Definition of the precise appearance and location of the ulcer or other source of bleeding by endoscopy gives important information about the risk of rebleeding and the indications for surgery. In some instances injection therapy with vasoconstrictors or sclerosing agents may be successfully used to treat the source.[8] Rebleeding rates are approximately twice as high for ulcers greater than 1 cm in diameter as compared with those smaller in size (12% versus 25%).[9] In addition, patients who have stigmata of recent hemorrhage on endoscopic examination are three times as likely to rebleed.

Angiography may be used in those instances where the source of bleeding remains unclear after endoscopy is performed and will likely be successful if the rate of bleeding is between 0.5 and 2 ml/min. It may also be useful in patients with gastritis who are hemorrhaging diffusely from the gastric mucosa. In this instance intra-arterial vasopressin may successfully control bleeding. Alternatively, if bleeding is occurring from a specific site, selective embolization of the bleeding vessel may be used to obtain vascular control. However, selective embolization techniques risk peripheral embolization to major organs such as the liver, as well as ischemic necrosis of neighboring tissues that could ultimately result in perforation. Acute gastroduodenal hemorrhage (or perforation) that occurs in the postoperative period is usually caused by underlying chronic peptic ulcer disease or the use of ulcerogenic drugs.[10] True stress gastritis or ulceration that requires operation is a rare event.

Occasionally, scanning of technetium-labeled red blood cells is used in an effort to identify the source of upper (or lower) gastrointestinal tract bleeding. The technique is very sensitive and can detect as little bleeding as 0.1 ml/min. However, it may not accurately demonstrate the exact source of bleeding.

In the majority of patients, upper gastrointestinal tract bleeding does stop. However, when operative intervention is required for patients with massive life-threatening hemorrhage, it is both diagnostic and therapeutic. A general rule of thumb is that operative management is needed for patients with persistent or repeated episodes of bleeding who have required transfusion of 4 or 5 U of blood. However, rebleeding alone is associated with an increased risk of mortality.[9] Elderly patients, patients with gastric ulcers or chronic duodenal ulcers, or patients who have a visible vessel in the base of the ulcer on endoscopy are most likely to bleed uncontrollably and require early operative intervention. In patients who are older than 60 years, hypotension on admission is associated with an increased risk of death. Ulcers larger than 1 cm in diameter occur more frequently in these individuals and carry an increased risk of rebleeding and mortality.[11]

The aim of surgery is first to control the site or active sites of hemorrhage and thereafter to control the release of gastric acid. Ligation of the bleeding point alone, in the absence of diffuse gastritis, is an unreliable method of managing patients with gastrointestinal tract bleeding because it is associated with a high rate of recurrence. Ideally, the situation is managed by ligating the bleeding vessel, usually a branch of the gastroduodenal artery, proximally and distally, closing the duodenal stump, resecting the antrum, and performing a truncal vagotomy. Intestinal continuity is restored by gastrojejunostomy. This is an extensive operation used infrequently for unstable, high-risk patients. Ligation combined with pyloroplasty and vagotomy may also provide satisfactory results in critically ill patients who will not be able to tolerate the more extensive procedure, even though the rate of early recurrent hemorrhage with this procedure is higher. Proximal gastric vagotomy may also be performed as primary surgical treatment for patients with bleeding duodenal ulcer disease with a low risk of mortality or morbidity and acceptable recurrence rates ($\sim$12%).[12] However, considerable experience is required for this procedure. Because of the usual length of the operation, it should be restricted to low-risk, hemodynamically stable patients.

ZOLLINGER-ELLISON SYNDROME

Patients with gastrinomas may present with a broad range of symptoms. Besides chronic peptic ulcer, diarrhea and acid-induced esophagitis may also be presenting findings. Once the diagnosis is confirmed, tumor localization is critically important in identifying patients with localized disease who are potentially curable.[13] Preoperative evaluation using computerized tomography and intravenous contrast or other imaging modalities are often helpful. Exploratory laparotomy is indicated for all patients who do not have evidence of metastatic disease after preoperative evaluation. At operation, the abdomen is carefully examined, including the duodenum. Intraoperative ultrasound and intraoperative endoscopy with transillumination of the duodenal wall are frequently helpful in localizing the lesions. Approximately 20% of patients with the syndrome can be cured using this approach. For patients with unresectable disease, the H^+-K^+ ATPase inhibitor omeprazole is highly effective in controlling symptoms related to the hypersecretion of gastric acid.

PERFORATION

Once the diagnosis of perforated viscus is made, a decision must be made whether or not to operate. This decision-making process may be quite difficult and is somewhat controversial. In patients who are diagnosed as having a gastrointestinal perforation, most surgeons would advocate prompt operation as soon as the patient is maximally prepared. The efficacy of nonoperative management has been debated since most reports of its use have not been randomized trials. Rather, these studies have often included high proportions of elderly, seriously ill patients. Nonoperative management would not seem to be the treatment of choice for patients whose premorbid health was good, nor should this management technique be expected to significantly improve outcome in patients who are morbidly ill at the time of diagnosis. The critical decision point is whether sealing of the perforation can be reasonably and accurately determined. In a recent investigation, Berne and Donovan reported their experience with the nonoperative treatment of perforated ulcer.[11] This treatment modality was employed in 12% of 294 patients with perforated duodenal, pyloric channel, or prepyloric ulcers who ranged from 19 to 62 years of age (mean 34.9 years). These patients were treated with intravenous fluids, broad spectrum antibiotics, nasogastric suction, and H_2 blockers. Upper gastrointestinal tract radiographs using water-soluble media were used to determine which ulcers were leaking and which had sealed spontaneously. This concept of self-sealing is critical to the successful implementation of nonoperative management. The mean hospital stay was 7.9 ± 3.3 days for these patients, and their mortality was not significantly different from those patients who were managed operatively. Thus, in the best circumstances, when sealing of the ulcer perforation can be conclusively and unequivocally demonstrated, nonoperative management can be successfully employed. However, one must question the rationale for nonoperative management in patients who are good operative risks and who are diagnosed early, especially given the likelihood that a definitive surgical procedure may be needed to control their disease if the ulcer diathesis is long-standing. In some series of patients with acute ulcers, as many as 75% have no further ulcer symptoms after simple closure of the perforation. In the case of chronic ulcers, it is the reverse; 75% of patients have subsequent ulcer symptoms following simple closure.

Most patients with perforated duodenal ulcer are treated by simple closure of the perforation alone or in combination with primary definitive operation. The major controversy concerning treatment of perforated ulcer is which of these two methods is best. Surgeons who prefer definitive therapy usually reserve this form of therapy for patients with "chronic" ulcers and simple closure for those with "acute" ulcers. A definitive operation not only takes care of the immediate problem of perforation, but also provides protection against the occurrence of further ulcer disease. Unfortunately, the differentiation between acute and chronic ulcers cannot always be made easily. There is no satisfactory way at the time of perforation to select precisely those patients who will eventually require or benefit from definitive therapy. Previous ulcer symptoms and the presence or absence of a chronic ulcer are not accurate predictors of the need for definitive ulcer operation. Some evidence suggests that in the absence of risk factors, mortality following simple closure and definitive surgery is the same and should be less than 2%. What are these risk factors? In a prospective study, Boey et al[14] evaluated the effect of major medical illnesses, preoperative shock and long-standing perforation (more than 24 hours) on mortality following surgery for perforated ulcers. Mortality increased progressively with increasing numbers of risk factors: 0%, 10%, 45.5%, and 100% in patients with zero, one, two, and three risk factors, respectively. It was concluded that simple closure is more prudent than definitive surgery if any risk factor is present. Other authors report a lower postoperative mortality in patients with perforated gastric ulcers who undergo definitive procedures.[15] The weight of available evidence would suggest that for selected patients the postoperative mortality after definitive surgery is at least equivalent to that seen after simple closure, but long-term recurrences are less with definitive surgery. For this reason, most surgeons would agree that definitive surgery is better than simple closure for the treatment of nonsealed perforated duodenal ulcer[16] when it can be safely performed.

Simple closure is preferred by most surgeons for all patients who represent an increased operative risk. For the elderly patient (>60 years of age) who is taking ulcerogenic medication, omental patch repair of a perforation may be very satisfactory.[17] Similarly for patients who present with gastric perforation, resectional therapy is indicated if the patient's condition permits.[18] Prepyloric ulcers behave like duodenal ulcers in this respect, but the surgeon must be cognizant of the higher risk of carcinoma in patients who present with a gastric perforation involving the gastric body or fundus.

The ideal operation for definitive treatment of perforated duodenal ulcers should have a negligible mortality, provide protection against recurrent ulcer, and not inflict undesirable gastric sequelae if it is performed on patients who would not have required definitive treatment to prevent recurrent ulcers. Age is a contraindication to definitive surgery only in the sense that coexisting severe disease that contraindicates such treatment occurs with increasing frequency with advancing age. Truncal vagotomy and pyloroplasty and truncal vagotomy and hemigastrectomy are acceptable definitive operations for perforated duodenal ulcer. The choice should depend on existing technical factors that govern the relative safety of the two operations. However, both operations are associated with an unacceptable rate of adverse postoperative sequelae for those patients who would not have required a definitive operation to prevent ulcer symptoms from returning.

At one time, truncal vagotomy with a pyloroplasty that incorporated the perforation was considered a more acceptable operation than vagotomy and hemigastrectomy for perforated duodenal ulcer. This operation was considered technically easier and therefore safer than vagotomy and hemigastrectomy. It was also expected that adverse sequelae would be less frequent and less severe than those following vagotomy and hemigastrectomy. In a prospective, randomized study by Boey et al[19] in 1982, recurrent symptoms occurred in 9% and reoperation was required in 6% of patients after truncal vagotomy and pyloroplasty, compared with 3% recurrence of symptoms and no reoperations after closure of the perforation and parietal cell vagotomy. In a prospective study by Ceneviva et al[20] in 1986, there was a 5% recurrence rate after parietal cell vagotomy compared with a 58% recurrence rate after simple closure. Jordan and Morrow[21] treated 88 patients with perforated ulcers by parietal cell vagotomy and closure of the perforation with an omental patch, without consideration as to whether the ulcers were acute or chronic. There was one operative death and a recurrent ulcer rate of 6%. In selected patients, the addition of parietal cell vagotomy to simple closure may be warranted even in patients without a prior history of peptic ulcer disease.[22] The recurrence rate with the addition of parietal cell vagotomy is clearly less, and it appears that a high percentage of the patients who have a recurring ulcer after this procedure can be successfully managed with H_2 blocker therapy alone. Thus, the available data suggest that patients without significant risk factors are ideal candidates for parietal cell vagotomy and omental patch closure.

OBSTRUCTION

Patients with ulcers who present with gastric distension and the inability to retain solids or liquids often require surgical intervention. A major issue for these individuals is whether the obstructive symptoms are secondary to benign or malignant disease. As part of the initial management, it is essential that adequate decompression of the stomach be achieved using irrigation as needed and continuous suction for at least 72 to 96 hours. Attempts to discontinue decompression prior to this time often only prolong the time needed before a definitive decision about the need for operation can be made. After 4 days a saline load test can be performed to aid the decision making.[23] Seven hundred fifty milliliters of isotonic saline are instilled into the stomach. A residual volume of more than 250 ml at the end of 30 minutes strongly suggests that surgical intervention is required during the current admission. Excluding patients with obstruction from other causes, the majority of patients who present with gastric outlet obstruction secondary to ulcer disease will require operation to correct the abnormality.[24] Smaller residual volumes suggest that the patient will be able to tolerate oral feedings and that the operation may be postponed. H_2-receptor blockers are discontinued at least 8 hours before the saline load test is performed since these drugs are known to slow gastric emptying. Serum gastrin levels should be requested on admission. If hypergastrinemia is detected, the presence of a gastrinoma must be determined before operation is performed. If elevated gastrin levels are found and a gastrinoma is excluded, the operation of choice may be an antrectomy with vagotomy, since G-cell hyperplasia may be present.

Some surgeons have advocated parietal cell vagotomy with dilation of the stenosed area of the pylorus or duodenum. Eighty percent of patients can be expected to have very good early postoperative results although the recurrence rate may be as high as 20% after 6 to 10 years of follow-up.[25] Most early advocates of intraoperative dilation and parietal cell vagotomy have withdrawn their support, citing an unacceptably high recurrence rate. Parietal cell vagotomy in combination with drainage performed by experienced surgeons and including a test for the completeness of gastric denervation can be expected to result in a good-to-excellent clinical course for some patients.[26] However, poor gastric emptying may still plague patients with edematous, hypomotile stomachs even if a pyloroplasty is performed in addition to parietal cell vagotomy. Truncal vagotomy with posterior gastrojejunostomy is an excellent procedure for elderly or debilitated patients since it can be performed expeditiously. For patients who are better risks, truncal vagotomy with antrectomy or gastroenterostomy can be expected to produce very good results. Performing an antrectomy, of course, provides additional protection against failure secondary to an incomplete vagotomy.

LONG-TERM COMPLICATIONS OF PEPTIC ULCER SURGERY INCLUDING CANCER

Up to 25% of patients have adverse postoperative sequelae after gastric surgery for benign or malignant conditions. By severely altering the normal physiology of the stomach and proximal small intestine, the operations can adversely affect gastrointestinal motor activity, digestion, and absorption. Fortunately, the majority of the problems, particularly the metabolic sequelae, can be managed by dietary or pharmacologic manipulation.

However, a small percentage of patients with complications following gastric operations will require reconstructive surgery. For enterogastric reflux, Roux-en-Y gastrojejunostomy is the procedure of choice. To slow the rapid gastric emptying responsible for dumping and diarrhea, jejunal interposition or the Roux-en-Y procedure is the most effective surgical choice. Intestinal pacing may prove to be useful in the future. Persistent gastric stasis following gastric surgery requires further gastric resection with gastroenteric anastomosis. When clearly documented, afferent limb syndromes are best treated surgically by reversing the gastrojejunal anastomosis or converting to a gastroduodenostomy. Overall, the results of the surgical treatment of these difficult postgastrectomy syndromes are not outstanding. Reconstructive gastric operations restore perfect or good health in 70% of patients, but 30% of patients are left moderately or severely disabled.[27] Therefore, the search has continued to develop more effective medical therapies for peptic ulcer disease and, in patients refractory to medical management, less physiologically disruptive operations. Of the currently available procedures, only parietal cell vagotomy eliminates most adverse postoperative sequelae; but, unfortunately, it is associated with a relatively high recurrence rate. Experimentally, the combination of mucosal antrectomy and proximal gastric vagotomy preserves both relatively normal gastric motor activity yet denervates the parietal cell mass and eliminates the gastrin-producing antral mucosa.[28,29]

One area of long-standing controversy has been the relative risk of long-term complications after surgical operations for chronic ulcer disease, especially the risk of gastric cancer. A recent retrospective study examined this issue in over 2500 patients with benign gastric or duodenal ulcers. The follow-up period ranged from 9 to 23 years. Thirty-eight patients developed biopsy-proven gastric carcinoma. In nine patients, carcinomas developed at the site of a benign ulcer. Only two of these patients had unequivocal evidence of disease that was initially benign. In these two individuals the carcinomas developed approximately 13 years after the benign ulcers were diagnosed. The overall incidence of gastric cancer in patients with benign gastric or duodenal ulcers was actually less than what would be expected for the general population.[30] Thus, malignant transformation of gastric ulcers would appear to be very rare.

This issue was addressed in a comprehensive follow-up study of 6459 patients by the Swedish Cancer Registry, the purpose of which was to determine the incidence of gastric cancer in patients who had undergone partial gastrectomy for biopsy-proven benign ulcer disease.[31] The overall risk of gastric cancer following gastrectomy was no different than that noted for age- and sex-matched controls. However, slight differences in risk were noted when the patients were subclassified. The adjusted risk was greater among women as compared with men, greater following partial gastrectomy for gastric ulcer than for duodenal ulcer, and greater following a Billroth II as compared with a Billroth I reconstruction. Somewhat similar findings were reported in a cohort study performed in Denmark.[32] In this study of 4164 patients who underwent peptic ulcer surgery between 1955 and 1960, the overall incidence of gastric cancer was not greater than expected. Unlike the Swedish study, the risk of cancer did not differ between patients with duodenal or gastric ulcers. In addition, two thirds of these patients had Billroth II reconstructions, which calls into question whether this particular subgroup of patients actually has an increased risk for the development of stomach cancers.

Similar observations have been made for residents in the United States.[33] Three hundred thirty-eight residents in Olmsted County, Minnesota, who had surgical treatment for benign peptic ulcer disease between 1935 and 1959 and who had no evidence of gastric cancer for 5 years following their initial operation, were followed for over 5635 person-years of observation. The risk of developing gastric cancer in this group was compared with the gastric cancer incidence for the local population. Carcinomas developed in the gastric remnant in only two of the patients followed as compared with an "expected" incidence of 2.6. These studies would suggest that there is no indication for routine endoscopic surveillance in asymptomatic patients who have previously had gastric surgery for benign peptic ulcer disease. Other large scale investigations have demonstrated that the risk of large bowel cancer after partial gastrectomy for benign ulcer disease is also not increased.[34]

INTRACTABILITY OR RECURRENCE

The availability of newer drugs, such as omeprazole, which by inhibiting the proton pump is a potent inhibitor of gastric acid secretion, to treat patients with ulcer disease may also affect the decision as to what patients should be operated on and when this operation should occur. For example, patients with duodenal ulcer disease who are treated with omeprazole tend to have better relief of their ulcer pain and tend to heal faster than those who are treated with standard doses of cimetidine.[35]

Although the introduction of cimetidine and other H_2 blockers has clearly changed the type of patients that are seen in the typical gastrointestinal surgeon's practice, they may also have decreased the need for reoperation in patients with recurrent ulcer disease. Medical therapy that includes cimetidine can be expected to achieve good results in about half of patients with recurrent ulceration, which is an improvement in the rate of reoperation compared with that seen in historic controls.[36]

Improvements in the medical care of patients with recurrent ulceration may also be a factor in the choice of elective operation. Some authorities have recommended parietal cell vagotomy (PGV) with or without pyloroplasty as the operation of first choice of patients with uncomplicated duodenal ulceration.[37,38] A recent follow-up study of 600 patients showed that ulceration recurred in 15% of those who had the operation (and most recurrences occurred within 5 years of operation). However, reoperation was necessary in only 29 of the patients. In 2 of these 29 patients, reoperation was required to treat gastric stasis. Very high satisfaction rates were reported for 92% of the individuals studied. The recurrence rate with this procedure is somewhat higher than that seen with more traditional operations such as truncal vagotomy and antrectomy. However, the increased morbidity associated with vagotomy and antrectomy (e.g., diarrhea, dumping, malabsorption), even when the operation is successful, and the fact that most patients who have parietal cell vagotomy and who have a recurring ulcer can be successfully managed medically, may influence the decision as to when reoperation is required and as to the procedure that is initially performed. Indeed, even those patients with relatively poor outcomes after primary or reoperative parietal cell vagotomy usually do not require any additional treatment or have no symptoms while they are being treated with antacids or H_2 blockers. Thus, ulcers that recur after parietal cell vagotomy typically have a benign course and respond well to treatment with H_2-receptor antagonists.

LAPAROSCOPIC TREATMENT

Recently, some reports have surfaced addressing the utility of laparoscopic approaches to the surgical management of patients with peptic ulcer disease. An initial report by Mouret and colleagues[39] evaluated the success of laparoscopy with fibrin sealant and an omental patch in five patients with perforated ulcers. The site of perforation was identified in four patients, three of whom had duodenal ulcers and one of whom had a gastric ulcer, and they were treated successfully. One patient required conversion to laparotomy for sepsis.

In a more extensive prospective, randomized, controlled trial, Taylor and colleagues[40] compared a laparoscopically performed anterior lesser curve seromyotomy and posterior truncal vagotomy with open truncal vagotomy and pyloroplasty in the treatment of patients with chronic duodenal ulcers. The mean duration of symptoms for all 146 patients studied was 7 years. These individuals were followed after surgery for periods ranging from 2 to 7.5 years with a mean interval of 4.5 years. Acid secretion was similarly decreased in the two groups of patients after operation. The ulcer recurrence rate was approximately twice as high in the patients who had laparoscopic surgery (6% versus 3%). However, overall Visick scores were higher in the patients who had lesser curve seromyotomies and posterior truncal vagotomies performed using the laparoscope.

Thus, laparoscopic techniques with which to treat peptic ulcer disease are still in the developmental stage. One reason for an increased recurrence rate with the technique of lesser curve seromyotomy with posterior truncal vagotomy is that nerve growth with reinnervation may occur at the sites where the seromyotomy was performed. This would lead to the reestablishment of some vagal innervation. Additional randomized controlled trials with lengthy follow-ups are needed to fully answer this question.

SUMMARY

Our understanding of the pathogenesis of peptic ulceration continues to improve and evolve. New treatment modalities that can favorably restore the balance between ulcerogenic and protective factors in the upper gastrointestinal tract are being introduced at a rapid pace. Surgical treatments also continue to be refined. Operative correction or obliteration must still be used to treat many complications and remains an important therapeutic option for selected patients with intractable or refractory disease.

REFERENCES

1. Ebell MH. Practical therapeutics: peptic ulcer disease. *Am Fam Physician.* 1992;46(1):217–227.
2. Gustavsson S, Nyren O. Time trends in peptic ulcer surgery, 1956 to 1986: a nationwide survey in Sweden. *Ann Surg.* 1989;210(6):704–709.
3. Paimela H, Tuompo PK, Perakyla T, Saario I, Hockerstedt K, Kivilaakso E. Peptic ulcer surgery during the H_2 receptor antagonist era: a population-based epidemiological study of ulcer surgery in Helsinki from 1972 to 1987. *Br J Surg.* 1991;78(1):28–31.
4. Welch CE, Rodkey GV, von Ryll GP. A thousand operations for ulcer disease. *Ann Surg.* 1986;204:454–467.
5. Glise H. Epidemiology in peptic ulcer disease: current status and future aspects. *Scand J Gastroenterol.* 1990; 175(suppl):13–18.
6. Gugler R. Current diagnosis and selection of patients for treatment of peptic ulcer disease. *Dig Dis Sci.* 1985; 30(suppl):30s–35s.
7. Donahue PE, Nyhus LM. Surgical excision of gastric ulcers near the gastroesophageal junction. *Surg Gynecol Obstet.* 1982;155:85–88.
8. Sugawa C, Joseph AL. Endoscopic interventional management of bleeding duodenal and gastric ulcers. *Surg Clin North Am.* 1992;72(2):317–334.
9. Branicki FJ, Boey J, Fok PJ, et al. Bleeding duodenal ulcer: a prospective evaluation of risk factors of rebleeding and death. *Ann Surg.* 1990;211:411–418.
10. Matthews JB, Tortella BJ, et al. Gastroduodenal hemorrhage and perforation in the postoperative period. *Surg Gynecol Obstet.* 1989;167:389–392.

11. Berne TV, Donovan AJ. Nonoperative treatment of perforated duodenal ulcer. *Arch Surg.* 1989;124:830–832.
12. Miedema BW, Torres PR, Farnell MB, et al. Proximal gastric vagotomy in the emergency treatment of bleeding duodenal ulcer. *Am J Surg.* 1991;161:64–68.
13. Berg CL, Wolfe MM. Zollinger-Ellison syndrome. *Med Clin North Am.* 1991;75(4):903–921.
14. Boey J, Choi SKY, Alagaratnam TT, et al. Risk stratification in perforated duodenal ulcers: a prospective validation of predictive factors. *Ann Surg.* 1989;205:22–26.
15. Hodnett RM, Gonzalez F, et al. The need for definitive therapy in the management of perforated gastric ulcers: review of 202 cases. *Ann Surg.* 1989;209:36–39.
16. Hay JM, Lacaine F, et al. Immediate definitive surgery for perforated duodenal ulcer does not increase operative mortality: a prospective controlled trial. *World J Surg.* 1989;12:705–709.
17. George RL, Smith IF. Long-term results after omental patch repair in patients with duodenal ulcers: a 5 to 10 year follow-up study. *Can J Surg.* 1991;34:447–449.
18. Turner WW Jr, Thompson WM Jr, et al. Perforated gastric ulcers: a plea for management by simple closures. *Arch Surg.* 1988;123:960–964.
19. Boey J, Lee NW, Koo J, et al. Immediate definitive surgery for perforated duodenal ulcers: a prospective controlled trial. *Ann Surg.* 1989;196:338–344.
20. Ceneviva R, de Castro e Silva O, Casteltranchi PL, et al. Simple suture with or without proximal gastric vagotomy for perforated duodenal ulcer. *Br J Surg.* 1986;73:427–430.
21. Jordan PH Jr, Morrow C. Perforated peptic ulcer. *Surg Clin North Am.* 1988;68:315–329.
22. Boey J, Branicki FJ, et al. Proximal gastric vagotomy: the preferred operation for perforations in acute duodenal ulcer. *Ann Surg.* 1988;208:169–174.
23. Silen W. Management of obstructing duodenal ulcer. In: Fischer JE, ed. *Common Problems in Gastrointestinal Surgery.* Chicago, Ill: Year Book Medical Publishers Inc; 1989:112–117.
24. Jaffin BW, Micheal D, Kaye DM. The prognosis of gastric outlet obstruction. *Ann Surg.* 1985;210:176–179.
25. Mentes AS. Parietal cell vagotomy and dilatation for peptic duodenal stricture. *Ann Surg.* 1990;212:597–601.
26. Donahue PE, Yoshida J, et al. Proximal gastric vagotomy with drainage for obstructing duodenal ulcer. *Surgery.* 1988;104:757–764.
27. Kelly KA, Becker JM, Van Heerden JA. Reconstructive gastric surgery. *Br J Surg.* 1981;68:687–691.
28. Becker JM, et al. Proximal gastric vagotomy and mucosal antrectomy: a possible operative approach to duodenal ulcer. *Surgery.* 1983;94:58–64.
29. Becker JM, et al. Complications of gastric surgery. *Practical Gastroenterol.* 1984;8(S4):17–24.
30. Lee S, Iida M, et al. Long-term follow-up of 2529 patients reveals gastric ulcers rarely become malignant. *Dig Dis Sci.* 1990;35:763–768.
31. Lundegardh G, Adami HO, et al. Gastric cancer after partial gastrectomy for benign ulcer disease. *N Engl J Med.* 1988;319:195–200.
32. Toftgaard C. Gastric cancer after peptic ulcer surgery: a historic prospective cohort investigation. *Ann Surg.* 1989;210:159–164.
33. Schafer LW, Larson DE, Melton LJ, Higgins JA, Ilstrup DM. The risk of gastric carcinoma after surgical treatment for benign ulcer disease: a population based study in Olmsted County, Minnesota. *N Engl J Med* 1983;309:1210–1213.
34. Lundegardh G, Adami HO, et al. The risk of large bowel cancer after partial gastrectomy for benign ulcer disease. *Ann Surg.* 1990;212:714–718.
35. Archambault AP, Pare P, et al. Omeprazole (20 mg daily) versus cimetidine (1200 mg daily) in duodenal ulcer healing and pain relief. *Gastroenterology.* 1988;94:1130–1134.
36. Kinney E, Goderwis D, Mullins RJ, et al. Management of recurrent duodenal ulcer disease. *Am Surg.* 1988;54:15–18.
37. Johnston GW, Spencer EFA, et al. Proximal gastric vagotomy: follow-up at 10–20 years. *Br J Surg.* 1991;78:20–23.
38. Emas S, Eriksson B. Twelve year follow-up of a prospective, randomized trial of selective vagotomy with pyloroplasty and selective proximal vagotomy with and without pyloroplasty for the treatment of duodenal, pyloric, and pre-pyloric ulcers. *Am J Surg.* 1992;164(1):4–12.
39. Mouret P, Francois Y, et al. Laparoscopic treatment of perforated peptic ulcer. *Br J Surg.* 1990;77(9):1006–1012.
40. Taylor TV, Lythgoe JP, et al. Anterior lesser curve seromyotomy and posterior truncal vagotomy versus truncal vagotomy and pyloroplasty in the treatment of chronic duodenal ulcer. *Br J Surg.* 1990;77:1007–1009.

SECTION IV

INTESTINAL TRACT

49
Eosinophilic Gastroenteritis
WILLIAM N. KATKOV and ROBERT H. SCHAPIRO

Eosinophilic gastroenteritis, first described by Kaijser[1] in 1937, is a rare disorder in which eosinophils infiltrate various segments and layers of the gastrointestinal tract. The different potential sites of eosinophilic infiltration account for the wide variety of clinical presentations seen with this disorder.[2,3] Although the cause of eosinophilic gastroenteritis is unknown, there is evidence that allergic phenomena, including the effects of activated eosinophils, may play a pathophysiologic role in some patients. Steroids are the mainstay of therapy, and the prognosis for persons with eosinophilic gastroenteritis is generally favorable.

CLINICAL FEATURES

Eosinophilic gastroenteritis can present with a variety of signs and symptoms. In 1970, Klein et al[4] classified eosinophilic gastroenteritis according to the intestinal layer involved (mucosa, muscularis, or serosa) and correlated this with the major clinical features of the disease.

Intestinal mucosal infiltration with eosinophils can lead to signs and symptoms of profound malabsorption including hypoalbuminemia, edema, iron-deficiency anemia, and weight loss. Patients may experience cramping, nausea, and diarrhea. Stools may be positive for occult blood. Pediatric patients, approximately 20% to 30% of those affected, may suffer from growth retardation.[5,6]

Predominant involvement of the muscularis is associated with luminal narrowing and symptoms of intestinal obstruction.[2,3,7] Associated symptoms can include pain, nausea, and vomiting. When the gastric antrum is involved, delayed gastric emptying is frequently encountered.

Isolated serosal or subserosal involvement with eosinophils is encountered in approximately 10% of patients with eosinophilic gastroenteritis. It is associated with a protein-rich exudative ascites that may contain large numbers of eosinophils.[2,3] This manifestation of eosinophilic gastroenteritis may be seen in combination with mucosal or muscular involvement.[8]

Peripheral eosinophilia is found in approximately 50% of patients with eosinophilic gastroenteritis. Although many case reports have identified a history of allergy in persons with eosinophilic gastroenteritis, an allergic diathesis is not a universal feature and is not required to establish a diagnosis.

DIFFERENTIAL DIAGNOSIS

Because the clinical features of eosinophilic gastroenteritis are so varied, a broad differential diagnosis must be entertained.[2] Malabsorption and obstruction are seen in a large number of disorders. Intestinal infiltration by eosinophils may be seen in a variety of conditions including eosinophilic granuloma, polyarteritis nodosa, parasitic infection, lymphoma, gastric cancer, Crohn's disease, and hypereosinophilic syndrome.[9]

Numerous conditions are characterized by peripheral eosinophilia. Some are accompanied by gastrointestinal tract infiltration with eosinophils, whereas others are not. The differential diagnosis of peripheral eosinophilia includes hypereosinophilic syndromes (including Löffler's syndrome, eosinophilic leukemia, and idiopathic hypereosinophilic syndrome), collagen vascular diseases (including rheumatoid arthritis, eosinophilic fasciitis, allergic angiitis, and eosinophilic granuloma), malignancies (including Hodgkin's disease and mycosis fungoides), allergies, and parasitic infections.[10] Of the diagnoses listed above, the most likely to be associated with both peripheral eosinophilia and intestinal mucosal eosinophilic infiltrates include hypereosinophilic syndrome, polyarteritis nodosa, eosinophilic granuloma, and intestinal parasitic infection.

The parasitic infections most often associated

with peripheral eosinophilia include schistosomiasis, hookworm, ascariasis, strongyloidiasis, toxicariasis, trichuriasis, intestinal capillariasis, and trichinosis. Infections with protozoa including amebiasis and giardiasis are *not* associated with an increased eosinophil count.

DIAGNOSIS

Mucosal biopsy confirms the diagnosis of eosinophilic gastroenteritis in a majority of cases in which mucosal infiltration predominates.[11] Because the lesion may be patchy, it is recommended that a minimum of eight biopsy specimens be examined when this diagnosis is suspected.[2] There are no precise histologic criteria for diagnosis in this disorder; however, the infiltrate, which may be diffuse or multifocal, consists typically of 10 to 50 eosinophils per high-powered field in the lamina propria.[12] Eosinophils are not necessarily restricted to one intestinal layer in a given patient. Biopsies may reveal involvement of the submucosa or muscular layers as well as the mucosa.

When mucosal disease predominates in eosinophilic gastroenteritis, contrast radiologic studies may show irregular and thickened intestinal folds, as well as edema of the intestinal wall. The radiologic pictures in these cases may suggest eosinophilic gastroenteritis, but similar findings may occur in a number of lesions that infiltrate the intestine or are associated with bowel edema or ischemia.[13]

Predominantly muscular involvement in the intestinal wall is associated with symptoms of intestinal obstruction. A typical radiographic appearance of antral irregularity and pyloric narrowing has been described in this form of the disease.[13] The small intestine is also frequently involved. The differential diagnosis in this form of eosinophilic gastroenteritis includes intestinal lymphoma, gastric carcinoma, and Crohn's disease.[14] In this setting, mucosal biopsy specimens may not be diagnostic. The need for a diagnosis, as well as the occurrence of obstruction, may lead to surgery and the opportunity to obtain a diagnostic full thickness intestinal biopsy.

Isolated serosal involvement is the least common form of eosinophilic gastroenteritis.[3,8] Radiographs may show no abnormalities, and the only abnormal clinical finding may be ascites. Ascites is characteristically exudative and contains large numbers of eosinophils.

In addition to the layer of intestine infiltrated by eosinophils, the involved segment(s) of the gastrointestinal tract significantly affects the clinical features of the disease. Gastric involvement is common (up to 40% in some reports) and may be accompanied by signs and symptoms of impaired gastric emptying, nausea, vomiting, and postprandial pain. Narrowing of the antrum has been described in a number of cases of eosinophilic gastroenteritis and in the setting of eosinophilic granuloma.[15,16] This condition can mimic lymphoma, Ménétrier's disease, and gastric carcinoma both clinically and radiologically.[13]

Other sites of involvement in eosinophilic gastroenteritis include the esophagus where the presentation may include dysphagia, heartburn, and nausea.[12,17,18] Manometric data may suggest achalasia. The small intestine is frequently involved in eosinophilic gastroenteritis. Signs and symptoms of malabsorption or intestinal obstruction are likely to predominate. Eosinophilic ileocolitis, as well as isolated colonic involvement, has also been reported in which the clinical and histologic features closely resemble inflammatory bowel disease.[19,20]

PATHOPHYSIOLOGY

Many patients with eosinophilic gastroenteritis exhibit features that point to an allergic basis for the disease. Peripheral eosinophilia is found in 40% to 50% of affected persons, and a history of allergic or atopic phenomena can be elicited in a similar proportion. The nature of the putative immunogen is unknown, and food allergy has not been established as a pathophysiologic factor. The efficacy of elimination diets in the treatment of eosinophilic gastroenteritis has been limited.[2,3] In one study seven patients with eosinophilic gastroenteritis and intestinal obstruction were carefully evaluated.[7] Two of the seven had normal peripheral eosinophil counts, and none had a history of allergy or food hypersensitivity. Serum immunoglobulin E (IgE) levels were normal in all the patients studied. It is postulated that nonallergic factors led to tissue eosinophilia in these patients.

The mechanism(s) by which eosinophils contribute to the clinical manifestations of this disorder remains unknown. One study evaluated the eosinophils in two siblings with mucosal eosinophilic gastroenteritis.[21] Evidence that eosinophils infiltrating the mucosa were activated suggests that products of eosinophilic activation and degranulation may play a primary role in bowel injury and pathology.

Tissue eosinophilia like that found in eosinophilic gastroenteritis may come about through different mechanisms including mast cell degranulation and the release of chemotactic factors attracting eosinophils.[22] Once present, eosinophils have the potential to cause tissue injury by mediating inflammatory responses and releasing cytotoxic proteins.[23] Four principal proteins are found in the granules of mammalian eosinophils, including major basic protein, eosinophil-derived neurotoxin, eosinophil cationic protein, and eosinophil peroxidase. All of these proteins are potent toxins for helminth larvae and mammalian cells. Therefore, although eosinophils may play a directly beneficial role as a host defense against parasitic infections, they have the potential to cause injury to host tissue. The deposition of major basic protein, in particular, has been associated with sites of inflammation and injury in a variety of disorders associated with peripheral or tissue eosinophilia.[23,24]

PROGNOSIS AND THERAPY

The prognosis for patients with eosinophilic gastroenteritis is generally favorable; however, isolated cases of fatal outcomes have been reported.[25,26] Spontaneous remission is rare, and treatment, which is effective, is usually indicated. While a trial of an elimination diet is warranted if an allergic history is prominent, the benefit, if any, is usually transient. Corticosteroids are the mainstay of therapy for patients with eosinophilic gastroenteritis. A 7- to 10-day course of 40 to 60 mg of prednisone usually leads to a remission of symptoms. The disease may recur when treatment is discontinued, and repeat courses of prednisone or low-dose long-term therapy may be required in some patients. There is no reported increased risk of malignancy associated with this disorder.

There are reports of patients treated successfully with oral sodium chromoglycate.[27,28] It is noteworthy that both of these case reports involved patients with systemic vasculitis, one a confirmed case of polyarteritis nodosa.

The use of ketotifen, a histamine (H_1) antagonist that inhibits mast cell degranulation, has been reported in six patients with eosinophilic gastroenteritis.[29] All participants in this open label study had peripheral eosinophilia and a history of allergic rhinitis. None of the patients had a history of food allergy, and only one had IgE antibodies to any food test antigens. Ketotifen therapy was associated with relief of symptoms and weight gain in all six patients.

SUMMARY

Eosinophilic gastroenteritis is a rare disorder with a variable clinical presentation. It most commonly affects the stomach and small intestine, presenting with symptoms of malabsorption or intestinal obstruction. The diagnosis is confirmed by documenting an eosinophilic infiltrate in the bowel wall and by excluding other conditions that may be associated with intestinal eosinophilia. The cause of this disorder remains unknown. Although many patients present with features suggesting an allergic basis for the disease, theses findings are not uniform. The prognosis for persons with eosinophilic gastroenteritis is generally favorable.

REFERENCES

1. Kaijser R. Zur Kenntnis der allergischen Affektioner desima Verdauungskanal von Standpunkt desima Chirurgen aus. *Arch Klin Chir.* 1937;188:36–64.
2. Cello JP. Eosinophilic gastroenteritis: a complex disease entity. *Am J Med.* 1979;67:1097–1104.
3. Talley NJ, Shorter RG, Phillips SF, et al. Eosinophilic gastroenteritis: a clinicopathological study of patients with disease of the mucosa, muscle layer, and subserosal tissues. *Gut.* 1990;31:54–58.
4. Klein NC, Hargrove RL, Sleisenger MH, et al. Eosinophilic gastroenteritis. *Medicine.* 1970;49:299–319.
5. Steffen RM, Wyllie R, Petras RE, et al. The spectrum of eosinophilic gastroenteritis: report of six pediatric cases and review of the literature. *Clin Pediatr.* 1991;30:404–411.
6. Kravis LP, South MA, Rosenlund ML. Eosinophilic gastroenteritis in the pediatric patient. *Clin Pediatr.* 1982;12:713–717.
7. Caldwell JH, Mekhjian HS, Hurtubise PE, et al. Eosinophilic gastroenteritis with obstruction: immunological studies of seven patients. *Gastroenterology.* 1978; 825–828.
8. McNabb PC, Fleming RC, Higgins JA, et al. Transmural eosinophilic gastroenteritis with ascites. *Mayo Clin Proc.* 1979;54:119–122.
9. Blackshaw AJ, Levison DA. Eosinophilic infiltrates of the gastrointestinal tract. *J Clin Pathol.* 1986;39:1–7.
10. Gallin JI. Eosinophils. In: Braunwald E, Isselbacher KJ, Petersdorf RG, et al, eds. *Harrison's Principles of Internal Medicine.* New York, NY: McGraw-Hill Book Co; 1987:282–283.
11. Katz AJ, Goldman H, Grand RJ. Gastric mucosal biopsy in eosinophilic (allergic) gastroenteritis. *Gastroenterology.* 1977;73:705–709.
12. Case Records of the Massachusetts General Hospital (Case 20-1992). *N Engl J Med.* 1992;326:1342–1349.
13. Marshak RH, Lindner A, Maklansky D, et al. Eosinophilic gastroenteritis. *JAMA.* 1981;245:1677–1680.
14. Shepherd NA. Pathological mimics of chronic inflammatory bowel disease. *J Clin Pathol.* 1991;44:726–733.

15. van Rensburg LCJ, Keet AD, Adams G. Eosinophilic granuloma of the stomach. *J Surg Oncol.* 1986;31:143–147.
16. Salmon PR, Paulley JW. Eosinophilic granuloma of the gastrointestinal tract. *Gut.* 1967;8:8–14.
17. Rumans MC, Lieberman DA. Eosinophilic gastroenteritis presenting with biliary and duodenal obstruction. *Am J Gastroenterol.* 1987;82:775–778.
18. Dobbins JW, Sheahan DG, Behar J. Eosinophilic gastroenteritis with esophageal involvement. *Gastroenterology.* 1977;72:1312–1316.
19. Tedesco FJ, Huckaby CB, Hamby-Allen M, et al. Eosinophilic ileocolitis: expanding spectrum of eosinophilic gastroenteritis. *Dig Dis Sci.* 1981;26:943–948.
20. Moore D, Lichtman S, Lentz J, et al. Eosinophilic gastroenteritis presenting in an adolescent with isolated colonic involvement. *Gut.* 1986;27:1219–1222.
21. Keshavarzian A, Saverymuttu SH, Tai P-C, et al. Activated eosinophils in familial gastroenteritis. *Gastroenterology.* 1985;88:1041–1049.
22. Wershil BK, Walker WA. Eosinophilic gastroenteritis. In: MacDermott RP, Elson CO, eds. *Gastroenterology Clinics of North America.* Philadelphia, Pa: WB Saunders Co; 1992:397–400.
23. Gleich GJ, Ottesen EA, Leiferman KM, et al. Eosinophils and human disease. *Int Arch Allergy Appl Immunol.* 1989;88:59–62.
24. Gleich GJ, Frigas E, Loegering DA, et al. Cytotoxic properties of the eosinophil major basic protein. *J Immunol.* 1979;123:2925–2927.
25. Tytgat GN, Grijm R, Dekker W, et al. Fatal eosinophilic gastroenteritis. *Gastroenterology.* 1976;71:479–483.
26. Konrad EA, Meister P. Fatal eosinophilic gastroenteritis in a two-year-old child. *Arch A Pathol Histol.* 1979;353:347–353.
27. Moots RJ, Prouse P, Gumpel JM. Near fatal eosinophilic gastroenteritis responding to oral sodium chromoglycate. *Gut.* 1988;29:1282–1285.
28. Heatley RV, Harris A, Atkinson M. Treatment of a patient with clinical features of both eosinophilic gastroenteritis and polyarteritis nodosa with oral sodium chromoglycate. *Dig Dis Sci.* 1980;25:470–472.
29. Melamed I, Feanny SJ, Sherman PM, et al. Benefit of ketotifen in patients with eosinophilic gastroenteritis. *Am J Med.* 1991;90:310–314.

50

Lactose Intolerance

RICHARD J. GRAND, ROBERT K. MONTGOMERY, and HANS A. BÜLLER

GENERAL CONCEPTS

Lactose intolerance is a common clinical problem. Low intestinal lactase levels may be due to mucosal injury, or, as in the majority of the world's adult population, to alterations in the genetic expression of the enzyme lactase-phlorizin hydrolase. In infants, carbohydrates account for 35% to 55% of daily calories ingested, and these are mainly as lactose. As weaning foods are introduced, lactose intake varies and approaches the quantity commonly ingested by adults. The average adult ingests 300 g of carbohydrates per day—approximately 52% of daily calories as starch (mainly cereals and potatoes), 37% as sucrose, 5% as lactose (mainly in milk), and 3% as fructose (in fruit and honey). Glycogen, glucose, and maltose are minor constituents of the diet, and cellulose accounts for approximately 4 g of carbohydrates per day.

LACTOSE DIGESTION

Lactose digestion is said to be slower than that of sucrose or maltose, and hydrolysis has been considered the rate-limiting step for the overall process of absorption. However, this concept needs further delineation. Lactose is hydrolyzed to glucose and galactose on the microvillus

---

Supported in part by National Institutes of Health Research Grant DK 32658, Grant P30 DK 34928 to the Center for Gastroenterology Research on Absorptive and Secretory Process, New England Medical Center Hospitals, Boston, Massachusetts, a grant from Nutricia, Zoetermeer, The Netherlands, and a NATO Collaborative Research Grant. Portions of this text are reproduced from Bayless T, ed. *Current Therapy in Gastroenterology and Liver Disease.* 4th ed. 1994:303–308, with permission of the publisher, Mosby–Year Book, St Louis, Mo, 63146.

membrane of the intestinal absorptive cells. Uptake of these monosaccharides is accomplished by the sodium-dependent glucose carrier.

COLONIC SALVAGE OF NONABSORBED LACTOSE

When lactose is not absorbed by the small bowel, it is passed rapidly into the colon as a consequence of the osmolarity of the intraluminal disaccharide. In the colon, lactose is converted to short-chain fatty acids and hydrogen gas by the bacterial flora, producing acetate, butyrate, and propionate. The short-chain fatty acids are absorbed by the colonic mucosa, and this route salvages malabsorbed lactose for energy utilization. This is a mechanism by which the newborn colon salvages lactose, and the adult who has low intestinal lactase activity may adapt to persistent lactose ingestion. This fermentative process not only conserves nutritionally important carbohydrate, but serves as the basis for the lactose breath hydrogen test (discussed below).

SYMPTOMS AND SIGNS OF LACTOSE MALABSORPTION

When clinical symptoms are induced by the ingestion of lactose, the term *lactose intolerance* is often applied. Lactose intolerance is characterized by abdominal pain, cramps or distension, nausea, flatulence, and diarrhea or vomiting. The abdominal pain may be crampy in nature and may be periumbilical or lower quadrant. Borborygmi may be audible on physical examination and to the patient. Lactose intolerance generally produces abnormal stools, which are usually bulky, frothy, and watery. In severe cases, mostly in infants, acidosis and dehydration may be a problem. Vomiting after lactose ingestion is often seen in adolescents.

Several factors account for the variability of symptoms produced by lactose ingestion in people who are intolerant. Important factors include the osmolarity and fat content of the food in which the sugar is ingested, rate of gastric emptying, sensitivity to intestinal distension produced by the osmotic load of unhydrolyzed lactose in the upper small bowel, rate of intestinal transit, and response of the colon to the carbohydrate load. In general, the higher the osmolarity of gastric contents and the higher the fat content of the diet containing the lactose, the slower the gastric emptying and the lesser the symptoms induced by sugar. Different individuals appear to have more or less sensitivity to abdominal distension, and they complain differently when ingested lactose stimulates an influx of water into the lumen of the small intestine or the production of gas leads to distension of the colon. Those with greater tolerance report fewer symptoms. These subjective responses are difficult to quantify. Patients with irritable bowel syndrome, who are also lactose intolerant, may have increased pain after lactose ingestion. Intestinal transit is also influenced by the quality of the diet and individual motility patterns. Accordingly, some lactose intolerant people experience very rapid movement of sugar to the cecum, whereas others have slower motility. Fecal flora are known to adapt to ingested carbohydrate. Thus, if lactose is provided slowly over a long period of time in many "intolerant" people, the flora may adapt to the load, and symptoms produced by gas and acid in the colon may be reduced or eliminated. This mechanism of lactose tolerance in people with low lactase levels accounts for the discrepancy between "lactase deficiency" and lactose intolerance.

The term *lactose malabsorption* is generally reserved for those patients for whom the intestinal malabsorption of lactose has been investigated using an appropriate test of absorption (e.g., lactose absorption test) or malabsorption (lactose breath hydrogen test).

CONFIRMATORY TESTS

The diagnosis of lactose malabsorption is based on the combination of clinical findings and results of appropriate tests. The presence of low fecal pH or reducing substances indicates lactose malabsorption, but these tests are only valid when lactose has been ingested, intestinal transit time is rapid, stools are collected fresh and assays are performed immediately, and bacterial metabolism of colonic carbohydrate is incomplete. In general, lactose malabsorption is best confirmed using more specific tests.

The capacity for sugar absorption can be measured using a lactose absorption test. In adults, it has a sensitivity of 75% and a specificity of 96%. However, in children, it is cumbersome, invasive, and time consuming and has largely been replaced by the lactose breath hydrogen test.

The breath hydrogen test really measures lactose nonabsorption (rather than lactose hydrolysis and monosaccharide uptake). Its sensitivity and specificity are superior to those for the absorption test, and it is simple and noninvasive. The lactose breath hydrogen test can be performed in people of all ages. The dose is customarily 2 g of lactose per kilogram body weight. Breath hydrogen is sampled before the ingestion of sugar and at 30-minute intervals following the ingestion of sugar for 3 hours. We customarily use a H$^+$ value of 10 parts per million as normal, comparing samples obtained after carbohydrate ingestion to the baseline value. H$^+$ values between 10 and 20 parts per million may be indeterminate unless accompanied by symptoms, but H$^+$ values over 20 parts per million are representative of lactose malabsorption. False-positive results are seen with inadequate pretest fasting or when the patient has smoked recently, and false-negative results are obtained when patients have recently used antibiotics or are nonhydrogen producers (approximately 1% of the population). In children less than 5 years of age an abnormal lactose breath hydrogen test always signifies abnormal intestinal mucosa or bacterial overgrowth, both of which require further definition by appropriate diagnostic tests. A normal breath hydrogen test does not rule out an intestinal mucosal lesion, and it cannot be used to avoid an intestinal biopsy.

The assay of disaccharidase activity in small bowel biopsy samples establishes the presence of disaccharidase deficiency and has been used to define populations at risk for low lactase levels. However, while low lactase activity accompanies intestinal injury, the lesion may be focal or patchy; consequently, intestinal biopsy samples may not yield an abnormal result. Clinical and biochemical data must always be compared to obtain the correct diagnosis.

APPROACH

Patients who have symptoms and signs of lactose intolerance should be evaluated in a systematic fashion. The clinical findings may not immediately suggest a diagnosis of lactose malabsorption as many patients with this diagnosis actually have a clinical pattern more like that seen in irritable bowel syndrome. Secondary causes for lactose malabsorption must be searched for, and appropriate confirmatory tests obtained. When considering lactose malabsorption, especially in infants and young children, the possibility of milk protein allergy must be ruled out.

It is important to remember that lactose malabsorption may occur in patients with other disorders (for example, the irritable bowel syndrome); thus, a lactose breath hydrogen test should be part of the evaluation of patients suspected of having irritable bowel syndrome so that appropriate therapy can be instituted.

PRIMARY LACTOSE MALABSORPTION

Lactose malabsorption occurs in three clinical settings: (1) racial or ethnic lactose malabsorption, (2) developmental lactase deficiency, and (3) congenital lactase deficiency (Table 50–1).

Racial or ethnic lactose malabsorption is the most common form of genetically determined reductions of lactase activity. This clinical finding has been termed *lactase deficiency,* although this term is really a misnomer, as the great majority of the world's populations develop low intestinal lactase levels during midchildhood (approximately age 5 years). This finding is most prominent in Asian, African, and indigenous populations (Table 50–2). Peoples of Scandinavian or Caucasian genetic background have acquired a high degree of lactose tolerance as adults, with preservation of intestinal lactase activity. The mechanisms underlying racial or ethnic lactase levels are now being elucidated. In the majority of people, a positive correlation exists between lactase levels and lactase messenger ribonucleic acid (mRNA) abundance, whether lactase activity is high or low. This indicates that molecular regulation of this enzyme is at the level of gene transcription. Furthermore, in most subjects with low lactase levels, individual intestinal absorptive cells that lack lactase enzyme also lack lactase mRNA.

TABLE 50–1. DISORDERS OF LACTOSE ABSORPTION

1. Primary
   a. Racial or ethnic
   b. Developmental
   c. Congenital
2. Secondary
   a. Bacterial overgrowth
   b. Infectious enteritis
   c. Mucosal injury
   d. Celiac sprue
   e. Drug-induced enteritis
   f. Inflammatory bowel disease
   g. Radiation enteritis
   h. Giardiasis

TABLE 50–2. DISTRIBUTION OF LACTASE PHENOTYPES IN SELECTED POPULATIONS

COUNTRY	POPULATION	LOW LACTASE (%)
Sweden	Swedes	1
Netherlands	Dutch	0
Austria	Austrians	20
France	French	32
	Southern French	44
Italy	Northern Italians	50
	Southern Italians	72
	Sicilians	71
United States	Northern European	7
	Whites	22
	Blacks	65
	American Indians	95
	Vietnamese	100

Data from Scrimshaw NS, Murray AB. The acceptability of milk and milk products in populations with a high prevalence of lactose intolerance. *Am J Clin Nutr.* 1988;48:1083–1085.

In the United States, lactase activity is normal in all children of any racial or ethnic group until approximately 5 years of age. Lactose intolerance detected in children before this age usually indicates an underlying mucosal lesion or bacterial overgrowth syndrome.

There is no evidence that lactase deficiency or lactose malabsorption is a normal part of the aging process. Thus, in the mixed population of Caucasian extraction, the normal aging process does not lead to lactase deficiency. However, alterations in motility secondary to other disorders, or intestinal injury, may produce lactose intolerance.

Developmental lactose malabsorption is a consequence of gestational age. During fetal development, lactase activity rises late in gestation so that premature infants born at 28 to 32 weeks' gestation have reduced lactase activity. If they are otherwise healthy, their colon can salvage unabsorbed carbohydrate so that these infants are not nutritionally compromised and do not have diarrhea.

Congenital lactase deficiency is characterized by the absence of lactase activity in the small intestine, with normal histologic findings and normal levels of other disaccharidases. This is a very rare syndrome associated with diarrhea from birth in affected infants. It was likely to have been a fatal process prior to the development of lactose-free infant formulas.

SECONDARY LACTOSE MALABSORPTION

Bacterial overgrowth or stasis syndromes may be associated with increased fermentation of dietary lactose in the small bowel. Clinical symptoms of lactose intolerance are often found. The diagnosis may be suspected when a very early peak of breath hydrogen is detected during lactose challenge.

Lactose malabsorption frequently occurs after mucosal injury of the gastrointestinal tract causing villus flattening or damage to the intestinal epithelium. Disorders that often produce this lesion are listed in Table 50–1. When the mucosa is damaged, lactase is usually the first affected disaccharidase, presumably because of its distal location on the villus. Treatment of the primary disorder is mandatory for the return of lactase activity, which often lags behind the return of normal intestinal morphology. Prolonged lactose intolerance, which may persist for months after healing starts, is unique to this disaccharidase, and its biochemical basis is unexplained.

TREATMENT OF LACTOSE MALABSORPTION

The treatment of lactose malabsorption includes four general principles: (1) reduction or restriction of dietary lactose, (2) substitution of alternative nutrient sources to avoid reduction in energy and protein intake, (3) regulation of calcium intake, and (4) the use of a commercially available enzyme substitute.

When lactose restriction is necessary, the patient must be instructed to read labels of commercially prepared foods, as hidden lactose may be difficult to identify. Table 50–3 summarizes the lactose content of selected foods. Complete restriction of lactose-containing foods should only be necessary for a limited period to ascertain the specificity of the diagnosis. As some patients can tolerate graded increases in lactose intake, small quantities of lactose may subsequently be reintroduced into the diet, careful attention being paid to associated symptoms. Because of its high sugar and fat content, ice cream may be a good way to introduce lactose into the diet. The diet should be reviewed with the patient to be certain that protein, fat, and other nutrients are supplied at appropriate levels.

Calcium is supplemented in the form of calcium carbonate; Tums is popular and effective. Standard preparations contain 500 mg of cal-

TABLE 50–3. LACTOSE CONTENT OF SELECTED FOODS

Product	Unit	Lactose (Approx g/U)
Milk	244 g (1 cup)	11
Low-fat milk, 2% fat	244 g (1 cup)	9–13
Skim milk	244 g (1 cup)	12–14
Nonfat dry milk, instant	91 g (1½ cup)	46
Whipped cream topping	3 g (1 tbs)	0.4
Light cream	15 g (1 tbs)	0.6
Cheese		
Cheddar	28 g (1 oz)	0.4–0.6
Cream	28 g (1 oz)	0.8
Parmesan, grated	28 g (1 oz)	0.8
Cheese, pasteurized, processed		
American	28 g (1 oz)	0.5
Swiss	28 g (1 oz)	0.4–0.6
Cottage cheese	210 g (1 cup)	5–6
Ice cream		
Vanilla, regular	133 g (1 cup)	9
Sherbet, orange	193 g (1 cup)	4
Ice, orange	100 g	0

From Bayless T, ed. *Current Therapy in Gastroenterology and Liver Disease.* 4th ed. St Louis, Mo: Mosby–Year Book; 1994:303–308.

TABLE 50–4. SOME COMMERCIAL "LACTASE" SUBSTITUTES

Name	Dose Form	Supplier
LactAid	Liquid or tablets	LactAid, Inc.
Lactrase	Capsules	Kremers-Urban
LactAce	Capsules	Nature's Way Products, Inc.
DairyEase	Tablets	Glenbrook Laboratories
Lactrol	Caplets	Advanced Nutritional Technology

From Bayless T, ed. *Current Therapy in Gastroenterology and Liver Disease.* 4th ed. St Louis, Mo: Mosby–Year Book; 1994:303–308.

cium carbonate equivalent to 200 mg of elemental calcium, which is 20% of the United States Recommended Daily Allowance (USRDA) for adults. In infants and young children, liquid calcium gluconate is readily tolerated and available. When complete lactose restriction is recommended, the USRDA for calcium should be provided as a supplement.

Commercially available "lactase" preparations are actually bacterial or yeast b-galactosidases. When added to lactose-containing food or when ingested with meals containing lactose, these are effective in reducing symptoms and breath hydrogen values in many lactose intolerant subjects. However, these products are not capable of completely hydrolyzing all dietary lactose, and the results achieved in individual patients are variable. Some of the commercial "lactase" preparations are listed in Table 50–4. LactAid liquid may be added to milk (14 drops/qt) which is then refrigerated overnight before use. The resulting hydrolysis of lactose (which is virtually 100% effective) produces a sweeter taste than milk containing lactose. Lactrase capsules may be sprinkled on or taken orally with lactose-containing foods, as can some of the other products listed in Table 50–4, but the individual doses required and responses to individual products must be tested in each patient. It should be noted that "acidophilus milk" is not sufficiently lactose depleted. Live culture yogurt, which contains endogenous b-galactosidase, is a useful alternative source of calcium and calories, and may be well tolerated by a number of lactose-intolerant patients. However, yogurts that contain milk or milk products added back after fermentation may produce symptoms. While consumption of yogurt alone by individuals with low lactose tolerance reduces symptoms, consumption of yogurt together with additional lactose does not reduce symptoms.

CONFOUNDING SITUATIONS

Patients demonstrating symptoms compatible with the diagnosis of lactose malabsorption, but for whom specific testing fails to reveal an abnormality, may have symptoms related to other carbohydrate ingestion. A careful dietary history should be obtained and appropriate breath hydrogen testing performed. The custom of eating extremely high-fiber foods may predispose some people to symptomatic carbohydrate malabsorption. Adjustment of carbohydrate intake alleviates symptoms.

SUMMARY

No matter what the origin, lactose intolerance represents an important source of clinical symptoms. Appropriate evaluation, often including specific absorption or breath hydrogen testing, usually indicates the correct therapeutic strategy.

Acknowledgments

The authors wish to thank their colleagues Drs. Menno Verhave, Stephen Krasinki, and Edmond Rings for fruitful collaboration and helpful comments.

REFERENCES

1. Büller HA, Grand RJ. Lactose intolerance. In: Creger WP, Coggins CH, Hancock EW, eds. *Annual Review of Medicine: Selected Topics in the Clinical Sciences.* Palo Alto, Calif: Annual Reviews Inc; 1990:(41)141–148.
2. Escher JC, de Koning ND, van Engen CGJ, et al. Molecular basis of lactase levels in adult humans. *J Clin Invest.* 1991;89:480–483.
3. Montgomery R, Büller HA, Rings EHHM, Dekker J, Grand RJ. Lactose intolerance and regulation of small intestine lactase activity. In: Berdanier CD, Hargrove JL, eds. *Nutrition and Gene Expression.* Boca Raton, Fla: CRC Press; 1992:23–53.
4. Rosado JL, Solomons NW, Lisker R, et al. Enzyme replacement therapy for primary adult lactase deficiency: effective reduction of lactose malabsorption and milk intolerance by direct addition of β-galactosidase to milk at mealtime. *Gastroenterology.* 1984;87:1072–1082.
5. Mobassaleh M, Montgomery RK, Biller JA, Grand RJ. Development of carbohydrate absorption in the fetus and newborn. *Pediatrics.* 1985;75(suppl):160–166.
6. Scrimshaw NS, Murray AB. The acceptability of milk and milk products in populations with a high prevalence of lactose intolerance. *Am J Clin Nutr.* 1988;48:1083–1085.
7. Maiuri L, Raia V, Potter J, et al. Mosaic pattern of lactase expression by villus enterocytes in human adult-type hypolactasia. *Gastroenterology.* 1991;100:359–369.

51
Celiac Sprue

KEVIN J. HORGAN

Celiac sprue, also known as celiac disease or gluten-sensitive enteropathy, is a chronic disease in which there is an abnormal jejunal mucosa that improves morphologically when treated with a gluten-free diet and deteriorates again with gluten ingestion. Gluten is a protein derived from cereal grains. Celiac sprue is believed to result from an aberrant immunologic response to gluten and its alcohol-soluble component gliadin. The mucosal abnormality primarily affects the small intestine more severely proximally than distally with occasional patchy involvement. The disease may present with a wide range of symptoms. In adults the clinical presentation generally is either with steatorrhea or malabsorption manifested by iron and folate deficiency. Recently, it has become clear that the disease may present with quite subtle manifestations, and the features of classic advanced celiac sprue have become less common. Hence, it is important to consider the diagnosis when the cause of diarrhea or steatorrhea, weight loss, abdominal pain, oral ulceration, or anemia is not apparent. The spectrum of symptoms seen probably relates to individual variability in gluten sensitivity. Also because celiac sprue is mainly a proximal enteropathy, the remaining normal small bowel can compensate to a certain extent. The disease is frequently diagnosed in patients with minimal symptomatology when the key diagnostic clue is the finding of a raised mean corpuscular volume (MCV) or a low red cell folate level.

DIAGNOSIS

The diagnosis depends on an adequate mucosal biopsy specimen from the distal duodenum or jejunum. The characteristic histologic findings are subtotal villous atrophy with crypt hyperplasia, a chronic inflammatory cell infiltrate of the lamina propria, and flattening of the surface epithelial cells. Between the epithelial cells an increase in the number of intraepithelial lymphocytes is seen. The mucosal abnormalities may be patchy, and in equivocal cases the biopsy should be repeated. Because of the long-term implications of a diagnosis of celiac sprue it is important, if possible, to firmly establish a diagnosis by a biopsy *before* treatment is initiated. However, in some patients ingesting a regular gluten-containing diet the mucosal abnormality may be mild with only partial villous atrophy. In such cases the only way to confirm the diagnosis is often to start treatment and assess the clinical and histologic response on follow-up. In equivocal cases a gluten challenge may help confirm the diagnosis. When the diagnosis is confirmed, it is important to explain the nature of the disease to the patient emphasizing that it is generally not a serious condition. They can be told that there is no reason why they should not lead a normal life if they are compliant with the gluten-free diet.

TREATMENT

The essence of the treatment of celiac sprue is lifelong adherence to a gluten-free diet. In practice the avoidance of gluten is quite difficult to achieve because gluten is present in so many foods. To avoid gluten patients must omit foods containing wheat, rye, barley, and oats. The essential items to be avoided include breads, cakes, cookies, and pasta. Soups and canned food also contain gluten and are more difficult to avoid. Although frequently patients are told to avoid mustard, white pepper, and gravy, this is generally not warranted as these items contain negligible amounts of gluten. The patients can be reassured that they can eat a relatively normal diet with meat, potatoes, green vegetables, salads, rice, and corn. Most problems arise from the large amount of processed and "junk" foods to which gluten is added. Beer is usually well tolerated because the gluten is generally destroyed during the manufacturing process. For a patient to adhere to the diet regimen, it is essential for them to consult a clinical dietician. It is also highly advisable that the patient join one of the lay self-help groups such as the American Celiac Society (58 Musano Court, West Orange, NJ 07052 and 201-325-8837), the Celiac Sprue Association (PO Box 31700, Omaha, NE 68131 and 402-558-0600), or the Gluten Intolerance Group of North America (PO Box 23053, Seattle, WA 98102 and 206-325-6980). These are excellent resources for general information as well as much practical advice concerning gluten-free products, gluten-free recipes, and access to gluten-free products while traveling. A gluten-free diet frequently results in constipation because of the dearth of bran. Defatted rice bran or soya bran and bulk agents such as methylcellulose are helpful in this context.

The lifelong avoidance of dietary gluten has widespread implications especially for teenagers and young adults who find the restrictions particularly irksome. With a gluten-free dietary regimen the patients generally feel much better, and the morphology of their jejunal mucosa returns to near normal. A gluten-free diet in older, apparently asymptomatic patients who present with minor nutritional or hematologic abnormalities may not always be warranted. However, it is only when a gluten-free diet is started that many patients become aware of the degree of their prior ill health. Patients usually begin to feel better within 1 to 2 weeks of starting the gluten-free diet. If there are profound nutritional disturbances, iron, folic acid, and vitamin D may be prescribed. If severe steatorrhea is a problem, then a low-fat diet may be necessary temporarily. In exceptional cases there may be vitamin B_{12} deficiency requiring correction. Some adult patients with celiac sprue have evidence of hyposplenism (Howell-Jolly bodies and thrombocytosis), and if this persists despite compliance with a gluten-free diet, then immunization with polyvalent pneumococcal vaccine is recommended.

Compliance with an absolutely gluten-free diet is not practical. It is clear that patients on a gluten-free diet often eat gluten-containing foods having discovered that such dietary indiscretion usually does not result in any diminution in their sense of well-being. This is despite documented induction of small intestinal mucosal abnormalities with dietary noncompliance. Some patients are able to tolerate a "low"-gluten diet without significant clinical deterioration. At present there is little evidence that such a "low"-gluten diet is harmful. It is important to follow patients relatively closely as subtle deterioration may occur that is avoidable. In teenagers this may mean failure to attain their full physical and intellectual development. The rationale for strict dietary compliance is not only to maintain short-term optimal health but also to prevent the development of celiac sprue–associated malignancies in the long-term. There is a wide spectrum in the degree of sensitivity of celiac sprue patients to gluten. Some remain well despite considerable dietary indiscretions, whereas others have to avoid even minimal gluten ingestion to avoid symptoms (even to the extent of avoiding communion wafers). At present we have no way of predicting an individual patient's sensitivity to gluten.

Following the diagnosis the patient should receive lifelong follow-up, and ideally a return to near normal mucosal morphology with gluten withdrawal should be confirmed. At present there is no preferable method for assessment of therapeutic response than subjective assessment of histologic findings. The timing of mucosal recovery is variable, and some features such as increase in villous height or crypt depth can take many months or even years. In some cases clinical improvement has occurred in the absence of any discernible mucosal response. Given that patients should receive lifelong follow-up, there is no consensus as to how frequently they must be evaluated. Once patients are well, annual visits should suffice when red cell folate, alkaline phosphatase, albumin, and a fasting serum carotene can be measured. A good case can be made for performing a follow-up biopsy every few years to detect noncompliance and also to help motivate patients in maintaining a rigorous approach to avoiding gluten. Antiendomysial immunoglobulin A (IgA) antibodies may be useful in assessing dietary compliance as an alternative to repeating a mucosal biopsy.

The vast majority of patients lead a normal life on a gluten-free diet. It has been suggested that some children may "grow out of the disease," but this is not valid. Celiac sprue (correctly diagnosed) is a lifelong condition.

If evidence of malabsorption persists 3 months after initiation of a gluten-free diet or if there is progression of symptoms before that, then the patient may have refractory celiac sprue. The most common cause by far of apparently refractory celiac sprue is failure to adhere to an adequately gluten-free diet. If diet noncompliance is not the problem then a systematic search for colonic disease, a complication of celiac sprue, or another cause of malabsorption and diarrhea must be made.

Dietary compliance should be assessed by a well-informed dietician. In North America where celiac sprue is not so common as in Europe, many dieticians are unfamiliar with the details of the gluten-free diet and may not be able to track down the sources of small amounts of gluten in the diet. It is helpful for the patient to contact one of the branches of the celiac societies. They can have their diet reviewed and also obtain up-to-date lists of gluten-free foods and the names of dieticians well versed in the intricacies of a gluten-free diet. Not only is there considerable variability between patients in their sensitivity to gluten, but also in a given patient the sensitivity may vary considerably with time. Some remain well for long periods on a "low"-gluten rather than a gluten-free diet. However, for unknown reasons these patients may abruptly become sensitive to small amounts of gluten that were previously well tolerated.

The omission of lactose in a milk-free diet may be helpful in some patients because of a prolonged lactase deficiency analogous to that seen in some children after self-limited gastroenteritis. If deficiencies of zinc and magnesium are found they should be corrected. There has been a report of zinc repletion resulting in resolution of symptoms in a case of refractory celiac sprue. However, this has not been a consistent finding with other refractory patients with zinc deficiency.

At this point, if an adequate therapeutic response has not been achieved, a trial of antibiotics for presumed bacterial overgrowth is warranted. Intestinal pseudoobstruction has been reported due to celiac sprue, so it is possible that more subtle motility disturbances might predispose to bacterial overgrowth. A 2-week course of antibiotics should be tried. Some refractory celiac sprue patients have transient responses with periodic courses of antibiotics.

ASSOCIATED DISEASES

A subset of patients with apparent refractory celiac sprue have concurrent colonic disease, which may independently cause diarrhea but not steatorrhea, creating an illusion of refractory disease. Colonic disease is suggested by the presence of an improved small bowel mucosa on rebiopsy despite continued diarrhea. The most important colonic disease associated with celiac sprue is collagenous colitis. Several cases of concomitant collagenous colitis and either celiac sprue or collagenous sprue (less commonly) have been reported. Concomitant collagenous colitis is frequently responsive to therapy with sulfasalazine. If collagenous colitis is a diagnostic consideration and flexible sigmoidoscopic biopsy specimens from several different levels are normal, then a colonoscopy should be done because the abnormalities may be confined to the ascending and transverse colon. At colonoscopy ideally ileal biopsies should be taken to exclude pathology there. There are not enough reported cases to know if the course of collagenous colitis is any different in the presence of celiac sprue or collagenous sprue than its usual benign outcome.

Lymphocytic colitis may be found in 30% of celiac sprue patients, but it does not give rise to symptoms in most. However, if evidence of it is found in a patient with refractory celiac sprue, then a trial of sulfasalazine is warranted.

In the face of a lack of response it is important to consider if the original diagnosis was correct and exclude alternative explanations of a flat jejunal mucosa such as giardiasis, tropical sprue, and Zollinger-Ellison syndrome. Giardiasis should be excluded by duodenal-jejunal aspirates and stool examination. Tropical sprue patients give a history of travel to an endemic area, and in contrast to celiac sprue the histologic lesion is present throughout the small bowel.

The next step in a refractory case is to exclude the two major complications of celiac sprue: intestinal lymphoma and collagenous sprue. The original biopsy specimens that provided the diagnosis of celiac sprue should be reviewed again to see if there was evidence of either complication that may have been missed. The number of lamina propria plasma cells should be checked to see if there is a dearth consistent with common variable immunodeficiency. An immunoglobulin determination should be done as common variable immunodeficiency is not invariably accompanied by a reduction in plasma cell number. This may also reveal selective IgA deficiency, which is increased in frequency in celiac sprue. The prognosis of celiac sprue associated with selective IgA deficiency is no different than without. Another potential finding is a high IgA level associated with lymphoma.

The next phase of investigations in the evaluation of refractory celiac sprue should include both enteroclysis and repeat duodenal-jejunal biopsies looking for evidence of lymphoma or collagenous sprue. The diagnosis of these complications may be difficult and remain elusive for a long period. The enteroclysis may demonstrate localized abnormality suggestive of lymphoma or a smooth, featureless, and occasionally narrowed small bowel referred to as a toothpaste-like pattern. It is useful to use a colonoscope in refractory celiac sprue patients to obtain biopsies from an adequate distance beyond the duodenal-jejunal junction. Biopsies should be taken from multiple sites as well as any abnormal-appearing areas as lymphoma may rarely occur in normal-appearing mucosa. Patchy involvement is typical in collagenous sprue. The proximal small bowel may remain abnormal for a prolonged period despite distal improvement. Accordingly, the presence of abnormality in the proximal small bowel on a gluten-free diet does not necessarily indicate refractory disease. Another potential pitfall in the evaluation of these patients is the finding of mesenteric adenopathy by computed tomography. Mesenteric adenopathy is occasionally seen in celiac sprue and usually regresses with a gluten-free diet; it is not of prognostic significance.

Small intestinal lymphomas (usually T cell) are recognized complications of celiac sprue. Although some patients on a strict diet occasionally present with lymphoma, there is evidence that dietary compliance reduces the risk. Lymphoma complicating celiac sprue may present with pain, bleeding, or obstruction. In some cases the lymphoma is associated with refractory celiac sprue, raising the question that these patients have a low-grade lymphoma de novo that cannot be currently differentiated from the lesions of celiac sprue.

When jejunal or ileal ulcers are found in celiac sprue patients it should be assumed that they are due to lymphoma until proven otherwise. Many, perhaps all, patients with small bowel ulcers have or will develop lymphoma. Because the diagnosis of lymphoma in the presence of ulceration may be difficult, a second opinion should be obtained from a pathologist with the appropriate expertise. Failure to confirm a diagnosis of lymphoma in a celiac sprue patient with jejunal or ileal ulcers mandates close follow-up for its subsequent development.

Previously it was recommended to perform a full thickness small bowel biopsy at laparotomy to rule out lymphoma. This is rarely done now because the yield is marginal in the absence of a radiologic or endoscopic abnormality directing attention to a suspicious area. Laparoscopic surgery is likely to be useful in the diagnosis of intestinal lymphoma in the future.

The prognosis of intestinal lymphoma complicating celiac disease is dismal. The benefit of chemotherapy in a patient malnourished from long-standing malabsorption may be marginal at best.

Collagenous sprue is a rare condition that usually occurs in the setting of partially responsive celiac sprue. The deposits of subepithelial collagen are patchy and may be missed if adequate biopsy specimens of the duodenum and jejunum are not taken. The diagnosis of collagenous sprue should only be made if the subepithelial deposit is unequivocally thicker than the basement membrane of celiac disease. The finding of trapped capillaries or inflammatory cells within the deposit clinches the diagnosis. Collagenous sprue has a poor prognosis. Coexisting collagenous colitis should be excluded.

There are case reports of celiac disease in association with pancreatic insufficiency. When pancreatic disease is suspected in the setting of refractory celiac disease, a 72-hour fecal fat determination may be obtained. This can be used to assess the benefit of pancreatic enzyme replacement. Diabetes mellitus and celiac sprue frequently coexist. Diarrhea or malabsorption in the presence of both conditions may result primarily from the complications of diabetes.

It is vital to emphasize to the patient with refractory celiac sprue that an improvement in symptoms is to be expected with appropriate management.

Steatorrhea should be treated with a low-fat diet. Antidiarrheal therapy may be helpful. A lactose-free diet should be continued if rechallenge makes symptoms worse. Nutritional deficiencies should be corrected. If an initial course of empiric antibiotic therapy for bacterial overgrowth is unsuccessful, then a second should be tried at some point.

For more severe symptoms the usual practice is to try a course of corticosteroid therapy, although there is frequently a relapse of symptoms when the dose is tapered. If doses significantly in excess of 10 mg of prednisone are required long term, other options should be considered.

For these patients the safest long-term approach is parenteral nutrition via a central line. This allows the patient adequate nutritional support with the opportunity to evaluate the efficacy of alternative therapies. While receiving parenteral nutrition, patients can eat as much as they can tolerate without worrying about starvation.

Next, an attempt can be made to eliminate all proteins from the patient's diet to determine if the patient has a multiple protein sensitivity. While on parenteral nutrition, all protein intake is stopped and then gradually resumed one protein at a time. Although some patients cannot tolerate such a rigorous approach, it is occasionally successful.

Finally, if the patient continues to do badly, it may be reasonable to use either cyclosporine or azathioprine as there are reports of therapeutic success with both of these immunosuppressive agents.

Because of the well-documented tendency for celiac sprue to occur in relatives (10% to 20% of first-degree relatives with severe mucosal abnormalities of which 50% are asymptomatic), it is common for patients and their relatives to ask about the risk of another family member's being affected. If the family member is symptomatic, then clearly they should be investigated with a small intestinal biopsy. If the family member is asymptomatic, a screening test (or tests) can be employed (folate or antigliadin and antiendomysial antibodies). However, given the limitations of screening tests, a cogent case for mucosal biopsy as the initial test can be made. This is especially so given the evidence that adherence to a gluten-free diet protects against the development of malignancy.

Patients with dermatitis herpetiformis frequently have abnormal jejunal mucosa, although usually the changes are minor in degree and are not associated with significant malabsorption. A gluten-free diet allows the mucosal lesion to resolve and also helps the skin eruption. However, it may take several years before any benefit on the skin is discernible from a gluten-free diet. It is recommended that a jejunal biopsy be performed on all patients with dermatitis herpetiformis.

REFERENCES

1. Holmes GKT, Prior P, Lane MR, Pope D, Allan RN. Malignancy in celiac disease: effect of a gluten free diet. *Gut.* 1989;30:333–338.
2. Loft DE. The epidemiology and diagnosis of celiac disease. *Eur J Gastroenterol Hepatol.* 1993;5:69–72.
3. Logan RFA, Rifkind EA, Turner IJ, Ferguson A. Mortality in celiac disease. *Gastroenterology.* 1989;97:265–271.
4. Marsh MN, ed. *Celiac Disease.* Cambridge, Mass: Blackwell Scientific Publications; 1992.
5. Murray JA. Celiac disease: pathogenesis and serologic tests. *Clin Immunol Newsletter.* 1993;13:105–112.
6. Trier JS. Medical progress: celiac sprue. *N Engl J Med.* 1991;325:1709–1719.
7. Weinstein WM. Intractable celiac sprue: management, maintenance and maladies. In: Barkin J, Rogers A, eds. *Difficult Decisions in Digestive Diseases.* 2nd ed. St. Louis, Mo: Mosby–Year Book Inc; 1994.

52
Toxigenic Diarrheas

VONDA G. REEVES-DARBY and JOHN R. MATHIAS

Annually, millions of people are affected by diarrhea caused by various toxigenic microorganisms. In well-developed countries diarrhea is commonly self-limited and nonfatal, causing only various degrees of morbidity. In underdeveloped countries diarrhea is the most common cause of death. Worldwide, approximately 5 million children die annually from diarrheal diseases. Extensive research is being conducted to understand the pathophysiology of toxin-induced diarrhea in the hope of finding more effective treatment. Most toxigenic diarrhea is food borne, ingested in contaminated food, either as a preformed toxin or as a microorganism, in which instance the toxin is produced in the lumen of the bowel. Enterotoxins are usually the cause of self-limited disease. Besides producing enterotoxins, other formed toxins, e.g., neurotoxins, can cause extraintestinal manifestations that aid in the differentiation of causative toxins.

Host factors, such as mucus secretion, pH, intestinal peristalsis, secretory antibodies (immunoglobulin A [IgA]), and phagocytes, are important defensive mechanisms against bacterial toxins. These factors protect against microorganism survival in the bowel lumen and consequent toxin production. Virulence factors, such as adherence to the intestinal mucosa, colonization, alteration of intestinal motility, or ability to invade the mucosa and cause mucosal inflammation, determine the onset and severity of disease.[1,2]

Enterotoxins are bacterial products that bind to membrane receptors and act directly on the mucosal epithelium of the small intestine. Secretion of fluid, malabsorption of electrolytes and water, and altered end-nerve and muscle function result in watery diarrhea. Fluid secretion is related to the enterotoxin's binding to specific receptors and activating intracellular second messengers that phosphorylate proteins through kinases A, G, and C. Cholera toxin is the prototype of an enterotoxin. In general, toxigenic diarrheas such as these are characterized by little or no fever and profuse watery diarrhea.

Cytotoxins refer to a group of bacterial products that can lyse cellular membranes or kill epithelial cells, or both. This process is largely accomplished by inhibiting protein synthesis in the cell, causing absorptive and secretory mechanisms of the cells to be destroyed. Fluid loss occurs because of impaired absorption and extravasation of fluid from the mucosa and submucosa. The prototype of a cytotoxin is *Shigella,* or Shiga toxin.

Microorganisms that penetrate the gastrointestinal mucosa often induce bloody diarrhea, or "dysentery"; they can also cause sepsis and "enteric fever syndromes." Stool analysis helps distinguish whether invasion or a break in the integrity of the mucosa has occurred. Stool leukocytes are present in diarrhea caused by invasive microorganisms. Other disorders, such as ulcerative colitis or Crohn's disease, must be considered. When stool leukocytes are found, other nonmicrobial toxin-mediated diseases, such as heavy metal poisoning, mushroom poisoning, and marine toxins, must be included in the differential diagnosis.

VIBRIO TOXINS

VIBRIO CHOLERAE

Cholera, an infection of the small intestine, is caused by a gram-negative toxigenic bacterium, *Vibrio cholerae* 01. The illness is characterized by the sudden onset of watery diarrhea, vomiting, and dehydration, often leading to death. Most cholera outbreaks have been traced to contaminated drinking water.

Cholera toxin, the classic example of a heat-labile toxin, is composed of noncovalent-bonded proteins. The B subunit, composed of five identical units that form a ring or pentamer struc-

TABLE 52–1. ASSESSMENT OF FLUID DEFICIENCY OR DEHYDRATION IN CHOLERA

Signs and Symptoms	Mild	Moderate	Severe
General	Alert, thirsty, restless	Thirsty, restless, irritable, postural changes	Drowsy, cold, sweaty extremities, muscle cramps
Pulse	Normal rate, volume	Rapid, weak	Feeble, unpalpable
Respiration	Normal	Deep, rapid	Deep, rapid
Systolic blood pressure	Normal	Low	Low, unrecordable
Skin turgor	Normal retraction	Retracts slowly	Retracts >2 s
Eyes	Normal	Sunken	Very sunken
Voice	Normal	Hoarse	Not audible
Total fluid loss	4%–5% body weight	6%–9% body weight	>10% body weight

ture, binds to the GM_1 sialoganglioside receptor on the epithelial cell membrane. The A subunit consist of two chains: A_1 penetrates the mucosal membrane and facilitates the attachment of A_2 to the cytosol of the epithelial membrane. A_2 causes adenosine diphosphate ribosylation of the G protein and activates adenylate cyclase. Adenylate cyclase converts adenosine triphosphate to adenosine 3′, 5′-cyclic monophosphate and active secretion of chloride with a concomitant passive flow of water.

Laboratory diagnosis of cholera permits early isolation of the patient and initiation of control measures. Stool analysis for vibrios in the range of 10^6 to 10^9/ml of fecal material is simplest, but rapid laboratory diagnosis using direct hemagglutination, dark-field microscopy, or fluorescent-tagged antibodies is both sensitive and specific. Treatment should begin as rapidly as possible to prevent dehydration, acidosis, and potassium depletion. Accurate assessment of dehydration and the amount of fluid loss (Table 52–1) is essential to clinical management of patients with cholera (Table 52–2).

Use of oral rehydration therapy restores volume losses, reduces losses of intestinal fluid, and may shorten the course of the disease. Oral rehydration fluid is composed (in grams per liter of clean water) of 3.5 g sodium chloride with 20 g of glucose or 40 g of sucrose, *or* 50 to 80 g of rice powder cooked for 2 or 3 minutes to make a thickened solution; when using the glucose or sucrose base, 2.5 g sodium bicarbonate *or* 2.9 g of trisodium citrate dihydrate (the latter is more stable in tropical conditions) and 1.5 g of potassium chloride must be added; the additional salts are helpful but not critical with the rice solutions. For appropriate replacement therapy, patients should consume 2 to 5 L of this solution every 24 hours. A version of this formula with glucose or sucrose is available in ready-made packets and may be obtained from the World Health Organization. Replacement solutions may also be prepared with simple ingredients from the kitchen: The Center for Disease Control has suggested using two glasses. The first glass has 8 oz (240 ml) of apple, orange, or pineapple juice (potassium source); ½ teaspoon of honey or corn syrup (sugar source); and 1 pinch of table salt (sodium chloride source). The second glass has 8 oz (240 ml) of boiled or carbonated water and ½ teaspoon of baking soda (bicarbonate source). For appropriate replacement therapy, alternate the glasses, having the patient consume a total of 2 to 5 L/24 h.

TABLE 52–2. SUMMARY OF CLINICAL MANAGEMENT OF PATIENTS WITH CHOLERA

1. *Rehydrate:* Estimate degree of dehydration and, if severe, rapidly replace lost water and electrolytes with oral or intravenous solution.
2. *Maintain hydration:* Track output and replace stool losses with oral rehydration therapy, considering normal insensible losses.
3. *Oral antibiotics:* Administer to lessen severity and shorten duration of diarrhea.
4. *Nutrition:* Begin oral feeding as soon as patient is able to retain food—usually within 6 hours of initiating hydration.
5. *Antidiarrheal and antisecretory agents:* Avoid. No proven benefit.

The best intravenous fluid is Ringer's lactate because lactate yields bicarbonate to correct acidosis. Potassium concentration is low but more than that in normal saline. With either Ringer's lactate or normal saline, prompt initiation of oral rehydration must complement maintenance intravenous therapy.

The purpose of antibiotic therapy in cholera is to reduce the number of organisms in the lumen that are producing toxin.[2,3] Toxins are produced during log phase growth. Tetracycline or doxycycline will reduce the duration of diarrhea by 50% for an average of about 2 days, reduce the diarrheal volume by about 60%, and reduce the duration of *Vibrio* excretion to 24 to 48 hours. Antibiotics should be given orally and started after completing initial rehydration. Injectable forms are not beneficial. The following antibiotics are effective in the listed adult dosage—tetracycline, 500 mg every 6 hours for 72 hours; doxycycline, 300 mg for one dose; furazolidone, 100 mg every 6 hours for 72 hours; trimethoprim-sulfamethoxazole, (Septra DS) one tablet every 12 hours for 72 hours. Prophylactic antibiotics are recommended for prevention of secondary cases. Use of antidiarrheal and antisecretory agents in the clinical management of cholera is not supported by clinical research.

V. cholerae 01 oral vaccines have been developed and tested but are not uniformly available, provide only a moderate degree of protection for a few months, and therefore are not yet practical. Attenuated strains of *V. cholerae* 01 prepared by recombinant deoxyribonucleic acid (DNA) techniques offer greater promise for the future.[4]

Vibrio parahaemolyticus

Vibrio parahaemolyticus, a gram-negative halophilic hemolytic bacillus, is usually found in marine waters. Outbreaks are most common in the summer months. The illness is characterized by explosive missile watery diarrhea, vomiting, abdominal cramps, and headache, after an incubation period of usually 12 to 48 hours. Headache is a useful clinical clue to this infection. Abdominal pain and cramps may be moderate to severe, and low-grade fever is not uncommon. Chills are present in 25% of all patients. The food-borne toxin has been implicated in raw or cooked seafood that has been improperly refrigerated. The diagnosis is confirmed by culture on TCBS (thiosulfate-citrate-bile salt-sucrose) agar. The mode of action is through cytotoxic activity. All three *V. parahaemolyticus* strains show cytotoxic activity.

Other *Vibrio* species, such as *V. vulnificus, V. fluvialis, V. mimicus, V. hollisae,* and *V. furnissii,* can involve the gastrointestinal tract and cause gastroenteritis.[5] Complicated cases are usually treated with oral tetracycline, but the disease is self-limited and therapy is supportive. There is no direct evidence that *V. vulnificus* causes gastroenteritis, but it is associated with potentially lethal wound infections and sepsis in patients who are immunocompromised or diabetic or have liver disease.

ESCHERICHIA COLI TOXINS

The types of *Escherichia coli* that cause diarrhea are listed in Table 52–3. They are enterotoxigenic, enteroinvasive, enteropathogenic, enterohemorrhagic, and enteroadherent. A further subclassification of the enterotoxigenic *E. coli* includes organisms that secrete heat-labile toxins. Heat-stabile toxins (STa and STb) can cause fluid secretion in the small intestine.

ENTEROTOXIGENIC *ESCHERICHIA COLI* HEAT-LABILE ENTEROTOXINS

Diarrhea caused by enterotoxigenic *E. coli* usually comes from contaminated water or foods. Enterotoxigenic *E. coli* secretes a heat-labile toxin similar to cholera toxins and binds to similar GM_1 receptors. A subclinical illness may be the only manifestation, which usually follows a 1- to 3-day incubation period. The clinical disease resembles mild cholera. There is no vomiting, but mild diffuse abdominal pain may accompany the diarrhea. "Traveler's diarrhea" is the common manifestation of enterotoxigenic *E. coli*. The diagnosis is clinical. Stool cultures do

TABLE 52–3. TYPES OF *ESCHERICHIA COLI* RESPONSIBLE FOR DISEASE

Organism	Disease	White Blood Cell Count	Toxin Type
Enterotoxigenic *E. coli**	Watery diarrhea	−	Enterotoxin
Enteroinvasive *E. coli*	Bloody diarrhea	+++	Cytotoxin
Enteropathogenic *E. coli*	Watery diarrhea	−	Cytotoxin
Enterohemorrhagic *E. coli*	Bloody diarrhea	++	Cytotoxin
Enteroadherent *E. coli*	Watery diarrhea +/− fever	±	Unknown

*Subclasses of organisms include heat-labile and heat-stabile toxins.

TABLE 52–4. RECOMMENDATIONS FOR PREVENTION OF TRAVELER'S DIARRHEA

1. *Lactobacillus* preparations: metabolize dietary carbohydrate to lactic acid and other organic acids thereby reducing intraluminal pH and inhibiting the growth of enteropathogens.
2. Bismuth subsalicylate: short-term intraluminal antimicrobial actions; only effective if given four times a day; not to be used in conjunction with doxycycline because it can prevent the absorption of doxycycline.
3. Avoid uncooked foods (leafy green salads and vegetables).
4. Be sure of the source of the ice used in drinks; drink only pasteurized beverages.
5. Chemoprophylactic drugs: doxycycline, 100 mg twice daily; trimethoprim-sulfamethoxazole (Septra DS), 1 tablet twice daily; and norfloxacin, 500 mg twice daily—any of preceding for 3 days.

not specifically identify what type of *E. coli* is present, but they do help exclude other organisms. The illness is self-limited and resolves in 1 to 3 days with adequate replacement of fluid and electrolytes. Antibacterial drugs protect against traveler's diarrhea. Prophylactic therapy is controversial in the 1990s; in general it is not routinely recommended. Doxycycline, trimethoprim-sulfamethoxazole, and most recently, the fluoroquinolones (norfloxacin and ciprofloxacin) have been used successfully.[3] No significant resistance to the fluoroquinolones has been noted in areas of high risk. Other therapeutic recommendations that may help to prevent disease when traveling are included in Table 52–4. Table 52–4 also lists all current chemoprophylactic drugs. Routine use of chemoprophylactic drugs is not advocated.

ENTEROTOXIGENIC ESCHERICHIA COLI HEAT-STABILE ENTEROTOXINS

Heat-stabile enterotoxins, in contrast to heat-labile enterotoxins, stimulate guanylate cyclase, resulting in increased levels of cyclic guanosine monophosphate. This response suppresses uptake of fluids and electrolytes by intestinal epithelial cells and seems to cause some secretion as well.

ENTEROINVASIVE ESCHERICHIA COLI

Invasion of the mucosa by *E. coli* causes dysentery or bloody diarrhea. These organisms are serologically and biochemically similar to shigellae. The pathogenicity is directly related to bacterial invasion and destruction of intestinal mucosa. The colon is the primary site of involvement of these bacteria. They do not produce enterotoxins, but do produce small quantities of a cytotoxin that serves as a virulence factor, enhancing invasion.

The initial symptoms of fever, toxemia, severe abdominal cramps, and watery diarrhea are followed by bloody mucous stools. The diagnosis of enteroinvasive *E. coli* includes serotypic identification of the strands and enzyme-linked immunosorbent assay (ELISA) testing to detect outer membrane proteins associated with invasiveness. To date, these tests are mainly research tools and are not widely available.

ENTEROHEMORRHAGIC ESCHERICHIA COLI

The prototype of enterohemorrhagic *E. coli* is *E. coli* serotype 0157:H7. This type has been associated with outbreaks of hemorrhagic colitis most commonly noted in nursing homes and day care centers. In most cases, the spectrum of illness included nonbloody or bloody diarrhea, asymptomatic infection, hemolytic uremic syndrome, and possibly, thrombotic thrombocytopenic purpura.[6]

Taking a careful history is important in patients with diarrhea from *E. coli* 0157:H7. Specific examples include ingestion of rare ground beef that has evidence of a bloody, red center. Hamburgers were implicated in the recent outbreak in Oregon at a Jack-In-the-Box restaurant that had received a tainted shipment of beef. Consumption of raw milk before the onset of illness is another common finding. Recent travel, animal exposure, or exposure to other family members with diarrhea are not associated factors. Diarrhea may last for as long as 3 weeks. Nausea and vomiting, along with abdominal cramps and fever, can occur in 25% to 50% of patients. Endoscopic examination can show a variety of findings, from ulcerations to inflammation or hemorrhage of the sigmoid colon or rectum. Friable mucosa can also be seen to extend to the ascending colon. The duration of disease after initiation of antibiotics is approximately 10 days.

The diagnosis of *E. coli* 0157:H7 is accessible through the Center for Disease Control Enteric Reference Laboratory. Waterborne *E. coli* 0157:H7 has been reported in the United States and was traced to drinking water from an unchlorinated municipal water system.

ENTEROPATHOGENIC ESCHERICHIA COLI

In infants in both developed and undeveloped countries, enteropathogenic E. coli is a common cause. The most significant clinical characteristic of enteropathogenic E. coli infection is that it occurs in infants less than 2 years of age. Pathophysiologically, the strands adhere to the mucosa of the small intestine and cause characteristic destruction and effacement of microvilli. By using Hep-2 cells, these pathogens can be seen adhering to the membrane, which distinguishes them from other types of E. coli. The clinical illness is characterized by prolonged watery diarrhea, emesis, and no fever. Antibiotic therapy is not routinely necessary because the clinical course is self-limited. Aggressive replacement of fluid and electrolytes and supportive care is the mainstay of therapy.

ENTEROADHERENT ESCHERICHIA COLI

Enteroadherent E. coli, or diffuse adhering E. coli, produce a poorly characterized clinical disease. Minimal changes in stool consistency are noted in volunteers given 10^7 to 10^{10} of enteroadherent E. coli. This implies no or low virulence. It is not clear whether these bacteria are etiologic agents or unrecognized pathogens that produce diarrhea in studies with adults. In developing countries, enteroadherent E. coli is implicated in persistent diarrhea in children.

PLESIOMONAS SHIGELLOIDES

Plesiomonas shigelloides, a member of the family Vibrionaceae, has recently become recognized by the medical community as a clinically important pathogen. Infection by P. shigelloides causes gastroenteritis and, infrequently, extraintestinal disease. Extraintestinal illnesses, which are more common in immunodeficient persons, include septicemia, cholecystitis, endophthalmitis, septic arthritis, meningitis, and cellulitis. Exposure of the general population to this environmental pathogen occurs through recreational use of water facilities, consumption of raw shellfish, and ingestion of certain foods or untreated water during foreign travel. The isolation of a large number of plesiomonads in the stools of a patient with diarrhea is clinically significant. Both adult and pediatric populations are affected by *Plesiomonas* gastroenteritis. The symptoms associated with the disease can vary but usually include fever, abdominal pain, nausea, vomiting, headaches, and dehydration. Fewer than 6% of cases have required hospitalization, because most are self-limited and resolve with antimicrobial therapy. Interestingly, several forms of diarrhea have been reported with plesiomonads—a secretory gastroenteritis, an invasive disease resembling shigellosis, and a choleralike illness. Prolonged diarrhea is most likely to be associated with the secretory form and can exist for more than 3 weeks. As many as 30 stools per day can occur at the peak of disease, and heavy concentrations of P. shigelloides organisms have been recovered from duodenal aspirates of patients in concentrations of up to 3×10^8/ml. The dysenteric or invasive form is much rarer and has accompanying abdominal pain and evidence of microscopic blood and mucus in the stool. A diarrhea resembling cholera in one patient who was coinfected with P. shigelloides and *Aeromonas sobia* has been reported.

The most frequently described extraintestinal disease is meningitis. In neonates, this is associated with a high fatality rate (approximately 80%) and is thought to be linked to immunocompromised states or nutritional status, or both. Route of entry of the organism in many instances is difficult to determine. It is believed that hematogenous spread of P. shigelloides occurs from the gastrointestinal tract or that systemic dissemination occurs after trauma in association with environmental contact with the organism.[7]

P. shigelloides is found primarily in fresh water or in estuarine environments in predominantly temperate and tropical climates. Disease outbreak is usually during warm weather months. Food, water, and animals are the primary vehicles of transmission. Asymptomatic carrier rates for humans are extremely low and depend on geographic locale and the sampling of the population. The frequency of P. shigelloides as stool enteropathogens varies from 0.2% to 15%. The rate is slightly higher in association with epidemics of diarrheal disease.

The presence of both an enterotoxin and a cytotoxin have been confirmed. Unfortunately, several issues remain undefined in infections caused by this organism. The ecology of this organism is not clearly understood, and further research is also needed to address its pathogenicity and epidemiology. Antimicrobial therapy is accepted as a way of eradication of P. shigelloides infections.[7]

SHIGELLA CYTOTOXINS

Four species of disease-causing *Shigella* are known. They are *Shigella dysenteriae, S. flexneri, S. boydii*, and *S. sonnei*. All invade the intestinal mucosa and cause an inflammatory diarrhea.[8] The clinical characteristics of the illness include high fever, abdominal cramps, and watery diarrhea, which are followed after 24 to 48 hours by bloody mucoid stools and severe tenesmus. Of interest is the frequent presence of neurologic complications, which have included seizures, lethargy, and confusion. Pathophysiologically, neurologic symptoms of the shiga neurotoxin are secondary to vascular changes and not to direct damage to neurons.

The mode of action of *Shigella* toxin involves binding of the B subunit to a 1-4 galactose residues of a glycolipid receptor on intestinal microvillus membranes. Shiga toxin inhibits protein synthesis identical to that of heat-labile *E. coli*. The second biologic activity of shiga toxin is severe bloody diarrhea and abdominal pain, which is predominantly caused by *S. dysenteriae* type 1. Damage to cells destroys the absorptive functions of the gut. The third clinical manifestation caused by shiga toxin is the hemolytic uremic syndrome. The mechanism by which these presentations occur has not been fully defined.[9] Serum and secretory antibodies to *Shigella* have been demonstrated in patients experimentally inoculated and in populations that have high natural occurrence of shigellosis. It is assumed that secretory IgA antibody is the primary mechanism of immunity. The significance of serum antibody levels to *Shigella* is unknown.

Treatment with antibiotics is complicated by rapidly developed drug resistance. *S. flexneri, S. boydii,* and *S. dysenteriae* are more likely to be multidrug resistant than *S. sonnei,* which is the predominant strain in the United States. Antibiotics that reduce the duration of diarrhea and eliminate *Shigella* from the stool include tetracycline, 500 mg four times daily for 5 days, or tetracycline, 2.5 g as a single dose, in adults. Ampicillin, 500 mg four times daily, and trimethoprim, 160 mg, with sulfamethoxazole, 800 mg, twice daily for 5 days, are also effective. Norfloxacin and ciprofloxacin at 500 mg twice daily for 5 days are as effective as trimethoprim with sulfamethoxazole. Treatment of dehydration and electrolyte imbalance must also be combined with antibiotic therapy. Medications that impair motility (antidiarrheal medications), such as diphenoxylate (Lomotil), loperamide (Immodium), or opiates, in general, are contraindicated because they can prolong intestinal clearance of pathogens and enhance intestinal invasion.

SALMONELLA TOXINS

Three species of *Salmonella* have been reported to be associated with human disease. They are *S. typhi, S. enteritidis,* and *S. choleraesuis. S. enteritidis* is the most common species to cause salmonellosis. Four clinical syndromes are noted in humans—gastroenteritis, enteric fever, bacteremia, and an asymptomatic carrier state. Gastroenteritis symptoms are fever, watery diarrhea, abdominal cramps, and inflammation causing blood and mucus in the stool. Enteric fever and sometimes focal extraintestinal infections may be caused by *S. typhi*.

The toxin binds to GM_1 receptors of the intestinal mucosa, activating the adenylate cyclase cascade. Cytotoxin from *Salmonella* is responsible for its invasiveness and the associated inflammatory diarrhea. *S. enteritidis* and *S. typhi* strains are associated with cytotoxin production. As with other cytotoxins, the organism inhibits protein synthesis. Indications for antimicrobial therapy are listed in Table 52–5.

Treatment with trimethoprim-sulfamethoxazole (Septra DS) twice daily, ampicillin, 500 mg four times daily, or ciprofloxacin, 500 mg twice daily for 10 to 14 days, is effective. For typhoid carriers, trimethoprim-sulfamethoxazole or amoxicillin is given for 4 to 6 weeks. Norfloxacin or ciprofloxacin for 4 weeks will also eliminate the carrier state. However, antibiotic usage is discouraged as it may prolong the intestinal carriage of nontyphoidal *Salmonella*. Maintenance therapy is often necessary for patients that are immunocompromised or who are seropositive

TABLE 52–5. INDICATIONS FOR ANTIMICROBIAL THERAPY FOR *SALMONELLA*

1. Presence of complicating, predisposing factors: sickle cell disease, acquired immunodeficiency syndrome (AIDS), malignancies, or aortic or iliac aneurysms.
2. Signs and symptoms of sepsis.
3. Chronic typhoid carrier states.
4. Infections with species associated with bacteremia: *S. typhi, S. paratyphi, S. choleraesuis.*
5. Focal infections such as osteomyelitis or abscess diseases.

for human immunodeficiency virus type 1 (HIV-1). Antimotility drugs are not used in patients with fever or dysentery.

STAPHYLOCOCCAL ENTEROTOXINS

Food poisoning caused by staphylococci is the most common disorder in humans. The most frequent symptoms are nausea, vomiting, and diarrhea. Typically appearing between 1 and 6 hours after contaminated food is eaten, the disease is caused by preformed enterotoxin. Staphylococcal food intoxication is self-limited and lasts only about 24 hours. Fever is not usually present. Abdominal pain, if present, is moderate in intensity and usually diffuse. Not everyone who consumes tainted food is affected. The staphylococci are usually introduced into food by food handlers. The organisms multiply and produce the toxin if food is kept at room temperature and not refrigerated immediately. Foods that are classically associated with staphylococcal food poisons are coleslaw and potato salad. Although these foods are kept cool, the inner part may be warm enough to promote toxin production. Salad dressings, milk products, and cream pastries also provide an excellent medium for staphylococcal multiplication. The main preventive measure is adequate refrigeration of food immediately after preparation. The food should be stored in containers that are designed to rapidly cool all parts of the food equally. Unfortunately, food contaminated with staphylococci is normal in color, taste, and appearance. The diagnosis is based on a classic clinical syndrome. More than 10^5 colony-forming units of staphylococci per gram can be cultured from contaminated food. As with most toxigenic diarrheal diseases, antimicrobial therapy is not indicated. If necessary, outline therapy for rehydration and intractable vomiting may be initiated on a case-by-case basis.

YERSINIA ENTEROCOLITICA ENTEROTOXIN

Yersinia enterocolitica causes acute gastroenteritis, mesenteric lymphadenitis, and some extraintestinal infections. It usually occurs in cooler climates like Europe and Canada. The gastroenteritis involves bloody diarrhea, vomiting, abdominal pain, and fever. Enterotoxin production is very common. The two most typical features of infection are diarrhea and abdominal pain.

Yersinia infection can mimic either acute appendicitis, resulting in an unnecessary appendectomy, or Crohn's ileitis. Other common symptoms include a combination of fever, vomiting, dysentery, or arthritis. Pharyngitis may be the first symptom in some children. The disease is self-limited, with patients having a *Shigella*-like illness of blood-streaked watery stools accompanied by abdominal pain, low-grade fever, and constitutional symptoms that improve by the second or third day of illness. Stool examination discloses fecal leukocytes and red blood cells. Complete recovery usually occurs in the second week in uncomplicated cases.

In some young adults and children a more aggressive infection may occur with fulminant ulcerative enterocolitis, mesenteric adenitis, peritonitis, and rarely, small bowel gangrene and massive intestinal hemorrhage.

Septicemia due to *Y. enterocolitica* can occur in patients who have a predisposing illness such as hemochromatosis, hemosiderosis, cirrhosis, or hemolytic anemia. These disorders suggest that *Yersinia* may use iron as a virulence factor. Other extraintestinal lesions can involve the meninges, bones, sinuses, and pleural spaces. Postinfection complications may be reactive arthritis, erythema nodosum, skin rashes, ankylosing spondylitis, and inflammatory bowel disease. Antimicrobial therapy for *Yersinia* enteritis is controversial; treatment is not generally advocated, which is in sharp contrast to therapy for infections that cause sepsis and high rates of morbidity and mortality. If therapy is contemplated, aminoglycosides, tetracycline, chloramphenicol, or trimethoprim-sulfamethoxazole are often chosen.[10]

AEROMONAS TOXINS

Aeromonas species are nonlactose-fermenting, facultatively anaerobic gram-negative rods that grow well in nonselective media. Three species have been identified—*A. hydrophila, A. sobia,* and *A. caviae*—all in the family Vibrionaceae. *Aeromonas* has been isolated in both adults and children. The organism produces both heat-stabile and heat-labile enterotoxins. The illness characteristic of *A. hydrophila* usually is self-limited and occurs in the warmer months. The disease includes symptoms of watery diarrhea (containing blood or mucus in up to a quarter of all cases), mild fever, and vomiting. Chronic dysentery and a choleralike diarrhea may occur in association with this organism. Usually, symptoms last about 1 week, but can persist for as long as 1 year in cases of chronic illnesses. The role of antimicrobial therapy in this illness is undefined. In vitro studies have shown that the organisms can be sensitive to aminoglycosides, trimethoprim-sulfamethoxazole, tetracycline, or chloramphenicol.

CLOSTRIDIUM TOXINS

Clostridia are involved in a wide variety of human infections related to extracellular toxins. Enteric diseases caused by clostridial organisms are divided into three clinical presentations. The first is that of clostridial food poisoning, caused by an enterotoxin produced by *Clostridium perfringens* type A. This is the most common form of toxin-induced diarrhea in the United States. Disease activity is related to the cytotoxic action of the enterotoxin on the intestinal epithelial cells. The *C. perfringens* enterotoxin binds to the mucosal cells and causes structural damage, inducing loss of intracellular substances like sodium chloride, protein, and fluid. Further damage to the cell causes death of the cell. Outbreaks are most common in the fall and winter months and are usually associated with specific foods. The infection rate is high and is most often associated with contaminated meat or meat products. A 6- to 24-hour incubation period is common. The key clinical symptom is crampy abdominal pain; nausea and watery diarrhea in the range of two to four stools per day may also occur. The disease is self-limited, and recovery is within 24 hours. The type of *C. perfringens* food poisoning cannot be distinguished easily from other noninfectious enterotoxigenic intoxications such as those caused by *Bacillus cereus* and *Staphylococcus aureus*. Since diarrhea is self-limited, supportive care and rehydration are the mainstay of therapy rather than antibiotics.

The second clinical spectrum of clostridia is that of pseudomembranous colitis. A severe necrotizing colitis, it is associated with cytotoxin production by *C. difficile*. The disease is related to antibiotic therapy, which enhances the overgrowth of *C. difficile*. Most antibiotics have been associated with pseudomembranous colitis. The more commonly implicated antimicrobials include ampicillin, clindamycin, and cephalosporins. The clinical manifestations include fever, abdominal cramps, and perfuse watery diarrhea that is sometimes bloody. Treatment of this clinical spectrum is effective with oral vancomycin or oral or intravenous metronidazole, or both. The toxins of *C. difficile* are the main cause of pseudomembranous colitis. At least two toxins are elaborated that are totally unrelated immunologically. The first is designated as toxin A, which causes fluid accumulation in animal ileal loop models and has been designated as an enterotoxin. Toxin A causes cytotoxic effects to Chinese hamster ovarian (CHO) cells in vitro. Toxin B does not affect CHO cells in vitro and is not associated with significant fluid accumulation in ileal loops. Both toxins A and B seem to be necessary to induce disease; synergy has been demonstrated between the two toxins. The toxins are found in 80% to 95% of patients affected by pseudomembranous colitis. A course of antimicrobial therapy to eliminate the organisms that are producing the toxins in the stool resolves the symptoms and lesions.[11]

The third clinical spectrum is that of necrotizing enteritis, a severe disease of the small intestine. Consumption of poorly cooked pork or canned meats is the source of infection. *C. perfringens* type C and the beta toxin it produces are the pathogenic factors. This disease is characterized by abdominal cramps, bloody diarrhea, vomiting, shock, and high mortality rates.

CAMPYLOBACTER TOXINS

Campylobacter jejuni, the leading cause of bloody diarrheal disease worldwide, is usually associated with self-limited diarrhea that occasionally contains blood or leukocytes and sometimes can be prolonged or recurrent. The most common subspecies are *C. fetus, C. jejuni, C. coli, C. fecalis*, and *C. sputorum*. *C. jejuni* is the major enteric pathogen of this genus and accounts for approximately 95% of the enteric infections. Identifying *Campylobacter* in stool cultures is easy using selective media and microaerophilic conditions. *Campylobacter* is similar to *Salmonella* in its mode of transmission, fecal and oral being the most common. It is also associated with ingestion of raw or contaminated milk, exposure to sick pets, and ingestion of contaminated poultry or eggs. Reservoirs are common in both domesticated and wild animals. Children and young adults are usually affected. The pathogenesis of *C. jejuni* is possibly related to two virulence factors—invasiveness and toxin production. Its actual mechanisms of pathophysiology, however, are unknown.

The clinical features of acute *Campylobacter* infection are predominately bloody diarrhea and crampy abdominal pain. The spectrum of disease ranges from asymptomatic carriers to severe life-threatening colitis with toxic megacolon. The incubation period is 1 to 6 days. Fatigue and myalgia may precede the onset of diarrhea; nausea, anorexia, lower abdominal cramping, and diarrhea follow. The diarrhea can be watery or bloody, with 10 or more stools per day. Abdominal pain and tenesmus may mimic acute appendicitis. Tenesmus is present in 25% of patients, and up to 80% of patients have a proctocolitis. Stool analysis discloses fecal leukocytes and red blood cells. A complete blood count shows leukocytosis. Examination of fresh stools gives a tentative diagnosis of *C. jejuni*. Complications of an infection of *Campylobacter* enteritis include pseudomembranous enterocolitis with toxic megacolon, Reiter's syndrome, and hemolytic-uremic syndrome. Therapy for *Campylobacter* infection involves supportive care and replacement of depleted fluid and electrolytes. Most infections are self-limiting. Erythromycin is the drug of choice in protracted *Campylobacter* diarrhea. Several studies have shown a lack of correlation with antibiotic therapy in reduction and duration of disease or symptoms. The only benefit of erythromycin therapy compared with placebo has been a decrease in the shedding of *C. jejuni* in the stools.[12] An alternative treatment is ciprofloxacin, 500 mg twice daily.

TOXINS ASSOCIATED WITH SEAFOOD CONSUMPTION

Three clinical entities have been described in association with neurologic abnormalities after ingestion of toxin-containing fish. Tetrodotoxin, saxitoxin, and ciguatoxin are associated with puffer fish, paralytic shellfish, and ciguatera poisoning, respectively. They are neurotoxic and cause alterations of sodium conduction in myelinated and nonmyelinated nerves. A fourth entity, scombroid fish poisoning, is caused by histamine production from bacteria in spoiling fish.[13] Treatment of tetrodotoxin poisoning includes gastric lavage and cardiorespiratory support. Prognosis is greatly improved if the patient survives the first 6 hours of illness. Saxitoxin, although not associated with diarrhea, is treated similarly to tetrodotoxin poisoning. Ciguatera is the most common form of fish intoxication in the United States. ELISA assay is available for detection of the toxin. Treatment with amitriptyline and mannitol are suggested.

Scombroid fish intoxication may or may not be associated with diarrhea. Spoiled fish have large amounts of preformed histamines, which cause symptoms of flushing, erythema, and vertigo. Treatment with antihistamines is usually effective.

REFERENCES

1. Harrison LA, Andersson B, Carlsson B, et al. Defense of mucous membranes by antibodies, receptor analogues and nonspecific host factors. *Infection.* 1984;12:111–117.
2. Gianella RA. Importance of intestinal inflammatory reaction on *Salmonella*-mediated intestinal secretion. *Infect Immun.* 1979;23:140–145.
3. Gorbach SL, Kean BH, Evans DG, et al. Travelers' diarrhea and toxigenic *Escherichia coli. N Engl J Med.* 1975;292:933–936.
4. Molla AM. Cholera. In: Rakel ED, ed. *Conn's Current Therapy.* Philadelphia, Pa: WB Saunders Co; 1989:48–51.
5. Ketyi I. Toxins as virulence factors of bacterial enteric pathogens. *Acta Microbiol Hung.* 1985;32:299–304.
6. Ryan CA, Tule RV, Hosek GW, et al. *Escherichia coli* 0157:H7 diarrhea in a nursing home: clinical, epidemiological and pathological findings. *J Infect Dis.* 1984;154:631–638.
7. Brenden RA, Miller MA, Janda JM. Clinical disease spectrum and pathogenic factors associated with *Plesiomonas shigelloides* infections in humans. *Rev Infect Dis.* 1988;10:303–316.
8. Levine MM, DuPont HL, Formal SB, et al. Pathogenesis of *Shigella dysenteriae* 1 (Shiga) dysentery. *J Infect Dis.* 1973;127:261–270.
9. Cantey JR. Shiga toxin—an expanding role in the pathogenesis of infectious diseases. *J Infect Dis.* 1985;i:503–506.
10. Cover TL, Aber RC. *Yersinia enterocolitica. N Engl J Med.* 1989;321:16.
11. Bartlett JG, Chang T-W, Gurwith M, et al. Antibiotic-associated pseudomembranous colitis due to toxin-producing *Clostridia. N Engl J Med.* 1978;298:531–534.
12. DuPont HL, Ericsson CD, Robins A, et al. Current problems in antimicrobial therapy for bacterial enteric infection. *Am J Med.* 1987;82(suppl 4A):324.
13. Miranda AG, DuPont HL. In: Yamada T, ed. *Textbook of Gastroenterology, 2.* New York, NY: JB Lippincott Co; 1991:1452–1456.

53
Invasive Pathogens
DAVID C. WOLF and RALPH A. GIANNELLA

Bacterial infections of the large and small bowel are important causes of diarrheal disease worldwide. The increased fluid secretion that follows infection with an invasive bacterial species is not due solely to an increase in mucosal permeability or the formation of an inflammatory exudate. Rather, the acute inflammation that follows intestinal invasion induces the production of intestinal secretagogues. These substances, including arachidonic acid metabolites, kinins, and other vasoactive substances, may be the final common pathway in the pathogenesis of these diarrheal disorders.[1]

This review concentrates on current recommendations for treatment of diarrheal diseases caused by invasive pathogens (Table 53–1) and also briefly reviews their epidemiology and natural history.

SHIGELLA

Man and the great apes are the only natural reservoirs for the four species of *Shigella* organisms: *S. dysenteriae, S. flexneri, S. boydii,* and *S. sonnei.* In the United States, between 13,000 and 19,000 cases of shigellosis are reported each year, primarily affecting children. Most infections are the result of person-to-person transmission of *S. sonnei.* The disease tends to run a mild course. In contrast, shigellosis is a major cause of morbidity and mortality in the third world. Poor sanitation results in the waterborne and foodborne transmission of infection, primarily because of aggressive strains of *S. flexneri.* Central America and India are also affected by a *S. dysenteriae* pandemic. In these areas, the mortality for shigellosis patients is as high as 2% to 10%.[2]

Within 12 hours of ingestion, *Shigella* bacteria multiply in the small intestine, reaching a concentration of 10^7 to 10^9/ml. Abdominal pain, cramping, and fever correlate with the localization of bacteria in the small intestine. Over the next few days, there is increased localization of bacteria in the colon, with a corresponding decreased density of bacteria in the small bowel. There is also evidence for colonic mucosal invasion. Clinically, the fever may subside, but the patient may suffer increasing lower abdominal pain and tenderness. Furthermore, the patient may experience the onset of fecal urgency, tenesmus, and the passage of bloody mucoid stools. Endoscopic evidence for colitis, ranging from proctitis to pancolitis, is seen in all patients with dysentery. Dysentery is not an invariable finding, however, appearing in about one half of adult patients presenting with shigellosis.[3]

In general, the symptoms of *Shigella* infection last about 1 week, although the duration of illness ranges between 1 day and 1 month. Infrequently, patients experience extraintestinal manifestations of infection including meningism and seizures in children, pneumonitis, and hemolytic-uremic syndrome (associated with *S. dysenteriae* infection). Reiter's syndrome, marked by peripheral arthritis, back pain, urethritis, and conjunctivitis, is described in 1% to 2% of patients, generally in those bearing the HLA-B27 histocompatibility antigen.

Shigellosis may be managed most often with oral rehydration, only. Kaolin-pectin and bismuth compounds are ineffective. Antimotility agents have the potential to worsen symptoms and may predispose to toxic dilation of the colon. Antibiotic therapy should only be used in patients with moderate or severe symptoms, given the self-limited nature of most cases and the potential for the development of antibiotic resistance. Indeed, antibiotic resistance has been noted following the introduction of new drug regimens for the treatment of *Shigella* infection: sulfonamides in the 1950s, tetracycline in the 1960s, ampicillin in the 1970s, and trimethoprim-sulfamethoxazole (TMP-SMX) in the 1980s. Nonetheless, antibiotics play an invaluable role in patients with severe symptoms. Treatment im-

TABLE 53–1. ANTIBIOTIC THERAPY FOR INVASIVE ENTERIC PATHOGENS

Organism or Syndrome	Adult Recommendation	Pediatric Recommendation	Alternate Drug

Shigella	TMP-SMX, 160 mg/800 mg b.i.d. for 5 d	TMP, 10 mg/kg/d, plus SMX, 50 mg/kg/d, in two divided doses for 5 d	Ciprofloxacin, 500 mg b.i.d. for 5 d
			Nalidixic acid for 5 d
			  Adults: 1 g t.i.d. or q.i.d.
			  Children: 55 mg/kg/d in four divided doses (considered drug of choice in Bangladesh and other third world nations)
			Ceftriaxone (IV/IM)
			  Adults: 1–2 g/d
			  Children: 50 mg/kg/d
			Tetracycline, 2.5 g single oral dose (may discolor teeth in children under 8 y)

Salmonella			
Gastroenteritis (for severe symptoms or immunocompromised patients)	Ciprofloxacin, 500 mg b.i.d.	Ampicillin, 50–100 mg/kg/d (four divided doses), or Amoxicillin, 40 mg/kg/d (three divided doses), for 5 d	Tetracycline, 500 mg q.i.d. TMP-SMX, 160 mg/800 mg b.i.d. Other β-lactam antibiotics

Bacteremia and localized infection	Bacteremia treated for 10–14 d; endocarditis and osteomyelitis treated for 4–6 wk or longer
	Chloramphenicol, 50 mg/kg/d in four divided doses (not for use in vascular infections)
	Ampicillin, 1 g q4–6h
	Amoxicillin, 1 g q6–8h
	TMP, 10 mg/kg/d, plus SMX, 50 mg/kg/d, in four divided doses
		Chloramphenicol, 50 mg/kg/d in four divided doses
		Ampicillin, 100 mg/kg/d (IV/PO) in four divided doses
			Cefotaxime, especially in meningitis or vascular infections
			  Adults: 2 g q4–6h
			  Children: 200 mg/kg/d, four divided doses
			Ciprofloxacin, 750 mg b.i.d., especially long-term therapy for prevention of bacteremia relapse in AIDS patients

Enteric fever	Chloramphenicol, 50 mg/kg/d in four divided doses for at least 2 wk
	Alternate: chloramphenicol, 1 g q8h until defervescence, followed by 500 mg q8h for at least 2 wk
		Same as adults	Ampicillin, 100 mg/kg/d in four divided doses (IV/PO) for at least 2 wk
			Amoxicillin, 1 g q.i.d. for 2 wk
			TMP-SMX, 160 mg/800 mg 1–2 tablets b.i.d. for 2 wk
			Cefotaxime (IV)
			  Adults: 2 g q4–6h for 2 wk
			  Children: 200 mg/kg/d in four divided doses for 2 wk; maximum dose 12 g/d
			Ciprofloxacin, 500 mg b.i.d. for 2 wk

Carrier state	Ciprofloxacin, 750 mg b.i.d. for 2–4 wk	Not formally studied	Ampicillin, 1 g q.i.d. for 1 mo Amoxicillin, 1.5 g q.i.d. for 1 mo TMP-SMX, 160 mg/800 mg b.i.d., plus rifampin, 600 mg q.d. for 1 mo

TMP-SMX = trimethoprim-sulfamethoxazole.

TABLE 53-1. ANTIBIOTIC THERAPY FOR INVASIVE ENTERIC PATHOGENS *Continued*

Organism or Syndrome	Adult Recommendation	Pediatric Recommendation	Alternate Drug
Campylobacter jejuni	Erythromycin, 250 mg q.i.d. for 5 d	Erythromycin, 30–50 mg/kg/d in four divided doses	Ciprofloxacin, 500 mg b.i.d. Norfloxacin, 400 mg b.i.d. Tetracycline, 500 mg q.i.d. Aminoglycosides Clindamycin, 150–450 mg q.i.d. Chloramphenicol, 250–750 mg q.i.d. Furazolidone, 100 mg q.i.d. TMP-SMX, 160 mg/800 mg b.i.d.
Campylobacter fetus	Ampicillin and gentamicin (IV)	Same as adults	Erythromycin, 0.25–1 g q6h
Yersinia enterocolitica	Tetracycline, 500 mg q.i.d. TMP-SMX, 160 mg/800 mg b.i.d. Chloramphenicol, 50 mg/kg/d in four divided doses Aminoglycosides	Same as adults, with exception of tetracycline (may discolor teeth in children under age 8 y)	Possibly cefotaxime, despite bacterial elaboration of β-lactamases
Escherichia coli			
Enteroinvasive	(No controlled studies) Consider empiric therapy with: Ampicillin, 1 g q6h TMP-SMX, 160 mg/800 mg b.i.d. Ciprofloxacin, 500 mg b.i.d. Norfloxacin, 400 mg b.i.d.	Same as adults, with exception of ciprofloxacin and norfloxacin; (quinolone antibiotics not yet recommended for children)	
Enterohemorrhagic	Unclear if antibiotics are effective; consider empiric therapy	Same as adults	Consider using immune globulin (contains antibodies to Shiga-like toxin 1)
Vibrio parahaemolyticus vulnificus and *alginolyticus*	Supportive therapy, only Tetracycline, 500 mg q.i.d. or 0.5–1 g IV q12h	Supportive therapy, only Chloramphenicol, 50 mg/kg/d in four divided doses Penicillin G, >75,000 U/kg/d in two to three divided doses	Chloramphenicol, 50 mg/kg/d in four divided doses Penicillin G, >20 million U/d IV in divided doses
Aeromonas hydrophila	(No controlled studies) TMP-SMX, 160 mg/800 mg b.i.d. Gentamicin, 3 mg/kg/d in three divided doses Chloramphenicol, 50 mg/kg/d in four divided doses Third-generation cephalosporins Ciprofloxacin, 500 mg b.i.d. Norfloxacin, 400 mg b.i.d.	Same as adults, with exception of ciprofloxacin and norfloxacin; (quinolone antibiotics not yet recommended for children)	

proves the clinical course of the disease, shortens the duration of fecal carriage of the organisms, and reduces the chance for person-to-person transmission.

In Bangladesh, where multiresistant *Shigella* species are common, nalidixic acid, an early quinolone agent, is now the drug of choice for shigellosis.[4] In the United States, TMP-SMX remains the first-line agent for suspected *Shigella* infection, save in areas where resistant strains are prevalent.

The newer quinolone agents, including ciprofloxacin and norfloxacin, appear to be highly efficacious, leading to rapid reduction in diarrhea and fever and a near 100% rate of bacteriologic cure.[5] Enthusiasm for their use is tempered by their expense and potential neurologic and rheumatologic side effects in children. More experience is required before these drugs can be recommended routinely for treatment of shigellosis worldwide.

Other drugs that may prove to be useful in *Shigella* infections are ceftriaxone, the b-lactam agent pivampicillin-pivmecillinam, single large dose (2.5 g) tetracycline, nonabsorbable oral gentamicin, and nonabsorbable bicozamycin.

SALMONELLA

Salmonellosis is a common disease. The more than 40,000 cases of salmonellosis reported to the Centers for Disease Control each year may represent only 1% to 5% of the actual incidence of the disease in the United States. Contaminated poultry, eggs, dairy products, and processed meats are the major sources of human *Salmonella* infection in this country. Patients may be affected by a number of distinctive clinical syndromes.

GASTROENTERITIS (ENTEROCOLITIS)

Gastroenteritis is the most common manifestation of infection with nontyphi *Salmonella*. This diarrheal illness is usually self-limited, beginning 6 to 48 hours after ingestion of bacteria and persisting for up to 1 week. Other accompanying symptoms include fever, chills, headache, myalgia, nausea, vomiting, and cramping lower abdominal pain. Mortality is less than 1%. Although fecal leukocytes and erythrocytes are discovered in about one third of patients, dysentery is infrequent in *Salmonella* infection. Still, endoscopically documented colitis, with histologic evidence for edema, inflammation, and microabscess, is relatively common.

As with shigellosis, rehydration therapy should be offered and antibiotic therapy should be avoided in patients with mild and moderate disease. Antibiotics should be administered to patients with severe symptoms, patients at the extremes of age, pregnant women, and patients with severe underlying illness or immunocompromise. Unfortunately, the antibiotics traditionally used to treat *Salmonella* infection (tetracycline, TMP-SMX, and b-lactam antibiotics) do not appear to reduce the duration of gastroenteritis symptoms. Chloramphenicol and ampicillin may actually prolong the duration of fecal carriage of organisms. Recent studies suggest that ciprofloxacin and norfloxacin improve the clinical course of illness. There are conflicting data regarding their effect on fecal carriage of *Salmonella*. Overall, ciprofloxacin and norfloxacin appear to be superior to traditional regimens for the treatment of severe *Salmonella* gastroenteritis in adults.

NONTYPHI *SALMONELLA* BACTEREMIA AND LOCALIZED INFECTIONS

In contrast to shigellosis, bacteremia is relatively common in salmonellosis, occurring in about 5% to 10% of cases. Patients with inadequate complement levels or diminished phagocytic activity (as in sickle cell disease), as well as infants and patients with acquired immunodeficiency syndrome (AIDS) and other immunosuppressed states, are particularly susceptible to bacteremia and extraintestinal *Salmonella* infection. *Salmonella* infections (most notably osteomyelitis, pneumonia, arteritis, and meningitis) are reported in virtually every organ in the body. Aggressive medical therapy with chloramphenicol, ampicillin, amoxicillin, or TMP-SMX for 10 to 14 days is indicated, although chloramphenicol may not be effective treatment for endocarditis or infected vascular aneurysms. Third-generation cephalosporins may also be beneficial.[6]

Patients with AIDS are subject to recurrent or breakthrough *Salmonella* bacteremia, despite appropriate antibiotic treatment. Long-term therapy with ciprofloxacin, 750 mg orally two times a day, may help prevent the relapse of bacteremia in such patients.[7]

ENTERIC FEVER (TYPHOID FEVER)

Enteric fever is caused by *S. typhi*, *S. paratyphi*, and related organisms. The diagnosis is made after isolation of *Salmonella* species from blood, bone marrow, or bile.

Remittent fever, often accompanied by headache, malaise, and anorexia, develops gradually following a 1- to 3-week incubation period. Fever becomes sustained during the second and third weeks of the illness. Diarrhea occurs in fewer than one half of patients. An altered level of consciousness, dizziness, or seizures occur in about 10% of patients. Indeed, the word *typhoid* is derived from the Greek term for "cloudy."

Without antimicrobial therapy, uncomplicated enteric fever usually resolves in 3 to 4 weeks. However, patients may suffer myocarditis, liver and bone marrow damage, and extraintestinal infection. Intestinal and colonic ulceration, bleeding, and perforation are well described. In the preantibiotic era, typhoid relapse occurred in about 8% to 12% of patients; death occurred in 12% to 16%.

The introduction of chloramphenicol in 1948 significantly reduced the morbidity and mortality of enteric fever, producing defervescence in 3 to 5 days. Chloramphenicol is still used commonly throughout the third world, although it does predispose to a high rate of disease relapse and has potentially life-threatening hematologic side effects.

In the United States high-dose ampicillin and amoxicillin are commonly recommended for *S. typhi* infection. Other drugs that have proved useful in clinical trials include TMP-SMX, third-generation cephalosporins,[6] ciprofloxacin, and ofloxacin.[8] High-dose steroids may be of benefit in severely ill patients with altered mental status or shock.

CARRIER STATE

Up to 4% of patients following enteric fever, and 1% of patients following nontyphoid illness may continue to shed bacteria more than 1 year after the resolution of acute salmonellosis. Thus, these asymptomatic patients potentially place others at risk. The Centers for Disease Control currently recommend that health care workers be excluded from direct contact with high-risk patients until stool cultures are documented to be negative for *Salmonella*. Traditional antibiotic regimens are about 70% effective in their ability to produce a bacteriologic cure in chronic carriers. In the past, cholecystectomy was recommended for some chronic *Salmonella* carriers with concurrent cholelithiasis, given the potential for bacteria to be sequestered in gallstones. Recently, several small studies used ciprofloxacin, 750 mg orally twice daily for 2 to 4 weeks in patients with chronic carriage; the bacteriologic cure rate averaged 90%. Ciprofloxacin appears to be the drug of choice for treatment of *Salmonella* carriage, despite reports that quinolone antibiotics used in acute infection may actually predispose to a prolonged carrier state.

CAMPYLOBACTER

Campylobacter species have long been recognized to be pathogens in domestic animals. Only during the past 20 years has *Campylobacter* been shown to play a major causative role in diarrheal diseases in the United States and Europe. Blaser and Reller[9] documented a 5% incidence of *C. jejuni* infection in outpatients presenting with diarrheal complaints. The peak incidence for infection is seen in children under age 5 years and young adults. *C. jejuni* may account for the complaints of 20% of children and 80% of college students with diarrhea containing fecal leukocytes. Undercooked poultry is the source of 50% to 70% of human cases of campylobacteriosis in developed countries. Consumption of contaminated meats, raw clams, and water and unpasteurized milk and contact with infected farm animals, dogs, cats, rodents, and birds account for most other human cases. Direct person-to-person contact is probably not an important means of transmission.

Campylobacteriosis may present as either an enteric or extraintestinal illness. *C. jejuni* is most often associated with the former; *C. fetus* subsp. *fetus* is most often associated with the latter.

Diarrhea is the hallmark of *Campylobacter* enteritis. Stools range in consistency from loose to watery to grossly bloody. Cramping abdominal pain and tenesmus are frequently noted. Prodromal symptoms of fever, headache, myalgia, and malaise are also common. Typically, symptoms last from 1 day to 1 week but can relapse or persist for longer periods of time. Endoscopy often reveals colitis, with histologic evidence for reduced mucus production, acute and chronic inflammation of the lamina propria, and crypt abscesses. Thus, *Campylobacter* enteritis may be difficult to differentiate from acute idiopathic inflammatory bowel disease.

C. jejuni infection is frequently accompanied by bacteremia or extraintestinal infection. Septic abortion, a wide variety of focal infections, and Guillain-Barre syndrome can occur, as well as a postinfection reactive arthritis in HLA-B27-positive patients.

C. fetus subsp. *fetus* is an infrequently encountered organism that characteristically produces opportunistic infections in immunocompromised individuals, infants, and pregnant women. Bacteremia is a common manifestation of *C. fe-*

tus infection. Mortality from bacteremia may range up to 43% in the setting of concurrent meningoencephalitis, septic arthritis, pneumonia, carditis, thrombophlebitis, or mycotic aortic aneurysm. *C. fetus* is also associated with septic abortion and a syndrome of relapsing fevers, chills, and myalgias.

Severe enteritis symptoms, enteritis persisting beyond 1 week, and certainly, systemic infection due to *C. fetus* necessitate antibiotic therapy. However, data on medical therapy for campylobacteriosis primarily arises from in vitro work and case reports. *C. jejuni* is sensitive to erythromycin, the tetracyclines, the aminoglycosides, clindamycin, chloramphenicol, and furazolidone in vitro. Erythromycin is the drug of choice for *C. jejuni* infection. Most authors agree that erythromycin shortens the duration of fecal carriage of *Campylobacter*. However, there is considerable debate whether antibiotic therapy actually speeds the resolution of symptoms. Quinolone antibiotics may speed clinical recovery in patients with enteritis, but their impact appears to be relatively modest.

C. fetus infection should be managed with intravenous ampicillin and gentamicin. Erythromycin is a second-line agent.

YERSINIA

Yersinia enterocolitica is a relatively uncommon cause of infectious colitis in the United States, but it is a frequent cause of diarrheal disease in northern Europe. Most cases of illness can be traced to ingestion of contaminated foods, especially milk products and raw pork. *Yersinia* has a propensity to invade epithelial cells of the ileum and colon.[10]

Children and infants typically suffer from symptoms of fever, diarrhea, and abdominal pain, in a syndrome not unlike other forms of infectious colitis. Stools may be streaked with blood. Symptoms may last from 1 to 3 weeks, although a chronic ileocolitis resembling Crohn's disease can occur.

Older children and young adults may experience invasion of *Yersinia* into mesenteric lymph nodes and intestinal lymphoid tissue, with resulting mesenteric adenitis and terminal ileitis. Patients may present with fever, right lower quadrant pain, and leukocytosis in a syndrome resembling acute appendicitis. Adults may suffer a variety of other problems following *Yersinia* infection including polyarthritis, Reiter's syndrome (most common in HLA-B27-positive patients), erythema nodosum (females predominate), and exudative pharyngitis. Septicemia and extraintestinal infection are rare occurrences. Septicemia is usually described in patients suffering from immunocompromise, cirrhosis, or iron-overload states, especially those individuals treated with deferoxamine.

Y. pseudotuberculosis is encountered less frequently than *Y. enterocolitica* and is most often associated with mesenteric adenitis.

Yersinia species are sensitive to tetracycline, TMP-SMX, chloramphenicol, the aminoglycosides, and ciprofloxacin. Anecdotal reports suggest that these antibiotics may be efficacious in the treatment of enteritis, mesenteric adenitis, and even erythema nodosum and arthritis. One controlled trial showed no advantage of TMP-SMX over placebo in the treatment of *Y. enterocolitica* diarrhea, but therapy was instituted relatively late in the course of illness.

ESCHERICHIA COLI

Diarrheagenic *Escherichia coli* bacteri are classified into five major categories. The first three categories of *E. coli* are not invasive pathogens. Enterotoxigenic *E. coli* (ETEC) causes a toxin-mediated syndrome of watery diarrhea in travelers. Enteropathogenic *E. coli* (EPEC) and enteroadherent *E. coli* (EAEC) alter the microvillous architecture of the small intestine and colon by tightly adhering to the brush border membrane. EPEC is an important cause of infantile diarrhea throughout the world but is infrequently seen in the United States and Canada. EAEC-induced diarrhea is less well defined.[1]

The two remaining categories of *E. coli* produce diarrheal disease marked by fecal leukocytes or frank blood. Enteroinvasive *E. coli* (EIEC) is a true invasive pathogen but does not produce bacteremia. The biochemical properties of EIEC and the clinical syndrome it produces resemble *Shigella* infection. EIEC-induced disease is rare in the United States but can cause sporadic outbreaks of self-limited diarrhea of mild or moderate severity. EIEC infection is also marked by fever, nausea, and abdominal pain. Unlike *Shigella* infection, true dysentery is rarely part of the clinical picture. Although there are no controlled studies, therapeutic recommendations for significant illness include ampicillin, TMP-SMX, and quinolone antibiotics.

Enterohemorrhagic *E. coli* (EHEC) was first described after an outbreak of hemorrhagic colitis in Oregon and Michigan in 1982 following the consumption of contaminated hamburgers. Since then, there have been many reports of sporadic cases and outbreaks attributable to *E. coli* O157:H7 and other EHEC serotypes. EHEC adheres to colonic mucosa but is not a true invasive pathogen. The bacterium produces two cytotoxins that are 60% to 99% homologous with the Shiga toxin produced by *Shigella dysenteriae* type 1. It is unclear if the cytotoxins are important in disease pathogenesis. Asymptomatic carriage of the organism appears to be a rare event.

EHEC infection is usually marked by watery diarrhea, which progresses to bloody diarrhea in 75% of cases. Other common symptoms include abdominal cramping and vomiting. In contrast to shigellosis, fever is often low grade or absent. The illness is generally self-limited but may persist for several weeks. About 10% of EHEC infections are accompanied by development of thrombotic thrombocytopenic purpura or hemolytic-uremic syndrome (HUS). Young children and elderly patients are particularly at risk for HUS, with a high mortality seen in the elderly.[11]

Despite sensitivity to a wide variety of antibiotics in vitro, it remains unclear whether antibiotic therapy influences the course of EHEC-induced diarrhea. Immune globulin preparations contain antibodies to Shigalike toxin 1, which is elaborated by EHEC. Administration of immune globulin preparations may ameliorate the course of HUS.

VIBRIO

The best-known *Vibrio* is *V. cholerae* O1, the etiologic agent for epidemic cholera. It is a small bowel pathogen that does not invade the intestinal mucosa. In contrast, *V. parahaemolyticus* induces diarrheal disease following invasion of colonic mucosa. This bacterium may also elaborate an enterotoxin. It is a major cause of diarrheal outbreaks in Japan and in coastal regions of the third world. It is also associated with outbreaks on the Atlantic and Gulf coasts of the United States. A 51% attack rate is described. *V. parahaemolyticus* produces self-limited explosive or bloody diarrhea, often following the ingestion of undercooked seafood. Therapy is supportive.[1]

V. vulnificus and *V. alginolyticus* infections occur after contact with contaminated seawater or ingestion of tainted seafood. Infection by these vibrios may result in cellulitis or otitis media, rather than diarrhea, in healthy individuals. Septicemia and a high mortality occur in patients with cirrhosis or immunocompromise, especially with *V. vulnificus*. Thus, patients with cirrhosis should be cautioned against eating uncooked seafood.

Tetracycline is the antibiotic of choice for most severe *Vibrio* infections, including *V. vulnificus* and *V. cholerae*. Chloramphenicol and penicillins may be used as alternative agents.

AEROMONAS AND PLESIOMONAS

Aeromonas hydrophila[12] and *Plesiomonas shigelloides*[13] are associated with outbreaks of diarrhea following ingestion of contaminated water and shellfish. Although these gram-negative rods are most likely true enteric pathogens, their role in the pathogenesis of diarrhea is unclear. The clinical spectrum of disease ranges from mild diarrhea to dysentery to sepsis and extraintestinal infection, especially in patients with chronic liver disease.

Although clinical studies are lacking, both organisms are sensitive in vitro to TMP-SMX, gentamicin, chloramphenicol, third-generation cephalosporins, and quinolones. *Plesiomonas* is sensitive to tetracycline, where *Aeromonas* demonstrates variable sensitivity to this drug. Both organisms are resistant to penicillin-like drugs.

REFERENCES

1. Cohen MB, Giannella RA. Bacterial infections: pathophysiology, clinical features, and treatment. In: Philips SF, Pemberton JH, Shorter RG, eds. *The Large Intestine.* New York, NY: Raven Press Ltd; 1991:395–428.
2. Herrington DA, Taylor DN. Bacterial enteritides. In: Field M, ed. *Diarrheal Diseases.* New York, NY: Elsevier Science Publishing Co Inc; 1991:239–291.
3. DuPont HL. *Shigella* species (bacillary dysentery). In: Mandell GL, Douglas RG Jr, Bennett JE, eds. *Principles and Practice of Infectious Diseases.* New York, NY: Churchill-Livingstone; 1990:1716–1722.
4. Salam MA, Bennish ML. Therapy for shigellosis. I. Randomized, double-blind trial of nalidixic acid in childhood shigellosis. *J Pediatr.* 1988;113:901–907.
5. Bennish ML, Salam MA, Haider R, et al. Therapy for shigellosis. II. Randomized, double-blind comparison of ciprofloxacin and ampicillin. *J Infect Dis.* 1990;162:711–716.
6. Soe GB, Overturf GD. Treatment of typhoid fever and other systemic salmonelloses with cefotaxime, ceftriaxone, cefoperazone, and other newer cephalosporins. *Rev Infect Dis.* 1987;9:719–736.
7. Jacobson MA, Hahn SM, Gerberding JL, et al. Ciprofloxacin for salmonella bacteremia in the acquired immunodeficiency syndrome (AIDS). *Ann Intern Med.* 1989;110:1027–1029.
8. Pithie AD, Wood MJ. Treatment of typhoid fever and infectious diarrhoea with ciprofloxacin. *J Antimicrob Chemother.* 1990;26(suppl F):47–53.

9. Blaser MJ, Reller B. *Campylobacter* enteritis. *N Engl J Med.* 1981;305:1444–1452.
10. Marks MI, Pai CH, LaFleur L, et al. *Yersinia enterocolitica* gastroenteritis: a prospective study of clinical, bacteriologic and epidemiologic features. *J Pediatr.* 1980; 96:26–31.
11. Griffin PM, Ostroff SM, Tauxe RV, et al. Illnesses associated with *Escherichia coli* O157:H7 infections: a broad clinical spectrum. *Ann Intern Med.* 1988;109:705–712.
12. Holmberg SD, Schell WL, Fanning GR, et al. *Aeromonas* intestinal infections in the United States. *Ann Intern Med.* 1986;105:683–689.
13. Holmberg SD, Wachsmuth IK, Hickman-Brenner FW, et al. *Plesiomonas* enteric infections in the United States. *Ann Intern Med.* 1986;105:690–694.

54
Schistosomiasis

EUGENE SUN and JAMES H. McKERROW

Schistosomiasis is a major parasitic disease caused by various species of the blood fluke *Schistosoma*. It is also known as *bilharziasis,* in honor of Theodor Bilharz, the German pathologist who discovered the cause of the disease in 1851. It is estimated that there are currently over 200 million cases worldwide, with over 70 countries involved.[1] Despite the availability of effective chemotherapy, control of schistosomiasis has proved elusive, and this difficulty in controlling the disease will likely persist well into the chemotherapeutic era; in fact, the number of cases has grown significantly in recent years. With increasing international travel and immigration from endemic areas, many more US physicians will encounter patients in whom schistosomiasis is a valid diagnostic concern and not an exotic tropical disease.

EPIDEMIOLOGY

Two populations in the United States are at risk for schistosomiasis: immigrants from endemic areas and US residents returning from travel to these areas. Although cases in the latter group have been widely publicized,[2] the former probably accounts for the majority of cases in this country. An accurate quantitation is difficult because of rapid fluxes in the at-risk population, but it has been estimated to approach 500,000.[3]

Determining the risk of infection, therefore, depends on knowing the geographic distribution of schistosomiasis. Four major species of schistosomes, *S. mansoni, S. haematobium, S. japonicum,* and *S. mekongi,* infect man, and each has its distinct distribution. *S. mansoni* is found throughout Africa, the Mideast, South America, and the Caribbean; *S. haematobium* is found in Africa and the Mideast; *S. japonicum* occurs in China, Japan, and the Philippines; and *S. mekongi* is concentrated along the Mekong River and its tributaries in Laos, Cambodia, and Thailand. A fifth species, *S. intercalatum,* appears to be restricted to West and Central Africa. Little is known about *S. intercalatum* infection, and it is not considered in the following discussion.

Often, in assessing exposure risk or in advising travelers, it is helpful to know the more detailed local epidemiology within individual countries. This information is available from the Centers for Disease Control (CDC) publication *Health Information for International Travel* which is updated annually, or by calling the CDC International Health telephone hotline at (404) 332-4559.

THE ORGANISM AND ITS LIFE CYCLE

Schistosomes belong to the large class of helminths called *flukes,* or *trematodes,* of which several other organisms can infect humans and cause disease. These include the lung fluke *Para-*

gonimus westermani, the liver flukes *Clonorchis sinensis, Fasciola hepatica,* and *Opisthorchis* species, and the intestinal fluke *Fasciolopsis buski.* All flukes share certain features such as waterborne transmission with snails as intermediate hosts and human infection involving tissue migration to a site of chronic infestation. Although schistosomes are commonly associated with liver disease, they are actually blood flukes, as their adult forms reside in the venous beds of the intestines or bladder. Schistosomiasis is one of the oldest infections known to man, described in records from ancient Egyptian and Chinese civilizations; parasite eggs have been found in mummies from the twelfth century BC.

The life cycle of schistosomes, which in broad scheme is shared by other parasitic flukes, reflects the organism's successful adaptation to both man and his environment. Although the nonparasitologist typically recalls little of the life cycle other than its exceeding complexity, a rational approach to diagnosis and management rests on an understanding of the host-parasite relationship.

Man is infected during contact with fresh water inhabited by infected snails. The infective larval forms, known as cercariae, are shed from snails during daylight hours, and are thermally attracted to humans in the water. Contact with skin stimulates the release of a proteolytic enzyme, which facilitates penetration through the epidermis. Once in the dermis, the larvae transform into preadult forms (schistosomulae), and migrate hematogenously to the lungs and then the liver, where they mature into adults and mate. The adult worms measure up to 26 mm in length and form pairs, with the female cradled in a groove in the male, then migrate finally to either the mesenteric or vesical venous plexus. *Schistosoma mansoni* lodge in the superior and inferior mesenteric veins; *S. haematobium* in the vesical, prostatic, rectal, and uterine plexi; and *S. japonicum* and *mekongi,* typically in the inferior mesenteric and superior hemorrhoidal veins.

On reaching their final destination, the fertilized female worms begin laying eggs, which penetrate the vascular bed into the intestinal lumen or lower urinary tract, thus gaining access to the environment and their next host, the freshwater snail. It is estimated that the average survival of adult worms is 5 to 10 years, based on declining egg counts in infected individuals after leaving endemic areas; however, eggs have been found in such individuals for up to 30 years. Egg production depends on the species, the worm burden, and probably a variety of host factors. In experimental infections, a single female of *S. mansoni* and *S. haematobium* can produce 200 to 300 eggs per day, whereas *S. japonicum* can produce several thousand.

CLINICOPATHOLOGIC SYNDROMES

Clinical disease in man results from immunopathologic responses to particular stages of the parasite and their associated antigens. It should be noted that the majority of infected individuals are asymptomatic or develop manifestations late in the course of infection. Unfortunately, the late stages of disease usually signify irreversible pathology, thus the rationale for screening and early treatment in endemic areas.

The clinical syndromes associated with schistosomiasis are each correlated with a specific stage of the parasite's development in man. In chronologic order, they are cercarial dermatitis, a local response to cercarial skin invasion; Katayama fever, a transient systemic illness corresponding to worm maturation and egg deposition; and chronic schistosomiasis, which results from the host response to eggs retained in tissues surrounding the adult worms.

Cercarial Dermatitis

Cercarial dermatitis, also known as *swimmers' itch, rice paddy itch,* and *clam-diggers' itch,* is a cutaneous response to skin penetration by cercariae and is seen with variable frequency depending on the schistosome species. It is most commonly the result of abortive invasion of the skin by nonhuman schistosome species, especially those of birds and lower mammals. In the United States most reports come from the Great Lakes region; worldwide, the distribution is cosmopolitan and occurs in both freshwater and marine environments. The cercariae of these species are able to penetrate the epidermis of human skin, but can progress no further in their life cycle. They die there and incite an acute inflammatory response characterized by edema and infiltration by neutrophils, eosinophils, and mononuclear cells. The inflammatory reaction is magnified in individuals previously sensitized to cercariae of the same or related species.

The clinical manifestations of cercarial dermatitis in the sensitized individual are biphasic. Immediately on contact with the cercariae, a tingling or prickling sensation becomes apparent, accompanied by erythema and pruritus. Several hours or even days later, a characteristic maculopapular, intensely pruritic rash erupts, which may become vesicular, or if secondarily infected, pustular in appearance. Purpuric lesions have also been described. Systemic symptoms are generally absent, and the rash typically resolves after several days, although hyperpigmentation can persist for weeks.[4-6]

ACUTE SCHISTOSOMIASIS (KATAYAMA FEVER)

The syndrome of acute schistosomiasis resembles serum sickness in its manifestations and may be mediated in part by immune complexes[7]; however, the pathogenesis is not well understood. It appears to coincide with the final maturation phase of the worms and the initiation of egg deposition. Symptoms roughly correlate with the intensity of infection and generally occur in previously uninfected individuals. The syndrome is distinctly uncommon among individuals living in endemic regions; it is mainly described in visitors and expatriates to these areas.[2] It is rarely seen in *S. haematobium* infection.

The onset of symptoms occurs as early as 2 weeks after cercarial exposure and as late as 10 weeks, with a mean incubation period of 4 to 5 weeks. The clinical severity is quite variable (Table 54–1), but symptoms usually include fever, sweats, abdominal pain or discomfort, headache, and constitutional symptoms. Diarrhea is common and may be bloody, presumably resulting from the extrusion of eggs into the intestinal lumen. A dry cough is also observed in many patients, which may be related to the transient pulmonary migration of the immature worms. Hepatosplenomegaly and lymphadenopathy may accompany the symptoms, but the physical examination is usually otherwise unrevealing.

Given this relatively nonspecific presentation and the frequent omission of a careful travel history, the diagnosis of acute schistosomiasis can be easily missed, and the symptoms attributed to a "viral syndrome," but for the invariable presence of peripheral eosinophilia, which may occasionally exceed 10,000/mm³. Other standard laboratory parameters, except for mild elevations in alkaline phosphatase, aspartate aminotransferase, and lactic dehydrogenase, are typically normal. Despite the suspected role of immune complexes, abnormalities in renal function and urine are usually not detected.

The clinical course can last from a few days to several months and is generally self-limited, although fatal cases have been described. The subsidence of symptoms does not indicate resolution of infection but merely a waning of the host response. Indeed, eggs begin appearing in the stool (or urine) during the course of the illness and continue long after the disappearance of symptoms, indicating established infection that can lead to chronic schistosomiasis.[8-10]

TABLE 54–1. FREQUENCY OF SIGNS AND SYMPTOMS IN ACUTE SCHISTOSOMIASIS

SYMPTOM OR SIGN	FREQUENCY (%)
Fever	96
Anorexia	92
Weight loss	85
Abdominal pain	85
Headache	81
Weakness	81
Diaphoresis	77
Chills	73
Myalgias and arthralgias	73
Diarrhea	65
Nausea	65
Dry cough	65
Vomiting	50
Tenesmus	50
Hepatomegaly	35
Bloody diarrhea	31
Splenomegaly	19
Periorbital edema	12

From Hiatt TA, Sotomayor AR, Sanchez G, Zambrana M, Knight WB. Factors in the pathogenesis of acute schistosomiasis mansoni. *J Infect Dis.* 1979;139:659.

CHRONIC SCHISTOSOMIASIS

Chronic schistosomiasis, by far the most important syndrome, is a constellation of pathologic lesions and clinical manifestations, which are a consequence of a cascade of host-mediated responses to the presence of schistosome eggs, as depicted in Figure 54–1. A significant proportion of the hundreds to thousands of eggs produced daily by the worms are not successfully extruded from the host, and are trapped in various tissues, inciting a characteristic inflammatory response. Disease manifestation is a function of the egg burden, their location, and the vigor of the individual's immune response to their presence. In the case of *S. haematobium* infection, pathology centers around the lower urinary tract initially and may later involve the genitals, rectum and upper urinary tract. Infection with *S. mansoni* and *japonicum* causes direct pathology in the intestines and liver with result-

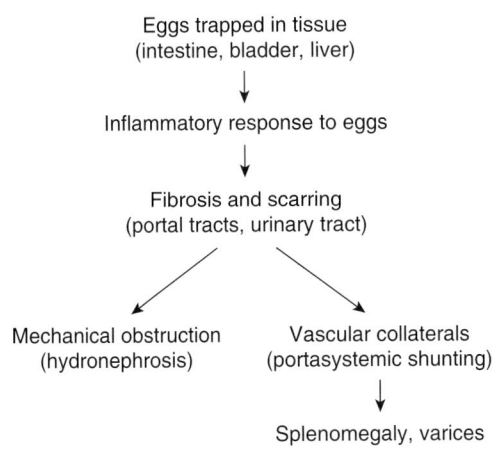

FIGURE 54–1. Pathophysiology of chronic schistosomiasis.

ing splenomegaly and esophageal varices. Distant egg embolization may occur in both urinary tract and hepatointestinal schistosomiasis.

Two points regarding the clinical presentation of chronic schistosomiasis deserve emphasis. First, it should be recognized that the majority of infected individuals are asymptomatic during most of their course. This does not necessarily indicate a benign course, as the clinical presentations of late disease are associated with irreversible pathology. More importantly, the asymptomatic stage is nonetheless associated with constant fecal or urinary egg passage, an integral part of the parasite life cycle, thus contributing to the maintenance of transmission within the community. Secondly, the endemic areas of schistosomiasis are generally found in the third world, where numerous other conditions such as hepatitis, malaria, typhoid fever, and intestinal helminths frequently coexist. Thus, the patient at risk for schistosomiasis is generally at risk for a number of other conditions as well, and the principle of Ockham's razor is not applicable.

INTESTINAL SCHISTOSOMIASIS

Approximately 10% to 20% of chronically infected individuals develop intestinal lesions. Eggs trapped in the intestinal wall give rise to "sandy patches," areas of mural thickening composed of eggs, fibrous tissue, and atrophic mucosa. Colonic polyposis is a distinct syndrome with a peculiar predilection for Egyptian patients; the polyps represent masses of eggs together with inflammatory cells and glandular proliferation. They are not adenomatous, and no association with colonic carcinoma has been demonstrated.[11] Intestinal lesions are more common with *S. mansoni* and *S. japonicum* than with *S. haematobium* infection; the majority of lesions are found in the rectosigmoid area. Clinical manifestations reflect the extent of pathologic involvement; typical symptoms are chronic bloody diarrhea and abdominal pain, with severe cases resulting in iron deficiency anemia and malnutrition.

HEPATOSPLENIC SCHISTOSOMIASIS

Hepatosplenic schistosomiasis is the major form of schistosomiasis due to *S. mansoni*, *S. japonicum*, and *S. mekongi* species. Because the adult worms of these species live in the mesenteric venous system, their eggs embolize via the portal vein to lodge in the hepatic presinusoids. Granuloma formation ensues, eventually progressing to a unique lesion described by Symmers[12] as *pipestem fibrosis*. Pathologic changes are limited to the portal tract, which becomes fibrotic, with extensive hepatic arterialization and a variable cellular infiltrate. In contrast to cirrhotic liver disease, the parenchyma is spared, the lobular architecture is preserved, and regenerative nodules are not observed. Fibrous obliteration of the portal area results in portal hypertension, although hepatic blood flow is maintained by arteriolar proliferation, and the hepatic venous wedge pressure is minimally elevated.[13]

Portal hypertension leads to two major clinical manifestations, congestive splenomegaly and esophageal varices. Often the first manifestation of disease is abdominal distension from massive splenomegaly or life-threatening variceal hemorrhage. Because hepatic, and thus coagulative, function is usually intact in schistosomiasis, the mortality from variceal bleeding may be better than in patients with cirrhotic liver disease. Decompensation of hepatic function is generally not seen until the terminal stage of disease, and it is unclear whether it is related to schistosome infection or comorbid conditions.

URINARY TRACT SCHISTOSOMIASIS

Involvement of the urinary tract results from infection with *S. haematobium*, which has a geographic distribution in Africa and the Mideast that overlaps with *S. mansoni*. The adult worms tend to reside in the vesical plexus but can also be found in the venous drainage of the genital tract and the lower gastrointestinal tract. Clinical manifestations of early *S. haematobium* infection include hematuria, dysuria, and frequent urinary tract infections; chronic infection may lead to obstructive uropathy and, ultimately, renal failure.[14,15]

ECTOPIC EGG SYNDROMES: PULMONARY AND CENTRAL NERVOUS SYSTEM SCHISTOSOMIASIS

In *S. haematobium* infection involving the vesical plexus and in advanced hepatosplenic disease associated with portal hypertension and portasystemic shunting, egg embolization to the pulmonary circulation can occur. Eggs lodged in the lung incite the same fibrotic tissue reaction as elsewhere in the body and, if hemodynamically significant, result in pulmonary hypertension and cor pulmonale.

An uncommon but potentially catastrophic site of egg embolization is the central nervous system (CNS).[16] Eggs, and rarely errant adult worms, can reach the brain and spinal cord by arterial embolization or through venous anastomoses, as are present between the pelvic and vertebral veins. *S. haematobium* and *S. mansoni* usually cause spinal cord syndromes, while *S. japonicum* has an unusual predilection for the brain. As might be expected, a variety of clinical presentations are associated with CNS involvement, depending on the location of the lesion and the magnitude of the inflammatory response. The most common spinal cord syndrome is transverse myelitis; other presentations include lower extremity radiculopathy and, rarely, spinal artery syndrome. Brain lesions can present as seizures, focal neurologic deficits, or generalized encephalopathy. The diagnosis of CNS involvement is difficult, as the underlying schistosomiasis may be unrecognized.

DIAGNOSIS

The first step in the diagnostic workup of suspected schistosomiasis in returning travelers or immigrants is a careful history with regard to water exposure in an endemic area, the absence of which effectively excludes the diagnosis. In travelers to endemic areas, elicitation of symptoms resembling cercarial dermatitis or Katayama fever may be helpful, although numerous conditions may produce similar nonspecific symptoms.

The cornerstone of diagnosis is the demonstration of eggs in the stool, urine, or, if necessary, a biopsy specimen. It is difficult to dogmatically recommend a minimum number of samples to examine, as egg excretion is at best a crude reflection of the worm burden. For screening purposes, three stool or urine samples should suffice. For patients in whom schistosomiasis is strongly suspected, three negative samples should not exclude the diagnosis, since clinical illness is not only a function of the parasite load but also of the individual immune response. An aggressive diagnostic workup should include multiple stool and urine samples and appropriate biopsies if necessary. Midday stool and urine samples should be collected on different days and examined after concentration for characteristic egg morphology. *S. mansoni* eggs are about 140 μm in length and have a diagnostic lateral spine. *S. haematobium* eggs have a terminal spine, and *S. japonicum* eggs are shorter (60 to 70 μm) and lack a visible spine. *S. mekongi* eggs are difficult to distinguish from those of *S. japonicum*. In patients from the Mideast or Africa, both stool and urine should be obtained, as dual infections with *S. mansoni* and *S. haematobium* are common.

Scrapings or biopsy specimens of the rectal mucosa may reveal eggs in some cases when stool and urine samples are negative and are indicated in suspected cases before more invasive procedures are performed. The specimen can be examined directly for eggs after compression between two glass slides. Liver biopsy is rarely indicated but may reveal eggs that are diagnostic or characteristic portal tract pathology that is strongly suggestive of schistosomiasis.

Serologic diagnosis of schistosomiasis has a limited role. The most commonly used tests detect antibody to egg proteins but do not distinguish active infection from past exposure. However, serology can be useful in two circumstances: (1) In cases of suspected acute schistosomiasis, egg excretion may be sparse, and a positive serology in a previously unexposed person can be diagnostic; (2) in the difficult cases where CNS involvement is suspected but eggs cannot be recovered, serologic results can be helpful in the diagnostic workup.

THERAPY

Treatment is indicated for all forms of schistosomiasis, even in the absence of symptoms, to prevent progression to chronic disease. Several agents are effective against the parasite; in the United States, praziquantel is readily available and is the drug of choice against all species of schistosomes.

Praziquantel (pyrazino-isoquinoline) has been

in clinical use since 1978.[17] The drug appears to paralyze the parasite's musculature and interfere with calcium ion transport, leading to disintegration of the worm surface. There is extensive worldwide experience with the drug; it appears to be at least as effective as other agents and has a very low incidence of toxic side effects. The drug has an oral bioavailability of 80% to 100% and reaches peak serum concentrations within 2 hours. Hepatic metabolites are renally secreted, with an elimination half-life of 4 to 6 hours. In patients with hepatic dysfunction, peak levels are elevated and result in a higher incidence of side effects.[18]

Extensive clinical trials, performed under the direction of the World Health Organization, have established the efficacy, toxicity, and optimal dosage regimens of praziquantel against *S. mansoni*, *S. haematobium*, and *S. japonicum*.[19] Cure rates range between 70% to 100%, and in those with residual egg excretion, mean egg counts are reduced by 95%. Current recommendations for adult and pediatric patients are two doses of 20 mg/kg 4 hours apart for *S. mansoni* and *S. haematobium* infections and three doses of 20 mg/kg four hours apart for *S. japonicum* and *S. mekongi* infections.[20]

Side effects of praziquantel are usually transient and limited to malaise, headache, dizziness, nausea, abdominal discomfort, and fever. No effect on renal, hepatic, or hematopoietic function has been observed. Although no teratogenic effects have been reported, usage in pregnancy has not been thoroughly studied, and it seems prudent to postpone therapy in pregnant patients in the absence of life-threatening disease.

Oxamniquine has been used extensively in Africa and South America in the treatment of *S. mansoni*.[21] There is a difference in susceptibility among geographically divergent strains of *S. mansoni*, and the drug is inactive against other schistosome species. For American strains of *S. mansoni*, the adult dosage is 15 mg/kg given once, and the pediatric dosage is 20 mg/kg in two doses given 4 hours apart. For African strains, the dosage should be increased to 15 mg/kg twice daily for two consecutive days, for a total dose of 60 mg/kg. Oxamniquine's efficacy is comparable to that of praziquantel, and it is also well tolerated, although there have been several reports of neuropsychiatric disturbances and seizures following administration of the drug.

Other drugs currently in use against schistosomiasis but unavailable in the United States include metrifonate, which is active against only *S. haematobium*, and two broad spectrum agents, amoscanate and niridazole, which are active against all schistosome species.

REFERENCES

1. *The Control of Schistosomiasis.* Geneva: World Health Organization; 1985. WHO technical report series, no. 728.
2. Centers for Disease Control. Acute schistosomiasis in U.S. travelers returning from Africa. *MMWR.* 1990;39:141.
3. Warren KS. Helminthic diseases endemic in the United States. *Am J Trop Med Hyg.* 1974;23:723.
4. Hoeffler DF. Cercarial dermatitis: its etiology, epidemiology, and clinical aspects. *Arch Environ Health.* 1974;29:225.
5. Centers for Disease Control. Cercarial dermatitis outbreak at a state park: Delaware, 1991. *MMWR.* 1992;41:225.
6. Kuntz RE. Cercarial dermatitis. In: Heyneman D, Goldsmith R, eds. *Tropical Medicine and Parasitology.* Norwalk, Conn: Appleton & Lange; 1989.
7. Lawley TJ, Ottesen EA, Hiatt RA, Gazze LA. Circulating immune complexes in acute schistosomiasis. *Clin Exp Immunol.* 1979;37:221.
8. Nash TE, Cheever AW, Ottesen EA, Cook JA. Schistosome infections in humans: perspectives and recent findings. *Ann Intern Med.* 1982;97:740.
9. Hiatt TA, Sotomayor AR, Sanchez G, Zambrana M, Knight WB. Factors in the pathogenesis of acute schistosomiasis mansoni. *J Infect Dis.* 1979;139:659.
10. King CH. Acute and chronic schistosomiasis. *Hosp Pract.* 1991;26:117.
11. Ayad El-Masr N, Farid Z, Bassily S, Kilpatrick ME, Watten RH. Schistosomal colonic polyposis; clinical, radiological and parasitological study. *J Trop Med Hyg.* 1986;89:13.
12. Symmers WSC. Note on a new form of liver cirrhosis due to the presence of the ova of *Bilharzia haematobia*. *J Pathol Bacteriol.* 1904;9:237.
13. Amaury C. Hemodynamic studies of portal hypertension in schistosomiasis. *Am J Med.* 1968;44:547.
14. Cheever AW, Kamel IA, Elwi AM, Mosimann JE, Danner R, Sippel JE. *Schistosoma mansoni* and *Schistosoma haematobium* infections in Egypt. *Am J Trop Med Hyg.* 1978;27:55.
15. King CH, Keating CE, Muruka JF, et al. Urinary tract morbidity in schistosomiasis haematobia: associations with age and intensity of infection in an endemic area of coast province, Kenya. *Am J Trop Med Hyg.* 1988;39:361.
16. Case records of the Massachusetts General Hospital 21-1985. *N Engl J Med.* 1985;312:1376.
17. King CH, Mahmoud AAF. Drugs five years later: praziquantel. *Ann Intern Med.* 1989;110:290.
18. Watt G, White NJ, Padre L, et al. Praziquantel pharmacokinetics and side effects in *Schistosoma japonicum*-infected patients with liver disease. *J Infect Dis.* 1988;157:530.
19. Davis A, Wegner DHG. Multicentre trials of praziquantel in human schistosomiasis: design and techniques. *Bull WHO.* 1979;57:767.
20. Drugs for parasitic infections. *Med Lett Drugs Ther.* 1993;35:111.
21. Shekhar KC. Schistosomiasis drug therapy and treatment considerations. *Drugs.* 1991;42:379.

55
Tropical Sprue: A Disappearing Enigma

LESLIE H. BERNSTEIN and VANDANA NEHRA

Although tropical malabsorption was probably first mentioned in a papyrus written in India before the birth of Christ and referred to as a "visit from the Goddess of Distension," its occurrence in the Western hemisphere was documented by Hillary[1] during the 18th century on the island of Barbados. During the centuries of colonization, the disease became well recognized by Europeans in China, India, Bengal, and the Philippines, as well as certain islands of the Caribbean, and the term *Indische Sprouw* (Dutch for sore mouth) was anglicized to *sprue* by Manson.

During the conflicts of the Spanish American War and World War II and among American troops serving in Vietnam, tropical sprue became a recognized problem for the fighting forces and in the 1950s, 1960s, and 1970s superb epidemiologic work by Sheehey[2] among the military in Puerto Rico, Klipstein and colleagues[3] in the barrios of Puerto Rico, and Baker and Mathan[4] in the villages of India, such as Aryapadi, provided much new data on the extent of this persistent problem.

Concurrently, the advent of diagnostic measures and laboratory procedures that allowed the sampling of the intestinal mucosa during life, the measurement of serum folate, B_{12}, and stool fat, and the use of aerobic and anaerobic bacterial cultures, yielded clinical data that allowed consistent diagnosis and explained the pathophysiology of the disease but as yet has not pinpointed the cause of this disease.

Since the disease remits with vitamin therapy and is cured with antibiotic therapy in expatriates who do not return to tropical areas, the treatment of the disease has been established without the cause ever having been elucidated. Theories that have been advanced regarding cause generally fall into one of three groups, singly or in combination. They are (1) a deficiency disease due to inadequate diet, (2) an infectious agent that is prevalent in tropical areas, and (3) a toxic agent (ingested with the diet) that forms because of inadequate refrigeration and sanitation in tropical areas. Nonetheless, no theory as yet has stood the test of time.

The deficiency disease theories have usually blamed inadequate folate in the diet, inadequate ingestion of vitamin B_{12}, or inadequate protein in the diet.[5] The occurrence of the disease among groups fed adequate diets in established military institutions or prison camps, away from the theater of war, has not lent credence to such reports.[2,6] Additionally, theories based on infections caused by yeast, viruses spread by insects, and bacterial overgrowth by common species of *Enterobacteriaceae,* have failed to explain why the disease is never transmitted outside of tropical areas, even from mother to child or husband to wife. Theories regarding dietary toxins arising in the tropics such as the "peroxidation" of unsaturated food fats in tropical heat,[7] although attractive, have failed to stand the test of time for they fail to offer adequate explanation for the recurrence of this disease decades after leaving the tropical area.

Nonetheless, tropical sprue seems to be disappearing from the medical scene, and the number of papers written on the subject and the number of investigators working in the field diminish decade by decade as sanitation, vitamin supplementation, antibiotics, and refrigeration penetrate the tropical areas of the world. Similarly, the number of cases diagnosed by US medical centers that treat expatriates or cases involving citizens traveling for prolonged periods in tropical areas has fallen dramatically, despite improved diagnostic methods and increasing awareness of tropical malabsorption syndromes. Certainly the recent discovery in Nepal of a *Coccidia*-like organism,[8] which was probably responsible for recurrent episodes of summer diarrhea and was found within the lumen but not within the enterocyte only after modern endoscopic methods were employed, lends some hope that the agent(s) responsible for tropical sprue will yet be elucidated.

CLINICAL HISTORY

Although it has been known for several hundred of years that sprue may occur in endemic or epidemic forms, be confined to houses or villages, and certainly to islands within a geographic area (sprue occurs in Puerto Rico, both halves of the island of Hispaniola, and Cuba but not Jamaica, Bermuda, or the Virgin Islands at the present time), tropical sprue has never been contracted by travelers who have not remained resident or traveled within the endemic area for a period usually of weeks or months.

The consultant in gastroenterology is likely to be called to assess a patient who is suffering from marked weight loss, diarrhea, or anemia. A careful history (as always) is essential to the diagnosis. Among the points that should be sought from the patient are the following:

1. *Where has the patient traveled in the last 30 years?* We have seen relapse of tropical sprue in an elderly patient who had not returned to Puerto Rico for 27 years.
2. *How long a period of time did the patient reside in these areas?* Tropical sprue has been reported in patients resident for 2 weeks or more in the endemic areas.
3. *In what type of facility was the patient resident?* Tropical sprue probably has never been transmitted among European or European-Americans in the resorts or the hotels of the Caribbean.
4. *Was the patient well during the period of tropical stay, and, if not, in what way was he ill?* Tropical sprue not uncommonly begins with low-grade fever and watery diarrhea, settling into a more chronic diarrhea with associated weight loss and anemia only after some weeks to months.
5. *How much weight has the patient lost and what has occurred to the patient's energy level and appetite?*
6. *What is the patient's genetic background? Are there any signs that a genetic predisposition to celiac disease exists in the patient or his family?* It is not uncommon in this era of world travel, to see in consultation, patients of northern European or Mediterranean ancestry who have spent periods of time (usually short) in a tropical area and who are referred because of folate deficiency, steatorrhea, and flat biopsy results. Not infrequently, a history of feeding problems in childhood, diagnosis of "a celiac condition" in infancy, or the fact that the patient has had dermatitis herpetiformis or is by far the shortest of a group of siblings will lead to the proper diagnosis of celiac sprue.
7. *Has the patient noted an increased darkening of the sun-exposed areas of the skin, loss of muscle tone particularly abdominal, sore tongue, or recurrent aphthae in the weeks preceding consultation?*
8. *Has the patient recently varied his dietary habits?* Tropical sprue that has been dormant for years to decades has been noted to be recrudescent in patients who have suddenly diminished their intake, for example, in an attempt to lose weight or because of clinical depression or coexistent illness. The mechanism for this late relapse has not been elucidated and appears to be much more common in patients of European ancestry who have returned from the Caribbean than among Europeans who have returned from Asia, where they presumably contracted the disease, although late relapses of sprue among British servicemen who have served in India have been noted.[9]
9. *What has the patient noted in regard to his stools?* The patient with tropical sprue usually notices an increase in volume, loosening of consistency, a lightening in color, and a marked increase in the foul odor of the stools. Patients whom we have treated have remarked, when questioned, that they occasionally carry spray cans of deodorant because of embarrassment when it is necessary for them to use a bathroom outside their own home. Other patients have reported repeatedly lighting matches in the lavatory to mask the foul odor of their stools. This foul odor is associated with protein and fat malabsorption. The former gives rise to increased amounts of hydrogen sulfide from cystine, taurine, and methionine and skatoles and indoles derived from unabsorbed tryptophane; whereas the latter engenders increased amounts of rancid smelling fatty acids such as butyric and caproic.

PHYSICAL EXAMINATION

The physical examination of a patient suffering from tropical sprue is variable but at times the cachexia is startling. Family members are frequently convinced that patients are suffering from terminal malignancy or acquired immunodeficiency syndrome. Patients usually are noted to have marked muscle wasting, and rarely tetany will be noted on application of the sphygmomanometer cuff. The skin may be normal or reveal darkening in the sun-exposed areas including the face, blush area of the neck, and backs of the hands. Hair may be fine and decreased in quantity. In women the breasts may be atrophic. Mucous membranes may show pallor, and glossitis is extremely common with atrophy first of the papilla on the lateral sides of the tongue spreading to the center, and with advanced disease, frequently associated with mucosal erosion. The examination of the abdomen usually reveals some degree of distension, which is out of character with the wasting noted on the rest of the physical examination and is probably related to the loss of abdominal muscular tone. Peristalsis may be visible from the side of the bed or examining table. In some advanced cases, edema of the extremities may be present and even pellagranous dermatitis of the extremities has been noted. Examination of the nails may show transverse ridges associated with hypoproteinemia that has occurred during the present relapse.

LABORATORY MANIFESTATIONS

Examination of the peripheral blood in patients with tropical sprue in relapse, usually reveals macrocytic anemia associated with hypersegmentation of the polymorphonuclear cells. Red cells not uncommonly show basophilic stippling due to retained strands of ribonucleic acid (RNA) and occasional Howell-Jolly bodies. Platelet counts may be mildly low.

Abnormal chemistry findings usually include hypoalbuminemia, hypocholesterolemia (usually between 90 and 120), hypohaptoglobinemia, and elevated lactate dehydrogenase (as is commonly seen in megaloblastic anemia) and, less commonly, hypokalemia and hypocalcemia and rarely hypoprothrombinemia. Serum and red cell folate levels are usually subnormal, and nearly as frequently, hypovitaminosis B_{12} is present. Oral D-xylose loading shows urinary secretion of less than 20% of the test dose or failure of blood levels to rise to the normal range. When fat balance studies are done, patients usually secrete between 20 to 55 g of fat per 24 hours.

RADIOLOGY AND HISTOLOGY

When tropical sprue is associated with weight loss and steatorrhea, oral barium studies usually manifest some abnormalities, but these are frequently mild and nondiagnostic. Because present-day barium preparations are manufactured to be nonflocculating, the classic moulage patterns are not seen. In general one notes only mild dilation of loops, prominence of valvulae conniventes, and a "wet" pattern, which consists of a graying of the barium preparation as it progresses distally. This is due to dilution of the contrast by the considerable fluid and mucus secretion within the lumen. *Quite frequently, no abnormality is noted. Diagnosis of tropical sprue should never be excluded on the basis of normal study findings.*

Colonoscopy is unrevealing except for mild megaloblastosis of the colonic epithelium on biopsy, but upper endoscopy is more helpful. In addition to providing small bowel mucosa for diagnosis, the endoscopist may note scalloping of the valvulae seen tangentially (also seen in celiac sprue).[10]

Recent studies have shown that large cup forceps biopsies, if handled properly, are useful for studying the histology of mucosal malabsorptive states. Suction biopsies taken with steerable catheters and Rubin or Crosby capsules are easier to orient, however, and may be taken without analgesia if the operator is proficient. If endoscopic biopsies of the second or third portion of the duodenum are taken, a more generous specimen may be taken by grasping the mucosa with the biopsy forceps and then backing the scope into the stomach, thus stripping the mucosa before pulling the specimen into the scope with the forceps. Specimens that can be oriented and flattened on gelfoam or paper will allow better sections to be examined. Sections that are cut tangentially rather than perpendicular to the mucosa are a source of misdiagnosis since the villi appear falsely elongated instead of showing the subtotal atrophy that is characteristic of tropical sprue. The atrophy is continuous from pylorus to ileocecal valve and does not show the patchiness and distal improvement seen in celiac disease. This may also explain the higher incidence of vitamin B_{12} malabsorption in tropical sprue.

Light microscopy reveals subtotal to total villus atrophy with the lamina propria crowded with inflammatory cells, usually mononuclear with some sprinkling of eosinophils and granulocytes. The epithelial cells are megaloblastic.

Electron microscopy reveals microvillous abnormalities and an increase in lysosomes and other cytoplasmic dense organelles. Also the subepithelial collagen layer is slightly thickened, as is seen in other malabsorptive states, but does not approach that of collagenous sprue.

If the patient has been treated with folate or vitamin B_{12}, rapid return of villus size is to be expected, but the inflammatory infiltrate may take months to disappear and, in our experience, does so only when antibiotic therapy is used (see below).

TREATMENT

One of the most dramatic and gratifying experiences in medicine awaits the medical consultant who makes the diagnosis of tropical sprue. Unlike celiac disease in which the response to folic acid consists of a reticulocyte response alone, the patient with tropical sprue usually responds with a remarkable improvement in the feeling of well-being within 24 hours. Patients note a return of energy after the administration of pharmacologic oral doses of folic acid (5 mg two or three times a day) and a dramatic increase in appetite. In view of demonstrated hypokalemia noted in pernicious anemia when treated, it is probably advisable to administer supplementary intravenous potassium to patients who are cachectic during the initial therapy, although hypokalemic crises have not been reported in tropical sprue. Diarrhea usually responds within 48 hours, although there are reports of the Indian form of the disease being less responsive to folate alone.

Unfortunately, the response to folate alone may not be maintained or will be lost when other stresses supervene including diminished intake from any cause, increased demand as in pregnancy,[11] or simply because of inability of the injured gut to absorb the daily requirement. *Antibacterial therapy is required for cure.*

Early reports with sulfa preparations used because of the suspicion of enteric infection indicated that tropical sprue responded to these compounds, and although nearly every antibiotic preparation has been used, the mainstay of therapy has been the cheap, widely available, and effective tetracyclines. Unlike Whipple's disease, where failure to cross the blood-brain barrier is associated with late neurologic relapse, tropical sprue yields slowly and completely to therapy with tetracycline. Response is associated with progressive restoration of serum and intracellular folate levels toward normal and the disappearance of the inflammatory cell infiltrate, which permeates the lamina propria. Additionally, absorption of labeled folate and vitamin B_{12} responds with return of normal coefficients of absorption. Response is permanent, unless the patient returns to the endemic area for an additional stay. This occurs with great frequency among expatriates in our large metropolitan population. Patients should be warned that "reinfection" is a distinct possibility on resumption of a tropical habitat, particularly since most of these patients return to family domiciles in the villages and not to the tourist hotels of the areas.

Follow-up visits after treatment need not be closely spaced, but every attempt should be made to impress on patients the chance of relapse if the course of antibiotics is abbreviated. A general recommendation is to start with 2 g of tetracycline daily in four divided doses, followed by 250 mg twice daily for six months.

If antibiotics are used as a "diagnostic test" (not recommended) in the absence of a complete workup for malabsorption, confusion may arise in patients with undiagnosed immunoproliferative small intestinal disease (IPSID)[12] or stagnant loop due to undiagnosed stricture, fistula, or diverticulae. Both will respond to tetracycline, but cure will not occur unless tetracyclines are maintained indefinitely in the former and correction of the underlying motility problem that prevents clearing of the gut is achieved in the latter. Occasionally, a high serum folate level associated with bacterial overgrowth is a clue to the diagnosis of stagnant loop syndrome.

Neither corticosteroids nor a gluten-free diet has any place in the treatment of tropical sprue. We have never encountered celiac sprue in a native-born expatriate of Puerto Rico, the Dominican Republic, Haiti, or the Indian subcontinent, although gluten has been noted to worsen tropical sprue and several other malabsorptive states.

REFERENCES

1. Hillary W. *Observations on the Changes of the Air and the Concomitant Diseases in the Islands of Barbados.* 2nd ed. London: Hawkes, Clorhe, Collins; 1766.
2. Tropical Sprue: Studies of the U.S. Army's sprue team in Puerto Rico. *US Army Medical Sciences Publication* 1958;5:55–56.
3. Klipstein FA, Beauchamp I, Corcino JJ. Nutritional status and intestinal function among rural populations of the West Indies. II. Barrio Nuevo, Pr. *Gastroenterology.* 1972;63:758–767.
4. Baker SJ, Mathan VI. Tropical sprue in southern India.

In: *Tropical Sprue and Megaloblastic Anemia.* London: Churchill Livingstone; 1971:189–260.
5. Walters JH. Dietetic deficiency syndromes in Indian soldiers. *Lancet.* 1947;1:861–865.
6. Stefanini M. Clinical features and pathogenesis of tropical sprue. *Medicine.* 1948;27:379–427.
7. French JM. *The influence of dietary triglyceride and fatty acids on intestinal absorption with special reference to the products of rancidity.* Birmingham, Ala: University of Birmingham; 1949. Thesis.
8. Connor BA, Shlim DR, Scholes JV, et al. Pathologic changes in the small bowel in nine patients with diarrhea associated with coccidia-like body. *Ann Intern Med.* 1993;119:377–382.
9. Mollin DL, Booth CC. Chronic tropical sprue in London. In: *Tropical Sprue and Megaloblastic Anemia.* London: Churchill Livingstone; 1971:61–128.
10. Tawil S, Brandt LJ, Bernstein LH. Scalloping of the valvulae conniventes in tropical sprue. *Gastrointest Endosc.* 1991;37:365–357.
11. Lawrence C, Klipstein FA. Megaloblastic anemia of pregnancy in New York City. *Ann Intern Med.* 1967;66:25–34.
12. Gilinsky NH, Novis BH, Wright JP, et al. Immunoproliferative small intestine disease: clinical features and outcome in 30 cases. *Medicine.* 1987;66:438–446.

56

Blind Loop Syndrome

FRED C. FOWLER and JAMES J. CERDA

The gastrointestinal tract is a complex microenvironment characterized by variations in pH, secretory products, and bacterial inhabitants. Alterations in the flora of the small intestine can result in the blind loop syndrome, a disorder characterized by malabsorption, steatorrhea, and vitamin B_{12} deficiency.[1] This disorder is also known as bacterial overgrowth, the stagnant bowel syndrome, the contaminated bowel syndrome, and small intestinal stasis. Each name emphasizes a different aspect of the pathophysiology of the disorder in which some defect in structure or function allows inappropriate proliferation and colonization of bacteria in the small intestine.

The first hint of this disorder was in 1890 when White reported a megaloblastic anemia associated with an intestinal stricture.[2] Seyderhelm later demonstrated that surgical correction of an intestinal stricture reversed megaloblastic anemia.[2] Cameron, Watson, and Witts[3] demonstrated the role of bacteria in this disorder by creating blind jejunal loops in rats. The rats developed vitamin B_{12} deficiency and diarrhea and weight loss. The blind loops were found to be colonized with large numbers of bacteria not usually found in the small intestine, including anaerobes.[3] Subsequent studies that have demonstrated the correction of malabsorption and diarrhea have confirmed the bacterial role in this disorder.

INTESTINAL FLORA

Traveling from the mouth to the anus, the type and numbers of bacteria present change dramatically as demonstrated in Figure 56–1.[4] Saliva contains approximately 10^6 organisms per milliliter with a mixture of aerobes and anaerobes. Most organisms are rapidly killed by the acid environment of the stomach.[4] The proximal small intestine contains no more than 10^5 organisms per milliliter in which streptococci, staphylococci, and lactobacilli and fungi are the primary constituents. Anaerobes are absent.[5] In the distal ileum the bacterial concentration increases to 10^7 to 10^8 organisms per milliliter with the appearance of anaerobes and coliforms. On crossing the ileocecal valve the anaerobic population rises to 10^{11} ml, whereas aerobes are present in a concentration of 10^8/ml.[6,7]

Patients with bacterial overgrowth have small bowel bacterial concentrations between 10^6 and 10^{11}/ml with multiple species present including anaerobes and coliforms.[1,8,9]

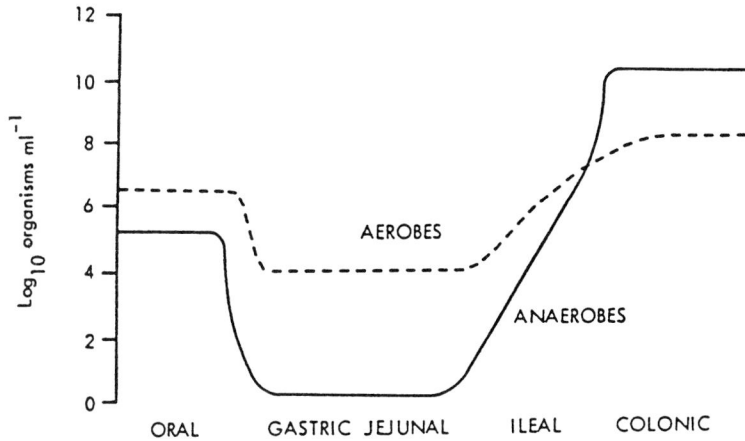

FIGURE 56–1. Schematic profile of normal gut flora. (From Isaacs PT, Kim YS. Blind loop syndrome and small bowel bacterial contamination. *Clin Gastroenterol.* 1983;12:395–414.)

PATHOPHYSIOLOGY OF THE BLIND LOOP SYNDROME

There are several aspects of the normal physiology of the gastrointestinal tract that keep the bacterial population in balance, the disruption of which can lead to overgrowth of bacteria in the small intestine.

Reduction in the acidity of the stomach allows more bacteria to survive passage through the stomach and produce bacterial overgrowth. The bacterial concentration in the stomach increases as the pH approaches neutral.[10] Gastric surgery aimed at acid reduction is frequently associated with bacterial overgrowth. Truncal vagotomy with pyloroplasty and partial gastrectomy with gastroduodenal anastomosis are frequently associated with bacterial overgrowth.[11,12] Altered motility or structure may play a role in the case of surgery, but patients with chronic gastric acid suppression with H_2-receptor antagonists have developed symptomatic bacterial overgrowth with no other risk factors.[13,14]

Normal motility is essential to keeping the bacterial population low in the small intestine. The migrating motor complex (MMC), also known as the *intestinal housekeeper*, is a cyclic wave of contractile activity that occurs every 2 hours in the fasting state and serves to maintain flow through the intestine.[15] Abnormalities of the MMC have been described in association with bacterial overgrowth.[16] Intestinal pseudo-obstruction with faulty MMCs are seen in up to half of patients with scleroderma, and this is frequently accompanied by bacterial overgrowth.[17,18] The hypomotility seen with diabetic autonomic neuropathy can also lead to bacterial overgrowth.[19] Medications that slow the gut should also be considered a potential predisposing factor.

Structural abnormalities are probably the most consistently troublesome source of bacterial overgrowth. Small intestinal diverticula are found in up to 5% of the population and are frequently an unsuspected source of bacterial proliferation.[20,21] The surgical creation of blind pouches in the proximal intestine often are followed by bacterial overgrowth. This is a frequent complication of antrectomy with a Billroth II anastomosis, and is especially prevalent if a gastrojejunostomy is performed.[22,23] The problem is also encountered when side-to-side or end-to-side anastomoses are performed.[24] Stricture may be encountered in association with adhesions, Crohn's disease, or previous abdominal irradiation and may produce slowed intestinal transit with consequent bacterial proliferation.[25,26] Fistulas are an especially troublesome problem, as they may allow continuous bacterial seeding of the proximal gastrointestinal tract. Bacterial overgrowth is a particularly troublesome cause of malabsorption in the elderly population and frequently is seen without any other predisposing factor.[27,28]

CLINICAL FEATURES

The main clinical features of bacterial overgrowth are steatorrhea, vitamin B_{12} deficiency, malnutrition, abdominal pain, and weight loss. The presentation can be quite variable, depending on the predisposing factors, the types of bacteria colonizing the intestine, and the duration of the disorder.

The primary cause of steatorrhea is thought to be deconjugation of bile acids in the intestine.[29] This permits premature absorption of the bile acids and thus lowers the luminal concentration below the critical micellar concentration necessary for lipid digestion.[30,31] This mechanism is supported by studies that demonstrate correction of steatorrhea by orally administered bile salts[31] and normalization of the luminal conjugated bile acid concentration by administration of oral antibiotics.[30] Unconjugated bile acids act as an irritant to mucosal cells and may hinder their function, thus compounding the problem. They impair transport of electrolytes and water in both the small intestine and colon, prompting diarrhea.[32,33] Also, unconjugated bile acids have been demonstrated to impair the transport of carbohydrate in the proximal small intestine.[34] It has also been suggested that bacterial enzymes such as proteases or glycosidases may cause mucosal injury.[35]

The vitamin B_{12} deficiency associated with bacterial overgrowth is mediated primarily by bacterial sequestration of the vitamin.[36] This leaves it unavailable for absorption in the patient. Anaerobes have an especially high affinity for vitamin B_{12}, including the intrinsic factor-cobalamin complex.[37] It has also been demonstrated that treatment with antibiotics that does not include anaerobic coverage fails to correct the vitamin B_{12} malabsorption.

Hypoalbuminemia and protein malnutrition that is out of proportion to the patient's diarrhea are often seen.[38] Intraluminal deamination of protein by bacteria is a major factor in this problem.[39] It has also been found that protein synthesis by the liver is diminished in the setting of bacterial overgrowth, and this problem is reversed by antibiotic treatment.[39] Both decreased absorption of protein and loss of endogenous protein have been demonstrated in the rat model of the blind loop syndrome, suggesting two other sources of protein malnutrition.[40]

Other nutritional deficiencies have been noted with bacterial overgrowth including vitamin D deficiency.[41] Both folate deficiency and folate excess have been described.[42]

DIAGNOSTIC TESTING

Quantitative culture of jejunal aspirate was once considered the gold standard for making the diagnosis of bacterial overgrowth.[43] The test results are considered positive if the bacterial concentration in aspirated secretion is greater than 10^5/ml. Also, positive cultures demonstrate a variety of organisms, including *Bacteroides* and the coliforms. The use of quantitative culture of jejunal aspirate has a number of limitations. The test requires peroral jejunal intubation with meticulous attention to sample collection and culturing techniques. The process is uncomfortable for the patient and time consuming. Furthermore, there is an inherent time delay in making the diagnosis while waiting for cultures. Also, it has been demonstrated that bacterial overgrowth may occur in a patchy fashion; thus, a false-negative result can occur if an uninvolved area of the intestine is cultured.[44]

As an alternative to culturing, a number of breath tests have been devised to detect bacterial overgrowth.[45] These are based on the ingestion of a substance that the normal human small intestine absorbs intact but that may be metabolized by displaced bacteria in the small intestine. A breakdown product of the metabolism of the substance can then be absorbed into the bloodstream and exhaled if it is volatile.

The first breath test described in 1971 was the ^{14}C-cholylglycine breath test.[46] It is based on the bacterial deconjugation of a bile acid that would otherwise be absorbed intact in the terminal ileum. Bacterial metabolism results in the production of [^{14}C]O_2 which is detectable in the breath. The test lacks both sensitivity and specificity.[47,48] If rapid intestinal transit is present or if the terminal ileum is diseased, intact cholylglycine may reach the colon where it is metabolized by bacteria and a false-positive result may be obtained. In clinical trials, there has been as high as a 40% false-negative rate in patients with culture-proven bacterial overgrowth.

Currently, the optimal breath test for the detection of bacterial overgrowth is the [^{14}C]-*d*-xylose breath test.[49] Xylose is minimally metabolized by humans and is readily absorbed in the proximal small intestine. If bacteria are present in the small intestine, they promptly metabolize the sugar, thus making it an ideal substrate for the test. The subject ingests 10 1Ci of [^{14}C]-*d*-xylose and 1 g of unlabeled xylose. Elevated levels of [^{14}C]O_2 can be detected in the breath of 85% of patients with bacterial overgrowth within 60 minutes of administration of the [^{14}C]-*d*-xylose. If delayed gastric emptying is present, samples may need to be taken for 180 minutes to ensure adequate evaluation.

Although less sensitive and specific than the [^{14}C]-*d*-xylose breath test, the hydrogen breath test is a simple and economical alternative. Unlike humans, bacteria metabolize carbohydrate to produce hydrogen gas. Some patients with bacterial overgrowth will have a baseline elevation in breath hydrogen.[50] Following the ingestion of lactulose, a nonabsorbable sugar, a rise in exhaled hydrogen is noted when the lactulose reaches the bacteria of the colon. In the presence of bacterial overgrowth, an additional peak is noted much sooner.[51] The distinction between the two peaks may not be entirely clear, thus rendering the test uninterpretable.[52] A similar test uses a 50- or 80-g glucose challenge followed by breath hydrogen measurement. Using the 50-g dose, the test has demonstrated a positive predicted value of 86% and a negative predictive value of 88%.[53] This test is based on the premise that bacteria colonizing the small intestine produce hydrogen; up to 27% of the population lack hydrogen-producing bacteria and thus present a false-negative hydrogen breath test.[54]

Urinary excretion of the metabolic products of bacteria, including indican, phenol, and p-cresol, have been suggested as a test for bacterial overgrowth but have been found to lack specificity.[8,55]

DIAGNOSIS

One must maintain a high index of suspicion for the blind loop syndrome. The presentation is often insidious, and the patient frequently has other medical problems to which the symptoms may be attributed. Patients with known Crohn's disease who develop bacterial overgrowth are often mistakenly treated for an exacerbation of their inflammatory bowel disease. Likewise, patients with motility problems, adhesions, or surgical changes from treatment of peptic ulcer disease are frequently considered to have a manifestation of their primary disease when in fact they have bacterial overgrowth. Thus, it is important to consider the diagnosis of blind loop syndrome in any patient who has the risk factors for the disorder described earlier in the setting of diarrhea, abdominal pain, weight loss, bloating, and macrocytic anemia.

The patient's first complaint is often diarrhea. This should prompt the clinician to look for evidence of malabsorption by measurement of quantitative fecal fat and serum vitamin B_{12}. A history of previous abdominal surgery suggests the need for contrast studies of the upper gastrointestinal tract to look for evidence of strictures, fistulae, or blind pouches. At that point, one may choose to further document the presence of malabsorption with a d-xylose absorption test in which the urinary excretion of orally ingested d-xylose is measured.[56] A small bowel biopsy may also be performed to rule out other causes of malabsorption such as celiac sprue. Biopsy results should be interpreted with caution, however, as bacterial overgrowth has been associated with some blunting of the villi.

Specific testing for bacterial overgrowth is limited by the resources available to the clinician, and referral may be necessary. Although an empiric trial of antibiotics is frequently used without a firm diagnosis, this approach may complicate the clinical picture.

TREATMENT

There are two basic approaches to the treatment of bacterial overgrowth. The first is to correct the structural or functional defect that predisposes to bacterial overgrowth. The other is to treat with antibiotics. Although surgical correction of a stricture, diverticulum, or fistula has the potential to cure the problem, this is true only in the minority of patients seen.[8,57]

Prokinetic agents may help to clear the structurally normal but sluggish intestine of unwanted bacteria. A series of patients with scleroderma and bacterial overgrowth were treated with daily injections of 50 g of octreotide to stimulate intestinal motility.[58] After 3 weeks of treatment, the patients' symptoms were significantly improved, and breath hydrogen testing demonstrated a marked reduction in bacterial overgrowth.

The choice of antibiotics is empiric; culture and sensitivity testing has no significant role. The antibiotic(s) chosen should have a broad spectrum of activity, have good gram-negative coverage, and have good anaerobic coverage. Tetracycline, 250 mg four times a day for 10 to 14 days, is an established treatment.[59] A combination of cephalexin, 250 mg four times a day, and metronidazole, 250 mg four times a day, is a rational choice that is associated with fewer treatment failures.[60] If monotherapy is desired, our institution has had excellent success with amoxicillin clavulanate. Although its potential side effects deter some clinicians, chloramphenicol has been used with success.[8] It must be remembered that relapse is quite common after treatment with antibiotics. Thus, it is not unusual to treat patients repeatedly. Rotation of antibiotic regimens can decrease the development of resistant strains and decrease the frequency of relapse episodes. Rarely, a patient may require continuous treatment.[60]

Appropriate nutritional support is important in the treatment of the patient with bacterial overgrowth. Intramuscular vitamin B_{12} injections, 50 μg per day for 2 weeks, should be given to those patients with a documented deficiency.[61] If bacterial overgrowth cannot be successfully eradicated, continued injections of 100 μg per month should be given. Supplementing the diet with medium-chain triglycerides that are not dependent on bile salts for their absorption may be useful in controlling steatorrhea and supplementing calories.[62] If significant malnutrition appears to be present, supplementation of vitamins, calcium, phosphorus, and trace elements may be necessary.[61] Finally, patients may not tolerate food containing lactose because of loss of the brush border enzymes from chronic diarrhea, and restriction of dairy products may be necessary.[8]

REFERENCES

1. Donaldson RM. Small bowel bacterial overgrowth. *Adv Intern Med.* 1970;16:191–212.
2. Ellis H, Smith SM. The blind loop syndrome. *Monogr Surg Sci.* 1967;4:193–227.
3. Cameron PG, Watson GM, Witts LJ. The experimental production of anaemia by operations on the intestinal tract. *Blood.* 1949;4:803–805.
4. Isaacs PT, Kim YS. Blind loop syndrome and small bowel bacterial contamination. *Clin Gastroenterol.* 1983;12:395–414.
5. Drasar BS, Shiner M, McLeod GM. Studies on the intestinal flora; the bacterial flora of the gastrointestinal tract in healthy and achlorhydric persons. *Gastroenterology.* 56:71–79.
6. Kalser MH, Cohen R, Arteaga I, et al. Normal viral and bacterial flora of the human small and large intestine. *N Engl J Med.* 1966;274:500–505, 558–563.
7. Gorbach SL, Plaut AG, Nahas L, et al. Studies of intestinal microflora: microorganisms of the small intestine and their relations to oral and fecal flora. *Gastroenterology.* 1967;53:856–867.
8. King CE, Toskes PP. Small intestine bacterial overgrowth. *Gastroenterology.* 1979;76:1035–1055.
9. Gorbach SL. Intestinal microflora. *Gastroenterology.* 1971;60:1110–1129.
10. Gray JD, Shiner M. Influence of gastric pH on gastric and jejunal flora. *Gut.* 1967;8:574–581.
11. Greenlee HB, Vivil R, Paez J, et al. Bacterial flora of the jejunum following peptic ulcer surgery. *Arch Surg.* 1971;102:260–265.
12. Browning GC, Buchan KA, Mackay C. The effect of vagotomy and drainage on the small bowel flora. *Gut.* 1974;15:139–142.
13. Ruddell WS, Losowsky MS. Severe diarrhea due to small intestine bacterial overgrowth during cimetidine treatment. *Br Med J.* 1980;281:273.
14. Milton-Thompson G, Lightfoot MF, Ahmet Z, et al. Intragastric acidity, bacteria, nitrite and N-nitroso compounds before, during, and after cimetidine treatment. *Lancet.* 1982;1:1091–1095.
15. Thompson DG, Wingate DL, Archer L, et al. Normal patterns of human upper small bowel motor activity recorded by prolonged radio-telemetry. *Gut.* 1980;21:500–506.
16. Van Trappen G, Janssens J, Hellemans J, et al. The interdigestive motor complex of normal subjects and patients with bacterial overgrowth of the small intestine. *J Clin Invest.* 1977;1158–1166.
17. Peachy RG, Creamer B, Pierce JW. Sclerodermatous involvement of the stomach and the small and large bowel. *Gut.* 1969;10:285–292.
18. Kahn I, Jeffries GH, Sleisenger MH. Malabsorption in intestinal scleroderma: correction by antibiotics. *N Engl J Med.* 1966;274:1339–1344.
19. Goldstein F, Wirts EC, Kowlessar OD. Diabetic diarrhea and clinical observations. *Ann Intern Med.* 1970;72:215–220.
20. Scudamore CH, Harrison RC, White TT. Management of duodenal diverticula. *Can J Surg.* 1982;25:311–314.
21. Doing A, Girdwood RG. The absorption of folic acid and labeled cyanocobalamin in intestinal malabsorption with observations on the fecal excretion of fat and nitrogen and the absorption of glucose and xylose. *Q J Med.* 1960;29:333–342.
22. Drasar BS, Shiner M. Studies on the intestinal flora: bacterial flora of the small intestine in patients with gastrointestinal disorders. *Gut.* 1969;10:812–819.
23. Wirts WC, Goldstein F. Studies of the mechanism of postgastrectomy steatorrhea. *Ann Intern Med.* 1963;58:25–31.
24. Schlegel DM, Maglintine DT. The blind pouch syndrome. *Surg Gynecol Obstet.* 1982;155:541–544.
25. Beeken WL, Kanish RE. Microbial flora of the upper small bowel in Crohn's disease. *Gastroenterology.* 1973;65:390–396.
26. Swan RW. Stagnant loop syndrome resulting from small-bowel irradiation injury and intestinal by-pass. *Gynecol Con.* 1974;2:441–445.
27. McEvoy A, Dutton J, James OFW. Bacterial contamination of the small intestine is an important cause of occult malabsorption in the elderly. *Br Med J.* 1983;287:789–793.
28. Montgomery RD, Haboubi NY, Mike NH, Chesner IM, Asquith P. Causes of malabsorption in the elderly. *Age Ageing.* 1986;15:235–140.
29. Dawson AM, Isselbacher KJ. Studies of lipid metabolism in the small intestine with observations on the role of bile salts. *J Clin Invest.* 1960;39:730–740.
30. Kim YS, Spritz N, Blum M, et al. The role of altered bile acid metabolism in the steatorrhea of experimental blind loop. *J Clin Invest.* 1966;45:956–962.
31. Tabaqchali S, Hatzioannou J, Booth CC. Bile salt deconjugation and steatorrhea in patients with the stagnant-loop syndrome. *Lancet.* 1968;2:12–16.
32. Phillips SF. Diarrhea: a current view of the pathophysiology. *Gastroenterology.* 1972;63:495–518.
33. Mekhjian HS, Phillips SF, Hoffman AF. Colonic secretion of water and electrolytes induced by bile acids: perfusion studies in man. *J Clin Invest.* 1971;50:1569–1577.
34. Gracey M. Intestinal absorption in the contaminated small bowel syndrome. *Gut.* 1971;12:403–410.
35. Jonas A, Krishnan C, Forstner GG. Pathogenesis of mucosal injury in the blind loop syndrome: release of disaccharidases from brush border membranes by extracts of bacteria obtained from intestinal blind loops in rats. *Gastroenterology.* 1978;75:791–795.
36. Dawson AM, Isselbacher KJ. Studies of lipid metabolism in the small intestine with observations on the role of bile salts. *J Clin Invest.* 1965;39:730–740.
37. Welkos SL, Toskes PP, Baer H. Importance of anaerobic bacteria in the cobalamin malabsorption of the experi-

mental rat blind loop syndrome. *Gastroenterology.* 1981; 80:313–320.
38. Cooke WT, Cox EB, Fone DJ, Gaddie R. The clinical and metabolic significance of jejunal diverticula. *Gut.* 1963;4:115–131.
39. Jones EA, Craigie A, Tavill AS, et al. Protein metabolism in the intestinal stagnant loop syndrome. *Gut.* 1968; 9:466–469.
40. Nygaard K, Rootwelt K. Intestinal protein loss in rats with blind segments on the small bowel. *Gastroenterology.* 1968;54:52–55.
41. Thompson GR. A case of osteomalacia, osteoporosis and hypercalcemia. *Br Med J.* 1967;1:219–225.
42. Neale G, Gomperttz D, Schjonsby H, et al. The metabolic and nutritional consequences of bacterial overgrowth in the small intestine. *Am J Clin Nutr.* 1972;25: 1409–1417.
43. Corazza GR, Menozzi MG, Strocchi A, et al. The diagnosis of small bowel bacterial overgrowth: reliability of jejunal culture and inadequacy of breath hydrogen testing. *Gastroenterology.* 1990;98:302–309.
44. Tillman CR, King CE, Toskes PP. Continued experience with the xylose breath test: evidence that the small bowel culture as the gold standard for bacterial overgrowth may be tarnished. *Gastroenterology.* 1981;80:1304. Abstract.
45. King CE, Toskes PP. The use of breath tests in the study of malabsorption. *Clin Gastroenterol.* 1983;12:591–610.
46. Sherr HP, Sasak Y, Newman A, et al. Detection of bacterial deconjugation of bile salts by a convenient breath-analysis technique. *N Engl J Med.* 1971;285:656–659.
47. James OFW, Agnew JE, Bouchier IAD. Assessment of [14C]-glycocholic acid breath test. *Br Med J.* 1973;3:191–195.
48. King CE, Toskes PP, Guilarte TR, et al. Comparison of the one-gram d-[14C]xylose breath test to the [14C] bile acid breath test in patients with small-intestine bacterial overgrowth. *Dig Dis Sci.* 1980;25:53–58.
49. King CE, Toskes PP, Spivey JC, et al. Detection of small intestine bacterial overgrowth by means of a [14C]-d-xylose breath test. *Gastroenterology.* 1979;77:75–82.
50. Ramakrishna BS, Mathan VI. Water and electrolyte absorption in the colon in tropical sprue. *Gut.* 1982;23: 843–849.
51. Bond JH, Levitt MD. Use of pulmonary hydrogen (H_2) measurements to quantitate carbohydrate absorption: study of partially gastrectomized patients. *J Clin Invest.* 1972;51:1219–1225.
52. King CE, Toskes PP. Comparison of the 1-gram [14C]xylose, 10-gram lactulose-H_2, and 80-gram glucose-H_2 breath test in patients with small intestine bacterial overgrowth. *Gastroenterology.* 1986;91:1447–1451.
53. Kerlin P, Wong L. Breath hydrogen testing in bacterial overgrowth of the small intestine. *Gastroenterology.* 1988;95:982–988.
54. Ravich WJ, Bayless TM, Thomas M. Fructose: incomplete intestinal absorption in man. *Gastroenterology.* 1983;84:26–29.
55. Aarbakke J, Schonsby H. Impaired oxidation of antipyrine in stagnant loop rats. *Scan J Gastroenterol.* 1978; 12:929–935.
56. Finlay JM, Hogarth J, Wightman KJR. A clinical evaluation of the *d*-xylose tolerance test. *Ann Intern Med.* 1964;61:411–416.
57. Donaldson RM. Small bowel bacterial overgrowth. *Adv Intern Med.* 1970;16:191–212.
58. Soudah H, Hasler WL, Owyang C. Effect of octreotide on intestinal motility and bacterial overgrowth in scleroderma. *N Engl J Med.* 1991;325:1461–1467.
59. Kahn IJ, Jeffries GH, Sleisenger MH. Malabsorption in intestinal scleroderma: correction by antibiotics. *N Engl J Med.* 1966;274:1339–1344.
60. Donaldson RM, Toskes PP. The blind loop syndrome. In: Sleisenger MH, Fordtran JS, eds. *Gastrointestinal Disease.* Philadelphia, Pa: WB Saunders Co; 1989:1289–1297.
61. Banwell JG. Small intestinal bacterial overgrowth syndrome. *Gastroenterology.* 1981;80:834–845.
62. Gracey G. The contaminated small bowel syndrome: pathogenesis, diagnosis, and treatment. *Am J Clin Nutr.* 1979;32:234–243.

57
Clostridium difficile Diarrhea

KENNETH D. FLORA and CLIFFORD S. MELNYK

Clostridium difficile, a constituent of normal colonic flora, causes a host of clinical syndromes in patients who are predisposed because of antibiotic use or debility. In this chapter we review the bacteriologic characteristics of *C. difficile,* the clinical spectrum of disease it causes, and its therapy and prevention.

HISTORICAL PERSPECTIVE

The original case of pseudomembranous colitis was reported in 1893 by Finney, who had removed a gastric tumor from a patient of Dr. William Osler. After surgery the patient died of complications resulting from diarrhea, with a subsequent autopsy revealing a bowel with a "diphtheritic membrane." Subsequent to this report, large hospitals noted 4 to 6 cases each year in patients having had similar procedures. With the increased use of antibiotics in the 1950s and 1960s, pseudomembranous colitis became a more frequent problem. Originally it was attributed to *Staphylococcus,* and therefore oral vancomycin became the antibiotic used most often in this therapy. In 1974, Tedesco noted that 42 out of 200 patients he studied developed diarrhea after being given clindamycin. Ten percent of these patients had pseudomembranous colitis on sigmoidoscopy. In retrospective studies, stools from these patients were later found to be positive for *C. difficile* toxin. Other studies reported in the 1970s characterized *C. difficile* and identified its production of a cytopathic toxin. At present, *C. difficile* and the toxins it produces are recognized as a major factor in antibiotic-associated diarrhea and colitis.

BACTERIAL CHARACTERISTICS

C. difficile is a gram-positive anaerobic bacillus that is 15 to 20 µm in diameter. It forms spores that are highly resistant to environmental conditions and solvents, with the exception of glutaraldehyde. The organism is found widely in the environment, in soil, hay, sand, and mud. In institutions it has been isolated from gowns, walls, toilets, beds, and wheelchairs. *C. difficile* is also present in animals such as horses, goats, cows, donkeys, and camels. Clostridia are a major constituent of human intestinal flora, being present in a concentration between 10^9 and 10^{10} organisms per gram of fecal material. *C. difficile* is a minor constituent after *C. ramosum* and *C. perfringens.*

C. difficile produces several toxins; a hemorrhagic enterotoxin, a cytotoxin, a nonhemorrhagic enterotoxin, a high molecular weight protein that changes membrane potentials and alters gastrointestinal peristalsis, and an adenosine diphosphate (ADP) ribosyl transferase. The first two toxins are clinically important. Toxin A, the enterotoxin, binds to receptors on the colonic mucosa causing changes in the intracellular tight junctions, increasing mucosal permeability, and promoting fluid loss into the bowel lumen. This results in intestinal fluid secretion and a hemorrhagic enteritis. Toxin B, a cytotoxin, induces alteration of cell shapes by acting on intracellular actin microfilaments. Its primary effect is the formation of a hemorrhagic enteritis. Toxin B is the toxin identified in standard laboratory assays, whereas toxin A is more clinically significant.

C. difficile is present in the colons of 30% to 70% of healthy infants, 3% to 6% of healthy adults, and 13% to 25% of ward patients. Colonization may be maintained for several months in infants, with or without the toxins, and low prevalence rates persist even when the "adult flora" becomes established at age 6 to 12 months. Older children rarely develop *C. difficile*–induced enteric disease, despite frequent exposure to antibiotics. Adults are the most susceptible for reasons that are not apparent. *C. difficile* toxin is present in 25% to 50% of healthy infants, less than 2% of healthy adults, but 2% of adults who are taking antibiotics. Despite the high frequency of *C. difficile* colonization and the elaboration of toxins, infants do not appear to suffer any ill effects.

SPECTRUM OF DISEASE CAUSED BY *C. DIFFICILE*

C. difficile diarrhea must be distinguished from the diarrhea caused by intolerance of antibiotic agents or "antibiotic-associated diarrhea," which is extremely common and is benign. The mechanism of this diarrhea is secretory with no mucosal abnormalities, and the frequent stools resolve with discontinuation of the offending antibiotic.

The mildest form of *C. difficile* diarrhea is self-limited and uncomplicated and serves as a nuisance to affected patients. This accounts for 15% to 25% of diarrhea in the hospital setting but less than 5% of outpatient diarrhea. Fevers are infrequent, and there is occasional abdominal discomfort. However, the serum white blood cell count and the colonic mucosa are normal.

Antibiotic-associated *colitis* refers to a more severe infection with *C. difficile.* Symptoms are more intense, and the watery diarrhea is of longer duration and increased frequency. Abdominal discomfort, fever, and leukocytosis is common, and 20% of patients pass occult blood in their stools. Flexible sigmoidoscopy reveals an erythematous colonic mucosa that is friable and occasionally hemorrhagic. Antibiotic-associated colitis affects from 0.1% to 1% of inpatients and 0.001% of outpatients.

Pseudomembranous colitis represents the most severe form of antibiotic-associated colitis, affecting between 0.1% and 10% of patients receiving "high-risk" antibiotics. Bloody diarrhea is more common in these patients, occurring in 5% to 10%. It is usually accompanied by crampy abdominal pain, high fever, high serum white blood cell count, with a significant "left shift," and the presence of fecal leukocytes in 60% to 70% of patients. The colonic mucosa is hemorrhagic with adherent white-yellow plaques of fibrin, mucin, neutrophils, and cellular debris. If these plaques coalesce, they form the classic pseudomembrane. The presentation of pseudomembranous colitis may resemble an acute abdomen and may be complicated by the development of toxic megacolon or visceral perforation.

Unusual presentations of *C. difficile* infection include a nonspecific postoperative fever, diarrhea with arthralgias, reactive pancreatic abscesses, and a cecal colitis similar to neutropenic typhlitis presenting as an acute appendicitis.

PATHOGENESIS

The development of diarrhea from *C. difficile* depends on four factors: (1) disruption of "colonization resistance" provided by normal colonic flora, (2) exposure to the *C. difficile* organism, (3) elaboration of virulence factors (toxins), and (4) alteration of host factors.

Older patients are most susceptible to *C. difficile* infection, especially those over 60 years of age. Age, however, does not predict the severity of the presentation of the disorder. Patients with debilitating illness are at increased risk. Such illnesses as diabetes, uremia, cardiovascular disease, chronic lung disease, neoplasms, immunosuppression, chemotherapy, and prolonged hospitalization or institutionalization increase a patient's risk for contracting the bacteria. Patients who have undergone abdominal surgery are also in the high-risk group. The most important host factor is having received antibiotic therapy.

Almost every antibiotic has been associated with the development of *C. difficile* infection. The most commonly associated antibiotics are ampicillin, clindamycin, and the second- and third-generation cephalosporins. The degree of an agent's activity against anaerobes appears the most important factor predisposing to *C. difficile* infection. The total dose of the antibiotic given, duration of therapy, and route of administration do not appear important. *C. difficile* diarrhea has developed after short, preoperative courses of antibiotics and up to 6 weeks after the discontinuation of a therapeutic course of antibiotics. The antibiotic appears to alter the normal intestinal flora, allowing *C. difficile* to proliferate. In vitro, *C. difficile* is inhibited by lactobacilli, *Bacteroides* species, group D *Enterococcus*, *C. bifermentins*, *Escherichia coli*, and *Peptostreptococcus*, with the suppressive effect of anaerobes being the most important. Therapies that use enemas containing mixtures of these bacteria have been shown to be effective in suppressing *C. difficile* infections.

DIAGNOSIS

Patients with *C. difficile* diarrhea should meet the definition of diarrhea (greater than or equal to three stools per day for longer than 2 days). Other causes for diarrhea must be excluded, and there should be a temporal association of the diarrhea with a positive toxin test result for *Clostridium difficile*.

The tests used most often for the identification of *C. difficile* are stool toxin assays. The classic test uses an epithelial cell monolayer onto which is poured a bacteria-free stool effluent, presumed to contain the cytotoxin (toxin B of *C. difficile*). If the cytotoxin is present, the cell monolayer is disrupted. The cytotoxic activity can be halted by the addition of antisera to *C. difficile* toxin B. This test is sensitive and highly specific, is less time consuming than cultures, and is most commonly used by clinical laboratories. Using the cytotoxin assay, toxin B is found in 15% to 25% of patients with *C. difficile* diarrhea, 50% to 75% of patients with antibiotic-associated colitis, and 90% to 100% of patients with antibiotic-associated colitis and pseudomembranes.

The gold standard for the diagnosis of *C. difficile* infection is culture of the organism. This is a time-consuming test because the organism is fastidious and requires a special agar containing cycloserine, fructose, and cefoxitin. *C. difficile* forms yellow-green colonies, which fluoresce under ultraviolet light on this agar, and patients with colitis may have between 10^4 to 10^5 colony-forming units per gram. Culture of the organism has been reported to be 97% sensitive and 93% specific.

The newest tests to identify *C. difficile* toxin involve a rapid, inexpensive ELISA test that can be used to identify both toxin A and toxin B. Sensitivity of this test ranges from 80% to 90%; however, it is recommended that it still be used in combination with culture or the older cytotoxin assay for confirmation of a positive value.

Flexible sigmoidoscopy can be the most rapid

means to diagnose *C. difficile* colitis, especially when pseudomembranes are present. Studies in patients with pseudomembranous colitis have shown that 95% of biopsy specimens obtained with flexible sigmoidoscopy yield positive cultures. Characteristic findings on endoscopy include multiple, discrete, slightly elevated plaques, 2 to 10 mm in diameter, which are yellow-white in color. The intervening mucosa is hyperemic and edematous (Fig. 57–1). Microscopically, pseudomembranous lesions have a "mushroom cap" or "erupting volcano" appearance, with necrotic material consisting of fibrin, mucin, neutrophils, and sloughed colonic epithelial cells attached to an area of mucosal ulceration (Fig. 57–2). There is an acute or chronic inflammatory infiltrate within the lamina propria. Careful flexible sigmoidoscopy allows for the rapid diagnosis of *C. difficile* without significantly increasing morbidity. In patients with toxic megacolon, sigmoidoscopy should be done with caution since overinsufflation of air can increase the risk of colonic perforation.

Barium enema examination should be avoided because the findings are usually nonspecific and the risk of colon perforation is relatively high. Computed tomography (CT) scan has been reported to show diffusely thickened or edematous colonic mucosa with pericolonic inflammation, with reactive lymph node enlargement and fatty tissue stranding. These findings are nonspecific, since they may occur with any form of colitis.

THERAPY

Diagnosis of *C. difficile* infection involves a high index of suspicion, and the degree of clinical aggressiveness depends on the severity of the patient's presentation. Therapy for those patients with uncomplicated "nuisance" diarrhea involves merely stopping the offending antibiotic and maintaining fluids and electrolytes. For those patients with stool positive for *C. difficile* toxin, cholestyramine or colestipol may be used as "toxin binders." Opiates are avoided, as are antiperistaltic agents, because of the risk of progression to more serious forms of colitis or toxic megacolon. This conservative approach allows for the resolution of symptoms in the majority of patients.

For patients presenting with more severe symptoms or antibiotic-associated colitis, the administration of oral antibiotics against *C. difficile* is appropriate. Both metronidazole and vancomycin have been shown to be efficacious. However, recent reports have demonstrated that metronidazole has a lower level of drug concentration in the colon than that achieved by the administration of vancomycin. In addition, there has also been the development of some metronidazole-resistant strains of *C. difficile*. Metronidazole still retains a good response profile and is less expensive and better tasting than vancomycin; however, patients with more severe disease should be given vancomycin as the first line of therapy.

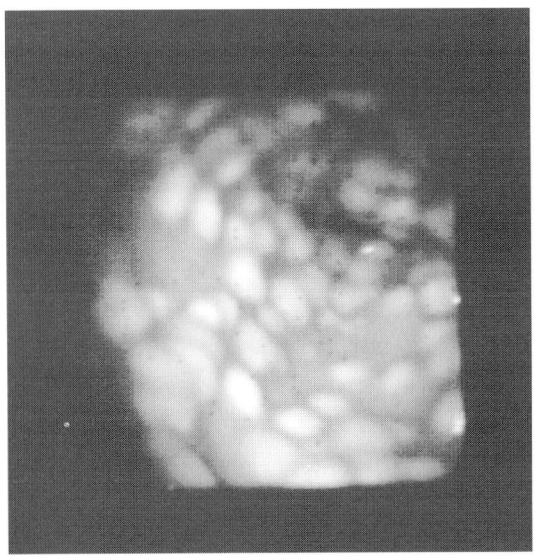
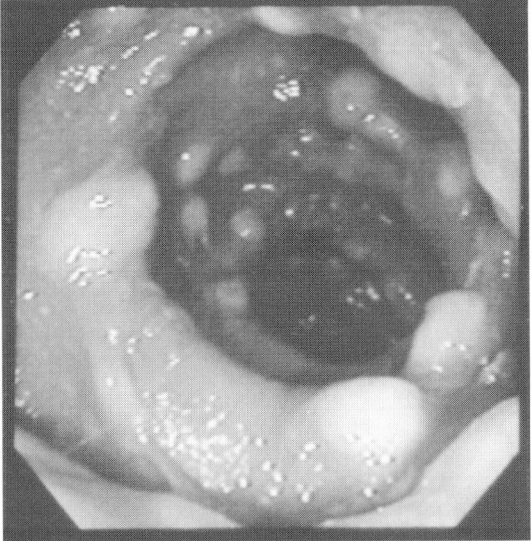

FIGURE 57–1. Flexible sigmoidoscopy revealing white-yellow, raised mucopurulent plaques, "pseudomembranes." Note the hyperemic, granular underlying mucosa.

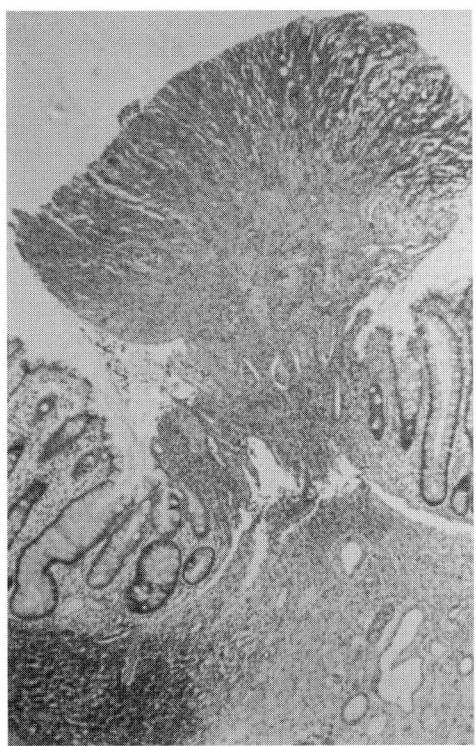

FIGURE 57–2. Microscopic photograph of a pseudomembrane attached to a mucosal ulcer. Note that the surrounding epithelium has only mild inflammation and edema.

Metronidazole is given in dosages of 250 to 500 mg orally four times daily for 10 days, whereas vancomycin may be given as 125 mg orally four times daily for 7 to 14 days or 500 mg orally four times daily for 5 to 10 days. Both antibiotics are poorly absorbed by the small bowel, which results in high concentrations in the colon. Intraluminal concentration of the antibiotic is important, as the clostridia rarely invade the mucosa. For severe antibiotic-associated colitis, vancomycin should be administered for at least 10 days in the higher dosage form. Metronidazole has some teratogenic effects and should be avoided in patients who are pregnant or in pediatric patients. Vancomycin has an exceedingly bitter taste, so the capsule form is usually preferred over the oral suspension by most patients. These antibiotics have been associated with prompt defervescence (24 to 48 hours) and resolution of diarrhea in 1 to 13 days (mean, 4½ days). If the patient has not responded within 7 days, the alternate antibiotic should be tried. Unfortunately, both drugs have been associated with relapse of *C. difficile* infection, with the rate after metronidazole higher than that after vancomycin. Relapses occur between 2 and 21 days after cessation of drug therapy. The use of a "toxin binder," such as cholestyramine given four times daily for 2 weeks after the antibiotic course of therapy, may decrease this relapse rate.

Patients with severe colitis and a clinical picture of ileus present a clinical challenge. Vancomycin is the oral "drug of choice" in these cases. Since the disease process is a toxin-mediated intraluminal process, all means to get the antibiotic to the bowel lumen must be explored. This may be achieved by tube irrigations, enemas, or instilling the antibiotic into any stomal opening (i.e., ileostomy, colostomy). In these desperate situations high-dose parenteral therapy with metronidazole as adjunctive therapy can be helpful.

Ten to twenty percent of patients suffer a relapse of antibiotic-associated colitis, with most patients having one relapse. It is unknown whether this represents persistent organism or that the organism has been reacquired from the environment. One theory is that *C. difficile* spores survive the high levels of antibiotic in the colon only to germinate once the antibiotic has been discontinued. Fortunately, these "offspring" organisms remain sensitive to vancomycin. Most relapses occur within a few weeks and are spontaneous. Patients with diverticular, functional, or organic bowel abnormalities are predisposed to multiple relapses.

Unfortunately, there is no satisfactory regimen in the treatment of a relapse. Repeating a course of the same antibiotic given, using the ultimate antibiotic (vancomycin), and longer courses of the same antibiotic have been advocated. Studies using longer courses of vancomycin with a gradual tapering of the dosage, alternating vancomycin and metronidazole (5 to 7 days each), and intermittent short courses of vancomycin as "pulses" have been found to be beneficial. Other antibiotics such as bacitracin, 25,000 U four times daily for 7 to 10 days, and rifampin, 600 mg orally twice daily, may have some synergistic effect with vancomycin. Bacitracin is poorly tolerated because of a very unpleasant taste.

Other, more creative methods of therapy have been reported. These include supplementation of antibiotics with yogurt or oral preparations of *Lactobacillus* organisms or capsules of *Saccharomyces boulardii* have been found to be beneficial. The instillation of "fecal enemas" that can introduce mixtures of normal flora constituents has also been found to suppress *C. difficile* infections. It is important to keep in mind that cholestyramine or colestipol will effectively bind any antibiotics administered to the patient, so they should be used only after completion of the antibiotic therapy.

Studies suggest that patients requiring antibiotics for life-threatening infectious diseases can be effectively treated with oral vancomycin while continuing the original offending agent. In vitro studies show no antagonism to the effectiveness of vancomycin on the *C. difficile* by other antibiotics.

PREVENTION

The most important therapy for *C. difficile* is the prevention of the acquisition of the organism. Such measures as using gloves and gowns and handwashing between every patient, sterilizing equipment, washing down contaminated rooms and beds constitute universal precautions that have been shown to be effective in decreasing the spread of *C. difficile*. The prudent use of antimicrobials is important; however, one must keep in mind that prior antibiotic therapy is not necessarily required, especially in those who have been institutionalized for prolonged periods or are severely debilitated or immunosuppressed. Physicians should be alert to the development of diarrhea in patients receiving antibiotics, and conservative measures should be begun immediately. It is controversial as to whether inpatients excreting *C. difficile* in the feces should be isolated. Unfortunately, there is no immunity to either the toxin or the disease. There are no good antitoxins currently available because it is difficult to purify the toxin and develop an immunogen.

REFERENCES

1. Anand A, Bashey B, Mir T, et al. Epidemiology, clinical manifestations, and outcome of *Clostridium difficile*–associated diarrhea. *Am J Gastroenterol.* 1994;89(4):519.
2. Bartlett J. *Clostridium difficile:* clinical considerations. *Rev Infect Dis.* 1990;12(2):A243.
3. Bowden T, Mansberger A, Lykins I. Pseudomembranous enterocolitis: mechanism of restoring floral hemostasis. *Am Surg.* 1981;47(4):180.
4. Fekety F, Shah A. Diagnosis and treatment of *Clostridium difficile* colitis. *JAMA.* 1993;269(1):71.
5. Gerdine D, Olson M, Peterson L, et al. *Clostridium difficile*–associated diarrhea and colitis in adults. *Arch Intern Med.* 1986;146:95.
6. Gerding D. Epidemiology and management of *Clostridium difficile* disease. *Contemp Int Med.* September 1990:55.
7. Hannonen P, Hakola M, Mottonen T, et al. Reactive oligoarthritis associated with *Clostridium difficile* colitis. *Scand J Rheumatol.* 1989;18:57.
8. McFarland L, Mulligan M, Kwok R, et al. Nosocomial acquisition of *Clostridium difficile* infection. *N Engl J Med.* 1989;320(4):204.
9. McFarland L. The epidemiology of *Clostridium difficile* infections: AGA viewpoints on infectious diseases. 1990;22(5).
10. Megibow A, Streiter M, Balthazar E, et al. Pseudomembranous colitis: diagnosis by computed tomography. *J Comput Assist Tomogr.* 1984;8(2):281.
11. Morris J, Zollinger R, Stellato T. Role of surgery in antibiotic-induced pseudomembranous enterocolitis. *Am J Surg.* 1990;160:535.
12. Tvede M, Rask-Madsen J. Bacteriotherapy for chronic relapsing *Clostridium difficile* diarrhoea in six patients. *Lancet.* 1989;1156.

58

Active Crohn's Disease

FERGUS SHANAHAN

Because the cause(s) of Crohn's disease is (are) unknown, a specific treatment is not yet possible. Therefore, the emphasis is on supportive measures, symptomatic remedies, and judicious use of antiinflammatory and immunomodulatory drugs.[1,2] While consensus guidelines may be followed, the management of patients with Crohn's disease should be individualized and cannot be algorithmic. The most important aspect of the management of this complex disorder is accessibility to a physician who is interested in the disease, sympathetic, and committed to long-term care of the patient.

The therapeutic considerations for the acutely active but uncomplicated case of Crohn's disease include (1) patient education and support, (2) diet and nutrition, (3) symptomatic therapy, and (4) antiinflammatory and immunomodulatory drug therapy. Although surgery is generally reserved for the management of complications of Crohn's disease or where medical therapy fails to control symptoms, a medical-surgical team approach is desirable. Early surgical consultation is wise so that the surgeon has an opportunity to assess the patient at more than one stage of the illness. The general principles of our management strategy are summarized below. Management of complications and specific aspects of Crohn's disease, including fistula and stricture formation, is covered in a separate chapter.

PATIENT EDUCATION AND SUPPORT

Physician-patient relationships are strengthened when patients are given sufficient information to alleviate fear of the unknown. It is too often forgotten that while the initial management of chronic illness may be routine for the physician, it is crisis for the patient. All patients need reassurance. The patient with Crohn's disease should be equipped with a simple but specific discussion regarding the nature of the disease and its clinical spectrum. Expectations of the outcome of treatment should be reasonable and not overstated. In encouraging patients with Crohn's disease to adopt a positive and hopeful attitude, we promote the advice of the late Norman Cousins to patients: "Don't deny the diagnosis, defy the verdict."

Many patients and their families benefit from a support group or patient advocate group. In the United States, physicians should encourage patients to enroll with the Crohn's & Colitis Foundation (444 Park Avenue South, New York, NY 10016). The Foundation publishes several excellent brochures and books for patients about inflammatory bowel disease. Similar foundations or associations exist in Canada and Europe.

DIET AND NUTRITIONAL CONSIDERATIONS

Although dietary factors have little, if any, role in the cause and pathogenesis of inflammatory bowel disease, patients with these disorders are frequently disappointed if physicians do not provide specific dietary instructions. This is not surprising, since diet is one area where patients feel they have some control. In general, we encourage as normal a diet as possible with minimal restrictions. The emphasis should be on maintaining adequate caloric intake and avoiding severely restrictive diets. The possibility of food allergy is often raised but is rarely a cause of disease relapse.[3]

Dietary and nutritional considerations are particularly relevant to the management of Crohn's disease in children and adolescents where inadequate caloric intake is the major cause of growth retardation. In adult patients, the specific nutritional factors that may require attention include dietary lactose and fiber intake, iron and vitamin supplementation, and the role of elemental diets as a therapeutic adjunct.

Lactose intolerance is always a potential confounding factor and should be considered if diarrhea is a prominent symptom. Specific diagnostic tests for this are seldom necessary, and a therapeutic trial of lactose restriction supplemented with lactose-digested dairy products, if desired, is usually adequate. Otherwise, there is no reason to advise patients to avoid milk or dairy intake. Patients with stricture formation should understand that a large bolus of dietary fiber may precipitate obstructive symptoms. Soluble fiber is preferred, and dietary residue should generally be limited in such patients. Specific instructions regarding avoidance of foods that are particularly high in fiber should be given.

Common indications for specific dietary supplements include iron for patients with chronic intestinal blood loss, calcium for patients receiving long-term corticosteroid therapy, and parenteral vitamin B_{12} for patients with extensive terminal ileal disease or previous ileal resection. Supplementation with additional vitamin and trace elements may be required for patients with extensive small bowel disease. However, in the absence of documented deficiency or susceptibility, we do not routinely prescribe multivitamin preparations and discourage indiscriminate use of "megavitamin therapy." Folic acid deficiency has been reported as a rare consequence of long-term sulfasalazine therapy, and some clinicians supplement folate prophylactically.

The role of nutritional replenishment for the malnourished patient with acutely active Crohn's disease is self-evident. However, whether parenteral or elemental diets or any form of nutrition can reduce intestinal inflammation and have a primary therapeutic effect is doubtful.[4] A recurring weakness of studies of elemental diet therapy for Crohn's disease has been the failure to include controls to account for the natural history of the disease and the large placebo effect associated with the treatment of the disease. Despite this, many physicians would regard a trial of dietary therapy as a reasonable option for patients who are intolerant or resistant to corticosteroids. At issue is whether an expensive elemental diet is required or whether a cheaper, more palatable, polymeric dietary formulation may be used instead. Our interpretation of the results of studies to date is that polymeric diets appear to be just as good as elemental diets.[4]

SYMPTOMATIC THERAPY

Symptomatic therapy should not merely imply the use of a nonspecific remedy for symptoms such as pain or diarrhea. Rather, a methodical and individualized approach to the management of symptoms in each patient will often reveal a simple and specific treatment and preclude the need to resort to more aggressive therapy with corticosteroids or immunosuppressants. Indeed, the value of attempting to understand the mechanism(s) of symptom production in each patient is well illustrated in the case of diarrhea in Crohn's disease. As shown in Table 58–1, there are several potential mechanisms (other than acute inflammation) by which diarrhea may occur in Crohn's disease. Bacterial overgrowth in a dilated segment or a bypassed loop of bowel may result in bile acid deconjugation with steatorrhea and diarrhea. Treatment is a broad spectrum antibiotic. In patients with disease in the terminal ileum or after surgical resection of the terminal ileum, reduced absorption of bile acids may lead to diarrhea due to a secretagogue effect of bile acids in the colon. This will usually respond promptly to cholestyramine. In contrast, other patients with more extensive disease or where there has been extensive resection of the terminal ileum (usually greater than 100 cm), a deficiency of bile acids may arise and lead to steatorrhea. Cholestyramine would exacerbate this; such patients require a low-fat diet. Other causes of diarrhea or steatorrhea include lactose intolerance, short bowel syndrome, and enteroentero or enterocolic fistula formation. Treatment differs in each case, and in some patients there may be more than one mechanism of diarrhea involved.

TABLE 58–1. MULTIPLE MECHANISMS OF DIARRHEA IN CROHN'S DISEASE

Bacterial overgrowth	→ Bile acid deconjugation
Bile acid diarrhea	→ Secretion in colon
Bile acid deficiency	→ Steatorrhea
Lactase deficiency	→ Osmotic overload
Short bowel syndrome	→ Malabsorption
Internal fistula	→ Bypass and altered transit time

There is a role for antidiarrheal drugs such as diphenoxylate (Lomotil) or loperamide (Immodium). In selected patients, these nonspecific antidiarrheals may be of temporary benefit. We prefer loperamide because it does not cross the blood-brain barrier and appears to have a lower frequency of side effects. However, because of the risk of toxic megacolon, these drugs should not be given to patients with acute severe colitis.

Symptomatic relief of pain is an important issue in the management of Crohn's disease. There is a significant risk of iatrogenic drug addiction. In our view, it is rarely necessary to prescribe long-term opiates. A requirement for opiates for pain relief should prompt a search for a complication of Crohn's disease such as a tight stricture or abscess formation. As a general principle, the best management of pain is to treat the underlying mechanism; suboptimal pain control usually implies suboptimal control of the underlying disease.

ROLE OF ANTIBIOTICS

We reserve the use of antibiotics for patients with fulminant colitis and those with complications such as intraabdominal or perineal sepsis. Although the use of broad spectrum antibiotics has been advocated by some clinicians for uncomplicated disease, there have been no convincing controlled trials (with the exception of metronidazole) of their use in Crohn's disease. In addition, there is a substantial risk of producing diarrhea by altering bowel flora or by predisposing to *Clostridium difficile* toxin-induced diarrhea.

Metronidazole (orally 10 to 20 mg/kg/d) has been shown in controlled studies to have a beneficial effect in patients with Crohn's colitis and ileocolitis, but it appears to lack efficacy in the small bowel.[5] However, many clinicians feel that its efficacy is not sufficiently impressive to recommend routine use. The most impressive therapeutic effects of metronidazole are in the management of perianal Crohn's disease.[6,7] Although metronidazole is regarded by many as the drug of first choice for this indication, it is curious that a controlled trial of metronidazole has never been conducted in this context. For patients with perianal disease who are intolerant or refractory to metronidazole, we recommend a trial of ciprofloxacin and, if unsuccessful, the initiation of immunosuppressive therapy with 6-mercaptopurine.

ANTIINFLAMMATORY DRUG THERAPY

SULFASALAZINE AND THE AMINOSALICYLATES

Sulfasalazine has proven efficacy in the management of Crohn's colitis but lacks efficacy in the small bowel. This is because exposure to the metabolic activity (azoreductase) of colonic bacteria is required for the release of sufficient amounts of the therapeutically active moiety 5-aminosalicylic acid (5-ASA), from sulfapyridine (the carrier molecule). The development of stable preparations of 5-ASA without the sulfa carrier has been an important advance. These preparations are a new option for patients who are allergic to sulfas and also permit site-specific delivery of 5-ASA to inflamed areas of the gastrointestinal tract.[8] Thus, the availability of sustained release preparations (e.g., Pentasa) enables the delivery of 5-ASA to the upper intestine, whereas the delayed pH-dependent release of Asacol allows delivery of 5-ASA to the distal ileum and colon. These delivery mechanisms represent a new option for the majority of patients with Crohn's disease. For patients with disease confined to the colon, prodrugs such as olsalazine (Dipentum) and balsalazine permit the release of 5-ASA exclusively in the colon, and topical preparations (enemas and suppositories) are available for treatment of local disease in the distal colon and rectum.

CORTICOSTEROIDS

Systemic corticosteroids remain a cornerstone treatment for acute severe relapses of Crohn's disease.[9,10] Their potent and relatively rapid acting antiinflammatory effects are particularly useful in patients with obstructive symptoms due to inflammatory strictures in the small bowel. When promptly administered in high dosage, a reduction in edema and inflammatory infiltration can have a profound alleviating influence on symptoms of bowel obstruction. Since the cross-sectional area of the intestinal lumen is a factor of the square of its radius (pr^2), it follows that a relatively small increase in the radius of the lumen (due to reduced intramural swelling) can substantially improve transit through the inflamed segment of bowel. Similarly, a short therapeutic trial of high-dose prednisolone (40 to 60 mg/d) may be helpful in distinguishing inflammatory (partially reversible) strictures from those that are fibrotic and fixed. However, long-term use of steroids is limited by significant toxicity, and these agents have no role in maintenance of remission.

Topical (enema) steroid therapy is associated with substantially reduced toxicity and is suited for patients with left-sided Crohn's colitis. Steroid foams (Cortifoam) are as efficacious as enemas (e.g., Cortenema) and tend to be better tolerated because they are easier to retain in the bowel. New topical formulations that are currently under study are associated with an improved toxicity profile because they have reduced systemic absorption, extensive first-pass metabolism, and little systemic bioactivity. Examples include budesonide, beclomethasone diproprionate, tixocortol pivalate, and prednisolone metasulfobenzoate. Although enema preparations of these agents are indicated for patients with distal colitis, a more exciting prospect is the potential role of oral formulations of topically active steroids for patients with extensive small bowel Crohn's disease.

IMMUNOSUPPRESSIVE AND IMMUNOMODULATORY DRUGS

PURINE ANALOGS

Despite the negative results in the National Cooperative Crohn's Disease Study,[11] the efficacy of the immunosuppressive purine analogs, azathioprine and its active metabolite, 6-mercaptopurine, is now generally accepted.[12,13] The role of these agents in both treatment of active disease[14,15] and maintenance of remission[16] has been convincingly demonstrated in well-designed controlled trials. These drugs are particularly useful in chronically active Crohn's disease that is uncontrolled by corticosteroids and in patients requiring persistently high doses of steroids for control of disease activity.[15] It is important to recognize that these drugs are slow acting. The mean clinical response time is approximately 3 months. Therefore, they should not be expected to produce prompt relief in acutely ill patients, and steroid therapy should be continued until sufficient time has elapsed for the immunosuppressant effect to become established.

A single daily dose of 50 to 100 mg/d is used. At the lower dose bone marrow suppression is rare. Indeed, purine analogs are remarkably well tolerated by patients with Crohn's disease. In a study of 396 patients observed over 18 years with a mean of 5 years, a very low level of toxicity was found.[17] Pancreatitis occurs in approximately 3% of patients. This is probably a hypersensitivity event and precludes further use of either form of purine analog. Occasionally these drugs produce a debilitating flulike illness that also appears to be a hypersensitivity phenomenon. A serious drug interaction may occur if purine analogs are given to patients taking the xanthine oxidase inhibitor, allopurinol. Because purine analogs are metabolized by this enzyme, the concomitant use of allopurinol leads to dangerously high drug levels. The major theoretical risk with long-term administration of immunosuppressives is the possibility of opportunistic infections or neoplasia. However, the degree of risk remains to be demonstrated and may not be a problem at the low doses currently used.[17] It is our practice to provide patients with a pamphlet that attempts to place in perspective the real and theoretical risks associated with these drugs in addition to the benefits.

Cyclosporine

Because of the delayed induction of clinical response associated with the purine analogs, other immunomodulatory agents that might have a more rapid onset of clinical efficacy are now being investigated. Cyclosporine has a rapid onset of action and suppresses the induction and amplification of the immune response by inhibiting cytokine gene activation.[12,13] Although cyclosporine appears to have a rapid and dramatic beneficial effect in patients with acute severe ulcerative colitis,[18] its role in Crohn's disease is less clear. Of 37 patients, 22 (59%) improved with cyclosporine (5 to 7.5 mg/kg/d for 3 months), compared with 11 of 34 (32%) receiving placebo.[19] Noteworthy was the fact that the improvement was evident after only 2 weeks. Although serious side effects did not arise in this study, the well-documented toxicity of cyclosporine remains a concern. Because of this, many clinicians feel that cyclosporine is unlikely to have a role in Crohn's disease on a long-term basis. However, the short-term use of cyclosporine in patients with active severe disease, as an interim measure before more slow-acting drugs such as 6-mercaptopurine take full effect, needs to be assessed. This cautious view is supported by the results of a second placebo-controlled trial that have been reported.[20] This large Canadian study found that cyclosporine at a dosage of 4.8 mg/kg is ineffective as therapy of Crohn's disease and may even have an adverse effect on disease activity in patients in remission.

Other Immunosuppressants

Continuing developments in the field of organ transplantation have maintained the search for safer and more effective immunosuppressive agents.[12,13] Newer agents include the macrolides, rapamycin and FK506, which may eclipse cyclosporine in clinical use during the next decade.[21] Studies of FK506 in inflammatory bowel disease are already underway. Its mode of action is similar to that of cyclosporine, but it is approximately one hundred-fold more potent. Toxicity is likely to be similar also, although early data have suggested that it occurs with a lower frequency than with cyclosporine.

The folic acid antagonist, methotrexate, has been reported in an open study to have a marked beneficial effect in some patients with inflammatory bowel disease, particularly Crohn's disease.[22] Some of these patients were refractory to other treatments including steroids and 6-mercaptopurine and responded to high-dose methotrexate (25 mg/intramuscularly) over a 12-week period. Controlled trials with lower doses of methotrexate have since been initiated. Other modes of immunosuppression include T-cell apheresis and monoclonal antibody therapy. These have not been subjected to controlled trials and are expensive, cumbersome, and not suited to long-term management for outpatients.

PROSPECTS FOR FUTURE DRUG DEVELOPMENT

Drug therapy for inflammatory bowel disease has traditionally been introduced on the basis of empiric observations in patients, followed by pharmaceutical modifications or improved delivery systems. It is likely that future development of novel drugs for Crohn's disease will be based on concepts that emerge from an improved understanding of pathogenesis. Thus, the identification of specific pathogenic mechanisms and inflammatory mediators of mucosal inflammation provides a glimpse of several new potential approaches to drug therapy. Major classes of drugs that are likely to emerge in the near future include inhibitors or antagonists of leukotrienes, cytokines, oxygen radicals, and nitric oxide. In addition, blockade of surface adhesion molecules and selective modulation of the mucosal immune system are attractive targets for therapeutic intervention.

REFERENCES

1. Shanahan F, Targan S. Medical treatment of inflammatory bowel disease. *Annu Rev Med.* 1992;43:125–133.
2. Shanahan F, Targan S. Inflammatory bowel disease. In: Kelley WN, et al, eds. *Textbook of Internal Medicine.* 2nd ed. Philadelphia, Pa: JB Lippincott Co; 1992:489–502.
3. Duerr R, Shanahan F. Food allergy. In: Targan S, Shanahan F, eds. *Immunology and Immunopathology of the Liver and Gastrointestinal Tract.* New York, NY: Igaku-Shoin; 1990:507–533.
4. Bernstein C, Shanahan F. Braving the elementals in Crohn's disease. *Gastroenterology.* 1992;103:1363–1364.
5. Bernstein C, Shanahan F. Metronidazole in Crohn's disease: what's the score? *Gastroenterology.* 1992;102:1435–1436.
6. Bernstein LH, Frank MS, Brandt LJ, Boley SJ. Healing of perineal Crohn's disease with metronidazole. *Gastroenterology.* 1980;78:357–365.
7. Brandt LJ, Bermsteom LH, Boley SJ, Frank MS. Metronidazole therapy for perineal Crohn's disease: a follow-up study. *Gastroenterology.* 1982;83:383–387.
8. Shanahan F. Clinical use of the new aminosalicylates in ulcerative colitis. *Practical Gastroenterol.* 1992;16:47–54.
9. Kuritzkes R, Shanahan F. Corticosteroid therapy. In: Gitnick G, ed. *Inflammatory Bowel Disease.* New York/Tokyo: Igaku-Shoin; 1991:299–321.
10. Jewell DP. Corticosteroids for the management of ulcerative colitis and Crohn's disease. *Gastroenterol Clin.* 1989;18:21–34.
11. Summers RW, Switz DM, Sessions JT Jr, et al. National Cooperative Crohn's Disease Study: results of drug treatment. *Gastroenterology.* 1979;77:847–869.
12. Bernstein CN, Shanahan F. Immunosuppressive and immunomodulatory therapy for inflammatory bowel disease. *Can J Gastroenterol.* 1993;7:115–120.
13. Bernstein CN, Shanahan F. Immunomodulatory therapy of inflammatory bowel disease. In: Targan S, Shanahan F, eds. *Inflammatory Bowel Disease: From Bench to Bedside.* Baltimore, Md: Williams & Wilkins; In press.
14. Present DH, Korelitz BI, Wisch N, Glass JL, Sacher DB, Pasternack BS. Treatment of Crohn's disease with 6-mercaptopurine: a long term randomized double blind study. *N Engl J Med.* 1980;302:981–987.
15. Ewe K, Press AG, Singe CC, et al. Azathioprine combined with prednisolone or monotherapy with prednisolone in active Crohn's disease. *Gastroenterology.* 1993;105:367–372.
16. O'Donoghue DP, Dawson AM, Powell-Tuck J, Brown RL, Lennard-Jones JE. Double-blind withdrawal trial of azathioprine as maintenance treatment of Crohn's disease. *Lancet.* 1978;2:955–957.
17. Present DH, Meltzer SJ, Krumholz MP, Wolke A, Koerlitz BI. 6-Mercaptopurine in the management of inflammatory bowel disease: short- and long-term toxicity. *Ann Intern Med.* 1989;111:641–649.
18. Lichtiger S, Present DH, Kornbluth A, Hanauer SB. Cyclosporine A in the treatment of severe refractory ulcerative colitis: a double blinded placebo controlled trial. *Gastroenterology.* 1993;104:A732.
19. Brynskov J, Freund L, Rasmussen SN, et al. A placebo-controlled double-blind randomized trial of cyclosporine therapy in active chronic Crohn's disease. *N Engl J Med.* 1989;321:845–850.
20. Archambault A, Feagan B, Fedorak R, et al. The Canadian Crohn's relapse prevention trial (CCRPT). *Gastroenterology.* 1992;102:A591.
21. Macleod AM, Thomson AW. FK506: an immunosuppressant for the 1990's? *Lancet.* 1991;337:25–27.
22. Kozarek RA, Patterson DJ, Gelfand MD, Botoman VA, Ball TJ, Wilske KR. Methotrexate induces clinical and histologic remission in patients with refractory inflammatory bowel disease. *Ann Intern Med.* 1989;110:353–356.

59
Benign Tumors of the Small Bowel
CAROL ANN BURKE and ROSALIND U. VAN STOLK

Small bowel tumors are rare. The small intestine is the site of less than 6% of all gastrointestinal neoplasms and 1.2% to 1.6% of all gastrointestinal malignancies. The prevalence varies according to the population studied. In two large reviews of 17,070 autopsies and 392,000 surgical pathology cases, the prevalence was 0.4% and 0.5%, respectively.[1,2] Twenty-five to seventy-five percent of small bowel tumors are benign.[3,4] Usually a greater percentage of malignancies are found in clinical studies and a greater percentage of benign tumors are found in autopsy reviews.[1] The paucity of small bowel tumors is surprising considering that the small bowel accounts for 75% of the total length of the gastrointestinal tract and 90% of its mucosal surface.

Following are the most common types of benign tumors, in decreasing order of frequency:

- Leiomyomas
- Adenomas
- Lipomas
- Hemangiomas

These four types comprise about 90% of all small bowel tumors. Less frequently reported benign tumors include

- Brunner's gland lesions
- Neurogenic tumors
- Fibromas
- Hamartomas
- Lymphangiomas

Most small bowel tumors are solitary, but multiple neoplasms are seen especially in the intestinal polyposis syndromes (Table 59–1). Reports of the location of benign small bowel tumors suggest an increase distally; however, considering that the length of the duodenum is only 20 to 30 cm and the jejunum and ileum are 2.5 and 3.5 m respectively, the duodenum has more tumors per unit area (Table 59–2).

ETIOLOGY AND PATHOGENESIS

The pathogenesis of small bowel neoplasms is not known. Purported mechanisms to account for the rarity of small bowel tumors include:

1. Alkaline pH of small intestinal fluid.
2. Rapid transit time decreasing exposure time to potential carcinogens.
3. Liquidity of small bowel contents with less mechanical irritation of the gut lining.
4. Relative sterility of the intestinal milieu with lower rates of formation of carcinogenic compounds from bacterial metabolic breakdown products.
5. Protective microsomal enzyme systems that detoxify potential carcinogens: These enzyme systems have been studied in animals and man. One enzyme system, benzpyrene hydroxylase, is produced in response to an exogenous inducer and converts the potent carcinogen benzpyrene, present in small quantities in food, to weakly carcinogenic or noncarcinogenic hydroxy and quinone derivatives.

TABLE 59–1. CLASSIFICATION OF THE POLYPOSIS SYNDROMES WITH SMALL BOWEL INVOLVEMENT

Familial
Neoplastic
Familial adenomatous polyposis
  Gardner's syndrome
  Turcot's syndrome

Nonneoplastic: Hamartomatous
Peutz-Jeghers syndrome
Neurofibromatosis
Cowden's syndrome
Familial juvenile polyposis

Nonfamilial
Nonneoplastic: Hamartomatous
Cronkhite-Canada syndrome
Juvenile polyposis of infancy

TABLE 59-2. LOCATION AND FREQUENCY OF BENIGN SMALL BOWEL TUMORS (%)

TUMOR	NUMBER	DUODENAL	JEJUNAL	ILEAL
Leiomyoma	161 (36)	31 (19)	79 (49)	51 (32)
Adenoma	108 (24)	35 (32)	29 (27)	44 (41)
Lipoma	77 (17)	22 (29)	11 (14)	44 (57)
Hemangioma	39 (9)	2 (5)	23 (59)	14 (36)
Neurogenic	28 (6)	7 (25)	9 (32)	12 (43)
Fibroma	13 (3)	2 (15)	4 (31)	7 (54)
Lymphangioma	11 (2)	1 (9)	4 (36)	6 (55)
Brunner's gland	6 (1)	6 (100)	—	—
Hamartomas	5 (1)	0	4 (80)	1 (20)
TOTAL	448	106 (24)	163 (36)	179 (40)

Data from clinicopathologic studies by Darling and Welch, 1959; Nordkild and Kjaergard, 1986; Aranha et al, 1979; Croom and Newsome, 1975; Cohen et al, 1971; Gupta et al, 1976; Moertel et al, 1961; Elias et al, 1954; Ostermiller et al, 1966; Herbsmann et al, 1980; Wilson et al, 1975.

6. Increased immunologic surveillance with abundant lymphoid tissue and immunoglobulin production: Evidence of these protective mechanisms stems from the greater incidence of small bowel cancer in immunocompromised patients such as organ transplantation recipients and patients with cancer or AIDS. It is known that patients with small bowel cancers have an increased frequency of second primary malignancies (15.6% to 25% versus a 3% to 6% incidence of second tumors in patients with other malignancies).[4,5]
7. Lower proliferation rates: The use of tritiated thymidine reveals that fewer small intestinal cells retain their proliferative potential at the luminal surface, possibly reducing neoplastic change in the small intestine.[6]

In spite of the myriad of speculative evidence for the protection of the small bowel against neoplastic transformation the pathogenesis of tumors is not well understood. Studies of the cause of small bowel tumors are hampered by small bowel neoplasm rarity, many histologic cell types, protean symptoms, and the relative inaccessibility of the small intestine to diagnostic methods.

SMALL BOWEL ANATOMY

A brief review of the anatomy of the small bowel is salient to the understanding of tumors of the small bowel because virtually all the histologic layers of the intestine are represented in small bowel neoplasms (Table 59–3). The small intestinal lining is thrown into a series of folds, plicae circulares or Kerckring's valves, composed of mucosa and submucosa. The mucosa consists of epithelium and loose connective tissue, blood vessels, lymphatics, nerves, and smooth muscle cells referred to as *lamina propria*. The smooth muscle cells of the muscularis mucosa separate the mucosa and submucosa. The submucosa contains Brunner's glands (duodenum), Peyer's patches (greater in ileum), connective tissue, fibrocytes, blood vessels, lymphatics, and a network of nerves, the Meissner's plexus. The next layer is the muscularis propria with an inner circular and outer longitudinal smooth muscle layer separated by Auerbach's plexus. The outermost layer is serosa.

TABLE 59-3. CLINICOPATHOLOGIC CORRELATES OF SMALL BOWEL TUMORS

HISTOLOGY	TUMOR
Mucosa	
Epithelium	Adenoma
Lamina propria	
Muscularis mucosa or propria	Leiomyoma
Submucosa	Brunner's gland lesions
	Lipoma
	Hemangioma
	Fibroma
	Neurogenic tumor
	Lymphangioma
Mixed	Hamartoma

SYMPTOMS

The majority of small bowel tumors are clinically silent. Generally, 50% of benign tumors are found incidentally during operations for other reasons or at autopsy.[7,8] If symptoms are present, they usually are vague. Hancock[9] stated that half of patients with small bowel tumors seeking a medical opinion were labeled neurotic, often repeatedly. The peak age of presentation is in the fifth to seventh decade. Symptoms are often chronic and intermittent and can include abdominal pain, nausea, weight loss, and bleeding. Because of the paucity of physical findings the symptoms are frequently dismissed and the diagnosis is delayed. Some series report a median interval between the onset of symptoms and operation of 9 weeks to 3 years.[4,10] This is important when considering the delay in diagnosis of malignant small bowel tumors, 75% of which are widely metastatic at the time of diagnosis.

Symptoms vary according to the size, location, blood supply, and type of growth pattern. The most frequently reported complications include bleeding (which is usually chronic, although massive bleeding has been reported), obstruction, and intussusception. Intussusception is the most common cause of obstruction due to small bowel tumors. The demographics, cause, and presentation of intussusception are different in children and adults. Greater than 90% of all intussusceptions occur in children, and 80% of these are idiopathic. The classic presentation in children is sudden abdominal pain, vomiting, and currant jelly stools. In contradistinction, only 5% of intussusceptions occur in adults, and an organic cause is found in 80% of these. Greater than 70% are due to benign small bowel tumors.[11] The course is chronic with nonspecific or intermittent obstructive symptoms. Therefore, intussusception in adults should alert the clinician to the diagnosis of a small bowel tumor.

TABLE 59-4. DIAGNOSTIC MODALITIES

Radiographic
Upper gastrointestinal tract and small bowel series
Enteroclysis (small bowel enema)
Abdominal computed tomography scan
Abdominal ultrasound
Angiography

Endoscopic
Esophagogastroduodenoscopy
Enteroscopy, push or passive
Interoperative enteroscopy
Colonoscopy with intubation of the terminal ileum
Endoscopic ultrasound

Surgical
Exploratory laparotomy

DIAGNOSIS

The diagnosis of small bowel tumors is difficult. The symptoms are vague, and access to the small intestine is limited. Even if patients are symptomatic, the preoperative diagnosis is made in only 19% to 41% of patients.[3,4] Other than surgery, there are two major modalities, radiographic and endoscopic, to evaluate the small intestine (Table 59-4).

The sensitivity of an upper gastrointestinal tract radiograph with small bowel series varies widely and is reported to be diagnostic in 30% to 70% of patients with small bowel tumors (Fig. 59-1). The small bowel enema or enteroclysis may increase the diagnostic yield. Computed tomography (CT) scans have occasionally been used to detect small bowel neoplasms, in particular lipomas, on the basis of their characteristic features and Hounsfield units[12] (Fig. 59-2). Angiography is useful for detecting actively bleeding lesions and nonbleeding hemangiomas and leiomyomas.

Endoscopy seems to have the highest sensitivity for detecting lesions within its reach (Fig. 59-3). Standard upper endoscopes are usually able to be passed into the third portion of the duodenum and occasionally past the ligament of Treitz into the proximal jejunum. The last 20 cm

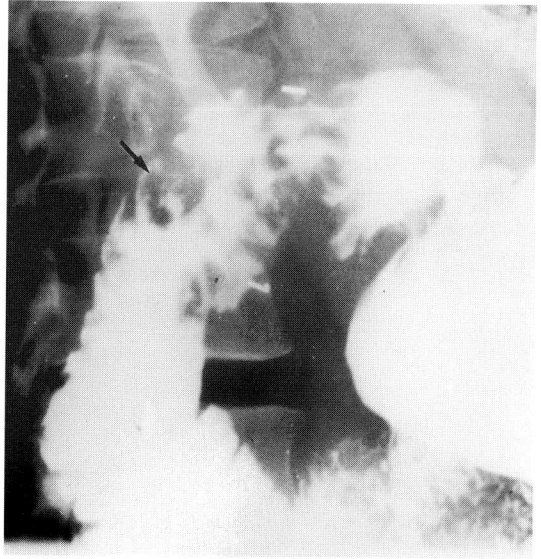

FIGURE 59-1. Upper gastrointestinal tract series demonstrating multiple polypoid filling defects in the duodenum (*arrow*). Endoscopic biopsy confirmed that they were Brunner's gland lesions. (Courtesy S. Shay, MD.)

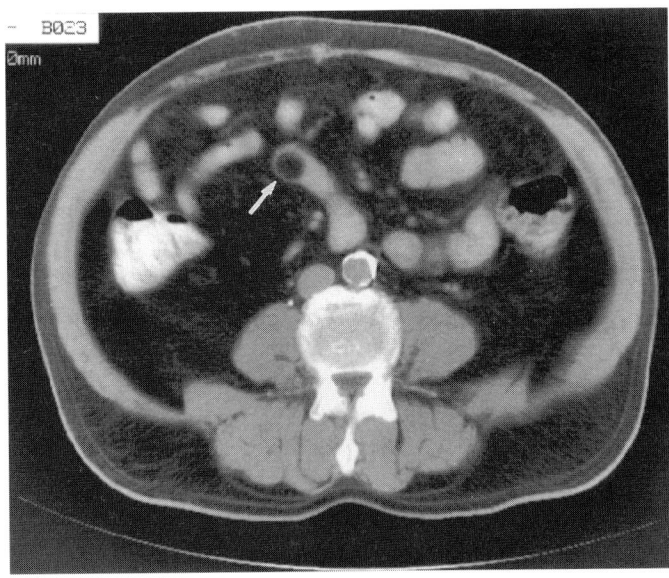

FIGURE 59–2. Computed tomography scan of the abdomen demonstrating a jejunal lipoma *(arrow)*. Note that the tumor is the same density as the subcutaneous fat. (Courtesy D. Einstein, MD.)

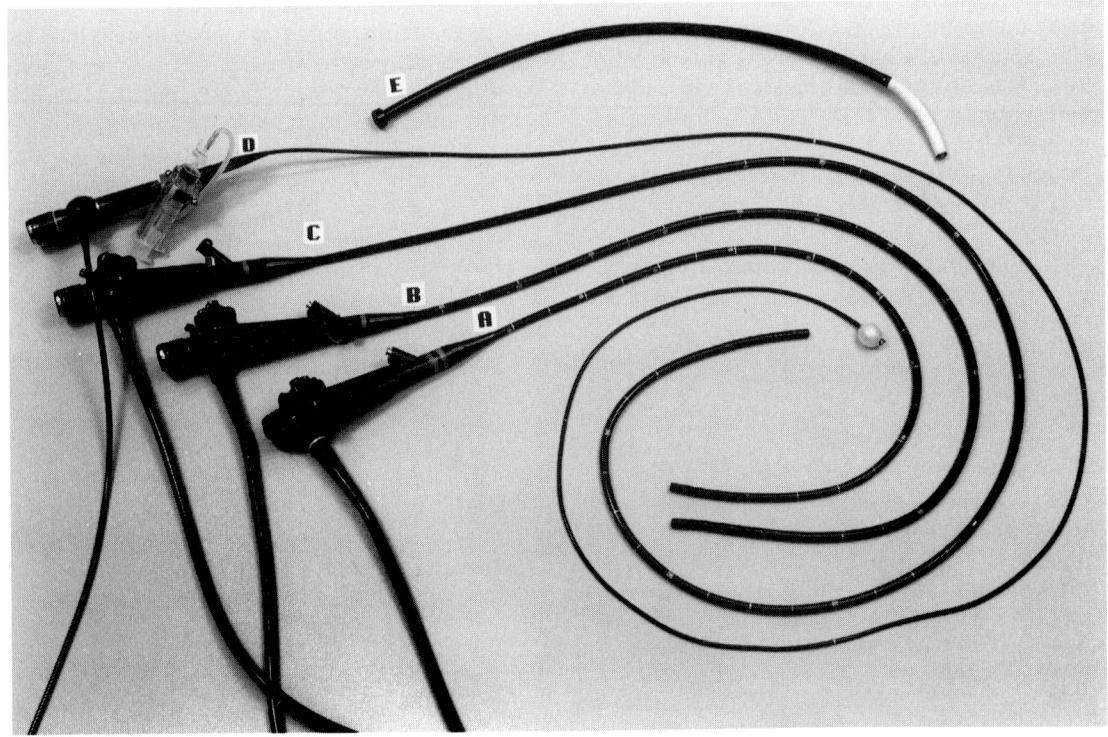

FIGURE 59–3. Comparative lengths of commonly used endoscopes for small bowel endoscopy. **A**, Standard upper endoscope, 100 cm. **B**, Pediatric colonoscope, 130 cm. **C**, Push enteroscope, 200 cm. **D**, Sonde-type passive enteroscope, 274 cm. **E**, Overtube, used for push enteroscopy.

of the terminal ileum may be seen at colonoscopy after negotiation through the ileocecal valve. Direct access to the rest of the small intestine may be obtained by the technique of "push enteroscopy," which refers to the use of a longer endoscope passed through the mouth. Many clinicians use a 130-cm pediatric colonoscope, although dedicated 2175-mm enteroscopes with therapeutic and angling capabilities are available. Special overtubes can be used during push enteroscopy to decrease intragastric looping and facilitate passage of the endoscope into the jejunum.[13]

A variety of longer enteroscopes up to 2864 mm are used for passive enteroscopy. One of the most common enteroscopes is the sonde-type, which is passed transnasally or orally.[14,15] A balloon cuff at the tip is inflated and allows passage of the scope by peristalsis into the distal part of the ileum. The drawbacks to passive enteroscopy are the time it takes for the instrument to reach the ileum, the limited biopsy capabilities and angling mechanisms, and the diminished views obtained on withdrawal of the scope.

Endoscopic ultrasonography provides ultrasound images of the gut wall. Interfaces between the histologic layers of the bowel create characteristic echo-rich or echo-poor bands. Endoscopic ultrasound is very accurate and sensitive in characterizing smooth muscle tumors (Fig. 59–4). It is also useful in elucidating invasion of mucosal tumors and features of submucosal tumors.[16,17]

TREATMENT

The treatment of solitary benign small bowel tumors should be undertaken if there are symptoms or the lesion is a malignant precursor, i.e., an adenoma. Local surgical resection is the most common therapy. In the hands of skilled endoscopists, endoscopic electrosurgical polypectomy has been proven to be safe and effective for tumors in the upper gastrointestinal tract.[18] The treatment of symptomatic hemangiomas includes endoscopic electrocautery, laser photocoagulation, angiographic embolization, or surgical resection.[19] The treatment of polyps, as seen in the polyposis syndromes, deserves special attention because of the number of polyps and the risk of carcinoma. Therapy in these syndromes is discussed later in this chapter.

SPECIFIC TYPES OF SMALL BOWEL TUMORS

LEIOMYOMAS

Leiomyomas are the most frequently reported and symptomatic small bowel tumor, composing 22% to 43% of collected series. They are usually solitary, submucosal, and well-circumscribed lesions but may be lobulated, sessile, or pedunculated. They may arise from any muscle layer but most commonly originate in the muscularis propria. Symptoms are dependent on the growth

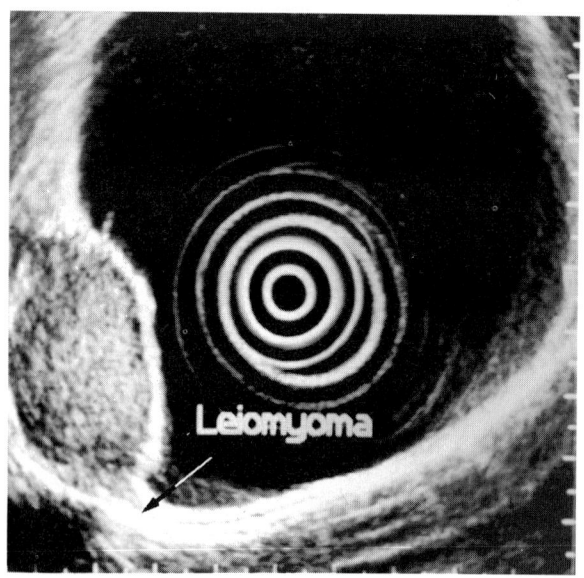

FIGURE 59–4. Endoscopic ultrasound of a leiomyoma. It can be visualized arising from the hypoechoic muscular layer *(arrow)*.

pattern. There are four types of growth patterns.[20] Greater than two thirds are extraluminal or subserosal. Intraluminal, intramural, and "dumbbell"-shaped (with extraluminal and intraluminal growth) leiomyomas occur with decreasing frequency. Bleeding or anemia are the most common symptoms.

Leiomyomas are difficult to diagnose noninvasively. Since the most common type of growth pattern is extraluminal, there may be no abnormality of the lumen on endoscopic or radiologic examination. A small bowel series may show only displacement of loops of bowel. Margulis and Burhenne[21] found that barium studies were normal in 50% of cases. The endoscopic appearance of a lesion with a central umbilication is an indication of the submucosal nature of the lesion. Other diagnostic techniques include celiac or mesenteric angiograms, which demonstrate hypervascular, intense collection of contrast during the capillary and early venous filling stage. Scintigraphy has been useful for diagnosis of bleeding[22,23] and nonbleeding leiomyomas.[23]

Microscopically, whorls of smooth muscle with palisading nuclei are seen. It is difficult to predict the malignant potential of leiomyomas except in the cases of obvious spread. The number of mitotic figures is the most characteristic feature of malignant lesions. One study suggested that two microscopic features are diagnostic of malignancy. These include greater than 5 mitoses per 10 high-power field (HPF) or moderate or marked cellular atypia in tumors greater than 5 cm. Lesions with tumor cell necrosis and fewer than 5 mitoses per 10 HPF should be viewed with a high index of suspicion.[24] A recent study found that stromal cell tumors could be characterized as benign or malignant on the basis of the number of mitotic figures, <2 or >10/10 HPF, respectively. DNA aneuploidy by flow cytometry was useful in predicting prognosis in the stromal cell tumors that had intermediate mitotic counts.[25]

ADENOMAS

Adenomas of the small bowel comprise about 20% to 30% of benign small bowel tumors. They are premalignant epithelial neoplasms most commonly found in the duodenum and in particular in the periampullary region. The majority produce no symptoms, but their periampullary location may result in obstructive jaundice or pancreatitis. They share the same gross and histologic features as their colonic counterparts. They are usually solitary, polypoid, or villous-appearing lesions that are sessile or pedunculated. They are infrequent both in clinical and necropsy studies, except in the familial adenomatous polyposis syndrome where they have been reported in 80% to 100% of cases screened[26–28] (see below). Histologically, crowded tubular or villous glands containing uniform but hyperchromatic, pencil-shaped nuclei are seen to involve the full thickness of the mucosa.

The importance of diagnosing adenomas is because of their high risk of malignancy. Cancer has been detected in up to 65% of adenomas with an increased incidence of malignancy in larger, villous, and ampullary lesions.[2] Importantly, endoscopic or surgical biopsy missed 15% to 56% of the carcinomatous lesions that were discovered when the total specimen was resected.[29,30] There is a high risk of malignant degeneration regardless of whether the tumors are symptomatic or picked up incidentally. Therefore, total excision of adenomas is required. The type of excision, local or radical is dependent on the pathology. In situ and intramucosal carcinomas have almost no risk of metastasis and can be managed by local resection. If invasive carcinoma is detected, a radical excision is required. Currently there are not recommendations regarding surveillance; however, there is approximately a 17% chance of recurrent adenoma after excision, and yearly endoscopic screenings for the first few years after removal may be warranted.[31]

LIPOMAS

Lipomas comprise 8% to 20% of all small bowel tumors, and the majority are found in the ileum. Most often they are incidental, but one third of symptomatic patients present with obstruction or intussusception. The majority of lipomas are submucosal, solitary, and yellowish. The easy indentation of the fatty tissue after compression with a closed biopsy forceps has given rise to the name "cushion" or "pillow sign."[32,33] Tenting of the overlying mucosa as it is pulled with the biopsy forceps away from the underlying mass is known as the "tenting sign."[32] These signs can help distinguish lipomas from other submucosal tumors. Directed biopsies of the lipomas often result in protrusion of fat from beneath the overlying denuded mucosa. This is called the "naked fat sign" and considered pathognomonic of a lipoma.[34] Histologically, lipomas are masses of adult adipose tissue with a delicate collagen capsule. Growth is by expansion and luminal compression. Barium radiographs may demonstrate a solitary, intraluminal defect that conforms to the shape of the small bowel lumen.

HEMANGIOMAS

The majority of benign vascular tumors are found in the skin, but they can also affect the gut. Hemangiomas comprise about 10% to 12% of benign small bowel tumors. There are no precise definitions for vascular lesions of the intestine; however, *hemangiomas*, also known as *angiomas*, refer to benign vascular neoplasms, whereas *arteriovenous malformations* refer to dilation of existing vascular structures.[35] They are usually jejunal and submucosal. Histologically, hemangiomas contain a discrete mass of blood vessels and are named according to their components. Capillary hemangiomas are thin-walled, blood-filled capillaries lined by a single layer of endothelial cells. If the capillaries are widely dilated, they are termed *cavernous hemangiomas*. Venous hemangiomas have thicker walls containing smooth muscle. These benign tumors are found more commonly in several rare disorders including Turner's syndrome, tuberous sclerosis, blue-rubber-bleb nevus syndrome, and Rendu-Osler-Weber syndrome. As expected, bleeding is the most common symptom. The diagnosis of vascular tumors is difficult. Occasionally, abdominal films disclose calcium deposits, which represent calcifications within thrombosed hemangiomas. Endoscopy, angiography, and scintigraphy may also be helpful diagnostically.

BRUNNER'S GLAND LESIONS

Abnormalities of Brunner's glands were first described in 1679 by Wepfer[36] from an autopsy of a beheaded woman. With the widespread use of endoscopy they are found to comprise 10% to 30% of all benign duodenal tumors. The incidence derived from esophagogastroduodenoscopy (EGD) has been found to be approximately 0.08%.[37] The majority of Brunner's glands abnormalities are asymptomatic. Bleeding is the most common symptom, occurring in 50% of symptomatic patients, but intestinal and biliary obstruction have also been reported. Microscopically, these tumors are abnormal growths of branched, acinotubular, mucin-secreting submucosal glands found almost exclusively in the duodenum. They are located between the pylorus and the papilla of Vater and are usually absent beyond the duodenojejunal junction. Feyrter[38] in 1934 analyzed more than 2800 duodenums and classified the proliferation of Brunner's glands abnormalities into three distinct types. The localized and diffuse nodular hyperplasias are more common than solitary polypoid lesion, which are the rarest. The polypoid tumors have been termed *Brunner's gland adenomas*. Since these polyps are essentially protrusions of normal tissue without the usual histologic features or premalignant connotation of adenoma, we feel that the term *Brunner's gland adenoma* is a misnomer. The absence of features such as loss of normal architecture, cellular immaturity, loss of cellular or nuclear polarity, or increased mitotic figures indicates that they are not cancer precursors. Histologically, these lesions are more appropriately labeled *hamartomas*.[39]

Diagnostic measures include the barium radiograph, which demonstrates solitary or multiple smooth, sessile, or polypoid lesions giving the appearance of cobblestoning or Swiss cheese. The endoscopic appearance is that of localized or diffuse, smooth-surfaced, rounded, polypoid, or nodular defects that are sessile or pedunculated (Fig. 59–5, see Color Plate IV). Hypoechoic features have been noted on endoscopic ultrasound.[17]

NEUROGENIC TUMORS

Neurogenic tumors compose 3.2% to 6.4% of benign small bowel tumors. There are a number of histologic types including the well-known and commonest neurofibroma, and rarer ganglioneuroma, neurilemoma (benign schwannoma), granular cell tumor, paraganglioma, and gangliocytic paraganglioma. The tumors are usually jejunal, solitary, smooth polypoid masses that can occur in any nervous tissue in any histologic layer including the submucosa, muscularis, or serosa. In the gastrointestinal tract they are said to arise more commonly from the myenteric than the submucosal nerve plexus. If nerve cell tumors are multiple and diffuse, they are usually associated with neurofibromatosis or von Recklinghausen's disease. Twenty-five percent of patients with generalized neurofibromatosis have involvement of the gastrointestinal tract. The small bowel is most frequently involved.

Grossly, endoscopically, and radiographically, these tumors may be indistinguishable from other mesenchymal neoplasms. The microscopic appearance of nerve cell tumors is variable and sometimes difficult to distinguish from smooth muscle tumors. Neurofibromas and many other neurogenic tumors contain a variety of nerve cell components and a mixture of other cell types that would justify their occasional classification as hamartomas.

FIBROMAS

Fibromas are one of a number of synonyms for inflammatory fibroid polyps. Seventy-five percent of these lesions are found in the ileum. Symptoms are rare, but when they occur, intussusception and intestinal obstruction account for 65%. The tumors are well circumscribed and submucosal. They appear as solitary or multiple polypoid masses. Their gross appearance most frequently mimics an ulcerated leiomyoma.[39] Histologically, these polyps contain a myxoid stroma with reactive blood vessels, mature-appearing fibroblasts, and a variable number of inflammatory cells.

LYMPHANGIOMA

Lymphangiomas can occur anywhere in the body and occasionally are found in the gastrointestinal tract. Their appearance at endoscopy and barium meal are very similar to lipomas. The histologic findings of multiple lymphatic channels and variable-sized vascular spaces lined by endothelial cells differentiate them from other small bowel tumors. The vessel lumens are empty or contain lymph. Biopsies of these lesions do not carry the same risk of bleeding as biopsy of hemangiomas.

HAMARTOMAS

Hamartomas are rare, nonneoplastic polyps. Histologically, these tumors are malformations of tissue indigenous to the organ in which they are located but present in improper proportions and with an excess of one tissue type. Hamartomas of the intestine are not common and usually coexist with similar malformations in other areas of the body. Hamartomas may be solitary and sporadic or associated with familial or nonfamilial syndromes (Table 59–2).

POLYPOSIS SYNDROMES WITH ASSOCIATED SMALL BOWEL TUMORS

Although small bowel tumors are extremely rare in the general population, they are a frequent and important finding in four of the polyposis syndromes. The polyposis syndromes are a diverse group of disorders characterized by the presence of multiple polyps affecting the gastrointestinal tract. They may be classified by their mode of inheritance and by the histologic type of polyp (Table 59–1). The familial polyposes are predominantly autosomal dominant diseases. Small bowel polyps are a prominent feature of familial adenomatous polyposis and three of the hamartomatous polyposes: Peutz-Jeghers syndrome, generalized juvenile polyposis, and Cronkhite-Canada syndrome.

FAMILIAL ADENOMATOUS POLYPOSIS

Familial adenomatous polyposis (FAP) and *Gardner's syndrome* are expressions of a single genetic disease characterized primarily by numerous adenomas of the colon and 100% risk of colon cancer without colectomy. The gene has been localized to the long arm of chromosome 5. Polyposis affecting the stomach and duodenum is now known to occur in the majority of patients with FAP. Numerous small hamartomatous polyps, called fundic gland polyps, involving the fundus and body of the stomach may be seen in up to 80% of patients. They carry no malignant potential. Once the diagnosis is established by multiple biopsy specimens, observation alone is appropriate.[26]

Adenomas of the small bowel are found in 80% to 100% of patients with FAP and are premalignant. They are most numerous in the periampullary region (Fig. 59–6), and their number and size tend to increase with age. They can appear as subtle, 2- to 3-mm lesions, noted only with careful endoscopic examination, to virtual carpeting of the mucosa by irregular flat areas of villous tissue. The mucosa of the duodenal papilla has adenomatous tissue in at least 50% of patients, even when it appears normal endoscopically. The appearance of the papilla ranges from normal size with a small periorifice polyp to gross enlargement, ulceration, and a frank mass. Periampullary cancer is the most common cancer death in patients with FAP who have had colectomy.

The adenomas of the duodenum and periampullary region in FAP are a manifestation of a generalized growth disorder imparted by the genetic disease. Removal of all adenomas is neither practical nor safe. The polyps are usually too numerous, and removal of a polyp does nothing to prevent polyp growth of the adjacent mucosa. Prostaglandin-inhibiting agents, which have been shown to have tumor-inhibiting properties, are being actively studied to determine if

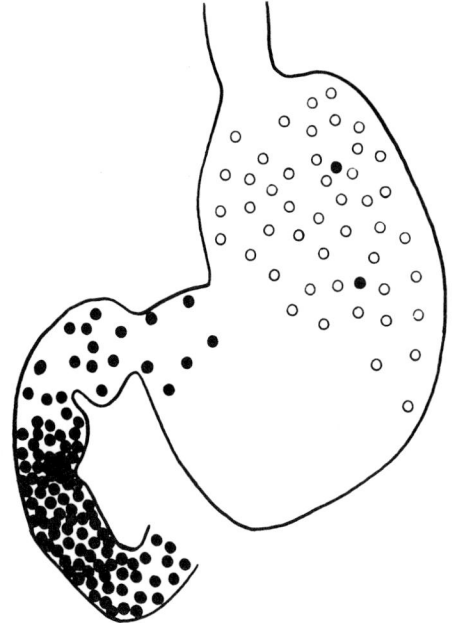

FIGURE 59–6. Representation of sites affected by upper gastrointestinal tract polyps in the familial adenomatous polyposis syndromes. Each circle represents one patient. *Open circles,* fundic gland polyps, and *solid circles,* adenomas. (From Spigelman A, Williams C, Talbot J, et al. Upper gastrointestinal cancer in patients with familial adenomatous polyposis. *Lancet.* 1989;2:784. With permission.)

their use might either halt the growth or cause regression of adenomas in the upper gastrointestinal tracts of patients with FAP.[40]

Surveillance upper endoscopy with forward viewing and side viewing endoscopes and multiple biopsies is recommended to identify patients with polyps exhibiting features suggesting high risk of malignant degeneration. Biopsy of the papilla must be taken at each examination regardless of the endoscopic appearance. Surveillance intervals are empiric. A 3-year interval has been recommended for patients with no adenomas and is probably appropriate for patients with gross duodenal polyps with *no* advanced pathologic features (progressive enlargement, high grade dysplasia). An enlarging mass, ulceration, or high-grade dysplasia should prompt surgical referral.[41]

Endoscopic attempts at adenoma ablation have been reported but are investigational. Laser, contact thermal, and bipolar electrocautery have been used. Standard monopolar polypectomy such as that used for colonic polypectomy and laser ablation are hazardous because of the depth of burn and risk of perforation. The contact cautery probes appear to be safe, and polyp tissue of the duodenum and the papilla can be ablated.[42] Unfortunately, because of the diffuse mucosal expression of this genetic disease, the polyp tissue always recurs. Endoscopic treatment should not be considered standard but may be applied in selected patients who carry a high surgical risk. Surgical treatment should be advised when high-grade dysplasia or cancer is found on biopsy. A limited duodenectomy with duct reimplantation is preferable to a Whipple's procedure. Surgery in these patients should be performed at referral centers with a large experience with patients with FAP.

PEUTZ-JEGHERS SYNDROME

Peutz-Jeghers syndrome is a syndrome of diffuse hamartomatous gastrointestinal polyps and mucocutaneous pigmentation that usually present in adolescence. The mucocutaneous pigmentations are glabrous, brown to green-black macules of melanin found on the lips and perioral and buccal areas. The distal limbs and perianal and genital areas can also be affected. The macules tend to fade at puberty. The polyps have a characteristic lobulated, cerebriform appearance. They are most common in the jejunum and ileum. Histologically, an arborizing core of smooth muscle is seen folded into fronds and lined by normal intestinal epithelial cells.

The most common symptoms are bleeding and obstruction, usually secondary to intussusception. Polyp-induced complications result in high relaparotomy rates, and multiple surgeries at short intervals are not unusual. Therefore, an attempt to remove all significant polyps during surgery should be made. Intraoperative endoscopy has been used as an adjunct for the detection and removal of polyps.

The risk of cancer developing in Peutz-Jeghers polyps is debated. Many authors believe the malignancies develop from synchronous adenomas rather than from hamartomas. The risk is estimated to be about 2% and develops after the age of 30 years.[43] Surveillance protocols are not established but should be based on the findings of adenomatous tissue.

GENERALIZED JUVENILE POLYPOSIS

Juvenile polyps are most commonly single and found in the colorectum. Generalized juvenile polyposis can be inherited or sporadic, and multiple polyps may be found anywhere in the gastrointestinal tract. Histologically, juvenile polyps are classified as hamartomas and are characterized by inflammatory expansion of the lamina propria. The risk of gastrointestinal cancer in patients with generalized juvenile polyposis seems to be elevated.[44] Colonoscopic surveillance of the colon has been recommended, but there are no clear recommendations for management of the small bowel tumors. If surgery is undertaken for polyp-related symptoms, it is advisable to remove any and all polyps.

CRONKHITE-CANADA SYNDROME

The Cronkhite-Canada syndrome is an acquired disorder characterized by multiple gastrointestinal polyps, diarrhea, protein-losing enteropathy, alopecia, and hyperpigmentation. The polyps are inflammatory with large cystic dilated spaces and are primarily found in the small intestine. A variety of treatments have been used including steroids, antibiotics, and surgical resection. Spontaneous remissions have been reported.[45] Aggressive nutritional support is the mainstay of therapy.

SUMMARY

Benign tumors of the small bowel are rare, and the majority produce no symptoms. They may arise from anywhere in the small intestine and from any histologic layer. A high index of suspicion should be maintained to make the diagnosis. Adenomas should be removed, either endoscopically or surgically, because they are premalignant. Other benign tumors should be resected only if they are symptomatic. The clinical features, diagnostic modalities, and therapeutic approach to small bowel tumors including the polyposis syndromes are reviewed.

REFERENCES

1. Darling R, Welch C. Tumors of the small intestine. *N Engl J Med.* 1959;260:397.
2. Perzin K, Bridge M. Adenomas of the small intestine: a clinicopathologic review of 51 cases and a study of their relationship to carcinoma. *Cancer.* 1981;48:799.
3. Freund H, Lavi A, Pfeffermann R, et al. Primary neoplasms of the small bowel. *Am J Surg.* 1978;135:757.
4. Nordkild P, Kjaergard H. Primary tumors of the small intestine: the diagnostic problems. *Ann Chir Gynaecol.* 1986;82:215.
5. Aranha G, Reyes C, Lindert D, et al. Primary tumors of the small intestine. *Am Surg.* August 1979:495.
6. Bone G, Wright N. The rarity of small bowel tumors: an alternative hypothesis. *Lancet.* 1968;1:618.
7. Croom R, Newsome J. Tumors of the small intestine. *Am Surg.* March 1975:160.
8. Cohen A, McNeill D, Terz J, et al. Neoplasms of the small intestine. *Dig Dis.* 1971;16:815.
9. Hancock R. An 11 year review of primary tumors of the small bowel including the duodenum. *Can Med Assoc J.* 1970;102:1177.
10. Gupta S, Udupa K, Gupta S. Intussusception in adults. *Int Surg.* 1976;61:231.
11. Pang L. Intussusception revisited: clinicopathologic analysis of 261 cases with emphasis of pathogenesis. *South Med J.* 1989;82:215.
12. Taylor A, Stewart E, Dodds W. Gastrointestinal lipomas: a radiologic and pathologic review. *AJR.* 1990;155:1205.
13. Shimizu S, Tada M, Kawai K. Development of a new insertion technique in push-type enteroscopy. *Am J Gastroenterol.* 1987;82:844.
14. Lewis B, Waye J. Small bowel enteroscopy in 1988: pros and cons. *Am J Gastroenterol.* 1988;83:799.
15. Tada M, Kawai K. Small bowel endoscopy. *Scand J Gastroenterol.* 1984;19(suppl 102):39.
16. Yasuda K, Cho E, Nakajima M. Diagnosis of submucosal lesions of the upper gastrointestinal tract by endoscopic ultrasonography. *Gastrointest Endosc.* 1990;36:S17.
17. Tio T, Tytgat G, den Hartog-Jager F. Endoscopic ultrasonography for the evaluation of smooth muscle tumors in the upper gastrointestinal tract: an experience with 42 cases. *Gastrointest Endosc.* 1990;36:342.
18. Bruns D, Jacobs W. Endoscopic electrosurgical polypectomy of the gastrointestinal tract. *South Med J.* 1977;70:926.
19. Shahed M, Hagenmuller F, Rusch T, et al. A 19 year old female with Blue-Rubber-Bleb-Nevus Syndrome: endoscopic laser photocoagulation and surgical resection of gastrointestinal angiomata. *Endoscopy.* 1990;22:54.
20. Gourtsoyiannis N, Bays D, Malamas M, et al. Radiologic appearances of small intestinal leiomyomas. *Clin Radiol.* 1992;45:94.
21. Margulis A, Burhenne H. *Alimentary Tract Roentgenology.* St. Louis, Mo: The CV Mosby Co; 1973.
22. Winzelberg G, McKusick K, Froelich J, et al. Detection of gastrointestinal bleeding with ^{99m}Tc-labelled red blood cells. *Semin Nucl Med.* 1982;12:139.
23. McDonald K. Technetium-99m RBC scintigraphy in the evaluation of small bowel leiomyoma. *Clin Nucl Med.* 1987;12:131.
24. Ranchod M, Kempson R. Smooth muscle tumors of the gastrointestinal tract and retroperitoneum: a pathologic analysis of 100 cases. *Cancer.* 1977;39:255.
25. Cooper P, Hardy G, Dixon M. A flow cytometric, clinical and histologic study of stromal neoplasms of the gastrointestinal tract. *Am J Surg Pathol.* 1992;16:163.
26. Sarre R, Frost A, Jagelman D, et al. Gastric and duodenal polyps in familial adenomatous polyposis: a prospective study of the nature and prevalence of upper gastrointestinal intestinal polyps. *Gut.* 1987;28:306.
27. Watanabe H, Enjoji M, Yao T, et al. Accompanying gastroenteric lesions in familial adenomatosis coli. *Acta Pathol Jpn.* 1977;27:823.
28. Church J, McGannon E, Hull-Boiner S, Jagelman D, Sivak M, van Stolk R. Upper gastroduodenal polyps in familial adenomatous polyposis. *Dis Colon Rectum.* 1992;35:1170.
29. Blackman E, Nash S. Diagnosis of duodenal and ampullary epithelial neoplasms by endoscopic biopsy: a clinicopathologic and immunohistochemical study. *Hum Pathol.* 1985;16:901.
30. Ryan D, Schapiro R, Warshaw A. Villous tumors of the duodenum. *Ann Surg.* 1986;103:301.

31. Bjork K, Davis C, Nagorney D. Duodenal villous tumors. *Arch Surg.* 1990;125:961.
32. Debeer R, Shinya H. Colonic lipomas: an endoscopic analysis. *Gastrointest Endosc.* 1975;22:90.
33. Rand A. Colonic lipoma. *Gastrointest Endosc.* 1982;27:40.
34. Messer J, Waye J. The diagnosis of colonic lipomas: the naked fat sign. *Gastrointest Endosc.* 1982;28:186.
35. Richardson J. Vascular lesions of the intestines. *Am J Surg.* 1991;161:284.
36. Wepfer J. Circutae Aquaticae Historia et Noxae. Basilae: Genathius JR Imprimebat; 1679.
37. Bastlein C, Decking R, Voeth C, et al. Giant brunneroma of the duodenum. *Endoscopy.* 1988;20:154.
38. Feyrter F. Über Wucherungen der Brunnerschen Drusen. *Virchows Arch [A].* 1934;293:509.
39. Fenoglio-Preiser C, Pascal R, Perzin K. *Tumors of the Intestines.* Washington, DC: Armed Forces Institutes of Pathology; 1990.
40. Waddel W, Ganser G, Cerise E, et al. Sulindac for polyposis of the colon. *Am J Surg.* 1989;157:175.
41. van Stolk R. Endoscopic surveillance for polyposis syndromes. *Gastrointest Endosc Clin North Am.* 1992;2:509.
42. van Stolk R, Sivak M, Petrini J, et al. Endoscopic management of upper gastrointestinal polyps and periampullary lesions in familial adenomatous polyposis and Gardner's syndrome. *Endoscopy.* 1982;19:19.
43. Panos R, Opelka F, Noguerus J. Peutz-Jeghers syndrome: a call for intraoperative enteroscopy. *Am Surg.* 1990;56:331.
44. Jass J, Williams C, Bussey H, et al. Juvenile polyposis: a precancerous condition. *Histopathol.* 1988;13:619.
45. Sleisenger M, Fordtran J. *Gastrointestinal Disease,* 4th ed. Philadelphia, Pa: WB Saunders Co; 1989.
46. Moertel C, Sauer W, Doherty M, et al. Life history of the carcinoid tumors of the small intestine. *Cancer.* 1961;14:901.
47. Elias W, Lund C, Yonemoto R. Neoplasms of the small intestine. *Am J Surg.* 1954;88:384.
48. Ostermiller W, Joergenson E, Weibel L. A clinical review of tumors of the small bowel. *Am J Surg.* 1966;111:403.
49. Herbsmann H, Wetstein L, Rosen Y, et al. Tumors of the small intestine. In: Ravitch M, ed. *Curr Probl Surg.* 1980;17:125.
50. Wilson J, Melvin D, Gray C, et al. Benign small bowel tumors. *Ann Surg.* 1975;181:247.

60

Vascular Malformations of the Gastrointestinal Tract

WILLIAM N. KATKOV

Intestinal vascular malformations, once thought to be rare, constitute an important group of lesions that can lead to gastrointestinal (GI) tract hemorrhage. Advances in our understanding of intestinal vascular malformations are a consequence, in large part, of progress in the fields of endoscopy and radiology. The availability of endoscopy and angiography and greater attention to previously undiagnosed cases of obscure intestinal bleeding have led to an appreciation for the significance of these lesions. These fields have, in turn, led to an array of therapeutic opportunities for the treatment of gastrointestinal tract hemorrhage.

Endoscopy and barium studies play a central role in the diagnosis of GI tract bleeding. Endoscopy, in particular, has tremendous diagnostic potential in identifying common sources of bleeding including peptic ulcer disease, gastritis, varices, and diverticular disease. The utility of colonoscopy in assessing the causes of lower GI tract bleeding is well established.[1,2]

Angiography has emerged as a vital tool in the evaluation of patients with gastrointestinal tract bleeding of obscure origin whether it be the patient with chronic recurrent bleeding or with acute hemorrhage. Intestinal bleeding of obscure origin is especially relevant to the subject of vascular malformations, for in this subset of patients, vascular malformations in general and angiodysplasia in particular are common diagnoses. This chapter reviews the topic of vascular malformations with an emphasis on approaches to diagnosis and treatment.

CLASSIFICATION

Any discussion of vascular malformations in the intestine is clouded by overlapping nomenclature and poorly defined categories. The interchangeable use of terms such as *hemangioma, telangiectasia, arteriovenous malformation, angiodysplasia,* and *angioma* is often encountered. Prior to the era of endoscopy and angiography, intestinal vascular lesions were classified on a pathologic basis as benign (including telangiectasias), malignant, or hemangiomatous.[3] Although these classification schemes do not emphasize the histologic characteristics of intestinal vascular lesions, endoscopy and angiography have focused on the appearance and clinical setting in which these lesions occur.

In 1976, Moore et al[4] described three categories of arteriovenous malformations (AVMs) as follows: type 1 AVMs are solitary, acquired, found in older patients, and localized to the right colon; type II AVMs are congenital, found in patients under 50 years of age, and are larger than type I lesions; type III AVMs are found in patients who, on physical examination and by history, meet criteria for hereditary hemorrhagic telangiectasia. A modification of this classification has been proposed by Richardson[5] in which these categories are expanded to account for the variety of clinical settings in which intestinal arteriovenous malformations are found (Table 60–1).

ANGIODYSPLASIA

In recent years, angiodysplasia has been recognized as one of the most common causes of gastrointestinal tract bleeding.[6,7] In the past, many cases of lower GI tract hemorrhage ascribed to diverticulosis were probably angiodysplastic in origin. Angiodysplasia is most likely an acquired lesion and is usually found in persons over the age of 50 years. Boley and Brandt[8] have postulated that these vascular ectasias develop in normal colonic mucosa and are a consequence of chronic constriction of veins draining the submucosal plexus leading to back pressure and formation of arteriovenous shunts.

There is some evidence that angiodysplasia may be associated with aortic stenosis; however, this relationship has not withstood rigorous analysis.[9] Angiodysplasia is frequently the implicated lesion in patients with chronic renal failure who experience gastrointestinal tract bleeding, and these lesions are also found in patients with von Willebrand's disease.[10,11] Angiodysplasia corresponds to the type I AVM in the classification scheme developed by Moore and colleagues.

Although angiodysplasia is usually found in older patients, similar lesions occur in other segments of the intestinal tract. After the large intestine, angiodysplasia is most commonly located in the stomach and small intestine. Just as endoscopy greatly increased the awareness of the prevalence and significance of angiodysplasia in the upper gastrointestinal tract and colon, the recent development of enteroscopy (discussed below) has identified angiodysplasia in the small bowel as a lesion frequently associated with cases of obscure intestinal bleeding.[12] In some reports, congenital angiodysplasia in children and infants corresponds to the type II lesion in Moore and colleagues' scheme and remains a rare diagnosis.[13] Histologically, angiodysplasia is characterized by clusters of thick-walled veins, sometimes associated with arteries and capillaries.

Several systemic diseases, often with cutaneous findings, are associated with intestinal vascular abnormalities. These include the CREST variant of progressive systemic sclerosis (scleroderma) that includes calcinosis, Raynaud's phenomenon, esophageal dysmotility, sclerodactyly, and telangiectasias.[14] The CREST syndrome also occurs in some patients with primary biliary cirrhosis, and intestinal telangiectasias have been described in such patients in the absence of portal hypertension and its effects on the gastrointestinal tract.

TABLE 60–1. TYPES OF INTESTINAL VASCULAR LESIONS

TYPE	DESCRIPTION
1	Acquired lesions limited to mucosa and submucosa
1A	Limited to cecum and right colon (most common type)
1B	Multiple lesions in colon or right colon lesion with involvement of other portion of the gastrointestinal tract
2	Congenital arteriovenous malformations that may be found throughout the gastrointestinal tract
3	Hereditary hemorrhagic telangiectasia (Rendu-Osler-Weber syndrome)
4	Multiple acquired vascular lesions usually found in elderly patients with associated diseases

Adapted from Richardson JD. Vascular lesions of the intestines. *Am J Surg.* 1991;161:284. Reprinted with permission from American Journal of Surgery.

Endoscopy is useful in identifying vascular ectasias; however, angiodysplasia may be variable in appearance. At colonoscopy, these lesions have the appearance of a tuft of bright red irregular vessels. Distinguishing angiodysplasia from vascular malformations associated with other diseases depends on an awareness of the underlying systemic disease and its extraintestinal findings.

Angiography plays an important role in the diagnosis of angiodysplasia especially in the setting of active bleeding. Because the endoscopic appearance of these lesions is variable and often subtle, angiography can confirm their presence particularly in the distal small intestine, cecum, and right colon. At the same time, angiography can demonstrate additional lesions not recognized by colonoscopy. This is important if surgical resection is planned. Several angiographic features have been described as characteristic of angiodysplasia.[15] These include a densely opacified, slowly emptying draining vein that is seen in the venous phase of the study. An early filling vein or vascular tuft may be detected in the arterial phase of the study.

Angiography has also emerged as a therapeutic modality in the management of some cases of gastrointestinal tract hemorrhage. The selective catheterization of a mesenteric branch feeding a bleeding site can allow for transcatheter embolization using gelfoam or coils. Occasionally, this procedure is associated with significant complications.[16]

Surgery has a traditional and prominent role in the management of active or recurrent lower gastrointestinal tract bleeding including that due to angiodysplasia. Series of patients undergoing surgical management of hemorrhage from these lesions always report a significant risk of recurrent bleeding.[17] With the emerging role of endoscopic therapy, surgery is usually reserved for those patients who experience ongoing massive bleeding or recurrent bleeding requiring frequent blood transfusions.

There has been great interest in recent years in the potential of hormonal therapy for angiodysplasia.[18] The efficacy of hormonal therapy in this setting remains controversial. Numerous reports of the use of estrogen-progesterone combinations in patients with recurrent intestinal bleeding due to angiodysplasia suffer from a lack of controls and a confounding mix of patients. These studies often include significant numbers of patients with associated medical conditions including renal failure, Rendu-Osler-Weber syndrome, and von Willebrand's disease. Although the mechanisms by which hormonal therapy may benefit these patients remain unclear, estrogen is known to shorten the bleeding time in patients with renal failure. There is, in addition, evidence that estrogen may thicken the mucosa overlying angiodysplastic lesions.[19]

In the small controlled experiences employing hormonal therapy for patients with angiodysplasia the results are mixed. A randomized crossover study by Van Custem et al[20] included patients with Rendu-Osler-Weber syndrome as well as idiopathic angiodysplasia. There was a significant reduction in the transfusion requirement in those patients receiving therapy. However, a study by Lewis et al[21] from Mt. Sinai Hospital in New York found no benefit when measured by similar rebleeding rates during follow-up among treated and control patients. Although hormonal therapy, a relatively low-risk and inexpensive treatment, is an attractive option for the treatment of patients with angiodysplasia, its efficacy has not been clearly demonstrated.

Octreotide, a long-acting analog of the gastrointestinal hormone somatostatin, is known to reduce splanchnic blood flow. Its use in various settings of gastrointestinal tract bleeding is being investigated. Anecdotal reports suggest that octreotide may be efficacious for the treatment of angiodysplasia.[22]

The endoscopic era has allowed for a firsthand assessment of intestinal vascular malformations in the upper GI tract proximal to the ligament of Treitz, colon, and terminal ileum. The recognition of vascular lesions in the small intestine relied on angiography. Patients with obscure and repeated episodes of bleeding often undergo multiple upper endoscopies and colonoscopies. In such patients, enteroscopy is an emerging diagnostic option. Long endoscopes or colonoscopes can be advanced up to 60 cm (2 feet) beyond the ligament of Treitz. Conventional endoscopes can be employed for intraoperative enteroscopy wherein the small intestine is "telescoped" over the endoscope by a surgeon assisting the endoscopist. Lesions can be marked with a serosal suture if resection is to be carried out.

A novel technique of enteroscopy, "sonde" endoscopy, uses an endoscope placed transnasally that has a balloon at its tip and passes by peristalsis throughout the entire length of the small intestine.[12] The mucosa is then examined during a careful withdrawal of the endoscope. The procedure is time consuming and labor intensive. Although the field of vision with these enteroscopes is limited and allows for examination of only 50% to 70% of the mucosa, there is a significant yield when the goal is to find potential sources of bleeding in carefully selected patients. These endoscopes provide additional diagnostic potential when colonoscopy and gastroscopy are unrevealing and may be complementary to intraoperative studies.

Endoscopic treatment is the mainstay of therapy for the majority of patients with angiodysplasia. There are few controlled trials, and the variety of therapeutic techniques employed makes comparisons difficult. Options available to the endoscopist include monopolar electrocoagulation, injection sclerotherapy, contact probes, and laser therapy. Jensen and Machiado[23] used a variety of therapeutic modalities (BICAP, Heater Probe, or argon laser) in 39 patients with colonic angiodysplasia. The patients were followed for a mean of 15 months. The mean number of bleeding episodes fell and mean hematocrits rose.[23] Cello and Grendell[24] achieved similar results using the argon laser in 38 patients with angiodysplasia who were followed for 6 months after treatment.

The decision whether to treat any individual lesion is difficult. Studies of the natural history of angiodysplasia have demonstrated that multiple lesions are common and rebleeding rates are high.[25] Conversely, incidentally identified angiodysplasia is not likely to bleed, and the identification of such lesions does not warrant intervention. Although the risk of endoscopic therapy is relatively low, reports of perforation accompany most series of electrocoagulation or laser therapy especially in the cecum and right colon. In the appropriately selected patient, however, endoscopic therapy is an attractive option.

HEMANGIOMAS

Hemangiomas are benign hamartomatous vascular tumors found throughout the gastrointestinal tract. These neoplasms are most commonly located in the small intestine with approximately one third occurring in the large intestine, usually in the rectum and sigmoid colon.[3,26] Gastric hemangiomas are rare. The most common clinical manifestation of hemangiomas is rapid, large-volume hemorrhage, which can recur over many years. Associated features may include calcification within a hemangioma, thrombocytopenia, and microangiopathic hemolytic anemia.

Aside from rare multisystem syndromes hemangiomas are not hereditary. Blue rubber bleb nevus syndrome is a rare condition in which cutaneous hemangiomas are associated with similar intestinal lesions that can lead to hemorrhage.[27] Cutaneous findings are common in the form of blue lesions on the lips, oral mucosa, and perianal skin. Diffuse cavernous hemangiomas have been described in the Klippel-Trénaunay syndrome, which is characterized by cutaneous hemangiomas or lymphangiomas, soft tissue and bone hypertrophy of an extremity, and varicose veins. The hemangiomas in this disorder are usually found in the distal colon and rectum but have been reported in the small intestine as well. The options for management of these lesions include surgery and laser therapy.[28,29]

Visceral hemangiomatosis of the colon and peritoneum has been reported without associated cutaneous involvement. Multifocal and even diffuse intestinal vascular malformations have been described in the absence of any associated systemic disease. When hemangiomas are recognized clinically, almost always because of substantial or recurrent bleeding, surgical resection is the most successful therapeutic intervention.

HEREDITARY HEMORRHAGIC TELANGIECTASIA (RENDU-OSLER-WEBER SYNDROME)

Hereditary hemorrhagic telangiectasia (Rendu-Osler-Weber syndrome) is an inherited autosomal dominant disorder in which telangiectasia may be found throughout the intestine and on the skin and mucous membranes.[30] The telangiectasias in this disorder are composed of dilated and tortuous, thin-walled vessels with scanty smooth muscle fibers, principally capillaries or venules. The clinical hallmarks of Rendu-Osler-Weber syndrome are its inheritance pattern, the presence of telangiectasia on the skin and in the mucous membranes of the nose and mouth, and the occurrence of repeated episodes of hemorrhage. Approximately one third of patients with this syndrome require treatment in their lifetime. Although the most common type of bleeding is recurrent epistaxis, hemorrhage from lesions throughout the intestinal tract can occur. It must be noted, however, that the cutaneous telangiectasias seen in Rendu-Osler-Weber syndrome are usually not identified before the second or third decade of life. Although epistaxis is the most common initial presentation, the clinical picture may be dominated by bleeding from intestinal telangiectasias.

Most of the therapeutic approaches employed in the treatment of angiodysplasia have been attempted in hereditary hemorrhagic telangiectasia including hormonal therapy and endoscopic coagulation. The obstacle to effective therapy in this disorder is that, by definition, the lesions are numerous and occur throughout the intestine. Consequently, patients with hereditary hemorrhagic telangiectasia are often faced with numerous hospitalizations and multiple blood transfusions.

DIEULAFOY'S VASCULAR MALFORMATION

Dieulafoy's vascular malformation, a lesion subjected to confusing nomenclature in the past, has also been called *caliber-persistent artery of the stomach*. Dieulafoy's vascular malformation can cause massive, usually painless, upper gastrointestinal tract hemorrhage and is associated with a high mortality.[31,32] The lesion is most commonly found in the stomach within 6 cm of the gastroesophageal junction along the lesser curvature. However, Dieulafoy-like vessels have been described in the small intestine and colon as well. Histologically, Dieulafoy's vascular malformation is a tortuous and enlarged artery found in the submucosa that persists into the overlying mucosa. The involved vessel is vulnerable to hemorrhage due to focal gastritis or the effect of the artery's pushing into overlying mucosa.

Bleeding from Dieulafoy's lesion, while often massive, is intermittent and unpredictable. Although endoscopy is the typical means of making this diagnosis, the findings may be subtle, and repeat procedures may be necessary before a definitive bleeding site is established. Whereas experience dictates that surgical wedge resection is the mainstay of therapy for Dieulafoy's lesion, viable endoscopic approaches have been reported including local injection of epinephrine, heater probe coagulation, bipolar electrocoagulation, and Nd:YAG laser photocoagulation.[32] Endoscopic therapy may be especially useful as part of an initial diagnostic study prior to surgery or in patients who are considered extremely poor operative candidates. There is no controlled experience comparing endoscopic and surgical management of a bleeding Dieulafoy lesion, and perforation as a complication of endoscopic management has been reported.[33]

GASTRIC ANTRAL VASCULAR ECTASIA (WATERMELON STOMACH)

Watermelon stomach, or gastric antral vascular ectasia, is a lesion distinct from angiodysplasia. This vascular malformation occurs in older patients and has a female predominance.[34] Although it is almost certainly acquired, no definite association with systemic disease has been established. The most common clinical manifestation of gastric antral vascular ectasia is iron deficiency anemia refractory to iron supplementation and requiring repeated transfusions. The endoscopic appearance of red linear streaks on the crests of longitudinal folds explains the term *watermelon stomach*. Histologically, findings include a mobile mucosa and dilated vascular channels in the submucosa with some penetration to the mucosa. The lesion consists of dilated, tortuous thin-walled veins and is restricted to the gastric antrum.

Gastric antral vascular ectasia is a diagnosis established by its distinctive endoscopic appearance. Angiography is generally not useful in making this diagnosis. Endoscopic biopsy results, in addition to the distinctive gross appearance of this lesion, demonstrate characteristics that contribute to establishing a definitive diagnosis.

Antrectomy with Billroth I anastomosis is the traditional surgical treatment for gastric antral vascular ectasia.[18] Although several endoscopic techniques have been reported, laser therapy is emerging as a potentially significant advance in the nonsurgical treatment of this lesion.[23,24] Gostout et al[35] reported the use of endoscopic laser therapy (Nd:YAG) in 13 patients, 12 of whom were available for follow-up for a median period of 6 months. Laser therapy was effective as measured by a rise in serum hemoglobin levels obviating the need for ongoing transfusions. No major complications were encountered.[35] A similar experience has been reported by Labenz and Borsch[36] in five patients with gastric antral vascular ectasia.

CONCLUSION

Endoscopy, as a diagnostic and therapeutic tool, has had a dramatic effect on the understanding and management of gastrointestinal tract bleeding. The recognition of the spectrum of intestinal vascular malformations has broadened the differential diagnosis and approach to patients with bleeding of obscure origin. Whereas many abnormal vascular lesions remain unusual diagnoses, angiodysplasia is common. The array of medical, endoscopic, and angiographic therapeutic options continues to expand, but surgery often remains the definitive treatment of choice for relentless hemorrhage.

REFERENCES

1. Brand EJ, Sullivan BH Jr, Sivak MV Jr, Rankin GB. Colonoscopy in the diagnosis of unexplained rectal bleeding. *Ann Surg.* 1980;192:111.
2. Jensen DM, Machiado GA. Diagnosis and treatment of severe hematochezia: the role of urgent colonoscopy after purge. *Gastroenterology.* 1988;95:1569.
3. Gentry RW, Dockerty MB, Clagett OT. Vascular malformations and vascular tumors of the gastrointestinal tract. *Int Abstr Surg.* 1949;88:281.
4. Moore JD, Thompson NW, Appleman HD, Foley D. Arteriovenous malformations of the gastrointestinal tract. *Arch Surg.* 1976;111:381.
5. Richardson JD. Vascular lesions of the intestines. *Am J Surg.* 1991;161:284.
6. Boley SJ, Sammartano R, Adams A, DiBiase A, Kleinhaus S, Sprayregen S. On the nature and etiology of vascular ectasias of the colon: degenerative lesions of aging. *Gastroenterology.* 1977;72:650.
7. Richter JM, Hedberg SE, Athanasoulis CA, Schapiro RH. Angiodysplasia: clinical presentation and colonoscopic diagnosis. *Dig Dis Sci.* 1984;29:481.
8. Boley SJ, Brandt LJ. Vascular ectasias of the colon. *Dig Dis Sci.* 1986;64:259.
9. Imperiale TF, Ransohoff DF. Aortic stenosis, idiopathic gastrointestinal bleeding and angiodysplasia: is there an association? *Gastroenterology.* 1988;95:1670.
10. Zuckerman G, Cornett G, Clouse R, Harter H. Upper gastrointestinal bleeding in patients with renal failure. *Ann Intern Med.* 1985;102:588.
11. Ramsay DM, Macleod DAD, Buist TAS, et al. Persistent gastrointestinal bleeding due to angiodysplasia of the gut in von Willebrand's disease. *Lancet.* 1976;2:278.
12. Lewis B, Waye J. Small bowel enteroscopy for obscure GI bleeding. *Gastrointest Endosc.* 1991;37:277. Abstract.
13. Sasaki K, Nakagawa H, Takahashi T, Sato E. Bleeding ectatic vascular lesion involving the sigmoid colon, endoscopically indistinguishable from angiodysplasia, in an 8-year-old boy. *Am J Gastroenterol.* 1991;86:105.
14. Rosekrans PC, de Rooy DJ, Bosman FT, Eulderink F, Cats A. Gastrointestinal telangiectasia as a cause of severe blood loss in systemic sclerosis. *Endoscopy.* 1980;12:200.
15. Boley SJ, Sprayregen S, Sammartano RJ, et al. The pathophysiologic basis for the angiographic signs of vascular ectasias of the colon. *Radiology.* 1977;125:615.
16. Uflacker R. Transcatheter embolization for treatment of acute lower gastrointestinal bleeding. *Acta Radiol.* 1987;28:425.
17. Hutcheon DF, Kabelin J, Bulkley GB, Smith GW. Effect of therapy on bleeding rates in gastrointestinal angiodysplasia. *Am Surg.* 1987;53:6.
18. Moshkowitz M, Arber N, Mir N, Gilat T. Success of estrogen-progesterone therapy in long-standing bleeding gastrointestinal angiodysplasia: report of a case. *Dis Colon Rectum.* 1993;36:194.
19. Lewis B. Obscure gastrointestinal bleeding. *Mt Sinai J Med.* 1993;60:208.
20. Van Custem E, Rutgeerts P, Vantrappen G. Treatment of bleeding gastrointestinal vascular malformations with oestrogen-progesterone. *Lancet.* 1990;335:953.
21. Lewis BS, Salomon P, Rivera-MacMurray S, Kornbluth AA, Wenger J, Waye J. Does hormonal therapy have any benefit for bleeding angiodysplasia? *J Clin Gastroenterol.* 1992;15(2):99.
22. Rossini FP, Arrigoni A, Pennazio M. Octreotide in the treatment of bleeding due to angiodysplasia of the small intestine. *Am J Gastroenterol.* 1993;88:1424.
23. Jensen DM, Machiado GA. Bleeding colonic angioma: endoscopic coagulation and follow-up. *Gastroenterology.* 1985;88:1433. Abstract.
24. Cello JP, Grendell JH. Endoscopic laser treatment for gastrointestinal vascular ectasias. *Ann Intern Med.* 1986;104:352.
25. Richter JM, Christensen MR, Colditz GA, Nishioka NS. Angiodysplasia: natural history and efficacy of therapeutic interventions. *Dig Dis Sci.* 1989;34:1542.
26. Wilson JM, Melvin DB, Gray G, Thorbjarnarson B. Benign small bowel tumour. *Ann Surg.* 1975;181:247.
27. Sandhu KS, Cohen H, Radin R, Buck FS. Blue rubber bleb nevus syndrome presenting with recurrences. *Dig Dis Sci.* 1987;32:214.
28. Telander RL, Ahlquist D, Blaufuss MC. Rectal mucosectomy: a definitive approach to extensive hemangiomas of the rectum. *J Pediatr Surg.* 1993;28:379.
29. Myers BM. Treatment of colonic bleeding in Klippel-Trénaunay syndrome with combined partial colectomy and endoscopic laser. *Dig Dis Sci.* 1993;38:1351.
30. Reilly PJ, Nostrant TT. Clinical manifestations of hereditary hemorrhagic telangiectasia. *Am J Gastroenterol.* 1984;79:363.
31. Case Records of the Massachusetts General Hospital (Case 41-1991). *N Engl J Med.* 1991;325:1086.
32. Stark ME, Gostout CJ, Balm RK. Clinical features and endoscopic management of Dieulafoy's disease. *Gastrointest Endosc.* 1992;38:545.
33. Bedford RA, van Stolk R, Sivak MV, Chung RS, Van Dam J. Gastric perforation after endoscopic treatment of a Dieulafoy's lesion. *Am J Gastroenterol.* 1992;87:244.
34. Borsch G. Diffuse gastric antral vascular ectasia: the "watermelon stomach" revisited. *Am J Gastroenterol.* 1987;82:1333.
35. Gostout CJ, Ahlquist DA, Radford CM, Viggiano TR, Bowyer BA, Balm RK. Endoscopic laser therapy for watermelon stomach. *Gastroenterology.* 1989;96:1462.
36. Labenz J, Borsch G. Bleeding watermelon stomach treated by Nd-YAG laser photocoagulation. *Endoscopy.* 1993;25:240.

61
Radiation Colitis
FREDERICK FALLICK and ROBERT BURAKOFF

Approximately 50% of all patients presenting with malignancy eventually receive radiation therapy. Acute intestinal injury affects an estimated 50% of patients receiving abdominal or pelvic radiotherapy (APRT). In 20% of those patients, symptoms are serious enough to interrupt the therapeutic schedule and may be severe enough to actually impact the chance for a cure. Chronic radiation injury to the intestine occurs in at least 10% of patients receiving APRT.[1]

In one series, overall 5-year survival was 42%. Sixty-two percent of the deaths that occurred were attributable to radiation-induced intestinal injury, either directly or indirectly.[2] In a series of 1801 patients with uterine cancer treated with radiation over a 20-year period, 95% of the radiation-induced bowel injuries involved the rectum or sigmoid colon. Intracavity radiation was used in 92% of the patients who subsequently developed this problem,[3] suggesting that the more frequent use of this modality in recent years has resulted in increased morbidity.

PREDISPOSING FACTORS

The following factors appear to contribute to the development of radiation colitis:

1. *Excessive radiation:* The *rad* is the most common term used to report radiation dosage. One rad is the amount of radiation that results in absorption of 100 ergs of energy per gram of tissue. Damage incurred by radiation is dose dependent. Different areas of the gastrointestinal (GI) tract have differing tolerances to radiotherapy. $TD_{5/5}$ and $TD_{5/50}$ represent the minimum and maximum tolerance dose range within which 5% to 50% of patients will develop clinically evident tissue injury. That range is 4500 to 6500 rads for small bowel and colon and 5500 to 8000 rads for rectum.[4] These doses actually overlap with therapeutic dosages required to effectively treat certain tumors. Patients who experience more severe acute injuries are more likely to develop chronic colitis.[5] However, many patients who develop chronic colonic injury have no history of prior acute radiation-induced injury.
2. *Chemotherapy:* Chemotherapeutic agents given during or after radiotherapy enhance the effect of the radiation, producing greater damage. Drugs most commonly implicated include 5-fluorouracil, dactinomycin (Actinomycin D), doxorubicin (Adriamycin), and methotrexate.[6]
3. *Prior surgery:* Prior abdominal and pelvic operations predispose to the development of adhesions that can fix intestinal loops in a set position within the field of radiotherapy. Hence, the same segments of intestine are repeatedly exposed to radiation, increasing the risk of injury.
4. *Vascular occlusive disease:* Hypertension, diabetes, and cardiovascular disease are associated with an increased risk of radiation injury.[7]

ACUTE COLITIS

The mechanism of acute gut injury involves the depletion of crypt cells, which normally migrate and differentiate into villous cells. Villi become blunted, and a constellation of functional disorders ensues, notably associated with the classic symptoms of diarrhea, nausea, vomiting, abdominal pain, and tenesmus. The diarrhea has recently been shown to be linked with decreased absorption of bile acids, vitamin B_{12}, lactose, and fat in the presence of rapid small intestinal transit time.[8]

DIAGNOSIS

Because the above-mentioned symptoms occur frequently in patients receiving radiation, or shortly after treatment, extensive diagnostic testing is usually unnecessary. Plain films of the abdomen may show an ileus or evidence of ischemia, i.e., mucosal edema with thumbprinting. When severe, edema may cause separation of intestinal loops or thickening and straightening of mucosal folds. Barium studies may show severe rectal spasm. Haustral markings may disappear, producing the "lead pipe" appearance of ulcerative colitis.[9]

If the patient should exhibit signs of peritonitis, perforation should be suspected, and the appropriate workup should be instituted beginning with surgical consultation and plain films to look for free intraabdominal air. Sigmoidoscopy and colonoscopy should be avoided when possible because of the risk of perforation.

TREATMENT

The acute phase usually begins during the first or second week of therapy and resolves completely shortly after radiotherapy is completed. Treatment is primarily symptomatic. If symptoms occur during radiotherapy, a 10% reduction in the daily dose of radiation may be of value. Mild sedatives, antispasmodic agents such as psyllium to increase stool bulk, topical analgesics, and warm sitz baths are the cornerstone of therapy and will relieve symptoms in the majority of patients. Diarrhea can be treated with loperamide, often very effectively. Suspected choleraic diarrhea secondary to bile salt malabsorption often responds well to empiric cholestyramine. A lactose- and fiber-restricted diet might also be of benefit. Glutamine is an amino acid that is widely available in the powdered, crystalline form and could easily be added to dietary liquids to provide enrichment. A glutamine-enriched diet has been shown to improve small bowel histologic findings and decrease morbidity and mortality in rats. Rarely, total parenteral nutrition (TPN) or an elemental diet needs to be temporarily employed to treat patients who cannot tolerate oral intake.

CHRONIC OR LATE-ONSET RADIATION COLITIS

The mechanism underlying chronic radiation-induced colitis involves the development of a progressive obliterative vasculitis. Subendothelial proliferation and medial thickening within small vessels gradually depletes the blood supply to the affected tissue. This process may take from weeks to several years before becoming clinically evident. The usual time frame is 6 months to 2 years. However, cases have been described as occurring as early as 3 months to as late as 31 years postirradiation, and this diagnosis should be considered in any patient who has ever received radiotherapy and subsequently presents with abdominal complaints.

The ischemic area of the bowel often initially ulcerates. This ulceration may progress through the full thickness of the bowel wall and result in perforation or fistulization, or healing may occur resulting in stricture formation.

Symptoms depend on the underlying pathology. The most common problem encountered in the colon is proctosigmoiditis, which affects 30% to 75% of patients with radiation-induced GI lesions.[1,8,9] Proctosigmoiditis often produces symptoms of tenesmus and a mucoid rectal discharge often mixed with blood. Partial or complete healing of proctosigmoid disease can produce stricture of the colonic lumen resulting in chronic constipation, bloating, and occasionally, a persistent decrease in stool caliber. Discrete ulceration occurs in 10% to 15% of cases, most commonly seen on the anterior wall of the rectum within 10 cm of the anal verge.[2] Feculent vaginal discharge, pneumaturia, or the rapid evacuation of undigested food can indicate the presence of a fistula.[10] Both strictures and enterocolonic fistulas predispose to bacterial overgrowth, which can lead to steatorrhea and vitamin B_{12} deficiency.

Diagnostic studies should also be geared to the clinician's index of suspicion. For the patient with obstructive symptoms, barium studies may help to differentiate mechanical obstruction from obstruction secondary to dysmotility. Strictures with proximal bowel dilation or straightened, ahaustral colonic segments similar to those seen in patients with chronic ulcerative colitis may also be observed.

Barium studies can also disclose fistulas and recurrence of malignancy. Nonspecific findings should be followed-up with computed tomography (CT) or colonoscopy. A CT scan of the abdomen and pelvis may help in demonstrating localized perforation and abscess formation or the extent of tumor recurrence. Cautious colonoscopy often reveals numerous submucosal telangiectatic vessels and provides the opportunity to perform a biopsy on suspicious strictures or ulcerations. Biopsy specimens taken from affected mucosa may contain characteristically bizarre radiation fibroblasts or, in the subacute stage, diagnostic, large, subintimal foam cells. It should be remembered, however, that the biopsy procedure can cause severe bleeding and perforation of already compromised tissue.

MANAGEMENT

Mild to moderately symptomatic problems can usually be managed conservatively. For patients with proctitis or proctosigmoiditis who experience tenesmus, pain on defecation and minor rectal bleeding, stool softeners, sedatives, bulking agents, antispasmodics, warm sitz baths, and a low-residue diet are often enough to adequately relieve the symptoms. A poor response suggests some loss of internal anal sphincter function due to radiation damage to the myenteric plexus. Steroid retention enemas and 5-aminosalicylic acid–containing compounds such as sulfasalazine, mesalamine enemas, and the newer site-specific mesalamine agents such as Pentasa and Asacol, which dissolve in the small and large bowel, respectively, may provide some relief, but their efficacy has not really been demonstrated in controlled clinical trials. Mild rectal bleeding from telangiectasias can often be controlled using Nd:YAG laser cauterization or the more common forms of electrocautery. More recently, argon laser therapy has been employed[11] and might prove to be a better and safer tool for the job because of its 1-mm penetration depth, in contrast with the 3- to 5-mm depth of the Nd:YAG laser and its selective photoabsorption by hemoglobin.

A single case report on the use of hyperbaric oxygenation in the treatment of radiation colitis reported successful abatement of gross hemorrhage and reversal of endoscopic bowel findings.[12] If massive bleeding occurs and cannot be controlled, surgical intervention is indicated.

Ulcers that do not heal can progress to perforation or fistula. Rectovaginal fistulas may close spontaneously, although this is rare. Diversion of the fecal stream can be helpful. Enterovesical, rectovesical, enterocolic, and many rectosigmoid fistulas require surgical revision.

Symptomatic strictures can often be dilated manually or endoscopically with good results. Extensive, long-standing strictures should be approached with caution because of the high risk of perforation. Surgical resection is often the only solution. Ulcerative rectosigmoid lesions may respond to sucralfate enemas, 2 g in 20 ml tap water twice daily. A small study reported encouraging initial results.[13]

Surgery should always be considered as the treatment of last choice. Healing is generally impaired in devitalized, devascularized radiation-damaged tissue. Sometimes however, when fistulas do not close and strictures progress to obstruction, surgery is unavoidable. An extensive discussion concerning the surgical procedures involved is beyond the scope of this text, but often these problems are acutely managed by diversion of the fecal stream, preferably with a transverse colostomy. Anastomosis with construction of a coloanal J-reservoir seems to help avoid the urgency and frequency symptoms associated with the coloanal sleeve anastomosis.[14]

Colorectal radiation injury is a serious, progressive disease whose best treatment is prevention. Preventive modalities include proper positioning during radiotherapy to maximally exclude uninvolved viscera from the therapeutic window, bladder distension with fluids to push the ileum out of the pelvis, ensuring good nutritional status prior to initiating therapy, and implementing intraoperative protective measures when possible. The recent use of biodegradable mesh slings to keep small bowel out of the pelvis appears promising.

Recent research involving antioxidants and free-radical scavengers, such as superoxide dismutase and betacarotene, may be useful in the prevention of radiation injury. However, the fundamental therapeutic effect of ionizing radiation involves the production of destructive free radicals. Radiation more effectively destroys well-oxygenated tumor tissue, and the use of the protective systemic antioxidants might significantly nullify the beneficial effects of radiotherapy. Other promising, but at present experimental, agents include prostaglandins (a prostaglandin E_2 analog is presently used to protect gastric mucosa from injury incurred by nonsteroidal anti-inflammatory drugs), the use of an elemental diet during the treatment period, and the use of topical radical scavengers such as sulfhydryl compounds and phosphorothioates during treatment to prevent local injury.

Hopefully, new preventive modalities in tandem with older, proven techniques will reduce the incidence of this severe complication of a potentially life-saving therapeutic modality.

REFERENCES

1. Russel JC, Welch JP. Operative management of radiation injuries of the intestinal tract. *Am J Surg.* 1979;137:433.
2. Galland RB, Spencer J. The natural history of clinically established radiation enteritis. *Lancet.* 1985;1:1257–1258.
3. Allen-Mersh TG, Wilson EJ, Hope-Stone HF, et al. Has the incidence of radiation-induced bowel damage following treatment of uterine carcinoma changed in the last 20 years? *J R Soc Med.* 1985;79:387–390.
4. Galland RB, Spencer J. Natural history and surgical management of radiation enteritis. *Br J Surg.* 1987;74:742–747.
5. Buchler DA, Kline JC, Peckham BM, et al. Radiation reactions in cervical cancer therapy. *Am J Obstet Gynecol.* 1971;111:745.
6. Shehata WM, Meyer RL. The enhancement effect of irradiation by methotrexate: report of 3 complications. *Cancer.* 1980;46:1349.
7. DeCosse JJ. Radiation injury to the intestine. In: Sabiston DC, ed. *Textbook of Surgery.* Philadelphia, Pa: WB Saunders Co; 1991:880.
8. Yeoh E, Horowitz M, Russo A, et al. Effect of pelvic irradiation on gastrointestinal function: a prospective longitudinal study. *Am J Med.* 1993;95:397–406.
9. Earnest OL, Trier JS. Radiation enteritis and colitis. In: Sleisenger MH, Fordtran JS, eds. *Gastrointestinal Disease.* 5th ed, Philadelphia, Pa: WB Saunders Co; 1993; 2:1257–1270.
10. Kimose HK, Fischer L, Spjeldnaes N. Late radiation injury of the colon and rectum: surgical management and outcome. *Dis Colon Rectum.* 1989;32:684–689.
11. Taylor JG, Disario JA, Buchi KN. Argon laser therapy for hemorrhagic radiation proctitis: long term results. *Gastrointest Endosc.* 1993;39:641–644.
12. Nakada T, Kugota Y, Sasagawa I. Therapeutic experience of hyperbaric oxygenation in radiation colitis. *Dis Colon Rectum.* 1993;36:961–965.
13. Kochhar R, Mehta SK, Aggarwal R, et al. Sucralfate enema in ulcerative rectosigmoid lesions. *Dis Colon Rectum.* 1990;33:49–51.
14. Luccarotti ME, Mountford RA, Bartolo DC. Surgical management of intestinal radiation injury. *Dis Colon Rectum.* 1991;34:865–869.

62

Chronic Intestinal Ischemic Syndrome

CHRISTIAN de VIRGILIO and BRUCE E. STABILE

Chronic mesenteric ischemia is rare. In fact, the largest surgical series spanning three decades included only 74 patients.[1] Recognition of chronic mesenteric ischemia is nevertheless crucial because it may progress to intestinal gangrene and death. Occlusion of the mesenteric vessels was first noted over 100 years ago, but the association between chronic mesenteric occlusion, abdominal angina and intestinal infarction was not made until 1936 by Dunphy.[2] The first successful thromboendarterectomy of the superior mesenteric artery (SMA) was performed in 1958 by Shaw and Maynard.[3]

CLINICAL PRESENTATION

The classic triad consists of postprandial abdominal pain, weight loss, and fear of eating. The pain is usually midabdominal, with an onset 30 to 45 minutes after a meal. Unlike other forms of atherosclerotic occlusion, the majority of patients in most series are women. The classic symptoms are not always present nor always recognized. Less typical presentations of chronic visceral ischemia as noted by Hallett and associates[4] included diffuse superficial gastric erosions, acalculous cholecystitis, and unexplained elevation of the liver chemistries. In the Mayo clinic experience, the average duration of symptoms prior to diagnosis was 12 months, the mean weight loss was 32 pounds, 34% had evidence of atherosclerosis in other peripheral arteries, and 75% had an abdominal bruit.[5] The differential diagnosis of chronic mesenteric ischemia should include malignancy, particularly pancreatic and gastric, and peptic ulceration.

DIAGNOSIS

Duplex ultrasonography is emerging as a potential screening tool for chronic visceral arterial occlusive disease. The Duplex scan can measure peak systolic velocity and diastolic velocity in the proximal 3 cm of the celiac axis or SMA. It can also detect diastolic flow reversal that is normally present in the SMA because of the high resistance in its vascular bed. Loss of diastolic flow reversal in the SMA is a result of a decrease in the vascular resistance and is indicative of a significant stenosis in the proximal SMA. A doubling of the peak systolic velocity in the celiac axis or SMA as compared with the aorta is also considered significant.[6] Spectral broadening, which is indicative of turbulent flow, further supports the diagnosis of a stenosis. If the diagnosis is in doubt, the study can be repeated after a test meal. Flow velocities in the celiac axis and SMA normally increase after a meal, but in the presence of a fixed stenosis, flow velocity fails to increase.[6]

Aortography is the diagnostic procedure of choice. It is essential to obtain both anteroposterior and lateral views of the aorta (Fig. 62–1). The lateral view allows visualization of orificial lesions of the celiac artery and SMA that might otherwise be missed (Fig. 62–1*B*). Identification of such lesions is critical for operative planning. Up to one third of patients are found to have concomitant significant stenoses of one or both renal arteries on arteriography.[7] In addition, the finding of a meandering mesenteric artery on arteriography signifies mesenteric occlusive disease. This artery is an ascending branch of the left colic artery that enlarges and provides collateral flow to the SMA. It forms an arcade with the left branch of the middle colic artery, which is known as Riolan's arch.

Occlusive disease causing a greater than 50% diameter reduction in two of the three mesenteric vessels is generally considered necessary to produce symptoms of chronic mesenteric ischemia. Proper patient selection prior to operative intervention is imperative, as patients with significant mesenteric stenosis observed on arteriography may be asymptomatic. Crawford and associates[8] noted that one third of patients studied with lateral aortography for other indica-

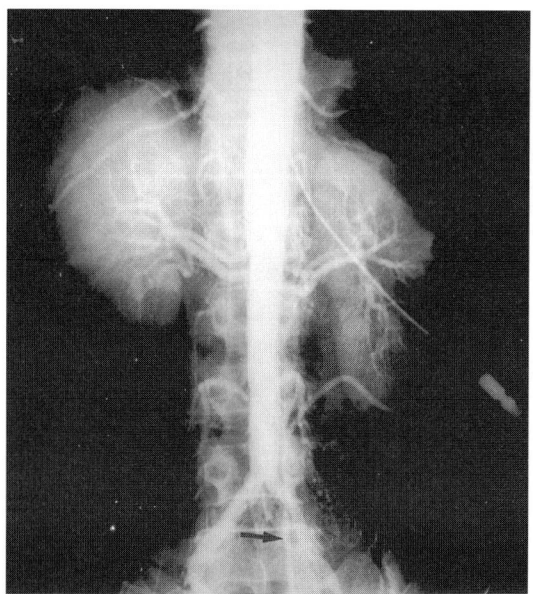
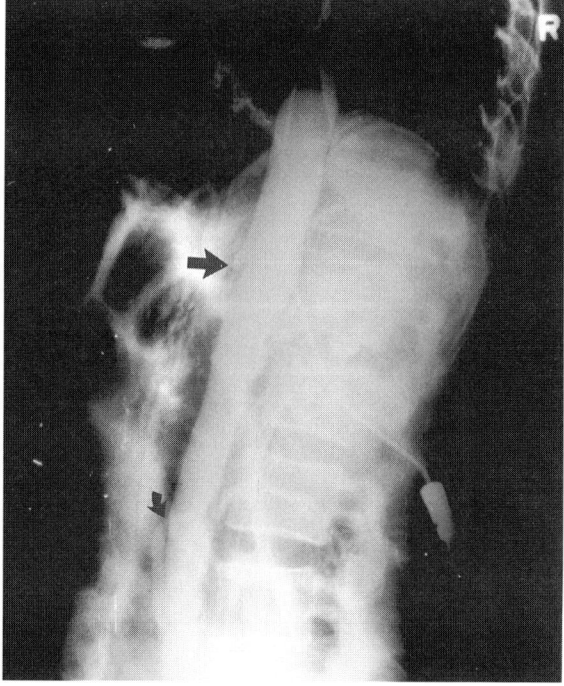

FIGURE 62–1. A, Anteroposterior aortogram demonstrates lack of visceral artery branches from the celiac axis and superior mesenteric artery (SMA), suggesting occlusive disease in these vessels. The inferior mesenteric artery (IMA) is faintly visible *(arrow)*. **B,** Lateral aortogram in the same patient shows an occluded SMA *(upper arrow)* and a stenotic origin of the IMA *(lower arrow)*. The origin of the celiac axis is occluded and not visualized.

tions were found to have asymptomatic high-grade stenoses of the celiac axis. Most vascular surgeons agree that no intervention is warranted for asymptomatic mesenteric lesions. Surgical intervention is therefore indicated if arteriography demonstrates significant stenosis or occlusion of at least two mesenteric vessels in association with appropriate symptomatology. There are, however, exceptions to this principle. Patients with single vessel stenosis and previous abdominal surgery may have mesenteric ischemia on the basis of interruption of gastroduodenal, pancreaticoduodenal, Riolan's arch, or hemorrhoidal collaterals. Another exception is the celiac compression syndrome. These patients typically complain of postprandial epigastric abdominal pain in association with angiographic demonstration of celiac axis compression just beyond its origin by the median arcuate ligament. It is unclear why isolated stenosis of the celiac axis in the absence of SMA or inferior mesenteric artery (IMA) stenosis causes abdominal pain. Theories include intestinal ischemia as a result of steal from the SMA or pain from compression of the celiac ganglia.[9]

PERCUTANEOUS TRANSLUMINAL ANGIOPLASTY

A potential alternative to surgical intervention in the management of chronic mesenteric ischemia is percutaneous transluminal angioplasty (PTA), a procedure particularly applicable to high-risk patients. Golden and coworkers[10] reported successful PTA of the SMA in six of seven patients who presented with typical abdominal symptoms. Odurny and associates[11] performed PTA on 19 arteries in 10 patients with chronic mesenteric ischemia. They reported a 90% success rate. Five patients with recurrent symptoms underwent redilation, with relief of symptoms in three. The only complication was an asymptomatic intimal SMA dissection. Lesions arising from the arterial ostia or from the celiac compression syndrome are less amenable to PTA. Long-term results following PTA do not approach those of surgical reconstruction, and thus PTA is reserved for patients with high operative risks.

PREOPERATIVE PREPARATION

Patients with chronic mesenteric ischemia do not typically require urgent operation, and thus proper attention should be given to preoperative preparation. These patients often have multiple medical problems including coronary artery disease, hypertension, and diabetes, as well as marked nutritional depletion. Optimization of cardiac and nutritional status, as well as adequate hydration, should be ensured prior to operation.

SURGICAL THERAPY

Several operative approaches are currently acceptable in the management of chronic intestinal ischemia. The decision as to which technique to use is based largely on the distribution of the disease as seen on arteriography, and in part, on the preference of the surgeon.

It is controversial whether it is most advisable to revascularize only one or all diseased arteries. Revascularization of a stenotic SMA alone generally relieves symptoms of mesenteric ischemia. However, the incidence of postoperative bowel infarction and symptom recurrence has been reported to be higher if only one stenotic vessel is revascularized.[5,12] Thus, it would seem prudent to revascularize all stenotic arteries whenever possible.

TRANSAORTIC ENDARTERECTOMY

Transaortic endarterectomy is ideal for patients in whom the disease is limited to the origins of the celiac axis and SMA. The procedure requires rotation of all the viscera from left to right to expose the supraceliac aorta. A cross clamp is placed on the aorta proximal to all the visceral vessels, and the aorta is incised longitudinally in a trap door fashion as described by Stoney and coworkers.[1] A local endarterectomy of the ventral aorta and the orificial atheromas is then performed (Fig. 62–2). The advantage of this technique is the avoidance of a synthetic graft and the attendant risks of graft infection and thrombosis. However, transaortic endarterectomy is a more technically demanding procedure, requires a more extensive operative exposure, and is performed in only a few centers.

AORTOMESENTERIC BYPASS

Aortomesenteric bypass is a more commonly used technique. The bypass can originate from the aorta above the celiac axis (antegrade) or from below the renal arteries (retrograde). The conduit is either a synthetic graft or saphenous vein.

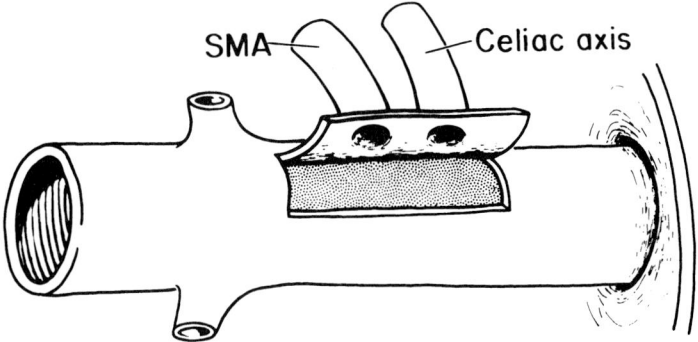

FIGURE 62–2. A trap door incision is made in the aorta, and a transaortic endarterectomy of the celiac axis, superior mesenteric artery (SMA), and adjacent aorta is performed.

Antegrade bypass using a Dacron graft is considered by some to be superior to retrograde bypass.[13] The antegrade graft originates from a relatively disease-free segment of the supraceliac aorta, diminishing the likelihood of future atherosclerotic occlusion of the graft. The bifurcated graft is then anastomosed to the celiac axis and the proximal SMA (Fig. 62–3). Because of its straight configuration, the antegrade graft has less tendency to kink and produce turbulent flow than the retrograde graft, thus decreasing the development of late neointimal hyperplasia and subsequent graft occlusion.[13] The advantage of the retrograde graft is that it requires less operative exposure and the aortic cross clamp can be applied below the renal arteries, thereby avoiding renal and visceral ischemia during reconstruction.

Results

Mortality following elective mesenteric reconstruction varies from 5% to 17%.[12] In the Mayo Clinic series, three of the five deaths (9% overall mortality) were due to complications of bowel infarction following graft occlusion.[5] Interestingly, in all three deaths revascularization was performed on fewer than the total number of stenotic mesenteric arteries.[5] The University of California at San Francisco (UCSF) group reported a 12% operative mortality with postoperative bleeding being the most common complication leading to death.[1] They compared results in patients undergoing transaortic endarterectomy versus antegrade aortomesenteric bypass and found no significant differences in overall mortality (15% versus 8%) or in overall complication rates. However, multiple complications and pulmonary complications were more common in the transaortic endarterectomy group.

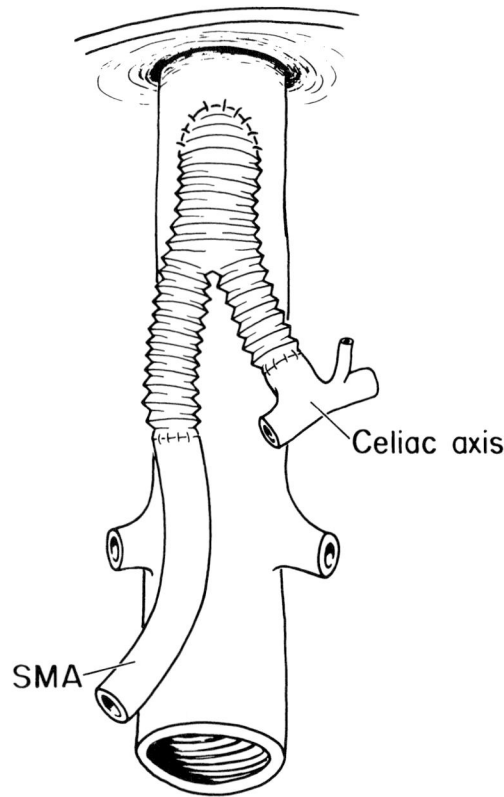

FIGURE 62–3. Antegrade aortomesenteric bypass from the supraceliac aorta to the celiac axis and superior mesenteric artery (SMA) using a bifurcated Dacron graft.

Multiple organ dysfunction is known to occur following mesenteric revascularization.[12] It is unclear whether this is due to reperfusion of ischemic bowel or due to the hepatic and renal ischemia following supraceliac aortic cross clamping. Supraceliac aortic clamping has been shown experimentally to cause hepatic dysfunction with prolongation of clotting times and thrombocytopenia.[12]

Long-term relief of symptoms following successful revascularization has been excellent. In the UCSF study, 96% of patients were symptom free at 1 year after surgery (87% at 5 years) and only 5% had fatal recurrent visceral ischemia.[1]

RECURRENT ISCHEMIA

Following mesenteric revascularization, close follow-up is recommended to detect stenosis of the graft and symptoms of recurrent intestinal ischemia. In the UCSF series, 12% of patients developed recurrent symptoms of mesenteric ischemia from 4 to 98 months postoperatively.[1] Repeat revascularization was performed and was successful in more than one half of those patients. In the Mayo Clinic series, recurrent symptoms occurred in 26% of patients.[5] The authors noted that symptom recurrence was related to the completeness of revascularization. If only one of three or one of two stenotic mesenteric arteries was revascularized, the recurrence rate was 50%. If two of three arteries were revascularized, the recurrence rate was 29%; if all stenotic vessels were revascularized (two of two or three of three), the recurrence rate was only 11%.

Surveillance Duplex scanning following aortomesenteric grafting or transaortic endarterectomy is recommended at regular intervals postoperatively to detect recurrent stenosis.

SUMMARY

Chronic mesenteric ischemia is rare. Recognition of the classic triad of postprandial abdominal pain, weight loss, and fear of eating should prompt a diagnostic evaluation. Duplex ultrasonography of the celiac axis and SMA holds future promise as a noninvasive screening tool but is not yet routinely available. Arteriography is the gold standard for diagnosis of mesenteric vascular occlusion and should include anteroposterior and lateral views. Demonstration of significant disease in two or three mesenteric vessels in association with appropriate symptomatology warrants treatment. PTA should be reserved for high-risk patients, as the recurrence rate is high. Antegrade aortomesenteric bypass from the supraceliac aorta to the celiac axis and SMA using a bifurcated Dacron graft or saphenous vein is the most commonly performed operation. Analysis of the reported results indicates that the operative mortality is approximately 10%. Long-term relief of symptoms is excellent; however, close follow-up is necessary to detect graft stenosis or occlusion.

REFERENCES

1. Cunningham CG, Reilly LM, Rapp JH, et al. Chronic visceral ischemia. *Ann Surg.* 1991;214:276–288.
2. Dunphy JE. Abdominal pain of vascular origin. *Am J Med Sci.* 1936;192:109–113.
3. Shaw RS, Maynard EP. Acute and chronic thrombosis of mesenteric arteries associated with malabsorption: report of two cases treated successfully by thromboendarterectomy. *N Engl J Med.* 1958;258:874–878.
4. Hallett JW, James ME, Ahlquist DA, Larson MV. Recent trends in the diagnosis and management of chronic intestinal ischemia. *Ann Vasc Surg.* 1990;4:126–132.
5. Hollier LH, Bernatz PE, Pairolero PC, et al. Surgical management of chronic intestinal ischemia: a reappraisal. *Surgery.* 1981;90:940–946.
6. Yao JT. Mesenteric vascular disease: Duplex scanning in diagnosis of splanchnic artery occlusive disease. In: Ernst CB, Stanley JC, eds. *Current Therapy in Vascular Surgery.* 2nd ed. Toronto: BC Decker Inc; 1991.
7. Cunningham CG, Reilly LM, Stoney R. Chronic visceral ischemia. *Surg Clin North Am.* 1992;72:231–244.
8. Crawford ES, Morris GC, Myhre HO, Roehm JO Jr. Celiac axis, superior mesenteric artery, and inferior mesenteric artery occlusion: surgical considerations. *Surgery.* 1977;82:856–866.
9. Evans WE, Hayes J. Celiac compression syndrome. In: Ernst CB, Stanley JC, eds. *Current Therapy in Vascular Surgery.* 2nd ed. Toronto: BC Decker Inc; 1991:747.
10. Golden DA, Ring EJ, McLean GK, Freiman DB. Percutaneous transluminal angioplasty in the treatment of abdominal angina. *AJR.* 1982;139:247–249.
11. Odurny A, Sniderman KW, Colapinto RF. Intestinal angina: percutaneous transluminal angioplasty of the celiac and superior mesenteric arteries. *Radiology.* 1988;167:59–62.
12. Harward TR, Brooks DL, Flynn TC, Seeger JM. Multiple organ dysfunction after mesenteric artery revascularization. *J Vasc Surg.* 1993;18:459–469.
13. Pairolero PC, Cherry KJ Jr. Bypass grafting for chronic splanchnic arteriosclerotic occlusive disease. In: Ernst CB, Stanley JC, eds. *Current Therapy in Vascular Surgery.* 2nd ed. Toronto: BC Decker Inc; 1991.

63
Chronic Intestinal Pseudoobstruction in Adults

SINN ANURAS and JITRA ANURAS

Chronic intestinal pseudoobstruction (CIP) is a term used to indicate a clinical syndrome in which patients have recurrent symptoms and signs of intestinal obstruction without detectable mechanical obstruction.[1] The syndrome is caused by severely abnormal gastrointestinal motility including either intestinal hypomotility (from smooth muscle dysfunction) or incoordinated hyperactive motility (from enteric nerve dysfunction) depending on the underlying causes. Although the term *intestinal pseudoobstruction* implies only small intestinal dysmotility, other parts of the gastrointestinal tract are often involved. Dysphagia, gastroparesis, and colonic dysfunction may also be present.

CLINICAL MANIFESTATIONS

CIP can be caused by many diseases. Regardless of the underlying cause of CIP, patients usually present with similar clinical manifestations. These include recurrent symptoms and signs of intestinal obstruction that are indistinguishable from those of mechanical obstruction. Figure 63–1 shows a plain abdominal roentgenogram of a patient with intestinal pseudoobstruction from scleroderma during an attack. Multiple air-fluid levels and dilation of the small intestine can be seen. The incidence and severity of recurrent obstructive episodes vary from patient to patient and from time to time. In a few patients, obstructive episodes may only occur once every few years. In the most severe cases, obstructive episodes may be persistent. Physical examination reveals cachectic and malnourished patients. Weight loss is due to malnutrition (inadequate intake) and malabsorption (from bacterial overgrowth). The abdomen is usually distended with mild tenderness but no guarding. Bowel sounds are usually inactive and infrequent. Succussion splash may be heard in patients with gastric distension. Borborygmi can be detected in most patients.

Between the recurrent intestinal obstructive episodes, patients may have postprandial abdominal pain and bloating. The abdominal pain is usually epigastric or periumbilical. Patients may have nausea and occasional vomiting. Dysphagia and heartburn from esophagitis are commonly seen in patients with scleroderma and

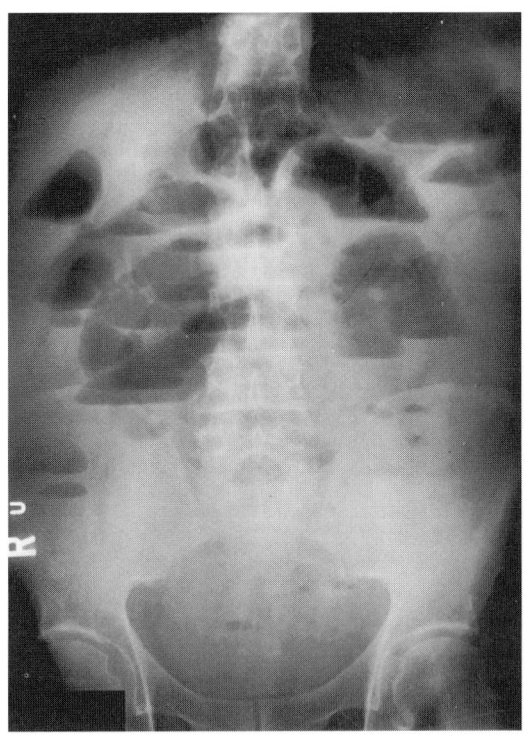

FIGURE 63–1. A plain abdominal x-ray film of a patient with scleroderma during an intestinal pseudoobstruction episode. Note multiple air-fluid levels and dilation of the small intestine.

type I familial visceral myopathy. Constipation is also common in patients with scleroderma and type I familial visceral myopathy. Diarrhea may occur in patients with bacterial overgrowth in the small intestine. Alternating constipation and diarrhea may occur in some patients.

Extragastrointestinal manifestations may be found in some patients depending on the underlying disease. Megacystis and megaureters are common in visceral myopathy patients who may have urinary retention and infection. Mydriasis, ptosis, and external ophthalmoplegia may occur in certain forms of familial visceral myopathies. Ataxia, dysautonomia, and neurologic symptoms may occur in patients with certain forms of visceral neuropathies. In the secondary form of CIP, patients also exhibit systemic manifestations of the underlying disease such as scleroderma or muscular dystrophies.

CIP can occur at any age, depending on the underlying disease. Therefore, it must be considered in the differential diagnosis in any patient with recurrent symptoms and signs of intestinal obstruction.

DIAGNOSIS

The diagnosis of CIP can be made by ruling out mechanical obstructing lesions in patients with recurrent symptoms and signs of intestinal obstruction. Figure 63–2 outlines the diagram of sequence of events in approaching CIP patients. It is important to objectively confirm ileus or gaseous distension and air-fluid levels in the small intestine by plain abdominal roentgenograms. Table 63–1 lists the features that are useful in differentiating CIP from true mechanical small bowel obstruction.

Patient Presentation

Patient presents with recurrent symptoms and signs of intestinal obstruction or ileus.

Documentation of Signs of Intestinal Obstruction

Plain abdominal roentgenograms to document intestinal obstructive findings such as gaseous dilatation of the intestine and air-fluid levels.

Rule out Mechanical Obstruction

Barium enema, upper gastrointestinal tract and small bowel x-ray studies, enteroclysis to rule out mechanical obstruction. When mechanical obstruction is ruled out, the diagnosis of intestinal pseudoobstruction is made.

Search for the Cause of Chronic Intestinal Pseudoobstruction

1. With appropriate tests, search for any systemic diseases (as listed in Table 63?2) that may cause chronic intestinal pseudoobstruction.

2. The findings on gastrointestinal contrast roentgenograms may give clues to underlying diseases (as listed in Table 63?3).

3. Family history must be obtained.

4. If the patient has surgery, a full-thickness biopsy must be obtained to examine for smooth muscle and myenteric plexus abnormalities.

Treatment

FIGURE 63–2. Sequence of events in approaching patients with chronic intestinal pseudoobstruction.

TABLE 63–1. FEATURES DIFFERENTIATING CHRONIC INTESTINAL PSEUDOOBSTRUCTION FROM TRUE MECHANICAL OBSTRUCTION

Chronic Intestinal Pseudoobstruction	Mechanical Obstruction
1. Patient experiences diarrhea or constipation.	1. Patient experiences constipation and obstipation.
2. Patient may have other gastrointestinal symptoms (e.g., dysphagia or symptoms of gastric atony).	2. Patient has no esophageal or gastric problems.
3. Patient has symptoms of abdominal pain, nausea, vomiting, or dysphagia between the attacks.	3. Patient is usually symptom-free between the attacks.
4. Patient has cachectic appearance.	4. Patient is seldom cachectic.
5. Patient may have urinary retention and infection.	5. Patient has no urinary symptoms.
6. Patient will have symptoms and signs of systemic disease (e.g., scleroderma or muscular dystrophies) if chronic intestinal pseudoobstruction is secondary.	6. There is no underlying systemic disease.
7. Patient may have family history of similar problems.	7. There is no family history.
8. Plain abdominal roentgenograms may show air throughout the small bowel and colon.	8. Plain abdominal roentgenograms show no air beyond the point of obstruction.
9. Esophagram may show esophageal aperistalsis and dilation.	9. Esophagram findings are normal.
10. Roentgenograms may show gastric atony and megaduodenum.	10. Upper gastrointestinal tract series may show dilation of proximal small bowel if the obstruction is in proximal bowel.
11. Small bowel roentgenograms may show dilation of entire small bowel with or without multiple diverticula.	11. Small bowel roentgenograms show dilation of bowel proximal to the obstructing lesion.
12. Enteroclysis shows no obstructing lesion.	12. Enteroclysis may show obstructing lesion.
13. Barium enema may show redundant colon or wide-mouthed diverticula.	13. Barium enema may show obstructing lesion.
14. Intravenous pyelogram may show megacystis or megaureter.	14. Intravenous pyelogram findings are normal.
15. Esophageal manometric studies may show diminished esophagogastric sphincter tone and low amplitude of contractions of lower two thirds of esophagus.	15. Esophageal manometric studies are normal.
16. Jejunal manometric studies: Fasting—one or more phases of migrating motor complexes are absent; there is low amplitude of contractions or retrograde and simultaneous contractions; fed—contractions are inactive after patient has eaten.	16. Jejunal manometric studies show clusters of contractions during both fasting and fed periods, but migrating motor complexes are present during fasting.
17. No obstructing lesion is found during exploratory laparotomy.	17. Obstructing lesion can be identified during exploratory laparotomy.

CAUSES

After the diagnosis of CIP is made in a patient, we must attempt to identify the underlying cause of CIP in that patient. The tests for identifying the causes are discussed in the latter part of this chapter. Table 63–2 lists the causes of CIP.[2] Table 63–3 lists characteristic gastrointestinal lesions seen in the various types of diseases. All the diseases listed in Table 63–2 can cause CIP in adults with a few exceptions such as childhood visceral myopathies (chronic intestinal pseudoobstruction in young children and megacystis microcolon–intestinal hypoperistalsis syndrome) and a type of familial visceral neuropathy. We will briefly describe some diseases that can cause CIP in adults.

Familial Visceral Myopathies

Several families with familial visceral myopathies (FVM) have been reported.[3-29] Familial visceral myopathies are characterized by degeneration and fibrous replacement of the smooth muscle of the gastrointestinal tract and, in some families, the urinary tract. Based on gross lesions of the gastrointestinal tract, which are unique and specific for each type of FVM, and patterns of inheritance in these families, at least three types of FVM have been identified (Table 63–4).

Type I FVM, the most common type, is transmitted by an autosomal dominant gene.[3-16] Patients with this disease have an atonic esophagus, megaduodenum (Fig. 63–3), redundant colon, and megacystis. Type II FVM is transmitted by

TABLE 63–2. CAUSES OF CHRONIC INTESTINAL PSEUDOOBSTRUCTION

1. Primary chronic intestinal pseudoobstruction
   a. Familial type
      (1) Familial visceral myopathies
      (2) Familial visceral neuropathies
      (3) Childhood visceral myopathies
         (a) Chronic intestinal pseudoobstruction in young children
         (b) Megacystis microcolon–intestinal hypoperistalsis syndrome
   b. Nonfamilial (or sporadic) type
      (1) Visceral myopathies
      (2) Visceral neuropathies
2. Secondary chronic intestinal pseudoobstruction
   a. Disease involving the intestinal smooth muscle
      (1) Collagen diseases: scleroderma, dermatomyositis, and systemic lupus erythematosus
      (2) Muscular dystrophies: myotonic dystrophy, Duchenne's muscular dystrophy
      (3) Amyloidosis
   b. Neurologic diseases
      (1) Chagas' disease
      (2) Ganglioneuromatosis of the intestine
      (3) Visceral neuropathy in carcinomatosis
   c. Endocrine disorders
      (1) Myxedema
      (2) Hypoparathyroidism
   d. Pharmacologic agents
      (1) Phenothiazines
      (2) Tricyclic antidepressants
      (3) Antiparkinsonian medications
      (4) Ganglionic blockers
      (5) *Amanita* (mushroom) poisoning
      (6) Narcotics (morphine and meperidine)
   e. Miscellaneous
      (1) Nontropical sprue
      (2) Jejunoileal bypass
      (3) Small intestinal diverticulosis
      (4) Porphyria
      (5) Eosinophilic gastroenteritis
      (6) Radiation enteritis
      (7) Sclerosing mesenteritis
      (8) Diffuse lymphoid infiltration of the small intestine

an autosomal recessive gene.[17-25] In this disease, gastric dilation and a slight dilation of the entire small intestine with numerous diverticula are present. Patients also have ptosis and external ophthalmoplegia. Type III FVM is transmitted by an autosomal recessive gene.[26-29] This type is characterized by marked dilation of the entire digestive tract from the esophagus to the rectum. Neither type II nor III appear to involve the urinary tract. Symptoms in these patients vary from none to gastrointestinal obstructive symptoms (intestinal pseudoobstruction syndrome) and dysuria. These three types of FVM cannot be distinguished by histologic examination of the muscularis propria of the gastrointestinal tract.

FAMILIAL VISCERAL NEUROPATHIES

Several families with familial visceral neuropathies (FVN) have been reported.[30-39] Thus far, there are at least two types of manifestations based on gross lesions, histologic findings, and pattern of inheritance (Table 63–5). Type I FVN[30-32] is transmitted by an autosomal dominant gene. The patients have dilation of distal small bowel and colon, and some patients may have gastroparesis. Type II FVN[33-39] is transmitted by an autosomal recessive gene. The patients have hypertrophic pyloric stenosis, dilated short small intestine, and malrotation of small intestine.

Schuffler et al[40] reported FVN in two siblings, which did not fit into either type of FVN described above. Both patients had a dilated esophagus and small intestine and extensive diverticulosis of the colon. In addition, the patients also had some abnormal neurologic findings.

CHILDHOOD VISCERAL MYOPATHIES

Childhood visceral myopathy is a unique type of visceral myopathy that involves only infants and young children.[41-44] Histologic changes of degenerated smooth muscle cells are indistinguishable from those found in familial visceral myopathies. Nearly all reported cases have no family history, although two of the patients reported by Anuras et al[41] are cousins, which raises the possibility of heredity in this type of visceral myopathy. The age at the onset of CIP varies from newborn to 5 years of age. Recurrent urinary tract infections occur in most cases. All patients have marked dilation of the small intestine and the colon. Megacystis is detected in all cases and megaureters in some cases.

In some infants, the colon may be small. Thus, a term *megacystis microcolon–intestinal hypoperistalsis syndrome* has been created for such

TABLE 63–3. CHARACTERISTIC GASTROINTESTINAL LESIONS SEEN IN THE VARIOUS TYPES OF DISEASES

DISEASE	OROPHARYNX	ESOPHAGUS	STOMACH	SMALL INTESTINE	COLON	ANORECTUM
Smooth Muscle Diseases						
Familial visceral myopathies						
Type I	Not involved	Dilation	Not involved	Megaduodenum	Redundant colon	Not involved
Type II	Not involved	Not involved	Dilation	Multiple diverticula	Not involved	Not involved
Type III	Not involved	Dilation	Dilation	Dilation	Dilation	Dilation of rectum
Infantile and childhood visceral myopathy	Not involved	Not involved	Dilation	Dilation	Dilation	Not involved
Connective tissue disease						
Scleroderma	Not involved	Dilation, aperistalsis of lower two thirds, incompetent lower esophageal sphincter	Gastroparesis occurs less frequently	Megaduodenum, diffuse dilation of small intestine may occur	Dilation with loss of haustral markings, wide-necked diverticula	Incompetent internal anal sphincter
Dermatomyositis, polymyositis	"Vallecular" sign, nasopharyngeal regurgitation, tracheal aspiration	Dilation, decreased peristalsis of entire esophagus	Gastroparesis (occurs seldom)	Megaduodenum, dilation of small intestine seldom occurs	Dilation of the colon	Not involved
Systemic lupus erythematosus	Not involved	Aperistalsis	Not involved	Megaduodenum	Not involved	Not involved
Mixed connective tissue disease	Not involved	Dilation of lower two thirds, aperistalsis	Not involved	Megaduodenum	Diverticula	Not involved
Muscular dystrophies						
Myotonic dystrophy	Incoordination of upper esophageal sphincter relaxation and pharyngeal contractions	Decreased peristalsis	Delayed emptying, dilation	Dilation	Dilation	External sphincter dysfunction
Duchenne's muscular dystrophy	Not involved	Dilation	Dilation	Dilation	Dilation	Not involved
Amyloidosis	Not involved	Aperistalsis, incomplete lower esophageal sphincter relaxation	Delayed emptying	Dilation	Dilation	Not involved
Metabolic disease						
Hypothyroidism	Hypertensive upper esophageal sphincter with incomplete relaxation	Decreased peristalsis of lower two thirds, incompetent lower esophageal sphincter	Dilation	Dilation	Dilation	Not involved
Hypoparathyroidism		Not involved	Not involved	Dilation	Not involved	Not involved

Disease	Deglutition	Esophagus	Stomach	Small intestine	Colon	Anorectum
Enteric Nerve Disease						
Familial visceral neuropathies						
Autosomal dominant	Not involved	Not involved	Dilation	Dilation	Dilation	Not involved
Autosomal recessive	Not involved	Dilation	Dilation	Dilation	Dilation, redundant colon, diverticulosis	Not involved
Congenital disorders						
Aganglionosis-Hirschsprung's disease	Not involved	Not involved	Not involved	Not involved	Dilation	Internal anal sphincter dysfunction
Infectious visceral neuropathy						
Chagas' disease	Not involved	Dilation, aperistalsis, incomplete lower esophageal sphincter relaxation	Dilation	Dilation of proximal small intestine	Dilation	Incompetent internal anal sphincter
Viral infection	Not involved	Not involved	Gastroparesis	Dilation	Dilation	Not involved
Drug-induced visceral neuropathy						
Phenothiazine	Not involved	Not involved	Not involved	Not involved	Dilation	Not involved
Tricyclic antidepressants	Not involved	Not involved	Not involved	Dilation	Dilation	Not involved
Paraneoplastic visceral neuropathy	Not involved	Dilation	Gastroparesis	Dilation	Dilation	Not involved
Parkinson's disease	Impaired deglutition	Diffuse spasm, dilation, aperistalsis	Gastroparesis occurs less frequently	Dilation	Dilation, sigmoid volvulus	Not involved
Extrinsic Nerve Disease						
Diabetes mellitus	Not involved	Diffuse spasm, decreased peristalsis	Dilation, delayed emptying	Delayed transit time	Dilation	Incompetent internal anal sphincter
Multiple sclerosis	Not involved	Not involved	Gastroparesis	Not involved	Dilation	Incompetent anal sphincter
Spinal cord injury	Not involved	Not involved	Not involved	Not involved	Dilation	Internal anal sphincter dysfunction

TABLE 63-4. CLASSIFICATION OF FAMILIAL VISCERAL MYOPATHIES

	Type I	Type II	Type III
Reported families	3–16*	17–25	26–29
Mode of transmission	Autosomal dominant	Autosomal recessive; isolated cases	Autosomal recessive
Gross lesions	Esophageal dilation, megaduodenum, redundant colon, and megacystis	Gastric dilation, slight dilation of the entire small intestine with numerous diverticula	Marked dilation of the entire digestive tract from the esophagus to the rectum
Microscopic changes	Degeneration and fibrosis of both muscle layers of digestive tract	Indistinguishable from type I	Indistinguishable from type I
Age at onset	After the first decade of life	Teenage and middle age	Teenage and middle age
Percentage of symptomatic cases	50%	75%	75%
Symptoms	Variable from dysphagia and constipation to intestinal pseudo-obstruction	Severe abdominal pain and intestinal pseudo-obstruction	Intestinal pseudoobstruction
Treatment and prognosis	Symptomatic relief with appropriate operation (side-to-side duodeno-jejunostomy or partial resection of duodenum); prognosis is good	Does not respond to medical treatment; no effective surgical procedure; prognosis is poor	Same as type II
Extragastrointestinal manifestations	Megacystis, uterine inertia, mydriasis, dysplastic nevus syndrome	Ptosis and external ophthalmoplegia, mild degeneration of striated muscle, peripheral neuropathy, and deafness	None observed

*The numbers are references of the reported families.

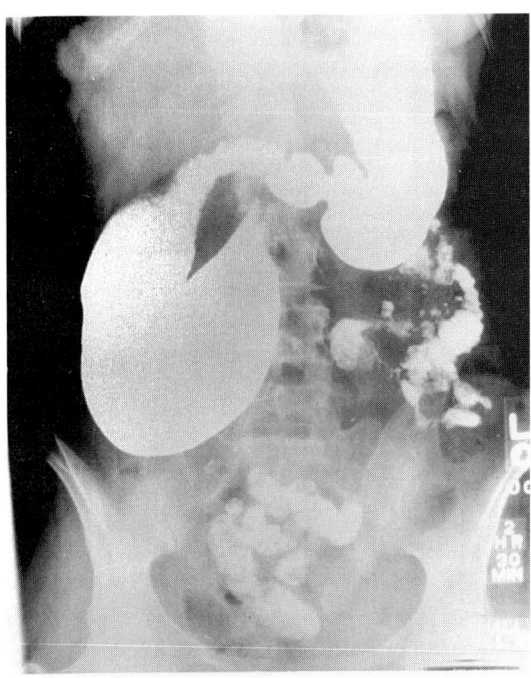

FIGURE 63-3. An upper gastrointestinal tract x-ray film showing megaduodenum in a type I familial visceral myopathy patient.

TABLE 63-5. CLASSIFICATION OF FAMILIAL VISCERAL NEUROPATHIES

	TYPE I	TYPE II
Reported families	30–32	33–39
Mode of transmission	Autosomal dominant	Autosomal recessive
Gross lesions	Dilation of various length of small intestine usually beginning from distal small bowel, megacolon, gastroparesis in one fourth of patients	Hypertrophic pyloric stenosis, dilated short small intestine, malrotation of small intestine
Microscopic changes	Degeneration of argyrophilic neurons and decrease in numbers of nerve fibers	Deficiency of argyrophilic neurons and increase in neuroblasts
Age of onset	Any age	Infancy
Percentage of symptomatic cases	>75%	100%
Symptoms	Early satiety; recurrent abdominal pain and distension; diarrhea or constipation; two thirds have intestinal pseudoobstruction	All patients have intestinal pseudo-obstruction
Treatment and prognosis	No effective medical or surgical treatments, but severely symptomatic patients are uncommon; prognosis is fair	No effective medical or surgical treatments; prognosis is poor because patients are severely ill
Extragastrointestinal manifestations	None	Malformation of central nervous system in some cases; patent ductus arteriosus

cases.[43,44] All patients in this group have died of intestinal pseudoobstruction during infancy.

CONNECTIVE TISSUE DISEASE

Connective tissue disease as a group (especially scleroderma) is the most common cause of CIP in adults.[45] Dilated loops of small intestine are seen in up to 50% of patients with scleroderma, but CIP occurs less frequently. Abnormal small intestinal motility occurs less commonly in other types of connective tissue disease such as dermatomyositis, systemic lupus erythematosus, and mixed connective tissue disease.

DIAGNOSTIC TESTS

RADIOLOGY TESTS

In patients with severe abnormal gastrointestinal motility, initial efforts should be directed toward ruling out mechanical obstruction. Only after this possibility has been eliminated should further investigation of the cause of CIP be undertaken. Plain abdominal roentgenograms must be obtained in symptomatic patients complaining of abdominal distension and pain. This often provides clues to enable localization of the abnormal organ. Air trapped in the diseased organ and air-fluid levels may be seen. In patients with gastroparesis, retained food and air are visible in the enlarged stomach. In intestinal pseudoobstruction, gaseous distension of the small bowel with air-fluid levels can be seen. In colonic pseudoobstruction, gaseous distension of the colon with air-fluid levels is visible. If the patient has generalized involvement of the gastrointestinal tract, a combination of all of the above may be noted. Barium contrast studies including esophagogram, upper gastrointestinal tract series, small bowel follow-through, or enteroclysis of the small bowel and barium enema may rule out mechanical obstruction.

BLOOD TESTS

A complete blood cell count may reveal anemia due to malabsorption from bacterial overgrowth syndrome. Blood chemistry values may also reflect malnutrition and malabsorption. Diabetic patients may have hyperglycemia. Thyroid diseases can be diagnosed by measuring serum triiodothyronine (T_3), thyroxine (T_4), and thyroid-stimulating hormone (TSH) levels. Elevated antinuclear antibody (ANA) levels indicate the need for collagen vascular disease workup. Patients with muscular dystrophies have elevated creatine phosphokinase (CPK) and isoenzyme levels. If Chagas' disease is suspected in patients from South America, hemagglutination and complement fixation tests should be obtained. Urinary porphyrins are positive in patients with porphyria.

Manometric Studies

Esophageal manometric studies are useful in evaluating patients with abnormal esophageal motility and dysphagia. Small intestinal manometric study is most useful and accurate at detecting small intestinal dysmotility; however, it cannot be used to diagnose any clinical syndrome or underlying disease. Anorectal and colonic manometric studies are useful in detecting abnormal motility of the anorectal area and the colon.

Histologic Studies

Full-thickness biopsy specimens taken from the dysfunctional part of the gastrointestinal tract, if available, usually distinguish muscle from nerve disease. Careful pathologic examination is important, and special study with silver stain for the myenteric plexus using Smith's method should be carried out if available.[46]

TREATMENT

Medical Treatment

Intestinal obstructive symptoms (abdominal distension, pain, and nausea and vomiting) occur intermittently in most patients. Only a small number of patients (approximately 10%) have persistent symptoms. These obstructive symptoms are directly related to meals. Therefore, by manipulating the amount, the nature, and the frequency of meals, patients with intermittent obstructive symptoms will become less symptomatic. Patients should consume 25 kcal/kg of ideal body weight per day divided into three or four equal amounts. At least half the calories should come from total feeding formulas such as Ensure, Isocal, or Vivonex because liquid empties faster from the stomach than a solid meal and probably progresses through the small bowel easier. A dietician can educate patients about the amount of calories in each type of food and ask patients to sample various types of feeding formulas to find some that are palatable. Carbonated beverages should be avoided to prevent adding excessive gas to the digestive tract. Fruit juice should be drunk instead. If patients have no appetite after the first meal, they should not force themselves to eat subsequent meals, because an obstructive episode can develop. In such cases, patients may need to fast, except for taking some fluid for that day. Occasionally, nasogastric suction and intravenous fluid are needed when obstructive symptoms are present. Persistent obstructive symptoms or the occurrence of symptoms several times a week despite diet manipulation requires the initiation of long-term parenteral nutrition to improve the patient's symptoms and nutritional status.

Abdominal pain unrelated to eating is uncommon in patients with CIP. During obstructive episodes, patients may require parenteral injection of narcotics such as morphine or meperidine. Long-term use of narcotics must be discouraged because of their addictive potential and their ability to further disturb gastrointestinal motility.

Oral antibiotics should be given to patients who have diarrhea and malabsorption from bacterial overgrowth. Alternating courses of tetracycline, ampicillin, trimethoprim-sulfamethoxazole (Bactrim), or metronidazole are recommended.

The prognosis of intestinal pseudoobstruction due to generalized involvement of the small intestine is poor because no effective medical treatment is available. Bethanechol, neostigmine, metoclopramide, cisapride, and domperidone are some of the prokinetic agents that have been tried, without good results.

Treating Underlying Systemic Disease

A few types of systemic disease causing gastrointestinal dysmotility, such as myxedema and celiac sprue, can be treated with thyroid replacement and gluten-free diets, respectively. Drug-induced gastrointestinal dysmotility can be improved by discontinuing the drug responsible for the adverse effect. Unfortunately, there is no effective medical treatment for patients with connective tissue disease or muscular dystrophies.

Surgical Treatment

Patients who have short segmental dysmotility of the small intestine, such as megaduodenum, have a better prognosis, because the dysfunctional segment can be resected or bypassed. Megaduodenum, which is commonly seen in type I FVM, scleroderma, and systemic lupus erythematosus, can be drained by a side-to-side duodenojejunostomy, and this procedure usually gives symptomatic relief to most patients. In some patients with a massively dilated duodenum, a side-to-side duodenojejunostomy may be inadequate to drain the duodenum. In such cases, subtotal duodenectomy and end-to-end duodenojejunostomy[47] may be required. For patients with long segmental dysfunction of the small intestine (over 1.2 m [4 ft] long), there is no effective surgical treatment. Any unnecessary surgery must be avoided in such patients, because it may create adhesions and more difficulties.

REFERENCES

1. Anuras S. Intestinal pseudoobstruction syndrome. *Annu Rev Med.* 1988;39:1.
2. Chokhavatia S, Anuras S. Neuromuscular disease of the gastrointestinal tract. *Am J Med Sci.* 1991;310:201.
3. Schuffler MD, Pope CE II. Studies of idiopathic intestinal pseudoobstruction. II. Hereditary hollow visceral myopathy: family studies. *Gastroenterology.* 1977;73:339.
4. Lewis TD, Daniel EE, Sarna SK, et al. Idiopathic intestinal pseudoobstruction: report of a case, with intraluminal studies of mechanical and electrical activity, and response to drugs. *Gastroenterology.* 1978;74:107.
5. Faulk DL, Anuras S, Gardner GD, et al. A familial visceral myopathy. *Ann Intern Med.* 1978;89:600.
6. Shaw A, Shaffer H, Teja K, et al. A perspective for pediatric surgeons: chronic idiopathic intestinal pseudoobstruction. *J Pediatr Surg.* 1979;14:719.
7. Weiss WW. Zur Atiologie Des Megaduodenums. *Dtsch Ztschr Chir.* 1938;251:317.
8. Law DH, Ten Eyck EA. Familial megaduodenum and megacystis. *Am J Med.* 1961;33:911.
9. Newton WT. Radical enterectomy for hereditary megaduodenum. *Arch Surg.* 1968;96:549.
10. Schuffler MD, Rohrmann CA, Chaffer RG, et al. Chronic intestinal pseudoobstruction: a report of 27 cases and review of the literature. *Medicine (Baltimore).* 1981;60:173.
11. Ducastelle T, Tranvouez JL, Lerebours E, et al. Myopathie viscérale héréditaire: une entité au sein des pseudo-obstructions intestinales idiopathiques. *Gastroenterol Clin Biol.* 1986;10:355.
12. Rodrigues CA, Shepherd NA, Lennard-Jones JE, et al. Familial visceral myopathy: a family with at least six involved members. *Gut.* 1989;30:1285.
13. Anuras S, Baker CRF Jr, Carter J, et al. Subtotal duodenectomy for massive dilatation of duodenum in patients with type I familial visceral myopathy. *Gastroenterology.* 1990;98:A323.
14. Eaves ER, Schmidt GT. Chronic idiopathic megaduodenum in a family. *Aust N Z J Med.* 1985;15:1.
15. Jones SC, Dixon MF, Lintott DJ, et al. Familial visceral myopathy: a family with involvement of four generations. *Dig Dis Sci.* 1992;37:464.
16. Bannister R, Hoyes AD. Generalised smooth-muscle disease with defective muscarinic-receptor function. *Br Med J.* 1981;282:1015.
17. Anuras S, Mitros FA, Nowak TV, et al. A familial visceral myopathy with external ophthalmoplegia and autosomal recessive transmission. *Gastroenterology.* 1983;84:346.
18. Ionasescu VV, Thompson HS, Aschenbrener C, et al. Late on-set oculogastrointestinal muscular dystrophy. *Am J Med Genet.* 1984;18:781.
19. Anuras S. A new family of small intestinal diverticulosis and external ophthalmoplegia. *Gastroenterology.* 1986;90:1328.
20. Faber J, Fich A, Steinberg A, et al. Familial intestinal pseudoobstruction dominated by a progressive neurologic disease at a young age. *Gastroenterology.* 1987;92:786.
21. Igarashi M, MacRae D, O-Uchi T, et al. Cochleo-saccular degeneration in one of three sisters with hereditary deafness, absent gastric motility, small bowel diverticulosis and progressive sensory neuropathy. *ORL J Otorhinolaryngol Relat Spec.* 1981;43:4.
22. Mulder NH, Que GS, Bartelink A, et al. Triad of duodenal megabulbus, diverticula and gastric atony in four siblings. *Neth J Med.* 1983;26:120.
23. Bardosi A, Creutfeldt W, DiMauro S, et al. Myo-, neuro-, gastrointestinal encephalopathy (MNGIE syndrome) due to partial deficiency of cytochrome-c-oxidase: a new mitochondrial multisystem disorder. *Acta Neuropathol (Berl).* 1987;74:248.
24. Cervera R, Bruix J, Bayes A, et al. Chronic intestinal pseudoobstruction and ophthalmoplegia in a patient with mitochondrial myopathy. *Gut.* 1988;29:544.
25. Cave DR, Compton CC. Case records of the Massachusetts General Hospital, Case 12-1990. *N Engl J Med.* 1990;322:829.
26. Anuras S, Mitros FA, Milano A, et al. A familial visceral myopathy with dilatation of the entire gastrointestinal tract. *Gastroenterology.* 1986;90:385.
27. Jacobs E, Ardichvili D, Perissino A, et al. A case of familial visceral myopathy with atrophy and fibrosis of the longitudinal muscle layer of the entire small bowel. *Gastroenterology.* 1979;77:745.
28. Alstead EM, Murphy MN, Flanagan AM, et al. Familial autonomic visceral myopathy with degeneration of muscularis mucosae. *J Clin Pathol.* 1988;41:424.
29. Strosberg JM, Peck B, Harris JR, eds. Scleroderma with intestinal involvement: fatal in two of a kindred. *J Rheumatol.* 1977;4:46.
30. Roy AD, Bharucha H, Nevin NC, et al. Idiopathic intestinal pseudoobstruction: a familial visceral neuropathy. *Clin Genet.* 1980;18:291.
31. Mayer EA, Schuffler MD, Rotter JI, et al. Familial visceral neuropathy with autosomal dominant transmission. *Gastroenterology.* 1986;91:1528.
32. Anuras S, Mukherjee SK, Dunn D, et al. A new family with autosomal dominant transmitted visceral neuropathy. *Gastroenterology.* 1988;94:A10.
33. Royer P, Ricour C, Nihoul-Fekete C, et al. Le syndrome familial de grêle court avec malrotation intestinale et stenose hypertrophique du pylore chez le nourrisson. *Arch Fr Pediatr.* 1974;31:223.
34. Tanner MS, Smith B, Lloyd JK. Functional intestinal obstruction due to deficiency of argyrophil neurones in the myenteric plexus: familial syndrome presenting with short small bowel malrotation, and pyloric hypertrophy. *Arch Dis Child.* 1976;51:837.
35. Laugier MMJ, Mercier C, Robert M, et al. Syndrome du grêle court avec malrotation intestinale et stenose hypertrophique du pylore. *Bordeaux Med.* 1975;8:419.
36. Nezelof C, Jaubert F, Lyon G. Syndrome familial associant grêle court, malrotation intestinale, hypertrophie du pylore et malformation cérébrale: étude anatomoclinique de trois observations. *Ann Anat Pathol.* 1976;21:401.
37. Sansaricq C, Chen WJ, Manka M, et al. Familial congenital short small bowel with associated defects. *Clin Pediatr.* 1983;23:453.
38. Harris DJ, Ashcraft KW, Beatty EC, et al. Natal teeth, patent ductus arteriosus and intestinal pseudo-obstruction: a lethal syndrome in the newborn. *Clin Genet.* 1976;9:479.

39. Kern IB, Harris MJ. Congenital short bowel. *Aust N Z J Surg.* 1973;42:283.
40. Schuffler MD, Bird TD, Sumi M, et al. A familial neuronal disease presenting as intestinal pseudoobstruction. *Gastroenterology.* 1978;75:889.
41. Anuras S, Mitros FA, Soper RT, et al. Chronic intestinal pseudoobstruction in young children. *Gastroenterology.* 1986;91:62.
42. Schuffler MD, Pagon RA, Schwartz R, et al. Visceral myopathy of the gastrointestinal and genitourinary tracts in infants. *Gastroenterology.* 1988;94:892.
43. Berdon WE, Baker DH, Blanc WA, et al. Megacystic-microcolon–intestinal hypoperistalsis syndrome. A new cause of intestinal obstruction in the newborn: report of radiologic findings in five newborn girls. *Am J Roentgenol Rad Ther Nucl Med.* 1976;126:856.
44. Young LW, Yunis EJ, Girdany BR, et al. Megacystis-microcolon–intestinal hypoperistalsis syndrome: additional clinical, radiologic, surgical and histopathologic aspects. *Am J Roentgenol.* 1981;136:749.
45. Chokhavatia S, Anuras S. Gastrointestinal smooth muscle dysfunction in systemic disease. In: Anuras S, ed. *Motility Disorders of the Gastrointestinal Tract.* New York, NY: Raven Press Publishers; 1992:211.
46. Smith BF. *The Neuropathy of the Alimentary Tract.* London: Edward Arnold; 1972.
47. Anuras S, Baker CRF Jr, Carter J, Stovall G, Shirazi SS, Novick DM. Subtotal duodenectomy for massive dilatation of duodenum in patients with type I familial visceral myopathy. *Gastroenterology.* 1990;98:A353.

64

Chronic Intestinal Pseudoobstruction in Childhood

PAUL E. HYMAN

Chronic intestinal pseudoobstruction is a term referring to a heterogeneous group of disorders that share a common constellation of symptoms and signs.[1] Pseudoobstruction describes a recurring symptom complex that may include abdominal pain, abdominal distension, nausea, vomiting, and constipation or diarrhea. Pseudoobstruction is a clinical diagnosis based on signs and symptoms of mechanical bowel obstruction in the absence of a physical obstruction. Many children with pseudoobstruction undergo multiple exploratory laparotomies in an effort to determine the anatomic cause for symptoms. It is now clear that pseudoobstruction describes a number of familial and nonfamilial disorders of gastrointestinal smooth muscle and the enteric nervous system. Pediatric forms of chronic intestinal pseudoobstruction encompass a number of conditions different from those that cause pseudoobstruction in adults and some forms that overlap. The primary forms of pseudoobstruction are both familial and nonfamilial, but in primary pseudoobstruction there is no identifiable causal systemic disease or drug.

Most forms of childhood pseudoobstruction are primary. Secondary forms of pseudoobstruction are more common in adults. (For example, causes of pseudoobstruction such as scleroderma and the muscular dystrophies are well recognized in adults.[1] Drugs such as opiates and anticholinergics are common causes of pseudoobstruction in adults.) Children and adults differ also in the severity of symptoms and signs. Of children born with pseudoobstruction, one third die in the first year of life because of complications related to the treatment of their condition. One third of infants and children with pseudoobstruction require total parenteral nutrition, and another one third require some form of tube feeding.[2] In children, pseudoobstruction is rarely a slowly degenerative disease, as it is in most adults. Because the newborn has little time to adapt or perhaps because of the effects of the disease on the developing intestine, in most cases pseudoobstruction appears to be a more malignant disease in children and infants than in adults.

ETIOLOGY

Most primary congenital forms of both neuropathic and myopathic pseudoobstruction are sporadic. That is, there is no family history, no associated syndrome, and no evidence of other predisposing factors such as toxins, infections, ischemia, or autoimmune disease. In a minority of cases chronic intestinal pseudoobstruction may result from a familial inherited disease. There are reports of autosomal dominant and recessive neuropathic and dominant and recessive myopathic patterns of inheritance.[3] In the autosomal dominant disease there is variability in expressivity and penetrance. Some of those affected die in childhood, but those less handicapped are able to reproduce.

Pseudoobstruction may result from in utero exposure to drugs or toxins during critical developmental periods. A few children with fetal alcohol syndrome and a few with narcotic-abusing mothers have neuropathic forms of pseudoobstruction. Presumably any substance that alters neuronal migration or maturation might affect the development of the myenteric plexus and cause pseudoobstruction. Secondary pseudoobstruction occurs in children with chromosomal abnormalities or syndromes. Children with Down syndrome may have abnormal esophageal motility, neuronal dysplasia in the myenteric plexus, and a higher incidence of Hirschsprung's disease than the general population. A few children with Down syndrome have a myenteric plexus neuropathy so generalized and so severe that they present with pseudoobstruction. Children with successfully treated neuroblastoma may present with pseudoobstruction long after measurable levels of circulating peptides are normal. Presumably a myenteric plexus abnormality represents just one part of the neurologic disorder that first presented as neuroblastoma. Children with neurofibromatosis, multiple endocrine neoplasia type 2b, and other chromosomal aberrations and autonomic neuropathies may suffer from severe neuropathic constipation. Children with Duchenne's muscular dystrophy sometimes develop pseudoobstruction, especially in the terminal stages of life. Esophageal manometry and gastric emptying test results are abnormal in Duchenne's muscular dystrophy, suggesting that the myopathy includes gastrointestinal smooth muscle, even in asymptomatic children.

In childhood, pseudoobstruction may be acquired following acute viral gastroenteritis. *Rotavirus*, the most common cause of viral gastroenteritis in children, is probably the most common offender. Other observations have implicated Epstein-Barr virus and cytomegalovirus infections of the myenteric plexus. Many acquired cases of pseudoobstruction might have resulted from myenteric plexus viral neuritis.

Perinatal asphyxia is a well-recognized cause of psychomotor retardation and developmental delay. The majority of children with cerebral palsy do not show evidence of pseudoobstruction. In the few that do have pseudoobstruction the myenteric plexus may have been injured by the same insult that resulted in central nervous system neuron death. Very preterm infants often have prolonged feeding difficulties. These difficulties may be in part related to immature motility patterns or to ischemia induced by the failure to meet the increased need for blood flow following feeding. Some infants with bronchopulmonary dysplasia appear to have severe gastrointestinal motility abnormalities. Their preterm birth and stormy courses including chronic hypoxemia and ischemia are consistent with the development of pseudoobstruction due to myenteric plexus injury or maturational arrest. A few children develop pseudoobstruction following neonatal necrotizing enterocolitis or gastroschisis, presumably for similar reasons of local ischemia and neuronal injury or maturational arrest.

It is possible that some cases of pseudoobstruction may be mediated by an abnormality of the immune system. Many affected infants and toddlers have food allergies, and a few older children have pseudoobstruction associated with autoimmune features such as persistently positive antinuclear antibodies (ANA) or systemic rhabdomyolysis.

PATHOLOGY[4,5]

The pathology of chronic intestinal pseudoobstruction typifies the heterogeneity of these conditions. The histopathology of tissues from patients with pseudoobstruction may be divided into three subclassifications: (1) myopathy, (2) neuropathy, and (3) no observable abnormalities. Smooth muscle degeneration and fibrosis are characteristics of myopathy. Often, but not always, the circular muscle layer is more involved than the longitudinal muscle. The pathologic features may be patchy in some cases; abnormalities may be subtle even when function is severely impaired. Neuropathies are far more common than myopathies but are more difficult to evaluate. Myopathies are evident in routine cross-sectional studies with metachromatic dyes like hematoxylin and eosin. Neuropathic abnormalities require tangential sections of the gut wall and special stains such as silver impregnation or immunohistochemistry for nerve-specific protein receptors and peptide neurotransmitters. Only a few centers specializing in neurohistopathology of the gut accept specimens for evaluation. These special stains may reveal abnormalities in nerve cell number or morphology. Occasionally, there are intranuclear inclusions within neurons.

In a number of infants and children with severe pseudoobstruction, no histologic abnormalities are discovered. Presumably these children have a defect in a receptor or neurotransmitter or other protein that has no effect on tissue histology but alters function.

The specific histopathologic diagnosis does not alter supportive care or drug therapy (see below). Therefore, it is not advisable to plan laparotomies specifically for the purpose of obtaining a full thickness biopsy for histopathologic evaluation. However, histopathology may add information that complements other diagnostic tests such as intestinal manometry. If laparotomy is planned for a purpose that includes enterotomy, such as a feeding jejunostomy, it may be useful to obtain a full thickness biopsy specimen for careful histopathologic evaluation at a center that specializes in the evaluation of the intestinal neuropathies. The appendix and gallbladder are not satisfactory tissues for evaluation of myenteric plexus abnormalities.

DIAGNOSIS

Rarely an early diagnosis of chronic intestinal pseudoobstruction occurs when a fetal ultrasound examination demonstrates abdominal distension, bladder distension, and polyhydramnios. With urinary tract obstruction alone, amniotic fluid is decreased. With intestinal obstruction alone, amniotic fluid is increased. The unique combination of polyhydramnios and bladder distension suggests a diagnosis of the megacystis-microcolon–intestinal hypoperistalsis syndrome.

The most severe phenotype of congenital chronic intestinal pseudoobstruction is the megacystis-microcolon–intestinal hypoperistalsis syndrome. In this disorder there is a functional obstruction of the gastrointestinal and urinary tracts' smooth muscle. The severe abdominal distension may impair respiratory efforts, and children with this condition require immediate surgical intervention. A vesicostomy is placed to relieve the bladder distension and to serve as a conduit for urine. A gastrostomy may be placed to provide gastric and intestinal decompression. A central venous catheter is necessary for provision of total parenteral nutrition. Megacystis-microcolon–intestinal hypoperistalsis syndrome is a particular phenotype that may result from either hollow visceral myopathy or hollow visceral neuropathy. Mortality in these newborn infants is high, but a number of children with this condition have gained at least partial bladder and bowel function as they grow older.

Over half the affected children develop symptoms at or shortly after birth. Approximately two thirds of children with congenital symptoms are born preterm. Intestinal malrotation is found in about 40% of children with congenital forms of pseudoobstruction regardless of whether it is neuropathic or myopathic. In some children symptoms are mistakenly attributed to the malrotation, but the intrinsic motility disturbance is recognized after correction of the malrotation fails to relieve symptoms.[6] In the most severely affected infants, including those with megacystis-microcolon–intestinal hypoperistalsis syndrome, symptoms of acute bowel obstruction appear within the first hours of life. Less severely affected infants present during infancy with symptoms of vomiting and diarrhea and failure to thrive. Over 75% of children develop symptoms by the end of the first year, and the remainder present sporadically through the next two decades.

There is great individual variation in the number and intensity of signs and symptoms. Signs and symptoms change with age and with medical intervention. Abdominal distension and vomiting are the most common features and are found in about three quarters of the patients. Constipation, abdominal pain, and poor weight gain are features in 60%. Diarrhea is a complaint in one third. Anorexia or early satiety occurs in a third. Urinary tract smooth muscle is affected in those with both hollow visceral neuropathy and hollow visceral myopathy, about one fifth of all pseudoobstruction patients. Chronic intestinal pseudoobstruction is frequently characterized by relative remissions and exacerbations. Parents are frequently able to identify factors that precipitate deterioration in the affected children. These factors include intercurrent infections, general anesthesia, psychologic stress, and poor nutritional status.

The radiographic signs are those of intestinal

obstruction. Plain x-ray films of the abdomen demonstrate gaseous distension and, in upright films, the presence of fluid levels in distended bowel loops. In those studied at birth microcolon is frequently found. The absence of propagating motility in chronic intestinal pseudoobstruction may be responsible for prolonged stasis of contrast material placed into the affected bowel. Therefore it is prudent to plan a means to evacuate nonsoluble contrast or to use a nontoxic isotonic water-soluble contrast to prevent residual barium from solidifying and presenting a true anatomic obstruction. Some children who are feeling well still show radiographic evidence of bowel obstruction on plain x-ray films. The greater problem arises when children develop an acute deterioration. Plain films showing air-fluid levels do not differentiate between anatomic and functional obstruction. In children who have had previous abdominal injury, it may be difficult to discriminate between physical obstruction related to adhesion and exacerbation of pseudoobstruction. At such time an enteroclysis study may be useful, but laparotomy is occasionally required.

Pseudoobstruction is commonly misdiagnosed in infants and children, despite the dramatic life-threatening clinical presentation in many children.[7] The time between the onset of symptoms and the diagnosis has averaged about 3 years, as physicians mistakenly contribute the symptoms to more common conditions. Delayed diagnosis could frequently be attributed to the primary physician's conviction that a psychiatric diagnosis was at the root of symptoms that were unexplainable by the common laboratory and radiographic investigations. Pseudoobstruction with intractable vomiting has been mistakenly diagnosed as a conversion disorder—a psychologic process whereby a physical symptom is substituted for an intrapsychic conflict resulting in the temporary loss of physical functioning.

Somatization is the process whereby psychologic distress is expressed in physical symptoms. A somatoform disorder is one in which somatic symptoms suggest a physical disorder, but for which no organic cause can be demonstrated. In somatoform disorder there is presumptive evidence of a psychologic basis for the disorder. In patients with pseudoobstruction who have been diagnosed as having a somatoform disorder, the appropriate testing has not been completed to demonstrate organic cause. In many patients and their families there is clear evidence of a maladaptation to the child's chronic illness, which is misinterpreted as a primary psychiatric

TABLE 64–1. WARNING SIGNS OF MUNCHAUSEN SYNDROME BY PROXY

Unexplained persistent or recurrent illness
Rare disorder as the primary diagnosis
Experienced physicians state they "have never seen a case like it!"
Investigations at variance with the health of the child
Overattentive mother who will not leave the child
Treatments not tolerated (IV lines get infected; drugs are vomited)
Mother complains that too little is being done to help the child

Adapted from Reece RM: Unusual manifestations of child abuse. *Pediatr Clin North Am.* 1990;37:905–921.

problem's being the root of the child's symptoms. Instead it is the anxiety, depression, and anger related to an inability to find appropriate diagnosis and treatment that cause secondary psychiatric symptoms.

Munchausen syndrome by proxy is a particularly malignant form of psychiatric disorder in which a parent uses her own children to provide dramatic entry into the health care system. The involved parent appears to be a highly involved, motivated, caring parent, eliciting sympathetic interest and involvement from hospital staff. The sociocultural setting of Munchausen syndrome by proxy and pseudoobstruction have much in common (see Table 64–1). To differentiate Munchausen syndrome by proxy from chronic intestinal pseudoobstruction is difficult. First, it is necessary to demonstrate that studies of intestinal transit and contraction are normal. Next, one separates the child from the mother and determines if symptoms resolve. Rarely, in cases of Munchausen syndrome by proxy masquerading as chronic intestinal pseudoobstruction, it has been possible to demonstrate the particular poison in use, such as ipecac.[8]

DIAGNOSTIC TESTING: RADIONUCLIDE SCINTIGRAPHY AND MANOMETRY

In mildly affected individuals, the gastric emptying of a solid nutrient meal is the best single screening test for gastroparesis. However, infants do not eat solids, and in severely affected children very delayed gastric emptying is found even with liquids. Radionuclide tests of intestinal or colonic transit have not been used in a clinical setting for pediatric patients.

Approximately half the children affected by pseudoobstruction have abnormalities in esophageal manometry. In children with myopathy, contractions are low amplitude but coordinated in the distal two thirds of the esophagus. Lower esophageal sphincter is low, and relaxation of the sphincter is complete. In children with neuropathy, the amplitude of contractions in the esophageal body may be high, normal, low, or absent. There may be simultaneous, spontaneous, or repetitive contractions. There may be incomplete relaxation of the lower esophageal sphincter.

Manometric studies of the gastric antrum and small bowel should not be used to diagnose pseudoobstruction. Chronic intestinal pseudoobstruction is a clinical diagnosis that is based on symptoms in the absence of a lesion that can be defined radiographically or at exploratory laparotomy. Before antroduodenal manometry is used to define the physiology of a motor disorder, it is imperative to eliminate the possibility of an anatomic blockage either with standard contrast radiography, enteroclysis "small bowel enema," or exploratory laparotomy. Although two patterns of antroduodenal manometry suggest mechanical obstruction in adults,[9,10] these patterns seem to be both insensitive and nonspecific in children. Thus, a sustained pattern of clustered contractions separated by periods of motor quiescence of variable duration is characteristic of mechanical obstruction in adults, but is normal in preterm infants and suggests neuropathic pseudoobstruction in older infants. The second pattern, repetitive simultaneous prolonged contractions in the proximal small bowel, is likewise neither a specific nor sensitive marker of anatomic obstruction in children.

Antroduodenal manometry is useful for characterizing the pathophysiology of undiagnosed chronic intestinal motility disorders. Moreover, it can be useful in determining the absence of physiologic abnormalities in Munchausen syndrome by proxy and in demonstrating characteristic increases in intraabdominal pressure without intestinal abnormalities in children with the "adult" rumination syndrome of repetitive gentle regurgitations.

Manometric studies are more sensitive than radiographic tests to evaluate the strength and coordination of contraction and relaxation in the gastrointestinal tract. Antroduodenal manometry is always abnormal in intestinal pseudoobstruction involving the upper gastrointestinal tract. In most cases the manometric disorganization correlates with the clinical severity. Visual inspection of the manometric record is usually sufficient to determine presence or absence of various features. Healthy features include the presence of the migrating motor complex (MMC) during fasting. The MMC consists of three different phases that cycle continuously from the stomach to the ileum during fasting. Phase 1 is a period of no contraction. Phase 2, a period of random contractions varying in amplitude and periodicity, is indistinguishable from the normal postprandial pattern. Phase 3 is a distinctive pattern of high-amplitude contractions that repeat at a rate of three per minute in the antrum and 11 to 13 per minute in the duodenum, persisting for 3 to 7 minutes and migrating from proximal to distal (Fig. 64–1A). The duration of the full cycle varies from an average of 45 minutes in the newborn to 100 minutes in children and adults. The presence of the MMC during fasting and the replacement of the MMC by a phase 2–like pattern (Fig. 64–1B) after a meal are the features of a study with normal results. The absence of either of these features or the presence of unexpected patterns of contraction define the features of the intestinal manometry.[11] Abnormal features during fasting include:

1. Absence of phase 3 of the MMC after 4 hours of recording
2. Absence of phase 2 of the MMC
3. Nonpropagating bursts of duodenal contractions (Fig. 64–2A)
4. Nonpropagated tonic duodenal contractions (Fig. 64–2B)
5. Absent or persistently low-amplitude contractions
6. Retrograde phase 3–like contractions

Postprandial abnormalities include phase 3–like contractions within the first 40 minutes after completion of a meal, persistent phase 1–like activity, and postprandial hypomotility. Neuropathic disorders yield results in which the contractions are normal in amplitude but disorganized. Myopathic pseudoobstruction results in contractions that are persistently low amplitude and coordinated. The presence of the MMC predicts the ability of the patient to eat. That is, 90% of children with phase 3 of the MMC are able to be fed enterally, and 90% of those without phase 3 of the MMC require parenteral nutritional support.[12] Antroduodenal manometry may be useful in explaining the child's condition to the parents. In addition, the manometric result may be useful in predicting the efficacy of specific drug therapy or nutritional support.

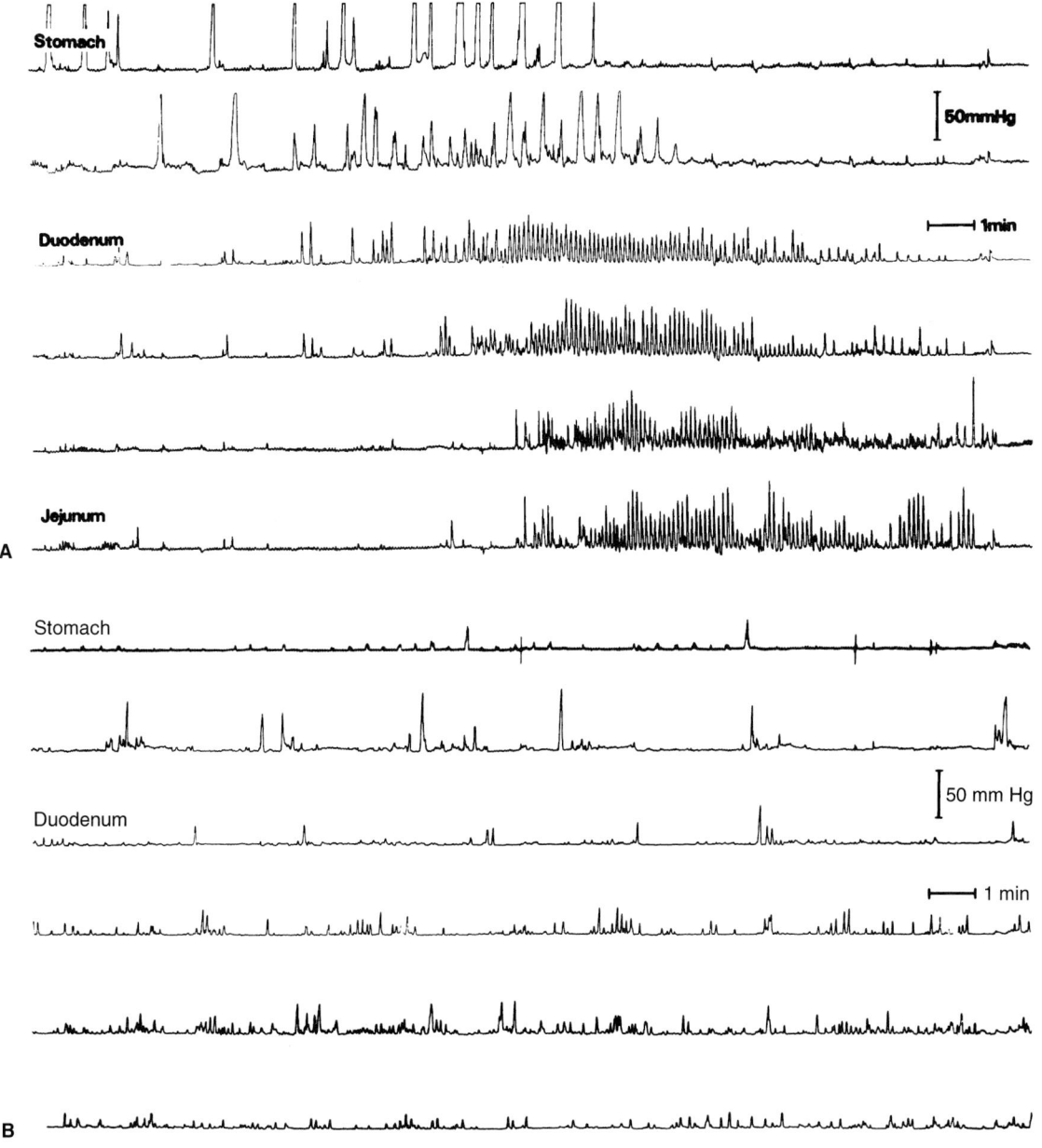

FIGURE 64–1. Examples of normal antroduodenal manometry. **A,** Phase 3 of the migrating motor complex. **B,** Phase 2 of the migrating motor complex, consisting of random, variable-amplitude, intermittent contractions.

Colonic manometry is useful for determining the pathophysiology of intractable constipation.[13] There are two characteristics of colon manometry that indicate a normal study. First is the presence of high-amplitude propagating contractions (HAPCs), defined as contractions with an amplitude of >60 mm Hg propagating aborally for 30 cm or more. Second, the total motor activity or motility index increases following a meal, a characteristic known as the gastrocolonic response. The presence of HAPCs and the gastrocolonic response indicate a patient with constipation that is of behavioral origin. On the other hand, the total absence of contrac-

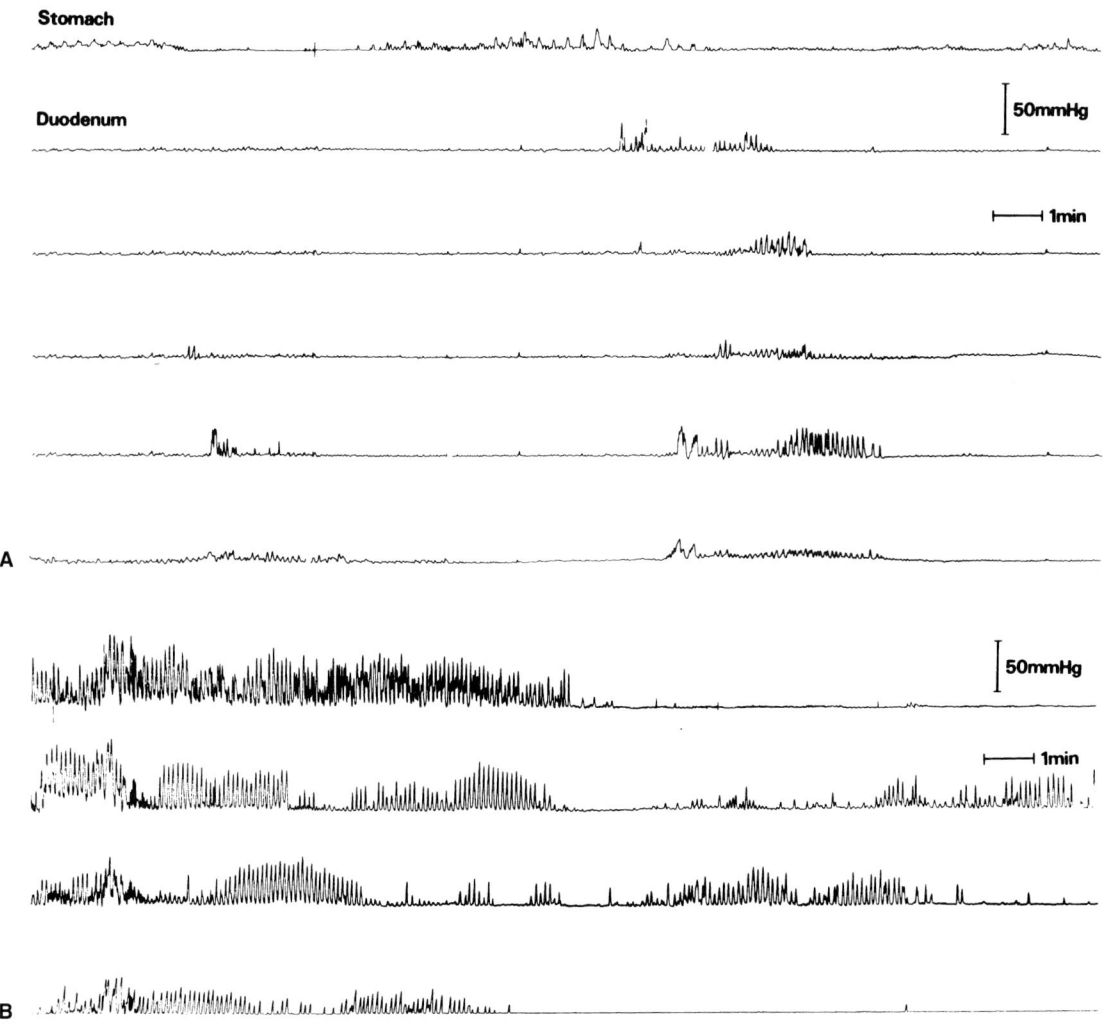

FIGURE 64-2. Examples of abnormal antroduodenal manometry. **A,** Persistently low amplitude coordinated contractions in the absence of dilated bowel is characteristic of myopathy. Here phase 3 is present, but amplitude is low. **B,** Clusters of nonpropagating contractions are characteristic of some neuropathies.

tion is typical of hollow visceral myopathy. The absence of HAPCs and a gastrocolonic response and the presence of tonic and phasic contractions are characteristic of neuropathic disease.

TREATMENT

Once the diagnosis of pseudoobstruction is established, it is generally accepted that there is no cure to this chronic illness. In some cases there are long spontaneous remissions. In other cases the condition appears to be static. In a number of children and adolescents there are episodes lasting weeks or months, with a spontaneous return to baseline. Finally in a few cases, there is slow but inexorable deterioration. Therapeutic measures are aimed chiefly at providing superior nutritional support and reducing symptoms to improve the quality of life.

About a third of children with pseudoobstruction require parenteral nutrition, and another third require some form of enteral tube feeding. In patients with megacystis-microcolon–intestinal hypoperistalsis syndrome, total parenteral nutrition (TPN) has been a mainstay of supportive care. The severity of TPN-associated cholestatic liver disease is correlated with the maturation of the liver at the time when TPN was initiated and the duration of TPN. Thus, a number of children born prematurely with hollow visceral myopathy or hollow visceral neuropathy develop cirrhosis in the first year of life and succumb to liver failure in the first 5 years of life. It has been a clinical observation that providing 10% to 20% of the total calorie requirement through enteral feeding prevents or delays the onset of TPN-associated liver disease. Since TPN has become readily available throughout North America, deaths from pseudoobstruction rarely occur as a direct consequence of the disease but are most often related to complications of parenteral nutrition. Thus, bacterial or fungal sepsis, TPN-associated liver disease including cholelithiasis, and other catheter-related complications such as perforation of a great vessel or malfunction of an infusion pump are the most frequent causes of death in children with chronic intestinal pseudoobstruction. For this reason every effort should be extended to provide nutritional support via the enteral route.

Children are more likely to adapt to enteral feeding if the bowel is not dilated and the migrating motor complex is present. In adults a gastrostomy for decompression decreases hospital admissions for chronic intestinal pseudoobstruction.[14] Gastrostomy for decompression in children may be useful for the treatment of dilated bowel. Some bowel function may return as the bowel diameter decreases. The gastrostomy tube may be used for continuous drip or bolus enteral feeding, as well as for decompression. TPN-dependent children may have aversion to food placed in their mouths in the first few years of life. Therefore a gastrostomy tube may be placed to establish a route to initiate enteral feedings, as well as to simplify administration of medications.

When gastroparesis is severe but small intestinal involvement is not, it is possible to use the gastrostomy tube for decompression and to place a jejunostomy tube for feeding. In a subset of infants and children without distal bowel dilation, there has been excellent success with jejunostomy tube feedings. In infants and toddlers, when gastrostomy tube feedings failed, the placement of a jejunostomy tube bypassed severe gastroparesis and allowed 10% to 20% or more of the total caloric requirements to be received enterally. The experience with jejunostomy in children is different from that published for adults in terms of success.[14] This discrepancy may be a result of subject selection, the pathophysiology of the underlying disorders, or improving technical skills. A surgically placed jejunostomy tube is superior to a jejunal feeding tube placed through a gastrostomy. The underlying motility disorder frequently causes reflux of a jejunal feeding tube, so that surgically placed tubes offer the only secure access in most cases.

Gastrostomy and jejunostomy provide access for decompression and feeding. Subtotal enterectomy may improve the quality of life for patients disabled by a massively dilated abdomen or those with severe unrelenting abdominal pain. Enterectomy may be an appropriate treatment for those receiving TPN after repeated central venous catheter infections with bowel flora. Subtotal enterectomy may be performed months or years prior to small bowel transplantation without complicating the latter procedure. Colectomy is an alternative for those with intractable constipation and fewer signs and symptoms of upper gastrointestinal tract involvement. However, an abnormality of the myenteric plexus may not recognize anatomic boundaries and often extends proximal to the colon in children with intractable constipation. Postcolectomy complications of continuing obstruction and pain may require further bowel resection in a substantial proportion of children selected for colectomy. Unfortunately, at this time there is no way to evaluate ileal motility in children. Prolonged periods of colonic diversion are not desirable because of the frequency of diversion colitis.[15]

Repeated exploratory laparotomies usually accrue in the first year of life before pseudoobstruction is considered in the differential diagnosis.

When performed in children with gastroparesis, fundoplication to stop vomiting often results in a constellation of signs and symptoms characterized by postprandial repeated retching, abdominal distension, abdominal pain, and diaphoresis, followed by stupor. Fundoplication should be avoided in children with pseudoobstruction.[16]

Small bowel transplantation is the curative surgery for chronic intestinal pseudoobstruction. Bowel transplantation is now performed at a number of transplantation centers in North America. Small bowel transplantation is often performed in tandem with liver transplantation. It appears as though immunologic factors are more favorable when the liver is transplanted with small bowel. Small bowel and liver transplantation may be especially important in children with TPN-associated liver disease. In such cases it is the liver transplant that is lifesaving, even though the small bowel allograft is curative. Several children with pseudoobstruction have undergone small bowel transplantation at different centers. Long-term results are unavailable at this time. There is great hope that small bowel transplantation will be effective.

Treatment with prokinetic drugs, especially cisapride, has been a useful adjunct to therapy in a sizable minority of children with chronic intestinal pseudoobstruction. Response to cisapride in children has been linked to the presence of the MMC and the absence of dilated bowel.[12] Cisapride appears to act by increasing the number and strength of intestinal contractions.[17] It is most effective for postprandial hypomotility, a condition that is diagnosed manometrically as normal fasting motility but displays a paucity of duodenal contractions after eating. Children with postprandial hypomotility frequently advance from continuous drip feedings to oral feedings with initiation of cisapride treatment. Children with postprandial hypomotility account for 3% to 5% of those diagnosed with chronic intestinal pseudoobstruction in childhood. In other types of enteric neuromuscular disorders cisapride sometimes increases appetite, decreases abdominal distension, and increases the frequency of spontaneous bowel movements. Half the children with pseudoobstruction do not respond to cisapride. Because oral forms of the drug may not be absorbed from children with severe gastroparesis, cisapride may be useful when used in combination with a jejunal feeding tube, thus bypassing the stomach. Recommended doses are 0.15 to 0.30 mg/kg/dose given three to four times daily with doses spaced at least 4 hours apart. There are anecdotal reports from Europe that much higher doses may be useful. The motilin agonist erythromycin in doses of 1 to 3 mg/kg intravenously or 3 to 5 mg/kg orally two or three times a day may be useful in cases of isolated gastroparesis. Erythromycin stimulates high-amplitude (three per minute) contractions in the gastric antrum. These are propagated as phase 3 of the MMC in children who have spontaneous phase 3 episodes but not in children without the MMC.

Other prokinetic agents such as bethanechol, neostigmine, and metoclopramide are not effective in chronic intestinal pseudoobstruction.

Antibiotic treatment for small bowel overgrowth is sometimes useful for eliminating diarrhea and decreasing abdominal distension.

Treatment of chronic visceral pain in children is difficult. Narcotics are to be avoided for chronic pain, because narcotics reduce bowel transit, and withdrawal is associated with pain that cannot be differentiated from the pain of pseudoobstruction. Relaxation techniques and self-hypnosis may be taught to older compliant children. Amitriptyline (Elavil) may increase the pain threshold in a minority of children.

REFERENCES

1. Christensen J, Dent J, Malagelada J-R, Wingate DL. Pseudo-obstruction. *Gastroenterology Int.* 1990;3:107–119.
2. Vargas JH, Sachs P, Ament ME. Chronic intestinal pseudo-obstruction syndrome in pediatrics: results of a national survey by members of the North American Society of Pediatric Gastroenterology and Nutrition. *J Pediatr Gastroenterol Nutr.* 1988;7:323–332.
3. Krishnamurthy S, Schuffler MD. Pathology of neuromuscular disorders of the small intestine and colon. *Gastroenterology.* 1987;93:610–639.
4. Lake BD. Observations on the pathology of pseudo-obstruction. In: Milla PJ, ed. *Disorders of Gastrointestinal Motility in Childhood.* New York, NY: John Wiley & Sons Inc; 81–90.
5. Schofield ED, Yunis EJ. Intestinal neuronal dysplasia. *J Pediatr Gastroenterol Nutr.* 1991;12:182–189.
6. Devane SP, Coobes R, Smith VV, et al. Persistent gastrointestinal symptoms after correction of malrotation. *Arch Dis Child.* 1991;218–221.
7. Glassman M, Spivak W, Mininberg D, Madara J. Chronic idiopathic intestinal pseudo-obstruction: a commonly misdiagnosed disease in infants and children. *Pediatrics.* 1989;83:603–608.
8. McClung HJ, Murray R, Braden NJ, Fyda J, Myers RP, Gutches L. Intentional ipecac poisoning in children. *Am J Dis Child.* 1988;142:637–639.
9. Summers RW, Anuras S, Green J. Jejunal manometry patterns in health, partial intestinal obstruction, and pseudo-obstruction. *Gastroenterology.* 1983;85:1301–1306.
10. Camilleri M. Jejunal manometry in distal subacute mechanical obstruction: significance of prolonged simultaneous contractions. *Gut.* 1989;30:468–475.
11. Hyman PE, Napolitano JA, Diego A, et al. Antroduodenal manometry in the evaluation of chronic functional gastrointestinal symptoms. *Pediatrics.* 1990;86:39–44.
12. Hyman PE, DiLorenzo C, McAdams L, Flores AF, Martin S, Tomomasa T. Predicting the clinical response to cisapride in children with chronic intestinal pseudoobstruction. *Am J Gastroenterol.* In press.
13. DiLorenzo C, Flores A, Reddy SN, Hyman PE. Colonic manometry differentiates causes of intractable constipation in children. *J Pediatr.* 1992;120:690–695.
14. Pitt HA, Mann LL, Berquist WE, et al. Chronic intestinal pseudo-obstruction: management with total parenteral nutrition and a venting enterostomy. *Arch Surg.* 1985;120:614–618.
15. DiSario JA, Foutch PG, Sanowski RA. Poor results with percutaneous endoscopic jejunostomy. *Gastrointest Endosc.* 1990;36:257–260.
16. Ordein J, DiLorenzo C, Flores A, Hyman PE. Diversion colitis in children with pseudo-obstruction. *Am J Gastroenterol.* 1992;87:88–90.
17. DiLorenzo C, Reddy SN, Villanueva-Meyer J, et al. Cisapride in children with chronic intestinal pseudoobstruction: an acute, double-blind crossover placebo controlled trial. *Gastroenterology.* 1991;101:1564–1570.

65
Short Bowel Syndrome

ROBERT G. GISH and EMMET B. KEEFFE

The term *short bowel syndrome* refers to a complex group of clinical signs and symptoms caused by significant reduction in the functional absorptive surface of the small intestine, typically as a result of Crohn's disease or major small bowel resection.[1] Small segments of jejunum or ileum can be resected with few sequelae, but removal of large segments of small bowel results in significant malabsorption requiring specialized treatment. Advances in medical and surgical management have resulted in an increased number of long-term survivors after extensive bowel resection leaving a short residual length of intestine.[2] Management of individuals with the short bowel syndrome requires understanding of the syndrome's pathophysiology and awareness of the complications that may result from a short bowel. Small bowel transplantation is a new treatment that may allow some individuals to become independent of total parenteral nutrition (TPN) and be spared many of the complications of the short bowel syndrome.[3]

PATHOPHYSIOLOGY

To plan therapy for patients with short bowel syndrome (Table 65–1), it is important to determine three factors:

1. The anatomic segment that has been resected
2. The approximate length of intestine that has been resected
3. The indication for small bowel resection

The two most common disorders resulting in short bowel syndrome are Crohn's disease with multiple bowel resections and massive intestinal resection following bowel infarction from compromised mesenteric arterial or venous blood flow. Other causes of short bowel syndrome are less common, and some conditions occur exclusively in infants and children. Factors other than the site and extent of resection that account for the severity of malabsorption in patients with short bowel syndrome are the presence or absence of the ileocecal valve, degree of adaptation in the remaining intestine, and the presence of any residual bowel disease (e.g., Crohn's disease). Removal of part of the stomach and the presence or absence of residual disease in the remaining small bowel will influence the patient's postoperative course. The contribution of these pathophysiologic factors are reviewed briefly in this section to provide a framework for discussion of therapy.

SMALL BOWEL

Although it is often difficult to estimate the actual length of bowel resected, removal of up to one half of the small intestine is associated with satisfactory nutrient absorption. The small bowel and colon that remain after intestinal resection both undergo an adaptive response. Up to a fourfold increase in the absorptive area of the small bowel may occur from villous hyperplasia. The full adaptive response takes up to 2 years to occur. Proximal small bowel resection results in a more extensive intestinal adaptive response than distal resection. In patients undergoing jejunoileal bypass surgery, the length of remaining intestine increases (80% to 120%), and the luminal diameter also increases (40% to 50%). The added absorptive surface increases the absorption of most nutrients. In fact, oral feeding with secretion of pancreatic and biliary juices into the intestinal lumen promotes this process; thus, early feeding is an important goal of therapy. Patients with short bowel syndrome who have undergone ileal resection have been divided into two subgroups: (1) individuals with an end-jejunostomy and (2) individuals with the jejunum in continuity with the colon. Patients with an end-jejunostomy and residual length of small bowel less than 100 cm almost always require long-term TPN. These patients, who lack a

TABLE 65–1. CONDITIONS LEADING TO MAJOR INTESTINAL RESECTION AND SHORT BOWEL SYNDROME

Compromised mesenteric arterial blood supply or venous thrombosis with bowel infarction secondary to
  Volvulus
  Intestinal strangulation
  Antithrombin III deficiency
  Protein C or S deficiency
  Antiphospholipid antibody syndrome
Crohn's disease
Radiation enteritis
Strangulated hernias
Trauma
Obesity treated by
  Jejunoileal bypass
  Gastric-intestinal bypass
Inadvertent gastric bypass to ileum
Resection of small bowel tumors
Desmoid disease
Pediatric conditions:
  Aganglionosis
  Neonatal necrotizing enterocolitis
  Abdominal wall defect (gastroschisis)
  Intestinal atresia
  Malrotation with midgut volvulus
  Segmental volvulus

TABLE 65–2. COMPLICATIONS OF THE SHORT BOWEL SYNDROME

Dehydration
Electrolyte abnormalities
  Hypokalemia
  Hypocalcemia
  Hypomagnesemia
Zinc deficiency
Selenium deficiency
D-lactic hyperchloremic acidosis
Chronic bacterial overgrowth
Steatorrhea
Bile acid malabsorption
  Choleretic diarrhea
Fat-soluble vitamin deficiency
Vitamin B_{12} malabsorption
Renal oxalate stones
Lithogenic bile and gallstones
Gastric acid hypersecretion
Rapid gastric emptying of liquids
TPN-induced liver disease
  Cholestatic liver disease
  Cirrhosis with liver failure
Malabsorption of medications
  Antibiotics
  Cyclosporine
Chronic hypoglycemia with sinus bradycardia

TPN = total parenteral nutrition.

colon, may present with a wide variety of complications (Table 65–2).

ILEOCECAL VALVE AND COLON

The presence of the colon in continuity with the small bowel significantly improves the ability of patients to maintain an adequate volume status, normal electrolyte balance, and satisfactory nutrition. Hyperplasia of the colonic mucosa also occurs after intestinal resection and may lead to an increase in fluid absorption with a subsequent decrease in daily fluid requirements. This adaptive response in the colon allows adult patients to survive with as little as 50 cm of remaining small bowel. The colon also plays an important role in slowing gastric emptying and inducing hyperplasia of the small bowel mucosa. The presence of an ileocecal valve and colon does not seem to correlate with the ability to ultimately discontinue TPN, but it does decrease the mean time for stopping intravenous nutrition in those individuals who can permanently be weaned from TPN. The absence of an ileocecal valve is associated with an increased incidence of bacterial overgrowth in the small intestine. Identification of this problem can be documented by the use of the breath hydrogen test or by improvement in diarrhea by an empiric trial of broad spectrum antibiotics.

Colonic preservation results in an increased incidence of renal (oxalate) stones but does not change the high prevalence of gallstones in patients with short bowel syndrome (40%). A special low-oxalate diet may decrease the frequency of renal stones in this setting, but there is no evidence that ursodeoxycholic acid has any clinical utility in preventing gallstone disease.

MOTILITY DISORDERS

The stomach and intestine have an integrated motility system that requires an intact enteric nervous system and feedback from the colon. With removal of the colon, gastric motility is altered and leads to early emptying of liquids from the stomach. The arrival of liquid in the colon normally promotes slowing of gastric emptying, which maintains a steady pace in the delivery of gastric contents into the small bowel and improves absorption. Removal of the "colon brake" and resultant rapid gastric emptying demonstrates the importance of the feedback loop from the colon and explains the higher ostomy volume and electrolyte losses in patients with an end-jejunostomy.[4] The small bowel transit time for both liquids and solids is increased in patients without a colon. Reduction in the amount of free water consumed orally may reduce the impact of rapid gastric emptying. Also, acid exposure to the small intestine is a determinant in the slowing of gastric emptying.[5] In addition, agents that decrease intestinal motility, such as fiber, loperamide, or anticholinergic agents, may decrease rapid fluid delivery to the distal small bowel.

Pediatric Patients

Pediatric patients with short bowel syndrome may present with a special group of problems. These patients have a lower absorptive surface per unit of energy intake and a smaller total intestinal surface area. Infants with less than 6 cm of small bowel beyond the ligament of Treitz generally do not survive. If the ileocecal valve is removed, the length of small intestine required to sustain life is 15 cm. In a national study of infants with short bowel syndrome, medical and surgical treatment could be predicted to be successful only if there was more than 20 cm of remaining small bowel in patients with an intact ileocecal valve or 30 cm of small bowel in patients without an ileocecal valve.

TREATMENT

The management of short bowel syndrome is different in the early postoperative period when patients are kept fasting compared with the later stages of recovery when some variety of feeding is initiated. Thus, combinations of parenteral and enteral therapy are used to provide nutrient requirements during the postoperative recovery phase and occasionally during the long term, although many patients can maintain satisfactory nutrition with oral feedings.[6]

Parenteral and Enteral Nutrition

The postsurgical course of patients with short bowel syndrome can be divided into three phases. The first phase involves the initiation of TPN therapy as the sole treatment for 7 to 10 days to allow healing of intestinal anastomoses and return of bowel function. During this phase, it is common practice to place an indwelling central venous catheter. Management of fluids and electrolytes is the major focus during this initial phase. In the second phase, continuous enteral feeding is begun slowly with an elemental formula via a nasogastric or nasoenteral tube at a low infusion rate. The enteral feeding rate is increased depending on patient tolerance. The osmolality of the liquid supplement and the "threshold of absorption" (the functional surface area of the gut) are important in determining early outcome of dietary supplementation. In the third phase, oral feeding with a modified diet is initiated after tolerance to the instillation of nutrients has been demonstrated by successful enteral feeding. For children, Pregestimil, Nutramigen, and Alimentum could be considered as the initial feeding supplement. Two formulas for adults that are useful in the short bowel syndrome are Vital and Vivonex. In each phase of the refeeding process, adequate carbohydrate, protein, and lipids, as well as electrolyte and vitamin supplements, must be administered. Ideally, all daily nutritional requirements should be administered using continuous or intermittent enteral or oral feedings, although this end-point of therapy is not possible in all patients. Bolus feedings may stimulate gallbladder emptying and decrease the risk of cholecystitis. Laboratory monitoring with glucose, electrolytes, blood urea nitrogen (BUN), calcium, magnesium, phosphorus, and liver enzymes is important during the early phases of recovery after bowel resection.

Chronic home medical care is an essential part of current medical practice. The complex vitamin, electrolyte, and metabolic deficiencies that may be seen in patients receiving long-term home TPN therapy can be predicted and treated appropriately. In the majority of patients, body weight can be maintained within the normal range. In a recent study, 78% of patients were able to return to a near-normal quality of life, but rehospitalization was necessary in 73% of the patients.[7] The most common reason for readmission was central line complications, particularly catheter sepsis. The incidence of septic complications depends on the type of indwelling catheter used and the maintenance of strict sterility. PercuCath and Landmark catheters can be placed through a peripheral vein and can be used for intermediate time periods of supplementation. Advances in central line design include the advent of the Port-a-Cath, where there is no external device and intravenous administration is transcutaneous into a reservoir. A practical problem for patients with short bowel syndrome is the frequent loss of health insurance.

Cyclic TPN may have a favorable effect on lipid oxidation and is a potential method of managing hospital and home TPN therapy and can also be recommended to improve the functional level of patients. This method of administering TPN more closely parallels the normal fed and fasting metabolic pattern of substrate supply, oxidation, and storage in individuals receiving a normal oral diet.

After a thorough assessment of the success of refeeding, low-dose or full-dose TPN can be continued long term to complete daily nutritional requirements that are not met by oral feedings. The current nutritional treatment options are listed in Table 65–3. The presence or absence of the colon, daily ostomy, or fecal volume and the original length of residual small bowel should be taken into account when formulating an ongoing treatment and diet plan for a given patient.

New oral dietary supplements are being developed to increase treatment options for nutritional therapy in patients with the short bowel syndrome. An oral protein hydrolysate, Peptamen, with short-chain peptides (molecular size less than 1000) markedly improves amino acid absorption and nitrogen balance. Many of the new supplements, including Peptamen, contain a higher concentration of glutamine, a conditionally essential amino acid, which has a favorable effect on the intestinal adaptive response, diminishes villous atrophy, and decreases gut permeability. This combination of effects improves the overall nutritional profile of patients. Oral hypoosmolar polymeric glucose preparation, a complex carbohydrate, can significantly improve carbohydrate absorption. This glucose preparation, as a dietary supplement, may allow patients to consume and absorb up to the 3000 kcal/d required to maintain an adequate energy intake.

Historically, medical therapy for short bowel syndrome has included a low-fat diet. Some clinicians now question this practice. Total caloric absorption and volume of diarrhea are often equivalent on either a low-fat, high-carbohydrate or high-fat, low-carbohydrate diet. Since patients have problems with the poor palatability of a strict low-fat diet, more liberal fat intake is currently recommended for patients with short bowel syndrome. If a patient has weight loss on an adequate caloric diet, it may be beneficial to increase the total carbohydrate intake to offset intestinal losses due to malabsorption using the polymeric glucose preparation described above.

TABLE 65–3. SPECIFIC NUTRITIONAL TREATMENT OPTIONS FOR SHORT BOWEL SYNDROME

Cyclic home TPN
Continuous nasoenteral feeding
Nocturnal nasoenteral feeding
Oral diet
   Moderate-fat diet
   Protein hydrolysate
   Medium-chain triglyceride oil
   Complex carbohydrate diet
   High-calorie diet
   Low-oxalate diet
Nutritional supplements
   Calcium
   Vitamin B_{12}
   "Water-soluble" fat-soluble vitamins
      Vitamin A
      Vitamin D
      Vitamin E
Antisecretory medications
   H_2-receptor antagonists
   Omeprazole
   Clonidine
Broad spectrum antibiotics
Octreotide
Intestinal pacing

TPN = total parenteral nutrition.

HEPATIC AND BILIARY DISEASE

A known complication of TPN therapy is a cholestatic syndrome that may eventually be complicated by cirrhosis. The use of oral feedings to supplement TPN or changing the carbohydrate content and minimizing lipids in the standard TPN formula may decrease the incidence and severity of TPN-induced cholestasis or liver failure. Some lipids are required, however, to prevent a cholestatic syndrome that occurs because of the presence of unopposed carbohydrate supplementation. The type of lipid preparation used as part of the daily TPN formula is important. Ivelip 20%, a formerly available commercial product, may rapidly produce cholestasis, a complication that has been attributed to the presence of toxic plant–derived fatty acids. This problem can be reversed by substituting Intralipid or Liposyn therapy.

Administration of ursodeoxycholic acid has been reported to decrease the severity of cholestasis in the setting of chronic TPN. The use of ursodeoxycholic acid to treat or prevent gallstones in patients with short bowel syndrome has not been described. Chronic liver disease, including cirrhosis, has been caused by long-term TPN, especially in children. Finally, some patients with short bowel syndrome have problems with malabsorption of medications. Administration of ursodeoxycholic acid has been demonstrated to increase the absorption of cyclosporine.

PHARMACOLOGIC THERAPY

Antisecretory agents that reduce gastric acid secretion, such as omeprazole, have been found to decrease volume of ostomy output by up to 1.5 L/d in some patients.[8] If a decrease in ostomy output is documented, this medication may allow patients to decrease requirements for intravenous fluid supplementation. Omeprazole has not been shown to have an effect superior to that of H_2-receptor antagonists but may be considered if these agents such as cimetidine, ranitidine, or famotidine initially fail to reduce ostomy output. Since omeprazole is inactivated in an acid environment, its absorption may be decreased when the pH in the stomach and proximal small bowel is low, a condition often seen with rapid gastric emptying.

Somatostatin and octreotide, a somatostatin analog, have been used to treat patients with short bowel syndrome.[9] These agents decrease bowel motility and the volume of intestinal secretions and reestablish a more normal intestinal motility pattern. Both compounds have a beneficial effect on the regulation of the migrating motor complex. The maximum effective dose appears to be 50 1g of octreotide administered twice a day. Both somatostatin and octreotide, unfortunately, may increase fat malabsorption. The use of octreotide is considered a reasonable option in the treatment of patients with short bowel syndrome and a high-volume ostomy or stool output. Choleretic diarrhea, induced by the presence of bile acids in the colon, may be reduced by the use of cholestyramine.

SURGICAL THERAPY

Surgery, excluding small bowel transplantation, is currently only considered in a few selected patients to achieve a specific outcome. Small bowel tapering and lengthening procedures have been proposed but have not been subjected to extensive clinical trials.[10] In patients with a dilated segment of small bowel, a tapering procedure with sequential narrowing and lengthening of the small bowel segment may result in an increased absorptive area. Colon interposition or the creation of intestinal valves may benefit patients with rapid intestinal transit. The interposition of a segment of colon can also be used to allow an anastomosis between the small bowel and colon when direct bowel approximation is not possible. The role of intestinal pacing has not been determined in humans; however, in animals with an electrically paced excluded loop of small bowel, studies have shown a significant modulation of the small bowel motility index and fluid secretion.[11] Future research in adults, infants, and children with short bowel will determine the role for this type of device. Finally, the most important role of the surgeon in the management of short bowel syndrome is to maintain intestinal length and avoid undue intestinal resection.

Small bowel transplantation has recently been instituted at a few institutions as a treatment option for patients with short bowel syndrome, particularly patients with difficulty with intravenous access and patients with TPN-induced liver failure. In the few reported cases of combine liver and small bowel transplantation, patients with short bowel syndrome and TPN-induced liver failure have had marked improvement in their clinical status. The surgical technique of intestinal transplantation uses conventional intestinal anastomoses. The complex immunology of the intestine with the subsequent risk of rejection and graft-versus-host disease has kept this therapy from being more widely used. However, the availability and use of the potent immunosuppressive agent, FK506, should improve the results of small bowel transplantation and possibly increase its application. The long-term survival of the small bowel graft is approximately 50% in patients who undergo small bowel transplantation. Finally, the cost of small bowel transplantation is not inconsequential, and patients may require up to 3 months of hospitalization. Once a patient who may benefit from small bowel transplantation is identified, a consultation with a center experienced with this therapeutic modality could be considered. Fetal intestinal transplantation may also be a useful option in the future.[12]

REFERENCES

1. Galea MH, Holliday H, Carachi R, et al. Short-bowel syndrome: a collective review. *J Pediatr Surg.* 1992;27:592.
2. Nightingale JMD, Lennard-Jones JE. The short bowel syndrome: what's new and old. *Dig Dis.* 1993;11:12.
3. Todo S, Tzakis AG, Abu-Elmagd K, et al. Intestinal transplantation in composite visceral grafts or alone. *Ann Surg.* 1992;216:223.

4. Nightingale JMD, Kamm MA, van der Sijp JRM, et al. Disturbed gastric emptying in the short bowel syndrome: evidence for a 'colonic brake'. *Gut.* 1993;34:1171.
5. Lin HC, Doty JE, Reedy TJ, et al. Inhibition of gastric emptying by acids depends on pH, titratable acidity and length of intestine exposed to acid. *Am J Physiol.* 1990;259:G1025.
6. Green JH, Heatley RV. Nutritional management of patients with short-bowel syndrome. *Nutrition.* 1992;8:182.
7. Burnes JU, O'Keefe SJ, Fleming CR, et al. Home parenteral nutrition: a 3-year analysis of clinical and laboratory monitoring. *J Parenter Enteral Nutr.* 1992;16:327.
8. Nightingale JMD, Walker ER, Burnham WR, et al. Effect of omeprazole on intestinal output in the short bowel syndrome. *Aliment Pharmacol Ther.* 1991;5:405.
9. Nightingale JMD, Walker ER, Burnham WR, et al. Octreotide (a somatostatin analogue) improves the quality of life in some patients with a short intestine. *Aliment Pharmacol Ther.* 1989;3:367.
10. Thompson JS, Pinch LW, Murray N, et al. Experience with intestinal lengthening for the short-bowel syndrome. *J Pediatr Surg.* 1991;26:721–724.
11. Teiser SB, Schusdziarra V, Bollschweiler E, et al. Effect of enteric pacing on intestinal motility and hormone secretion in dogs with short bowel. *Gastroenterology.* 1991;101:100.
12. Kellnar S, Schreiber C, Rattanasouwan T, et al. Fetal intestinal transplantation: a new therapeutic approach in short-bowel syndrome. *J Pediatr Surg.* 1992;27:799.

Acknowledgments

The authors would like to thank William Berquist, MD, for his review of this chapter and constructive comments.

66

Acute, Recurrent, and Chronic Appendicitis

BENJAMIN N. SMITH, NORMAN D. GRACE, and PARDON R. KENNEY

In 1886, Reginald Fitz, Professor of Pathologic Anatomy at Harvard, first used the term *appendicitis* to clearly identify the vermiform appendix as the culprit in most instances of right lower quadrant inflammation formerly thought to originate in the cecum and referred to as *perityphilitis*.[1] He stressed the importance of surgical therapy. Soon thereafter, in 1889, McBurney described the clinical manifestations of appendicitis, including the point of maximal tenderness that now bears his name.[1] In the century that has elapsed since these initial descriptions of appendicitis, the literature has emphasized early diagnosis and surgical intervention for this entity. It is this emphasis on prompt surgical intervention, perhaps more than any of the advances in medical diagnostics and therapeutics, that has improved the prognosis in appendicitis from an often fatal disease 100 years ago to one in which death is currently quite uncommon.

The past decade has seen the introduction and development of interventional radiology and laparoscopic surgery. These techniques may offer attractive alternatives to the traditional surgical approach with the potential benefit of reduced complications and cost.

DEVELOPMENTAL ANATOMY AND FUNCTION

At birth the appendix is shaped like an inverted pyramid and arises from the inferior tip of the cecum. Differential growth of the cecum during childhood rotates the base of the appendix to its adult position on the posteromedial aspect of the cecum, about 3.0 cm below the ileocecal valve.

The adult appendix is usually about 10 cm in length. The position of the tip of the appendix has important clinical implications, as it may influence the presenting symptomatology in acute appendicitis. The most common position is behind the cecum but still within the peritoneal cavity.

The human appendix appears to be a functional, although not indispensable, immunologic organ that is part of the secretory immune system of the gut.[1]

ACUTE APPENDICITIS

INCIDENCE

Acute appendicitis is the most common abdominal surgical emergency, afflicting 7% of Americans during their lifetime. Interestingly, the incidence of acute appendicitis has been declining over the past three to four decades.[1] Explanations have included changing dietary habits, antibiotics, better nutrition, and improved diagnostic capability.[1,2] The incidence varies with age: it is rare in infants, most likely because the appendix is a conical structure with a wide orifice in this age group. The incidence rises steadily in childhood and peaks in the teens and twenties. Thereafter, the incidence declines. This trend in incidence roughly parallels the amount of lymphoid tissue in the appendix, which peaks during the teen years and then diminishes after age 30 years.[1,2] However, in the elderly, the incidence has increased in parallel to the increased life expectancy for this age group.

ETIOLOGY

The precipitating event in acute appendicitis appears to be obstruction of the appendiceal lumen. The most common cause is hyperplasia of submucosal lymphoid follicles (60%), followed by fecaliths (35%), other foreign bodies (4%), and strictures or tumors (1%).[2] The amount of lymphoid tissue peaks during the teen years, then diminishes after age 30 years.[1,2] Hyperplasia of the follicles may be triggered by infections and other diseases that specifically stimulate lymph tissue. Presumably, an enlarged follicle obstructs the appendiceal lumen at some point along its length, initiating the series of events that characterize acute appendicitis. Foreign bodies include vegetable matter and fruit seeds, parasites such as pinworms *(Enterobius vermicularis)* and *Taenia* and *Ascaris* organisms, and even inspissated barium. In 1% of cases, the obstruction is secondary to tumors or strictures of the appendix or cecum.[2] The most common tumors are carcinoid tumors in young adults and cecal carcinomas in the elderly, although metastatic carcinoma, usually from a primary breast cancer, is also encountered.[2]

PATHOPHYSIOLOGY

Obstruction of the appendiceal lumen triggers a sequence of physiologic events characterized by progressive inflammation and infection. Early in the course of appendicitis, intraluminal pressure rises as mucus secretion continues distal to the obstruction. This rising pressure eventually interrupts lymphatic drainage and promotes bacterial proliferation and diapedesis. The appendiceal distension with stimulation of visceral afferent nerve fibers is experienced by the patient as vague, diffuse, midabdominal pain with anorexia, nausea, and occasional vomiting and corresponds to the surgical stage of acute focal appendicitis. If the obstruction is not relieved, a progressive rise in intraluminal pressure results in venous obstruction with further ischemia, edema, and transmural bacterial invasion. This corresponds to the surgical stage of suppurative appendicitis. The patient experiences the classic shift and localization of pain in the right lower quadrant as somatic nerves in the parietal peritoneum are directly irritated by the inflamed appendix. If the obstruction is not relieved or the appendix removed surgically by this point, a complicated course is likely to occur, as the arterial blood supply of the appendix is interrupted, infarcts with gangrene develop, and local or free perforation ensues.

The degree of peritoneal soilage depends on the rate of progression of the above sequence of events. In about 98% of cases, the process proceeds slowly enough for inflammatory adhesions between the appendix and omentum or loops of intestine to wall off the process. However, in 1% to 2% of patients (usually a very young, a very old, or an immunocompromised host), the process may proceed too rapidly for sealing off to occur and generalized peritonitis ensues.[2]

CLINICAL MANIFESTATIONS

Acute appendicitis usually presents with the following sequence of symptoms[3]:

1. Diffuse abdominal pain, frequently worse in the periumbilical area
2. Anorexia, nausea, and vomiting
3. Shift of pain to the right lower quadrant
4. Fever

The order of symptom appearance has some differential diagnostic significance.[1,2] For example, if vomiting precedes the onset of abdominal pain, the diagnosis of acute appendicitis should be questioned. Shift of the pain from the periumbilical region to the right lower quadrant typically occurs within 4 to 6 hours. Although 95% of patients experience nausea, vomiting, and anorexia, the vomiting is generally not prolonged, and most patients vomit only once or twice.

Pain in acute appendicitis may be atypical in almost 50% of patients. In some patients it may begin in the right lower quadrant from the start, whereas in other patients the pain never becomes localized. Factors that seem to predispose to atypical pain include chronic antibiotic therapy and older age.[2]

Temperature elevation is normally about 1°C. Localized tenderness is detected by gentle palpation over McBurney's point. There may be local hyperesthesia in the right lower quadrant that can be best elicited by gently pinching the skin between thumb and forefinger.[1] Rebound tenderness may be present, but it is not essential to making a diagnosis of acute appendicitis. Sometimes pressure in the left lower quadrant produces pain in the right lower quadrant (Rovsing's sign), and it adds additional support to the diagnosis of acute appendicitis.[2]

The rectal examination is critical in every patient suspected of having appendicitis. Patients with acute appendicitis may have pain on palpation high in the right side of the rectal cavity. Occasionally a mass or fullness is appreciated in cases of appendicitis complicated by abscess or phlegmon. In patients whose appendix is located within the pelvis, pain on rectal examination may be the only physical sign elicited.[2] Every woman with right lower quadrant pain should have a pelvic examination to help exclude other pelvic pathology such as an ovarian cyst or tubal abscess.[2]

The pattern of abdominal pain is key to the diagnosis of acute appendicitis. However, the position of the appendix may vary, and this may cause the physical signs to deviate from the classic pattern and location. A retrocecal or retroileal location of the appendix may prevent contact of the inflamed appendix with the anterior parietal peritoneum. Pain may be less intense and remain poorly localized, and muscular rigidity may be absent. Back or right flank pain may be the sole presenting symptom. Pelvic appendicitis is a treacherous disease. Pain tends to localize more frequently in the left lower quadrant than on the right. Patients may experience urinary urgency and the urge to defecate. Although pain is a constant symptom in pelvic appendicitis, there are generally no peritoneal signs. The site of origin of pain is best detected by serial rectal and pelvic examinations.

LABORATORY FINDINGS

The white blood cell (WBC) count usually ranges from 10,000 to 16,000/mm^3 in acute appendicitis. Ninety-six percent of patients have an elevated WBC count, a left shift, or both.[4] However, a normal WBC count does not rule out appendicitis.[1] If the inflamed appendix lies near the bladder or ureter, red cells or white cells may appear in the urinalysis. Bacilluria does not result from acute appendicitis.[1,2]

RADIOGRAPHIC FINDINGS

Radiographic studies may be helpful in atypical cases and in patients who are very young or old.[3] Plain films may show a localized ileus or soft tissue density in the right lower quadrant. In complicated appendicitis, abdominal films may show absence of the right psoas shadow, scoliosis to the right, or an abnormal right flank stripe.[2] A fecalith in the right lower quadrant is a strongly supportive sign in a patient suspected of having acute appendicitis.

A barium enema examination can be safely performed in patients with acute appendicitis.[5] Its use is advocated only when the diagnosis is unclear and avoidance of negative results from laparotomy is critical. Positive findings include nonfilling or partial filling of the appendix and extrinsic pressure on the cecum (e.g., from an abscess) resulting in a "reverse 3" configuration of the cecum. However, "partial filling" is sometimes difficult to define radiologically. Consequently, the barium enema examination has a false negative rate of 10%.[5]

DIFFERENTIAL DIAGNOSIS

The differential diagnosis is essentially that of the acute abdomen. It may be helpful to prioritize the differential diagnosis by age. Infants less than 2 years old are especially susceptible to intussusception, although all ages may be afflicted. In children and young adults, acute mesenteric adenitis, regional enteritis, Meckel's diverticulitis, *Yersinia* and *Salmonella* infections, and viral gastroenteritis should be considered. In young women the gynecologic conditions of acute salpingitis (pelvic inflammatory disease), mittelschmerz, ruptured ectopic pregnancy, and endometriosis are prevalent. All ages are susceptible to salmonella enteritis, ureteral colic, and pyelonephritis. In older adults, diverticulitis and perforating cecal carcinoma become more prevalent.[2]

SURGICAL MANAGEMENT

As noted above, removal of the appendix represents safe, effective, and accepted therapy for this disease. Early diagnosis and surgical intervention are imperative to prevent the complication of perforation, a potentially fatal event if not treated in a timely fashion.

The surgical approach to the appendix is through a small right lower quadrant muscle splitting incision that is well tolerated by most patients. When the diagnosis is in doubt after examination of the appendix, it may be necessary to extend this incision medially to evaluate more fully the distal small bowel. Perforation commonly leads to abscess formation. In the traditional approach, abscess cavities are thoroughly debrided and drained with closed suction drainage.

Retrocecal appendixes present special problems in both diagnosis and surgical therapeutics. Because these appendixes can be extremely long, extensive mobilization of the right colon may be necessary to adequately free the appendix into the wound itself.

Ten percent to forty percent of explorations for appendicitis may reveal a normal appendix.[3] In this setting, a variety of other potentially surgically treatable diseases must be excluded. These include a search for Meckel's diverticulum, evaluation for Crohn's disease and mesenteric adenitis, evaluation for tumor in the right side of the colon, and evaluation of the right adnexa. In a small percentage of patients, no clear-cut cause for the right lower quadrant pain is found, and the most appropriate management after exploration is to close the incision.

An acceptable rate of negative exploration is between 15% and 20%. Because the majority of patients who undergo the procedure are young and healthy, the exploration itself carries little morbidity. Furthermore, the appendix is removed even if it is normal so that recurrent symptoms in the right lower quadrant cannot be attributed to appendicitis.

There is an inverse relationship between the incidence of perforation and the incidence of negative exploration. In institutions with a very high negative exploration rate (approaching 30%), the incidence of perforation is very low, implying very early surgical intervention in patients with right lower quadrant pain. Where the negative exploration rate is lower, the perforation rate is higher, implying a delayed, observational philosophy toward right lower quadrant pain. These numbers may be altered in the future by the more liberal use of laparoscopy.

ANTIBIOTICS

The use of preoperative prophylactic antibiotics is generally recommended in both operative and laparoscopic appendectomy. Antibiotics that are effective against the human colonic microflora are appropriate and must have both aerobic and anaerobic spectra of activity, including efficacy against *Bacteroides fragilis* and *Escherichia coli*.[6] Cefoxitin has been the mainstay of treatment over the past 10 years, but other antibiotics are equally efficacious. Acceptable single agent therapy also includes cefotetan and cefmetazole, ticarcillin-clavulanic acid, ampicillin sulbactam, and cilastatin-imipenem for severe infections.[6] Appropriate combination therapy includes clindamycin or metronidazole plus an aminoglycoside or a third-generation cephalosporin. The combination of clindamycin plus a monobactam (e.g., Aztreonam) is also effective.[6] The oral regimens of trimethoprim-sulfamethoxazole plus metronidazole, amoxicillin plus clavulanic acid, or metronidazole plus a quinolone (e.g., Ciprofloxacin) demonstrate suitable in vitro activity but have not been tested in vivo.[6]

In cases of nonperforated appendicitis, there is no need to continue antibiotics for more than one dose postoperatively. However, when perforated appendicitis is found, antibiotics should be continued until the patient is afebrile, the WBC count has fallen below 12×10^3, and bowel function has returned. This usually requires a full 5-day course.[6]

MANAGEMENT OF THE APPENDICEAL MASS

Acute appendicitis is a surgical disease. Medical management has been attempted with some success in remote places where surgical intervention was not accessible. The treatment of appendicitis with a palpable mass is an exception to this rule and remains controversial. This complication occurs in 2% to 6% of cases of acute appendicitis.[7] Some surgeons have advocated an initial period of observation and antibiotic treatment, followed by interval appendectomy. Others have advised immediate surgery and, if possible, appendectomy. The traditional approach includes surgical drainage of appendiceal abscesses, despite a postoperative complication rate of 15% to 50%.[7]

Ultrasound and computed tomography (CT) scans make it possible to reliably distinguish periappendiceal phlegmons from abscess collections preoperatively. This distinction is critical, as most failures of conservative therapy involve periappendiceal abscesses, not phlegmons. Recent studies suggest that almost all patients with appendicitis and phlegmonous inflammation recover without surgery.[7]

Percutaneous drainage of periappendiceal abscesses is felt to be safe and effective therapy.[8] Simple needle evacuation of abscess cavities under ultrasound or CT guidance, in conjunction with appropriate antibiotic therapy, appears to be adequate treatment in many cases. Percutaneous insertion of an indwelling pigtail catheter is required when abscess cavities cannot be completely decompressed by needle aspiration, as can occur in the presence of appendiceal fistulas.[8] Overall, percutaneous drainage of periappendiceal abscesses is successful 85% of the time, with an immediate complication rate of ≤3.5%.[7,8] Approximately 15% of abscesses require operative intervention when they cannot be drained percutaneously for technical reasons (e.g., inaccessible or loculated) or run a complicated course (e.g., perforate or cause intestinal obstruction).[7,8]

Opinion differs regarding the optimal management of the appendix after successful medical treatment of an appendiceal phlegmon or abscess. Some investigators advocate interval appendectomy, citing a 10% to 20% risk of recurrent appendicitis and the need to exclude malignancy in older individuals. Opponents of interval appendectomy can cite an operative complication rate as high as 16% to 23%.[8] One third of appendixes are normal or cannot be found. Almost all instances of recurrent appendicitis occur within 1 year. Most proponents of interval appendectomy recommend a follow-up barium enema to help exclude a malignancy in elderly patients. Some authors advocate a CT scan or ultrasound evaluation as well.

LAPAROSCOPIC APPENDECTOMY

Although operative laparoscopy is an established diagnostic and therapeutic modality in gynecologic surgery, its use in general surgery has been quite limited until recently. Increased use of the laparoscope has paralleled technologic advances in laparoscopic equipment and increased third-party interest in "minimally invasive surgery" with short length of hospital stay and speedy return to normal activity. The experience with laparoscopic appendectomy is not nearly as extensive as the widely accepted laparoscopic cholecystectomy. The role of laparoscopic appendectomy is unclear, since the surgical approach to acute appendicitis is generally straightforward, efficient, involves minimal morbidity or mortality, and requires only a 1- to 2-day hospital stay. There is an understandable reluctance on the part of many surgeons to add maneuvers that might delay definitive surgical therapy and thereby risk a complicated course.

Patient Selection

The laparoscope can be very helpful in clarifying the diagnosis in atypical presentations of acute appendicitis. For example, in women of reproductive age, it may be very difficult to distinguish acute appendicitis from gynecologic conditions with overlapping manifestations. The negative appendectomy rate in these women approaches 40%, which far exceeds the 15% to 20% negative appendectomy rate in the general population.[9] Some investigators have found alternative diagnoses in 40% to 60% of patients using this technique.[9,10]

In all patients, inability to visualize the appendix may necessitate surgical exploration. The accuracy of diagnosis using this technique is operator dependent, with a significant learning curve.

Laparoscopic Versus Open Appendectomy: Morbidity and Mortality

Early experience suggests that laparoscopic appendectomy may have an advantage over surgical appendectomy in terms of morbidity and mortality. The complication rate for surgical removal of an appendix is about 15% and may include pneumonia, wound infections, intestinal obstruction, or spontaneous abortion. The mortality for surgical appendectomy is approximately 0.1% to 0.2%.[10] The complication rate of laparoscopic appendectomy is approximately 3% and the mortality about 0.01%.[9]

Economic Considerations

Since the average length of hospital stay for laparoscopic appendectomy may be less than that for open appendectomy, the potential economic savings in that regard are considerable. However, randomized, prospective trials are needed to ensure that these differences do not reflect patient selection.

McKernan and Saye[11] have reported a series of 32 laparoscopic appendectomies in which 94% were performed on an outpatient basis. However, only 13 of the 32 patients had acute appendicitis, for a negative appendectomy rate of 59%. No complications developed, and all patients resumed normal activity within 7 days. In a series of 100 incidental appendectomies performed at the time of videolaparoscopic evaluation for gynecologic complaints, the average hospital stay was 14 hours, and all patients were discharged within 24 hours.[12] These reports differ from traditional series involving surgical appendectomy, as they contain a paucity of acute cases. Furthermore, the cost of instrumentation for the laparoscopic procedure, much of which is disposable, may offset the potential savings in duration of hospital stay.

Potential Advantages and Disadvantages

Laparoscopic appendectomy has several other potential advantages over open appendectomy. These include decreased anesthesia time, a smaller incision and subsequent scar, decreased need for postprocedure analgesia, a shorter recuperative period, and decreased risk of adhesions.

On the negative side, widespread adoption of laparoscopic appendectomy, with its obligatory learning curve, may require the training of a new group of subspecialists for a procedure that is currently handled expertly by general surgeons and surgical house officers. Some advocates of laparoscopic appendectomy recommend delegating this approach only to specially trained surgeons, as the success rate for this technique may be very operator dependent.

Conclusions

Diagnostic laparoscopy may be justified in women of reproductive age (in whom the diagnosis of acute appendicitis is incorrect 40% of the time). In these women, laparoscopy frequently establishes an alternative gynecologic diagnosis, avoiding surgery in over 30% of cases.

Advantages to laparoscopic appendectomy over surgical appendectomy may include a shortened hospital stay, decreased postoperative pain, a shortened recuperative period, and reduced morbidity and mortality. Operative appendectomy remains the mainstay of treatment for acute appendicitis. The role for laparoscopic appendectomy remains to be defined by randomized, prospective trials.

RECURRENT AND CHRONIC APPENDICITIS

Even as the classic descriptions of acute appendicitis were being documented by Fitz and McBurney, their contemporaries were describing atypical presentations of appendiceal colic and suggesting the existence of recurrent and chronic disease. However, the entities of recurrent and chronic appendicitis remain controversial, with scant mention in most textbooks.

Resistance to the concepts of recurrent and chronic appendicitis is to some degree historical, part of a sustained backlash that began in the 1920s against the overzealous use of exploratory laparotomy for presumed appendicitis in many patients with chronic or recurrent abdominal pain. The great majority of these laparotomies yielded a normal appendix and no relief of symptoms. As a result, the diagnoses of chronic and recurrent appendicitis fell into disrepute. The entity of recurrent appendicitis has regained some legitimacy based on data showing that 10% to 20% of patients presenting with acute appendicitis give a history of at least one similar attack in the past.[13]

Definitions

There is lack of consensus regarding the definitions of recurrent and chronic appendicitis, which reflects, in large part, the absence of firmly established clinical and pathologic criteria. Crabbe et al[13] defined recurrent appendicitis as repeated self-limited attacks of right lower quadrant abdominal pain in patients eventually diagnosed with acute appendicitis. In their series the surgical specimens revealed acute inflammation of the appendix identical to that seen in acute appendicitis.

Chronic appendicitis was diagnosed in patients who related a history of persistent right lower quadrant pain for greater than 2 weeks, had findings at surgery and in the pathology specimen consistent with chronic inflammation (intramural lymphocytes and eosinophils), and experienced relief of symptoms after appendectomy.[13]

INCIDENCE

Crabbe et al[13] reported on 205 patients who underwent appendectomy over a 3-year period between January 1982 and December 1984. Twenty-one patients (10%) met their criteria for diagnosis of recurrent appendicitis, and three patients (1.5%) satisfied criteria for chronic appendicitis. These findings were consistent with previously reported statistics on the incidence of recurrent and chronic appendicitis.

SIGNS AND SYMPTOMS

A diagnosis of recurrent appendicitis may be applied to patients presenting with symptoms consistent with acute appendicitis who give a history of at least one similar, self-limited attack.[13] Because there is no pathologic difference between recurrent and acute appendicitis, the diagnosis is based on clinical presentation.[13]

The symptomatology of chronic appendicitis is less well defined. The finding of right lower quadrant tenderness on examination in a patient relating a history of pain in that region for more than 2 weeks is suggestive.

LABORATORY FINDINGS

The most useful examination for establishing the diagnosis of recurrent or chronic appendicitis is the barium enema.[13–15] Lee et al[14] documented abnormal findings in 85% of their patients with recurrent appendiceal colic, whereas Grossman[15] found that 100% of the patients with chronic symptoms who underwent barium enema had abnormal findings. The most common finding was an appendix that did not fill. Cecal abnormalities including a mass effect on the cecum and mild colitis were also seen.[14,16] However, nonfilling of the appendix occurs in 5% to 10% of normal appendixes.[16]

In infants and children, an upper gastrointestinal tract series with small bowel follow-through to evaluate the appendix may be preferable.[17] In one study, 80% of children with recurrent abdominal symptoms had abnormal findings on barium study, and 96% had complete resolution of their symptoms after appendectomy.[17] Nonfilling of the appendix may be an uncommon finding in infants and children with recurrent and chronic symptoms, occurring in less than 20% of cases.[16]

ETIOLOGY

Radiologic and histologic evidence supports partial or intermittent obstruction of the appendiceal lumen as the most plausible etiologic mechanism for recurrent and chronic appendicitis.[14,17] Schisgall[17] found inspissated casts of stool within the appendixes of many infants and children with recurrent attacks of appendiceal colic. He hypothesizes that these casts act as foreign bodies, producing intermittent partial obstruction or distension of the appendix. Lymphoid hyperplasia may initiate the process of appendicitis in some cases by narrowing the appendiceal lumen and trapping liquid stool. The water is then absorbed, leaving behind a partially obstructing cast.[17] Other reported causes of luminal obstruction include fecaliths, purulent material, luminal fibrosis, and malrotation of the appendix.[14]

TABLE 66–1. KEY CLINICAL, LABORATORY, AND PATHOLOGIC FEATURES OF RECURRENT AND CHRONIC APPENDICITIS

	RECURRENT APPENDICITIS	CHRONIC APPENDICITIS
Incidence	10%	1.5%
Symptoms	Symptoms of acute appendicitis with history of recurrent right lower quadrant pain	Right lower quadrant discomfort lasting at least 2 weeks
Signs	Signs equivalent to acute appendicitis	Tenderness over McBurney's point
Laboratory findings	Elevated WBC count and other laboratory findings of acute appendicitis	Often no abnormalities
X-ray examination	Nonfilling of the appendix on barium enema	Adults: nonfilling of appendix Children: partial obstruction, nonfilling of appendix, retained barium
Pathology	Acute inflammation	Chronic inflammation: eosinophils and lymphocytes

WBC = white blood cell.

PATHOLOGY

In patients who proceed to appendectomy for recurrent appendicitis, the histologic findings are generally the same as those for acute appendicitis. There is no evidence of chronic inflammation.[13] For patients diagnosed as having chronic appendicitis, a reliable correlation between clinical findings and chronic inflammatory changes of the appendix is required.[13]

TREATMENT

Recurrent appendiceal colic should be managed in the same manner as acute appendicitis. Many authors emphasize the point that a history of right lower quadrant pain in the past should never delay surgical intervention if current signs and symptoms suggest appendiceal colic.[13]

In patients with chronic right lower quadrant pain, the appropriate management is unclear. Several series support removal of the appendix in patients with more than 2 weeks of right lower quadrant pain, discomfort on palpation of McBurney's point, and an abnormal barium enema. For example, 17 of the 20 patients in Grossman's series experienced permanent relief of symptoms following appendectomy in follow-up ranging from 3 months to 7 years.[15] Note that Grossman's study excluded all women with "pelvic disorders."[15]

Recurrent and chronic appendicitis have yet to be generally accepted as clinical entities based on evidence of a well-defined and reproducible set of historical, diagnostic, and pathologic criteria (Table 66–1). Recurrent appendicitis is a much more common syndrome than chronic appendicitis. The minimal requirement to establish the diagnosis is a history of similar attacks in a patient presenting with symptoms consistent with acute appendicitis. The important caveat is not to let a history of similar attacks dissuade one from prompt surgical intervention.

The important criteria for making the diagnosis of chronic appendicitis include persistent right lower quadrant pain lasting at least 2 weeks, pain over McBurney's point, and an abnormal barium enema. In general, the appendixes removed from patients fulfilling these criteria are found to have evidence of chronic inflammation. More importantly, almost all patients will experience permanent relief of their symptoms following appendectomy.

REFERENCES

1. Schwartz SI. Appendix. In: Schwartz SI, Shires GT, Spencer FC, eds. *Principles of Surgery.* 5th ed. New York, NY: McGraw-Hill Book Co; 1989:1315–1326.
2. Concon RE, Telford GL. Appendicitis. In: Sabiston DC Jr, ed. *Textbook of Surgery: The Biological Basis of Modern Surgical Practice.* 14th ed. Philadelphia, Pa: WB Saunders Co; 1991:884–898.
3. Schrock TR. Acute appendicitis. In: Sleisenger MH, Fordtran JS. *Gastrointestinal Disease: Pathophysiology, Diagnosis, Management.* 4th ed. Philadelphia, Pa: WB Saunders Co; 1989:1382–1389.
4. Bower RJ, Bell MJ, Ternberg JL. Diagnostic value of the white blood count and neutrophil percentage in the evaluation of abdominal pain in children. *Surg Gynecol Obstet.* 1989;152:424–426.
5. Rajagopalan AE, Mason JH, Kennedy M, Pawlikowski J. The value of the barium enema in the diagnosis of acute appendicitis. *Arch Surg.* 1977;112:531–533.
6. Bohnen JMA, Solomkin JS, Dellinger PE, Bjornsen HS, Page CP. Guidelines for clinical care: anti-infective agents for intra-abdominal infection: a surgical infection society policy statement. *Arch Surg.* 1992;127:83–89.
7. Bagi P, Dueholm S, Karstrup S. Percutaneous drainage of appendiceal abscess: an alternative to conventional treatment. *Dis Colon Rectum.* 1987;30:532–535.
8. Shapiro MP, Gale ME, Gerzof SG. CT of appendicitis: diagnosis and treatment. *Radiol Clin North Am.* 1989;27:753–762.
9. Whitworth CM, Whitworth PW, Sanfillipo J, Polk HC Jr. Value of diagnostic laparoscopy in young women with possible appendicitis. *Surg Gynecol Obstet.* 1988;167:187–190.
10. Deutsch DA, Zelikovsky RR, Reiss R. Laparoscopy in the prevention of unnecessary appendectomies: a prospective study. *Br J Surg.* 1982;69:336–337.
11. McKernan JB, Saye WB. Laparoscopic techniques in appendectomy with argon laser. *South Med J.* 1990;83:1019–1020.
12. Nezhat C, Nezhat F. Incidental appendectomy during videolaseroscopy. *Am J Obstet Gynecol.* 1991;165:559–564.
13. Crabbe MM, Norwood SH, Robertson HD, Silva JS. Recurrent and chronic appendicitis. *Surg Gynecol Obstet.* 1986;163:11–13.
14. Lee AW, Bell RM, Griffen WO Jr, Hagihara PF. Recurrent appendiceal colic. *Surg Gynecol Obstet.* 1985;161:21–24.
15. Grossman EB Jr. Chronic appendicitis. *Surg Gynecol Obstet.* 1978;146:596–598.
16. Sakover RP, DelFava RL. Frequency of visualization of the normal appendix with the barium enema examination. *AJR.* 1974;121:312–317.
17. Schisgall RM. Appendiceal colic in childhood: the role of inspissated casts of stool within the appendix. *Ann Surg.* 1980;192:687–693.

67
Hirschsprung's Disease
DAVID L. GEIER and PHILIP B. MINER, JR.

HISTORICAL PERSPECTIVE

In 1886 at a meeting in Berlin, Harold Hirschsprung (1830–1916), a Professor of Pediatrics at the University of Copenhagen, described the disease that today bears his name. He presented case summaries of two children who died in the first year of life.[1] They had clinical symptoms of intestinal obstruction, and their physical examination revealed a distended abdomen. Autopsy studies showed markedly dilated sigmoid and transverse colonic segments; however, the rectum was not dilated. A flurry of case reports followed his presentation, and in 1901 Tittel[2] described the pathologic basis for Hirschsprung's disease, the absence of ganglion cells in the rectum. The pathology of congenital aganglionosis was further emphasized by Robertson and Kernohan[3] in 1938, and between 1948 and 1964 three major surgical techniques were described as definitive treatment of Hirschsprung's disease. The Swenson, Duhamel, and Soave techniques continue to be the mainstay of surgical management today.[4–6]

ETIOLOGY

Hirschsprung's disease (congenital megacolon) represents the congenital absence of parasympathetic ganglion cells in the colon. The cause of this aberrancy is unknown; however, many interesting observations have been made. It often occurs in association with genetic anomalies, especially Down syndrome and Waardenburg's syndrome (white forelock, widened root of the nose, and cochlear deafness) (Table 67–1). Hirschsprung's disease appears in approximately one out of 5000 live births (0.02% incidence) and with an overall frequency of 3.6% among siblings of index patients.[7]

The associated genetic anomalies provide insight into this developmental problem.[8] The problem appears to arise in the neural crest as the enteric nervous system evolves in utero. Because patients with Hirschsprung's disease most frequently have an aganglionic distal colonic segment (while more proximal colon has ganglion cells), many authorities believe this represents developmental arrest of the normal cranial-caudal migration of the neural crest.[9] However, the development of the enteric nervous system is more complex; microenvironment influences on the bidirectional migration of the neural crest likely play a vital role in healthy development of the enteric nervous system.[10] This could explain the rare cases of zonal aganglionosis and hypoganglionosis.

CLINICAL PRESENTATION

There are three important clinical presentations of Hirschsprung's disease (Table 67–2). The earliest presentation occurs in the neonate with Hirschsprung's disease who typically does not pass meconium within the first 24 hours of life. They have abdominal distension and may have bilious vomiting. A rectal examination reveals no stool in the rectum, and as the examining finger is withdrawn, there is a "gush" of meconium. Failure to diagnose Hirschsprung's disease in the early neonatal period may result in devastating consequences such as Hirschsprung's associated enterocolitis (HAEC), bowel perforation, and death.

The second presentation is perhaps more common. The infant has constipation since birth and may require daily enemas. Infants often are labeled as "failure to thrive." A high index of suspicion with the proper diagnostic studies provides the correct diagnosis in these cases.

TABLE 67-1. ASSOCIATED ANOMALIES

Cardiac
Defects in cardiac septation
Tetralogy of Fallot
Ventricular septal defect
Patent ductus arteriosus

Central Nervous System
Down syndrome
Waardenburg's syndrome
Neuroblastoma
Piebaldism
Gross skull malformations
Neurofibromatosis

Endocrine
Pheochromocytoma

Gastrointestinal
Malrotation of the gut
Bilateral inguinal hernias
Imperforate anus
Meckel's diverticulum
Polyposis syndromes

Genitourinary
Cystic deformities
Cryptorchidism
Hypoplastic uterus

Miscellaneous
Premature birth

TABLE 67-2. CLINICAL PRESENTATION OF HIRSCHSPRUNG'S DISEASE

AGE	HISTORY	PHYSICAL EXAMINATION
Neonate	Failure to pass meconium Abdominal distension Intestinal obstruction	No stool on rectal examination "Gush of meconium"
Infant	Failure to thrive Constipation	Distended abdomen
Adult	Chronic constipation Associated anomalies	Distended abdomen Fecaloma, tight sphincter

The final, uncommon presentation is that of the adolescent or adult.[11] These patients present with chronic constipation since birth. They typically have used daily laxatives, enemas, and digital disimpaction. They may also have associated congenital abnormalities. The clinical presentation of a young adult with Hirschsprung's disease is also referred to as congenital megacolon. The diagnosis can easily be overlooked in this population.

VARIANTS

Apart from the different clinical presentations in the various age groups, symptoms of Hirschsprung's disease depend on the length of the aganglionic segment. The majority of patients (80% to 90%) have short segment disease, which is by definition aganglionosis no further than the sigmoid colon.[12] Long segment disease involves colon beyond the sigmoid but no further than the cecum. Total colonic aganglionosis involves the entire colon, as well as varying lengths of small bowel and occasionally the stomach. Ultrashort segment disease involves only the anal sphincter, in which case the diagnosis is made by anorectal manometry and not by biopsy.

COMPLICATIONS

Multiple complications are possible in Hirschsprung's disease (Table 67-3). The most common complication is HAEC. This condition can be life threatening and warrants immediate attention. The focus should not only be on the enterocolitis but also on the underlying Hirschsprung's disease. HAEC causes abdominal pain, abdominal distension, watery diarrhea and fever.[13] HAEC results in more morbidity and more deaths than any other complication of Hirschsprung's disease.

Risk factors in the development of HAEC include a delayed diagnosis of Hirschsprung's disease and the presence of Down syndrome.[14] The pathogenesis of HAEC is not completely understood; however, there is evidence it may be related to mechanical dilation and fecal stasis, increased prostaglandin E_1 activity, and infections such as rotavirus and *Clostridium difficile*.[15] HAEC can occur prior to surgery, following a

TABLE 67-3. COMPLICATIONS OF HIRSCHSPRUNG'S DISEASE

COMPLICATION	ETIOLOGY	DIAGNOSIS	TREATMENT
HAEC	Unknown (? colonic dilation and stasis)	Endoscopy, clinical symptoms and signs	Supportive care, antibiotics, rule out PMC, definitive surgery
PMC	*Clostridium difficile*	Flexible sigmoidoscopy, biopsies, stool studies	Metronidazole or vancomycin
Fecal impaction	Stasis secondary to aganglionosis	Rectal examination, plain films	Bulk-forming laxatives, enemas, definitive surgery
Stercoral ulcers	Pressure necrosis from fecal impaction	Flexible sigmoidoscopy	Treat fecal impaction

HAEC = Hirschsprung's associated enterocolitis, PMC = pseudomembranous colitis.

diverting colostomy, and following definitive surgery. This is disconcerting because obstructive symptoms are relieved by surgery, but there continues to be a risk of developing HAEC following a definitive procedure. However, most experts believe that early diagnosis and early surgery prevent many cases of HAEC.

A subset of patients with the clinical picture of HAEC have *C. difficile* infections and pseudomembranous colitis (PMC). Thomas et al[16] first described this association when four out of six patients with clinical HAEC had high titers of *C. difficile* cytotoxin.[16] *C. difficile* was isolated in five of the six patients. Only two of four with available histologic tissue specimens had actual PMC, however. Because *C. difficile* may be isolated in up to 90% of healthy neonates, care must be taken before *C. difficile* can be implicated as a causative agent in HAEC.

Brearly and colleagues[17] also reported an association between HAEC and *C. difficile*.[17] In 26 patients with HAEC histologic data was available from 20. Thirteen of the 20 had nonspecific colitis, whereas 7 of the 20 had PMC. This data makes it clear that in patients with HAEC, stool studies should be performed to check for *C. difficile*, and appropriate follow-up treatment should be given.

Additional complications of Hirschsprung's disease include fecal impaction and ulcers of the colon associated with necrosis caused by fecal impaction (stercoral ulcers).

EVALUATION

A systematic approach to the diagnosis of suspected Hirschsprung's disease includes a detailed history and physical examination, radiographic studies, anorectal manometry, and histologic studies (Table 67–4). The salient features of the history and physical examination have been reviewed in the clinical presentation section of this chapter.

TABLE 67-4. DIAGNOSTIC STUDIES FOR HIRSCHSPRUNG'S DISEASE

Radiographic
Plain films show ileus, dilated colon, and absence of air in the rectum
Barium enema shows dilated proximal colon and a "transition zone"

Manometry
Absence of internal anal sphincter relaxation with balloon distension of the rectum

Histologic
Absence of ganglion cells in Meissner's and Auerbach's plexus
Hypertrophied smooth muscle
Increased and hypertrophied axons

Radiographic studies identify megacolon defined as a rectosigmoid colon diameter greater than 6.5 cm.[18] Studies include plain films and barium enemas. Plain films show an ileus with a dilated colon and absence of air in the rectum. The barium enema examination should be done with care. It is advisable to alert the radiologist to the suspected diagnosis of Hirschsprung's disease. It is often preferable not to use aggressive enemas or cathartic cleansing of the colon prior to the barium enema examination. Typically, the aganglionic segment is undilated and may even be narrowed by spasm. The ganglionic segment in the more proximal colon is dilated, and the area between the ganglionic and aganglionic segment is called the *transition zone*. In most patients the transition zone is in the rectosigmoid area (Fig. 67–1).

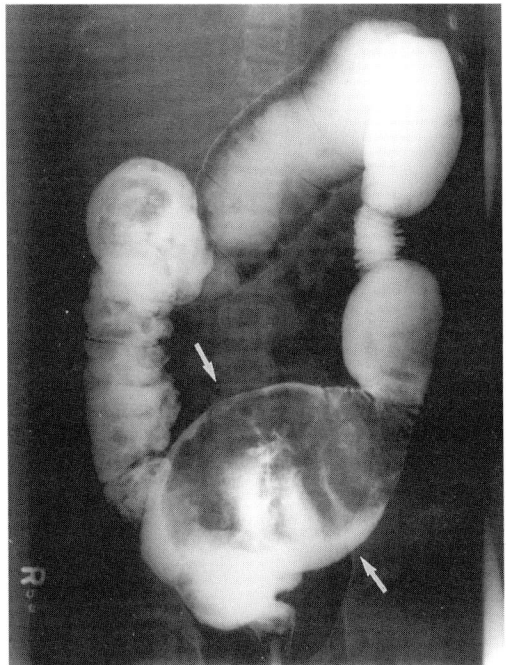 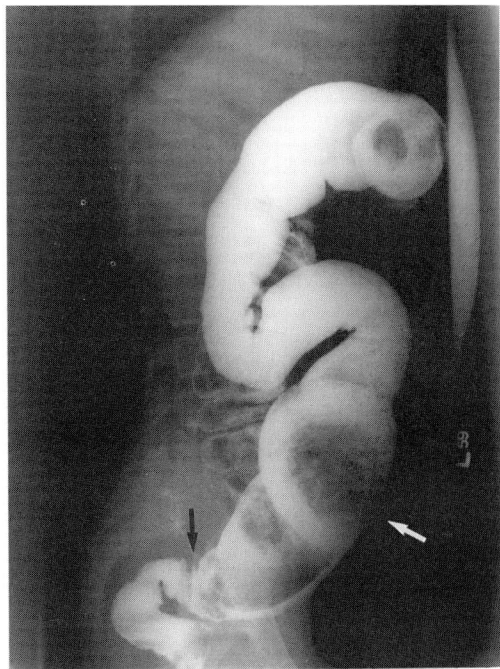

FIGURE 67–1. Hirschsprung's disease in a young child. Anteroposterior view **(A)** and lateral view **(B)** of a barium enema. Note the dilated proximal colon *(white arrows)* and the "transition zone" *(black arrow)*.

Anorectal manometry can help distinguish between Hirschsprung's disease and acquired megacolon as a cause of constipation. Yokoyama et al[19] successfully used anorectal manometry to diagnose Hirschsprung's disease in 268 constipated patients, 95 of which had documented Hirschsprung's disease. They found the reliability of manometry was 95%.

The classic manometric finding in Hirschsprung's disease is the absence of internal anal sphincter relaxation following balloon distension of the rectum (Table 67–4). Failure of relaxation is often accompanied by an increased basal pressure. There can be false-positive results with manometry. In several adults we have seen failure of relaxation of the internal anal sphincter in patients who have normal results from colonic biopsies. In this latter group, large volume distension (200 ml) often results in relaxation of the internal anal sphincter suggesting that the deficit in these patients is one of impaired relaxation at normal volumes. Manometric examples of a normal patient, an adult with impaired relaxation, and a patient with Hirschsprung's disease are shown in Figure 67–2.

To distinguish between congenital megacolon of Hirschsprung's disease origin and acquired megacolon due to other factors such as an anal fissure or sensitivity of the anal canal, it is important that the rectum is emptied prior to the manometric study. A distended rectum causes a number of anorectal abnormalities including chronic anal sphincter relaxation. Absence of a cutaneoanal reflex ("anal wink") suggests a spinal cord abnormality, but this reflex may be absent in patients with a markedly distended rectum. This may be due to competitive neurologic input from the distended rectum and cutaneous stimulation. Complete emptying of the rectum prior to anorectal manometry studies is also important because balloon distension may not be perceived in the presence of a large amount of stool. Also, a chronically distended rectum may not allow the balloon to come in contact with the rectal wall, therefore interfering with accurate manometry.

If manometric results indicate a high probability of Hirschsprung's disease, histologic verification of absence of ganglion cells is critical. We approach this problem by using flexible sigmoidoscopy and obtaining mucosal biopsy specimens with large forceps. Biopsy specimens are taken from at least two areas: 2 cm above the pectinate line and at least 5 cm above the pectinate line. Two biopsy specimens may improve the diagnostic yield of the test and provide information on

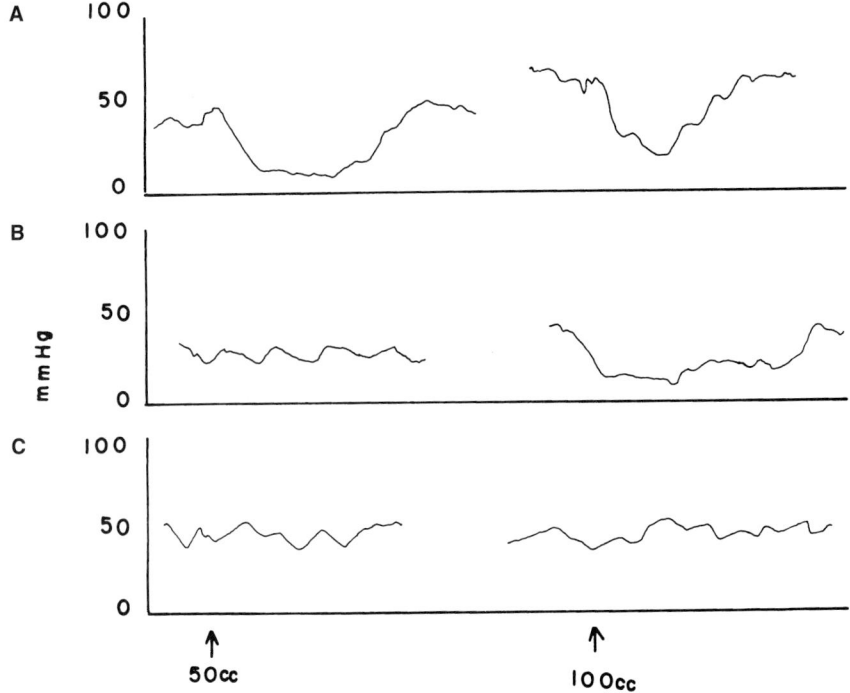

FIGURE 67–2. Anorectal manometry. **A,** A normal patient, with normal internal anal sphincter relaxation in response to balloon distension in the rectum. **B,** A patient with impaired relaxation to small volume distension (50 ml) but normal relaxation in response to 100 ml. **C,** A patient with Hirschsprung's disease with absence of internal anal sphincter relaxation to balloon distension.

the length of the aganglionic segment. A second technique not requiring general anesthesia is the suction biopsy. Suction biopsies or biopsies with the sigmoidoscope may reveal ganglion cells, which obviates the need for a full thickness biopsy.

In the absence of ganglion cells on suction biopsy or flexible sigmoidoscopy biopsy, it is imperative to obtain a full thickness biopsy to verify the absence of ganglion cells. Full thickness biopsies require general anesthesia. These biopsies should contain all three layers of the colonic wall and act as the gold standard in diagnosing Hirschsprung's disease.

In patients with Hirschsprung's disease biopsy specimens show absence of ganglion cells in Meissner's and Auerbach's plexus, hypertrophied smooth muscle, and increased and hypertrophied axons (Fig. 67–3). Different staining techniques such as hematoxylin and eosin, acetylcholinesterase, and neuron-specific enolase (NSE) may be used to aid in the diagnosis (Table 67–5).

TABLE 67–5. HISTOLOGIC STAINING TECHNIQUES

Hematoxylin and Eosin
Generally sufficient to identify ganglion cells

Acetylcholinesterase
Marked increase in coarse acetylcholinesterase-positive fibers
Quantitative acetylcholine usually increased

Neuron-specific Enolase (NSE)
NSE fibers in normal individuals; no NSE fibers in patients with Hirschsprung's disease

TREATMENT

Treatment for Hirschsprung's disease is primarily surgical. Nonsurgical management can be successful during the short-term evaluation of these patients. It seems obvious that patients with Hirschsprung's disease who seek medical care at 18 and 20 years of age have used medical management for the first 20 years of their life to

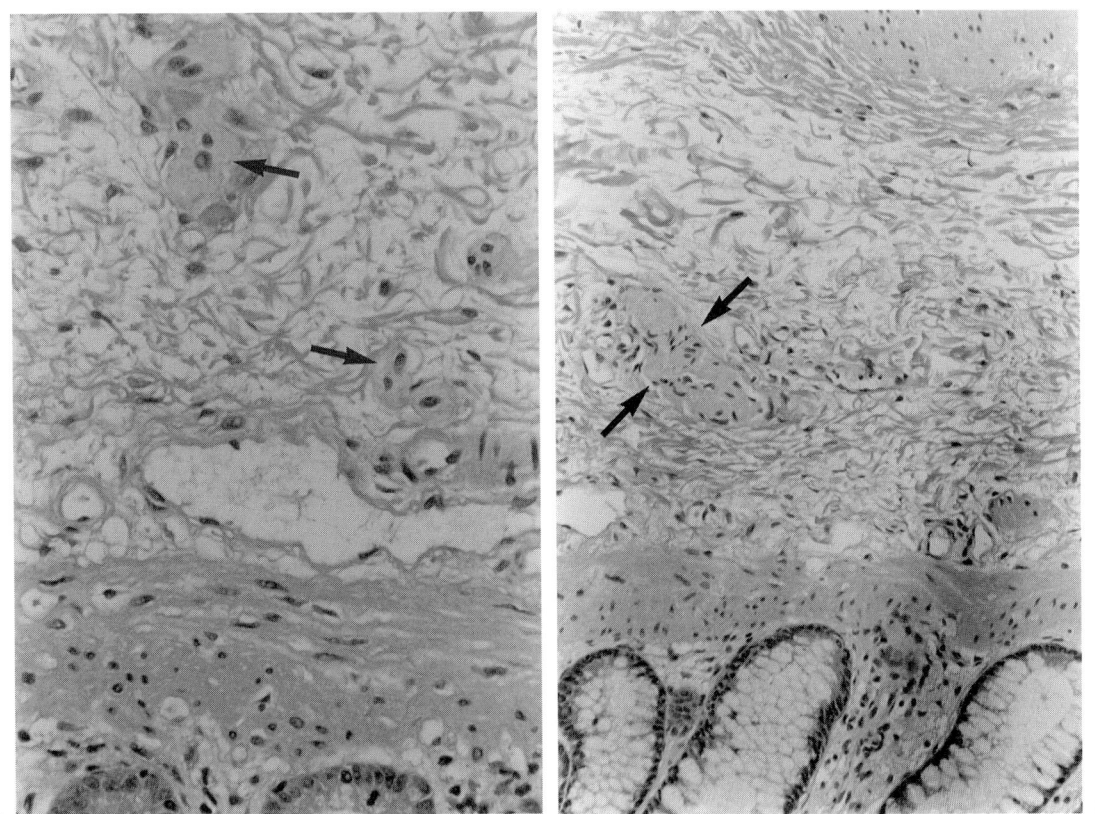

FIGURE 67-3. Histology. **A,** A patient with normal ganglion cells *(arrows)* in the colonic enteric nervous system. **B,** A patient with Hirschsprung's disease. Note the absence of ganglion cells and the presence of coarse nerve fibers *(arrows)*.

avoid surgery. As their constipation progresses or becomes more severe, the focus shifts to possible surgical management. Nonsurgical techniques are generally initiated early in childhood by the child's parents and consist of dietary or enema management protocols. These over-the-counter protocols include softening of the stool with mineral oil or osmotic agents and attempting to increase the motility of the large, dilated colon.

The definitive treatment for Hirschsprung's disease is surgical (Table 67-6). Goals of surgery are to relieve obstruction, to preserve normal bowel habits, to protect sexual function, and to maintain fecal continence. Many authorities favor a diverting colostomy as the initial procedure followed by a definitive procedure at a later date.[20] The initial use of a diversion procedure helps to prevent anastomotic leaks and abscess problems that frequently occur when the dilated proximal ganglionic segment is anastomosed too early.

Swenson introduced the first definitive procedure for Hirschsprung's disease in 1948.[1] The Swenson procedure involves resection of the aganglionic segment and direct end-to-end anastomosis of the proximal ganglionic segment to the anorectal canal. A second procedure is the Duhamel operation. This procedure leaves the aganglionic rectal segment in place, and the proximal ganglionic segment is anastomosed in a side-to-side fashion to the rectal stump.[5] The Soave procedure removes the rectal mucosa and leaves an aganglionic rectal cuff. The ganglionic segment is then "pulled through" and anastomosed to the aganglionic cuff.[6] Figure 67-4 illustrates the surgical techniques.

DIFFERENTIAL DIAGNOSIS (MIMICRY)

Mimicry of Hirschsprung's disease occurs in several clinical disease states (Table 67-7). Neuro-

TABLE 67-6. SURGICAL TREATMENT OF HIRSCHSPRUNG'S DISEASE

Procedure	Technique	Comments
Diversion	Ostomy to abdominal wall using ganglionic segment	Used in infants as the initial procedure
Anorectal myectomy	Muscularis is divided and strip excised	Useful in ultrashort segment disease
Swenson	Resection of the aganglionic segment with anastomosis near the dentate line	Original procedure, can be technically difficult because of extensive resection
Duhamel	Ganglionic proximal segment anastomosed end-to-side to aganglionic rectal cuff	The incidence of fecal impaction can be high following this procedure
Soave	Aganglionic rectum is stripped of its mucosa and the ganglionic segment is "pulled" through and anastomosed near the dentate line	Anastomotic strictures can occur following this procedure

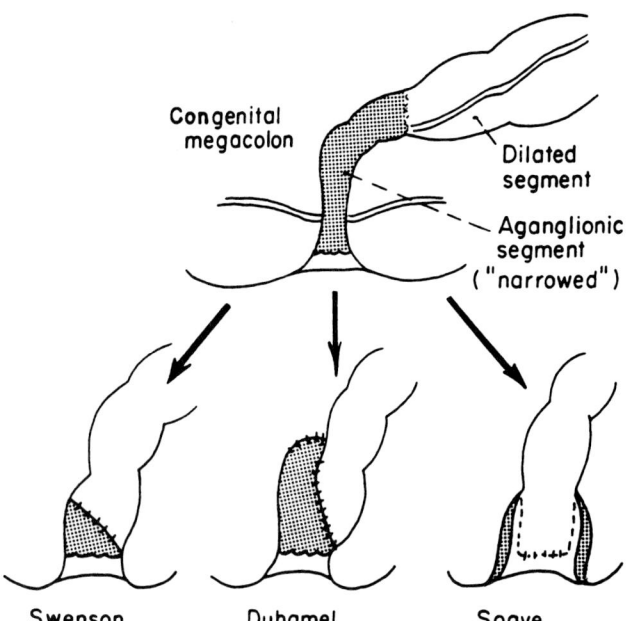

FIGURE 67-4. The three definitive surgical procedures available in Hirschsprung's disease. (From Phillips SE. Megacolon: congenital and acquired. In: Sleisenger MH, Fordtran JS, eds. *Gastrointestinal Disease*. 4th ed. Philadelphia, Pa: WB Saunders Co; 1989:1394.)

TABLE 67-7. DIFFERENTIAL DIAGNOSIS OF HIRSCHSPRUNG'S DISEASE

Neurogenic Origin
Hypoganglionosis
Hyperganglionosis (neuronal dysplasia)
Zonal aganglionosis
Short segment aganglionosis

Myopathic Origin
Familial visceral myopathies
Progressive systemic sclerosis
Muscular dystrophies
Amyloidosis

Miscellaneous
Intestinal atresia
Imperforate anus
Acquired megacolon (multiple causes)
Hypothyroidism
Medication-induced hypomotility
Spinal cord injuries
Inadequate diet

logic problems involving the gut that can be confused with Hirschsprung's disease include short segment aganglionosis, hypoganglionosis, hyperganglionosis (neuronal dysplasia),[21] and zonal aganglionosis.

Myopathic gut problems may also initially present with the same symptoms of Hirschsprung's disease. These pseudoobstructive lesions include familial visceral myopathies, progressive systemic sclerosis, myotonic dystrophy, muscular dystrophy, and amyloidosis.

Other problems that do not appear to have a neurogenic or muscular origin include idiopathic megacolon, intestinal atresia, and imperforate anus. Intestinal atresia and imperforate anus are emergencies of neonatal life. They may only be confirmed by immediate diagnostic tests, and they require surgical intervention.

Finally, other important causes of constipation in children and young adults are hypothyroidism, inadequate dietary intake, anal fissures resulting in anal canal pain, and voluntary pelvic floor contractility inhibiting motility into the rectum. Hypomotility associated with medications, diabetes mellitus, neonatal sepsis, adrenal insufficiency, brain injury, pituitary tumors with acromegaly, and sacral spinal cord injuries can all mimic Hirschsprung's disease.

In the vast context of constipation, Hirschsprung's disease is an uncommon cause that should be suspected in the neonate and young adult as the exclusion is simple and the discovery is rewarding. The increasing availability of anorectal manometry as a diagnostic tool will probably allow us to uncover more cases of Hirschsprung's disease at earlier ages and help avoid complications and discomfort in these patients.

REFERENCES

1. Ehrenpreis T. *Hirschsprung's Disease.* Chicago, Ill: Year Book Medical Publishers Inc; 1970.
2. Tittel K. Über eine angeborene Missbildung des Dickdarmes. *Wein Klin Wschr.* 1901;14:903.
3. Robertson HE, Kernohan JW. The myenteric plexis in congenital megacolon. *Proc Staff Meet Mayo Clin.* 1938;13:123.
4. Swenson O. My early experience with Hirschsprung's disease. *J Pediatr Surg.* 1989;24:839–845.
5. Duhamel B. Retrorectal and transanal pull-through procedure for the treatment of Hirschsprung's disease. *Dis Colon Rectum.* 1964;7:455.
6. Soave F. Hirschsprung's disease: a new surgical technique. *Arch Dis Child.* 1964;39:116.
7. Passarge E. The genetics of Hirschsprung's disease: evidence for heterogeneous etiology and a study of sixty-three families. *New Engl J Med.* 1967;276:138–142.
8. Ryan ET, Ecker JL, Christakis NA, Folkman J. Hirschsprung's disease: associated abnormalities and demography. *J Pediatr Surg.* 1992;27:76–81.
9. Krishnamurthy S, Schuffler MD. Pathology of neuromuscular disorders of the small intestine and colon. *Gastroenterology.* 1987;93:610–639.
10. Tam PKH. An immunochemical study with neuron-specific-enolase and substance P of human enteric innervation: the normal developmental pattern and abnormal deviations in Hirschsprung's disease and pyloric stenosis. *J Pediatr Surg.* 1986;21:227–232.
11. Crocker NL, Messmer JM. Adult Hirschsprung's disease. *Clin Radiol.* 1991;44:257–259.
12. Hirschsprung's disease and related disorders. In: *Gastrointestinal and Oesophageal Pathology.* New York, NY: Churchill Livingstone Inc; 1989:257.
13. Alexander BH, Chapman ND. The enterocolitis of Hirschsprung's disease: its natural history and treatment. *Am J Surg.* 1962;103:70–74.
14. Teitelbaum DH, Qualman SJ, Caniano DA. Hirschsprung's disease: identification of risk factors for enterocolitis. *Ann Surg.* 1988;207:240–244.
15. Imamura A, Puri P, O'Briain DS, Reen DJ. Mucosal immune defense mechanisms in enterocolitis complicating Hirschsprung's disease. *Gut.* 1992;33:801–806.
16. Thomas DF, Malone M, Fernie DS, Bayston R, Spitz L. Association between *Clostridium difficile* and enterocolitis in Hirschsprung's disease. *Lancet.* January 1982;9:78–79.
17. Brearly S, Armstrong GR, Nairn R, et al. Pseudomembranous colitis: a lethal complication of Hirschsprung's disease unrelated to antibiotic usage. *J Pediatr Surg.* 1987;22:257–259.
18. Preston DM, Lennard-Jones JE, Thomas BM. Towards a radiologic definition of idiopathic megacolon. *Gastrointest Radiol.* 1985;10:167.
19. Yokoyama J, Kuroda T, Matsufugi H, Hirobe S, Hara S, Katsumata K. Problems in diagnosis of Hirschsprung's disease by anorectal manometry. *Prog Pediatr Surg.* 1989;24:49–58.
20. Martin LW, Torres AM. Hirschsprung's disease. *Surg Clin North Am.* 1985;65:1171–1180.
21. Athow AC, Filipe MI, Drake DP. Hyperganglionosis mimicking Hirschsprung's disease. *Arch Dis Child.* 1991;66:1300–1303.

68
Slow Transit Constipation
ALAIN WATIER and GHISLAIN DEVROEDE

Constipation is neither a disease nor a sign, only a symptom. Symptoms cannot be measured objectively because they are the personal, subjective expressions of a dysfunctional disorder. Thus physicians have attempted to define constipation objectively, for instance, as two or fewer stools per week or as straining at stool more than 25% of the time.[1] But patients base their definition of constipation on what they view as a "normal" pattern of defecation: stools are too hard, too difficult to expel, too small, or too infrequent. Some also complain of a sensation of incomplete evacuation. Thus physicians and patients often do not "hear" each other when they talk.

Objective parameters like size, length, weight, consistency, and frequency may be evaluated, but they are influenced by sex, race and culture, age, diet, environment, emotions, stress, and personality.

Because these numerous variables do not permit us to define adequately what constitutes "normality," the definition of constipation should be based on self-report.[2] This should not deter us from describing the signs of constipation, however.

SUBTYPES OF CONSTIPATION

The most objective classification of constipation is usually made by an evaluation of the colonic transit time of radiopaque markers.[3,4] This technique of measurement is simple and reproducible[5] and can be done in any radiology department. Tracking the progression of markers along the colon by daily radiographs of the abdomen will reveal the type of constipation,[4] and will enable us to pinpoint specific areas of the bowel that are not functioning properly by calculation of segmental colonic transit time.[6] With techniques designed to minimize radiation, markers can be ingested repetitively; a single film of the abdomen is taken after a variable length of time.[5,7] These techniques, however, do not measure the mean transit time of a single marker but the mean transit time of the bolus of markers.[5] This is a potential source of error because these mean transit times are not reproducible from day to day. If one fails to understand this, he or she misses the point that the single-radiograph technique requires the establishment of a steady state condition with longer periods of ingestion as the severity of constipation increases.[5]

On the basis of radiopaque marker studies, patients with constipation may be divided into three groups. In the first group (propulsion defect) there is delay in the colon. In the second group, feces pass normally along the colon but are stored too long in the left colon (hindgut dysfunction) or in the rectum (outlet obstruction).[4] In the third group, transit time of markers is normal.

A simpler classification consists in separating constipation patients in whom radiopaque markers have delayed transit times (slow transit constipation, Arbuthnot Lane's syndrome)[8] from constipation patients in whom markers have normal transit times. Great care should be taken here to define what constitutes "normality." For instance, patients with "normal" overall large bowel transit time may have isolated delayed segmental transit time in the descending colon, or vice versa, some may have "normal" segmental transit times but overall delayed transit. Only one third of patients with "normal" colorectal transit time also have "normal" segmental transit time,[9] and in only four out of six constipated patients were both anorectal manometry findings and colorectal transit time normal. There is a link between the "normality" of bowel habits, as defined by stool frequency, and the "normality" of radiopaque marker transit times. Thus only 29% of patients with fewer than two stools per week and 50% of patients with fewer than three stools per week are considered to have "normal" transit time in the large bowel.[10] The type of healthy subjects selected as controls against which constipation is defined is important. Controls who say that stress does not modify their bowel habits and does not trigger abdominal symptoms will have shorter transit times than the other controls, thus making the other controls "abnormal." Radiologic evaluation is another important consideration. Compartmental analysis reveals subtle abnormalities in patients considered to have "normal" transit times. Delayed transit in the ascending colon is termed *colonic inertia*.[10,11] The incidence of colonic inertia is about 15% of the entire cohort complaining of constipation or 16% to 41% of those in whom colorectal transit is delayed. Right colonic stasis is seldom limited to that site and practically always is associated with overall colorectal delayed transit.

Some patients with delayed transit in the ascending colon have clear evidence of reflux from left to right colon as demonstrated on sequential plain films of the abdomen,[11] and in some the delay is not reproducible. A possible explanation would be that distal spasm slows down transit through the ascending colon. These patients probably belong to the group of subjects constipated by hindgut dysfunction. The diagnosis of colonic inertia should probably be reserved for the situation in which transit time in the ascending colon is prolonged and there is no reflux of markers from the left colon because there is little colonic motor activity.

Patients with hindgut dysfunction have normal right colon transit and distal delay; 33% of patients with fewer than two stools per week have such a pattern and are divided roughly into half with a delay in the left colon and rectosigmoid area and the other half with outlet obstruction.[10] Isolated stasis in the left colon occurs in 15% of a constipated cohort or 36% of those found to have delayed overall large bowel transit.

Some patients have normal colonic function but rectal stasis. They suffer from outlet obstruction.[4] This also is relatively rare and occurs in only 13% of a constipated cohort but in 31% of those found to have delayed overall large bowel transit.

Fifty-four percent of patients with slow transit constipation (STC) will also exhibit anismus on investigation.[12] Anismus, or rectosphincteric dyssynergia, is an abnormal defecatory mechanism in which there is contraction rather than relaxation of the striated muscle of the pelvic floor during straining. Transit studies do not suggest a difference between STC alone and STC with anismus (both were abnormal). Patients with anismus may have a normal transit time. Both groups complain of excessive straining at defecation and a feeling of incomplete evacuation and rarely have the urge to defecate. The incidence of abdominal pain and bloating is similar in the two groups. On anorectal physiologic assessment there was no difference between the groups with respect to resting or contracting anal pressures. Interestingly the incremental pressure difference (the ability to increase voluntary contraction as a percentage of resting pressure) was significantly higher in STC patients (143%) than in patients with STC-anismus (65%). In patients with anismus at defecography anorectal angles were significantly more acute and perineal descent was less than in those with simple STC.

Colonic scintigraphy provides accurate information about the transit times through individual colonic segments because it permits frequent observation and clearly delineates the entire colon.[13] Segmental transit[14] times in the colon can also be measured, but the optimum site for injection of a bolus is a technical problem that remains difficult to solve. The measurement of transit time with radiopaque markers is essentially a dye-dilution curve technique. Instead of having an intravenous injection as for blood flow, markers are instilled into the cecum, and it is only because gastrointestinal transit time is so much shorter than large bowel transit, that the technique is feasible: 20 ingested markers are within the colon the next day. The scintigraphy technique using a pill that dissolves in the cecum is an even better technique in this regard. But available radionuclear techniques have not yet solved the problem that transit through the left colon depends on that through the right colon and that transit through the rectum depends on that through the right and left colon. The mathematics used to solve the problem of radiopaque markers' transit time (Arhan segmental transit time) have not yet been applied to colonic scintigraphy, and thus its use is limited to differentiating slow transit from normal transit constipation; the method is not useful for calculating segmental constipation, particularly in the hindgut.

Dynamic scanning of the large bowel with either food or bisacodyl stimulation will most likely become essential to distinguishing patients with slow transit constipation who have a hypomotile colon from those who have a hypermotile colon.

Slow transit constipation and colonic inertia represent the most severe forms of constipation. Isolated chronic colonic pseudo-obstruction may be a label given to some patients with colonic inertia or slow transit constipation; most have severe constipation and few unequivocal abnormalities in either muscular or neural structures. Motor activity is less than normal in the fasting state. Contraction amplitude in the distal large bowel is lower after meals, and the rectal wall is much more inelastic (flaccid). One third have a family history. Radiographs usually show marked dilation of the colon.

Constipation is more severe in women with colonic inertia than in those with slow transit constipation and is usually resistant to all types of medical treatment.

CLINICAL MANIFESTATIONS AND PHYSICAL EXAMINATION

Symptoms are almost always confined to women of reproductive age[10,11] and usually appear before the age of 20. Problems begin in early childhood but may arise suddenly after intraabdominal or pelvic surgery[15] or injury to the perineum.[11,16] Several weeks may elapse between bowel movements. Malaise, nausea, abdominal distension, and pain are prominent features. Straining at defecation, anal pain, rectal bleeding, or a sense of incomplete rectal evacuation are associated symptoms. Assisted defecation by digital pressure in the vagina or manual extraction of stools in the rectum frequently are elicited spontaneously during the history. But they are not necessary for diagnosis.

Patients are disabled by their symptoms. They are obsessed with abdominal and defecatory symptoms. Laxative abuse is common (50% of these patients). Mean number of bowel movements varies from 1 ± 0.2 to 1.6 ± 0.2 weekly. Some patients may have a bowel movement only every 3 to 4 weeks.

At physical examination the abdomen is usually bloated, fecal masses are not palpable, and there is no excess gas on percussion. There is no soiling of the perineal skin. Fecal impaction is usually absent, and the rectum is commonly empty. Tone of the internal anal sphincter and voluntary contraction of the external anal sphincter are usually normal. Rectal prolapse may be seen. Anismus has also been found in these patients.

PATHOGENESIS

ARE COLONIC INERTIA AND SLOW TRANSIT CONSTIPATION LIMITED TO THE SMALL BOWEL?

Motor abnormalities often extend to other segments of the gastrointestinal tract. Dysphagia and gastroesophageal reflux are associated with hypertonic pharyngoesophageal and weak gastroesophageal sphincters in patients with colonic inertia. There is also a high incidence of simultaneous contractions of the esophagus (tertiary contractions).[11,17] Gastric emptying is delayed.[17] Mouth-to-cecum transit time is lengthened. The rectum is also hypersensitive to bethanechol, contracting more and faster than in controls. The anus may be hypertonic,[11] and the rectoanal inhibitory reflex may be abnormal in 75% of patients.[11] Terminal ileal motility is also abnormal in patients with chronic idiopathic constipation.

SEX-RELATED ETIOLOGIC FACTORS

Concomitant gynecologic, hormonal, urinary, and neurovegetative disturbances have been described. Menses tend to be irregular (45%). Some women describe changes in bowel habits at different times during their menstrual cycles.[18] In some patients transit seems to be prolonged during the luteal phase. In another study no difference in transit times was found between follicular and luteal phases.[18] Galactorrhea has also been described.[11,16] Female sex hormones are known to influence gastrointestinal function. Patients with constipation consistently demonstrated lower than normal serum levels of adrenal and ovarian steroid hormones.[19] Whether these abnormalities are due to an altered enterohepatic circulation of the steroid hormones or are of primary pathogenic importance remains to be determined.

The incidence of gynecologic operations (ovarian cystectomies, hysterectomies), other than terminations, sterilization, dilatation and curettage, and cesarean section, is much higher than in the general population. This is probably related to inappropriate surgery for abdominal pain.[11,20] On the other hand, ultrasonography reveals no abnormalities of pelvic structures in women with severe idiopathic constipation.

ENTERIC NEURONAL DISTURBANCES

Anatomic evidence of colonic abnormalities comes from histologic examination of colonic myenteric nerve plexus by silver staining. A distinctive abnormality in the myenteric plexus of the colon involving fewer than normal and morphologically altered argyrophilic neurons has been demonstrated in patients with slow transit constipation. Decreased neuronal processes (dendrites and axons) and clusters of variably sized nuclei within ganglia also have been described. A reduction in the ability of cholinergic nerve fibers within human colonic tissues to release acetylcholine on electrical stimulation has been reported in severe constipation.

CIRCULATING PEPTIDE HORMONES

Patients with severe idiopathic constipation have impaired motilin release in response to oral water stimulation.[21] Failure of normal gastrin, Motilin, and pancreatic polypeptide release after a standard meal has been demonstrated in slow transit constipation.[21]

INTESTINAL NEUROPEPTIDES

Earlier studies have shown that substance P and bombesin excite colonic motility, whereas galanin, vasoactive intestinal polypeptide (VIP), somatostatin, and enkephalin mainly inhibit intestinal motility.

Dolk et al[22] investigated the presence and density of neuropeptide immunoreactive nerve fibers in the resected colon wall from patients with severe idiopathic chronic constipation. Apart from a difference in the amount of the nerve fibers' immunoreactive calcitonin gene-related peptide (CGRP) in the myenteric ganglia, they could demonstrate neither total absence nor high density of any types of immunoreactive nerve fibers (enkephalins, substance P, somatostatin, neuropeptide Y, bombesin, motilin, tyrosine hydroxylase, dynorphin, galanin).

On the other hand, low levels of VIP (a nonadrenergic noncholinergic [NANC] inhibitory transmitter and of peptide-histidine-methionine (PHM) in the muscularis externa of the descending colon have been described. Levels of substance P, which stimulates muscle contractility in vitro, were lower than normal in mucosal biopsies. Other studies showed that substance P was present in normal concentrations in the descending colon of constipated patients.

Serotonin (5-hydroxytryptamine [5-HT]) stimulates both cholinergic excitatory and NANC inhibitory neurons in the gut, and it has been suggested that serotoninergic neurons are probably interneurons within the enteric nervous system.

Lincoln et al[23] showed that the serotonin content of the sigmoid colon was higher in patients suffering from severe idiopathic constipation than in controls. They also showed that the total indole levels were higher in the mucosa and circular muscle but not in the region consisting of the myenteric and submucosal plexus.

High levels of neuropeptide Y have also been shown.

NEUROIMMUNOCHEMISTRY

Abnormalities in monoclonal antibodies against neurofilaments have been demonstrated in patients suffering from severe constipation, suggesting an underlying neuropathy.

EXTRADIGESTIVE MANIFESTATIONS

Patients may have many urinary symptoms (nocturia, difficulty in straining), residual urine, abnormal urodynamic studies, and hypersensitivity of the bladder to bethanechol.[11,16,24,25] Pale cold fingers,[16] blackouts or epilepsy,[16] postural hypotension,[11,16] and Raynaud's phenomenon[16] have also been described. Abnormal acetylcholine sweat spot test results may be found in constipated patients, thus suggesting a subclinical autonomic neuropathy. A particular fingerprint pattern has also been described in these patients, suggesting a genetic component. Immune system abnormalities have also been defined.

CONVENTIONAL RADIOLOGY AND ENDOSCOPY

Barium enema is usually normal. There is no quantitative clinical way to recognize large-bowel length or volume, and dye-dilution curves have not been used outside of a research setting. A double contrast enema helps to exclude not only a structural lesion but also Hirschsprung's disease and idiopathic megarectum or megacolon.

At sigmoidoscopy small, hard stools are usually seen in a normal size rectal ampulla. In anismus, feces are packed solid at the level of the puborectalis muscle. Melanosis coli may be present. Its presence and concentration do not correlate to patterns of transit through the large bowel, bowel movements, and duration of symptoms.[26] The lumen may be enormous and contain stools of much smaller caliber. Atony of the bowel wall is demonstrated when the rectum remains wide open when it is exposed to atmospheric pressure. Rigid proctoscopy should be done twice: the first time without patient preparation and the patient in a nonfasting state to check for stool distribution and appearance, and the second time to evaluate prolapse after an enema has been given.

FUNCTIONAL EVALUATION

ANORECTAL MANOMETRY

The diagnostic usefulness of anorectal manometry for a single patient presently is limited to the differential diagnosis of idiopathic constipation and short-segment Hirschsprung's disease, which neither radiology nor pathology is able to diagnose, especially in the ultrashort forms of the disease, and to the diagnosis of anismus.[27] Few studies have focused on anorectal motility in patients with colonic inertia as opposed to slow transit constipation and with slow transit constipation as opposed to normal transit constipation. Resting pressure in the anal canal of patients with chronic idiopathic constipation may be above normal, normal, or below normal. In the original paper describing colonic inertia, pressure was found to be higher than normal in both the upper and lower anal canal.[11] Normally, anal pressure is higher in the upper than in the lower anal canal, but in 20% of constipated patients an inverted profile may be recognized. Instability of the anal pressure in constipation may be associated with slow or ultraslow waves. The rectoanal inhibitory reflex (RAIR) may be below normal, normal, or above normal in amplitude. An elevation in the threshold of the RAIR has also been recognized. In the original paper describing colonic inertia, 76% of patients had an abnormal RAIR, with at least one of the values indicating a reflex configuration outside the normal range.[11] Painful constipation is accompanied by an elevated anal maximum resting pressure and by an elevated RAIR amplitude; of note, painful constipation is also accompanied by a shorter colorectal transit time. Some patients with slow transit constipation or colonic inertia also appear to have anismus.[28-31]

BALLOON DEFECATION

In balloon defecation a water-filled balloon is used to investigate the rectoanal dynamics during defecation. Patients with anismus cannot expel a balloon from their rectum.[28,32-34]

DEFECOMETRY

Defecometry records the pressures within a balloon, over time, as it is defecated. This is the only technique capable of detecting the amount of work performed during defecation and may be helpful in evaluating abnormal defecatory patterns in patients with colonic inertia.[35]

BALLOON PROCTOGRAM

A balloon proctogram evaluates the level of the pelvic floor in relation to the pubococcygeal line; it also describes the change in the anorectal angle and the behavior of the anal sphincters.[36] Balloon topography, in addition, yields opening pressures of the anal canal during distension and permits evaluation of the anal canal length.

DEFECOGRAPHY

Defecography is another way to investigate anorectal morphology and dynamics during defecation.[37,38] Failure of the anorectal angle to widen on straining, pelvic floor descent, presence of rectocele, internal intussusception or mucosal prolapse, a longer than normal time to expel barium, incomplete rectal emptying, inability to defecate, and a nonrelaxing puborectalis have all been described. The clinical importance of these findings is, however, still unclear.

RECTAL SENSATION

Constipated patients usually have a higher mean rectal sensory threshold than a control group has. Evidence suggests that many patients with constipation but without obvious megarectum fail to appreciate small volumes of up to 50 ml in a rectal balloon, whereas this volume is felt by all normal adults. Rectal sensation tested by balloon distension (rectometrogram) is depressed in patients with de novo slow transit constipation. It is also depressed in children and in adults with chronic idiopathic constipation. Of note, many clinicians confuse hypoesthesia and atonicity of the rectal wall, a motor problem, with real lack of sensation. Rectal sensation may also be evaluated by application of a slowly increasing current to the rectal mucosa, noting the sensory threshold. Rectal mucosal electrosensitivity correlates well with values of rectometrogram.

RECTAL AND SIGMOID COMPLIANCE

The normal rectum demonstrates a receptive relaxation in response to distension, confirming its function as a reservoir. This ability is defined as compliance or distensibility of the rectum. There is as yet no generally accepted "gold standard" to evaluate rectal compliance.[39] In the rectometrogram technique, compliance represents the rectal pressure change that results from infusion of a given quantity of water. Reported findings from the use of this technique in constipated patients vary greatly. Barostat measurements allow evaluation of the pressure volume quotient at defined distension pressure intervals. This is a more objective measurement of rectal compliance because it has no association with the subject's perception of a rectal balloon. In chronic severe constipation, changes in rectal wall contractility in response to feeding, to neostigmine, and to glucagon are decreased. Greater rectal distension is required to generate rectal contractions in elderly patients admitted with fecal impaction and in chronically constipated patients with incontinence.

Barostat measurements in the sigmoid may provide a way to detect colonic tone and phasic events. The elastic properties of the sigmoid colon are different in constipated patients who have delayed left colonic transit. Maximum tolerable volumes are less than in health, with decreased compliance of the bowel wall. In health, contractile activity reaches a peak of half the maximum tolerable volume and then decreases because of muscle overstretch, whereas in constipation the maximum activity is reached at maximum distension.

COLONIC MOTILITY TESTS

There is some evidence that there are two distinct patterns of colonic motor activity in patients with constipation: some have little movement and little progression of feces from the cecum, whereas others have a pattern resembling that of normal subjects and respond to a number of stimuli.[40]

Studies of colonic motility have shown that in some constipated subjects, motor activity of the sigmoid colon increases to an abnormal degree after meals, suggesting spasticity. In others, it is the reverse and hypomotility is observed after meals.[41] This again suggests two groups of constipated subjects who have delayed transit in colon: the hypomotor and the hypermotor subjects.

Patients with slow transit constipation do not have colonic hypersegmentation and may have little spontaneous colonic activity or response to topical stimulation with bisacodyl, food, or edrophonium chloride. This latter finding suggests a possible abnormality of the myenteric plexus.

Usefulness of colonic motility tests (pressure studies) in daily practice is limited by such variables as normal ranges for colonic pressures, bowel preparations, variability and reproducibility of motor activity, and segmental differences.[42] In patients disabled by severe dysmotility syndrome, however, they sometimes provide the only objective evidence of abnormalities.

There seems to be no increase in intraluminal pressure during fasting in patients with severe constipation. There is also no movement of an intraluminal tracer (technetium-99m DTPA [diethylenetriaminopentaacetic acid]) during the same period.

Colonic motor response to eating is depressed in patients with slow transit constipation.[43] Patient response after ingestion of a meal is characterized by a shorter than normal period of contractile activity and by propagated contractions of well below normal amplitude.[44] Propulsive activity of the colon throughout 24 hours is not vigorous, and the urge to defecate is minimal.[45]

Twenty-four-hour manometric recordings reveal not only that chronically constipated patients have a significantly lower number of mass movements[44] but also that about 30% of them have no movement at all.[43,45] These mass movements are also of significantly shorter duration.

Prolonged ambulatory recording in patients with slow transit constipation shows that the rectal motility index and the frequency of anal canal contractions are below normal. In response to feeding, patients had significantly reduced motor activity in the distal bowel and anal canal.

COLONIC AND RECTAL ELECTROMYOGRAPHY

Despite considerable progress in the knowledge of human colonic motor function, the relationship between electrical and mechanical activity and their significance in regard to transit of the products of digestion and their daily distribution in health and disease remain uncertain.[46] Recording electrical activity of the large bowel is interesting and may be a key element in dictating conduct.

The basal colonic electrical rhythm may be altered in patients with constipation. There seems to be an increase in mean frequency of the slow waves. Bueno[46] found an increase in the frequency of short spike bursts (11 to 80 per hour, lasting 1.5 to 3.5 seconds) thought to be associated with segmental nonpropulsive contractions. The high pressure peristaltic waves are accompanied by electrical long spike bursts (20 to 26 per hour, lasting 17 to 21 seconds).

Slow propulsion of radiopaque markers does not necessarily indicate the absence of motility. Distal obstruction may be accompanied by retrograde propagation of peristaltic movements. Segmental nonpropulsive hypermotile zones may be present in painful constipation. This is accompanied by an increase in the number of nonpropagated action potentials.

In patients with prolonged colonic transit time the number of propagating electrical potentials is significantly decreased in fasting conditions, and no postprandial increase in their number is observed.[46] Myoelectrical evidence of the absence or reduction of migrating long spike bursts is pathognomonic for colonic inertia. Absence of these bursts revealed a rare congenital abnormality of the hindgut (Likongo syndrome).[47]

Rectal motor complexes[48,49] have also been described, but no pattern of cyclic motility in the anal canal has been reported. Patients complaining of slow transit constipation have impaired cyclic rectal activity. They have little rectal motility and display few rectal motor complexes (3.3 ± 1.3 per subject per 24 hours), which are irregularly distributed over time and respond weakly to ingestion of a standard meal. Rectal motor complexes occur as often in patients with slow transit constipation without anismus as they do in controls, but with a markedly reduced amplitude. This and the less frequent occurrence of sampling reflex (spontaneous fall of anal sphincter pressure of less than 1 minute duration), which is indicative of rectal filling, support the concept of reduced transit of feces to the rectum from the colon.

ELECTROMYOGRAPHY AND PUDENDAL NERVE MOTOR TERMINAL LATENCY

Slow transit constipation is frequently associated with anismus. Anal electromyography (EMG) and pudendal nerve motor terminal latency (PNMTL) assessment provide in-depth physiologic evaluation of disorders of defecation in these patients. Straining may damage the nerves that supply the pelvic floor.[50,51] Electrophysiologic evidence of reinnervation in the external anal sphincter and puborectalis muscle has been demonstrated.[52]

Severely constipated patients may have abnormally prolonged PNMTL.[52] Significant perineal descent seems to correlate with increased PNMTL, but some authors have refuted these findings. EMG of the puborectalis may also document paradoxical puborectalis syndrome (anismus) in chronic constipation,[53] but this may be limited to this muscle or to the external anal sphincter or encompass both muscles.

SACRAL REFLEX FUNCTION

Reflexes between the perineal skin and the pelvic floor can also be investigated to determine the integrity of the innervation to and from the cauda equina. Electrical stimulation of the dorsogenital nerve fails to elicit reflex activity in the external anal and urethral sphincters in most women defecating less than twice a week. In young women defecating from once a week to once every 5 weeks, fewer patients had complete absence of the reflex. They also had normal sensory thresholds and normal motor unit potentials, but there was a prolonged pudendoanal latency.[54]

In elderly patients of both sexes the reflex was absent in only 4 of 15 patients, and it was prolonged in 5. These studies suggest an impairment of the integration of sensory information in some patients with chronic idiopathic constipation.

Spinal evoked responses during electrical rectal stimulation or external anal sphincter contraction elicited by magnetic stimulation over the lumbosacral cord identifies patients with limited sacral neuropathies.

CONSTIPATION AS A BODY CLUE

The scientific approach to medicine does not take into account the subjective, often imaginary elements in the patient's body image. Physicians must constantly keep in mind that constipation involves not only the infrequent passage of hard stools but also the psychological effect this condition has on the patient. Physicians still find selfish pleasure in their practice of medicine: because of their curiosity about interesting "cases" and their desire to control the disease and the patient, they use many invasive procedures ("furor medicus") for the sake of reaching a high degree of diagnostic certainty. Often the constipated patient is not a "good," compliant patient, and this may trigger unpleasant feelings, frustration, and even anger in the physician and may lead to a break in the physician-patient relationship, to unnecessary surgery, or even to medicolegal difficulties between physician and patient.

Recording a life history as well as a case history is essential. An in-depth interview covering major life experiences serves this purpose. It may trigger marked emotional responses, which contribute to the release of long repressed conflicts. A cruder approach is to use the MMPI (Minnesota Multiphasic Personality Inventory) or another psychologic test and relate the findings and profile interpretation to the patients.[55] Some patients resent even the idea of having a psychologic problem, and caution must be exercised in this regard or the patient may go shopping for another doctor.

The possibility of sexual abuse in the past history must be recognized.[56-58] Disclosure of the trauma, particularly if it is accompanied by emotional release, may suddenly cure constipation associated with what has been labeled the "pathogenic secret."[59]

The relationship between emotions, personality, and bowel habits is poorly understood, although such a relationship was proposed over 50 years ago. Voluntary repression of defecation is said to lead to chronic rectal distension and megarectum, but this is simplistic. There is a relationship between stool output and personality. Healthy volunteers tend to produce more frequent and heavier stools if they display a good degree of self-esteem and are outgoing.[60]

Constipated patients found to have normal colorectal transit times have significantly more psychopathology than do those with delayed transit times in which the pathophysiologic signs correlate with the symptom of constipation.[61] Normal transit times in patients complaining of constipation is universally associated with evidence of psychosocial disturbances, including use of antidepressant medications, psychiatric counseling, and ongoing litigation. Patients complaining of constipation whose colorectal transit time is less than 70 hours have abnormally high scores of somatization, anxiety, and depression; interpersonal sensitivity, hostility, phobic anxiety, paranoid ideation, and psychosis scores are also higher than in controls and patients with constipation and delayed transit times.[61] Somatization of affect is the tendency to interpret anxiety as a physical symptom. Clinicians must recognize the "hidden agenda" of these patients. Not surprisingly, constipated patients fare poorly after surgery for their symptoms if they are anxious or depressed.[62]

Constipated patients with delayed transit through the ascending colon have a different personality than arthritic controls.[55] They score higher on several scales of the MMPI: hypochondria, hysteria, control, and low back pain. They score lower on the male-female (MF) scale, which means they are more feminine. They show a profile known as the "psychosomatic V" or "conversion valley": this profile indicates patients who are protected from depression by their constipation.

There is a close relationship between levels of anxiety and transit time in the ascending colon. In patients with constipation due to delayed colonic transit but with some evidence of motor activity in the large bowel, constipation might be the sole expression of anxiety.[55] Megacolon is found in psychiatric patients, which also suggests a link between mind and body. Similarly, in patients with constipation due to colonic inertia, transit times in the ascending colon correlate with the level of paranoia.[55] Cure from constipation by a psychologic approach demonstrates that the basic mechanism in some people is not organic.[63] Moreover the absence of a parallel between improvement of psychopathology and improvement of physiopathology is a potent argument that psychological disturbance is not simply a consequence of bowel dysfunction.[63] A disturbed childhood, psychosexual problems, and personality difficulties are commonly associated with constipation. Adult subjects who seek medical help for irritable bowel syndrome have been shown to have a recollection of significantly more painful childhood events. Memory is colored by intervening events, and what matters is not the event itself but its meaning to the person.

Available data thus concur on the need to include an appraisal of psychologic elements in the medical management of patients with chronic idiopathic constipation.

TREATMENT

DIET

A trial with a high-fiber diet (30 g of dietary fiber or 14.4 g of crude fiber) should be done before any diagnostic studies are made in constipated patients whose history and physical examination do not suggest organic disease. This type of diet usually does not work in patients suffering from slow transit constipation or colonic inertia. In fact, it makes symptoms even worse and thus should be abandoned.

BIOFEEDBACK

Biofeedback techniques (manometry, EMG) aimed at specific measurable functional abnormalities found in patients with chronic constipation may be useful. Numerous studies now provide evidence for this.[64,65] Biofeedback also may decrease (1) the force of contraction of the external anal sphincter, (2) the ultraslow waves, and (3) the sensory threshold for rectal distension and (4) can coordinate the contraction and relaxation of the pelvic floor. There is no question that anismus disappears and that constipation eases during and after biofeedback therapy. Associated symptoms such as abdominal pain and bloating may also regress. It remains to be discovered why and how this occurs and in whom. Many biofeedback protocols also include generalized relaxation techniques and increased body awareness of muscle relaxation.

PHARMACOLOGIC APPROACH

Changes in Bowel Content

Bulk laxatives may be recommended for long-term therapy of chronic idiopathic constipation. They may increase symptoms if there is a delayed transit through the colon[16] and are usually of no therapeutic value in slow transit constipation and colonic inertia. Magnesium hydroxide (Milk of Magnesia), mineral oil, and low-volume enemas are usually not successful in these patients.

Lactulose, a nonabsorbable synthetic disaccharide, is metabolized by colonic bacteria and has both an osmotic and a stimulation effect.

An oral colon washout solution (such as 250 to 500 ml of polyethylene glycol solution) daily has also been suggested as a relatively safe approach.

Changes in Motor Function

Colonic instillation of bisacodyl is associated with an increase in sporadic spike bursts recorded myoelectrically, which are, particularly the propagating ones, associated with abdominal cramping and an urge to defecate. However bisacodyl does not modify motor activity of the ascending or descending colon.

Bethanechol has been tried without success in patients with delayed transit in the ascending colon.

Cisapride, a gastrointestinal prokinetic agent without antidopaminergic or direct cholinomimetic effects, stimulates release of acetylcholine from the myenteric plexus and stimulates motility of the small and large bowel in humans. Cisapride accelerates colonic transit in the cecum and ascending and transverse colon and thus may be useful in the treatment of colonic inertia. It increases stool frequency and the number of stools of normal consistency while concomitantly reducing laxative use. It increases rectal motor activity and rectal compliance in constipated patients and reduces the sensory threshold to rectal distension.

Trimebutine (not available in the United States) interacts with opiate receptors in the intestine. It is useful in constipated patients who have evidence of delayed transit, probably by stimulation of propagated electrical activity. Naloxone, a specific opioid antagonist, has been used in severe constipation. It seems to accelerate gastric emptying and small bowel transit time.

Misoprostol (200 µg t.i.d.) may be useful in some patients.

Vasopressin, injected intramuscularly at a pharmacologic dose, increases propagated electrical activity and triggers defecation in patients with slow transit constipation who have less than one stool per week.

Erythromycin, a motilin agonist, has been shown to accelerate transit in normal volunteers. Cases of chronic intestinal pseudo-obstruction with a sustained response to erythromycin have been reported.

SURGICAL APPROACH

Surgery for intractable debilitating constipation is a radical step not to be taken without investigation[66] and until all other means of treatment have been exhausted. It does not provide a perfect solution.

Results of studies on the surgical treatment of constipation are difficult to analyze. Lack of uniform preoperative physiologic evaluation and random allocation of patients to a variety of surgical resections create a heterogeneous patient population. Different definitions of functional outcome and variable length of follow-up add to this lack of uniformity. Following an extensive algorithm of physiologic investigation is manda-

TABLE 68-1. RESULTS OF 18 STUDIES OF SMALL BOWEL OBSTRUCTION

Author	Year	Number of Patients	SBO (%)	Surgery for SBO (%)	Successful Functional Outcome (%)
Hughes	1981	10	50	100	80
Klatt	1983	9	–	–	100
Preston	1984	16	43	42	81
Gilbert	1984	6	NS	NS	100
Roe	1986	7	NS	NS	71
Beck	1987	11	7	100	100
Walsh	1987	21	29	59	57
Leon	1987	13	70	44	77
Grasslander	1987	6	–	–	100
Vasilevsky	1988	52	36	66	79
Kamm	1988	44	18	100	50
Zenilman	1988	12	8	0	100
Akerwall	1988	12	25	100	66
Yoshioka and Keighley	1989	40	10	75	58
Pemberton	1990	38	11	75	NS
Koremans	1990	11	–	–	60
Wexner	1991	16	19	0	94
Pena	1992	105	24	48	89

SBO = small bowel obstruction.

tory in the selection of patients with severe constipation for colectomy. This will reduce the number of candidates and possibly will predict a good outcome. Colonic transit time; evacuation proctography; anorectal manometry and EMG; rectal sensation and compliance; balloon expulsion test; esophageal, small bowel, and colonic manometry; gastric emptying studies; and colonic EMG are all putative tests to evaluate colorectal physiology in patients with intractable constipation.

The following criteria for election as a subtotal colectomy candidate were proposed by Rex et al[67]:

1. Documented colonic inertia
2. Absence of outlet obstruction
3. Adequate sphincter length
4. Absence of clinically apparent psychologic disturbances
5. Absence of diffuse gut dysmotility
6. Major interference with life activities

Several reports noted the outcome of segmental colectomy for chronic intractable constipation. Total abdominal colectomy with ileorectal anastomosis is the standard operation for the treatment of chronic intractable slow transit constipation. Table 68–1 is a compilation of results and complications of 18 published papers.

Total proctocolectomy with ileoanal reservoir has also been performed to help patients with severe intractable constipation.

Preoperative outcome predictors have been sought to improve some poor results. Yet they are unsubstantiated in long-term controlled trials. Some psychologic aspects (anxiety and depression) predict poor surgical outcome,[62] and up to one fourth of patients undergoing colectomy need psychiatric treatment.[68] The track record of most surgical procedures for disorders having a physiologic basis but with exaggerated psychiatric overtones is a dismal one of failed surgical endeavor.[69]

An abnormally high level of rectal sensation also predicts failure, and abnormal compliance may herald a poor postoperative result. Failure to expel preoperatively a rectal balloon filled with 50 ml of water predicts postoperative pain and need of laxatives, but neither defecography nor anismus at electromyography can predict those outcomes. Conversely, tailoring the large bowel resection to the extent of abnormal transit may be helpful.

Patients with colonic inertia or slow transit constipation who exhibit paradoxical puborectalis contraction should be treated with biofeedback to correct the aberrant muscle function before even thinking of surgery. After the training has been completed, if colonic inertia is again noted on repeat colonic transit time and the paradoxical contraction has been corrected, the patient may be a candidate for surgical treatment.[70]

Chronically constipated women should be questioned regarding physical or sexual abuse because they may benefit from specific therapy for this trauma and because abuse may be a marker for functional gut disorders. These patients are at risk of unnecessary surgery.[20,57,71] It is not clear, however, the extent to which such a history will influence the need for or appropriateness of surgery for intractable colonic inertia.[67]

A successful functional outcome has been reported in 80% of cases. However, there are many postoperative complications, such as persistent constipation, diarrhea (22%), and fecal incontinence (11%). A high reoperation rate of 27% and a high incidence of small bowel obstruction (25%) have been reported.[72] Subtotal colectomy for other indications is usually not associated with this incidence of small bowel obstruction. It is not clear why there are such different outcomes after identical surgical procedures.

Surgery remains a viable option in psychologically normal patients with objective evidence of diffuse colonic slowing and in the absence of a generalized intestinal motility disorder. In addition, candidates for surgery should be warned that a satisfactory clinical outcome is not guaranteed and that complications are not uncommon.

Psychological Approach

Although psychotherapy has proven useful in patients with irritable bowel syndrome, in a randomized trial[73] a notable exception was constipation. Yet there are anecdotal reports[74] that cure may occur during long-term follow-up and not because of organic medical treatment. It is only at that moment, in retrospect, that constipation is recognized as having underlying psychological and emotional factors. What can be said from these striking anecdotes, well documented in terms of pathophysiology, is that surgery should be performed with caution and that in the domain of constipation, very long term studies are needed before it can be asserted that surgery is better than psychotherapy.

REFERENCES

1. Drossman DA, Sandler RJ, McKee DC, Lovitz AJ. Bowel patterns among patients not seeking health care. *Gastroenterology.* 1982;83:529–534.
2. Whitehead WE, Chaussade S, Corazziari E, Kumar D. Report of an international workshop on management of constipation. *Gastroenterol International.* 1991;4(3):99–113.
3. Lanfranchi GA, Bazzocchi G, Brignola C, et al. Different patterns of intestinal transit time and anorectal motility in painful and painless chronic constipation. *Gut.* 1984;25:1352.
4. Martelli H, Devroede G, Arhan P, Duguay C. Mechanisms of idiopathic constipation: outlet obstruction. *Gastroenterology.* 1978;75:623–631.
5. Bouchoucha M, Devroede G, Arhan P, et al. What is the meaning of colorectal transit time measurement? *Dis Col Rect.* (In press).
6. Arhan P, Devroede G, Jehannin B, et al. Segmental colonic transit time. *Dis Col Rect.* 1981;24:625–629.
7. Metcalf AM, Phillips SF, Zinsmeister AR, et al. Simplified assessment of segmental colonic transit time. *Gastroenterology.* 1987;92:40–47.
8. Arbuthnot Lane W. Chronic intestinal stasis. *Br Med J.* June 1909:1408–1411.
9. Kuijpers H. Application of the colorectal laboratory in diagnosis and treatment of functional constipation. *Dis Col Rect.* 1990;33:35–39.
10. Wald A. Colonic transit and anorectal manometry in chronic idiopathic constipation. *Arch Intern Med.* 1986;146:1713.
11. Watier A, Devroede G, Duranceau A, et al. Constipation with colonic inertia a manifestation of systemic disease? *Dig Dis Sci.* 1983;28(11):1025–1033.
12. Wexner SD, Bartolo DCC. Slow transit constipation and anismus. In: Wexner SD, Bartolo DCC, eds. *Constipation: Etiology Evaluation and Management.* Oxford, England: Butterworth-Heinemann, Ltd. 1995:160–167.
13. Kamm MA, Lennard-Jones JE, Thompson DG, et al. Dynamic scanning defines a colonic defect in severe idiopathic constipation. *Gut.* 1988;29:1085–1092.
14. Stivland T, Camilleri M, Vassallo M, et al. Scintigraphic measurement of regional gut transit in idiopathic constipation. *Gastroenterology.* 1991;101:107–115.
15. Roe AM, Bartolo DCC, Mortensen NJMcC. Slow transit constipation. Comparison between patients with and without previous hysterectomy. *Dig Dis Sci.* 1988;33:1159–1163.
16. Preston DM, Lennard-Jones JE. Severe chronic constipation of young women: idiopathic slow transit constipation. *Gut.* 1986;27:41–48.
17. Reynolds JC, Ouyang A, Lee CA, et al. Chronic severe constipation. Prospective motility studies in 25 consecutive patients. *Gastroenterology.* 1987;92:414–420.
18. Kamm MA, Fasthing MJG, Lennard-Jones JE. Bowel function and transit rate during the menstrual cycle. *Gut.* 1989;30:605–608.
19. Kamm MA, Furthing MJG, Lennard-Jones JE, et al. Steroid hormone abnormalities in women with severe idiopathic constipation. *Gut.* 1991;32:80–84.
20. Denis P, Duval V, Roussignol C, Weber J. Anisme et aggression sexuelle. *Gastroenterol Clin Biol.* (In press).
21. Preston DM, Adrian TE, Christofides ND, et al. Positive correlation between symptoms and circulating motilin, pancreatic polypeptide and gastrin concentrations in functional bowel disorders. *Gut.* 1985;26:1059–1064.

22. Dolk A, Broden G, Holmstrom B, et al. Slow transit chronic constipation (Arbuthnot Lane's disease): an immunohistochemical study of neuropeptide-containing nerves in resected specimens from the large bowel. *Int J Colorect Dis.* 1990;5:181–187.
23. Lincoln J, Crowe R, Kamm MA, et al. Serotonin and 5-hydroxyindoleacetic acid are increased in the sigmoid colon in severe idiopathic constipation. *Gastroenterology.* 1990;98:1219–1225.
24. Bannister JJ, Lawrence WT, Smith A, et al. Urological abnormalities in young women with severe constipation. *Gut.* 1988;29:17–20.
25. Abdel-Rahman M, Toppercer A, Duguay C, et al. Urorectodynamics in patients with colonic inertia. *Urology.* 1981;18(4):428–432.
26. Badioli D, Marcheggiano A, Pallone F, et al. Melanosis of the rectum in patients with chronic constipation. *Dis Col Rect.* 1985;28:241–245.
27. Meunier PD. Anorectal manometry. A collective international experience. *Gastroenterol Clin Biol.* 1991;15:697–702.
28. Preston DM, Lennard-Jones JE. Anismus in chronic constipation. *Dig Dis Sci.* 1985;30:413.
29. Jones PN, Lubowski DZ, Swash M, Henry MM. Is paradoxical contraction of puborectalis muscle of functional importance? *Dis Col Rect.* 1987;30:667–670.
30. Barnes PRH, Lennard-Jones JE. Patients with constipation of different types have difficulty in expelling a balloon from the rectum. *Gut.* 1985;26:1049–1052.
31. Read NW, Timms JM, Barfield LJ, et al. Impairment of defecation in young women with severe constipation. *Gastroenterology.* 1986;90:53–60.
32. Barnes PRH, Lennard-Jones JE. Balloon expulsion from the rectum in constipation of different types. *Gut.* 1985;26:1049–1052.
33. Read NW, Timms JM, Barfield LJ, et al. Impairment of defecation in young women with severe constipation. *Gastroenterology.* 1986;90:53–60.
34. Kuijpers HC, Bleijenjerg G. The spastic pelvic floor syndrome. A cause of constipation. *Dis Col Rectum.* 1985;28:669–672.
35. Lestar B, Penninckx FM, Kerremans RP. Defecometry. A new method for determining the parameters of rectal evacuation. *Dis Col Rect.* 1989;32:197–201.
36. Preston DM, Lennard-Jones JE, Thomas BM. The balloon proctogram. *Br J Surg.* 1984;71:29.
37. Mahieu P, Pringot J, Bodart P. Defecography. I. Description of a new procedure and results in normal patients. *Gastrointest Radiol.* 1984;9:247.
38. Mahieu P, Pringot J, Bodart P. Defecography. II. Contribution to the diagnosis of defecation disorders. *Gastrointest Radiol.* 1984;9:253.
39. Madoff RD, Orrom WJ, Rothenberger DA. Rectal compliance: a critical reappraisal. *Int J Colorect Dis.* 1990;5:27–40.
40. Bazzochi J, Ellis J, Villanueva-Meyer J, et al. Postprandial colonic transit and motor activity in chronic constipation. *Gastroenterology.* 1990; 98:686–693.
41. Meunier P, Rochas A, Lambert R. Motor activity of the sigmoid colon in chronic constipation: comparative study with normal subjects. *Gut.* 1979;20:1095.
42. Jameson JS, Misiewicz JJ. Colonic motility: practice or research? *Gut.* 1993;34:1009–1012.
43. Narducci F, Bassotti G, Gaburri M, Morelli A. Twenty-four-hour manometric recording of colonic motor activity in healthy man. *Gut.* 1987;28:17–25.
44. Bassotti G, Betti C, Erbella GS, et al. Prolonged manometric investigation of the colon in research on chronic constipation. *Ital J Gastroenterol.* 1991;23(suppl 1):13–15.
45. Bassotti G, Gaburri M, Imbimbo BP, et al. Colonic mass movements in idiopathic chronic constipation. *Gut.* 1988;29:1173–1179.
46. Bueno L, Fioramonti J, Ruckebusch Y, et al. Evaluation of colonic myoelectrical activity in health and functional disorders. *Gut.* 1980;21:480–485.
47. Likongo Y, Devroede G, Schang JC, et al. Hindgut dysgenesis as a cause of constipation with delayed colonic transit. *Dig Dis Sci.* 1986;31:993–1003.
48. Kumar D, Williams NS, Waldron D, Wingate DT. Prolonged manometric recording of anorectal motor activity in ambulant human subjects: evidence of periodic activity. *Gut.* 1989;30:1007–1011.
49. Orkin BA, Hanson RB, Kelly KA. The rectal motor complex. *J Gastrointest Motility.* 1989;1:5–8.
50. Kiff ES, Barnes PRM, Swash M. Evidence of pudendal neuropathy in patients with perineal descent and chronic straining at stool. *Gut.* 1984;11:1279–1284.
51. Henry MM, Parks AG, Swash M. The pelvic floor musculature in the descending perineum syndrome. *Br J Surg.* 1982;69:470–472.
52. Snooks SJ, Barnes PRH, Swash M, Henry MM. Damage to the innervation of the pelvic floor musculature in chronic constipation. *Gastroenterology.* 1985;89:977–981.
53. Miller R, Duthie GS, Bartolo DCC, et al. Anismus in patients with normal and slow transit constipation. *Br J Surg.* 1991;78:690–692.
54. Varma JS, Smith AM. Neurophysiological dysfunction in young women with intractable constipation. *Gut.* 1988;29:963–968.
55. Devroede G, Roy T, Bouchoucha M, et al. Idiopathic constipation by colonic dysfunction: relationship with personality and anxiety. *Dig Dis Sci.* 1989;34(9):1428–1433.
56. Drossman DA. Sexual and physical abuse and gastrointestinal disorders in women: what is the link? *Med Aspects Hum Sexuality.* (In press).
57. Arnold RP, Rogers D, Cook DAG. Medical problems of adults who were sexually abused in childhood. *Br Med J.* 1990;300:705–708.
58. Leroi AM, Bernier C, Watier A, et al. Why do patients with functional motor disorders of the lower gastrointestinal tract complain more often of a past history of sexual abuse than patients with functional motor disorder of the upper gastrointestinal tract? Submitted to *Int J Colorectal Dis.*
59. Devroede G. Constipation and sexuality. *Med Aspects Hum Sexuality.* Feb. 1990:40–46.
60. Tucker DM, Sandstead HH, Logan GM Jr, et al. Dietary fiber and personality factors as determinants of stool output. *Gastroenterology.* 1981;81:879.
61. Wald A, Hinds JP, Camana BJ. Psychological and physiological characteristics of patients with severe idiopathic constipation. *Gastroenterology.* 1989;97:932–937.
62. Fisher SE, Breckon K, Andrews HA, Keighley MRB. Psychiatric screening for patients with faecal incontinence or chronic constipation referred for surgical treatment. *Br J Surg.* 1989;76:352–355.
63. Devroede G, Bouchoucha M, Girard G. Constipation, anxiety and personality: what comes first? In: "Stress and Digestive Motility" L. Bueno, S. Collins, J.L. Junior, John Libbey Eurotext, London, Paris. 1989; pp. 55–60.

64. Loening-Baucke V. Modulation of abnormal defecation dynamics by biofeedback treatment in chronically constipated children with encopresis. *J Pediatr.* 1990;116: 214–222.
65. Weber J, Ducrotte Ph, Touchais JY, et al. Biofeedback training for constipation in adults and children. *Dis Col Rect.* 1987;30:844–846.
66. Wexner SC, Jagelman DN. Colectomy for constipation: physiologic investigation is the key to success. *Dis Col Rect.* 1991;34:851–856.
67. Rex DK, Lappas JC, Goulet RC, Madura JA. Selection of constipated patients as subtotal colectomy candidates. *J Clin Gastroenterol.* 1992;15(3):212–217.
68. Kamm MA, Hawley PR, Lennard-Jones JE. Outcome of colectomy for severe idiopathic constipation. *Gut.* 1988;29:969–973.
69. Keighley MRB. Surgery for constipation. *Br J Surg.* 1988;75:625–626.
70. Schmitt SL, Wexner SD, Bartolo DCC. Surgical treatment of colonic inertia. In: Wexner SD, Bartolo DCC, eds. *Constipation: Etiology Evaluation and Management.* Oxford, England: Butterworth-Heinemann, Ltd. 1995: 153–159.
71. Longstreth GF, Preskill DB, Youketes L. Irritable bowel syndrome in women having diagnostic laparoscopy or hysterectomy. Relation to gynecologic features and outcome. *Dig Dis Sci.* 1990;35(10):1285–1290.
72. Kamm MA, Hawley PR, Lennard-Jones JE. Outcome of colectomy for severe idiopathic constipation. *Gut.* 1988;29:969–973.
73. Guthrie E, Creed F, Dawson D, Torrenson B. A controlled trial of psychological treatment for the irritable bowel syndrome. *Gastroenterology.* 1991;100:450–457.
74. Devroede G. Psychophysiological considerations in subjects with chronic idiopathic constipation. In: Wexner SD, Bartolo DCC, eds. *Constipation: Etiology, Evaluation and Management.* Oxford, England: Butterworth-Heinemann, Ltd. 1995:103–134.

69

Intestinal Obstruction

MICHAEL E. GLICK

Intestinal obstruction is a common problem defined by impaired transit of intestinal contents. This impaired transit may be due to mechanical obstruction or may be functional (ileus) due to an impairment of normal intestinal propulsion as a consequence of neuromuscular dysfunction.

CLASSIFICATION

Intestinal obstruction can be classified by mechanism, by site, by consequences, or by underlying pathology. The mechanism may be mechanical, due to a structural blockage of intestinal transit, or may be functional, due to absence or disorganization of the normal propulsive activity of the intestinal tract. Intestinal obstruction also may be classified as proximal small bowel obstruction, distal small bowel obstruction, or colonic obstruction (Table 69–1). It is also useful to classify mechanical obstruction by the physiologic consequences because these consequences alter management and prognosis. Intestinal obstruction may be classified as simple (uncomplicated) obstruction, closed loop obstruction, or strangulated obstruction. A simple or uncomplicated obstruction occurs when there are no superimposed consequences to the interference with intestinal transit. A closed loop obstruction impairs intraluminal flow both proximally and distally. Strangulated obstruction is a mechani-

TABLE 69–1. CLASSIFICATION OF INTESTINAL OBSTRUCTION

1. Uncomplicated (simple) intestinal obstruction
  a. High small bowel
  b. Low small bowel
  c. Colonic
2. Complicated intestinal obstruction
  a. Closed loop obstruction
  b. Strangulated obstruction

TABLE 69–2. ETIOLOGY OF INTESTINAL OBSTRUCTION

Mechanical
1. Intraluminal
  a. Foreign body
    (1) Gallstones
    (2) Bezoar
    (3) Meconium
    (4) Feces
    (5) Parasites
    (6) Barium
  b. Intussusception
  c. Polypoid neoplasm
2. Mural
  a. Congenital (atresia, bands, Meckel's diverticulum, stenosis, etc.)
  b. Inflammatory
    (1) Crohn's disease
    (2) Diverticulitis
    (3) Ischemic strictures
    (4) Radiation enteritis
    (5) Drug induced (nonsteroidal antiinflammatory drugs, potassium chloride)
  c. Neoplastic
    (1) Primary
    (2) Metastatic
    (3) Traumatic (hematoma)
3. Extrinsic
  a. Adhesions
    (1) Congenital
    (2) Postoperative
  b. Hernias
    (1) External (inguinal, femoral)
    (2) Internal
  c. Volvulus
  d. Mass
    (1) Abscess
    (2) Pancreas (annular, inflammation, or neoplasm)
    (3) Carcinomatosis
    (4) Endometriosis
    (5) Pregnancy
Functional
1. Acute pseudoobstruction
  a. Postoperative ileus
  b. Nonoperative ileus
    (1) Electrolyte disturbances
    (2) Inflammatory (cholecystitis, pancreatitis, abscess, pyelonephritis, sepsis)
    (3) Idiopathic (spinal cord injury, trauma, etc.)
    (4) Intestinal ischemia
2. Chronic pseudoobstruction
  a. Myopathy
  b. Neuropathy

cal obstruction complicated by interference with the blood supply to a segment of intestine that threatens ischemia or necrosis.

ETIOLOGY

While the two most common causes of mechanical small bowel obstruction are hernias and adhesions, the differential diagnosis is extensive and challenging (Table 69–2). Mechanical obstruction may be due to an *intraluminal* process such as a foreign body, intussusception, or polypoid neoplasm. Obstruction may also be due to a *mural* lesion of the gut wall that may be congenital or inflammatory (e.g., Crohn's disease or diverticulitis). Lastly, obstruction may be due to an *extrinsic* process such as adhesions, hernias, volvulus, or masses. An obstruction may be functional rather than mechanical, most often postoperative, or due to inflammation or electrolyte imbalance. Rarely, functional obstruction may be due to a neuromuscular process leading to a chronic impairment of gastrointestinal motility.

The most common causes of obstruction, in descending order, include adhesions or bands, hernias, cancer, volvulus, intussusception, inflammatory lesions, congenital malformations, and foreign bodies. The approximate frequencies of these causes are summarized in Table 69–3.

PATHOPHYSIOLOGY

The effects of intestinal obstruction are due to disturbances of normal intestinal transport, increased fluid secretion, decreased fluid absorption, and the consequences of the loss of the integrity of the bowel wall. Obstruction leads to impaired intestinal absorption and increased intestinal secretion with sequestration of fluid into the gut lumen, abdominal distension, increased intraluminal pressures with impaired vascular supply, nausea, and vomiting. Intestinal distension is not harmful unless it leads to impaired respiration, intravascular fluid depletion, or intraluminal pressures that constitute risk of ischemia or perforation. Simple obstruction may lead to massive sequestration of intraluminal fluid with intravascular depletion, dehydration, and shock. Intraluminal stasis leads to a rapid

TABLE 69-3. FREQUENCY OF CAUSES OF INTESTINAL OBSTRUCTION

Cause	Frequency of Occurrence
Adhesions and bands	50%
Hernias	21%
Cancer	13%
Volvulus	3%
Intussusception	2%
Inflammatory	1%
Congenital	1%
Foreign bodies	1%
Other	6%

proliferation of bacteria, which is harmless until impaired vascular supply or increased intraluminal pressures promote transluminal leakage of bacteria or bacterial toxins. Toxins reaching the peritoneal cavity are rapidly absorbed. Bacteria leaking into the peritoneal cavity produce peritonitis.

In a closed loop obstruction, increased intestinal secretion within the isolated segment of gut leads to increased intraluminal pressure, impaired circulation, ischemia, loss of intestinal integrity, necrosis, and perforation. In a strangulated obstruction, the early impairment of blood supply to a segment of intestine may lead to blood loss or leakage of bacterial toxins and bacteria into the peritoneal cavity. Therefore, it is critical to recognize the threat of strangulation, since early intervention is essential for preservation of life. Resection of the strangulated segment of bowel is essential to eliminate the source of bacteria and bacterial toxins. Although the consequences of fluid sequestration into the intestinal lumen and blood loss can be repaired by fluid, electrolyte, and blood replacement, the consequences of leakage of intestinal bacteria and their toxins can only be alleviated by surgical intervention.

CLINICAL PRESENTATION

The clinical presentation of intestinal obstruction is determined by the site of obstruction, the cause of the obstruction, and any complications associated with the obstruction (Table 69-4).

SYMPTOMS

The most frequent symptoms of obstruction are abdominal pain, vomiting, and obstipation. Initially, intestinal obstruction and distension lead to crampy abdominal pain. However, with increased intestinal distension, strangulation, or perforation, pain may become constant. Pain is often diffuse, but with a closed loop obstruction and transmural injury, the pain may become localized. Often, vomiting decompresses the intestine and relieves pain. Passage of intestinal contents through a partial obstruction may also relieve pain. The progression of pain with increased severity, localization, and constancy suggests strangulation and warrants urgent surgical intervention. With partial obstruction, there may be continued passage of stool and flatus.

Vomiting is also a frequent presentation. Vomiting occurs early in proximal intestinal obstruction and may not occur at all in distal intestinal obstruction or colonic obstruction. The quality of the vomitus may provide some clue to the level of obstruction. In a proximal obstruction, the vomitus may be bilious. In more distal obstruction, the vomitus may be "feculent" because of extensive bacterial overgrowth. Frequently, colonic obstruction occurs in the face of a competent ileocecal valve that prevents retrograde movement of colonic contents into the distal small bowel. Under such circumstances, distension may be extensive without vomiting. With a partial obstruction, there may be no vomiting, and some flatus may be passed. Key elements of the history should include a search for previous operations, prior symptoms of distension or crampy abdominal pain, prior change in stool habits, weight loss, and use of drugs.

TABLE 69-4. CLINICAL PRESENTATION OF INTESTINAL OBSTRUCTION

	Proximal Small Bowel	Distal Small Bowel	Colon
Vomiting	Frequent, bilious, relieves pain	Intermittent, feculent	Intermittent, feculent
Pain	Colicky, intermittent, relieved by vomiting	Intermittent or constant	Constant
Distension	Minimal	Moderate	Severe
Tenderness	Epigastric or periumbilical	Diffuse	Diffuse

PHYSICAL EXAMINATION

A search for abdominal scars is essential, and a careful examination to exclude hernias is imperative. Blood pressure and pulse monitoring performed while the patient is reclining and upright may be a guide to volume depletion. A fever may suggest impairment of intestinal wall integrity. Skin turgor may provide evidence of dehydration. Distension may be minimal or dramatic. On auscultation of the abdomen, there may be high-pitched peristaltic sounds, or a silent abdomen may suggest peritoneal inflammation or ileus. Abdominal examination may reveal distension, tenderness, or guarding. Localized distension may suggest a closed loop, and localized tenderness may suggest peritoneal irritation. Diffuse tenderness suggests strangulation, perforation, and peritonitis. A mass palpated within the abdomen may be due to closed loop obstruction or malignancy. Rectal and pelvic examination is essential in the search for a pelvic mass. The clinical presentation, including symptoms and physical findings, is summarized in Table 69–4. This table emphasizes the relationship between the site of intestinal obstruction and the presenting signs and symptoms.

LABORATORY STUDIES

Laboratory tests are not usually helpful in the diagnosis of intestinal obstruction but are essential in defining the metabolic consequences of obstruction. A marked increase in hematocrit and azotemia suggest hemoconcentration due to intravascular volume depletion. Volume depletion may lead to a contraction alkalosis, or sepsis may lead to a metabolic acidosis. Electrolyte derangements may be a consequence of fluid sequestration or fluid loss through vomiting. Emesis of gastric acid from proximal obstruction may deplete chloride. More distal obstruction may result in a more balanced loss of acid and base. A leukocytosis or shift in the white cell differential may be a consequence of volume depletion or may suggest intestinal strangulation or perforation. Elevated serum amylase may be due to intestinal amylase as a consequence of strangulation or may suggest pancreatic inflammation secondary to obstruction or an ileus as a consequence of pancreatitis. It is essential not to assume that hyperamylasemia is due to underlying pancreatitis. A urinalysis provides specific gravity as a guide to the state of hydration, and a positive result from a urine sediment test may suggest a retroperitoneal cause for ileus.

RADIOLOGIC STUDIES

Plain films of the abdomen, as well as an upright chest film, are the most important study for the initial evaluation and observation of patients with abdominal pain, distension, or vomiting. Recumbent films are essential to search for unusual gas patterns, seek evidence for the site of intestinal obstruction, and differentiate mechanical obstruction from paralytic ileus. In addition, these films may provide a clue as to the cause of the obstruction. An early feature of intestinal obstruction is the accumulation of intraluminal gas proximal to the level of obstruction. This accumulation of gas and intestinal secretions is visible as air-fluid levels. The fluid is the result of decreased intestinal absorption and increased intestinal secretion, and the gas is a consequence of impaired passage of swallowed air. Early in the course of intestinal obstruction, air-fluid levels are visible on recumbent films. It is usually possible to distinguish between distended small bowel and colon. Small bowel distension is marked by the smaller diameter of distended loops, central localization of the loops, stepladder pattern, and the valvulae conniventes that mark small bowel anatomy. In contrast, colonic obstruction can be distinguished by the location of the air-fluid levels and by the haustral markings in the colon. Occasionally, massive small bowel distension may be difficult to distinguish from colonic obstruction. In proximal small bowel obstruction, the findings on recumbent films may be much less dramatic. However, there will usually be a distended proximal loop of bowel and absence of distal gas, particularly absence of gas in the rectum. A distended colon with no air-fluid levels seen in the small bowel implies a competent ileocecal valve, whereas air-fluid levels seen throughout the small and large intestine imply an incompetent ileocecal valve, a less common condition. When obstruction is limited to the small bowel, the level of obstruction may be suggested by the amount of distended small bowel. If there are diffuse air-fluid levels with distension of the colon to the rectum and the rectal examination is unremarkable, a paralytic ileus is likely. A number of radiologic features may suggest specific complications. The finding of a "coffee"-bean sign suggests a closed loop obstruction marked by a localized dilation of a loop of intestine. Free air under the diaphragm, best seen in an upright chest film, may signify perforation. If an upright chest film is not possible because of patient debility, a lateral film of the abdomen should be obtained. Sequential films of the abdomen are essential as a tool to follow the progress of an intestinal obstruction.

Intraluminal contrast studies may be indicated. A water-soluble contrast enema may be helpful to distinguish between colonic obstruction and functional ileus. A contrast enema may also be important to seek a specific site of obstruction and a specific cause. This examination may also have therapeutic potential in patients with intussusception or volvulus. Water-soluble contrast should *not* be used in the upper gastrointestinal tract, since the hyperosmotic nature of this contrast agent may exacerbate fluid sequestration, and the large quantity of intraluminal fluid is likely to dilute the water-soluble agent, diminishing any diagnostic information.

Occasionally, an upper gastrointestinal tract barium study is indicated in an effort to differentiate obstruction from paralytic ileus, to determine the completeness of an obstruction, to seek a cause for recurrent obstruction, and to look for evidence of carcinomatosis. The passage of barium through the area of partial obstruction suggests that continued observation may be indicated.

MANAGEMENT

Patients with suspected intestinal obstruction should always receive early surgical consultation. Figure 69–1 outlines an algorithm for management of intestinal obstruction. Internist and surgeon should frequently reevaluate and reconsult with each other. The first goal is to correct fluid and electrolyte deficits. The second goal is the decompression of the gut by gastrointestinal intubation. The urgency for alleviation of obstruction is often a difficult judgment based on clinical suspicion of closed loop obstruction, intestinal strangulation, or intestinal infarction. Usually, fluid and electrolyte repletion are necessary prior to surgical intervention.

The degree of dehydration and electrolyte loss can be assessed by clinical signs with the help of calculations of hemoconcentration and azotemia. If there has been intraluminal bleeding, blood replacement may be necessary.

Every patient with intestinal obstruction should undergo nasogastric intubation. Intestinal decompression may alleviate discomfort and may provide definitive management. A postpy-

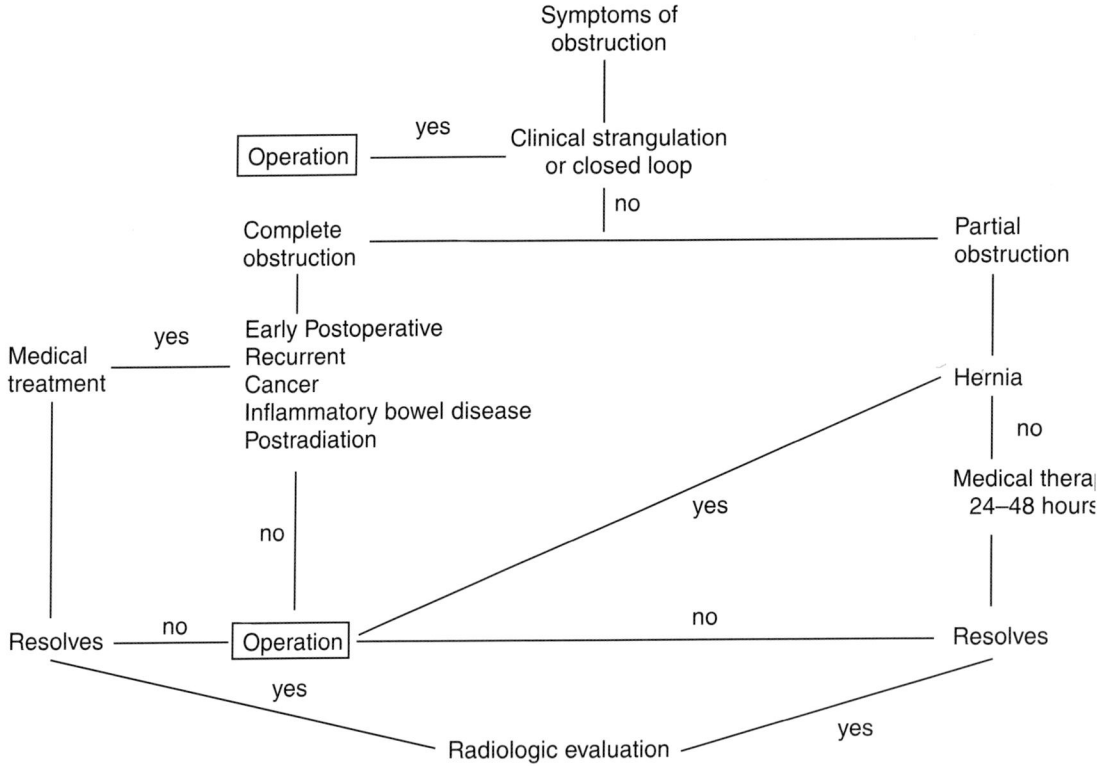

FIGURE 69–1. Management of intestinal obstruction.

loric or long intestinal tube is rarely necessary. However, a long tube may be of benefit in patients with prolonged ileus, known carcinomatosis, or an underlying disease process for which surgery is unlikely to be of benefit. The volume of nasogastric aspirate is helpful in assessing fluid status and should be monitored at frequent intervals. If the patient is improving with nasogastric suction, continued medical management may be justifiable. Throughout any period of observation, frequent reevaluation should include vital signs, temperature, abdominal examination (to assess pain, tenderness, or peritoneal inflammation), white cell count, and repeat abdominal x-ray examination.

Evidence of progressive abdominal distension, increasing abdominal pain, or increasing gut dilation on abdominal films are all indications for urgent surgical exploration. Patients with closed loop obstruction or large bowel obstruction with a competent ileocecal valve require urgent operation to prevent perforation. The closed loop cannot be decompressed with a nasogastric tube. In patients showing signs of nutritional depletion or requiring prolonged nasogastric intubation, parenteral nutrition should be considered. A more prolonged trial of management with intravenous fluid and intestinal suction may be warranted in patients who have had recurrent small bowel obstructions due to adhesive disease, known inflammatory bowel disease, known intraperitoneal cancer or carcinomatosis, or surgery. However, even these patients may require operative intervention if they do not show progressive improvement over several days' observation.

Definitive intervention includes operation to address the underlying problem. The specific intervention is dependent on the underlying cause of intestinal obstruction. Antibiotics are unnecessary unless there is clinical suspicion of strangulation or perforation with toxicity. Under these circumstances, antibiotics should include coverage for both aerobic and anaerobic intestinal and colonic organisms. Antibiotics in this setting are an adjunct to definitive resection and lavage of the contaminated peritoneal cavity.

Any trial of nonoperative treatment carries a risk of progressive gut injury, missed strangulation, perforation, or peritonitis. Evidence of the development of these complications must be sought diligently. However, patients with Crohn's disease, radiation enteritis, or carcinomatosis often improve without surgical intervention.

REFERENCES

1. Cohn I. Intestinal obstruction. In: Berk JE, ed. *Bockus Gastroenterology.* 4th ed. Philadelphia, Pa: WB Saunders Co; 1985.
2. Jones RS. Intestinal obstruction. In: Sabiston DC, ed. *Textbook of Surgery.* Philadelphia, Pa: WB Saunders Co; 1991.
3. McFadden DW, Zinner MJ. Manifestations of gastrointestinal disease. In: Schwartz SI, ed. *Textbook of Surgery.* New York, NY: McGraw-Hill Book Co; 1994.
4. Schuffler MD, Sinanan MN. Intestinal obstruction and pseudo-obstruction. In: Sleisenger MH, Fordtran JS, eds. *Gastrointestinal Disease.* 5th ed. Philadelphia, Pa: WB Saunders Co; 1993.
5. Summers RW, Lu CC. Approach to the patient with ileus and obstruction. In: Yamada T, ed. *Textbook of Gastroenterology.* New York, NY: JB Lippincott Co; 1991.

70
Irritable Bowel Syndrome and Constipation

ROBERT F. WILLENBUCHER

The irritable bowel syndrome (IBS) is a heterogenous group of functional gastrointestinal tract disorders involving the small intestine and colon. A functional gastrointestinal tract disorder is characterized by a chronic or recurrent symptom or symptom complex referable to the gastrointestinal tract without an identifiable anatomic cause. Central to the definition of IBS is abdominal pain. Therefore, IBS should be viewed as a functional gastrointestinal tract disorder with abdominal pain of colonic origin. Pain of colonic origin is that which is relieved by defecation or is associated with a discreet change in bowel habit (i.e., stool consistency or frequency). The focus of this chapter is on patients with IBS who have constipation as their primary bowel complaint.

PATHOPHYSIOLOGY

Some appreciation of the pathophysiologic processes that underlie IBS is necessary to adequately direct treatment. It is crucial to understand that even in patients with constipation-predominant IBS there is considerable heterogeneity in the pathophysiology. Understanding and identifying these variations in pathophysiology through careful history taking and simple diagnostic tests allows the development of a rational therapeutic approach.

Patients with constipation-predominant IBS may have some component of altered visceral sensation or altered colonic motility. In addition, many or most patients have a significant psychologic component of pathogenesis. In fact, it is likely that psychologic factors play a critical role in the modulation of visceral pain perception. In addition, psychologic factors appear to weigh heavily in patients with apparent misperceptions of their bowel habit. Because patients with constipation-predominant IBS have some component of disordered visceral sensation, colonic dysmotility, or psychopathology, each of these factors is discussed separately in this chapter.

Altered visceral perception in patients with IBS has been demonstrated using a technique of rectosigmoid balloon distension. IBS patients have a significantly lower pain threshold for rectosigmoid distension as compared with controls. This lowered pain threshold is specific to visceral sensation in that cutaneous pain sensation has not been found to differ from controls.[1] It has been hypothesized that the visceral hypersensitivity observed in patients with IBS is secondary to up-regulation of visceral afferent nerves or disordered central processing of afferent information.[2]

IBS is often defined as a motility disorder. Yet, despite extensive investigation by numerous investigators, no consistent abnormalities in colonic motility have been described. However, when the focus is instead directed toward constipation, independent of whether criteria for IBS (see below) are satisfied, recognizable motility patterns emerge. In patients with functional constipation (as defined by less than three bowel movements per week) two different abnormal patterns of colonic motility can be observed. Early studies showed that constipation could be associated with either increased or decreased colonic motility.[3] More recently, techniques have been developed to correlate colonic motility and intraluminal transit using simultaneous manometry and radionuclide transit. When applied to patients with constipation, this technique demonstrated two characteristic patterns of motility and transit.[4] One group of constipated patients had an increase in segmenting contractile activity with associated movement of tracer into the sigmoid and into the transverse colon, as described for normal controls. The second group of constipated patients had no increase in contractile activity and no associated transit of tracer. Neither group had the high-amplitude propagating contractions that were observed in the control patients. These propagating contractions, with their associated rapid transit of luminal contents to the sigmoid, seem to be necessary for a normal bowel habit. In addition, anorectal dysfunction may be present in up to 20% of selected patients with idiopathic constipation.[5]

From the first description of IBS by DaCosta in 1871, symptoms of psychologic distress in association with IBS have been noted. It has since been clearly demonstrated that IBS patients (those individuals with IBS who seek medical attention), particularly those referred to medical centers, frequently have psychiatric diagnoses including personality disorder, anxiety, depression, and somatization. This is different from individuals who meet diagnostic criteria for IBS that do not seek medical care. These individuals do not appear to differ psychologically from the general population. It has been asserted that in IBS patients, childhood reinforcement of the sick role and psychologic trauma (e.g., divorce of parents, sexual abuse) significantly affect the future likelihood of seeking (and repeatedly seeking) medical attention.[6]

DIAGNOSIS

The diagnosis of IBS involves not only the exclusion of organic disease but the careful characterization of the disordered bowel habit, patterns of pain, and the identification of psychosocial factors. As is the case with most medical illness, a reliable diagnosis can be made on the basis of a carefully performed history and physical examination with a limited diagnostic workup.

DEFINITION

Since Manning and coworkers' original paper,[7] a variety of symptom-based diagnostic criteria have been developed to aid in the diagnosis of IBS. These diagnostic schemata, whether used to define research study populations or for purposes of clinical diagnosis, fail to identify homogeneous groups of patients. The failure to identify homogeneous groups of patients results in treatment failure if simple fulfillment of diagnostic criteria is used to dictate cookbook thera-

TABLE 70–1. SYMPTOM CRITERIA FOR CONSTIPATION-PREDOMINANT IRRITABLE BOWEL SYNDROME

Continuous or recurrent symptoms (for at least 3 months) of:
1. **Abdominal pain:** relieved with defecation or associated with a change in stool frequency or consistency
2. **Disturbed defecation (constipation):** two or more of the following:
   Diminished stool frequency
   Hard stools
   Staining or incomplete evacuation
   Bloating or feeling of abdominal distension

NOTE: Evaluation should include exclusion of organic disease as described in the Diagnosis section.

Adapted from Wald A, Hinds JP, Caruana BJ. Psychological and physiological characteristics of patients with severe idiopathic constipation. *Gastroenterology.* 1989;97:932–937.

pies. Table 70–1 is a diagnostic scheme adapted for this chapter from an international working group.[8] It is readily apparent that this diagnostic scheme does not differentiate a patient with severe constipation (e.g., one bowel movement per week) from a patient with straining but normal stool frequency and an anxiety disorder. Both patients may fulfill criteria for diagnosis of constipation-predominant IBS, but treatment would be very different.

HISTORY AND PHYSICAL EXAMINATION

The history should be conducted in as nonjudgmental and open-ended manner as is possible. A major therapeutic maneuver is achieved in the first meeting if a good rapport is developed with the patient. An important goal of the history, however, is to obtain very specific information about the patient's bowel habit and pattern of pain. The onset and duration of symptoms are important pieces of information. The finding of long-term symptoms in a 35-year-old patient speaks less for organic disease than the new onset of symptoms in a 50-year-old patient. In addition, other indicators of organic disease such as weight loss and hematochezia should be pursued in the history.

Patients complaining of constipation should be carefully questioned as to the specifics of their constipation. Constipation can mean altered stool frequency, straining at bowel movements, or hard stools. Patients who state they are constipated may have any or all of these symptoms or their "constipation" may be limited to a sense of incomplete evacuation. Patients with decreased stool frequency should be questioned to establish whether they are aware of an urge to have a bowel movement and whether they routinely attend to that urge. Impaired rectal sensation may be a contributing factor in some patients with constipation. Impaired rectal sensation may result from a disease process (e.g., stroke, diabetes mellitus) or from chronic inattention to fecal urgency. In addition, all patients should be questioned about laxative use or abuse. A review of the patient's medications should be done to identify and possibly substitute constipating medications like calcium channel blockers or medications with anticholinergic side effects.

The abdominal pain associated with IBS can be quite variable in location, but it should be in association with a change in bowel frequency or consistency or relieved with defecation. Some patients with IBS have a prominent postprandial component to their pain pattern, but location and altered bowel habit point to IBS rather than biliary colic.

One of the most important parts of the history is the exploration of possible psychosocial factors. Frequently, it is the identification of the recent onset of a major psychologic stressor that clarifies why the patient has chosen to seek medical attention at a particular point in time after an extended period of seemingly unchanged chronic symptoms. As a rapport and trust develop between practitioner and patient, an increasingly deep exploration of psychologic factors can be undertaken. Some effort should be made to identify psychologic precipitators of discreet episodes of increased symptoms. In addition, further insight can be gained from a review of the patient's medical care–seeking behavior as it relates to IBS or other medical complaints.

The physical examination, which can serve to strengthen the physician-patient relationship, should be focused on the recognition of signs of organic disease—specifically, signs of nutritional deficiency, abdominal and rectal masses, and occult fecal blood.

Diagnostic Investigation

Generally, a limited investigation including a complete blood count, routine serum chemistries, and flexible sigmoidoscopy with an air contrast barium enema (or perhaps colonoscopy) is sufficient to exclude organic disease in patients with constipation-predominant IBS. There is a great tendency for certain IBS patients to seek medical care from multiple physicians and consequently undergo repetitive diagnostic testing. This phenomenon is not only costly but serves to reinforce the sick role. Wherever possible, it is prudent to obtain previous, reliable diagnostic information to avoid perpetuating this process.

In patients with decreased stool frequency who fail to respond to initial general measures (see below), it may be useful to do some further testing of colonic function. Assessing colonic transit with the use of radiopaque markers can be a very useful test in this setting. Twenty radiopaque markers (either made from 1.5-mm sections of nasogastric tubes or commercially available) are swallowed, and abdominal x-ray films are obtained on alternate days, with the first x-ray film being obtained on day 1 (24 hours after marker ingestion). Normally, at least 80% of the markers should be expelled by day 5, and all markers should be expelled by day 7. This test should be performed without the use of laxatives. In some patients with delayed colonic transit, markers may be distributed throughout the colon. This has been termed *colonic inertia*. In other patients with delayed transit, markers may accumulate in the rectum or rectosigmoid and may indicate anorectal dysfunction. These patients should undergo x-ray defecography or anorectal manometry to evaluate anorectal function. Use of ingested radiopaque markers will identify a significant number of patients with normal transit times who insist that they have infrequent bowel movements or even that they have not had a bowel movement at all during the study period. In a previous study measuring psychologic stress of patients who stated they had fewer than two bowel movements per week, patients who were found to have normal colonic transit times scored significantly higher than did patients with constipation and prolonged transit times or than asymptomatic controls did.[9] The finding of normal transit in patients who complain of severe constipation allows the careful discussion of misperceptions of bowel habit.

TREATMENT

After consideration of the previous two sections, it is possible to categorize patients by their underlying pathophysiology and predominant symptoms. This allows for more directed treatment, although most patients require some combination of treatment approaches.

GENERAL MEASURES

Establishing a good rapport with the patient is the cornerstone of effective treatment. Brief, but frequent, office visits that focus on the patient's overall well-being and daily functioning help to establish this relationship. Follow-up office visits should not focus primarily on specific symptoms, as this may encourage somatization and also convey to the patient that ongoing complaint about symptoms will assure continued interest by their physician. Office visits should begin with open-ended general questions like "How are things going for you?" rather than "Is your constipation any better?" Patients should be encouraged to talk about their work and home life before proceeding to specifics of their IBS.

Another important therapeutic maneuver is to provide reassurance. Frequently, patients with long-term symptoms choose to seek medical attention because of specific fear about an illness. Often this fear is triggered by illness in an acquaintance or information presented in the media. Concerns about cancer are quite common. Specific fears should be addressed, and the negative results of the diagnostic workup should be emphasized. Reviewing laboratory data and showing the patient the x-ray films often helps in this process and is appreciated by the patient. In addition, it provides more tangible proof of their good health.

Demanding patients who insist on additional diagnostic tests should have their demands judged primarily on medical need. Flatly refusing will likely result in the patient obtaining their workup elsewhere. Instead, deferring decision until results from previous workups can be obtained and reviewed on a subsequent visit allows for additional trust to develop in the relationship with the patient. At that point, the medical necessity of further diagnostic tests can be discussed with the patient more effectively.

During the first visit or two, some attempt should be made at identifying psychosocial stressors that trigger symptoms. A nonjudgmental discussion of how emotions, negative thoughts, and psychologic stress affects physiologic processes may help the patients to gain insight into potential triggers of their symptoms. The simple realization of this process may assist some patients in adopting more effective coping strategies. Other patients may benefit from some form of psychologic therapy (see below).

Some form of a nutritional survey should be performed with each patient. Effort should be made to identify symptom-triggering foods and to attempt to eliminate those foods. This is an ideal time to provide guidelines on a low-fat, low-cholesterol, high-fiber diet to aid in general health maintenance. Patients should be instructed to increase their dietary fiber, especially since constipation is a prominent symptom. This should be accomplished through increasing the amount of fiber-rich foods in the diet and through fiber supplements that may include bran or one of the many psyllium-containing products available on the market. The goal should be approximately 25 to 30 g of dietary fiber per day. This may require 10 to 15 g of supplementary fiber. A sudden increase in dietary fiber, particularly in IBS patients, frequently results in a marked increase in bloating symptoms and a dismayed or even irate patient. Psyllium should be added to the diet slowly, beginning with a dose of approximately 3 g a day and increasing slightly each week such that the target amount of fiber is achieved over a several-week period. Patients should be instructed to increase their water consumption as well.

Many patients respond quite favorably to these general measures. Patients with persistent symptoms should have further treatment directed at predominant symptoms as follows.

CONSTIPATION

Patients with constipation refractory to general measures and fiber should undergo a radiopaque marker transit study as described in the diagnostic investigation section. Normal results from a transit study in patients who claim to have infrequent bowel movements (less than two per week) are highly predictive of a significant psychologic component to the underlying disease process.[9] These patients are most likely to respond to some form of psychologic therapy rather than more intensive pharmacotherapy directed at constipation.

In patients with delayed colonic transit evidenced by radiopaque marker study, the possibility of anorectal and pelvic floor dysfunction should be excluded with anorectal manometry or sensation testing and x-ray defecography whenever available. This is particularly important in patients with delayed colonic transit who strain at their bowel movements. Patients with specific forms of anorectal dysfunction, like internal rectal prolapse or impaired internal anal sphincter relaxation, are more likely to respond to surgical measures.

In patients without anorectal or pelvic floor dysfunction, bowel habit should be carefully reviewed and a course of bowel retraining undertaken. This includes attending to all bowel movement urges and developing a daily routine with time set aside to sit on the commode regardless of urge. Patients who are impacted with hard stool should be disimpacted with a regimen of enemas and an oral osmotic laxative (e.g., magnesium citrate) or mineral oil. After disimpaction and during bowel retraining, oral osmotic laxatives (e.g., Milk of Magnesia or lactulose) should be used as needed. Elderly patients should be monitored for electrolyte abnormalities, and magnesium-containing laxatives should be avoided in patients with impaired renal function. Chronic use of senna- or phenolphthalein-containing laxatives should be avoided.

Patients with persistent symptoms may be treated with a trial of prokinetic agents. Metoclopramide is generally unsuccessful, as it has little effect on colonic motility. Cisapride, a prokinetic agent that increases myenteric cholinergic outflow through its effect on serotonin receptors, is currently approved in the United States for treatment of gastroesophageal reflux. At dosages of 10 to 20 mg orally four times a day, some patients with constipation or constipation-predominant IBS may respond favorably to cisapride.[10,11] Patients with refractory and debilitating symptoms of constipation may ultimately require abdominal colectomy and ileoproctostomy. This should only be undertaken after a careful assessment of upper gastrointestinal tract motility is carried out to exclude a diffuse gastrointestinal tract motility disorder.

Abdominal Pain, Gas, and Bloating

There is a distinct subset of patients who complain primarily of postprandial abdominal pain or discomfort and bloating without decreased stool frequency. Excessive intestinal gas is often an associated complaint. The majority of these patients do not have excessive production of intestinal gas but more likely have visceral hypersensitivity to normal degrees of gaseous bowel distension.

Exclusion or limitation of gas-producing foods may result in symptomatic improvement regardless of the actual degree of gas production. Lactase deficiency may contribute to gas and bloating, and a lactose-free diet may improve symptoms. A stepwise elimination of other gas-producing foods may identify other dietary factors. A partial list of "flatugenic" foods includes beans, the cabbage family, onions, and starches (except rice starch).

A variety of anticholinergic or spasmolytic medications are available for the treatment of the crampy abdominal pain associated with IBS. These medications have met with mixed results in placebo-controlled trials. This lack of success most likely is due to the lack of a clear correlation between increased gastrointestinal tract motility and pain symptoms and to the likelihood that symptoms are due to a sensory defect rather than hypercontractility. Some patients respond favorably to anticholinergic agents (e.g., dicyclomine 10 to 20 mg 30 minutes before meals), but anticholinergic side effects are frequently bothersome.

Patients with intractable pain may benefit from referral to a multidisciplinary pain center. Treatment with antidepressant medications that modulate serotonin levels in the central nervous system has been used with some success in other chronic pain syndromes. It is probable that psychologic therapies (see below) may modulate pain perception at the neurochemical level in selected patients. IBS, by definition, is a chronic disorder. Therefore, narcotics and sedative-hypnotics should be avoided because of their potential for addiction and abuse.

Psychologic and Behavioral Therapy

Patients with identifiable axis 1 psychiatric diagnoses (e.g., depression) should be referred to a psychiatrist for appropriate psychopharmacotherapy. Attention should be given to avoiding antidepressants with anticholinergic effects in constipated patients. Effective treatment of an underlying depression frequently results in marked improvement in coping with previously debilitating bowel symptoms.

A variety of behavioral and psychologic therapies have been investigated in the treatment of IBS.[6] These studies have suffered from methodologic flaws that have limited their interpretation, but anecdotal experience suggests that these therapies can be very successful.

Behavioral therapies include relaxation training and meditation, hypnosis, and biofeedback. These techniques are particularly useful when patients can recognize stressors that trigger their IBS symptoms and then institute an activity (e.g., meditation) that mitigates their response to the stressor.

A variety of psychotherapies may be useful in improving overall well-being in IBS patients. Insight-oriented psychotherapy (e.g., object relations psychotherapy) is useful for patients motivated to understand the effect of previous interpersonal relationships on their reaction to psychosocial stressors. Cognitive (cognitive behavior) therapy holds that faulty learning or misinterpretations of reality (e.g., feelings of worthlessness) lead to negative automatic thoughts or cognitions and subsequent dysfunctional behavior. Identifying and restructuring negative thoughts and misperceptions of reality are the goals of cognitive behavior therapy. Stress-coping training and stress management are examples of cognitive behavior therapy.

There is some evidence that a multicomponent approach involving relaxation techniques, biofeedback, and psychotherapy may be highly effective.[12] Most likely, studies of IBS do not consistently report efficacy of psychologic treatment because inadequate diagnostic criteria were used to define study groups. Commonly used diagnostic criteria (Table 70–1) fail to define homogeneous groups of patients. Individual patients will usually respond to a flexible, multicomponent treatment approach involving relaxation techniques and psychotherapy tailored to their individual needs.

The therapeutic approach to the constipation-predominant patient with IBS can be summarized as follows:

1. Develop an appreciation for the potential underlying pathophysiologic components including visceral hypersensitivity, impaired colonic motility, and psychopathology.
2. Perform a careful history and physical examination focused on interpreting symptoms in the context of the underlying pathophysiology.
3. Perform a limited diagnostic workup consisting of a complete blood count, routine serum chemistries, and flexible sigmoidoscopy or air contrast barium enema (or colonoscopy) to exclude organic disease.
4. Institute general treatment measures that include developing a therapeutic relationship, providing reassurance and education, and dietary interventions including fiber supplementation.
5. Patients who fail to respond adequately to general treatment measures should receive additional diagnostic testing and therapy directed at their predominant symptom(s).

REFERENCES

1. Whitehead WE, Holtkotter B, Enck P, et al. Tolerance for rectosigmoid distention in irritable bowel syndrome. *Gastroenterology.* 1990;98:1187–1192.
2. Mayer EA, Raybould HE. Role of visceral afferent mechanisms in functional bowel disorders. *Gastroenterology.* 1990;99:1688–1704.
3. Connell AM. The motility of the pelvic colon. II. Paradoxical motility in diarrhoea and constipation. *Gut.* 1962;342–348.
4. Bazzocchi G, Ellis J, Villanueva-Meyer J, et al. Postprandial colonic transit and motor activity in chronic constipation. *Gastroenterology.* 1990;98:686–693.
5. Martelli H, Devroede G, Arhan P, Duguay C. Mechanisms of idiopathic constipation: outlet obstruction. *Gastroenterology.* 1978;75(4):623–631.
6. Drossman DA, Thompson WG. The irritable bowel syndrome: review and a graduated multicomponent treatment approach (see comments). *Ann Intern Med.* 1992;116:1009–1016.
7. Manning A, Thompson WG, Heaton K, Morris A. Towards positive diagnosis of the irritable bowel. *Br Med J.* 1978;653–654.
8. Thompson WG, Dotevall G, Drossman DA, Heaton KW, Kruis W. Irritable bowel syndrome: guidelines for the diagnosis. *Gastroenterol Int.* 1989;2:92–95.
9. Wald A, Hinds JP, Caruana BJ. Psychological and physiological characteristics of patients with severe idiopathic constipation. *Gastroenterology.* 1989;97:932–937.
10. Van Outryve M, Milo R, Toussaint J, Van Eeghem P. "Prokinetic" treatment of constipation-predominant irritable bowel syndrome: a placebo-controlled study of cisapride. *J Clin Gastroenterol.* 1991;13:49–57.
11. Muller-Lissner SA. Treatment of chronic constipation with cisapride and placebo. *Gut.* 1987;28:1033–1038.
12. Neff DF, Blanchard EB. A multi-component treatment for irritable bowel syndrome. *Behav Ther.* 1987;18:70–83.

71

Irritable Bowel Syndrome and Diarrhea

DAVID J. ROBERTS and JOHN W. WILEY

This chapter is devoted to the management of diarrhea-prone irritable bowel syndrome. To effectively discuss the management of this disorder, we first provide some background regarding aspects of the history, physical examination, and initial laboratory evaluation that supports the diagnosis of this common presentation to the clinician.

Historically, irritable bowel syndrome (IBS) has been viewed appropriately as a diagnosis of exclusion. Although no pathognomonic marker has been identified, we feel that the presence of a relatively specific constellation of persistent, intermittent symptoms is highly supportive of the diagnosis of IBS. We encourage the practitioner to view and discuss the diagnosis IBS with the patient in a "positive" light, both to allay concerns regarding more serious diagnoses and to help remove the stigma that is frequently associated with so-called "functional" bowel disorders. Reassurance and insight are two key aspects to managing the patient with IBS. We favor performing a limited number of diagnostic tests, initially, to help build the patient's confidence in the physician and the diagnosis. Our diagnostic and initial therapeutic measures are outlined in Figure 71–1.

Our experience suggests that repeated diagnostic testing undermines the patient's confidence in both the physician and the diagnosis, as well as plays into a tendency of patients with IBS to seek opinions from multiple physicians. It is prudent to establish early in the treatment plan a realistic goal of reducing and not eradicating symptoms, emphasizing that the physician and patient share responsibility for management decisions. This also provides the patient with the appropriate psychosocial support that is an important component in the management of a chronic disorder such as IBS.

Although the differential diagnosis of IBS is quite extensive at first glance (Table 71–1), many possibilities can be excluded on the basis of the history alone. To this end, we feel that the most important aspect of the patient's initial evaluation is the history.

HISTORY

The history should focus on eliciting the presence of symptom patterns that are characteristic of IBS. A number of key historical features proposed by Manning and colleagues[28] support the diagnosis of IBS (Table 71–2). These include abdominal pain relieved by defecation, distension of the abdomen and abdominal pain associated with altered stool frequency or consistency. Additionally, a sense of incomplete evacuation and the presence of mucus in the stool support the diagnosis of IBS, as do chronic symptoms that are consistent in their pattern but variable in intensity. Flares in symptomatic IBS are frequently associated with periods of stress. The presence of persistent, painless, watery diarrhea, particularly when associated with weight loss, should alert the clinician to consider causes other than IBS.

Special attention should be paid to the pres-

TABLE 71–1. DIFFERENTIAL DIAGNOSIS OF DIARRHEA-PRONE IRRITABLE BOWEL SYNDROME

1. Inflammatory bowel disease
2. Colorectal cancer
3. Giardiasis and other parasitic disorders
4. Infectious diarrhea, including *Clostridium difficile*
5. Food intolerance: lactose, fructose, or sorbitol intolerance; wheat, bran products, and brassica vegetables
6. Small bowel bacterial overgrowth
7. Microscopic or collagenous colitis
8. Laxative abuse
9. Endocrinopathies: hyperthyroidism, carcinoid, vipomas, gastrinomas, somatostatinomas

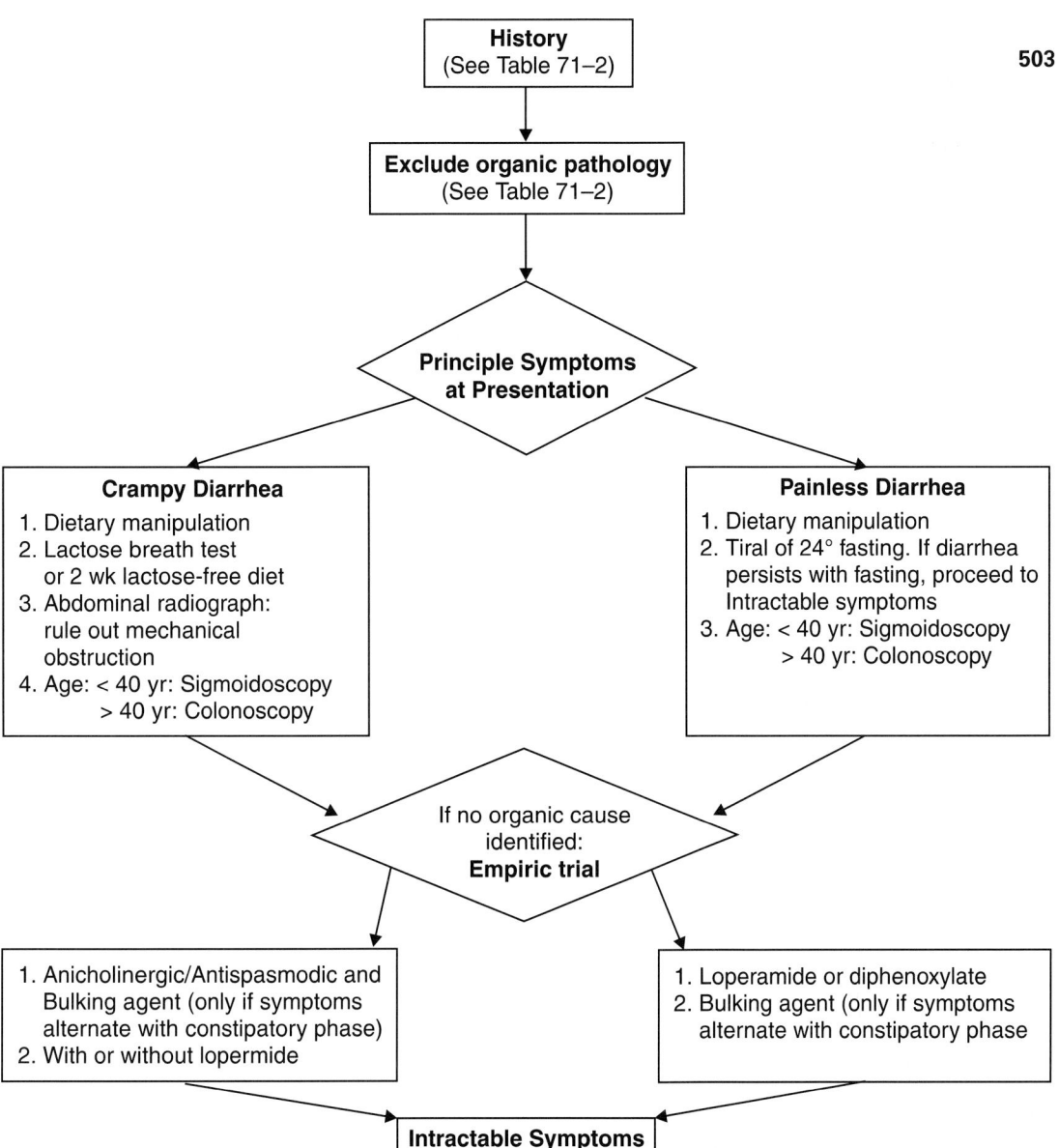

FIGURE 71–1. Algorithm for management of diarrhea-prone irritable bowel syndrome.

TABLE 71–2. KEY FEATURES OF THE HISTORY AND EVALUATION

Key Features of History
Consistent with Diagnosis of IBS
1. Longevity of illness: chronic history with waxing and waning symptoms
2. Abdominal distension
3. Abdominal pain associated with altered frequency or consistency of stools
4. Presence of mucus with defecation
5. Sense of incomplete evacuation
6. Absence of unintentional weight loss and constitutional symptoms and signs
7. Absence of blood with bowel movements
8. Exacerbations with psychologic distress
9. History of childhood sexual or physical abuse

Inconsistent with Diagnosis of IBS
1. Diet history: history of reproducible intolerance to specific food categories such as lactose, sorbitol, fructose, beans, wheat products
2. Water supply and travel history: rule out giardiasis and infectious diarrheas
3. Past medical history: inflammatory bowel disease or gastrointestinal neoplasia or systemic illness (diabetes mellitus, scleroderma, etc.)
4. Past surgical history: bile acid diarrhea, bacterial overgrowth, postvagotomy syndrome

Key Features of Diagnostic Evaluation
*1. Complete blood count
*2. Sedimentation rate
*3. Rectal examination: tone, pain, fissures, hemorrhoids, mucus, occult blood in stool
*4. Integument examination: signs of prior surgery or physical abuse
*5. Stool examination: ova and parasites, culture for enteric pathogens, leukocytes and *Clostridium difficile* toxin, if indicated by history
6. If history and physical examination are equivocal: flexible sigmoidoscopy or colonoscopy with biopsy to rule out inflammatory bowel disease, colorectal neoplasia, microscopic or collagenous colitis and melanosis coli
7. If indicated by history and symptoms: lactose hydrogen breath test or 2-week lactose-free diet; thyroid function testing; rule out hyperthyroidism
8. Intractable symptoms: jejunal aspiration for ova and parasites, endoscopy with small bowel biopsy, small bowel barium study
9. Rarely needed tests: small bowel manometry and gastrointestinal transit studies; assessment of bile acids; serum studies for gastrointestinal hormone-secreting tumors: vipoma, gastrinoma, somatostatinoma; rule out carcinoid syndrome and medullary thyroid carcinoma

*Recommended initial evaluation for all patients suspected of having diarrhea-predominant IBS.
IBS = irritable bowel syndrome.

ence of anal incontinence, systemic illness, prior hospitalizations, and surgical history. Inquiries should be made regarding other family members affected by similar symptoms, recent travel, and water supply. The family history should include pointed questions regarding a history of "spastic colitis," inflammatory bowel disease, and cancer. Recent studies by Drossman et al[10] suggest that individuals who have a history of psychologic trauma including divorce, alcoholism, and sexual or physical abuse are more likely to experience symptoms of IBS. Careful questioning may reveal that the patient is unduly concerned about cancer. A food and drug inventory are mandatory. Specific inquires should be made regarding the consumption of lactose-containing foods, bran products, wheat products, brassica vegetables (e.g., asparagus, broccoli, cauliflower), foods containing sorbitol or fructose, and the effect of high-fat meals on the patient's symptoms.

Features of a patient's history that do not support the diagnosis of IBS and suggest the need for additional diagnostic studies include onset in old age, progressive symptoms, nocturnal diarrhea, fever, weight loss not readily attributable to depression, rectal bleeding not associated with fissures or hemorrhoids, and steatorrhea.

PHYSICAL FINDINGS

The physical examination in IBS patients is characteristically unrevealing. The patient may complain of vague and poorly localized tenderness during the abdominal examination and a tender loop of bowel may be palpated. The presence of any structural abnormalities such as lymphadenopathy, masses, hepatosplenomegaly, ascites, jaundice, or occult blood in the stool argue against a diagnosis of IBS. The rectal examination is a particularly useful aspect of the physical examination. It is important to assess the tone of the sphincter, degree of pain and tenderness associated with the examination, and to document the presence of hemorrhoids or fissures. Assessing the presence of mucus or occult blood and confirming the consistency of stool in the rectal vault can be helpful. Occasionally, the integument examination can be informative if it reveals evidence for unmentioned prior surgery or physical abuse.

INITIAL LABORATORY AND DIAGNOSTIC EVALUATION

The initial laboratory evaluation should include a complete blood count and a sedimentation rate (Table 71–2). The combination of normal values on these two tests and the absence of findings on the history or physical examination that suggest organic dysfunction are 83% sensitive and 97% specific in supporting the diagnosis of IBS.[8]

Stool should be collected for occult blood, leukocytes, and culture for enteric pathogens. Specific clinical situations may warrant testing of the stool for *Clostridium difficile* toxin, ova and parasites (O&P), and fecal fat. Positive results in any of these tests would not be consistent with a diagnosis of IBS.

When the physician is faced with an equivocal initial history or physical examination, a sigmoidoscopy should be performed if the patient is less than 40 years old. We usually perform colonoscopy if the patient is over 40 years old. Endoscopy is useful to rule out gross inflammatory conditions, colorectal neoplasia, and melanosis coli, as well as microscopic and collagenous colitis with the aid of a biopsy. If the patient complains of anal incontinence, the physician should consider obtaining anal-rectal manometry and defecography studies.

INITIAL TREATMENT

When the history, physical examination, and initial laboratory studies are consistent with the diagnosis of IBS, we favor an empiric approach to treatment targeted at the patient's main complaint. The patient is actively encouraged to participate in all management decisions. Realistic goals should be established that focus on symptom diminution and not curing the IBS. Patient education regarding the possible pathophysiologic mechanism(s) underlying IBS, as well as available behavior, dietary, and pharmacologic interventions, should be discussed and is often quite helpful in alleviating the patient's concern that the symptoms of IBS are all "in my head."

In general, for the IBS patient with diarrhea and alternating constipation, we favor the gradual introduction of a fiber supplement to avoid the attendant bloating and cramping that are often experienced with the abrupt addition of high-dose fiber supplementation. The patient should gradually increase a fiber preparation (Metamucil, Konsil, L.A. Formula, Citracil, etc.) from 1 teaspoon in a glass of liquid followed by another glass of liquid once a day to a maximum dose of 1 to 2 tablespoons twice a day over a 2- to 3-week period. The timing of administering these hydrophilic colloids may be individualized. Ideally, they are best prescribed at mealtime to allow efficient mixing with the stool as it forms. However, obese individuals may benefit from its appetite-suppressant effects when taken before meals, and conversely, thin patients may wish to consume the fiber preparation after meals. Several studies have suggested that the efficacy of fiber supplementation in reducing symptoms in IBS is limited to those patients with the complaint of constipation.[4,30] For this reason we generally do not offer fiber to patients with "pure" functional diarrhea.

When the patient presents primarily with noncrampy diarrhea, we initiate treatment with an antidiarrheal agent such as loperamide (Imodium), 2 mg every 6 to 8 hours, or diphenoxylate (Lomotil), 2.5 to 5 mg every 6 hours. Loperamide has a longer duration of action than diphenoxylate and lacks the atropine found in Lomotil. In the subset of IBS patients who present with crampy diarrhea, we generally include an antispasmodic, typically an anticholinergic. It is important for the patient to realize that any relief associated with antispasmodics is usually incomplete. Either dicyclomine (Bentyl), 10 to 20 mg orally, hyoscyamine sulfate (Levsin), 0.125 mg sublingually or orally, or propantheline bromide (Pro-Banthine), 7.5 to 15 mg orally, are given 30 to 40 minutes before meals. Patients should be screened for the presence of disorders, such as glaucoma and obstructive uropathy, where the use of anticholinergics is contraindicated.

INTRACTABLE SYMPTOMS

Unfortunately, a sizable proportion of the IBS population continues to experience symptoms despite an empiric trial. In this subset we routinely repeat stool testing for O&P; if clinical suspicion of giardiasis remains, we either investigate with a jejunal aspirate for O&P or initiate an empiric trial with metronidazole. The physician should consider the possibility of thyroid dysfunction, particularly hyperthyroidism, which can present with diarrhea.

The subset of patients with intractable diarrhea generally requires quantification of stool volume, electrolytes, and osmolarity. These patients should fast for 24 hours, and stool volume should be documented to help to differentiate between secretory and osmotic diarrhea. Quantification of stool fat to document maldigestion or malabsorption and alkalinization of stool to detect phenolphthalein-containing laxative abuse may be helpful when routine tests fail to reveal a cause for the patient's symptoms.

Occasionally, a small bowel biopsy, dedicated small bowel barium study, or investigation into bacterial overgrowth is indicated. We hold these specialized tests in reserve for those patients who present with atypical features of IBS or who have a medical or surgical history that is supportive of alternative diagnoses. For example, the patient with long-standing diabetes mellitus may develop abdominal pain associated with diarrhea as a result of autonomic neuropathy or small bowel bacterial overgrowth.

If no organic disease is suggested by the initial history, physical examination, and routine laboratory studies, very few patients require extensive studies to confirm the diagnosis of IBS. Only in the face of severe and intractable symptoms do we obtain motility or transit studies or attempt to document the rare entities of bile salt malabsorption, gastrointestinal hormone-secreting tumors (such as gastrinomas, vipomas, and somatostatinomas), medullary thyroid carcinoma, and the carcinoid syndrome (which can present with diarrhea).

SPECIFIC TREATMENT OPTIONS

Diet and Bulking Agents

Many patients report exacerbation of symptoms with the ingestion of certain foods. In the absence of lactose intolerance, a reproducible intolerance to specific food items, or the unusual case of true excess intestinal gas production, it is unlikely that an exclusion diet will provide lasting symptomatic relief in IBS.

One of the mainstays in the management of IBS has been to increase stool bulk (Table 71–3). A study by Payler and colleagues[36] suggests a basis for this treatment. Colonic transit time was accelerated by wheat bran in healthy volunteers with an initial transit time of 3 days. However, the bran prolonged the transit time in a subgroup of IBS patients who had an initial transit time of 1 day.

A large number of clinical trials have been performed using various fiber preparations in IBS patients. Interpretation of these studies has been hampered by a large placebo response of 63% to 71% and the small number of patients enrolled.[23] Fiber supplementation is no better than placebo for the treatment of IBS patients with diarrhea-predominant symptoms.

Opiates

Both morphine and the endogenous enkephalins evoke atropine-resistant colonic motor activity. Multiple studies have demonstrated the ability of loperamide (Imodium) to significantly improve the symptoms of diarrhea and fecal urgency in both painful and painless IBS diarrhea.[5,19,25,47,48] Diphenoxylate (Lomotil) is also effective but has the potential for additional adverse side effects because commercial preparations often contain atropine in small doses. Additionally, the therapeutic half-life for loperamide is longer than diphenoxylate. Once the dietary assessment has been completed and organic illness has been excluded, we favor short-term use of antidiarrheal medications in treating diarrhea-prone IBS.

Anticholinergics

Although they are employed frequently, the role of anticholinergics in the treatment of IBS is unresolved. Numerous studies have shown improvement in certain symptoms including fecal urgency and pain[6,35,40,42]; however, no effect on diarrhea has been convincingly demonstrated. It has been suggested that the antispasmodic properties of these agents would offer the most relief to the subset of IBS patients with pain predominance or to those with postprandial symptoms. Several studies support this view and have demonstrated the effectiveness of clidinium and cimetropium in decreasing the postprandial increase in colonic and rectal motility.[6,26,40,42] This effect has been demonstrated only in constipation-predominate IBS and not in the diarrhea subtypes.[14]

Dicyclomine (Bentyl) is one of the most widely prescribed anticholinergic agents for IBS. In controlled trials, dicyclomine was associated with improvement in fecal urgency and pain but was associated with significant side effects.[35] Interpretation of the studies evaluating the use of anticholinergics in treating IBS is complicated by inadequate blinding of the treatment and placebo arms. Furthermore, some studies fail to show a global improvement in symptoms with anticholinergics compared with placebo.[37]

Empiric treatment with anticholinergics usually begins with small doses, followed by gradu-

TABLE 71–3. AGENTS AVAILABLE FOR TREATMENT OF DIARRHEA-PRONE IRRITABLE BOWEL SYNDROME

Class or Name	Dose	Reference
Diet and bulking agents		
Bran	Gradual increase up to 12 g/d	4, 18, 30, 32, 36
Opiates		
Diphenoxylate	1–2 tablets q8h prn	14
Loperamide	1–2 tablets q6h prn	5, 11, 19, 25, 47, 48
Anticholinergics		
Prifinium	90 mg/d × 4 wk	37, 40
Clidinium	2.5–5 mg PO q6–8h	42
Cimetropium	TRC	6, 26
Propantheline	7.5–15 mg PO q8h prn	21
Dicyclomine	10 mg PO q8h prn	35
Antispasmodics		
Mebeverine	TRC	7, 24
Peppermint oil	TRC	9, 39
Octylonium	TRC	33
Trimebutine	100 mg IV or PO q8h prn	12, 13, 27, 31
Calcium channel blockers		
Nifedipine	10–20 mg PO q12h prn	34
Nicardipine	To be determined	38
Verapamil	30 mg PO q8h prn	3
Allergy medicine		
Disodium cromoglycate	500 mg PO t.i.d.	1, 45
Anxiolytics		
Chlordiazepoxide	5–10 mg PO t.i.d.	15
Diazepam	2.5–5 mg PO t.i.d.	16
Buspirone	5–10 mg PO t.i.d.	49
Antidepressants		
Amitriptyline	10 mg PO b.i.d. to t.i.d., starting dose	14
Peptides and hormones		
Leuprolide acetate (Lupron: Gn-RH agonist)	Investigational	29
CCK-receptor antagonists	Investigational	22
Octreotide (somatostatin-receptor agonist)	Investigational	17, 43
Serotonin (5-HT$_3$)-receptor antagonist		
Ondansetron	10 mg IV 4–8 mg PO t.i.d.	41, 44

CCK = cholecystokinin, Gn-RH = gonadotropin-releasing hormone, TRC = titrate to clinical response.

ally increasing the dose to avoid the anticholinergic side effects of mydriasis, tachycardia, xerostomia, and difficulty with micturition. We commonly start with hyoscyamine, 0.125 mg sublingually, or dicyclomine, 10 to 20 mg orally 30 to 60 minutes before meals.

ANTISPASMODICS

Several agents that have antispasmodic properties but do not depend on inhibition of endogenous cholinergic tone have been evaluated in IBS. Mebeverine is one such agent similar to papaverine in structure and without anticholinergic side effects. It is very potent in inhibiting colonic motility and peristalsis in IBS patients.[7] Of three trials evaluating mebeverine, two studies[7,46] showed a small advantage of the drug over placebo, whereas the third showed no benefit over a 16-week period.[24] Octylonium, a calcium channel blocker, and trimebutine are two other antispasmodic agents that have been examined in IBS patients. The former was studied in 10 patients, not all of whom met the criteria for IBS,[33] and a controlled trial evaluating the latter found no significant differences in symptom improvement when compared with controls.[13]

PEPPERMINT OIL

Peppermint oil is a naturally occurring smooth muscle relaxant. Two small blinded studies demonstrated global improvement in symptoms but did not document improvement of specific symptoms such as diarrhea or fecal urgency.[9,39] In addition, both studies had an unusually low placebo response. Given the scarcity of side effects and the initial promise of these agents, larger controlled clinical trials are warranted.

CALCIUM CHANNEL BLOCKERS

Few reports exist on the use of calcium channel blockers in IBS, and at present no controlled studies support their use in the treatment of diarrhea-prone IBS.[3,34,38]

ALLERGY MEDICINE

A study involving patients with persistent idiopathic diarrhea demonstrated significant improvement of symptoms in a subset of eight patients treated with disodium cromoglycate.[1] This improvement did not correlate with the presence of other atopic diseases, a history of food intolerance, or the presence of lactase deficiency. The study has been repeated in an uncontrolled fashion.[45] Although the use of disodium cromoglycate in IBS patients requires further investigation, the possibility of food allergy as a contributing factor in diarrhea of unknown origin is provocative.

ANXIOLYTICS AND ANTIDEPRESSANTS

Anxiolytic and antidepressant compounds appear well suited for treating a subset of patients with IBS for several reasons. A significant percentage of IBS patients exhibit depression and anxiety.[14] Additionally, both anxiolytics and antidepressants alter intestinal motility.[14] The tricyclic antidepressants contain inherent anticholinergic activity, and the benzodiazepines are peripheral smooth muscle relaxants. However, despite the conceptual basis for their use as therapeutic agents, these agents have not been shown to be effective in the treatment of diarrhea-prone IBS,[49] and because of their abuse potential, they have a limited role in the treatment of most IBS patients.

PEPTIDES AND BIOGENIC AMINES

There is no clear evidence supporting a role for gastrointestinal peptides or hormones in the pathogenesis of IBS; however, certain peptides and biogenic amines may have a role in both the generation and treatment of symptoms in some IBS patients.

Leuprolide acetate (Lupron) is a gonadotropin-releasing hormone agonist that shows some promise in treating premenopausal women with symptoms of nausea and vomiting.[29] No effect on diarrhea-prone IBS has been reported.

Ondansetron, a serotonin (5-HT$_3$) receptor antagonist, slowed colonic transit in control subjects, and constipation was the most frequently reported side effect when this agent was used as an antiemetic during cancer chemotherapy.[41] Preliminary studies in patients with diarrhea-predominant IBS[44] demonstrated symptomatic improvement in loose stools and slowing of colonic transit time. However, until well-controlled trials are performed, routine use of this drug cannot be recommended.

Finally, a somatostatin-receptor agonist and specific antagonists of the gastrointestinal peptide cholecystokinin (CCK) have been touted as potential therapeutic agents in IBS patients with intractable symptoms. Octreotide, a synthetic analog of somatostatin, and various investigational CCK-receptor antagonists are not currently approved or recommended for IBS treatment, but these agents are conceptually interesting based on in vitro and in vivo studies demonstrating modulation of gut motility, secretion, and sensory neural pathways.[17,22,43]

CONCLUSION

The initial management of diarrhea-prone IBS is best approached with a thorough history and a limited number of diagnostic tests. In the absence of data that support the presence of organic disease, we believe that an exhaustive search for the cause of the diarrhea is not justified, initially, as this tends to undermine the patient's confidence in the diagnosis and often fosters undue concern that a malignancy underlies the symptoms.

IBS is a common disorder with essentially no mortality. Currently, a disproportionate amount of health care resources are being used during the initial evaluations of these patients to rule out unusual causes to explain the patient's symptoms. There is little doubt that improved understanding of the pathophysiology of IBS will lead to better treatments. Generally, after the initial history, physical examination, and laboratory studies exclude organic disease, we perform an empiric trial to control the patient's symptoms in conjunction with the cornerstones for management of these patients, insight and reassurance.

REFERENCES

1. Bolin TD. Use of oral sodium cromoglycate in persistent diarrhea. *Gut.* 1980;21(10):848.
2. Butrak E, Bartnik W. Results of treating chronic diarrhea with loperamide in patients with functional intestinal disorders. *Pol Tyg Lek.* 1979;34(11):437.
3. Byrne S. Letter: Verapamil in the treatment of irritable bowel syndrome. *J Clin Psychiatry.* 1987;48:388.
4. Cann PA, Read NW, Holdsworth CD. What is the benefit of coarse wheat bran in patients with irritable bowel syndrome? *Gut.* 1984;25:168.
5. Cann PA, Read NW, Holdsworth CD, Barends D. Role of loperamide and placebo in management of irritable bowel syndrome. *Dig Dis Sci.* 1984;29:239.
6. Centonze V, Imbimbo BP, Capanozzi F, et al. Oral cimetropium bromide, a new antimuscarinic drug, for long-term treatment of irritable bowel syndrome. *Am J Gastroenterol.* 1988;83:1262.
7. Connell AM. Physiological and clinical assessment of the effect of the musculotropic agent mebeverine on the human colon. *Br Med J.* 1965;2:848.
8. Crouch MA. Irritable bowel syndrome: toward a biopsychosocial system understanding. *Prim Care.* 1988;15:99.
9. Dew NJ, Evans BK, Rhodes J. Peppermint oil for the irritable bowel syndrome: a multicenter trial. *Br J Clin Pract.* 1984;38:394.
10. Drossman DA, Leserman J, Wachman G, et al. Sexual and physical abuse in women with functional or organic gastrointestinal disorders. *Ann Int Med.* 1990;1B:828.
11. Drossman DA, Thompson WG. The irritable bowel syndrome: review and a graduated multicomponent treatment approach. *Ann Int Med.* 1992;1626(12, pt 1):1009.
12. Fielding JF. Double blind trial of trimebutine in the irritable bowel syndrome. *Ir Med J.* 1980;73:377.
13. Frexions J, Fioramonti J, Bueno L. Effect of trimebutine on colonic myoelectrical activity in IBS patients. *Eur J Clin Pharmacol.* 1985;28(2):181.
14. Friedman G. Treatment of irritable bowel syndrome. In: Friedman G, ed. The irritable bowel syndrome: realities and trends. *Gastroenterol Clin North Am.* 1991;20(2):329.
15. Ibid., 327.
16. Ibid., 328.
17. Hasler W, Soudah H, Owyang C. Somatostatin analogue inhibits afferent response to rectal distension in irritable bowel patients with rectal urgency. *Gastroenterology.* 1992;102:A457.
18. Heaton KW. *Role of Dietary Fiber in Irritable Bowel Syndrome.* Philadelphia, Pa: Grune & Stratton Inc; 1985:203.
19. Hovdenak N. Loperamide treatment of the irritable bowel syndrome. *Scand J Gastroenterol.* 1987;130(suppl):81.
20. Ibid., 84.
21. Ivey KJ. Are cholinergics of use in the irritable colon syndrome? *Gastroenterology.* 1975;68(5, pt 1):1300.
22. Kellow JE, Miller LJ, Phillips SF, et al. Altered sensitivity of the gallbladder to cholecystokinin octa-peptide in irritable bowel syndrome. *Am J Physiol.* 1987;253(5, pt 1):G650.
23. Klein KB. Controlled clinical trials in the irritable bowel syndrome: a critique. *Gastroenterology.* 1988;5:232.
24. Kruis W, Weinzier M, Schussler P, et al. Comparison of the therapeutic effect of wheat bran, mebeverine and placebo in patients with irritable bowel syndrome. *Digestion.* 1986;34:196.
25. Lavo B, Stenstam M, Nielsen AL. Loperamide in treatment of irritable bowel syndrome: a double blind placebo controlled study. *Scand J Gastroenterol.* 1987;130(suppl):77.
26. Lanfranchi GA, Bazzochi G, Campiari M, et al. Reduction by cimetropium bromide of the colonic motor response to eating in patients with the irritable bowel syndrome. *Eur J Clin Pharm.* 1988;33:571.
27. Lattecke K. A trial of trimebutine in spastic colon. *J Int Med Res.* 1978;6:86.
28. Manning AP, Thompson WD, Heaton KW, et al. Towards positive diagnosis of the irritable bowel. *Br Med J.* 1978;2:G53.
29. Mathias JF, Ferguson L, Clench MH. Debilitating "functional" bowel disease controlled by leuprolide acetate, gonadotropin-releasing hormone (GnRA) analog. *Dig Dis Sci.* 1989;34:761.
30. Mortensen PB, Andersen JR, Arttmann S, Krag E. Short-chain fatty acids and the irritable bowel syndrome: the effect of wheat bran. *Scand J Gastroenterol.* 1987;22:198.
31. Moshal MG, Herron M. A clinical trial of trimebutine (Mebutin) in spastic colon. *J Int Med Res.* 1979;7:231.
32. Muller-Lissnev SA. Effect of wheat bran on weight of stool and gastrointestinal transit time: a meta-analysis. *Br Med J.* 1988;296:615.
33. Narducci F, Bassotti G, Granata M, et al. Colonic motility and gastric emptying in patients with irritable bowel syndrome: effect of pretreatment with octylonium bromide. *Dig Dis Sci.* 1986;31:241.
34. Narducci F, Bassotti G, Gaburri M, et al. Nifedipine reduces the colonic motor response to eating in patients with the irritable colon syndrome. *Am J Gastroenterol.* 1985;80:317.
35. Page JG, Dirnberger GM. Treatment of the irritable bowel syndrome with Bentyl (dicyclomine hydrochloride). *J Clin Gastroenterol.* 1981;3:153.
36. Payler DK, Pomare EW, Heaton KW, et al. The effect of wheat bran on intestinal transit. *Gut.* 1975;16:209.
37. Piai G, Mazzacca G. Prifinium bromide in the treatment of the irritable colon syndrome. *Gastroenterology.* 1979;77:500.
38. Prior A, Harris SR, Whorwell PJ. Reduction of colonic motility by intravenous nicardipine in irritable bowel syndrome. *Gut.* 1987;28:1609.
39. Rees WDW, Evans BK, Rhodes J. Treating irritable bowel syndrome with peppermint oil. *Br Med J.* 1979;2:835.
40. Sasaki T, Takekashi T, Okada T. Results of prifinium bromide therapy in irritable bowel syndrome. *Clin Ther.* 1985;7(4):512.
41. Smith RN. Safety of ondansetron. *Eur J Clin Oncol.* 1989;25(suppl):547.
42. Snape WJ, Wright SH, Battle WM, Cohen S. The gastrocolic response: evidence for a neural mechanism. *Gastroenterology.* 1979;77:1235.
43. Soudah HC, Hasler WL, Owyang C. Effect of octreotide on intestinal motility and bacterial overgrowth in scleroderma. *N Engl J Med.* 1991;325:1461.
44. Steadman CJ, Talley NJ, Phillips SF, et al. Trial of a selective serotonin type 3 receptor antagonist ondansetron (GR38032F) in diarrhea predominant irritable bowel syndrome. *Gastroenterology.* 1990;98:A394.
45. Stefanini GF, Prati E, Albini MC, et al. Oral disodium cromoglycate treatment on irritable bowel syndrome: an open study on 101 subjects with diarrheic type. *Am J Gastroenterol.* 1992;87(1):55.

46. Tasman-Jones C. Mebeverine in patients with the irritable colon syndrome: double blind study. *N Z Med J.* 1973;77:232.
47. Tytgat GN, Huibregtse K, Meuwissen SG. Loperamide in chronic diarrhea and after ileostomy. *Arch Chir Neerl.* 1976;28(1):13.
48. Verhaegen H, DeCree J, Schuermans SV. Loperamide (R 18553), a novel type of antidiarrheal agent. *Arneimittelforschung.* 1974;24(10):1657.
49. Wheatly D. Buspirone multicenter efficacy study. *J Clin Psychiatry.* 1982;43:92.

72
Diverticular Disease of the Colon

DILIP G. PATEL and W. GRANT THOMPSON

Diverticulosis coli is common in Western countries. Most of those with the condition are unaware of it. Some are found incidentally to have diverticula when undergoing a barium enema for other indications. A small minority suffer complications that include bleeding from an arteriole in the diverticulum or infection resulting from perforation. This chapter reviews the epidemiology of colonic diverticular disease and the management of uncomplicated and complicated disease.

EPIDEMIOLOGY

About one half of Europeans and North Americans can expect to develop colonic diverticula by retirement age. On the other hand, the disease is rare in native Africans. It seems to be less prevalent in vegetarians and in Britons on a wartime, high-fiber diet. Afro-Americans have acquired a susceptibility to diverticular disease similar to that of their white compatriots. These facts have led to the belief that the disease is one of western Europeans and Americans, and some claim that it is due to the lack of dietary fiber.

Most of those with colonic diverticula suffer no important consequences; in fact, most are unaware that they have diverticula. A few develop symptoms because of a coincident irritable bowel syndrome (IBS) or complications such as bleeding or infection (complicated diverticular disease) (Fig. 72–1). This minority suffers considerable disability and expense.

CLASSIFICATION OF DIVERTICULAR DISEASE

Colonic diverticula may be complicated or uncomplicated (Table 72–1). Those with uncomplicated disease have no symptoms due to the diverticula themselves but may have coincident IBS symptoms of abdominal pain and altered bowel habit. In a few cases, a nutrient arteriole that pierces the colonic muscle through the neck of the diverticulum becomes eroded and bleeds. Alternatively, the thin wall of the diverticulum, which contains no muscle layer, may burst resulting in local infection (diverticulitis, obstruction, fistula, abscess) or peritonitis.

TREATMENT

UNCOMPLICATED DIVERTICULAR DISEASE

Those with no symptoms require no treatment. Although the muscle hypertrophy and segmental contractions may be constipating, it appears that most of those with symptoms have a coexistent IBS. Like, diverticula, the IBS is apparently uncommon in rural Africa, and there may be a relationship to fiber deficiency. However, the one condition is not a precursor of the other. Therefore, treatment of the symptoms in uncomplicated diverticular disease is the same as that of IBS.

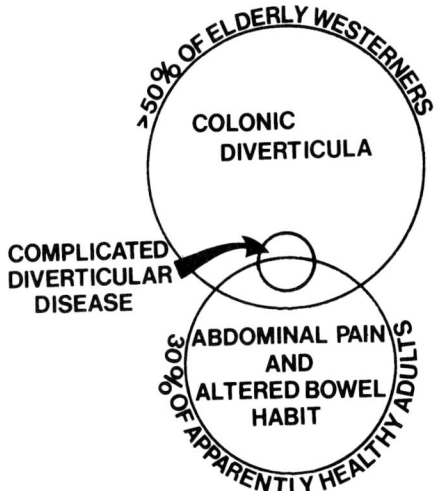

FIGURE 72–1. Venn diagram indicating the relationship of diverticular disease, functional bowel disease, and the complications of diverticular disease. (From Thompson WG, Patel DG. Clinical picture of diverticular disease of the colon. *Gastroenterol Clin North Am.* 1986;15:903–916.)

TABLE 72–1. CLASSIFICATION OF DIVERTICULAR DISEASE OF THE COLON

1. Uncomplicated diverticular disease
    a. Asymptomatic
    b. Symptomatic (coexistent irritable bowel syndrome)
2. Complicated diverticular disease
    a. Diverticular hemorrhage
    b. Diverticulitis
        (1) Peridiverticulitis
        (2) Bowel obstruction
        (3) Fistula
        (4) Abscess
        (5) Peritonitis

Complete reviews of IBS are available elsewhere (see references). The first task of management is a firm diagnosis based on history, physical examination, and a minimum of tests. On this basis, the patient may be reassured. The symptoms should not be blamed on the diverticula, and fears of cancer or inflammatory bowel disease should be set right. Aggravating factors such as lactose intolerance, drugs, alcohol, and caffeine should be identified. A high-bulk diet or supplements of bran or psyllium (three tablespoons daily and adjust) may help the constipation component of IBS, and fiber has an impressive placebo response.

Most of the 15% of adults who have IBS do not consult physicians, but many of those that do seek medical attention have psychosocial dysfunction, a previous life-threatening event, or abuse. Clearly such issues must be dealt with in any management plan. Drugs are of no proven benefit but might be used for certain specific indications in difficult cases, such as loperamide (Imodium) for incapacitating diarrhea or amitriptyline (Elavil) for chronic pain. A small number of troubled patients may be helped by psychologic or behavioral therapies, if available. IBS is chronic, so continuing care by the primary care physician is often required.

Another issue is whether or not the diverticula themselves require treatment. Those who believe that diverticula, and probably their complications, are related to fiber deficiency advocate a high-fiber diet. This makes sense, but efficacy is uncertain. A high-fiber diet is difficult to achieve, and mindful of our attempts to stamp out smoking, it seems unlikely that we can motivate those with asymptomatic diverticula to so radically alter their eating habits.

COMPLICATED DIVERTICULAR DISEASE

Diverticular Hemorrhage

Colonic bleeding occurs in up to 2.5% to 5.0% of cases with diverticulosis. Bleeding occurs in elderly patients and is often sudden. A large amount of blood can be stored in the colon so that a patient may present with the symptoms and signs of hypovolemic shock before the blood appears. This is followed by evacuation of red- to maroon-colored clots per rectum.

Bleeding results from perforation of the nutrient arteriole at the base of the diverticulum. Usually a single diverticulum is involved, and inflammation is conspicuously absent. Even though the majority of diverticula occur in the sigmoid colon, bleeding is usually from a right-sided diverticulum. The bleeding usually stops spontaneously. Repeated or continued bleeding requires intervention.

Persistent rectal bleeding with small amounts of blood mixed with or on the stool rarely results from diverticular disease. This type of bleeding is more likely with local trauma, proctitis, hemorrhoids, or polyps. Hyperemic and friable mucosa on prominent folds within the colonic segment containing the diverticula can cause minor bleeding. This is most likely due to local ischemia from compression of the folds by the hypertrophic colonic muscle.

An iron deficiency anemia is unlikely to be caused by diverticular disease, so a meticulous search for another cause of occult blood loss is in order. The differential diagnosis of diverticular hemorrhage includes acute infections, nonspecific inflammatory bowel disease, neoplasms, and vascular lesions such as angiodysplasia.

Management

Initial management requires prompt and adequate resuscitation. Intravenous access correction of hypovolemia and hypoperfusion reduce the morbidity and mortality from a significant bleeding episode.

If the bleeding stops, one may opt to do nothing immediately. Alternatively, one may clean the colon with an oral purgative to cleanse the clots from the colon in preparation for a colonoscopy. The examination may be incomplete, however, and a repeat colonoscopy or double contrast barium enema must be done at a later date to rule out a malignancy. It is usually more practical to pursue investigation later, when the colon is free of blood, either with a flexible sigmoidoscopy and barium enema or with a total colonoscopy. If brisk bleeding continues, a red blood cell scan can help to determine the site of the bleeding but does not disclose the cause. It rather serves as a guide for angiography. Mesenteric angiography should be done in the case of continued severe bleeding. If the bleeding site is determined by angiography, then vasopressin can be infused through the intraarterial catheter at 0.2 U/min, increasing to 0.4 U/min, if necessary. If it is successful and bleeding does not recur, surgery may be avoided. Vasopressin infusion is not without complications. Ischemic damage to myocardium, brain, and kidney can occur. Selective embolization can be tried in poor-risk patients but may produce bowel ischemia.

When the bleeding continues, surgery becomes imperative. If the site of bleeding has been determined, segmental resection is adequate. If there is doubt about the location of the bleeding, a subtotal colectomy with ileorectal anastomosis must be done.

Diverticulitis

Acute inflammation of the tissues surrounding the sigmoid colon follows a microperforation of one or more diverticula. The ensuing peridiverticulitis produces severe abdominal pain, usually in the left lower quadrant of the abdomen. Diverticulitis can be a severe illness with fever, pain, and malaise. If the disease progresses, abscess, fistula, obstruction, or peritonitis are likely complications.

An attack of diverticulitis presents with left lower quadrant pain and symptoms of peritoneal irritation. Urinary symptoms and minor changes in bowel function are common. The patient is usually elderly, and symptoms and signs of inflammation may be initially less pronounced than those of a younger patient.

Physical examination reveals an ill-looking patient with fever and signs of peritoneal irritation in the left lower quadrant of the abdomen. There is fever and leukocytosis. A plain film of the abdomen is not usually useful, but may help rule out other conditions. Diverticulitis due to disease located in the right side of the colon rarely presents with right-sided abdominal symptoms and signs, which may be difficult to distinguish from acute appendicitis. Peridiverticulitis in patients under the age of 40 years carries a high morbidity. Complications may require surgical intervention. Immunocompromised patients, patients on nonsteroidal antiinflammatory drugs (NSAIDs), and patients with renal failure or renal transplantation are more likely to develop generalized peritonitis. A grave outcome may be provoked by a delay in diagnosis, especially when the symptoms and signs are masked by an altered immune status.

Management

A mild attack can be managed at home with clear fluids and oral antibiotics. Ampicillin, 500 mg four times daily, tetracycline, 500 mg four times a day, or metronidazole (Flagyl), 500 mg four times a day, is commonly used. A patient with severe symptoms or signs requires hospitalization. The in-hospital treatment should include bowel rest, maintenance of fluid and electrolyte balance, adequate pain control, intravenous antibiotics, and nasogastric suction if there is vomiting. The antibiotics should be effective against the normal colonic flora: both anaerobes and enteric gram-negative bacteria. A commonly used combination is clindamycin (Cleocin), 600 mg every 6 hours, and an aminoglycoside such as gentamicin (Garamycin), 1.5 mg/kg every 8 hours. The dosage of gentamicin may have to be modified if renal function is impaired, and blood levels of the drug are helpful. Because of cost and the concern that clindamycin might become complicated by *Clostridium difficile* infection, metronidazole, 500 mg every 8 hours, is commonly substituted.

Intravenous antibiotics should be continued for 7 to 10 days. If there is no clinical improvement in the first 48 hours, progression of the disease or abscess should be suspected. Endoscopic examination is unhelpful and may be contraindicated. The single most useful test is a computed tomography (CT) of the abdomen. It is noninvasive and will help demonstrate an abscess or disease of surrounding structures.

Obstruction

Obstruction due to a peridiverticular inflammatory mass or scar tissue may be difficult to distinguish from a rectosigmoid carcinoma. A gentle, flexible sigmoidoscopy without preparation may help make a diagnosis of cancer. A single contrast barium enema, either with barium or gastrografin, usually localizes the obstruction. Since barium is toxic to the peritoneum, gastrografin is preferred if a perforation of the colon is suspected. The definitive treatment is surgical resection of the narrowed segment.

Fistula

Fistulas are inflammatory communications between the colon and skin (colocutaneous), bladder (colovesical), vaginal (colovaginal), and the small bowel (coloenteric). Colocutaneous and colovaginal fistulas are usually obvious. A colovesical fistula is suspected in diverticulitis when there is air with micturition (pneumaturia) or repeated multiorganism cystitis. A coloenteric fistula may bypass a long segment of the small bowel and result in malabsorption. Surgical treatment is usually required once the inflammation has subsided. The choice of the procedure depends on the site of the fistula.

Abscess

An abscess may be drained through a percutaneous needle guided by CT. Culture and sensitivity of the aspirated fluid help guide the selection of appropriate antibiotics. Drainage and antibiotics help control the infection pending a definitive surgical treatment.

Peritonitis

Peritonitis occurs following rupture of an abscess or free perforation of intestinal contents into the peritoneal space. It is fortunately rare, but it should be suspected if the patient with diverticular disease becomes very ill with high fever, signs of shock, and peritoneal irritation. The only option is resuscitation, antibiotics, and emergency surgery with resection of the involved segment, colostomy, and mucous fistula (Hartmann's procedure).

SUMMARY

Diverticulosis affects up to 50% of western Europeans and Americans by age 60. It usually is asymptomatic. When symptoms occur without complications, they are due to coincident functional bowel disorders. Treatment is therefore directed at them. The complications of colonic diverticula are bleeding usually from diverticula in the right side of the colon and infection due to perforation of a diverticulum in the sigmoid colon. The infection may be local (peridiverticulitis, abscess, fistula) or a generalized peritonitis. Fistulas may track into bladder, skin, vagina, or small bowel. Prompt management of these complications is essential to prevent serious consequences, especially in the elderly where the initial symptoms may be deceptively mild. Bleeding from a diverticulum usually stops and, once resuscitation is complete, may be investigated by colonoscopy. Infection must be managed by restricted oral intake and prompt antibiotic therapy. Severe cases require hospitalization for intravenous feeding and antibiotics. Investigation is directed toward the detection of abscess, obstruction, or fistula, and one must be alert to the possibility of peritonitis. Many of these hospitalized patients require an operation, so it is wise to promptly consult a surgeon.

REFERENCES

1. Boley SJ, Biase A, Brandt LJ, Sammartano RJ. Lower intestinal bleeding in the elderly. *Am J Surg.* 1979;137:57–64.
2. Casarella WJ, Kantor IE, Seaman WB. Right-sided colonic diverticula as a cause of acute rectal haemorrhage. *N Engl J Med.* 1972;286:540.
3. Detry R, James J. Acute localized diverticulitis: optimum management requires accurate staging. *Int J Color Dis.* 1992;7:38–42.
4. Drossman DA, Thompson WG. Irritable bowel syndrome: a graduated, multicomponent treatment approach. *Ann Intern Med.* 1992;116:1009–1016.
5. Eisenstat TE, Rubin RJ, Salvati EP. Surgical management of diverticulitis: the role of the Hartmann procedure. *Dis Colon Rectum.* 1983;26:429–432.
6. Jones DJ. Diverticular disease. *Br Med J.* 1992;304:1435–1437.

7. Labs JD, Sarr MG, Fishman EK, Siegelman SS, Cameron JL. Complications of acute diverticulitis of the colon: improved early diagnosis with computerized tomography. *Am J Surg.* 1988;155:331–335.
8. Sim GPG, Scobie BA. Natural history of diverticulosis of the colon. *N Z Med J.* 1982;95:611–613.
9. Thompson WG. *Gut Reactions.* New York, NY: Plenum; 1989.
10. Thompson WG. The irritable bowel syndrome: pathogenesis and management. *Lancet.* 1993;341:1569–1572.
11. Thompson WG, Patel DG. Clinical picture of diverticular disease of the colon. *Gastroenterol Clin North Am.* 1986;15:903–916.
12. Thompson WG, Patel DG, Tao H, Nair RC. Does uncomplicated diverticular disease produce symptoms? *Dig Dis Sci.* 1982;27:605–608.

73

Medical Management of Ulcerative Colitis

FRANK PROCACCINO and VIKTOR E. EYSSELEIN

The cause of ulcerative colitis remains elusive, hence directed medical therapy has not evolved. Medical therapy has focused on suppression and interruption of the operant amplification and maintenance events mediating inflammation. Hampering the development of novel therapeutic approaches has been our inability to reproducibly assess disease activity and response to therapy. Optimal medical therapy of this complex disease requires a comprehensive approach, challenging the physician to rationally select pharmacologic agents, recognize and treat problematic extraintestinal manifestations, accurately assess the nutritional status, and be cognizant of the psychologic needs of patients with chronic disease. Expanding the therapeutic options of ulcerative colitis are sphincter-sparing "curative" operations, which have become much more acceptable to patients. Physicians are now electing this approach earlier in the course of this disease. The chapter focuses on available therapeutic agents and a rational approach toward management of ulcerative colitis.

SULFASALAZINE

Sulfasalazine historically used in the management of rheumatoid arthritis and serendipitously found to be beneficial in the management of inflammatory bowel disease, consists of an antibiotic sulfapyridine and an antiinflammatory agent 5-aminosalicylic acid (5-ASA) linked by an azo bond.[1] Approximately 75% of the ingested sulfasalazine is ultimately delivered to the colon where bacteria cleave the azo bond yielding the carrier sulfapyridine and the therapeutic 5-ASA moiety.[2,3] Sulfapyridine is almost fully absorbed in the colon, metabolized by the liver, and renally excreted, whereas 5-ASA has limited colonic absorption, exerts primarily a topical effect, and then is excreted in the feces.[2,3] The precise mode of action of sulfasalazine and 5-ASA remains unrecognized, but these agents are known to have numerous antiinflammatory and immunologic actions including inhibition of the lipoxygenase pathway, inhibition of interleukin-1 production, oxygen-derived free-radical scavenging properties and impairment of lymphocyte responsiveness.[4,5]

Clinical trials have established the efficacy of sulfasalazine in patients with mild-to-moderate ulcerative colitis.[6] Sulfasalazine should be started at a low dosage of 500 mg orally twice daily, with a gradual increase in the dosage to 3 to 4 g/d over a period of 1 week to minimize potential adverse drug reactions. Generally, the desired response is achieved in nearly 80% of patients within 2 to 4 weeks, at which time maintenance therapy should be continued. Although doses of 5 to 6 g/d may occasionally be required, dose-related toxic effects are often prohibitive.

The efficacy of sulfasalazine in the prevention of relapses in ulcerative colitis is well established. In a placebo-controlled trial, over a course of a year, 24 of 33 placebo-treated patients relapsed, whereas 7 of 34 who had received sulfasalazine, 2 g/d, relapsed.[7] In a separate study, to determine the optimal dosage for maintenance treatment in ulcerative colitis, 170 patients were randomized to receive 1, 2, or 4 g daily and over 6 months were found to have relapse rates of 33%, 14%, and 9%, respectively.[8] Although a lower relapse rate is achieved at the higher dosage, this was at a considerable cost in terms of side effects of therapy, therefore 2 g/d is the recommended dosage for maintenance therapy.

The incidence of adverse reactions in patients treated with sulfasalazine approaches 30%.[9] These adverse reactions include hypersensitivity reactions and dose-related toxic effects that correlate to serum sulfapyridine levels. The predominant determinant of serum sulfapyridine levels is the rate of acetylation, which varies considerably among individual patients. Anorexia, dyspepsia, nausea, and headache are common adverse reactions and may be improved if sulfasalazine is taken with food in four divided dosages. Mild allergic reactions such as fever, rash, and arthralgias occur in 5% to 7% and may respond to a process of gradual desensitization.[10] Through its interference with the absorption of folic acid, sulfasalazine may predispose to the development of a megaloblastic anemia.[11] Serious reactions are rare but include hemolytic anemia, agranulocytosis, pancreatitis, hepatic dysfunction, fibrosing alveolitis, and peripheral neuropathy. Male infertility due to altered sperm morphology or oligospermia is common and reverses within 3 months of discontinuing therapy.[12] Exacerbations of the underlying colitis have been occasionally attributed to the use of sulfasalazine.[13]

AMINOSALICYLATES

Mesalamine (5-ASA) is a suitable, although a more costly, alternative in the treatment of patients with mild-to-moderate active ulcerative colitis and for maintenance therapy in patients who are intolerant of sulfasalazine.[14] Oral mesalamine is rapidly and extensively absorbed from the proximal gastrointestinal tract, and the challenge of developing effective oral preparations that deliver therapeutic quantities to the targeted distal tissue has been met with a variety of formulations. These include sustained release formulations in which 5-ASA is incorporated into inert granules that act as a semipermeable membrane dispersing 5-ASA in a time- and pH-dependent fashion (Pentasa) or into pH-dependent systems in which 5-ASA is coated with an inert polymer that dissolves according to luminal pH (Asacol, Rowasa, Claversal, Salofalk). An additional approach has been the development of "prodrugs" that link two molecules of mesalamine by an azo bond, and like sulfasalazine rely on colonic bacteria splitting for release of the active moiety (olsalazine, Ipsalazide, Balsalazide). For patients who find topical therapy acceptable, mesalamine enemas and suppositories (Rowasa) are effective in both the acute management of mild-to-moderate active left-sided ulcerative colitis and proctitis, respectively, and for maintenance therapy as well.[15–17] A favorable response rate of 63% has been reported with the use of topical 5-ASA products in limited ulcerative colitis, and over 50% of patients have cessation of rectal bleeding by 1 week.[18]

Pentasa is formulated to release approximately 50% of the 5-ASA into the small intestine and on theoretical grounds should constitute an advance in the treatment of patients with proximal Crohn's disease. Studies are under way to determine optimal dosage in Crohn's disease. Placebo-controlled trials have demonstrated Pentasa to be an effective monotherapy at dosages of 2 to 4 g/d in mild-to-moderate active ulcerative colitis with nearly 80% treatment benefit, 30% to 50% symptom relief, and 30% to 50% improvement of mucosal healing by 8 weeks.[19] In ulcerative colitis, Pentasa 1500 mg/d was as effective as sulfasalazine 3 g/d in the maintenance of remission, which over the course of 12 months was 54% and 46%, respectively.[20] Asacol has been effective in both the induction and maintenance of remission.[21,22] The 400-mg Asacol tablet provides the same amount of 5-ASA as 1 g of sulfasalazine, and when comparable dosages are used, the relapse prevention profile of Asacol is similar to that of sulfasalazine.[22] Although the optimal dosing profile has yet to be established, most advocate the use of 4.8 g/d in divided doses for active ulcerative colitis.[23] The prodrug olsalazine has a therapeutic efficacy similar to that of sulfasalazine in the treatment of mild-to-moderate flares of ulcerative colitis and in maintaining remission; however, use of this product is limited by diarrhea, which occurs in up to 15% of patients and requires discontinuation of therapy in up to 6%.[24] This adverse effect can be in part overcome by initiating therapy at a low dosage of 250 mg twice daily and gradually titrating up to 1 to 3 g/d. Topical preparations of mesalamine (Rowasa) are available in both an enema (4 g/60 ml) and suppository (500 mg) form and are effective in the treatment of proctosigmoiditis and proctitis, respectively.[15–18]

CORTICOSTEROIDS

Corticosteroids remain the mainstay of therapy of active ulcerative colitis. There is no evidence that corticosteroids are useful for maintenance therapy, and their use is limited by both short- and long-term systemic effects. Available in oral, parenteral, and topical form, the mode of administration is dictated by the severity of the exacerbation and the extent of disease.

In limited left-sided disease topical corticosteroids in the form of retention enemas or foams are effective.[25] In most patients, the 60-ml enema delivers 100 mg of hydrocortisone up to the mid-descending colon; administration is once a day at bedtime for 21 days, followed by a taper. Patients should be encouraged to retain the enema at minimum 1 hour and ideally overnight. If the disease extends less than 10 cm or if the patient has difficulty retaining an enema, hydrocortisone foam (Cortifoam), which delivers 80 mg of hydrocortisone, may be applied once or twice daily. A satisfactory response is typically seen within 5 to 7 days. Treatment is generally for 2 to 3 weeks followed by a gradual taper.

Systemic corticosteroid administration with oral prednisone is appropriate for the outpatient management of a mild-to-moderate flare of ulcerative colitis in patients with more extensive disease. Comparing the efficacy of 60-, 40-, and 20-mg daily dosages of prednisone in this outpatient setting, Baron et al[26] reported remission rates of 65%, 65%, and 30%, respectively. Adverse effects of treatment including acne, edema, dyspepsia, and moon facies were most frequent among patients given 60 mg daily, whereas there was no difference in adverse effects among the 40- and 20-mg groups.[26] In view of the therapeutic advantage, prednisone at 40 mg/d is regarded as the optimal starting dosage with a clinical response generally evident within 2 to 3 weeks.

Parenteral corticosteroid administration is indicated for a severe or fulminant flare of ulcerative colitis. Although there is no universally recommended dosage of parenteral corticosteroid administration in ulcerative colitis, most prefer hydrocortisone 300 mg daily either as a continuous infusion or in divided doses. Parenteral corticosteroids and parenteral adrenocorticotropic hormone (ACTH) for severe ulcerative colitis have been determined for the most part to be equally effective in comparison studies, although data suggest intravenous ACTH is more effective for those patients not previously treated with corticosteroids, whereas intravenous hydrocortisone seems preferable for patients already receiving steroid treatment.[27,28] Despite these results most clinicians opt to use parenteral hydrocortisone.

IMMUNOSUPPRESSIVES

Unlike the situation for Crohn's disease, enthusiasm for the use of immunosuppressive agents in ulcerative colitis has been tempered by two prevailing concerns: (1) fear of increasing the risk of colon cancer, a well-recognized complication in the natural history of ulcerative colitis, and (2) risk of potentially severe complications with immunosuppressive therapy in the face of increasing acceptability of sphincter-sparing "curative" operations. Nevertheless, subgroups of patients with ulcerative colitis and those in whom surgical options are unacceptable may benefit from immunosuppressive therapy.

In the management of acute active disease, azathioprine had no therapeutic advantage when compared to sulfasalazine,[29,30] nor did the adjunctive therapy with azathioprine to a corticosteroid regimen offer any benefit when compared to corticosteroids alone.[29,31] Azathioprine has been demonstrated to have a "corticosteroid-sparing" effect in chronic active ulcerative colitis.[32] 6-Mercaptopurine, the active metabolite of azathioprine, has been demonstrated to be effective in the induction and maintenance of remission and to have corticosteroid-sparing properties as well.[29,33] Response rates approach 60% for patients with left-sided disease and proctosigmoiditis.[34] Unfortunately, a clinical response may not be evident for 3 to 6 months after initiation of therapy, and there is a 4% incidence of pancreatitis.[35] Cyclosporine on the other hand, has a rapid onset of response and, in several uncontrolled trials using variable dosages and modes of administration, has been demonstrated to be effective in achieving and maintaining remission in 80% of patients with ulcerative colitis.[29,36] Through a mechanism that involves inhibition of synthesis or release of interleukin-2, cyclosporine depresses helper T-cell function.[29] The therapeutic window is relatively small for cyclosporine, and there is significant concern about its toxicity profile, which includes renal insufficiency, hypertension, seizures, and a malignant potential that makes long-term benefits of the use of this agent in ulcerative colitis questionable.

ANTIBIOTICS

There appears to be little role for antibiotics in the management of ulcerative colitis except in overt sepsis or empirically as part of the early intensive medical therapy of the potentially lethal complication, toxic megacolon. Although the antimicrobial and immunosuppressive properties of metronidazole have therapeutic applications in the management of Crohn's colitis and ileocolitis, metronidazole as either primary or adjuvant therapy in ulcerative colitis is not supported in clinical studies.[37]

ANTIDIARRHEAL AGENTS

Antidiarrheal agents (loperamide [Imodium], diphenoxylate hydrochloride [Lomotil]) may be effective adjuvant therapy to first-line agents in the symptomatic management of the distressing and potentially disabling diarrhea associated with ulcerative colitis. Use of these agents for chronic diarrhea in patients with stable disease and for diarrhea in those who have undergone intestinal resection may respond with a 30% to 40% reduction in stool weight, improved consistency of stool, and a reduction in frequency of bowel movements.[38] The potential for adverse effects including central nervous system (CNS) depression, physical dependence, and, of most concern, induction of toxic megacolon must be considered. Loperamide is relatively well sequestered from the cerebral spinal fluid by the blood-brain barrier and hence is relatively free of CNS effects. The potential for abuse of Lomotil exists, although the addictive properties are quite low. Antidiarrheal agents should not be administered in the acutely ill or unstable patient with ulcerative colitis because of the concern of inducing toxic megacolon and should be withdrawn immediately if signs of toxic megacolon develop.

PSYCHOSOCIAL ASPECTS

The psychosocial burden and the difficult adjustments made by patients with this chronic disease should not be underestimated by the physician. Sensitivity to the patient's emotional functioning can only enhance the management of the intestinal and extraintestinal manifestations. Therapy itself with sulfasalazine and corticosteroids may cause mood swings and alter behavior. A widely held misconception that psychologic factors influence disease activity is held by patients and physicians alike. An association between psychiatric factors and ulcerative colitis is reported in early studies; however, careful review reveals serious methodologic flaws, and several recent systematic studies using improved diagnostic techniques failed to confirm this association and failed to demonstrate that stressful life events precipitated exacerbations.[39,40]

DIETARY AND NUTRITIONAL ASPECTS

Numerous mechanisms contribute to the nutritional disturbances and malnutrition associated with inflammatory bowel disease, although these tend to be less problematic in ulcerative colitis than in Crohn's disease. Patients often seek a nutritional basis of therapy for their disease, since this is an aspect of therapy that they can manipulate the most. There are no universally recommended restrictions on diet. Foods should be eliminated only if they consistently and reproducibly precipitate symptoms. Dietary fish oil n-3-w-fatty acid supplementation, via the inhibition of leukotriene synthesis, has been reported in several small series to have modest clinical efficacy as adjunct therapy of mild-to-moderate ulcerative colitis.[41] Despite these results, dietary fish oil supplementation has not gained widespread clinical acceptance. Induction of remission in Crohn's disease with either total parenteral nutrition (TPN) or enteral diets has directed interest to the efficacy of parenteral and enteral nutrition as primary therapy for ulcerative colitis.[42-44] Total parenteral nutrition preserves protein nutrition and may be beneficial in patients with ulcerative colitis in whom there is a strong likelihood of surgical intervention; however, it should be recognized that TPN does not alter the course of ulcerative colitis.[42,43] As far as enteral nutrition is concerned, few reports address its efficacy in ulcerative colitis, and current evidence for a primary therapeutic role of enteral supplementation is not convincing.[45,46]

EXTRAINTESTINAL MANIFESTATIONS

In addition to the gastrointestinal manifestations, ulcerative colitis is associated with widespread involvement of other organ systems that are a considerable source of morbidity and mortality. Extraintestinal manifestations occasionally precede the development of overt bowel symptoms and may be more problematic than the bowel disease itself. Although the cause and pathophysiology of these extraintestinal manifestations remain obscure, it has been speculated that these represent immunologically mediated phenomena. Based on their clinical course, these extraintestinal manifestations can be divided into two groups: (1) those in which clinical activity correlates with the activity of the underlying intestinal disease and respond to medical or surgical therapy directed at the underlying bowel disease and (2) those in which clinical activity is independent of the activity of the underlying bowel disease.

Musculoskeletal

A spectrum of musculoskeletal manifestations such as peripheral and axial arthritides, osteomyelitis, and hypertrophic osteoarthropathy may complicate ulcerative colitis.[47,48] Peripheral or "colitic" arthritis is nonerosive, migratory, and asymmetric with a pauciarticular distribution that primarily involves the knees, hips, and ankles but may involve the elbows, wrists, and small joints of the hands and feet as well. Arthritic symptoms generally parallel the activity of the intestinal disease and may be a harbinger of a flare-up. Therapy is usually directed at the underlying bowel disease. Axial arthropathies include sacroiliitis and ankylosing spondylitis. Prevalence varies considerably based on mode of evaluation. Axial arthropathies are seen in approximately 20% of patients with ulcerative colitis on routine radiographic studies and in 50% with technetium pyrophosphate scans, although only a small fraction manifest with clinical symptoms of backache, morning stiffness, and stooping.[49] The HLA-B27 phenotype is present in up to 90% of patients with ankylosing spondylitis.[50] Ankylosing spondylitis may antedate the onset of intestinal disease. The course of the central arthritides does not correlate with that of the intestinal disease and is unaltered by proctocolectomy.[51,52] Treatment is directed toward management of symptoms and supportive care, with emphasis on physical therapy and preservation of range of motion. Nonsteroidal antiinflammatory drugs (NSAIDs) should be used judiciously, as they may exacerbate the underlying intestinal disease and precipitate a flare-up.[53] Sulfasalazine is the drug of choice.

Mucocutaneous

Aphthous ulcerations of the oral cavity parallel intestinal disease activity, and therapy is directed toward the underlying bowel disease with local symptomatic therapy with topical anesthetics if the lesions are painful.[54] The two most frequent cutaneous manifestations of inflammatory bowel disease are erythema nodosum and pyoderma gangrenosum. Erythema nodosum is a nonspecific dermatologic manifestation seen most frequently in the pediatric population and presents as red, raised, tender nodules commonly located on the extensor surfaces of the extremities. Erythema nodosum tends to parallel the activity of the intestinal disease but occasionally precedes the onset of bowel symptoms.[55] Pyoderma gangrenosum (PG) presents initially as an erythematous, tender, bluish-purple plaque or papule that may progress indolently or rapidly to a fully developed ulcer with a boggy, tender serpiginous border and surrounding erythema. PG has a tendency to heal centrally while continuing to spread peripherally and can be very destructive and disfiguring. This lesion is generally found on the lower extremities and trunk but may develop anywhere on the body. Manifestations of PG may be independent of underlying intestinal activity, but PG is not uncommonly seen with active bowel disease.[56] Treatment of PG is empiric and depends on the extent and course of the condition. PG exhibits pathergy; therefore aggressive surgical débridement is to be discouraged. Early lesions may respond to local injection of triamcinolone acetonide 10 to 40 mg/ml injected radially around the ulcer rim, but generally, systemic corticosteroids are required for extensive disease.[57] Dapsone, azathioprine, cyclophosphamide, cyclosporine, and clofazimine have also been reported to be efficacious in the treatment of PG.[58–60]

Ophthalmologic

The ophthalmologic manifestations of ulcerative colitis are uveitis and episcleritis.[61] Uveitis presents as blurred vision, headache, photophobia, and eye pain. Slit lamp examination is required for diagnosis. Although uveitis usually manifests during a flare-up of the underlying bowel disease, it may occur independent of this as well. Potential sequelae of uveitis include development of synechiae with scarring and blindness. Management with topical steroids and mydriatic agents is generally effective, although severe flare-ups may require additional systemic steroids as well. Episcleritis presents with burning eyes and scleral injection. Activity parallels that of the underlying bowel disease, and it is effectively treated with topical steroids.

HEMATOLOGIC

The most common hematologic abnormality seen in inflammatory bowel disease is anemia. Iron deficiency anemia is the most common anemia, but nutritional anemias, anemia of chronic disease, and autoimmune hemolytic anemia also occur.[62] Folate deficiency caused by sulfasalazine therapy can result in a macrocytic anemia.

A hypercoagulable state has been described in inflammatory bowel disease. Hypercoagulation as manifested by thrombocytosis, increased thromboplastin generation time, and an increase in fibrinogen and clotting factor VIII predisposes to peripheral venous thrombosis and pulmonary embolus. Thromboembolic complications in cerebral and retinal vessels, peripheral arteries, and in the portal vein have also been attributed to this hypercoagulation.[63]

HEPATIC

Patients with inflammatory bowel disease have a spectrum of hepatobiliary disorders that range from mild and insignificant to severe and life threatening. Macrovesicular fatty change is a common histologic finding in liver biopsy specimens of patients with ulcerative colitis and likely is due to malnutrition, bacterial metabolites, corticosteroids, and total parenteral nutrition.[64,65] Autoimmune chronic active hepatitis has been associated with ulcerative colitis and does not appear related to the severity or activity of the colitis.[66]

Primary sclerosing cholangitis (PSC), occurring in up to 4% of patients with ulcerative colitis, is a progressive, ultimately fatal, chronic hepatobiliary disorder for which no effective medical or surgical therapy now exists.[67] PSC is characterized by chronic fibrosing inflammation of bile ducts, usually affecting both extrahepatic and intrahepatic biliary ductal systems. The course is generally one of slow progression to cirrhosis, portal hypertension, and death caused by liver failure; however, the time course of this progression is unpredictable. Common clinical presentations of PSC are progressive fatigue and pruritus followed by jaundice, but the disease may be present for many years without symptoms and discovered because of a persistently elevated alkaline phosphatase level. Liver biopsy is frequently performed because of an abnormal biochemical profile, but this is of less diagnostic utility than endoscopic retrograde cholangiopancreatography (ERCP). Preliminary trials of ursodeoxycholic acid for PSC have demonstrated promising results with improvement of serum liver test results and liver histologic appearance, although long-term follow-up to learn whether ursodeoxycholic acid therapy leads to improved survival is pending.[68] At this time, the most successful therapy for severe sclerosing cholangitis is liver transplantation. Guidelines for timing of transplantation are difficult to determine, as many of the patients are young and have relatively well-preserved synthetic function until late in the disease. Proctocolectomy has not been associated with any beneficial effect on the clinical or biochemical features, on the associated cholangiographic abnormalities and histologic features, or on the overall progression of and survival with PSC.[69]

COMPLICATIONS OF ULCERATIVE COLITIS

TOXIC MEGACOLON

The term *toxic megacolon* indicates the cardinal features of this acute and potentially lethal complication of inflammatory bowel disease. Early in the course of ulcerative colitis, patients are at greatest risk for developing toxic megacolon. Toxic megacolon may even occur as the initial presentation. Toxic megacolon usually occurs in patients with pancolitis but has been reported in patients with limited disease as well. Overall, toxic megacolon complicates 1% to 18% of all cases of ulcerative colitis and 1% to 8% of cases of Crohn's disease.[70] Clinically, toxic megacolon presents as fever, tachycardia, leukocytosis, and anemia with accompanying dehydration, hypotension, mental status changes, and metabolic disturbances. The abdomen is distended and tender over the distribution of the colon, and bowel sounds are markedly hypoactive or absent because of the loss of colonic motility. Dilation may be total or segmental, and the transverse colon is usually the most dilated segment because gas tends to accumulate in the highest portion of the colon. Anticholinergics, antidiarrheals, and opiates inhibit the propulsive activity of the colonic musculature and have all been temporally associated with the development of toxic megacolon.[71] Toxic megacolon has also been temporally associated with the performance of barium enema examinations and colonoscopy in the setting of active ulcerative colitis.[72]

Medical therapy of toxic megacolon includes the use of high-dose intravenous corticosteroids, prompt and aggressive correction of fluid and electrolyte abnormalities, and broad spectrum antibiotic coverage, as disruption of the mucosal barrier may promote translocation of bacterial organisms and the development of peritonitis. Recovery from the acute episode of toxic megacolon with these aggressive measures may be achieved in up to 42% of patients within 48 to 72 hours; however, only 16% can be expected to have acceptable long-term results secondary to recurrences and fulminant disease.[73] Medical management of toxic megacolon should be regarded almost exclusively as preparation and optimization for imminent surgery. Prolongation of medical therapy beyond 48 to 72 hours without objective evidence of improvement may cause further transmural extension of the inflammatory process and predispose to colonic perforation at which point the operative mortality approaches 50%. In contrast, medical therapy directed toward resuscitation and preparation for surgery reduces the operative mortality in this condition to less than 5%.[72]

Dysplasia or Carcinoma

Patients with long-standing ulcerative colitis are at an increased risk for the development of colonic carcinoma compared with the general population. The risk of developing cancer becomes appreciable 8 to 10 years after diagnosis and increases with time, estimated as about 7% at 20 years of disease and 7% to 14% at 25 years of disease.[74] The risk of malignancy is a function of the anatomic extent of the disease, the risk much greater with pancolitis than with limited left-sided disease. Dysplasia is an unequivocal neoplastic change of the colonic epithelium without invasion into the lamina propria. Controversy exists as to the incidence of dysplasia, the chronology of its development, and the extent to which it is reversible. The morphologic diagnosis of dysplasia is difficult in the presence of inflammation, since there is considerable interobserver variability in interpreting dysplasia and the ability of endoscopic examination to detect dysplasia is uncertain. Colonoscopic surveillance for dysplasia once a year or every 2 years with random biopsies has been widely advocated, although there are significant limitations to this practice and the benefits and cost effectiveness of surveillance are less clear.[75,76]

APPROACH TO INDIVIDUAL PATIENTS

Ulcerative Proctitis and Distal Ulcerative Colitis

Sulfasalazine is the treatment of choice for patients with ulcerative proctitis and distal ulcerative colitis who wish to avoid topical therapy. Sulfasalazine therapy is initiated at 500 mg orally twice daily and gradually increased to 4 g/d over the course of 1 week. The desired response can be anticipated in 80% of patients within 2 to 4 weeks, and once there is clinical or sigmoidoscopic documentation of remission, a maintenance regimen of sulfasalazine at 2 g/d should be continued. Patients receiving long-term sulfasalazine therapy should be supplemented with folic acid 1 mg/d. Oral 5-ASA products such as Asacol and Pentasa or olsalazine (Dipentum) could be substituted for patients intolerant to sulfasalazine. Adjuvant topical corticosteroids, either as a suspension enema or as a foam is indicated if there is an unsatisfactory response to oral sulfasalazine or 5-ASA. For patients who find topical therapy acceptable, corticosteroids (hydrocortisone [Cortenema Cortifoam]) or 5-ASA (mesalamine [Rowasa enemas, Rowasa suppositories]) products are acceptable first-line agents as well. Topical therapy with corticosteroids or 5-ASA is generally administered once a day at bedtime until remission, at which point the frequency of administration can be gradually reduced and maintenance therapy continued with either sulfasalazine or an acceptable 5-ASA product. Adverse effects of topical steroid therapy are usually minimal, but patients who require sustained treatment with these agents may develop similar adverse effects as those seen with systemic corticosteroid use. Discontinuation of therapy is associated with a tendency to promptly relapse. Tapering schedules of 5-ASA to every other night, every third night, and so on are associated with predictable relapse rates, and generally remission can be maintained with approximately 2 to 3 enemas per week. Absence of response to any of these agents requires the use of oral prednisone beginning at a dosage of 30 to 40 mg/d.

DISEASE PROXIMAL TO THE SIGMOID COLON

Sulfasalazine is the current treatment of choice for patients with mild-to-moderate symptoms of ulcerative colitis that extends proximal to the sigmoid colon. Sulfasalazine should be started in a similar manner as in mild-to-moderate distal disease and oral 5-ASA agents substituted in sulfasalazine-intolerant patients. Prednisone should be considered in patients who do not satisfactorily respond to sulfasalazine or 5-ASA within 3 to 4 weeks. Optimal results with prednisone are achieved when treatment is initiated with adequate dosages, generally 30 to 40 mg/d. Corticosteroids are not effective as maintenance therapy. Once remission is achieved, prednisone should be tapered and maintenance therapy with sulfasalazine or 5-ASA continued. The dosage of prednisone can be tapered fairly rapidly (2.5 to 5 mg/wk) until a dosage of 20 mg/d is achieved. At this point, tapering should be slower (2.5 to 5 mg every other week). The schedule of tapering may need to be even slower and should be individualized on the basis of the patient's clinical condition and previous response to corticosteroids. Intractability and corticosteroid dependence may warrant the use of immunosuppressive therapy. Azathioprine or 6-mercaptopurine therapy at 50 mg/d can be started in these patients. A complete blood count should be monitored weekly for the initial month and then at monthly intervals for the duration of therapy. If treatment is tolerated and there are no untoward events, the dosage can be increased to 1 to 2 mg/kg/d after 1 month. Failure to achieve the desired therapeutic response within 4 to 6 months warrants discontinuation of therapy. If the desired therapeutic result is achieved, the drug can be continued for a minimum of 1 year. An attempt should then be made to discontinue use of the drug before committing the patient to indefinite long-term therapy.

SEVERE DISEASE

Severe diarrhea, abdominal pain, dehydration, fever, and inability to maintain adequate oral intake are indications for inpatient management. Bowel rest should be prescribed for the patient. Volume status and metabolic abnormalities should be assessed and appropriately managed, and the patient should be observed closely for the development of colonic dilation. Parenteral administration of corticosteroids with either hydrocortisone (300 mg/d), prednisolone (60 to 80 mg/d), or methylprednisolone (48 to 60 mg/d) should be initiated either via continuous infusion or as a bolus every 6 to 8 hours. There is no conclusive evidence to suggest that one form of corticoid or one mode of administration is superior to the other. The decision to start total parenteral nutrition is based on the patient's current nutritional status and the projected course of disease. The addition of broad spectrum parenteral antibiotics should be considered if there are signs of sepsis or in the severely ill patient with toxic megacolon. Early surgical consultation should be obtained. Parenteral administration of cyclosporine as a continuous infusion at dosages ranging from 2.5 to 5 mg/kg/d with close observation of renal function and blood levels is rapidly effective in the treatment of severe, resistant ulcerative colitis. For the patient with severe colitis who remains toxic, especially with ongoing signs of dilated colon, colectomy should be performed within 48 to 72 hours of admission to decrease the risk of perforation. For the patient who has a prompt response to therapy, oral alimentation can be started, antibiotics discontinued, prednisone administered orally, and sulfasalazine or 5-ASA instituted as long-term maintenance therapy.

PREGNANCY

The majority of patients with ulcerative colitis are of childbearing age; thus, the effect of ulcerative colitis on pregnancy is an important clinical issue. Fertility in women with ulcerative colitis is normal but may be impaired during periods of significant disease activity.[77] The incidence of prematurity, stillbirths, and developmental defects is similar to that of the general population.[78] The incidence of spontaneous abortions is slightly higher in women with inflammatory bowel disease than in the general population.[79] Pregnancy does not alter the risk for a patient with ulcerative colitis to experience a relapse. Recurrence of ulcerative colitis during pregnancy is approximately 33%, which is similar to the relapse rate for patients who are not pregnant.[80] Exacerbations tend to occur most frequently during the first trimester or in the postpartum period. The occurrence and severity of the exacerbations of ulcerative colitis are independent for each pregnancy. In general, it is quite reasonable to proceed with pregnancy while the disease is quiescent, but patients should be discouraged from becoming pregnant when their disease is active.

Sulfasalazine can cross the placental barrier and is also present in breast milk, but there is no evidence that it causes harm to the fetus or newborn.[81] It is important to emphasize that the patient should take 1 mg of folic acid daily to avoid folate deficiency, as sulfasalazine inhibits the absorption of folic acid. The safety of 5-ASA products in pregnancy has not been established, and detectable levels of parent compound have been found in cord serum and amniotic fluid.[82] Evaluation of 17 patients with inflammatory bowel disease who were maintained on 5-ASA during pregnancy supports the safety of 5-ASA, and the investigators suggested that 5-ASA therapy may be continued during pregnancy if the drug plays an important role in the treatment of the individual patient.[83] Corticosteroids cross the placental barrier and have resulted in increases in low birth weights, spontaneous abortion, and fetal abnormalities when administered to animals, although these effects have not been observed in human studies.[80] During pregnancy, corticosteroids may be used for moderate-to-severe disease to induce remission; however, corticosteroids should not be used in mild disease and should be withdrawn during pregnancy once remission is achieved. In general, it appears that the risks to the pregnancy of treatment with sulfasalazine and corticosteroids are less than the risks of allowing the disease activity to go untreated. Although women receiving immunosuppressive drugs have delivered normal infants, the risk of fetal damage makes it unwise to treat pregnant women with these agents. Usually, discontinuation of immunosuppressive therapy is recommended at least 6 months before the patient contemplates a pregnancy.

REFERENCES

1. Svartz N. Salazopyrin: a new sulfanilamide preparation. *Acta Med Scand.* 1942;110:577–596.
2. Schroder H, Campbell DES. Absorption, metabolism, and excretion of salicylazosulfapyridine in man. *Clin Pharmacol Ther.* 1972;13:539–551.
3. Azad Khan AK, Piris J, Truelove SC. An experiment to determine the active therapeutic moiety of sulphasalazine. *Lancet.* 1977;2:892–895.
4. Nielsen OH, Bukhave K, Elmgreen J, Ahnfelt-Ronne I. Inhibition of 5-lipoxygenase pathway of arachidonic acid metabolism in human neutrophils by sulfasalazine and 5-aminosalicylic acid. *Dig Dis Sci.* 1987;6:577–582.
5. Craven PA, Pfanstiel J, Saito R, DeRubertis FR. Actions of sulfasalazine and 5-aminosalicylic acid as reactive oxygen scavengers in the suppression of bile acid-induced increases in colonic epithelial cell loss and proliferative activity. *Gastroenterology.* 1987;92:1998–2008.
6. Dick AP, Grayson MJ, Carpenter RG, Petrie A. Controlled trial of sulphasalazine in the treatment of ulcerative colitis. *Gut.* 1964;5:437–442.
7. Dissanayake AS, Truelove SC. A controlled therapeutic trial of long-term maintenance treatment of ulcerative colitis with sulphasalazine (Salazopyrin). *Gut.* 1973;14:923–926.
8. Azad Khan AK, Howes DT, Piris J, Truelove SC. An optimum dose of sulphasalazine for maintenance treatment in ulcerative colitis. *Gut.* 1980;21:232–240.
9. Pullar T. Adverse effects of sulphasalazine. *Adverse Drug React Toxicol Rev.* 1992;11(2):93–109.
10. Holdsworth CD. Sulphasalazine desensitization. *Br Med J (Clin Res).* 1981;282:110–111.
11. Halsted CH, Gandhi G, Tamura T. Sulphasalazine inhibits the absorption of folates in ulcerative colitis. *N Engl J Med.* 1980;305(25):1513–1517.
12. Birnie GG, Mcleod TIF, Watkinson G. Incidence of sulphasalazine-induced male infertility. *Gut.* 1981;22:452–455.
13. Schwartz AG, Targan SR, Saxon A, Weinstein WM. Sulfasalazine-induced exacerbation of ulcerative colitis. *N Engl J Med.* 1982;306:409–412.
14. Brogden RN, Sorkin EM. Mesalazine: a review of its pharmacodynamic and pharmacokinetic properties and therapeutic potential in chronic inflammatory bowel disease. *Drugs.* 1989;38(4):500–523.
15. Biddle WL, Greenberger NJ, Swan JT, McPhee MS, Miner PB Jr. 5-Aminosalicylic acid enemas: effective agents in maintaining remission in left-sided ulcerative colitis. *Gastroenterology.* 1988;94:1075–1079.
16. Campieri M, Gionchetti P, Belluzzi A, et al. Optimum dosage of 5-aminosalicylic acid as rectal enemas in patients with active ulcerative colitis. *Gut.* 1991;32:929–931.
17. Campieri M, Gionchetti P, Belluzzi A, et al. 5-Aminosalicylic acid as enemas or suppositories in distal ulcerative colitis. *J Clin Gastroenterol.* 1988;10:406–409.
18. Sutherland LR, Martin F, Greer S, et al. 5-Aminosalicylic acid enema in the treatment of distal ulcerative colitis, proctosigmoiditis and proctitis. *Gastroenterology.* 1987;92:1894–1898.
19. Hanauer S, Schwartz J, Robinson M, et al. Mesalamine capsules for treatment of active ulcerative colitis: results of a controlled trial. *Am J Gastroenterol.* 1993;88(8):1188–1197.
20. Mulder CJJ, Tytgat GNJ, Weterman IT, et al. Double-blind comparison of slow release 5-aminosalicylate and sulfasalazine in remission maintenance in ulcerative colitis. *Gastroenterology.* 1988;95:1449–1453.
21. Sninsky CA, Cort DH, Shanahan F, et al. Oral mesalamine (Asacol) for mildly to moderately active ulcerative colitis. *Ann Intern Med.* 1991;115(5):350–355.
22. Riley SA, Mani V, Goodman MJ, Herd ME, Dutt S, Turnberg LA. Comparison of delayed release 5-aminosalicylic acid (mesalazine) and sulphasalazine in the treatment of mild to moderate ulcerative colitis relapse. *Gut.* 1988;29:669–674.
23. Schroeder KW, Tremaine WJ, Ilstrup DM. Coated oral 5-aminosalicylic acid therapy for mildly to moderately active ulcerative colitis. *N Engl J Med.* 1987;317:1625–1629.
24. Rao SS, Cann PA, Holdsworth CD. Clinical experience of the tolerance of mesalazine and olsalazine in patients intolerant of sulphasalazine. *Scand J Gastroenterol.* 1987;22:1038–1041.
25. Truelove SC. Treatment of ulcerative colitis with local hydrocortisone hemisuccinate sodium: a report on a controlled therapeutic trial. *Br Med J.* 1958;2:1072–1077.

26. Baron JH, Connell AM, Kanaghinis TG, Lennard-Jones JE, Jones FA. Outpatient treatment of ulcerative colitis: comparison between three doses of oral prednisone. *Br Med J.* 1962;2:441–443.
27. Kaplan HP, Portnoy B, Binder HJ, Amatruda T, Spiro H. A controlled evaluation of intravenous adrenocorticotropic hormone and hydrocortisone in the treatment of acute colitis. *Gastroenterology.* 1975;69:91–95.
28. Meyers S, Sachar DB, Goldberg JD, Janowitz HD. Corticotropin versus hydrocortisone in the intravenous treatment of ulcerative colitis: a prospective, randomized double-blind clinical trial. *Gastroenterology.* 1983;85:351–357.
29. Hawthorne AB, Hawkey CJ. Immunosuppressive drugs in inflammatory bowel disease: a review of their mechanisms of efficacy and place in therapy. *Drugs.* 1989;38(2):267–288.
30. Caprilli R, Carratu R, Babbini M. A double-blind comparison of the effectiveness of azathioprine and sulphasalazine in idiopathic proctocolitis. *Am J Dig Dis.* 1975;20:115–120.
31. Jewell DP, Truelove SC. Azathioprine in ulcerative colitis: final report on a controlled therapeutic trial. *Br Med J.* 1974;4:627–630.
32. Kirk AP, Lennard-Jones JE. Controlled trial of azathioprine in chronic ulcerative colitis. *Br Med J.* 1982;284:1291–1292.
33. Present DH, Chapman ML, Rubin PH. Efficacy of 6-mercaptopurine in refractory ulcerative colitis. *Gastroenterology.* 1988;94:A359.
34. Adler DJ, Korelitz BI. The therapeutic efficacy of 6-mercaptopurine in refractory ulcerative colitis. *Am J Gastroenterol.* 1990;85(6):717–722.
35. Present DH, Meltzer SJ, Krumholz MP, Wolke A, Korelitz BI. 6-Mercaptopurine in the management of inflammatory bowel disease: short and long term toxicity. *Ann Intern Med.* 1989;111:641–649.
36. Sandborn WJ, Tremaine WJ. Cyclosporine treatment of inflammatory bowel disease. *Mayo Clin Proc.* 1992;67:981–990.
37. Gilat T, Suissa A, Leichtman G, et al. A comparative study of metronidazole and sulfasalazine in active, not severe, ulcerative colitis: an Israeli multicenter trial. *J Clin Gastroenterol.* 1987;9:415–417.
38. Barrett KE, Dharmathaption K. Pharmacological aspects of therapy in inflammatory bowel diseases: anti-diarrheal agents. *J Clin Gastroenterol.* 1988;10:57–63.
39. North CS, Clouse RE, Spitznagel EL, Alpers DH. The relation of ulcerative colitis to psychiatric factors: a review of findings and methods. *Am J Psychiatry.* 1990;147:974–981.
40. North CS, Alpers DH, Helzer JE, Spitznagel EL, Clouse RE. Do life events or depression exacerbate inflammatory bowel disease: a prospective study. *Ann Intern Med.* 1991;114:381–386.
41. Stenson WF, Cort D, Rodgers J, et al. Dietary supplementation with fish oil in ulcerative colitis. *Ann Intern Med.* 1992;116:609–614.
42. Dickinson RJ, Ashton MG, Axon ATR, Smith RC, Yeung CK, Hill GL. Controlled trial of intravenous hyperalimentation and total bowel rest as an adjunct to the routine therapy of acute colitis. *Gastroenterology.* 1980;79:1199–1204.
43. McIntyre PB, Powell-Tuck J, Wood SR, et al. Controlled trial of bowel rest in the treatment of severe acute colitis. *Gut.* 1986;27:481–485.
44. Greenberg GR, Fleming CR, Jeejeebhoy KN, Rosenberg IH, Sales D, Tremaine WJ. Controlled trial of bowel rest and nutritional support in the management of Crohn's disease. *Gut.* 1988;29:1309–1315.
45. Rocchio MA, Mo Cha CJ, Haas KF, Randall HT. Use of chemical defined diets in the management of patients with acute inflammatory bowel disease. *Am J Surg.* 1974;127:469–475.
46. Axelson CK, Jarnum S. Influence of an elemental diet on protein exudation in chronic inflammatory bowel disease. *Digestion.* 1977;16:77–86.
47. Greenstein HJ, Janowitz HD, Sachar DB. The extra-intestinal complications of Crohn's disease and ulcerative colitis: a study of 700 patients. *Medicine.* 1976;55:401–412.
48. Allan RN. Extra-intestinal manifestations of inflammatory bowel disease. *Clin Gastroenterol.* 1983;12:617.
49. Levine JB. The arthropathies of IBD: more than meets the eye. *IBD News.* 1990;11(2):1.
50. Brewerton DA, Caffrey M, Nicholls A, et al. HLA-B27 and arthropathies associated with ulcerative colitis and psoriasis. *Lancet.* 1974;1(2):956–958.
51. Fernandez-Herlihy L. The articular manifestations of chronic ulcerative colitis: an analysis of 555 cases. *N Engl J Med.* 1959;261:259–263.
52. Miller MM. Ankylosing spondylitis, Reiter's syndrome, psoriatic arthritis and arthritis of inflammatory bowel disease. *Primary Care.* 1984;11:271.
53. Kaufmann HJ, Taubin HL. Nonsteroidal anti-inflammatory drugs activate quiescent inflammatory bowel disease. *Ann Intern Med.* 1987;107:513–516.
54. Basu MK, Asquith P. Oral manifestations of inflammatory bowel disease. *Clin Gastroenterol.* 1980;9:307.
55. Mir-madjlessi SH, Taylor JS, Farmer RG. Clinical course and evolution of erythema nodosum and pyoderma gangrenosum in chronic ulcerative colitis: a study of 42 patients. *Am J Gastroenterol.* 1985;80(2):615–620.
56. Hickman JG. Pyoderma gangrenosum. *Clin Dermatol.* 1983;1(1):102–113.
57. Moschella SL. Pyoderma gangrenosum: a patient successfully treated with intralesional injections of steroid. *Arch Dermatol.* 1978;114:1232–1233.
58. August PJ, Wells GC. Pyoderma gangrenosum treated with azathioprine and prednisone. *Br J Dermatol.* 1974;91(suppl):80–82.
59. Martin de Hijas C, del-Rio E, Gorospe MA, Velez A, Garcia del Pozo JA. Large peristomal pyoderma gangrenosum successfully treated with cyclosporine and corticosteroids. *J Am Acad Dermatol.* 1993;29:1034–1035.
60. Kark EC, Davis BR. Clofazimine treatment of pyoderma gangrenosum. *J Am Acad Dermatol.* 1981;5:346–347.
61. Petrelli EA, McKinley M, Troncale FJ. Ocular manifestations of inflammatory bowel disease. *Ann Ophthalmol.* 1982;14:356–360.
62. Altman AR, Maltz CR, Janowitz HP. Autoimmune hemolytic anemia in ulcerative colitis. *Dig Dis Sci.* 1979;24:282–285.
63. Talbot RW, Heppell J, Dozois RR, Beart RW. Vascular complications of inflammatory bowel disease. *Mayo Clin Proc.* 1986;61:141.
64. Eade MN. Liver disease in ulcerative colitis: analysis of operative liver biopsy in 138 consecutive patients having colectomy. *Ann Intern Med.* 1970;72:475–487.
65. Desmet VJ, Geboes K. Liver lesions in inflammatory bowel disorders. *J Pathol.* 1987;151:247–255.
66. Olsson R, Hulten L. Concurrence of ulcerative colitis and chronic active hepatitis: clinical course and results of colectomy. *Scand J Gastroenterol.* 1975;10:331–335.

67. LaRusso NF, Wiesner RH, Ludwig J, MacCarty RL. Primary sclerosing cholangitis. *N Engl J Med.* 1984;310:899–903.
68. Beuers U, Spenger U, Kruis W, et al. Promises, promises: ursodeoxycholic acid for primary sclerosing cholangitis. *Gastroenterology.* 1993;104:941–943.
69. Cangemi JR, Wiesner RH, Beaver SJ, et al. Effect of proctocolectomy for chronic ulcerative colitis on the natural history of primary sclerosing cholangitis. *Gastroenterology.* 1989;96(3):790–794.
70. Jalan KN, Sircus W, Card WI, et al. An experience of ulcerative colitis: toxic dilatation in 55 cases. *Gastroenterology.* 1969;57:68–72.
71. Brown JW. Toxic megacolon associated with loperamide therapy. *JAMA.* 1979;241(5):501–502.
72. Marshak RH, et al. Toxic dilatation of the colon in the course of ulcerative colitis. *Gastroenterology.* 1960;38:165.
73. Grant CS, Dozois RR. Toxic megacolon: ultimate fate of patients after successful medical management. *Am J Surg.* 1984;147:106–110.
74. Collins RH, Feldman M, Fordtran JS. Colon cancer, dysplasia and surveillance in patients with ulcerative colitis: a critical review. *N Engl J Med.* 1987;316:1654–1658.
75. Woolrich AJ, daSilva MD, Korelitz BI. Surveillance in the routine management of ulcerative colitis: the predictive value of low-grade dysplasia. *Gastroenterology.* 1992;103:431–438.
76. Bernstein CN, Shanahan F, Weinstein WM. Are we telling patients the truth about surveillance colonoscopy in ulcerative colitis? *Lancet.* 1994;343:71–74.
77. Willoughby CP, Truelove SC. Ulcerative colitis and pregnancy. *Gut.* 1980;21:469–474.
78. Nielson OH, Andreasson B, Bondesen S, Jaenum S. Pregnancy in ulcerative colitis. *Scand J Gastroenterol.* 1983;18:735–742.
79. Baiocco PJ, Korelitz BI. The influence of inflammatory bowel disease and its treatment on pregnancy and fetal outcome. *J Clin Gastroenterol.* 1984;6:211–216.
80. Magadam M, Korelitz BI, Ahmed SW. The course of inflammatory bowel disease during pregnancy and postpartum. *Am J Gastroenterol.* 1981;75:265–269.
81. Mogadam M, Dobbins WO, Korelitz BI, Ahmed SW. Pregnancy in inflammatory bowel disease: effect of sulfasalazine and corticosteroids on fetal outcome. *Gastroenterology.* 1981;80:72–76.'M
82. Azad Khan AK, Truelove SC. Placental and mammary transfer of sulphasalazine. *Br Med J.* 1979;2:1553.
83. Habal FM, Hui G, Greenberg GR. Oral 5-aminosalicylic acid for inflammatory bowel disease in pregnancy: safety and clinical course. *Gastroenterology.* 1993;105:1057–1060.

74

Surgery for Ulcerative Colitis

RICHARD L. GROTZ, JOHN H. PEMBERTON, and KEITH A. KELLY

The ultimate goals of surgery for ulcerative colitis are to eradicate the disease and to restore the patient to an excellent quality of life after operation. Past patients undergoing resection for colitis have usually had to face proctocolectomy with permanent ileostomy, an operation that eradicates the disease but that leaves the patient with a suboptimal quality of life. Today, ileal pouch–anal anastomosis (IPAA) with anal sphincter preservation has gained a primary role in surgical treatment. It not only eradicates the disease; it also restores an excellent quality of life.

ILEAL POUCH–ANAL ANASTOMOSIS

Early attempts at reestablishing intestinal continuity following proctocolectomy consisted of constructing an ileoanal anastomosis without a pouch; the terminal ileum was directly anastomosed to the anal canal.[1,2] However, excessive stool frequency due to the minimal storage capacity of the terminal ileum caused us to abandon this procedure. The use of a pouch proximal to the anal anastomosis has facilitated reliable preservation of voluntary transanal defecation, reasonable fecal continence, and an excellent quality of life in the majority of patients.

INDICATIONS AND CONTRAINDICATIONS

Appropriate candidates for restorative proctocolectomy are patients under the age of 65 years who are refractory to medical therapy or who have unremitting extraintestinal manifestations of the disease, growth retardation, persistent low-grade hemorrhage, stricture, or evidence of severe mucosal dysplasia. In obese or tall patients, the small bowel mesentery may not reach the anal canal, thus precluding IPAA. Absolute contraindications to IPAA are Crohn's disease, invasive carcinoma of the distal one half of the rectum, and an incompetent anal sphincter. Sometimes, depending on the degree of sphincter dysfunction, patients with incontinence preoperatively may still be considered for IPAA.

Indeterminate Colitis

In 5% to 10% of patients with inflammatory bowel disease, the pathologic features do not allow a clear separation between Crohn's disease and ulcerative colitis. These patients typically have clinical and radiologic features similar to ulcerative colitis, but at the time of colectomy, frozen section analysis shows transmural features of Crohn's disease. IPAA is safe in this situation.[3,4] However, an IPAA should not be done if Crohn's disease is suspected *preoperatively*. Moreover, patients with clinical features of ulcerative colitis and Crohn's disease, and who have significant perianal disease, should *not* undergo IPAA.

Toxic Megacolon

Toxic megacolon may be the first manifestation of ulcerative colitis. If significant clinical improvement is not evident with conservative management in 24 to 48 hours, surgical intervention is usually indicated. Patients should undergo excision of the cecum and colon, closure of the proximal rectum, and end-ileostomy. They may be candidates for IPAA later, when functional results comparable with those patients undergoing standard IPAA can be achieved.[5] In the rare emergency situation where rectal bleeding complicates toxic megacolon and is so severe that the distal rectal mucosa must be removed, the surgeon may elect to perform an IPAA in the emergency setting to preserve transanal defecation.

Patients with toxic megacolon who respond to medical management should still be considered for early elective resection. Grant and Dozois[6] demonstrated that nearly one third of patients with megacolon ultimately developed a second episode. In fact, early operative intervention has been attributed to an improved outcome in patients with fulminant colitis.[7–9] Moreover, in an earlier report on patients with toxic colitis treated only with proximal fecal diversion and no colectomy, 60% of patients failed to improve or developed recurrent toxic symptoms.[10] Thus, early surgical intervention should be strongly considered in patients with toxic megacolon.

Carcinoma

The risk of carcinoma with ulcerative colitis increases over time.[11–15] Onset of disease during childhood, duration of symptoms greater than 10 years, and total involvement of the large intestine are important factors predisposing to the development of cancer. The exact incidence is unknown, but population-based studies report the cumulative risk of cancer in ulcerative colitis to range from 1.3% at 18 years after onset of colitis to 14% at 20 years.[11,12] More recently, a multicenter report from Europe stated an overall 12% risk at 25 years after onset of colitis.[13]

In patients with chronic ulcerative colitis and a concomitant colonic cancer, adequate preoperative staging is critical; IPAA should be avoided in most patients with metastatic disease. The selection of the appropriate procedure at the time of operation is dictated by the location and extent of the cancer. Patients with advanced disease or low-lying invasive rectal carcinomas should not be considered for IPAA.[16] Importantly, technical concerns to consider during resection for ulcerative colitis and carcinoma include higher ligation of the ileocolic vessels, extensive lymphatic clearance of cecal tumors, and wider mesorectal excision for rectal tumors.

A conservative approach has been encouraged by some[17] who advocate initial total abdominal colectomy with rectal preservation and end-ileostomy for Dukes' B or C lesions. Adjuvant therapy is then considered, and if no recurrence has developed after an appropriate period of observation, IPAA is performed with subsequent ileostomy closure.

At Mayo Clinic, patients often undergo IPAA as the initial procedure for Dukes' B or C tumors.[16] In fact, of the eight patients with Dukes' C lesions who underwent concomitant colectomy and IPAA, only one patient has subsequently died of metastatic disease. Moreover, the functional results of IPAA in patients with cancer did not differ from those without cancer. Thus, this approach obviates a third operation and restores intestinal continuity earlier than the three-stage approach. In the situation of advanced disease and limited life expectancy, an ileorectostomy, if feasible, is a reasonable option.

Primary Sclerosing Cholangitis

Unfortunately, primary sclerosing cholangitis fails to improve following proctocolectomy for ulcerative colitis.[18] However, proctocolectomy may still be necessary because of intractable intestinal symptoms, severe bleeding, or premalignant colonic mucosal changes. When resection is indicated, a permanent abdominal stoma is discouraged, because of the possible development of peristomal varices and subsequent life-threatening hemorrhage from them. Instead, IPAA or ileorectostomy are recommended in these patients.[19] Although the risk of colonic resection is expected to be increased in cirrhotic patients, the morbidity is related primarily to the liver disease.[20]

Backwash Ileitis

Mucosal inflammation occurring proximal to the ileocecal valve is seen in approximately 10% of patients undergoing proctocolectomy for ulcerative colitis. The cause of backwash ileitis is unknown. Furthermore, constructing a reservoir using terminal ileum with mucosal ulcerations is somewhat of a concern. At Mayo Clinic, however, the risk of developing pouchitis in patients with backwash ileitis was 13% compared with 16% in patients with a normal terminal ileum.[21] The presence of nonspecific inflammatory changes in the terminal ileum did not result in more fistulas, abscesses, or other pouch complications than occurred in other patients without backwash ileitis. Thus, the presence of backwash ileitis is not a contraindication to IPAA.

OPERATIVE TECHNIQUE

An abdominal colectomy with proximal rectal mobilization is performed first. After the diagnosis of ulcerative colitis has been verified by the pathologist, the distal rectal dissection is continued. Transanal resection of the anal mucosa is started at the dentate line and continued proximally for 3 to 5 cm, preserving the anal sphincters and the distal rectal tunica muscularis. Above this, the full thickness of rectum is removed. The J pouch is constructed by stapling or sewing two 15-cm limbs of terminal ileum side to side. Additional methods of reservoir construction include using three limbs of terminal ileum to form an S pouch, four limbs to create a W pouch, two isoperistaltic ileal limbs to form an H pouch, and two limbs opened and folded back on themselves to form a K (Kock-type) pouch. The reservoir is brought through the proximal anal canal where a hand-sewn anasto-

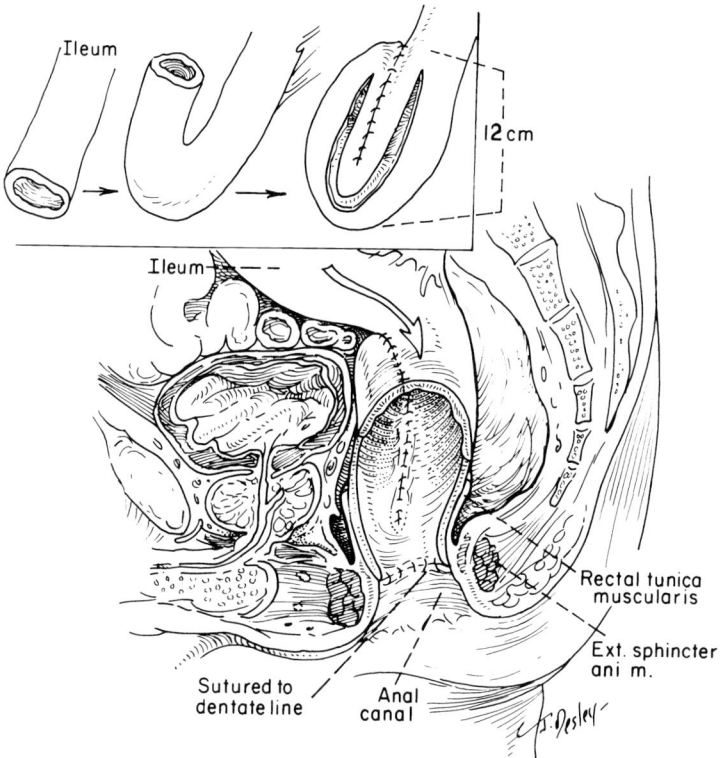

FIGURE 74–1. Ileal pouch-anal anastamosis. A J-shaped pouch is anastomosed to the dentate line with interrupted sutures. (Modified from Taylor BM, Beart RW Jr, Dozois RR, et al. Straight ileo-anal anastomosis versus ileal pouch-anal anastomosis. *Arch Surg.* 1983;118:696–701. By permission of Mayo Foundation.)

mosis is performed at the dentate line (Fig. 74–1). A temporary loop ileostomy is fashioned without tension on the ileal pouch.

Patients are hospitalized for 7 to 10 days after the initial operation and return 2 months later for closure of the loop ileostomy at a second operation.

Results

Short-term

Over 1400 patients have undergone IPAA at Mayo Clinic since 1981. The perioperative mortality was 0.2%.[22] Most complications occurred in the early postoperative period and did not result in loss of the pouch or long-term disability. Pelvic sepsis and transient urinary dysfunction complicated 5% and 6% of procedures, respectively. Impotency occurred in 1% of patients. Small bowel obstruction developed in 17% of patients and required exploration in 7.5%.[23] Failure, defined as pouch excision and/or permanent ileostomy, occurred in 6% of patients. These data support the statement that IPAA is a reasonably safe operation for patients with ulcerative colitis.

Concern over increased morbidity from the two operations necessary for the IPAA has led some surgeons to perform single-stage IPAA without proximal fecal diversion *selectively*.[24–26] At Mayo Clinic, approximately 4% of patients have undergone IPAA without a diverting ileostomy.[26] In the group without ileostomy, pouch-related complications were more common than in the group with ileostomy (22% vs 11%, respectively). However, functional results were similar at 28 months follow-up.

Long-term

Long-term results showed a mean stool frequency of seven stools every 24 hours with 91% of patients being completely continent during the day and 87% during the night at 3 years after operation.[22] Functional status improved over time with a reduction in nighttime soilage and the need for antidiarrheal medication and an increased ability to defer stooling (Table 74–1). The results from Mayo Clinic are similar to those from other institutions.[27–31] Not surprisingly, younger patients have a better result with fewer daily stools than patients over the age of 50 years (6.3 versus 8 stools every 24 hours, respectively). Moreover, patients with a higher stool frequency preoperatively were more likely to have a greater number of stools postoperatively as well.[22]

Stricturing of the anastomosis was one of the most common late complications of IPAA. Two causes of stricture formation are anastomotic tension and sepsis. The major sequelae of anastomotic stricturing was poor pouch emptying resulting in higher stool frequency. Most strictures were treated by dilation with the patient under anesthesia; rarely, correction of a stricture required longitudinal incision, mobilization and advancement of a perianal skin flap, complete pouch revision, or, ultimately, pouch excision.

Pouch-perianal fistulas developed in approximately 5% of patients, whereas pouch-vaginal fistulas occurred in 4% of women.[32] Most fistulas resolved with fistulotomy, drainage of perianal suppuration, and dilation of an accompanying anastomotic stricture. More difficult fistulas required fecal diversion to promote healing. Ultimately, approximately 20% of patients with pouch fistulas required excision of the pouch because of complications from the fistula.

Pouchitis, a frequent complication following IPAA, is characterized by the spontaneous onset of watery, often bloody stools, increased stool frequency associated with fecal urgency, incontinence, abdominal discomfort, malaise, and fever. The disorder affects 10% to 45% of patients with a pelvic reservoir,[22,27,33,34] with the incidence ris-

TABLE 74–1. FUNCTIONAL RESULTS OF ILEAL POUCH–ANAL ANASTOMOSIS FROM 6 MONTHS TO 5 YEARS POSTOPERATIVELY IN 389 PATIENTS

PARAMETER	FOLLOW-UP					
	6 MO	1 Y	2 Y	3 Y	4 Y	5 Y
Number of stools (mean±SD)						
Day	5±2	5±3	6±3	6±2	6±3	6±2
Night	1±1	1±1	2±2	2±1	1±1	1±1
Discriminate between gas and stool (percentage of patients)	69	77	73	84	77	86
Diphenoxylate (Lomotil) (percentage of patients)	26	19	17	25	6	4
Psyllium (Metamucil) (percentage of patients)	43	36	40	38	30	27

ing as the length of follow-up increases.[35,36] At Mayo Clinic the mean time between operation and first occurrence of pouchitis was 17 months.[35] Furthermore, of the patients at risk for recurrence of pouchitis, 61% developed at least one further episode.[35]

The etiology of pouchitis is unknown. It may be related to bacterial overgrowth or by-products from intraluminal bacterial colonization, a defect in pouch motility, ischemia and reperfusion injury, or a *de novo* type of inflammatory bowel disease. Unrelated factors are the type of pouch constructed, age and sex of the patient, or the association of postoperative pelvic sepsis or backwash ileitis.[35] Interestingly, patients with extraintestinal manifestations of inflammatory bowel disease are at increased risk.[35]

No distinguishing absorptive, histologic, or emptying abnormality has been found in patients with a history of recurrent pouchitis when compared with patients with no pouchitis.[37] Pouch endoscopy demonstrates friable mucosa with ulceration and edema, but the endoscopic findings do not always correlate with the clinical findings.[38] Importantly, pouchitis should be distinguished from perianastomotic inflammation, which is likely due to residual inflamed rectal mucosa or Crohn's disease.

Traditional therapy has been the use of an antibiotic directed against anaerobic bacteria (metronidazole). Patients refractory to antibiotics may respond to topical steroids or sulfasalazine enemas. Rarely, some patients require other medications or even pouch revision or excision for relief.

Failure

Pouch excision and conversion to a permanent ileostomy occurred in 6% of patients at Mayo Clinic.[22] The most common reasons were pelvic sepsis, gross nighttime fecal incontinence, excessive stool frequency, and the presence of Crohn's disease. Pouchitis accounted for only 2% of all patients who required pouch excision. Other large series report rates of failure following IPAA from 2% to 12%.[27,29,30,39,40]

Physiologic Changes After Ileal Pouch–Anal Anastomosis

Following IPAA, the major concern of most patients is maintaining adequate continence. Clearly, after IPAA, defecation is not normal. Factors such as diet, stool volume, and intestinal transit and absorption affect the frequency of defecation, and all of these are altered by IPAA. Changes in several physiologic parameters are responsible.

Typically, the resting anal canal pressure, determined by the tone of the internal anal sphincter, is only slightly decreased postoperatively compared with preoperative levels (71 versus 87 cm of water, respectively).[41] Anal canal squeeze pressure, reflective of external anal sphincter function, is usually preserved. Nonetheless, some patients do experience profound decreases in resting pressure at night or have an impaired squeeze response, and they are prone to incontinence.[42]

After IPAA, most patients discriminate between gas, liquid stool, and solid stool before and during fecal passage.[43] This suggests that the anal transitional zone, which is routinely removed during IPAA, is *not necessary* for maintaining anorectal sensation. Perhaps, instead, sensory and proprioceptive receptors located in the pelvic floor muscles or in the mucosa of the distal anal canal may be responsible.

In health, the rectoanal inhibitory response is manifested by relaxation of the proximal anal sphincter during rapid rectal distension. Fecal contents are able to enter the upper anal canal to be "sampled" by the anal canal mucosa. This response is almost always lost following IPAA, suggesting it is mediated by proprioceptive receptors in the excised rectal wall. However, the degree of continence after IPAA does not appear to correlate with the presence or absence of this reflex. Moreover, as previously mentioned, most patients retain the ability to discriminate the physical nature of the fecal content.

Pouch capacity and compliance are inversely related to frequency of defecation.[37,39] Retrospective comparisons suggest that triple (S) and quadruple loop (W) pouches have reduced stool frequencies compared with double loop (J) design.[44–46] However, the degree of improvement in neorectal function has not proven to be dramatic using the more complex reservoir designs. Indeed, the maximal capacity and distensibility of the J pouch and healthy rectum have been reported to be nearly identical.[37] Furthermore, the S and W pouches are not easy to construct and require increased operative time. The type of pouch constructed, providing it is constructed well, appears to have little impact on functional outcome. At Mayo Clinic, the double limb J-shaped design has been the predominant type of pouch used for reservoir construction with excellent functional results.

Following IPAA, defecation remains spontaneous and voluntary, provided no outlet obstruction is present distal to the reservoir. Conversely, incomplete pouch emptying is associated with a poor functional outcome. Such an outcome was especially common in the initial reports of the S pouch, when a long efferent limb was interposed between the reservoir and the anal canal.[47] Long-term follow-up revealed that only 40% of these patients evacuated spontaneously; the rest needed to catheterize the pouch to empty it. At Mayo Clinic, the efficiency of pouch emptying was measured using recovery of a semisolid artificial stool instilled into the pouch.[48] Most patients evacuated their pouches as efficiently as normal controls with a similar rate of fecal flow. Patients with higher stool frequencies emptied their pouches less completely than patients with good functional results. Thus, defecation is not greatly disturbed following IPAA in most patients with a J pouch.

In health, the anorectal angle contributes to continence by creating a flap-valve at the anorectal junction. The anorectal angle is formed by the puborectalis muscle pulling the anorectum anteriorly toward the pubis. Normally, the angle is about 100 degrees (range, 60 to 105 degrees) and is located below the pubococcygeal line.[49] During periods of increased intraabdominal pressure, the angle becomes more acute, thus preventing transanal passage of stool. Voluntary squeeze accentuates the angle, whereas, in contrast, during hip flexion and straining to defecate, the angle become more obtuse (>110 degrees), and the anorectal junction descends.[50] After IPAA, the anorectal angle is about 100 degrees and remains below the pubococcygeal line. During voluntary squeeze, although the angle narrows, it does not narrow to the same degree as in healthy subjects. Moreover, during sitting, the anorectal junction no longer descends.[50] Thus, IPAA does preserve the anatomy of the pelvic floor, yet the dynamic movements are disturbed to a certain degree. It is uncertain whether altered pelvic floor movements contribute to the functional outcome.

In health, coordination between rectal and anal motility is important to maintain continence. The high-pressure zone in the anal canal prevents transanal flow of stool until the sphincters are relaxed willfully at a socially acceptable time. Recently, a novel technique of studying neorectal and anal motility following IPAA has been developed at Mayo Clinic.[51] Using a six-channel microtransducer catheter placed in the ileal pouch and anal canal, prolonged ambulatory recordings were made by attaching the transducers to a portable digital recorder. Interestingly, resting anal canal pressures were similar in healthy controls and continent patients following IPAA, but patients had more frequent spontaneous episodes of anal canal relaxation than controls. Furthermore, large pressure waves in the pouch were invariably accompanied by a return to basal anal canal resting pressures and an increase in anal canal contractility. These data suggest that, at least in continent patients following IPAA, coordination of the neorectum and anal canal persists and may be important in facilitating continence.

After IPAA, about 650 ml of semisolid stool are passed daily; this is four times the amount of stool found in normal subjects with an intact, healthy colon. Dietary restrictions and bulk-forming agents have little effect on the volume excreted but may reduce fecal urgency and perineal irritation by making the stool less liquid and possibly by binding intraluminal bile salts. Agents such as loperamide hydrochloride may be helpful in that they improve intestinal absorption, reduce the volume and frequency of stool passed, and increase the anal canal pressure. It is interesting that small intestinal transit is slowed following IPAA compared with healthy controls.[52] The ileal "brake" effect is preserved after IPAA allowing sufficient time for small intestinal absorption and digestion.[53,54]

In summary, satisfactory fecal continence is preserved after IPAA, provided the high-pressure zone in the anal canal is competent and the ileal reservoir is distensible, capacious, and readily evacuable under voluntary control. Most patients are able to adapt to different signals suggesting the need for defecation. Certainly, the fact that the IPAA largely preserves the pelvic floor anatomy and movements contributes to the good results most patients achieve. Nonetheless, defecation is not perfect after IPAA.

QUALITY OF LIFE

Although the physiologic results following surgery for ulcerative colitis are important to understand, the quality of life experienced by these patients should not be neglected. Indeed, quality-of-life issues are often the primary motivating factor for patients choosing IPAA. Several studies have analyzed the outcome from surgery for ulcerative colitis.[55–60] Most patients lead a normal lifestyle and are satisfied with the operation regardless of the procedure.

The quality of life after Brooke ileostomy and IPAA for ulcerative colitis and familial adenomatous polyposis was reviewed at Mayo Clinic.[61]

With both operations, the patients were highly satisfied (93% Brooke ileostomy, 95% IPAA). However, 39% of Brooke ileostomy patients desired a change in the type of stoma they had. Furthermore, "performance scores" for daily activities (sexual life, sports, social, work, recreation, family relationships, and travel) were better for patients with an IPAA. These data confirm that patients with an IPAA experience a better quality of life than patients with a Brooke ileostomy and help to establish IPAA as an attractive option to Brooke ileostomy.

OTHER SURGICAL APPROACHES

BROOKE ILEOSTOMY

Proctocolectomy with Brooke ileostomy cures the patient of ulcerative colitis and does so with a predictable long-term outcome. At present, the best application for this operation is in patients who are not candidates for IPAA. This category includes patients over the age of 65 years, patients who are obese, and patients with an impaired anal sphincter or with severe perianal disease. In addition, some patients elect to have a permanent ileostomy, because they wish to undergo only one operation or because they do not want to defecate four to seven times in 24 hours.

Technique

Preoperative siting conducted by an enterostomal therapist facilitates correct placement of the stoma. The operation entails resection of the entire large intestine. An intersphincteric anal dissection is used to minimize injury to pelvic nerves during the perineal phase, leaving the external anal sphincter and puborectalis muscle intact. The ileum is transected 1 cm proximal to the ileocecal valve. The stoma is then "matured" in the right lower quadrant (Fig. 74–2).

Results

Permanent abdominal Brook ileostomy has several disadvantages that render it a displeasing option for most patients with ulcerative colitis. The stoma is completely incontinent; thus, an appliance must be worn day and night to collect the output. The ileostomy is unattractive because of its appearance and the uncontrollable noise and odor emanating from it. The appliance is uncomfortable and causes skin irritation. The appliance may also dislodge, causing soilage of clothing and embarrassment. Finally, stomal supplies are expensive. Although patients do recover their general health rapidly following proctocolectomy, the stigma of living with a permanent ileostomy is distressing to most patients.

Complications following proctocolectomy

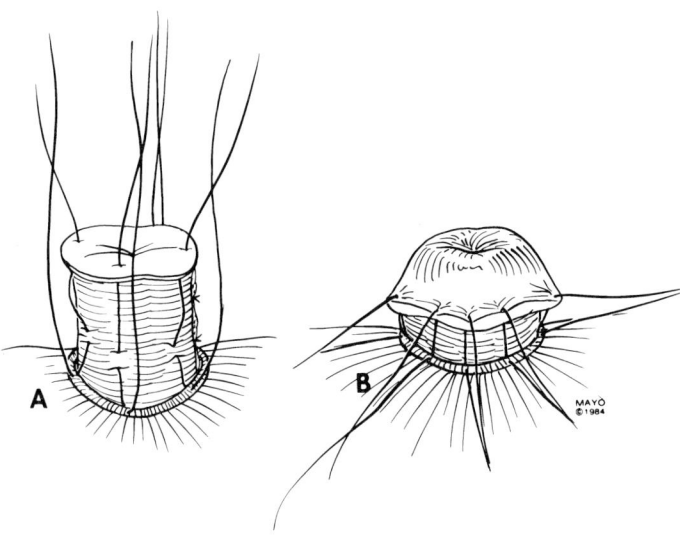

FIGURE 74–2. Construction of a Brooke ileostomy. **A,** Four quadrant sutures are placed between the cut end of the ileum, the seromuscular layer of the ileum at skin level, and the subcuticular layer of the skin. **B,** The ileum is everted immediately. Additional sutures are placed between the cut ileal end and the subcuticular layer of skin. (Reprinted with permission from Pemberton JH, Beahrs OH. Brooke ileostomy. In: Nelson RL, Nyhus LM, eds. *Surgery of the Small Intestine.* Norwalk, Conn: Appleton-Century-Crofts; 1987:449–458.)

and Brooke ileostomy are *common.* In reviewing the results of conventional ileostomies, Pemberton[62] found the incidence of stomal hernia and prolapse to be 1% to 6%; retraction, 5% to 15%; and overall stomal revision rate, 10%. Small bowel obstruction occurred in 12% to 15% of patients. Stomal stenosis is a rare complication today, because the technique of immediate maturation described by Brooke in 1952 almost always prevents it.[63]

An unhealed perineal wound persists in up to one third of patients following proctectomy for inflammatory bowel disease. The majority of perineal sinuses heal with conservative management and wound débridement. Ultimately, a chronic perineal wound may require closure with a myocutaneous flap.[64]

ILEORECTOSTOMY

Despite the popularity of IPAA for ulcerative colitis today, ileorectostomy remains an alternative for patients who refuse a proctocolectomy and permanent ileostomy, but who wish to avoid even the small chance of sexual or urinary dysfunction that might occur after IPAA. Additional indications for ileorectostomy are a *preoperative* diagnosis of indeterminate colitis, age over 65 years, and a body habitus that precludes IPAA. The appropriate candidate has a minimally diseased and relatively compliant rectum. Otherwise, incontinence and excessive stool frequencies inevitably result. The primary benefits of ileorectostomy are that the rectum is not disturbed and that no perineal wound is created. The rationale for ileorectostomy is that most of the large intestine is removed, thereby reducing the amount of disease and the risk of malignant degeneration.

Technique

The operation removes the cecum and colon and preserves the rectum. The ileum is divided just proximal to the ileocecal valve and anastomosed to the rectum in either an end-to-end or side-to-end fashion (Fig. 74–3). A diverting ileostomy is not necessary; should doubt exist about the integrity of the anastomosis, an ileorectostomy should not be performed.

Results

In distinct contrast to Brooke ileostomy and IPAA, the perioperative mortality following ileorectostomy ranges from 2% to 8%; most deaths are attributed to anastomotic dehiscence.[65] Small bowel obstruction develops in up

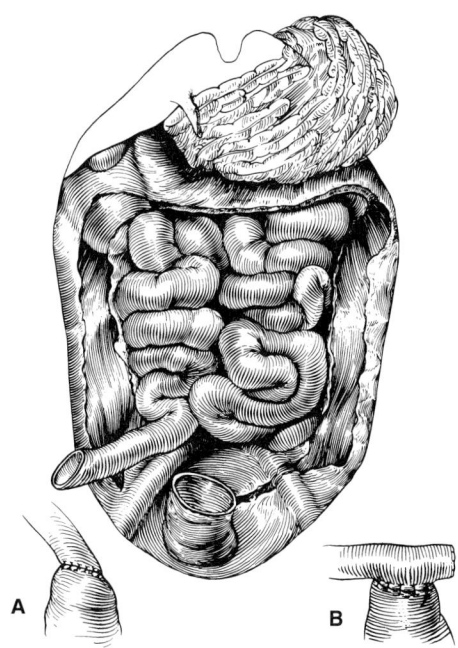

FIGURE 74–3. Ileorectostomy. *Above,* the abdominal colectomy has been completed, the specimen removed, and the ends of the bowel are ready for the anastomosis. Intestinal continuity is restored with either an end-to-end (**A**) or side-to-end (**B**) ileorectostomy. (Reprinted with permission from Farnell MB, Adson MA. Current results: the Mayo Clinic experience. In: Dozois RR, ed. *Alternatives to Conventional Ileostomy.* Chicago, Ill: Year Book Medical Publishers Inc; 1985:81–99.)

to 20% of patients. Rates of complete continence are good, and stool frequency is about four stools every 24 hours.[65–67]

The major risk of ileorectostomy is from the diseased rectum that remains. The reality of this operation is that patients are often troubled by unremitting bleeding and mucous discharge and the need for continued steroid medications. Long-term surveillance of the rectal stump is necessary. The prevalence of carcinoma developing in the retained rectum is about 5% at 15 to 20 years after surgery.[66,67] The incidence of the need for interval proctocolectomy for complications from the rectal remnant varies from 5% to 58% of patients.[68,69] At Mayo Clinic, the chance of achieving a good result with ileorectostomy is only 45%.[70] Importantly, however, conversion to an IPAA is still possible at a later date.

An interesting study was recently conducted at Mayo Clinic comparing the functional result of ileorectostomy with IPAA for familial adenomatous polyposis.[71] The overall complication rates were similar. The stool frequency for ileorectostomy was four stools per day compared with five stools per day with IPAA. Nighttime spotting and daytime soilage were similar between the groups; however, nighttime soilage was more frequent following IPAA than ileorectostomy (4% versus 0%, respectively). Although the patients in this series had familial adenomatous polyposis, the results of ileorectostomy would likely be even worse in patients with ulcerative colitis. These data support our belief that IPAA is the best operation for ulcerative colitis.

KOCK POUCH

The Kock pouch consists of an ileal pouch, a valve made by intussusception of the terminal ileum into the pouch to keep it continent, and an efferent limb leading from the pouch to a skin-flush stoma. Patients empty the pouch by intubation. The operation is performed in patients who desire control of fecal discharge but who have had their anal sphincters removed.

We discourage patients from proceeding with this operation because of the high probability that they may need reoperation to remain continent over time. Reoperations are frequent, because the valve responsible for continence often slips out of place. Reoperation is the only means of correcting this complication. The reoperation rate for valve slippage is about 20% in our hands.

ILEAL POUCH–DISTAL RECTAL ANASTOMOSIS

Problems with nighttime fecal incontinence in some patients after IPAA have led surgeons to study a new operation, the ileal pouch–distal rectal anastomosis, which preserves all the anal canal mucosa. The hypothesis is that the mucosa of the proximal portion of the anal canal, the anal transitional zone, is responsible for sensation; if this mucosa is spared and anal sensation maintained, fecal continence would be improved. Some authors have reported that this new approach not only preserves anal sensation but is faster and safer than traditional IPAA and maintains sphincter strength better.[24,31,36,72,73] However, prospective trials comparing ileoanal operations in which the anal transitional zone is excised with those in which the anal transitional zone is preserved have failed to find significant functional differences between the two approaches.[74,75] Furthermore, retaining the anal transitional zone leaves diseased mucosa behind, which predisposes the patient to the need for continued surveillance, risk of symptoms and need for therapeutic intervention, and risk of cancer.

SUMMARY

The criteria for an ideal operation for ulcerative colitis are complete excision of the disease, preservation of the transanal route of defecation and willful fecal continence, and restoration of an excellent quality of life after operation. At the present time, IPAA best satisfies these criteria. Unfortunately, IPAA is not a perfect operation. However, increasing experience with IPAA has demonstrated its safety and overall satisfactory outcome in the great majority of patients, such that permanent ileostomy, ileorectostomy, Kock pouch, and ileal pouch–distal rectal anastomosis are performed now in a distinct minority of our patients with ulcerative colitis. Moreover, future modifications of IPAA will likely reduce perioperative morbidity and improve long-term functional results, thereby increasing the already widespread acceptance of this operation.

REFERENCES

1. Ravitch MM, Sabiston DC. Anal ileostomy with preservation of the sphincter. *Surg Gynecol Obstet.* 1949;84:1095–1099.
2. Nissen R. Demonstrationen aus der operativen Chirurgie. Zunächst einige Beobachtungen aus der plastischen Chirurgie. *Zentralbl Chir.* 1933;60:883–888.
3. Wells AD, McMillan I, Price AB, et al. Natural history of indeterminate colitis. *Br J Surg.* 1991;78:179–181.
4. Pezim ME, Pemberton JH, Beart RW Jr, et al. Outcome of "indeterminate" colitis following ileal pouch-anal anastomosis. *Dis Colon Rectum.* 1989;32:653–658.
5. Galandiuk S, Pemberton JH, Tsao J, et al. Delayed ileal pouch-anal anastomosis. *Dis Colon Rectum.* 1991;34:755–758.
6. Grant CS, Dozois RR. Toxic megacolon: ultimate fate of patients after successful medical management. *Am J Surg.* 1984;147:106–110.
7. Hawley PR. Emergency surgery for ulcerative colitis. *World J Surg.* 1988;12:169–173.
8. Johnson WR, Hughes ES, McDermott FT, et al. The outcome of patients with ulcerative colitis managed by subtotal colectomy. *Surg Gynecol Obstet.* 1986;162:421–425.
9. Morgan B, Glenn D, Vickers C. Colectomy and ileostomy in the management of ulcerative colitis. *Can J Surg.* 1987;30:354–355.
10. Goligher JC, Hoffman DC, deDombal FT. Surgical treatment of severe attacks of ulcerative colitis with special reference to the advantages of early operation. *Br Med J.* 1970;4:703–706.
11. Gilat T, Fireman Z, Grossman A, et al. Colorectal cancer in patients with ulcerative colitis: a population study in central Israel. *Gastroenterology.* 1988;94:870–877.

12. Hendriksen C, Kreiner S, Binder V. Long-term prognosis in ulcerative colitis: based on results from a regional patient group from the county of Copenhagen. *Gut.* 1985;26:159–163.
13. Ekbom A, Helmick C, Zack M, et al. Ulcerative colitis and colorectal cancer: a population based study. *New Engl J Med.* 1990;323:1228–1233.
14. Devroede GJ, Taylor WF, Sauer WG, et al. Cancer risk and life expectancy with ulcerative colitis. *New Engl J Med.* 1971;285:17–21.
15. Lennard-Jones JE, Melville DM, Morson BC, et al. Precancer and cancer in extensive ulcerative colitis: findings among 401 patients over 22 years. *Gut.* 1990;31:800–806.
16. Taylor BA, Wolff BG, Dozois RR, et al. Ileal pouch-anal anastomosis for chronic ulcerative colitis and familial polyposis coli complicated by adenocarcinoma. *Dis Colon Rectum.* 1988;31:358–362.
17. Wiltz O, Hashmi HF, Schoetz DJ Jr, et al. Carcinoma and the ileal pouch-anal anastomosis. *Dis Colon Rectum.* 1991;34:805–809.
18. Wiesner RH, LaRusso NF, Dozois RR, et al. Peristomal varices after proctocolectomy in patients with primary sclerosing cholangitis. *Gastroenterology.* 1986;90:316–322.
19. Fucini C, Wolff BG, Dozois RR. Bleeding from peristomal varices: perspectives on prevention and treatment. *Dis Colon Rectum.* 1991;34:1073–1078.
20. Metcalf AM, Dozois RR, Wolff BG, et al. The surgical risk of colectomy in patients with cirrhosis. *Dis Colon Rectum.* 1987;30:529–531.
21. Gustavsson S, Weiland LH, Kelly KA. Relationship of backwash ileitis to ileal pouchitis after ileal pouch-anal anastomosis. *Dis Colon Rectum.* 1987;30:25–28.
22. Pemberton JH, Kelly KA, Beart RW Jr, et al. Ileal pouch-anal anastomosis for chronic ulcerative colitis: long-term results. *Ann Surg.* 1987;206:504–513.
23. Francois Y, Dozois RR, Kelly KA, et al. Small intestinal obstruction complicating ileal pouch-anal anastomosis. *Ann Surg.* 1989;209:46–50.
24. Sugerman HJ, Newsome HH, Decosta G, et al. Stapled ileoanal anastomosis for ulcerative colitis and familial polyposis without a temporary diverting ileostomy. *Ann Surg.* 1991;213:606–619.
25. Thow GB. Single-stage colectomy and mucosal proctectomy with stapled antiperistaltic ileoanal reservoir. In: Dozois RR, ed. *Alternatives to Conventional Ileostomy.* Chicago, Ill: Year Book Medical Publishers Inc; 1985: 420–432.
26. Galandiuk S, Wolff BG, Dozois RR, et al. Ileal pouch-anal anastomosis without ileostomy. *Dis Colon Rectum.* 1991;34:870–873.
27. Becker JM, Raymond JL. Ileal-pouch anal anastomosis: a single surgeon's experience with 100 consecutive cases. *Ann Surg.* 1986;204:375–381.
28. Schoetz DJ Jr, Coller JA, Veidenheimer MC. Ileoanal reservoir for ulcerative colitis and familial polyposis. *Arch Surg.* 1986;121:404–409.
29. Cohen Z, McLeod RS, Stern H, et al. The pelvic pouch and ileoanal anastomosis procedure: surgical techniques and initial results. *Am J Surg.* 1985;150:601–607.
30. Nasmyth DG, Williams NS, Johnston D. Comparison of the function of triplicated and duplicated pelvic ileal reservoirs after mucosal proctectomy and ileoanal anastomosis for ulcerative colitis and adenomatous polyposis. *Br J Surg.* 1986;73:361–366.
31. Sagar PM, Holdsworth PJ, Johnston D. Correlation between laboratory findings and clinical outcome after restorative proctocolectomy: serial studies in 20 patients after end to end pouch anal anastomosis. *Br J Surg.* 1991;78:67–70.
32. Wexner SD, Wong WD, Rothenberger DA, et al. The ileoanal reservoir. *Am J Surg.* 1990;159:263–302.
33. Fonkalsrud EW. Endorectal ileoanal anastomosis with isoperistaltic ileal reservoir after colectomy and mucosal proctectomy. *Ann Surg.* 1984;199:151–157.
34. Wong WD, Rothenberger DA, Goldberg SM. Ileoanal pouch procedures. *Curr Probl Surg.* 1985;22:1–78.
35. Lohmuller JL, Pemberton JH, Dozois RR, et al. Pouchitis and extraintestinal manifestations of inflammatory bowel disease after ileal pouch-anal anastomosis. *Ann Surg.* 1990;211:622–629.
36. Wexner SD, James K, Jagelman DG. The double-stapled ileal reservoir and ileoanal anastomosis: a prospective review of sphincter function and clinical outcome. *Dis Colon Rectum.* 1991;34:487–494.
37. O'Connell PR, Rankin Dr, Weiland LH, et al. Enteric bacteriology, absorption, morphology, and emptying after ileal pouch-anal anastomosis. *Br J Surg.* 1986;73: 909–914.
38. Di Febo G, Miglioli M, Lauri A, et al. Endoscopic assessment of acute inflammation of the ileal reservoir after restorative ileo-anal anastomosis. *Gastrointest Endosc.* 1990;36:6–9.
39. Nicholls RJ, Pezim ME. Restorative proctocolectomy with ileal reservoir for ulcerative colitis and familial adenomatous polyposis: a comparison of three reservoir designs. *Br J Surg.* 1985;72:470–474.
40. Morgan RA, Manning PB, Coran AG. Experience with the straight endorectal pullthrough for the management of ulcerative colitis and familial polyposis in children and adults. *Ann Surg.* 1987;206:595–599.
41. Heppell J, Kelly KA, Phillips SF, et al. Physiologic aspects of continence after colectomy, mucosal proctectomy and endorectal ileo-anal anastomosis. *Ann Surg.* 1982;195:435–443.
42. O'Connell PR, Stryker SJ, Metcalf AM, et al. Anal canal pressure and motility after ileoanal anastomosis. *Surg Gynecol Obstet.* 1988;166:47–54.
43. Beart RW Jr, Dozois RR, Wolff BG, et al. Mechanisms of rectal continence: lessons from the ileoanal procedure. *Am J Surg.* 1983;149:31–34.
44. Nicholls RJ. Restorative proctocolectomy with various types of reservoir. *World J Surg.* 1987;11:751–762.
45. Nasmyth DG, Johnston D, Godwin PG, et al. Factors influencing bowel function after ileal pouch-anal anastomosis. *Br J Surg.* 1986;73:469–473.
46. Tuckson WB, Fazio VW. Functional comparison between double and triple ileal loop pouches. *Dis Colon Rectum.* 1991;34:17–21.
47. Nicholls RJ, Pescatori M, Motson RW, et al. Restorative proctocolectomy with a three-loop ileal reservoir for ulcerative colitis and familial adenomatous polyposis. *Ann Surg.* 1984;199:383–388.
48. Stryker SJ, Borody TJ, Phillips SF, et al. Motility of the small intestine after proctocolectomy and ileal pouch-anal anastomosis. *Ann Surg.* 1985;201:351–356.
49. Hardcastle JD, Parks AG. A study of anal incontinence and some principles of surgical treatment. *Proc R Soc Med.* 1970;63(suppl):116–118.
50. Barkel DC, Pemberton JH, Pezim ME, et al. Scintigraphic assessment of the anorectal angle in health and after ileal pouch-anal anastomosis. *Ann Surg.* 1988;208: 42–49.
51. Ferrara A, Pemberton JH, Hanson RB. Coordination between ileal pouch and anal canal activity preserves continence after ileoanal anastomosis. *Am J Surg.* 1992; 163:83–89.

52. Soper NJ, Orkin BA, Kelly KA, et al. Gastrointestinal transit after proctocolectomy with the ileal pouch-anal anastomosis or ileostomy. *J Surg Res.* 1989;46:300–305.
53. Soper NJ, Chapman NJ, Kelly KA, et al. The ileal brake after ileal pouch-anal anastomosis. *Gastroenterology.* 1990;98:111–116.
54. Armstrong DN, Ballantyne G, Adrian TE, et al. Adaptive increases in peptide YY and enteroglucagon after proctocolectomy and pelvic ileal reservoir construction. *Dis Colon Rectum.* 1991;34:119–125.
55. Roy PH, Sauer WG, Beahrs OH, et al. Experience with ileostomies: evaluation of long-term rehabilitation in 497 patients. *Am J Surg.* 1970;119:77–86.
56. Morowitz DA, Kirsner JB. Ileostomy in ulcerative colitis: a questionnaire study of 1803 patients. *Am J Surg.* 1981;141:370–375.
57. Bone J, Sorensen FH. Life with a conventional ileostomy. *Dis Colon Rectum.* 1974;17:194–199.
58. Watts JMcK, de Dombal FT, Goligher JC. Long-term complications and prognosis following major surgery for ulcerative colitis. *Br J Surg.* 1966;53:1014–1023.
59. Gerber A, Apt MK, Craig PH. The improved quality of life with the Kock continent ileostomy. *J Clin Gastroenterol.* 1984;6:513–517.
60. McLeod RS, Fazio VW. Quality of life with the continent ileostomy. *World J Surg.* 1984;8:90–95.
61. Pemberton JH, Phillips SF, Ready RR, et al. Quality of life after Brooke ileostomy and ileal pouch-anal anastomosis. *Ann Surg.* 1989;209:620–628.
62. Pemberton JH. Management of conventional ileostomies. *World J Surg.* 1988;12:203–210.
63. Brooke BN. The management of an ileostomy including its complications. *Lancet.* 1952;2:102–104.
64. Anthony JP, Mathes SJ. The recalcitrant perineal wound after rectal extirpation. *Arch Surg.* 1990;125:1371–1377.
65. Parc R, Levy E, Frileux P, et al. Current results: ileorectal anastomosis after total abdominal colectomy for ulcerative colitis. In: Dozois RR, ed. *Alternatives to Conventional Ileostomy.* Chicago, Ill: Year Book Medical Publishers Inc; 1985:81–99.
66. Oakley JR, Lavery IC, Fazio VW, et al. The fate of the rectal stump after subtotal colectomy for ulcerative colitis. *Dis Colon Rectum.* 1985;28:394–396.
67. Leijonmarck CE, Lofberg R, Ost A, et al. Long-term results of ileorectal anastomosis in ulcerative colitis in Stockholm County. *Dis Colon Rectum.* 1990;33:195–200.
68. Aylett SO. Diffuse ulcerative colitis and its treatment by ileorectal anastomosis. *Ann R Coll Surg Engl.* 1960;27:260–284.
69. Lindham S, Lagercrantz R. Ulcerative colitis in childhood: should the rectum be preserved at surgery? Long-term results in 50 patients. *Scand J Gastroenterol.* 1980;15:123–127.
70. Farnell MB, van Heerden JA, Beart RW Jr, et al. Rectal preservation in nonspecific inflammatory disease of the colon. *Ann Surg.* 1980;192:249–253.
71. Ambroze WL, Dozois RR, Pemberton JH, et al. Familial adenomatous polyposis: results following ileal pouch-anal anastomosis and ileorectostomy. *Dis Colon Rectum.* 1992;35:12–15.
72. Lavery IC, Tuckson WB, Fazio VW, et al. Pouch surgery: the importance of the transitional zone. *Can J Gastroenterol.* 1990;4:428–431.
73. Johnston D, Holdsworth PJ, Nasmyth DG, et al. Preservation of the entire anal canal in conservative proctocolectomy for ulcerative colitis: a pilot study comparing end-to-end ileoanal anastomosis without mucosal resection with mucosal proctectomy and endo-anal anastomosis. *Br J Surg.* 1987;74:940–944.
74. Seow-Choen F, Tsunoda A, Nicholls RJ. Prospective randomized trial comparing anal function after hand sewn ileoanal anastomosis with mucosectomy versus stapled ileoanal anastomosis without mucosectomy in restorative proctocolectomy. *Br J Surg.* 1991;78:430–434.
75. Kmiot WA, Keighley MRB. Totally stapled abdominal restoration proctocolectomy. *Br J Surg.* 1989;76:961–964.

75

Toxic Megacolon

HENRYK PLUTA and KENNETH L. BOWES

Toxic megacolon is the most serious life-threatening complication of inflammatory bowel disease. It is associated with and probably due to extensive ulceration and thinning of the bowel wall from the inflammatory disease process. Clinically, it is characterized by the development of signs and symptoms of systemic toxemia, exacerbation of abdominal pain and diarrhea, and physical findings of the acute abdomen. The patient is in imminent danger from perforation of the colon or the development of massive hemorrhage.

Toxic megacolon develops in 6% to 13% of patients with ulcerative colitis and in 2% to 6% of those with Crohn's disease. It rarely occurs in a number of other conditions including ischemic colitis, amebiasis, typhoid fever, cholera, shigellosis, salmonellosis, and pseudomembranous colitis. A particularly virulent form has been described in acquired immunodeficiency syndrome (AIDS) patients with acute colitis induced by cytomegalovirus.

Pathologically, all coats of the colon, including the muscle, are markedly thinned. The gut has the consistency of wet blotting paper, and there is extensive mucosal ulceration most marked in the transverse colon. The bowel is markedly congested. There is often a relatively mild inflammatory cell response. Large areas of ulceration into the deep muscle coats are covered on the mucosal surface by only a thin layer of vascular granulation tissue. Auerbach's plexus is not directly affected, and dilation is felt to be due to a primary toxic atrophy or inhibition of muscle cells. The excised colon specimens frequently demonstrate single or multiple perforations.

In all cases of toxic megacolon the precipitating factor appears to be an extension of the ulceration and inflammatory process to involve colonic musculature and frequently serosa. Ultimately, the colon loses its ability to contract and becomes widely distended. This thinned wall is in danger of perforation, and the extensive associated ulceration is prone to massive hemorrhage. There is growing risk of systemic septic toxemia.

CLINICAL FEATURES

The clinical picture of toxic megacolon is often dramatic. Typically, a patient who is experiencing an exacerbation of inflammatory bowel disease over several days or weeks suddenly becomes acutely ill and develops rapid progression of symptoms. In some, a barium enema or administration of narcotics or anticholinergics appears to be the precipitating factor. The development of systemic toxemia, an acute abdomen, and extensive (often bloody) diarrhea are the clinical hallmarks. A dilated transverse colon is usually, but not inevitably, seen, and it should be emphasized that the colon can perforate without exhibiting marked dilation.

These patients are systemically acutely and severely ill. Fever ($>38°C$), tachycardia (>100), tachypnea, pallor, lethargy, anemia (<10 g), abdominal pain, and bloody diarrhea ($>6/d$) are usually the first ominous symptoms. Early in the course of the disease, the abdominal pain may be diffuse and colicky, reflecting powerful contractions of the bowel; but later with bowel paralysis, abdominal pain is constant and due to deep ulceration and actual or impending perforation. Distension is usually marked. The appearance of tenderness, guarding, and especially rebound tenderness raises the terrible specter of perforation. Disappearance of bowel sounds is an ominous finding.

Laboratory features include anemia (often <10 g); leukocytosis; hypoalbuminemia; elevated erythrocyte sedimentation rate; low serum levels of calcium, potassium, phosphate; and the presence of a metabolic alkalosis.

Abdominal radiographs usually reveal marked dilation of the transverse (and less commonly the sigmoid) colon. There is a paucity of haustral markings. This localization may be due to the more anterior situation of the transverse colon, but the transverse colon is also the area most marked by deep ulceration. Air in the small bowel may be a graver prognostic indicator as it indicates a more generalized ileus. The submucosal appearance of pneumatosis is a particularly serious prognostic sign. The appearance of free intraperitoneal air means perforation, and immediate operation is mandatory.

DIAGNOSIS

Some divide acute severe exacerbations of inflammatory bowel disease into two categories, fulminant colitis and toxic megacolon, the implication being that the first does not require operation but the second does. I believe the differentiation is artificial, as both are part of the same disease process. Both reflect exacerbation of the underlying inflammatory disease process. The appearance of systemic symptoms, bloody diarrhea, and abdominal distension and tenderness in a patient with known inflammatory bowel disease indicates a souring situation and the need for vigorous, supportive, and specific therapy. Although a dilated transverse colon gives credence to the diagnosis of toxic megacolon, perforation of the colon can certainly occur in its absence, and some dilation of the transverse colon can occur in a variety of acute and chronic abdominal conditions.

Patients with no previous inflammatory bowel disease pose a different problem. A history of tropical travel suggests a possible infectious cause. Recent antibiotic use raises the possibility of pseudomembranous enterocolitis. A possible AIDS diagnosis has serious prognostic implications.

Abdominal radiographs may suggest the diagnosis, indicate the severity, diagnose perforation, and help exclude other disease.

Laboratory tests for *Shigella, Salmonella, Campylobacter, Yersinia enterocolitica,* and ova and parasites help exclude an infectious origin.

Barium studies, colonoscopy, and full sigmoidoscopy are contraindicated, as they may exacerbate the situation. A limited distal rectal sigmoidoscopy may be of value in differentiating Crohn's disease and ulcerative colitis in patients with no previous inflammatory bowel history.

Evaluation of complete blood count, serum, electrolytes, proteins, and arterial blood gases is of significant value in diagnosis, assessment of severity, and early management of the disease.

MANAGEMENT

Management consists of supportive measures, specific therapy, and continuous frequent reassessment. Both a gastroenterologist and surgeon should be involved in the initial assessment and follow-up throughout the patient's hospitalization.

The gut should be rested by fasting and the passage of a nasogastric tube. Patient discomfort, vomiting, distension, and diarrhea will be lessened; possibly the inflammatory process will abate more quickly, and the contamination and risk of aspiration will be less should perforation and surgery be required.

Total parenteral nutrition is usually indicated. On admission of patients with toxic megacolon, malnutrition is seen in many, significant weight loss is common, and hypoalbuminemia is nearly universal. The illness often lasts for many days or weeks, and maintenance of nutrition is vital. Many patients are in a catabolic state and have high energy requirements to maintain the status quo.

Metabolic, fluid, and electrolyte abnormalities should be corrected. Fluid, electrolyte, and caloric replacement should be adjusted on the basis of daily estimations, and where possible, losses due to diarrhea, nasogastric suction, and third space shifts of extracellular fluid should be measured.

Antibiotics are of little value in arresting the inflammatory process of Crohn's disease and ulcerative colitis but should be administered to diminish the bacterial load of future perforation and to treat microperforations that may already be present. Metronidazole may be of significant value in the management of Crohn's disease.

Intravenous steroids are mandatory in all patients who have had steroids in the past and may be of value in recent-onset inflammatory bowel disease. Unfortunately, steroids tend to mask the clinical features of impending or frank perforation, and their use should color the weight given to systemic toxicity and signs of peritoneal inflammation. Frequent reassessment is mandatory. In the first 24 hours, clinical assessments should be made every few hours. Frequent assessment of vital signs (hourly in very ill patients) and often care in an intensive care unit may be advisable. Some advocate frequent (every 4 hours) x-ray examination of the abdomen, but the frequency of x-ray examinations depends on the clinical state of the patient. Assessment by both a surgeon and a gastroenterologist with continuing discussion of the situation is mandatory.

Some advocate repetitive rolling of the patient to attempt movement of the gas out of the transverse colon. I have no experience with this technique, but it appears to be derived from the false concept that the gas is somehow injurious to the bowel and causes a perforation from high intraluminal pressure. Surely elevated intraluminal pressure would result in movement of the gas to other parts of the colon long before it would tear the colon wall. The gas is merely a sign of local ileus and perhaps a partial indicator of the severity of the disease. The intraluminal pressure is, we suspect, low.

Surgery is indicated in all patients with present or impending perforation. The problem is in diagnosing those who will perforate if managed medically and sometimes in diagnosing those who have already experienced a microperforation. The administration of steroids compounds the diagnostic problem. There is little doubt that a high percentage of those with toxic megacolon will require colectomy in the year after diagnosis. Estimates vary from 30% to 100%, probably because of differences in diagnosing toxic megacolon by different clinicians.

Generally, all frank perforations, all patients who do not respond to good, vigorous medical treatment after 24 to 72 hours, and all patients who deteriorate while on medical treatment require surgery.

OPERATION

The operation of choice includes resection of all the abdominal colon, ileostomy, and closure of the rectal stump. Abscesses should be drained.

Lesser procedures are rarely indicated. A patient with multiple perforations may justify an ileostomy and creation of multiple colostomies ("blow holes"), but the improvement is often minimal. Resection of the rectum is indicated only if massive hemorrhage from the rectum is present.

MORTALITY

The mortality of elective colectomy in healthy subjects should be less than 2%. Reported mortality for total abdominal colectomy in toxic megacolon patients ranges from 14% to 30%. High mortality is due to procrastination often to the point of bowel perforation. Mortality will undoubtedly be lower the earlier the patient undergoes surgery. A more aggressive surgical approach would lead to lower mortality but would remove some colons that might be saved. A large percentage of patients who have recovered from an episode of severe fulminant colitis or toxic megacolon, however, require total abdominal colectomy for intractable disease within 1 year.

This dilemma faces the clinician in every patient. In many aspects early operation is in fact the more conservative and safest approach.

REFERENCES

1. Adams JT. Toxic dilation of the colon. *Arch Surg.* 1973;106:678–682.
2. Danovitch SH. Fulminant colitis and toxic megacolon. *Gastroenterol Clin North Am.* 1989;18(1):73–82.
3. Grant CS, Dozois RR. Toxic megacolon: ultimate fate of patients after successful medical management. *Am Surg.* 1984;147:106–110.
4. Jalan KN, Sircus W, Card WI, et al. An experience of ulcerative colitis. *Gastroenterology.* 1969;57:68–82.
5. McInnerney GT, Sauer WG, Baggenstoss AH, Hodgson JR. Fulminating ulcerative colitis with marked colonic dilation: a clinicopathologic study. *Gastroenterology.* 1962; 42:244–256.
6. Orkin BA, Telander RL, Wolff BG, Perrault J, Ilstrup DM. The surgical management of children with ulcerative colitis. *Dis Colon Rectum.* 1990;11:947–955.
7. Soyer MT, Aldrete JS. Surgical treatment of toxic megacolon and proposal for a program of therapy. *Am J Surg.* 1980;140:421–425.
8. Zenilman ME, Becker JM. Emergencies in inflammatory bowel disease. *Gastroenterol Clin North Am.* 1988;17(2): 387–407.

76

Infectious Colitis

ROBERT T. YAVORSKI and ROBERT W. SJOGREN

Infectious colitis encompasses a wide spectrum of illnesses ranging from acute self-limited diarrhea to severe life-threatening disease. The agents responsible for the associated manifestations are likewise varied, including many bacterial, viral, and protozoan enteropathogens. The patient's response to infection is dependent on multiple variables to include underlying risk factors for disease, age, and living conditions, as well as prompt recognition of the problem and institution of appropriate therapy.

In this chapter the approach to the patient with infectious diarrhea is discussed. Particular attention is directed toward the enteroinvasive pathogens that often result in a dysentery-type illness with acute colitis and the potential for significant morbidity. Both pharmacologic and nonpharmacologic therapeutic agents available for treatment of these infections are reviewed.

Acute infectious diarrhea is a common disorder in the United States and the leading infectious disease in third world countries, accounting for significant morbidity and mortality. Patient groups that appear particularly susceptible to infection include those who are at the extremes of age, use day care centers, are institutionalized, are in chronic health care facilities,

---

The opinions and assertions contained herein are the private views of the authors and are not to be construed as official or as reflecting the views of the Department of the Army or the Department of Defense.

have a history of travel to a foreign country, have a history of camping, or are immunocompromised (such as those with human immunodeficiency virus [HIV] infection).

When a patient presents with suspected infectious diarrhea, a careful history helps to suggest the etiologic agent responsible and to rule out a variety of noninfectious causes. For example, recent antibiotic use suggests the possibility of *Clostridium difficile*–induced diarrhea (pseudomembranous enterocolitis). Diarrhea developing in an American traveler to southern Asia, the Middle East, Africa, or Latin America 2 to 3 days after arrival at his destination is suggestive of enterotoxigenic *Escherichia coli* (ETEC) infection, although infections with *Shigella* sp., *Campylobacter* sp., enteroadherent *E. coli* (EAEC), and others are common as well. Diarrhea developing in infants in day care centers is often the result of a viral infection, particularly rotavirus. Other agents that commonly infect this population group include *Giardia lamblia* and *Campylobacter* sp., with occasional outbreaks of infection from *Salmonella* sp. and *Shigella* sp. reported as well. Diarrhea in a patient with a history of camping with ingestion of unpurified water is likely due to *Giardia lamblia*. Diarrhea in a patient with acquired immunodeficiency syndrome (AIDS) presents a more difficult diagnostic problem because a multitude of the usual pathogens may exist, as well as less common organisms. Examples include protozoal agents (*Cryptosporidium, Enterocytozoon bieneusi* or Microsporidia, *Entamoeba histolytica,* and *Isospora belli*), bacterial agents (*Neisseria gonorrhoeae* and *Chlamydia trachomatis*), and viral agents (cytomegalovirus, herpes simplex virus, and the HIV virus itself). Further questioning may also help to separate acute infectious diarrhea from the food poisoning syndromes, as well as diarrhea due to medications, inflammatory bowel disease, and an underlying malignancy.

The severity of the diarrheal illness in a particular patient is not generally predictive of the cause. However, a description of the stool characteristics (to include volume, consistency, and the presence of blood or mucus) is important. A history of grossly bloody bowel movements of either large or small volume associated with fever and abdominal cramping or pain is usually indicative of infection with an invasive enteropathogen, the prototype of which is *Shigella* sp. Other agents such as enteroinvasive *E. coli* (EIEC), *Campylobacter* sp., *Salmonella* sp., *Yersinia* sp., enterohemorrhagic *E. coli* (EHEC), *Chlamydia trachomatis, Neisseria gonorrhoeae,* and *E. histolytica* can also cause a frank colitis or proctocolitis with bloody diarrhea.

DIAGNOSTIC WORKUP

Since many cases of acute infectious diarrhea are of a self-limited nature, an aggressive search for the etiologic agent responsible is not always necessary and not cost effective. Such cases include patients with nonbloody diarrhea of less than 4 days' duration, who appear nontoxic without fever. In these patients, supportive care with oral rehydration therapy and perhaps an antimotility agent plus observation is all that is necessary. Conversely, obtaining a pathologic diagnosis is important in patients infected with enteroinvasive bacterial agents and parasites, as prompt treatment can result in a shorter duration of illness and lower morbidity. As a result, patients with diarrhea associated with fever, dehydration, prolonged duration of illness, abdominal pain, or tenesmus should have stools examined for gross blood and fecal white blood cells. If blood is present in the stools or there are fecal polymorphonuclear leukocytes, a liquid sample should be submitted for culture to rule out such infections as *Campylobacter, Shigella, Salmonella,* EHEC, *Aeromonas, C. difficile, Plesiomonas,* and *Yersinia.* Culture of many of these organisms, such as *C. difficile, Yersinia,* and EHEC, require special media, so proper coordination with the laboratory is important. If no fecal polymorphonuclear neutrophil leukocytes (PMNs) are identified, stool samples for examination for ova and parasites should be obtained to rule out *Giardia lamblia, E. histolytica,* and *Cryptosporidium.* If *Giardia* is strongly suspected, and upper gastrointestinal tract endoscopy with duodenal biopsy and aspirate or a "string test" (Entero-test, HDC Corporation, Mountain View, Calif.) may improve the diagnostic yield. If *Cryptosporidium* is strongly considered, a small bowel biopsy sample with fixation for electron microscopy may improve yield. Finally, amebiasis can be very difficult to diagnose and asymptomatic cyst passers should not be confused with patients with active disease demonstrating motile trophozoites. Appreciation of trophozoites requires an experienced technician. Serum titers (amebic enzyme immunoassay [EIA]) may be useful in diagnosing invasive disease, including dysentery, but cannot distinguish acute from remote infection.

If all the above studies are unrevealing, one

must consider either a false-negative test or infection with agents that are not identified on standard testing such as viruses, *Yersinia*, ETEC, enteropathogenic *E. coli* (EPEC), *Vibrio cholerae*, and *Vibrio parahaemolyticus*. As noted above, the history may suggest ordering other tests such as stool samples for *C. difficile* toxin titer in patients with a history of antibiotic exposure. An unprepped flexible sigmoidoscopy is often useful in the diagnostic evaluation to look for the degree and extent of inflammation and to obtain biopsies for histology and culture as needed.

TREATMENT

There are three main therapeutic options for the treatment of infectious diarrhea. These include replacement and maintenance of fluid and electrolyte losses, administration of nonantibiotic antidiarrheal agents, and antimicrobial therapy.

FLUID RESUSCITATION

The cornerstone of therapy for infectious diarrhea regardless of the cause is replacement of the extracellular fluid deficit. Before deciding on the type of fluid and its mode of administration (intravenous versus oral), a clinical assessment of the patient's hydration status should be made. This can be performed by bedside evaluation of vital signs (evaluating for increased respirations, orthostatic hypotension, and tachycardia), assessment of skin turgor, patient sensorium, and appearance of overall toxicity. In addition, evaluation of blood urea nitrogen and creatinine, urinary electrolytes, and arterial blood gases yields more information on the patient's volume and acid-base status. There is no one specific test to best predict the degree of fluid deficit, but acute weight loss appears to be the best quantitative indicator.

In patients with severe dehydration (>10% loss of body weight), intravenous fluid replacement is indicated. One suggested approach in adults is infusion of 5% dextrose in isotonic saline, usually starting at 10 to 20 ml/kg/h, with hourly monitoring to assess the adequacy of rehydration (return of pulse and blood pressure to normal, adequate urinary output, etc.). Physicians should be aware that improvement in the patient's volume status may increase stool volumes, and the fluid infusion rate should be adjusted accordingly. During this rapid fluid infusion, the patients must be observed carefully for signs of volume overload such as periorbital edema and pulmonary edema. Rates should be adjusted downward in patients with cardiac or renal insufficiency. Intravenous infusion rates in children are similarly based on weight and severity of dehydration and can be found in standard pediatric texts. As noted above, it is advised to include dextrose in the intravenous solution to prevent precipitation of hypoglycemia as a result of dilution. The infusion may also be supplemented as needed with bicarbonate and potassium. Serum electrolytes and glucose should be rechecked at 4- to 6-hour intervals during the rehydration phase.

For moderate (6% to 10% weight loss) dehydration in both children and adults, it is recommended to give the World Health Organization (WHO) oral replacement fluid (ORS) (see below) at a rate of 100 to 150 ml/kg over the first 4 to 6 hours (15 to 40 ml/kg/h). This initial volume may be repeated depending on clinical response. For mild (3% to 5% weight loss) dehydration, administer 40 to 50 ml/kg of ORS over the first 4 to 6 hours.

The WHO ORS is a safe and cost-effective means of treating diarrhea that is significantly underutilized in the United States. It was formulated to replace stool losses of Na^+, K^+, and HCO_3^- using oral solutions containing the proper balance of glucose, which when present in the small bowel facilitates sodium and water reabsorption from the intestinal lumen into the intravascular compartment. This rehydration solution is formulated as a powder, available in commercially prepared packets. When added to 1 L of water, the appropriate electrolyte balance is achieved. If the WHO ORS cannot be obtained, a similar rehydration formula can be prepared at home by mixing ¾ teaspoonful of table salt (3.5 g of NaCl), 1 teaspoonful of baking soda (2.5 g of $NaHCO_3$), and 4 heaping teaspoonfuls of table sugar (40 g sucrose) in 8 oz (240 ml) of orange juice (1.5 g KCl) and diluting to 1 L with clear water.

Table 76–1 lists the electrolyte composition of normal and diarrheal stools in comparison with various commercial oral and intravenous rehydration formulas and "traditional" home remedies. It is important to note that home remedies do not offer the proper balance of electrolyte replacement for patients with diarrhea. Furthermore, the solutions are hypertonic and, when present in the intestinal lumen, can promote net water movement from blood to lumen, potentially worsening the diarrhea.

There are few contraindications to oral re-

TABLE 76–1. COMPARISON OF ELECTROLYTE CONTENT OF DIARRHEAL STOOLS VERSUS ELECTROLYTE CONTENT OF ORAL AND INTRAVENOUS REHYDRATION FLUIDS

	Electrolyte Content (mEq/L)					Carbohydrate Content (g/L)
	Na^+	K^+	Cl^-	HCO_3^-	Citrate	
Stools						
Normal	32	75	16	32	–	–
Diarrheal	53–124	16–37	24–90	18–48	–	–
Intravenous rehydration fluids						
Normal saline	154	–	154	–	–	–
Ringer's solution	130	4	109	28*	–	–
Oral rehydration fluids						
World Health Organization formula	90	20	80	–	30	20
Pedialyte RS	75	20	65	–	30	25
Pedialyte	45	20	35	–	30	25
Resol	50	20	50	–	34	20
Ricelyte	50	25	45	–	34	30
Gatorade	23	<1	17	–	–	40
Coca-Cola	2	<1	–	–	13	100
Apple juice	<1	25	–	–	0	120
Orange juice	<1	50	–	–	120	
Chicken broth	250	8	–	–	0	0

*Equivalent from lactate conversion.
Adapted from Cheney CP, Wong RKH. Acute infectious diarrhea. *Med Clin North Am.* 1993;77:1169 and Powell DW, Szauter KE. Nonantibiotic therapy and pharmacotherapy of acute infectious diarrhea. *Gastroenterol Clin North Am.* 1993;22:683.

placement therapy: these include patients with uncontrollable vomiting, presence of ileus, or in patients with severe dehydration and altered sensorium. The goals of therapy include replacement of the fluid deficit already present plus replacement of losses due to continued diarrhea and insensible losses. When the initial rehydration phase is complete, the maintenance phase of fluid therapy begins.

There is some controversy over the best fluid to administer as maintenance therapy. Several authors are concerned that continued use of high Na^+-containing ORS (such as the WHO formula) is not indicated, as patients have been shown to develop periorbital edema and occasionally hypernatremia if the solution is continued. As a result, a general guideline to maintenance therapy is to alternate ORS with free water or to dilute it. In adults, one suggested method is to alternate 8 oz (240 ml) glasses of ORS with water at a rate equal to measured losses. In children, ORS can be alternated with breast milk, diluted nonhuman milk, or other commonly consumed beverages at a rate equal to measured losses. Although milk has traditionally been eliminated from the diet, there is no convincing evidence that milk is detrimental. Table 76–1 lists several commercially available solutions with Na^+ concentrations in the desired 50 mEq/L range. Finally, newer cereal-based ORS (primarily rice) appears to reduce the volume and duration of diarrhea by as much as 50% and may be even more efficacious than conventional forms of ORS.

Despite the fact that continued oral intake of food during the course of acute infectious diarrhea may increase the volume of diarrhea, most authors now recommend that patients be fed, not starved, during the episode, particularly children. This is based on studies indicating that most carbohydrate, fat, and protein are still absorbed during the illness, and these nutrients are important for postinfectious repair of the enterocyte. However, certain foods should still be avoided, such as soups with a high sodium concentration; foods with a high sugar content, as this may worsen diarrhea; and high-fiber foods such as fruits and vegetables, as they are difficult to digest.

Nonantibiotic Antidiarrheal Agents

Intraluminal Agents

Cholestyramine is a nonabsorbable anion exchange resin used primarily in patients with hypercholesterolemia. Its mechanism of action is to bind bile acids in the intestine, thereby disrupting micellar delivery of cholesterol for absorption. A common side effect of this medication is constipation, and thus, it has been tried in a number of diarrheal illnesses with varying success. In a number of toxin-induced diarrheas, including pseudomembranous colitis caused by *C. difficile,* cholestyramine is felt to act by binding luminal toxin and has been shown to reduce the duration of diarrhea. Hence, cholestyramine may have a role as an adjunct to treatment of resistant toxin-induced diarrheas. In *C. difficile*–related disease, it is recommended that treatment be given for 5 days past the end of the illness to prevent recurrences. However, it should be noted that some authors do not recommend cholestyramine or any agent with antidiarrheal activity for patients with infectious colitis, particularly those with fever and abdominal pain for fear of precipitating a toxic megacolon.

Kaolin-containing preparations are commonly used in diarrheal illness, primarily acting as an intraluminal adsorbent. However, the use of kaolin-containing preparations has not been shown to be efficacious in acute infectious diarrhea. Some animal studies even suggest Na^+ and K^+ losses may increase. Their routine use is therefore not indicated.

Antimotility Agents

Antimotility agents include the opiates and their synthetic derivatives. The two most common agents in use today include loperamide (Imodium) and diphenoxylate (when dispensed with atropine is marketed as Lomotil). They appear to have antisecretory activity and antimotility effects, but the latter is responsible for the major clinical effects. Prolongation of intestinal transit time is achieved by an increase in segmental contractions of circular muscles in the bowel wall, thereby decreasing forward propulsion. Loperamide appears to have greater efficacy than diphenoxylate with a lower incidence of central nervous system side effects and decreased addictive potential. Its efficacy in nondysenteric acute infectious diarrhea such as traveler's diarrhea has been illustrated in double-blind studies. The major concern with antimotility agents is that their mode of action on gut motility can increase bacterial colonization and potentially increase the risk of bowel wall invasion by enteroinvasive organisms, thereby prolonging the excretion of pathogenic bacteria. For these reasons, opiates are generally contraindicated in any patient with a dysentery-type illness or who appears toxic. Although some authors argue against the routine use of antimotility agents in infectious diarrhea, as the precise enteropathogen is often not known, it appears they can be safely used in mild, nondysenteric diarrheas. A general guideline is to limit their use to 48 hours, and if diarrheal symptoms persist, discontinue their use. The specific suggested treatment regimen for loperamide use is as follows: In adults, the initial dose is 4 mg, then 2 mg after each loose stool, not to exceed a dosage of 16 mg/d. In children 2 to 5 years old, the dosage is 1 mg three times daily; for children 6 to 8 years old, the dosage is 2 mg twice daily; and for children 8 to 12 years old, the dosage is 2 mg three times daily. Of note, some authors do not advocate the use of loperamide in infants and children because of the variability of responses and the potential to cause respiratory depression.

Diphenoxylate-atropine compounds contain "nonpharmacologic" amounts of atropine intended to limit the addictive potential. However, anticholinergic side effects are common. The medication is to be avoided in patients with asthma, chronic obstructive pulmonary disease, prostatic hypertrophy, or acute angle-closure glaucoma. The recommended dosage (2.5 mg/0.025 mg) is 2 tablets four times daily. Some authors recommend an initial dose of 5 to 10 mg.

Other preparations in this category include codeine phosphate, which can be given up to 60 mg three times daily, and paregoric, which is administered as a liquid, 1 to 2 teaspoonsful four times daily.

Antisecretory Agents

Bismuth subsalicylate (Pepto-Bismol) is an insoluble mixture of trivalent bismuth and salicylate. The precise mechanism of action is unclear, although several have been implicated to include bacteriostatic or bactericidal effects on organisms, preventing attachment of bacteria to the intestinal epithelium, and antisecretory action. Bismuth subsalicylate preparations have been shown to have efficacy in the treatment of traveler's diarrhea and acute diarrhea in children. Its efficacy in viral diarrhea has yielded conflicting results. The medicine appears to be safe. The specific suggested treatment regimen for bismuth subsalicylate is as follows: For adults, the dose is 30 ml q30–60min with an 8 dose per day maximum. The pediatric dose is 5 ml for children 3 to 6 years old, 10 ml for children 6 to 9 years old, and 15 ml for children 8 to 12 years old. The dosing schedule in children is the same as adults. As this medication is an aspirin-containing compound, some authors caution against potentiating gastritis, causing Reye's syndrome, or aggravating a bleeding condition. Finally, bismuth subsalicylate turns stools black, and this result should not be misinterpreted as melena.

The gut peptide somatostatin and its synthetic analogs, octreotide and vapreotide, are potent inhibitors of intestinal secretion. They have been effectively used in patients with chronic AIDS-related diarrhea of unknown cause and in patients with cryptosporidiosis who had failed other antimicrobial regimens. In one study, stool volumes were decreased by greater than 50% in approximately one half of the patients receiving octreotide. Side effects of octreotide may include nausea, pain at the injection site (usually delivered subcutaneously), abdominal pain, and long-term complications such as hyperglycemia and gallstone formation. At this time, the role of these medicines in the treatment of acute infectious diarrhea remains unclear.

Microbial Agents

In Europe, *Saccharomyces boulardii,* a nonpathogenic yeast, has been widely used to prevent antibiotic-associated diarrhea. Recent controlled, blinded studies in the United States in nearly 200 patients have shown clear efficacy in the prevention of antibiotic-associated diarrhea. In a smaller number of patients, prevention of relapses of *C. difficile* colitis and diarrhea in patients previously treated with vancomycin or metronidazole was achieved. Further study in the United States will likely precede the widespread use of this agent.

Antiinflammatory Agents

Several types of bacterial diarrheas are associated with elevated levels of prostaglandins, and prostaglandins (particularly those in the "E" series) can cause diarrhea. Studies in animal models suggest that treatment with cyclooxygenase inhibitors such as indomethacin can reduce intestinal secretion in experimental salmonellosis, cryptosporidiosis, amebiasis, and cholera. However, neither indomethacin nor aspirin was shown to significantly reduce the diarrhea associated with cholera, and controlled studies are lacking.

ANTIMICROBIAL AGENTS

Empiric Therapy

The diagnostic workup previously described was developed to isolate an infectious agent to help guide specific antibiotic therapy, which when applied, would hopefully shorten the patient's duration of illness. Unfortunately, tests such as fecal leukocytes, stool specimens for ova and parasites, stool cultures, and flexible sigmoidoscopies take time, and results may not be available for days. As a result, one often has to make a decision regarding antibiotic therapy based on history and clinical evaluation. Three of the main factors to consider before deciding on empiric therapy are the status of the host (adult versus child, immunocompetent versus immunosuppressed, degree of toxicity, etc.), the location from which the host arrived (urban or rural United States versus foreign country), and a best clinical estimate as to the cause of the offending agent (bacterial, viral, or parasitic). In general, patients who appear toxic and febrile without evidence of a self-limited process are suitable candidates for empiric antimicrobial therapy, especially if they present with bloody diarrhea. Antibiotics to consider at this time include ciprofloxacin, 500 mg twice daily for 3 to 5 days, or trimethoprim-sulfamethoxazole (TMP-SMX), 160/800 mg twice daily for 3 to 5 days, for a suspected bacterial infection, and metronidazole, 250 to 500 mg three times daily, if the history is highly suspicious for a protozoan infection.

Culture-Guided Therapy

There appears to be a general consensus regarding antimicrobial therapy for certain culture (or test)-proven enteric pathogens, as multiple studies have documented their efficacy. These pathogens include *Shigella, V. cholerae,* traveler's diarrhea (most commonly ETEC), *C. difficile,* and the protozoans *E. histolytica, G. lamblia,* and *I. belli.* The recommended treatment for these pathogens in adults and children is listed in Table 76–2 with an alternative agent in the event of a drug allergy.

There is another group of pathogens for which treatment with antimicrobial therapy is somewhat controversial, either because there is inconclusive evidence to document efficacy (most cases), antimicrobial therapy is recommended for a specific group of patients only, or isolated preliminary reports have suggested an actual harmful effect of the medicine. The pathogens in this group include EPEC, EHEC, EIEC, nontyphoidal *Salmonella, Campylobacter jejuni, Yersinia enterocolitica, V. parahaemolyticus,* and the noncholera vibrios. The controversies surrounding treatment of these pathogens is discussed below. Those pathogens for which antibiotic therapy is suspected to be efficacious but not clearly proven are also listed in Table 76–2.

EHEC infection was first identified in 1977, but the first human cases were not reported un-

TABLE 76–2. ANTIMICROBIAL THERAPY OF ACUTE INFECTIOUS DIARRHEA

Pathogen	Adult Dosage	Pediatric Dosage	Comments*
Bacterial			
Campylobacter	Erythromycin, 250–500 mg q.i.d. × 7 d, or ciprofloxacin, 500 mg b.i.d. × 7 d	Erythromycin, 40 mg/kg/d div q6h × 7 d, or chloramphenicol, 50–75 mg/kg/d div q6h	Treat dysentery and severe disease only; ciprofloxacin contraindicated in children
Clostridium difficile	Metronidazole, 250 mg q.i.d. × 10 d, or vancomycin (PO) 125–250 mg q.i.d. × 10 d	Vancomycin, 20–40 mg/kg/d PO q6h (max 2 g/d), or metronidazole, 35–50 mg/kg/d div q8h × 10 d	
Escherichia coli (traveler's diarrhea) presumed ETEC or EAEC	Ciprofloxacin, 500 mg b.i.d. × 5 d, or TMP-SMX, 160/800 mg b.i.d. × 5 d	4 mg TMP/20 mg SMX/kg/d div q12h	TMP-SMX not for use in children <2 mo
EPEC	As for Shigella	Neomycin, 30 mg/kg PO q8h × 5 d	Limited or lack of placebo-controlled studies documenting efficacy of antibiotics
EIEC	As for Shigella	As for Shigella	
Salmonella	Ciprofloxacin, 500 mg b.i.d. × 7 d, or ampicillin, 250–500 mg q.i.d.	Ampicillin, 50–100 mg/kg/d div q8h × 7–14 d, or chloramphenicol, 50–75 mg/kg/d div q6h	Treat only infants <12 wk, patients with bacteremia or "altered hosts" (see text)
Shigella	TMP-SMX, 160/800 mg b.i.d. × 5 d, or ciprofloxacin, 500 mg b.i.d. × 5 d	8 mg TMP/40 mg SMX/kg/d div q12h × 10 d, or ampicillin, 50–100 mg/kg/d div q8h	
Vibrio cholerae	Tetracycline, 500 mg q.i.d. × 3 d, or furazolidone, 100 mg q.i.d. × 3 d	Tetracycline, 50 mg/kg/d div q6h × 3 d, or 8 mg TMP/40 mg SMX/kg/d div q12h	Tetracycline not indicated for children <9 y
Noncholera vibrios	Tetracycline, 500 mg q.i.d. × 3 d, or furazolidone, 125 mg q.i.d. × 3 d	Furazolidone, 5 mg/kg/d PO q6h × 3 d	Treatment indicated only for severe illness
Yersinia	Tobramycin, 3–5 mg/kg/d div q8h, or ciprofloxacin, 500 mg b.i.d.	Tobramycin, 6.0–7.5 mg/kg/d div q6–8h, or chloramphenicol, 50–75 mg/kg/d div q6h × 10 d	Treatment indicated only for severe or prolonged illness
Protozoan			
Entamoeba histolytica	Metronidazole, 500 mg t.i.d. × 7 d followed by iodoquinol, 650 mg t.i.d. × 20 d	Metronidazole, 35–50 mg/kg/d div q8h × 7 d followed by iodoquinol, 40 mg/kg/d div q8h × 20 d	
Giardia lamblia	Quinacrine, 100 mg t.i.d. × 7 d, or metronidazole, 250 mg t.i.d. × 7 d	Quinacrine, 7 mg/kg/d div q8h (max 300 mg/d) × 5 d, or metronidazole, 35–50 mg/kg/d div q8h	Safety and efficacy of metronidazole not established in children for this indication
Isospora belli	TMP-SMX, 160/800 mg b.i.d. × 7–14 d, or pyrimethamine, 75 mg/d plus leucovorin (Folinic Acid), 10 mg/d × 14 d	8 mg TMP/40 mg SMX/kg/d div q12h	

*The list of comments is not comprehensive. Physicians should read the package insert for dosage adjustments, incompatibilities, and adverse reactions.
Adapted from Cheney CP, Wong RKH. Acute infectious diarrhea. *Med Clin North Am.* 1993;77:1169 and McQueen CE, Boedecker EC. Acute infectious diarrhea. In: Bayless TM, ed. *Current Therapy in Gastroenterology and Liver Disease.* 3rd ed. Philadelphia, Pa: BC Decker Inc; 1990:199.

til 1983. EHEC strain 0157 was recently the topic of national concern in the largest outbreak ever reported (>500 patients), when traced to contaminated hamburger in the Pacific Northwest. Greater than 90% of patients presented with bloody diarrhea, and some with hemolytic-uremic syndrome (HUS). The 0157 serotype is easily identified by stool culture and should be obtained in suggestive cases. Treatment of EHEC infection has not undergone double-blind placebo-controlled antimicrobial trials to date. However, anecdotal observations indicate that antibiotic therapy is not helpful, and it even appears to worsen the clinical course in the most recent cases. As a result, current treatment is supportive, and antibiotics and antimotility agents are not recommended.

Outbreaks of EIEC diarrhea are rarely reported and are usually food related. As a result, no therapeutic placebo-controlled trials have been performed. However, EIEC infection produces a clinical illness of diarrhea and dysentery very similar to shigellosis with similar virulence properties. It appears that the current opinion regarding this pathogen is to treat it in the same fashion as shigellosis.

Strains of EPEC may cause epidemic outbreaks of diarrhea, often in infants. Again, there is little data regarding the efficacy of antimicrobial treatment of this pathogen. In small studies, however, TMP-SMX, oral neomycin, and oral gentamicin have shown some effectiveness.

In salmonellosis, although multiple antibiotic trials proved efficacy of therapy, none of the trials altered the duration or severity of fever and diarrhea. As a result, treatment of nontyphoidal salmonellosis has only been recommended by some authors for infants less than 12 weeks of age. Others have expanded the treatment parameters to include patients who are at risk for developing secondary complications such as those with immunocompromised states, hemoglobinopathies, internal prostheses, or malignancies and the elderly. In situations where the pathogen has caused bacteremia, or in *Salmonella typhimurium* infection, treatment is always indicated, with ciprofloxacin being the treatment of choice. Ampicillin and chloramphenicol have proven effective as well.

C. jejuni is one of the most common enteric pathogens in the world. The data on the efficacy of antimicrobial therapy against this pathogen are mixed. However, two studies using erythromycin have demonstrated effective treatment. Ciprofloxacin has also been shown to clear *C. jejuni* diarrhea, but resistance to ciprofloxacin therapy and relapse have been reported. As a general rule, treatment is recommended if the illness is severe or prolonged or if dysentery is present.

Gastrointestinal disease due to *Y. enterocolitica* is mostly recognized in children, but patients of all ages can be infected. The two most common features of infection are diarrhea and abdominal pain, the latter often localizing in the right lower quadrant in patients over the age of 5 years. Most patients experience several days of watery, sometimes blood-streaked diarrhea, which tends to improve by the third day of the illness. No evidence has proven that antimicrobial therapy alters the course of this usually self-limited illness, and treatment is not commonly advocated. Treatment is recommended, however, for prolonged or septicemic illness, as mortality can approach 50% even with antibiotic therapy. Aminoglycosides, fluoroquinolones, chloramphenicol, and other agents have generally proven effective, although resistance is seen in rare strains.

V. parahaemolyticus is a major etiologic agent of bacterial diarrhea in Japan, but it has also been implicated as a causative agent of food poisoning in the United States, where nearly all cases have been associated with raw or improperly stored seafood or with contamination of food with seawater. Self-limited watery diarrhea is the most common form of the illness. Antibiotics have not been shown to alter the course of the illness. Two other members of the Vibrionaceae family include the nonvibrio Vibrionaceae, *Aeromonas* sp. and *Plesiomonas shigelloides*. Both have been implicated in traveler's diarrhea, and *P. shigelloides* has also been associated with food-borne outbreaks, particularly oysters. Although large clinical trials with antimicrobial agents are lacking, it appears that severe illness associated with these organisms may benefit from treatment with tetracycline, furazolidone, TMP-SMX, and others.

Enteric pathogens that should not be treated include suspected viral agents and cryptosporidiosis in AIDS patients. Although rotavirus and Norwalk agent virus account for a large percentage of gastrointestinal infections (the incidence of rotavirus in children around the world is thought to approach or surpass the incidence of ETEC), no effective antiviral agent currently exists. For *Cryptosporidium,* no single agent has been proven effective in its eradication to date, although bovine hyperimmune colostrum against *Cryptosporidium* has shown some efficacy in AIDS patients.

PREVENTION OF DIARRHEA

Most data on the effectiveness of prophylactic therapy in the prevention of diarrhea are derived from studies of traveler's diarrhea. Because the pathogens known to be associated with traveler's diarrhea are transmitted by fecally contaminated water and food, the best prevention is to avoid these substances. As this is a difficult and often impossible task in some foreign coun-

TABLE 76-3. PROPHYLAXIS OF TRAVELER'S DIARRHEA

Therapeutic Agent	Dose Frequency	Comments
Bismuth subsalicylate	2 tablets q.i.d.	Antibiotics should be started 1 day before the person travels and discontinued 1 day after departing the high-risk area. The National Institutes of Health Consensus Conference recommends against "routine" use of antibacterial agents; bismuth subsalicylate is acceptable.
Doxycycline	100 mg q.d.	
Trimethoprim-Sulfamethoxazole (TMP-SMX)	160 mg TMP/800 mg SMX q.d.	
Norfloxacin	400 mg q.d.	

Modified from Sack RB. Traveler's diarrhea. In: Bayless TM, ed. *Current Therapy in Gastroenterology and Liver Disease.* 3rd ed. Philadelphia, Pa: BC Decker Inc; 1990:208.

tries, other pharmacologic agents have been studied.

Specific agents that have been proven to decrease the attack rate of traveler's diarrhea are shown in Table 76–3. The only clinically useful nonantibiotic medication is bismuth subsalicylate (Pepto-Bismol). Regular dosing of this agent decreases the attack rate by 40% to 60%. The antibiotics norfloxacin, TMP-SMX, and doxycycline have also been shown to be effective, the former two agents conferring an approximate 90% anticipated protection. It is important to note that routine use of prophylactic antibiotics is not recommended by most experts because of the generally mild and self-limited nature of the disease, potential medication side effects, and potentially selecting resistant bacterial strains. Therefore, prophylactic antibiotics should be reserved for those travelers who are chronically ill or immunocompromised, in which a significant dehydrating illness may convey a high morbidity.

REFERENCES

1. Cantey JR. *Escherichia coli* diarrhea. *Gastroenterol Clin North Am.* 1993;22:609.
2. Cantey JR. Infectious diarrhea: pathogenesis and risk factors. *Am J Med.* 1985;78(6B):65.
3. Chak A, Banwell JG. Traveler's diarrhea. *Gastroenterol Clin North Am.* 1993;22:549.
4. Cheney CP, Wong RKH. Acute infectious diarrhea. *Med Clin North Am.* 1993;77:1169.
5. DiJohn D, Levine MM. Treatment of diarrhea. *Infect Dis Clin North Am.* 1988;2:719.
6. Gorbach SL. Bacterial diarrhoea and its treatment. *Lancet.* 1987;2:1378.
7. McQueen CE, Boedeker EC. Acute infectious diarrhea. In: Bayless TM, ed. *Current Therapy in Gastroenterology and Liver Disease.* 3rd ed. Philadelphia, Pa: BC Decker Inc; 1990:199.
8. Pothoulakis C, LaMont JT. *Clostridium difficile* colitis and diarrhea. *Gastroenterol Clin North Am.* 1993;22:623.
9. Powell DW, Szauter KE. Nonantibiotic therapy and pharmacotherapy of acute infectious diarrhea. *Gastroenterol Clin North Am.* 1993;22:683.
10. Sack RB. Traveler's diarrhea. In: Bayless TM, ed. *Current Therapy in Gastroenterology and Liver Disease.* 3rd ed. Philadelphia, Pa: BC Decker Inc; 1990:208.

77
Nonneoplastic Polyps
MARSHALL SPARBERG

Polyp refers to any visible, discrete tissue protruding above the surface into a hollow organ. Neoplastic polyps are true growths that are malignant or have malignant potential. Nonneoplastic polyps, on the other hand, do not have any potential for true growth, although they may enlarge because of the addition of normal structures, such as inflammatory cells or blood vessels.

For convenience, nonneoplastic polyps can be divided into those of the upper gastrointestinal tract and those of the small bowel and colon.

NONNEOPLASTIC UPPER GASTROINTESTINAL TRACT POLYPS

Gastric polyps in general are uncommon and usually are diagnosed incidentally during barium studies or at endoscopy.

These nonneoplastic polyps do not cause symptoms, such as abdominal pain or bleeding, and, after their benign nature is established, do not require removal. Although the surface of the polyp could be eroded and cause occult gastrointestinal blood loss, another source for occult bleeding should be sought.

Hyperplastic polyps are the most common type of polyp in the stomach, usually occurring in the antrum. These polyps are less than 2 cm, either sessile or pedunculated, and occasionally eroded, with inflammation seen histologically. Other histologic features are elongated and cystic gastric glands with bundles of invaginated muscularis mucosae. Occasionally, hyperplastic polyps tend to regress spontaneously. They do not have malignant potential. The relationship between these single hyperplastic polyps and diffuse hyperplastic gastric polyposis (Ménétrier's disease) is unclear.

Pedunculated gastric polyps may be resected with snare cautery, similar to colonoscopic polypectomy. Because of gastric peristalsis, glucagon should be administered prior to gastric polypectomy so that the specimen is not lost.

Unlike the colon, the stomach wall is much thicker, so that snare cautery of sessile polyps may be performed by creating a "pseudostalk," similar to the large particle biopsy, or using the morseling technique.

Pancreatic rests are the second most common causes of a gastric polypoid lesion. They are asymptomatic and primarily found as a filling defect on upper gastrointestinal tract radiologic studies or at upper endoscopy. They occur on the greater curvature aspect of the prepyloric antrum, are sessile, and usually less than 1 cm. Endoscopically, pancreatic rests are covered by normal-appearing mucosa and may have a central dimple. If a sufficiently deep biopsy is obtained, normal-appearing pancreatic tissue is seen.

NONNEOPLASTIC COLONIC POLYPS

The most important point about nonneoplastic colonic polyps is to distinguish them from adenomas or carcinomas. Occasionally, these polyps may produce symptoms in their own right, such as bleeding, anal prolapse, or abdominal pain. Many nonneoplastic polyps are observed at colonoscopy performed because of gross or occult bleeding, because of abdominal pain, or as a screening procedure for possible neoplasia.

Hyperplastic polyps are the most common colorectal polyp, particularly in the distal colon. Of those rectal polyps 3 mm or less, over 90% will be hyperplastic in nature. These polyps are usually sessile, tiny, and flat when viewed colonoscopically. Hyperplastic polyps biopsy specimens have a distinctive histologic appearance with elongated cysts and a micropapillary epithelium, without cytologic atypia.

Both neoplastic and hyperplastic polyps occur with increased age of the patient, and islands of adenomatous tissue or even adenocarcinoma have been seen within a hyperplastic polyp. These facts have been used to support the view that hyperplastic polyps seen on proctoscopy or flexible sigmoidoscopy are a sign that neoplastic polyps may be found on colonoscopy. There is no good evidence to support this view.

Juvenile polyps occur most frequently in patients less than 10 years of age but may occur in patients of any age and can be responsible for lower gastrointestinal tract bleeding because of their increased vascular supply. These polyps often are pedunculated and, if sufficient care is not taken during colonoscopic polypectomy with adequate cautery, may bleed profusely. Juvenile polyps may be as large as 2 cm in size and often occur in the rectum. Since they are pedunculated, prolapse of these polyps through the anus may be a presenting symptom.

Histologically, juvenile polyps consist of dilated mucus-filled cystic glands in an expanded lamina propria with normal epithelium. Although they are sometimes called *retention polyps,* they are probably hamartomas.

Inflammatory polyps are seen in patients with colitis, both due to specific pathogens, such as *Shigella* or ameba, or due to nonspecific inflammatory bowel disease. This type of polyp is frequently seen in patients with inflammatory bowel disease who have had significant mucosal destruction, leading to regeneration, or mucosa with inflammation and granulation tissue. They are often multiple and may be quite large, earning the name *giant pseudopolyps.* The term *pseudopolyp* also is used to describe inflammatory polyps, probably to distinguish them from true neoplasm, but the term should be abandoned, since pseudopolyps do fit the definition of a polyp given in the introduction to this section. Occasionally, bridging and bizarre configurations may be seen.

Inflammatory polyps have no malignant potential in themselves but can cause confusion in patients with chronic ulcerative colitis undergoing colonoscopy for dysplasia, since "dysplasia-associated lesion or mass" is a sign of carcinoma. Actually, other than dysplasia-associated polyps having a very irregular appearance, biopsy specimens for dysplasia in chronic ulcerative colitis are best taken from the intervening mucosa rather than the inflammatory polyps.

Lymphoid polyps are small, smooth, and sessile excrescences, often in the rectal area and frequently multiple. They appear paler than the hyperplastic polyps because of the marked infiltration of the lamina propria by mature lymphocytes, raising the normal overlying colonic epithelium.

Peutz-Jeghers polyps usually occur in the small bowel but may appear in the colon. They are true hamartomas with prominent branching bands of smooth muscle in the lamina propria. Although initially thought to be completely benign, malignancies in patients with Peutz-Jeghers syndrome have been reported.

Cap polyps are dark red, sessile, and located on mucosal folds. On biopsy, elongated and inflamed cysts are present, with a cap of inflammatory tissue.

Other rare causes of polypoid masses in the colon are *colitis cystica profunda* and *pneumatosis coli.* The former is caused by dilated, mucus-filled glands in the submucosa and must be distinguished from colloid carcinoma. Pneumatosis coli is characterized by air-filled submucosal cysts that are often discovered incidentally at sigmoidoscopy and surprise the endoscopist by deflating on biopsy. Usually pneumatosis coli is asymptomatic, but occasionally patients complain of tenesmus and require a more aggressive approach, even to the point of using hyperbaric chambers.

78
Complications of the Ileoanal Pullthrough Procedure and the Kock Continent Ileostomy

ERIC W. FONKALSRUD

Operations for treatment of medically intractable ulcerative colitis include proctocolectomy with permanent ileostomy, continent ileostomy (Kock pouch), subtotal colectomy with ileostomy and Hartmann's rectal pouch or ileorectal anastomosis, and colectomy with mucosal proctectomy and endorectal ileal pullthrough (ERP). During the past 10 years, ERP has emerged as the operation of choice for the definitive surgical treatment of ulcerative colitis and for patients with familial adenomatous polyposis. This operation cures the disease and obviates the unpleasant and cumbersome features of a permanent ileostomy, as well as the morbidity of proctectomy, and permits a near-normal lifestyle.

ERP is a modification of the rectal mucosa stripping operation described by Soave[1] in 1965 for the treatment of Hirschsprung's disease. This is the most successful and frequently used operation for the definitive treatment of Hirschsprung's disease with excellent long-term results having been reported at numerous large medical centers extending over a period of more than two-and-a-half decades.

For patients with ulcerative colitis or familial colonic polyposis, a standard total colectomy with removal of the upper rectum is performed, following which the mucosa is dissected free and removed from the lower rectum down to the anus, thus preserving an intact rectal muscle cuff and anal sphincter apparatus. The distal ileum is rarely involved with ulcerative colitis and should be preserved as close to the ileocecal valve as feasible. Continuity of the intestinal tract is reestablished by extending the distal ileum into the pelvis through the rectal muscle cuff and suturing it circumferentially to the anus. This operative procedure provides the following advantages:

1. It is a definitive operation with removal of all diseased colonic and rectal mucosa.
2. The parasympathetic innervation to the bladder and genitalia are preserved.
3. A permanent abdominal stoma is avoided.
4. The anorectal sphincter mechanism is preserved, and thus, continence is maintained.

With sphincter-sparing operations now available for most patients with ulcerative colitis refractory to medical therapy, it has become very important to inform patients of all surgical alternatives before proceeding with proctocolectomy whenever feasible and to carefully distinguish patients with ulcerative colitis from those with Crohn's disease who should not have an ileoanal pouch procedure. Because ERP is much more acceptable than other surgical procedures, patients with ulcerative colitis are being referred for operation earlier in the course of their disease than previously.

Although ERP was initially limited to patients who were young and with relatively quiescent disease, the indications have been greatly liberalized. The pullthrough procedure is currently withheld only from a small group of patients with concomitant major medical problems, such as coronary artery disease, stroke, and active cancer, and from occasional patients with very acute severe colitis, which might preclude a safe 4- to 6-hour operation. Obesity greatly increases the technical difficulty of the ileoanal anastomosis and is a relative contraindication to operation. The severity of the colitis has also increased the operative morbidity somewhat; however, those patients receiving long-term corticosteroid therapy and those who have been given cyclosporine, azathioprine (Imuran), 6-mercaptopurine, and other immunosuppressive medications have a considerably increased risk of postoperative complications. Patients with severe rectal inflammatory disease are more likely to experience postoperative rectal strictures and incomplete ileoanal anastomotic healing.

Removal of the entire rectal mucosa down to the dentate line has been shown not to interfere appreciably with anorectal sphincter function or the ability to discriminate between gas and liquid or solid luminal contents, providing the anal sphincter and rectal muscles are not permanently disturbed during the operative procedure.[2] The length of the anal sphincter and the mean resting pressure are generally well maintained at levels comparable with normal. The rectoanal inhibitory reflex may be abnormal, although continence after the ileoanal anastomosis does not appear to be hampered by the absence of this reflex.

Although the initial operations preserved a long rectal muscle cuff extending from peritoneal reflection to dentate line, it has subsequently been shown that the length of rectal muscle retained above the ileoanal anastomosis need not be longer than 5 cm.[3] Shorter muscle cuffs may increase the risk of bladder dysfunction, retrograde ejaculation, and impotence. Longer muscle cuffs may cause compression of the ileal pullthrough segment, are prone to contracture, may cause pouch angulation, and appear to provide no useful function. As long as the lower 4 cm of the rectal muscle cuff is not damaged, both the anal sphincter resting pressure and the squeeze pressure return to close to normal within 6 weeks. Recent reports indicate that a stapled anastomosis between the end of the pouch and the full thickness of rectum 2 to 3 cm above the dentate line may function well; however, they are more prone to complications, since almost all patients with ulcerative colitis continue to have active disease in the remaining rectum, the rectal muscularis is divided sufficiently low that injury to the seminal vesicles is more frequent, and a one-layer stapled anastomosis is not as strong as the ileoanal anastomosis through a rectal muscle cuff.

Early reports indicated that the straight ERP without reservoir produced satisfactory continence; however, long-term follow-up of these patients indicated that many experienced persistent stool frequency and urgency with moderate incontinence.[4] The straight ileal pullthrough procedure maintains peristaltic contractions down to the anal anastomosis. Most surgeons performing the pullthrough procedure have, therefore, constructed an ileal reservoir above the ileoanal anastomosis to reduce peristalsis in the distal ileum and to provide an area for fecal storage. Although occasional patients with a straight ERP may experience a favorable clinical result, those who continue to experience stool frequency and urgency may be reconstructed at a later time to a pullthrough procedure with ileal reservoir.[5] Those patients with polyposis who have undergone a previous colectomy with ileorectal anastomosis many years earlier are more likely to do well with a subsequent straight ileoanal anastomosis.

For most patients, the ileoanal pullthrough operation is performed in two stages. The first operation consists of colectomy, mucosal proctectomy, construction of an ileal reservoir, endorectal ileal pullthrough with ileoanal anastomosis, and cutaneous ileostomy. A completely diverting ileostomy is advisable for at least 3 months to minimize the risk of pelvic infection. Patients with chronic ulcerative colitis who receive long-term steroid therapy are often malnourished and frequently have a suppressed immune response, increasing the risk of postoperative infection and delayed wound healing. Many patients with polyposis and occasional highly selected patients with ulcerative colitis may undergo the entire ERP safely in one stage without ileostomy. A radiographic contrast enema and sigmoidoscopy are performed 2 months after surgery to assure that the pouch has healed well without sinus tracts or other complications. If sinus tracts, strictures, or other disorders are noted, closure of the ileostomy should be delayed a few weeks until the problem has been resolved.

At the second operation, performed 3 to 4 months after the initial procedure, the ileostomy is closed. Adhesions in the lower small intestine are lysed to minimize the risk of early postoperative obstruction. In our clinical experience, an end-ileostomy has fewer complications than have been reported with a loop ileostomy, and a stoma appliance can be used more easily. The ileoanal anastomosis is dilated to approximately a #20 Hegar while the patient is under anesthesia. Postoperative rectal dilation with a #18 Hegar is performed on a daily basis for 1 month, and then every other day for 2 months more. Oral metronidazole, 250 mg twice daily, is given for 6 weeks after operation to minimize pouch

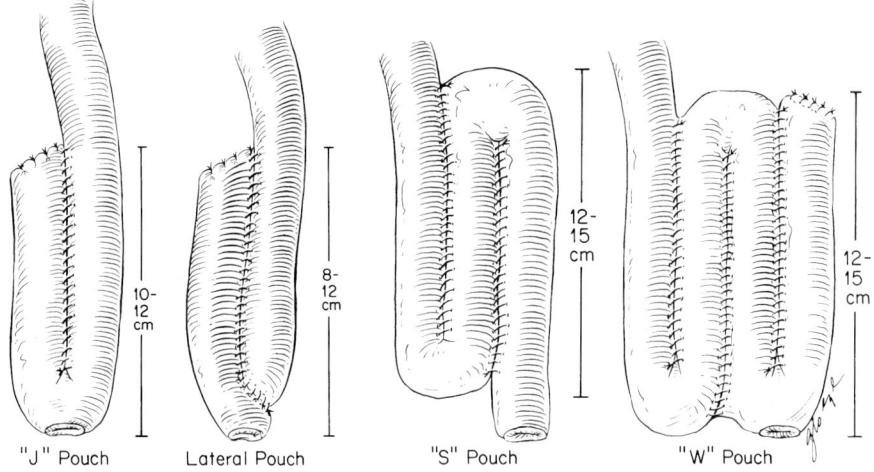

FIGURE 78–1. The most frequent ileal reservoir configurations used clinically in patients undergoing ileal pouch anal anastomosis.

mucosal inflammation as the reservoir adapts to the new function of fecal storage.

For occasional patients undergoing emergency colectomy, the operation has three stages, the first consisting of colectomy, cutaneous ileostomy, and Hartmann's pouch closure of the rectum. During the second procedure, completion colectomy, mucosal proctectomy, and construction of the ileoanal pouch procedure with diverting ileostomy are performed. At the third stage, approximately 3 months later, the ileostomy is closed. The three-stage operation is avoided whenever possible because of the increasing risk of adhesions and other complications with multiple operations.

Four types of reservoir configurations have been used clinically; the J-shaped reservoir, the lateral reservoir, the S-shaped reservoir, and the W-shaped reservoir (Fig. 78–1). The distal ileum is bent back on itself to form two (J and lateral), three (S), or four (W) loops, which are opened and sutured or stapled together to make a pouch. The lateral and S pouches have a short distal spout which is anastomosed to the anus, whereas the side of a loop in the J and W pouches is sutured to the anus. Although more than 4500 ileoanal pouch procedures have been performed in various medical centers throughout the world, there is no unanimity of opinion regarding which of the reservoir configurations provides the best long-term function with lowest risk of complications.[6] Nonetheless, we and most surgeons use the J pouch whenever feasible.

CLINICAL EXPERIENCE

During the past 14 years, 364 patients with ulcerative colitis, 47 with polyposis, and 3 with Hirschsprung's disease have undergone colectomy, mucosal proctectomy, and ileoanal pouch procedures in our hospital. Following the ileoanal pullthrough procedure with lateral or J-shaped reservoir, the average number of movements per 24 hours at 3 months after surgery is 6.2, and at 6 months is 5.2. From the last 220 consecutive patients, 11% have less than two episodes of staining or soiling per week, and 5% have more than two episodes per week at 6 months following surgery. At 9 months after surgery, 81% are able to delay defecation for more than 2 hours after the initial urge. Almost all patients indicate that they are able to empty the reservoir almost completely with each defecatory action with minimal straining. Residual fecal volumes in reservoirs rarely exceed 15 ml after defecation. Measurements of fecal bile salts and serum vitamin B_{12} levels have been within normal range in 30 of the patients in whom these studies were evaluated. None of the 192 men have had impotence, although one has had retrograde ejaculation. Twenty-nine women have delivered normal babies, 16 by vaginal route. There was a mean period of 3.2 weeks after ileostomy closure before patients returned to full school or work activities. Many patients participate in vigorous exercise including competitive running, football, swimming, skiing, and wrestling.

COMPLICATIONS OF ENDORECTAL ILEAL PULLTHROUGH

Major complications following the endorectal ileal pullthrough procedure in my personal experience with 367 patients include ileoanal stenosis or outflow obstruction in 25%, reservoir enlargement in 23%, steroid withdrawal symptoms in 16%, reservoir inflammation (pouchitis) in 11%, adhesions, internal hernias, intussusception in 9%, wound infection in 7%, ileostomy obstruction or dysfunction in 3%, pelvic sinus tracts in 4%, and intestinal leak or perforation in 0.5% (Table 78–1). During their period of immediate postoperative convalescence, three patients experienced perforation of duodenal or gastric ulcers related to corticosteroid therapy. Forty-three percent of patients experienced complications, and 36% required reoperation, almost half of which were performed more than 2 years following ileostomy closure (Table 78–2).

During the first 2 years after surgery, the most common complications requiring reoperation were intestinal adhesions (16), internal hernia (11), and intussusception (3). Eighteen patients underwent surgical repair or dilation of rectal strictures under anesthesia. Ileostomy revision was performed on three patients and drainage of infection on six patients. During the first 2 years after surgery, 12 patients underwent reconstruction of the ileal spout, or reservoir shortening, or conversion of a straight pullthrough into a reservoir because of delayed emptying and stasis. Five additional patients underwent various minor operative procedures while under anesthesia. Fifty-eight patients required reoperation more than 2 years following ileostomy closure for treatment of reservoir stasis with pouch enlargement and ileoanal stenosis or outflow obstruction. Ten of these patients had shortening of the ileal spout transanally; however, 34 required abdominoperineal mobilization of the pouch with reconstruction and performance of a new ileoanal anastomosis. Fourteen underwent reconstruction of a straight pullthrough into an ileoanal pouch.

TABLE 78–1. COMPLICATIONS FOLLOWING ENDORECTAL ILEAL PULLTHOUGH (ERP) IN 94 CHLDREN AND 273 ADULTS

	Number of Patients		
Complication	Children	Adults	Percent
Ileoanal stenosis, outflow obstruction	19	72	25
Reservoir enlargement	16	68	23
Steroid withdrawal symptoms	14	46	16
Pouchitis	9	32	11
Adhesions, internal hernia, intussusception	8	26	9
Wound infection	5	23	7
Fecal urgency, frequency (patients without pouch)	5	11	4
Peripullthrough sinus	3	14	4
Ileostomy obstruction	3	10	3
TOTAL COMPLICATIONS*	82	302	
TOTAL AFFECTED PATIENTS	42 (45%)	116 (42%)	43

*Sixty percent of complications occurred in first 115 patients.

TABLE 78–2. COMPLICATIONS REQUIRING REOPERATION FOR ENDORECTAL ILEAL PULLTHOUGH (ERP) IN 94 CHLDREN AND 273 ADULTS

Complication	Children	Adults	Percent
Patients with reoperation*	31	101	36
Less than 2 years postoperatively	20	54	20
More than 2 years postoperatively	11	47	16
Postoperative deaths (<90 d)	0	1	0.3
Permanent ileostomy (four with Crohn's disease)	4	7	3

*Nineteen of the last 185 patients have had a reoperation (10.3%).

Of the 367 patients, 11 returned to an ileostomy (3%); most of these were during our early clinical experience. Four of these patients who initially had indeterminate colitis proved to have Crohn's disease within 3 years after ileostomy closure. Sixty percent of all complications occurred in the first 115 patients. There was one postoperative death within 90 days because of acute adrenal insufficiency related to long-term high-dose steroid administration. Children have approximately the same incidence of complications as do adults.

Although functional results during the first postoperative year in most cases show a gradual reduction in stool frequency, occasional patients experience repeated episodes of pouch inflammation with persistent diarrhea, urgency, frequency, and occasional incontinence. For many years, these patients were managed by dietary restrictions, antiperistaltic medications, and rectal irrigations with tap water. During the past 6 years, we have used an increasingly aggressive surgical approach to management of patients with these symptoms, which are usually due to reservoir stasis resulting from reservoir outlet obstruction or to a large pouch that empties incompletely. This policy has resulted in only two patients from the last 175 consecutive patients returning to a permanent ileostomy following the pullthrough procedure.

The important features of optimal function following the pullthrough procedure appear to include (1) the use of a short rectal muscle cuff, (2) a short ileal reservoir, (3) a very short ileal spout, (4) removal of all rectal mucosa down to the dentate line, and (5) aggressive correction of postoperative rectal strictures. Routine use of a #18 Hegar dilator on a daily basis for the first 3 months postoperatively has virtually eliminated rectal strictures. Reconstruction of previously constructed ileoanal pouches that are not functioning optimally to conform to these characteristics has resulted in a marked improvement in intestinal function and has greatly reduced the occurrence of reservoir pouchitis or the need for a permanent ileostomy.[7] Less than 5% of our last 150 patients have experienced pouchitis following ERP. When pouchitis occurs, stool frequency, urgency, soiling, and persistent diarrhea are common. Treatment with oral metronidazole (Flagyl), 250 mg/day, combined with twice daily tap water irrigation and once daily mesalamine (Rowasa) enemas provide prompt remission in most patients who do not have pouch stasis.

DISCUSSION

Somewhat comparable early results with respect to stool frequency and satisfactory continence have been reported with each of the four major ileal reservoirs. Nevertheless, after a year or longer, several patients experience repeated episodes of pouch inflammation with persistent diarrhea and incontinence. Recent reports have indicated sufficiently severe symptoms a few years after ERP to warrant pouch removal and construction of a permanent ileostomy. From 6% to 13% of patients from two of the largest accumulated clinical experiences with J and S pouches were returned to a permanent ileostomy.[8,9] Failure of the ileoanal pouch procedure has been even higher in hospitals where the operation is performed on an infrequent basis. Functional results appear less related to the configuration of the reservoir than to certain other factors, including size.

The ileum, unlike the colon, is unable to store fecal contents for prolonged periods without developing chronic mucosal inflammation. Ileal reservoir mucosa becomes inflamed when stasis and bacterial overgrowth occur, leading to diarrhea, fecal urgency, frequency, and occasional incontinence. Recurrent pouchitis several months following ERP is much more common in large reservoirs that empty only partially with each defecatory movement. Reservoir stasis, whether due to a large, poorly contractile pouch, outflow obstruction from a true stricture, chronic rectal muscular spasm, or functional obstruction from an elongated ileal spout, results in rapid bacterial growth, decreased water absorption, development of chronic diarrhea, and chronic mucosal inflammation, which may extend to the muscularis and affect contractility. An ileal spout of more than 1 to 2 cm length appears to produce functional outflow obstruction, since there are no contractile movements in this segment of intestine.

Optimal function of an ileoanal reservoir is associated with almost complete emptying with each defecatory movement and with minimal straining. Since the 24-hour fecal output in the absence of diarrhea rarely exceeds 800 ml, reservoirs with a capacity of more than 250 ml are unnecessary and may be counterproductive. Four to five movements of 200-ml volume each are more effective than more frequent movements of smaller volume. Stool frequency and continence with a short lateral or J-shaped reservoir (2 × 10 cm) in our experience has been comparable to, if not better than, that reported with larger J pouches (2 × 15 cm), S pouches (3 × 15 cm), and W pouches (4 × 12 cm). The distal ileum loses normal peristaltic contractions and myoelectric waves when chronically distended or obstructed or when reconstructed with long vertical suture lines as with a Kock pouch or ileoanal reservoir. Since the normal ileum proximal to the ileal pouch serves an important function in fluid, ion, and substrate absorption, including bile acids and vitamin B_{12} absorption, it is beneficial to use as small a segment of distal ileum for the reservoir as is necessary for satisfactory function.

In the absence of outflow obstruction, small reservoirs are likely to empty almost completely four to five times per 24 hours and thus minimize stasis. If there is no obstruction to outflow, prompt complete emptying usually occurs. If there is partial outflow obstruction, the contraction of the pouch may not overcome the resistance, and only partial emptying may result, leading to the need for more frequent movements. If the pouch is very large or distended, the stimulating peristaltic wave from the proximal small intestine may initiate a less effective mass contraction, which even in the absence of outflow obstruction may result in incomplete pouch emptying and stasis. We have observed a very close relationship between the efficiency of reservoir emptying with each defecation and the functional result with the patient. Patients with a low residual reservoir volume after defecation rarely experience pouch inflammation and rarely require medications.

Among patients with reconstructed reservoirs, and those with short uncomplicated lateral ileal and J reservoirs in our clinical experience, less than 5% have developed chronic pouch inflammation, which is considerably less than that reported by other authors using larger reservoirs. Gradual enlargement of the ileal reservoir during the first year is anticipated regardless of the configuration. Enlargement of sufficient magnitude to produce chronic pouchitis may not become evident for several months or even years after operation; however, when the symptoms of stasis persist despite therapy, operative shortening of the reservoir and ileal spout may relieve the pouchitis permanently, as with more than 50 patients in our clinical experience. Medications to reduce peristalsis may provide transient benefit but are likely to be counterproductive with respect to increasing the symptoms of reservoir stasis.

Reservoir reconstruction is a formidable undertaking and should be reserved for the patient who is experiencing increasingly severe symptoms due to pouch stasis that is not relieved by rectal dilations or irrigations, dietary restrictions, and intermittent metronidazole administration. The close relationship between long, angulated, efferent conduits and severe evacuation difficulties has been well demonstrated.[10] Pelvic scarring with compression of the lower reservoir and spout is almost invariably associated with chronic pouchitis and marked enlargement of distal mesenteric lymph nodes, which further compound the obstruction. Pelvic débridement combined with reservoir reconstruction has provided long-lasting marked clinical improvement for the vast majority of such patients.

Long-term follow-up is necessary to recognize some of the more insidious complications of ERP. Almost all complications following ERP are surgically correctable when recognized and treated early. ERP appears to be an excellent alternative to proctocolectomy with permanent ileostomy for the treatment of ulcerative colitis refractory to medical therapy.

COMPLICATIONS OF THE KOCK CONTINENT ILEOSTOMY

In 1969, Kock described a new type of continent ileostomy that obviated wearing a stoma appliance and provided a more free lifestyle after total proctocolectomy for ulcerative colitis or polyposis coli. For construction of the pouch and the nipple valve, 45 to 50 cm of distal ileum are used. The proximal 35 cm are constructed into a pouch, somewhat similar to that described for the J-shaped ileoanal pouch. A nipple valve is made by intussuscepting the outflow segment from the pouch and then securing it in position with sutures or staples (Fig. 78–2). The pouch is stapled or sutured to the peritoneum and fascia of the abdominal wall with or without prosthetic material, and the efferent limb is brought through the abdomen as a flush stoma. The pouch is emptied by having the patient pass a large soft Silastic catheter through the valve via the stoma several times daily. For most patients a small gauze dressing without a stoma bag is kept over the ileostomy.

Complications related primarily to nipple valve malfunction have necessitated reoperation in up to 50% of patients with a Kock pouch in many large series. If the pouch is not emp-

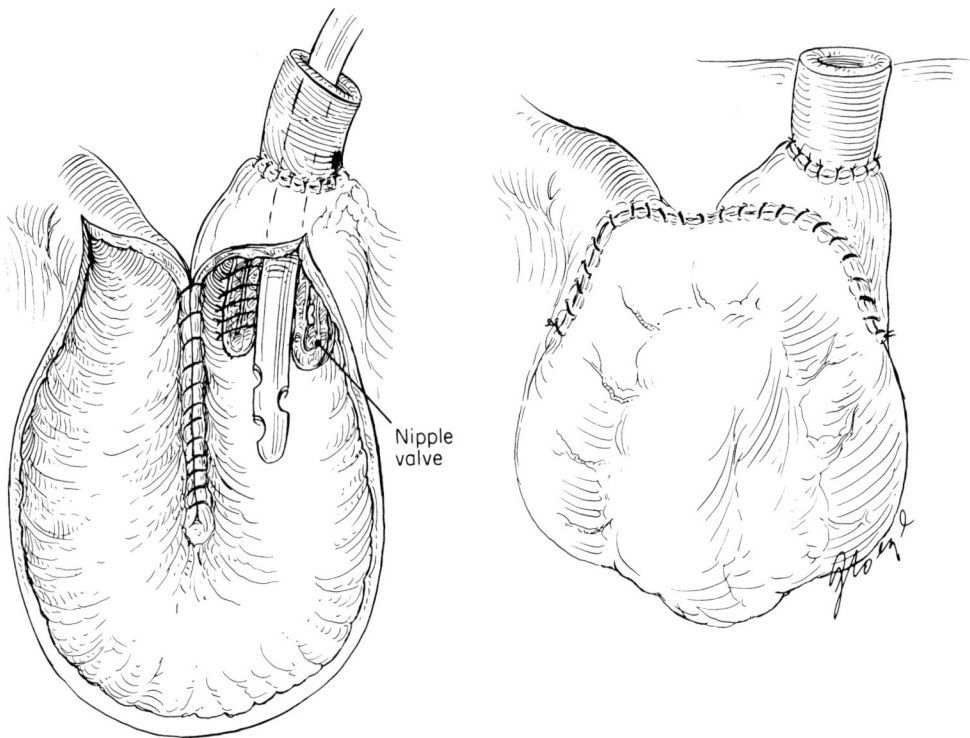

FIGURE 78–2. The continent ileostomy used most frequently consists of a distal ileal reservoir and nipple valve constructed by intussuscepting the efferent limb of ileum and suturing or stapling it in place. The distal efferent limb is brought through the abdominal wall as a flush stoma. The pouch is emptied by intermittently catheterizing through the stoma and nipple valve.

tied frequently or adequately, distension of the pouch occurs, placing tension on the nipple valve, which may cause it to slip or loosen and permit free drainage or incontinence.

Several syndromes of dysfunction related to the Kock pouch, variably called *stagnant loop syndrome, enteritis, nonspecific ileitis* and *pouchitis* have been reported on a frequent basis. Clinical features include diarrhea, malabsorption of fat and vitamin B_{12}, proliferation of anaerobic bacteria, inflammation of the pouch, abdominal cramps, malaise, fever, and incontinence. These symptoms are analogous to those of stasis with the ileoanal pouch procedure and may be temporarily relieved for most patients by emptying the pouch more frequently, irrigating with tap water or mesalamine (Rowasa) enemas, and giving oral metronidazole. Food particles that are not digested and that are too large to pass through the irrigating catheter may occasionally require removal through an endoscope. Thus, although the Kock continent ileostomy (or various modifications described by other authors) has many theoretical advantages over the permanent ileostomy, its high rate of mechanical, functional, and metabolic complications has limited its clinical usefulness. The number of continent ileostomy procedures, performed in major centers that offer all the current alternatives for treatment of ulcerative colitis has decreased markedly over the past 10 years. The continent ileostomy is currently most useful for patients with ulcerative colitis or colonic polyposis who have already undergone total proctocolectomy with ileostomy and who strongly desire a continence-restoring operation. As for the ileoanal pouch procedure, care must be taken to avoid performing the operation on patients with Crohn's disease.

REFERENCES

1. Soave F. A new surgical technique for treatment of Hirschsprung's disease. *Surgery.* 1964;56:1007–1012.
2. Dozois RR, Kelly KA, Welling DR, et al. Ileal pouch-anal anastomosis: comparison of results in familial adenomatous polyposis and chronic ulcerative colitis. *Ann Surg.* 1989;210:268–273.
3. Fonkalsrud EW, Loar N. Long-term results after colectomy and endorectal ileal pullthrough procedure in children. *Ann Surg.* 1992;215:57–62.

4. Morgan RA, Manning PB, Coran AG. Experience with the straight endorectal pullthrough for management of ulcerative colitis and familial polyposis in children and adults. *Ann Surg.* 1987;206:595–599.
5. Fonkalsrud EW, Stelzner M, McDonald N. Construction of an ileal reservoir in patients with a previous straight endorectal ileal pullthrough. *Ann Surg.* 1988;208:50–55.
6. McHugh SM, Diamont NE, McLeod R, Cohen Z. S-pouches vs. J-pouches: a comparison of functional outcomes. *Dis Colon Rectum.* 1987;30:671–677.
7. Fonkalsrud EW, Phillips JD. Reconstruction of malfunctioning ileoanal pouch procedures as an alternative to permanent ileostomy. *Am J Surg.* 1990;160:245–251.
8. Galandiuk S, Scott NA, Dozois RR, et al. Ileal pouch-anal anastomosis: reoperation for pouch-related complications. *Ann Surg.* 1990;212:446–454.
9. Wexner SD, Jensen L, Rothenberger DA, et al. Long-term functional analysis of the ileoanal reservoir. *Dis Colon Rectum.* 1989;32:275–281.
10. Liljeqvist L, Lindquist K, Ljungdahl I. Alterations in ileoanal pouch technique, 1980 to 1987: complications in functional outcome. *Dis Colon Rectum.* 1988;31:929–938.

79

Anal Fissure

THOMAS P. SOKOL

An anal fissure is a common anorectal condition, which comprises 6% to 15% of visits to a colon and rectal surgical practice. The presenting complaint of severe pain is in itself almost diagnostic.

An anal fissure is a cut or crack at the anal verge extending into the anal canal. It involves the skin known as the anoderm, which is rich with somatic nerves. The cut extends and may involve the dentate line.

The sex distribution is equal, and the age distribution runs the gamut from young to old. It is the most common cause of rectal bleeding in infancy. Many patients can recollect the inciting event by recalling the nature of the bowel movement that precipitated the acute pain. Although the condition might become episodic, it is the recurrence of symptoms that makes the patient consider "cancer" and thus seek medical consultation.

ETIOLOGY, PATHOGENESIS, AND PHYSIOLOGY

Most triggering events would relate the occurrence of the fissure to be at the time of a hard bowel action. Straining for a large or hard fecal bolus tears the anoderm. This tear occurs in the cutaneous portion of the anoderm between the level of the anal valves (dentate line) and the anal orifice. This tear is situated superior to the caudad border of the involuntary internal sphincter. In the acute phase one visualizes simply a linear, radial cut.

The most common site of an anal fissure in either sex is the posterior midline. Female patients form anterior midline fissures more commonly than male patients. Anterior fissures comprise 10% of fissures in female patients as opposed to 1% in male patients. The reason fissures tend to occur posteriorly may be multifactorial. When one considers the anatomy of the anal canal it is false to conceptualize a circular image. Shaftik's work involving the triple loop theory of muscular slings maps an ellipse axised in the anterior posterior planes.[1] In this model the most outer or subcutaneous external sphincter wraps about the anus from posterior to anterior. The next cephalad or superficial external sphincter wraps about the anus from anterior to posterior. The deep external sphincter, which may be confluent with fibers of the puborectalis muscle, is oriented posterior to anterior. This looping of the muscles lends a buttressing support of the anal canal laterally but potentiates areas of weakness both anteriorly and posteriorly. In the male, the transverse perineus muscle is well developed anteriorly. In the female, the attendant vaginal introitus fails to support the anus anteriorly. In addition, the male urogenital diaphragm and contents also lend support anteriorly; this likely explains the infrequence of anterior fissures in male patients.

Ischemia to the anoderm in the posterior midline may lend itself to traumatic insult. The vascular distribution of the inferior rectal artery was studied by postmortem arteriography.[2] The majority of specimens demonstrated that the posterior commissure of the anal canal is less well perfused than other regions. Additionally, the terminal branches coursing longitudinally within the sphincters may be more susceptible to occlusive insult during sphincter spasm. Recent blood flow studies indicate fissure healing after sphincterotomy in part may be due to an augmentation of mucosal blood flow.

Anal fissures are often reported following bouts of diarrheal episodes. It is postulated that continued anodermal irritation prevents adequate rejuvenation of the protective skin barriers and leads to breakdown.

If unhealed the superficial acute cut begins to deepen and eventually exposes the fibers of the internal sphincter. Thus, the internal sphincter often forms the floor of the fissure. As events progress, the edges of the fissure become more edematous and fibrotic. There forms a sentinel tag or pile at the outer edge of the fissure. It has been speculated this tag results from a low-grade infection that leads to lymphatic edema versus repetitive trauma to the area. With time the anal valve immediately above the fissure becomes edematous and fibrotic, resulting in an hypertrophied anal papilla. This is often referred to as the "internist" polyp but in actuality is not a true polyp. It has also been named Lane's polyp.

Thus, the classic findings of a chronic anal fissure are denoted by the triad of a sentinel tag, an anal fissure, and a hypertrophied anal papilla. This transition usually occurs over 6 weeks. I like to conceptualize an analogy for my patients as follows: Pretend you were to drag your heel through the sand at the beach. Then you abruptly raise your foot out of the sand. The trough or cut you have made is the fissure. The mound of sand you have displaced backwards is the sentinel tag, and the entry point mound is the hypertrophied anal papilla.

With increasing chronicity, cicatrization becomes more pronounced, leading to anal stenosis. This stenosis has been referred to as *pectenosis*. Microscopic examination of biopsy specimens of the internal sphincter at the fissure and remote from the fissure site reveals fibrosis.[3] The patient often resorts to long-term laxative or lubricant use, which promotes the stenosis.

Physiologic testing is not necessary in most cases of anal fissure. Manometric studies were done to compare a cohort of controls versus hemorrhoid versus fissure patients. Basal resting pressures were 71.2 mm Hg, 85.3 mm Hg, and 87.4 mm Hg, respectively. Squeeze pressures were relatively similar in the three groups, thus finding the internal sphincter responsible for differences in resting tone.[4]

Nothmann and Schuster[5] found the rectoanal inhibitory reflex (RAIR) to be present in fissure patients, but an abnormal overshoot contraction phenomenon was seen following relaxation induced by rectal distension. The cause of the overshoot is likely related to pain-induced contraction.

Cerdan and associates[6] documented a return of anal pressure to normal following healing induced by either anal dilation or internal sphincterotomy. This was sustained in the sphincterotomy group.

Anal manometry may be of significance when used in evaluation of patients who demonstrate fissure recurrence after sphincterotomy. It may be of use in the nonhealing fissure or ulcer patient who is immunocompromised. Caution should be employed in any human immunodeficiency virus (HIV) patient who suffers from diarrhea. Sphincterotomy should be avoided in this setting. In contrast, in patients who are immunocompromised, whose fissure has been excluded as a sexually transmitted disease (STD) and manometry (optional) confirms sphincter hypertension, then indeed a limited internal sphincterotomy may be curative.

SYMPTOMS AND PHYSICAL EXAMINATION

Symptoms of anorectal pain and bright red blood on defecation are classic for fissure. The pain often occurs during and after defecation and is described as a sharp, cutting, or tearing type. The pain can be so excruciating that fear of defecation is imposed and results in constipation or impaction.

The patient may complain of anal swelling and a discharge. This may be associated with pruritus ani. Spasm may translate to bladder symptoms of dysuria, retention, and increased urinary frequency.

Examination by visual inspection usually confirms the diagnosis. It is important to have good lighting and to reassure the patient vocally during the examination. Many patients are so apprehensive of the prospect of examination that buttock clench may make it impossible to see.

Patient rapport must be established quickly, and I have found this feasible by diagramming and discussing the probable diagnosis and mechanism of cause prior to the physical examination. Gentle separation of the buttocks and slow eversion of the perianum usually identifies the lesion.

It is important to inspect the fissure for features atypical of fissure in ano. One must always be suspicious for Crohn's disease, as 7% to 10% of patients with inflammatory bowel disease (IBD) present with anal pathology prior to proximal bowel manifestation. The base of an acute fissure has a filmy white covering due to the connective tissue of the submucosa and an absence of granulation tissue. A chronic fissure exposes the white underlying circular fibers of the internal sphincter. In contradistinction the Crohn's fissure is associated with ragged ulcer edges that are serrated, rolled, or everted. A pinkish, meaty, friable granulation base, which bleeds easily, is often seen.

One should be alert to the atypical fissure location found in other disease processes. Lateral fissures should raise concern over the following causes: trauma, IBD, syphilis, gonorrhea, tuberculosis, chancroid *(Haemophilus ducreyi)*, *Chlamydia,* cytomegalovirus (CMV), herpes simplex, neoplastic (squamous cell carcinoma, basal cell carcinoma, cloacogenic carcinoma, adenocarcinoma, and leukemia) and pruritus ani.

If an ulcer or fissure is not visible but symptoms are suggestive, a lubricated Q-Tip may be helpful. This 'Q-Tip' examination is accomplished by inserting a cotton tip applicator 1 to 2 cm inside the anal verge. It is initially directed away from the suspected locale of the fissure. With gentle pressure the sphincter may relax slightly in nonfissure-bearing zones. Finally, a flinch or wince when the suspected area is rubbed should pinpoint the fissure's location.

Gentle massage of a topical anesthetic may permit digital evaluation. If this is feasible, anoscopy can be performed. I prefer to use tetracaine 2% jelly (Dermocaine). Attention should be paid to proximal mucosa and where feasible proctoscopy should be done to exclude proctitis. Visualization of the classic triad of the sentinel tag, internal sphincter fibers in the fissure base, and hypertrophied anal papilla helps to prognosticate the condition for the patient. A chronic fissure may become infected and undermine as a submucosal or subcutaneous fistula. The internal sphincter usually serves as a buttressing base preventing transsphincteric extension of the fistula tract.

TREATMENT

The initial episode of an acute anal fissure will heal spontaneously in approximately 87% of cases. Conservative therapy including topical anesthetics and bran products healed chronic anal fissures in only 40% of cases.[7]

It is my practice to attempt conservative management initially in the vast majority of patients. A bulky yet soft stool is encouraged by the use of psyllium or bran products and stool softeners. The avoidance of "sharp foods" such as nuts, popcorn, chips, seeds, and hot spices makes common sense to the patient who is hoping to avoid a traumatic bowel movement. Topical anesthetic agents are often helpful if applied by gentle *external* massage preceding a bowel action. The patient is already often referred after insertion of suppositories have only served to induce more discomfort. Although some patients have reported benefit from suppositories, it is my practice to avoid them because insertion may be traumatic to the fissure. Additionally, the suppository melts in the rectum not in the anal canal where it is needed.

It has been my experience that most patients with anal fissures have enlarged internal hemorrhoids. This may be secondary to the increased intraluminal pressure or indeed a preexisting phenomenon. I have found gentle anoscopy often breaks the spasm, and injection sclerotherapy (5% phenol in oil) of the internal hemorrhoids is useful. As explained to the patient, intuitively, the reduction of the internal hemorrhoids allows for a relatively larger anal passage. The stool need not stretch the anus as far, resulting in less tearing of the fissure and thus triggering less internal sphincter spasm. In my practice this has become part of my conservative treatment of anal fissure disease and has contributed to a high success rate of nonoperative healing.

SURGICAL MANAGEMENT

Unlike the old dictum, "When all else fails, send them to the surgeon," surgical intervention for anal fissure is not only gratifying but curative. If medical management fails to relieve fissure pain or to promote healing, then surgery is curative in better than 90% of cases. The basis of surgery is to reduce internal anal sphincter pressure to normal and to promote healing by natural apposition of the fissure edges. This is achievable by internal sphincter manual stretch versus controlled surgical partial internal sphincterotomy.

Sphincter stretch was first employed by Récamier in 1838. Since then it has been championed by many, but the name most commonly associated today is the Lord procedure. This procedure is best performed while the patient is under general anesthesia and involves initial dilation, then slow forceful stretch of the sphincters, preferably in a lateral direction. Variations in technique are likely responsible for the wide variations in results and complications. Two fingers (index and long) are inserted from both hands and outward traction of four fingers is applied for 4 minutes. For the most part it is agreed that anal stretch, in this manner, is an uncontrolled fracturing of the internal sphincter. By juxtaposition, the voluntary external sphincters are innocent bystanders and affected. Recent work by Bartolo[8] using intrarectal ultrasound has documented perirectal trauma as hematoma and fracture of internal and external sphincters following manual stretch.

To avoid variation in the degree of sphincter stretch, Sohn and colleagues[9] have devised a hydrostatic balloon that delivers a reliable, consistent, and reproducible diameter of dilation, (40-mm balloon for 5 minutes).

Since it is difficult to quantify and qualify the finger manual stretch, a large variation in complication rates has been reported. In series performed by surgeons adept and proficient in the technique, results regarding fissure cure or recurrence are excellent. Complications are prejudiced by how carefully one defines incontinence and whether fecal soilage of undergarments is included.

In the United States, partial internal sphincterotomy has supplanted stretch and is standard in the surgical management of fissure disease. Eisenhammer in 1951 proposed midline internal sphincterotomy, within the fissure, but later changed to lateral sphincterotomy remote from the fissure.

Posterior midline sphincterotomy may potentiate a "keyhole" deformity like the skeleton key lock of old. A weakness emanates as a groove or slit posteriorly that can lead to anal soilage and a higher incidence of impaired flatus control. A lateral internal sphincterotomy is wrapped by the external sphincter, which can buttress any weakness of the anal canal. This is in contrast to the posterior midline, where external sphincter fibers may be decussating.

In 1969 Notaras described the closed, percutaneous, lateral internal sphincterotomy. The modification by Bonello in which a Smith Buie self-retaining retractor is employed to make the internal sphincter taut prior to cutting is my favored technique.[10] In this procedure a #11 blade is inserted submucosally at the level of the intersphincteric groove (junction between internal and external sphincter). The blade is inserted parallel to the sphincter, then turned perpendicular, and incised outward or laterally away from the anal canal. By having the sphincter taut, a simple pop is felt as the caudad third of the internal sphincter is divided. The external sphincter is avoided. The blade is returned to its parallel position and withdrawn. The small wound (a few millimeters) obviates the morbidity of the open technique. Walker et al[11] reviewed their series of various techniques (open, closed, multiple) of lateral internal sphincterotomy and concluded complications were lowest in the closed group.

Successful healing with lateral partial internal sphincterotomy ranges from 93% to 97%. Infection is seen in 1% and may be associated with a fistula usually due to unrecognized proximal mucosal penetration by the scalpel. Nonhealing, unless due to unrecognized IBD, is usually due to temerity with the extent of sphincterotomy. During the first 6 weeks, the incidence of fecal soilage or poor flatus control is high. Permanent soilage or difficulty with gas continence is low and less than 15%. Solid stool incontinence should not occur.

Fissurectomy remains controversial. Those in favor of the procedure tout the benefit in excising scarred edges of the chronic ulcer to promote healing. This also ensures proper biopsy to rule out neoplasm. No good evidence has supported the proposed benefit. Most surgeons, however, excise a large sentinel tag and papilla to obviate the mechanical barriers to healing.

Combining hemorrhoid surgery with fissure surgery is accepted in the setting of large hemorrhoids. The sphincterotomy site is incorporated within one of the hemorrhoid wounds.

Anal stenosis associated with fissure is often sufficiently relieved by the internal sphincter division. When sphincterotomy alone is insufficient, an anoplasty is employed to advance anoderm into the anal canal, thereby enlarging the anal aperture.

HIV

Today, the physician is frequently confronted with the HIV-positive patient with anorectal complaints. It is important to distinguish "benign" anal fissure from AIDS-specific "idiopathic" anal ulcer.[12] Viamonte developed characteristics to identify these patients. Benign anal fissures tend to occur low in the anal canal, the sphincter is normal to hypertonic, the fissure is noninvasive, a sentinel tag is present, and mucosal bridging is absent. In contradistinction the idiopathic (non-STD) anal ulcer occurs high, the sphincter is lax, invasion is present, a sentinel tag is absent, mucosal bridging is frequent, and the ulcer has a broad base. In the latter group Centers for Disease Control AIDS criteria occur in 100% and are present in only 50% of the benign anal fissure group.

In the anal ulcer group débridement, culture, and biopsy may be beneficial in promoting healing. In nonresponders the use of intralesional methylprednisolone (Depo-Medrol) (80 mg) has been preliminarily promising.

CONCLUSION

Anal fissure is one of the most common disorders of the anorectum. Conservative measures including bulking of the stool and topical anesthetics usually provide eventual spontaneous healing. Lateral fissures should raise a warning flag for vigilance to rule out other etiologic agents involving infectious, traumatic, neoplastic, and inflammatory causes.

Partial, lateral, internal sphincterotomy is usually curative of the chronic fissure. It can be accomplished with the patient under sedation and local anesthesia in the outpatient setting. Complication rates are low, and pain relief is rapid.

REFERENCES

1. Shaftik A. A new concept of the anatomy of the anal sphincter mechanism and the physiology of defecation—the external anal sphincter: a triple loop system. *Invest Urol.* 1975;12:412.
2. Klosterhalfen B, Vogel P, Rixen H, Mittermayer C. Topography of the inferior rectal artery: a possible cause of chronic, primary anal fissure. *Dis Colon Rectum.* 1989;32:43–52.
3. Brown AC, Sumfest J, Rozwadowski J. Histopathology of the internal anal sphincter in chronic anal fissure. *Dis Colon Rectum.* 1989;32:680–683.
4. Lin J-K. Anal manometric studies in hemorrhoids and anal fissures. *Dis Colon Rectum.* 1989;32:839–842.
5. Nothmann B, Schuster M. Internal anal sphincter derangement with anal fissure. *Gastroenterology.* 1974;67:216–230.
6. Cerdan FJ, Ruiz de Leon A, Azpiroz F, Martin J, Balibrea J. Anal sphincter pressure in fissure-in-ano before and after lateral internal sphincterotomy. *Dis Colon Rectum.* 1982;25:198–201.
7. Jensen S. Treatment of first episode of acute anal fissure: prospective randomized study of Lignocaine ointment verses hydrocortisone ointment or warm sitz baths plus bran. *Br Med J.* 1986;292:1167–1169.
8. Bartolo D. Personal Communication at Sansum/USC Colon Rectal Surgery Seminar, Pasadena, Calif. 1994.
9. Sohn N, Eisenberg M, Weinstein M, Lugo R, Ader J. Precise anorectal sphincter dilatation: its role in the therapy of anal fissures. *Dis Colon Rectum.* 1992;35:322–327.
10. Nadler L, Bonello J, Tangen L. A modified technique of subcutaneous lateral internal sphincterotomy in the treatment of chronic fissure-in-ano. *Contemp Surg.* 1991;39(5):26–29.
11. Walker W, Rothenberger D, Goldberg S. Morbidity of internal sphincterotomy for anal fissure and stenosis. *Dis Colon Rectum.* 1985;28:832–835.
12. Viamonte M, Dailey T, Gottesman L. Ulcerative disease of the anorectum in the HIV+ patient. *Dis Colon Rectum.* 1993;36:801–805.

80
Anorectal Abscess
PHILLIP R. FLESHNER and JONATHAN R. HIATT

Despite being one of the more common diseases affecting the anorectum and a source of considerable morbidity, anorectal abscess has received little attention in modern gastroenterologic literature. This chapter reviews the anatomic basis for this disease and presents current concepts of its clinical diagnosis and management.

PRACTICAL ANATOMY

Many clinicians are generally unaware of the complex spatial relationships of the anus and rectum. Nonetheless, understanding the anatomy of this region is critical to appreciating the origin and ramifications of anorectal abscess (Fig. 80–1).

The anal sphincter consists of two funnel-shaped muscle groups, one situated inside the other. The inner layer, also known as the internal sphincter, is really only an enlarged portion of the circular smooth muscle of the rectum. The outer layer (external sphincter) contains skeletal muscle fibers, and although composed of three separate parts, acts functionally as a single muscle group. The area between these two sleeves of muscle is called the intersphincteric space. Just above the external sphincter lies the puborectalis muscle, which wraps around the posterior aspect of the rectum. The levator muscles are immediately above the puborectalis muscle.

As the rectum merges with the upper anus, the mucosal lining is thrown into 6 to 12 vertical folds called the anal columns. Between the anal columns at the level of the dentate line is a space called the anal crypt. Arising from the bottom of the anal crypt are orifices of the ducts of anal glands. These ducts pass outward through the submucosa and internal sphincter to drain the glands that lie within the intersphincteric space. Thus, anal glands may be considered diverticula of the anal canal.

PATHOGENESIS

Anorectal abscesses were once thought to arise from infection penetrating the anal wall through a fissure or other anal wound. However, modern studies[1,2] have demonstrated that anorectal sepsis begins with infection of anal glands and the subsequent development of an intersphincteric abscess.

As with other diverticula of the gastrointestinal tract, the contents of anal glands are subject to stasis and secondary infection. Once an inflammatory process is initiated, the glands become obstructed by edema, and bacteria multiply rapidly. As this process extends to adjacent tissue, an early intersphincteric abscess develops. This abscess may spread in any direction; downward extension leads to a perianal abscess, outward spread results in an ischiorectal abscess, and upward spread causes a supralevator abscess. Maturation of the glandular abscess with proximal spread within the intersphincteric space results in a full-blown intersphincteric abscess (Fig. 80–2).

A collective review of the large reported series of anorectal abscess is shown in Table 80–1. Well over 90% of these infections involve one of the spaces below the levator muscles. Forward pull of the puborectalis muscle on the posterior anorectum, by acting as a barrier to upward extension of the intersphincteric abscess, may account for this observation. The far greater incidence of abscess in male patients is difficult to explain on an anatomic basis alone, since there is no difference in anal gland distribution between the sexes.[11] The reasons for this sex difference remain undefined.

CLINICAL FEATURES

The most common patient complaints relate to perianal pain and swelling (Table 80–2). The

ANORECTAL ABSCESS

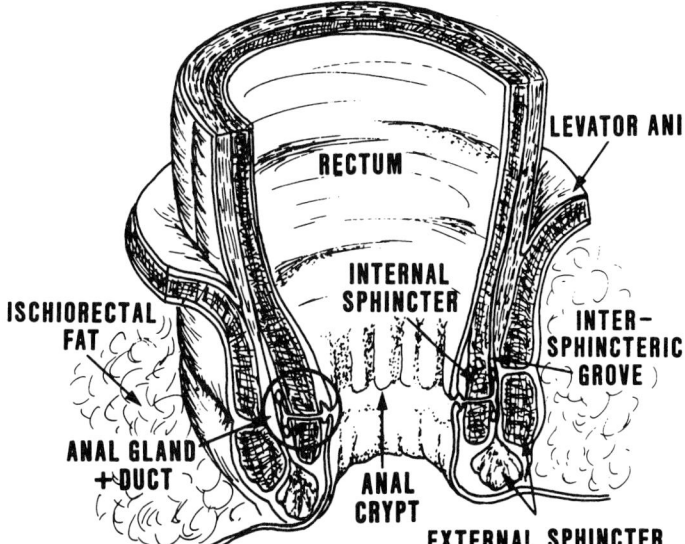

FIGURE 80–1. Anatomy of the distal rectum, anus, and anal sphincter

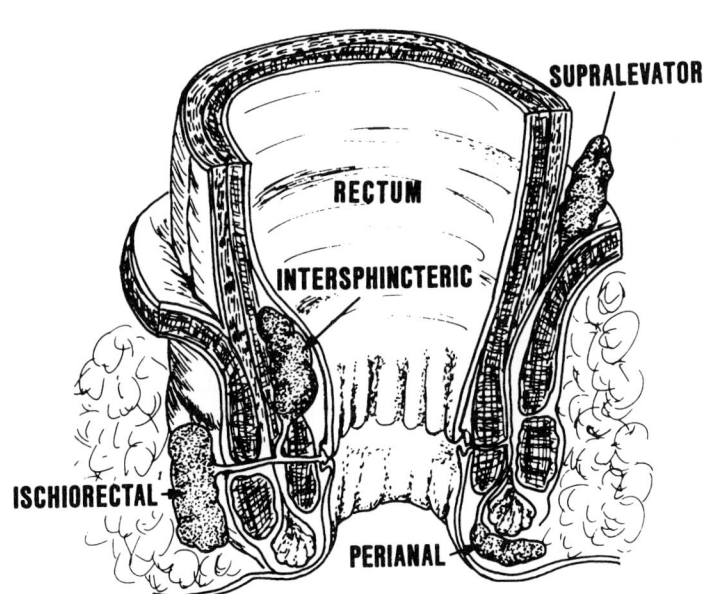

FIGURE 80–2. The four types of anorectal abscess depicting their common development from infected anal glands residing within the intersphincteric groove.

TABLE 80–1. SEX AND ANATOMIC DISTRIBUTION OF ANORECTAL ABSCESS

			ABSCESS LOCATION (%)			
AUTHOR	NUMBER	MALE (%)	PA	IR	IS	SL
Buchan and Grace[3]	183	78	56	42	1	0
Bevans and colleagues[4]	184	84	71	22	1	2
McElwain and colleagues[5]	1000	74	46	39	15	0
Kovalcik and colleagues[6]	174	72	65	29	7	0
Grace and colleagues[7]	165	75	76	22	2	0
Vasilevsky and Gordon[8]	117	77	19	61	18	2
Ramanujam and colleagues[9]	1023	66	43	23	28	7
Winslett and colleagues[10]	233	72	64	35	2	0

PA = perianal abscess, IR = ischiorectal abscess, IS = intersphincteric abscess, SL = supralevator abscess.

TABLE 80-2. SYMPTOMS OF ANORECTAL ABSCESS

AUTHOR	NUMBER	SYMPTOM (%)			
		PAIN	SWELLING	FEVER	DRAINAGE
Bevans and colleagues[4]	184	100	96	19	13
Kovalcik and colleagues[6]	174	NR	NR	28	6
Vasilevsky and Gordon[8]	117	93	50	6	6
Ramanujam and colleagues[9]	1023	90	NR	42	4

NR = not recorded.

pain of early infection in the intersphincteric space may be described as only a dull ache or throbbing deep within the perineum. However, with extension into the ischiorectal or perianal spaces, the pain becomes intense and is aggravated by sitting, coughing, sneezing, and straining. Associated anal sphincter spasm contributes to the discomfort.

Swelling is common in perianal and ischiorectal abscesses, and it is virtually never described in intersphincteric or supralevator abscesses. In the early abscess, fever may be slight; systemic signs and symptoms of sepsis develop as the abscess grows larger. Drainage, when present, may emanate from the perianal skin or the anus itself. Perianal drainage is due to spontaneous dermal erosion of the abscess, whereas anal drainage reflects small amounts of pus collecting within the anal canal.

Classic physical signs of inflammation, including erythema, swelling, induration, and tenderness, are usually present. A superficial tender mass just outside the anal outlet without tenderness above the dentate line is virtually diagnostic of a perianal abscess. When the mass lies further outward on the buttock, an ischiorectal abscess should be considered. However, in adults, the dermal reaction of a perianal abscess may extend laterally and could be easily confused with an ischiorectal abscess. Intersphincteric abscesses usually are noted as tender submucosal masses in the lower part of the rectum. Fluctuance and tenderness higher in the rectum or palpable through the vagina should alert the clinician to the possibility of a supralevator abscess.

The diagnosis of one variant of ischiorectal abscess, the deep postanal space abscess, deserves special attention.[12] These patients have severe perianal pain that may radiate to the sacrum, coccyx, or buttock, yet primary inflammatory skin changes are absent. Rectal examination reveals exquisite posterior rectal tenderness.

A high degree of suspicion is required for diagnosis and treatment, and early colorectal surgical consultation is mandatory.

ANCILLARY STUDIES

The diagnosis of anorectal abscess depends primarily on an adequate history and physical examination. Since leukocytosis is not a constant feature, a complete blood count (CBC) is generally unwarranted. Sigmoidoscopy can identify proctocolitis, and anoscopy may identify the primary rectal opening. However, in most patients these studies are unrewarding and painful. They should be reserved for the patient under anesthesia or, alternatively, after the abscess has resolved. Some investigators have advocated use of endorectal ultrasound (ERUS) as a helpful diagnostic adjunct.[13] Although 10 of 12 intersphincteric abscesses were correctly identified in the study by Law and colleagues,[13] none of the four supralevator or ischiorectal abscesses were seen. These results are not surprising, since ERUS provides superb anatomic detail of the anorectal wall. Although worthy of further study, the natural tendency of ERUS to aggravate pain in the inflamed anorectum combined with its poor definition of the supralevator and ischiorectal spaces will probably limit the clinical utility of this procedure.

MANAGEMENT

Once an anorectal abscess is suspected, immediate consultation with a colorectal surgeon is mandatory. Hot baths and antibiotics alone are uniformly unsuccessful and only prolong patient discomfort.[6,14-16] Delayed surgical drainage may also allow the suppurative process to extend to adjacent tissues. Such extension may lead to destruction of the anorectum and severe septic morbidity and mortality.[4]

OPERATIVE STRATEGY

Perianal Abscess

Most perianal abscesses (Fig. 80–3A) are small and can be drained with the generous use of local anesthesia in the office. Inadequate anesthesia only leads to incomplete drainage and increased morbidity. Bupivacaine with epinephrine is preferred, since it is long lasting and minimizes bleeding. The tissues around the abscess are infiltrated, a generous ellipse of skin over the abscess cavity is excised, and the pus is drained. After curettage, the cavity is loosely packed with iodoform wick gauze. In 24 hours the gauze is removed in a sitz bath. Three weeks later, sigmoidoscopy and anoscopy are performed to exclude any associated colorectal disease and to identify if the internal opening of an anal fistula is present.

Ischiorectal Abscess

These abscesses (Fig. 80–3B) are generally more extensive than the perianal type and consequently should be drained in the operating room

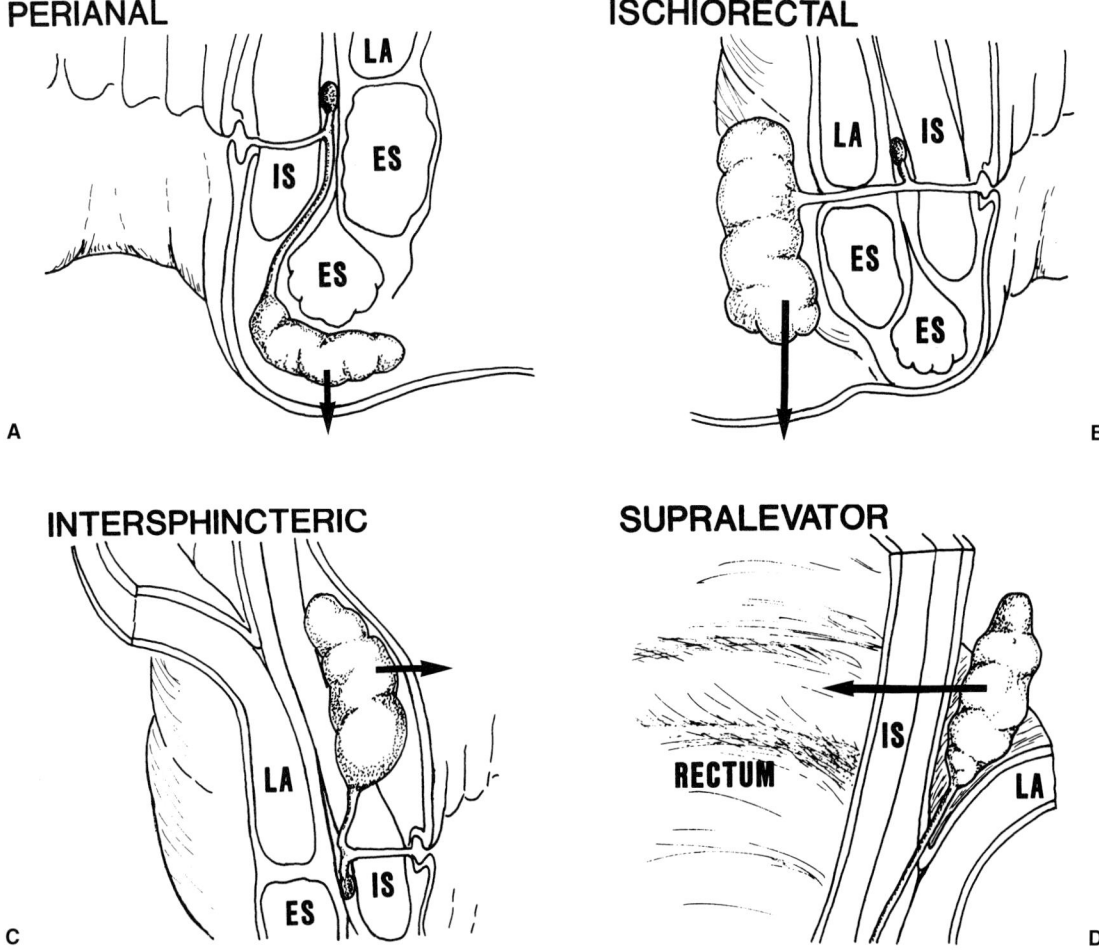

FIGURE 80–3. A, Relationship of a perianal abscess and the internal sphincter *(IS)*, external sphincter *(ES)*, and levator ani *(LA)*. The preferred route of drainage is through the perianal skin *(arrow)*. **B,** The ischiorectal abscess lies lateral to the internal sphincter *(IS)*, external sphincter *(ES)*, and levator ani *(LA)* muscles. This abscess should be drained via the perianal skin *(arrow)*. **C,** Intersphincteric abscesses lie medial to the external sphincter *(ES)* and levator ani *(LA)* muscles. These abscesses must be drained into the rectum *(arrow)*, thus sacrificing part of the internal sphincter *(IS)*. **D,** Supralevator abscesses are above the sphincter complex and should be drained internally by dividing a portion of the internal sphincter *(IS)*.

with the aid of adequate anesthesia. Sigmoidoscopy and anoscopy should be done with the patient asleep. Principles of operative management are similar to those for perianal abscess, except that (1) the incision should be placed as medially as possible; (2) all loculations of pus within the ischiorectal space must be broken; and (3) the abscess cavity should be drained with a soft plastic catheter rather than packing. This assures excellent drainage and obviates painful removal of packs.

Intersphincteric Abscess

To gain surgical exposure, intersphincteric abscesses (Fig. 80–3C) must be drained under regional or general anesthesia. The abscess is readily seen during sigmoidoscopy and anoscopy. The abscess must be unroofed and the internal sphincter removed with the offending anal crypt and gland.

Supralevator Abscess

With the patient under general anesthesia, sigmoidoscopy and anoscopy are performed to site a supralevator abscess (Fig. 80–3D). Transrectal drainage is preferred. The internal sphincter should be divided and the cut edges oversewn to control bleeding.

Additional Management Concerns

Additional management issues concern the role of antibiotics and the value of abscess cultures. Antibiotics during or after surgery should be only used in selected cases. Patients with diabetes, valvular heart disease, prosthetic heart valves, a history of endocarditis, or a compromised immune system should be treated with antibiotics whose spectrum covers both *Enterococcus* and gram-negative aerobes (e.g., ampicillin and gentamicin). Abscess cultures are done almost routinely, yet the results contribute little more than additional cost. Like antibiotics, abscess cultures should be used selectively. The culture does predict the likelihood of the development of an anal fistula. If the culture demonstrates skin bacteria, the chance of a subsequent fistula is negligible. If enteric bacteria are found, the incidence rises to over 50%.[7] Another clinical situation in which to consider abscess culture is the septic patient. An immediate Gram stain aids in identifying the offending organism and guides specific antibiotic treatment. Finally, if there is slow healing of the abscess cavity, cultures and biopsy of the abscess wall should be obtained, examining for conditions such as Crohn's disease, tuberculosis, actinomycosis, or leukemia.[17]

Few topics in colorectal surgery generate as much controversy as optimal management of the internal fistulous opening noted at the time of abscess drainage. Many investigators believe that the tract from the abscess to the internal opening should be laid open. They argue that this fistulotomy eradicates the origin of the fistula and lowers the incidence of postoperative anal fistula and recurrent abscess.[2,5,6,9,14] However, others contend that many such patients will not develop a fistula, and there is a considerable risk of seriously damaging the sphincter muscle in the presence of acute inflammation.[8,15,18] Until these issues are resolved with a controlled trial, no firm guidelines will exist. We believe that primary fistulotomy should be undertaken if the internal site is easily identified, except in patients with a first episode of anorectal suppuration or where the tract turns high to involve a significant portion of the sphincter mechanism.

ANORECTAL ABSCESS AND CROHN'S DISEASE

Perianal complications of Crohn's disease are frequent and carry considerable morbidity. Anorectal abscess, an important manifestation of this pathologic condition, is seen in 5% to 7% of patients.[19,20] Like the patient with inflammatory bowel disease, localized pain, drainage, and fever are prominent symptoms. However, management of the abscess is not routine. Since poor perineal wound healing is common in the patient with Crohn's disease, incisions should be avoided.[21] Second, any damage to the sphincter mechanism, as with fistulotomy, is ill advised in these patients who often have chronic diarrhea and require maximal sphincter function. Therefore, an anorectal abscess in association with Crohn's disease should be simply unroofed and drained through as small an incision as possible. In patients with a very early abscess, antibiotics and hot baths alone may be beneficial. The efficacy of this therapy is difficult to glean from the literature, although we have used it on occasion with satisfactory results. The use of metronidazole might also be considered, since it is somewhat effective.[22] If nonoperative treatment is chosen for the early abscess, the clinician must observe the patient closely and assure timely surgical intervention if needed.

ANORECTAL ABSCESS AND HIV DISEASE

Anorectal disease complicates the course of at least one third of patients who carry the human immunodeficiency virus (HIV).[23] This high incidence, combined with the exponential increase of HIV infection noted in the general population,[24] suggests that clinicians will face this difficult problem with increasing frequency. Early studies described poor healing of anorectal wounds, a high incidence of postoperative fecal incontinence, and perioperative mortality much greater than that seen in the HIV-negative patient population (Table 80–3). Although the data of one study was more encouraging, poor anal wound healing was still observed.[27] Levels of circulating T4 cells are generally predictive of operative morbidity. In one study, operative morbidity was 65% in patients with a T4 count below 200 versus 7% in the group of patients with T4 counts above 200.[28] These considerations mandate extreme conservatism in managing the HIV-positive patient with anorectal abscess. Hot baths and antibiotics are the mainstays of treatment, particularly in the patient with a markedly depressed T4 lymphocyte count. Surgery is reserved for ongoing sepsis and should be as limited as possible.

ANORECTAL ABSCESS AND LEUKEMIA

Anorectal infections are common in acute leukemia. In one series, perianal infections occurred in 60% of patients with acute monocytic leukemia and in 31% of those with acute myelomonocytic leukemia.[30] Since pus is not found in these neutropenic patients, fluctuance is often absent, and not unexpectedly the infection often goes undetected. Pain alone may be the predominant symptom. The delay in diagnosis in these immunocompromised patients may account for the overall mortality, which exceeds 20%.[31]

Because of concerns over the spread of infection into surrounding tissues in these immunocompromised hosts and the potential for bleeding and poor wound healing, many surgeons have avoided operative drainage. Two recent studies have confirmed that surgery has a higher mortality and morbidity than broad spectrum antibiotics and hot baths alone.[31,32] Thus, initial management of patients with leukemia and anorectal infections should be nonoperative, with surgery reserved for those patients who become overtly septic during treatment or those patients who develop a fluctuant abscess, which can be drained with certainty through a small incision. The recent availability of granulocyte-stimulating factors may impact on these management principles.

SUMMARY

In comparison with the complex anatomy that accounts for the pathogenesis and diagnosis of these infections, treatment of the patient with an anorectal abscess is rather straightforward. Consultation with a colorectal surgeon and prompt drainage is the best therapy for most patients. In special situations, such as Crohn's disease, leukemia, or HIV disease, antibiotics may be tried initially, with surgical drainage reserved for failures of this medical regimen.

TABLE 80–3. ANORECTAL SURGERY IN HIV DISEASE

		Complications (%)			Predictive Value
Author	Number	Wound	Incontinence	Death	of T-Cell Count
Wexner and colleagues[23]	51	88	>50	18	(+)
Carr and colleagues[25]	13	31	NR	NR	NR
Wolkomir and colleagues[26]	20	67	NR	5	(+)
Safavi and colleagues[27]	62	53	0	0	(−)
Moenning and colleagues[28]	39	NR	NR	NR	(+)
Orkin and Smith[29]	40	NR	NR	NR	NR

NR = not recorded.

REFERENCES

1. Parks AG. Pathogenesis and treatment of fistula-in-ano. *Br Med J.* 1961;1:463–469.
2. Eisenhammer S. The final evaluation and classification of the surgical treatment of the primary anorectal cryptoglandular intermuscular (intersphincteric) fistulous abscess and fistula. *Dis Colon Rectum.* 1978;21:237–254.
3. Buchan R, Grace RH. Anorectal suppuration: the results of treatment and the factors influencing the recurrence rate. *Br J Surg.* 1973;60:537–540.
4. Bevans DW Jr, Westbrook KC, Thompson BW, Caldwell FT. Perirectal abscess: a potentially fatal illness. *Am J Surg.* 1973;126:765–768.
5. McElwain JW, MacLean MD, Alexander RM, Hoexter B, Guthrie JF. Anorectal problems: experience with primary fistulotomy for anorectal abscess. *Dis Colon Rectum.* 1975;18:646–649.
6. Kovalcik PJ, Peniston RL, Cross GH. Anorectal abscess. *Surg Gynecol Obstet.* 1979;149:884–886.
7. Grace RH, Harper IA, Thompson RG. Anorectal sepsis: microbiology in relation to fistula-in-ano. *Br J Surg.* 1982;69:401–403.
8. Vasilevsky CA, Gordon PH. The incidence of recurrent abscesses or fistula-in-ano following anorectal suppuration. *Dis Colon Rectum.* 1984;27:126–130.
9. Ramanujam PS, Prasad ML, Abcarian H, Tan AB. Perianal abscesses and fistulas. *Dis Colon Rectum.* 1984;27:593–597.
10. Winslett MC, Allan A, Ambrose NS. Anorectal sepsis as a presentation of occult rectal and systemic disease. *Dis Colon Rectum.* 1988;31:597–600.
11. Hill MR, Shryock EH, ReBell FG. Role of the anal glands in the pathogenesis of anorectal disease. *JAMA.* 1943;121:742–751.
12. Hanley PH. Anorectal abscess fistula. *Surg Clin North Am.* 1978;58:487–503.
13. Law PJ, Talbot RW, Bartram CI, Northover JMA. Anal endosonography in the evaluation of perianal sepsis and fistula in ano. *Br J Surg.* 1989;76:752–755.
14. Lindell TD, Fletcher WS, Krippaehne WW. Anorectal suppurative disease. *Am J Surg.* 1973;125:189–194.
15. Scoma JA, Salvati EP, Rubin RJ. Incidence of fistulas subsequent to anal abscesses. *Dis Colon Rectum.* 1974;17:357–359.
16. Abcarian H. Acute suppurations of the anorectum. *Surg Annu.* 1976;8:305–333.
17. Goldberg SM, Gordon PH, Nivatvongs S. *Essentials of Anorectal Surgery.* Philadelphia, Pa: JB Lippincott Co; 1980:101.
18. Parks AG, Gordon PH, Hardcastle JD. A classification of fistula-in-ano. *Br J Surg.* 1976;63:1–12.
19. Fry RD, Shemesh EI, Kodner IJ, Timmcke A. Techniques and results in the management of anal and perianal Crohn's disease. *Surg Gynecol Obstet.* 1989;168:42–48.
20. Pritchard TJ, Schoetz DJ Jr, Roberts PL, Murray JJ, Coller JA, Veidenheimer MC. Perirectal abscess in Crohn's disease. *Dis Colon Rectum.* 1990;33:933–937.
21. Baker WNW, Milton-Thompson GJ. Management of anal fistulae in Crohn's disease. *Proc R Soc Med.* 1974;67:58–63.
22. Bernstein LH, Frank MS, Brandt LJ, Boley SJ. Healing of perineal Crohn's disease with metronidazole. *Gastroenterology.* 1980;79:357–365.
23. Wexner SD, Smithy WB, Milsom JW, Dailey TH. The surgical management of anorectal diseases in AIDS and pre-AIDS patients. *Dis Colon Rectum.* 1986;29:719–723.
24. CDC Update. Acquired immunodeficiency syndrome—United States. *MMWR.* 1989;39:81–86.
25. Carr ND, Mercey D, Slack WW. Non-condylomatous perianal disease in homosexual men. *Br J Surg.* 1989;76:1064–1066.
26. Wolkomir AF, Barone JE, Hardy HW III, Cottone FJ. Abdominal and anorectal surgery and the acquired immune deficiency syndrome in heterosexual intravenous drug users. *Dis Colon Rectum.* 1990;33:267–270.
27. Safavi A, Gottesman L, Dailey TH. Anorectal surgery in the HIV+ patient: update. *Dis Colon Rectum.* 1991;34:299–304.
28. Moenning S, Huber P, Simonton C, Odom C, Kaplan E, Nightengale S. Prediction of morbidity by T4 lymphocyte count in the HIV positive or AIDS anorectal outpatient. *Dis Colon Rectum.* 1991;34:P17. Abstract.
29. Orkin BA, Smith LE. Perineal manifestations of HIV infection. *Dis Colon Rectum.* 1992;35:310–314.
30. Schimpff SC, Wiernick PH, Block JB. Rectal abscesses in cancer patients. *Lancet.* 1972;2:844–847.
31. Carlson GW, Ferguson CM, Amerson JR. Perianal infections in acute leukemia. *Am Surg.* 1988;54:693–695.
32. Shaked AA, Shinar E, Freund H. Managing the granulocytopenic patient with acute perianal inflammatory disease. *Am J Surg.* 1986;152:510–512.

81
Pruritus Ani
EDWARD PIKEN

Pruritus ani is a common and troublesome symptom characterized by an unpleasant cutaneous sensation that induces the patient to scratch the skin around the anal orifice.

Pruritus ani is said to occur in 1% to 5% of the population. There is a male-to-female predominance of 4:1. The disorder can occur at any age but most often occurs in the fifth and sixth decades of life.[1] Pruritus ani has multiple origins. It may be idiopathic, caused by a local problem, or a dramatic presentation of a multisystemic or infectious disease. A careful history and physical examination is therefore mandatory.

CLINICAL FEATURES

The patient complains of itching around the anus sometimes associated with pain or other areas of pruritus. The symptoms may worsen with anxiety or stress or may be exacerbated by bowel movements or wiping. The symptoms may be acute or chronic and may be associated with local or systemic problems, depending on the cause of the disorder.

ETIOLOGIES

BOWEL DYSFUNCTION AND LOCAL DISEASE

A careful history should begin with an inquiry into bowel function and consistency. A history of either constipation or diarrhea can lead to hemorrhoidal irritation or prolapse and possible subsequent pain and itching. Bright red blood coating the outside of the stool or found on toilet paper after defecation is commonly associated with anal fissures, hemorrhoids, or polyps. Patients should be questioned regarding possible incontinence and asked to describe their usual wiping regimen after bowel movements. The history of a fullness or a rectal lesion bobbing in and out of the anus should be a clue for enlarged hemorrhoids, anal papillae, or rectal polyps. A history of previous rectal surgery causing disruption of the normal sphincter mechanism should be investigated.

Physical examination should include a search for the above-mentioned polyps, enlarged hemorrhoids, or papillae. The anus should be examined for normal afferent sensation. The sphincter should be examined for tightness and response to rectal squeezing. Abnormal sensory input, a loose sphincter, and weak sphincteric responses may all lead to fecal soiling, incontinence, and subsequent pruritus. Formal anal manometry studies were performed by Eyers and Thompson.[2] They found abnormal anal sphincter pressures in response to rectal distension. Allan and colleagues[3] documented increased rectal liquid leakage from the anal canal in pruritus patients as compared with age- and sex-matched controls.

The findings of anal hirsutism and folds are often a clue to a difficulty in cleansing on wiping. Local perianal malignancies and Bowen's and Paget's diseases may first present as pruritic problems.

INFECTIONS

Perirectal infections leading to pruritus can be a sign of localized infection or a sign of serious systemic illness; diabetes, immunocompromising illnesses such as human immunodeficiency virus (HIV) infection, myeloproliferative disorders, and recent use of antibiotics or chemotherapy predispose to subsequent rectal or perirectal infections. Infectious agents to be considered include bacteria, fungi, parasites, viruses, and spirochetes. High-risk sexual activity and receptive anal intercourse predispose to the development of sexually transmitted diseases.

Bacterial infections involving the perianal

skin are commonly found in patients with pruritus ani. These infections may be the primary cause of the disorder or secondary infections in areas of rawness, moisture, or excoriations. Bacterial infections can be diagnosed by appropriate cultures and smears. Fever, intense erythema, and tenderness often accompany such infections. The infections respond promptly to systemic antibiotics unless complicated by multisystemic illness.

Baral[4] cultured *Staphylococcus aureus* in six of seven patients with pruritus ani, whereas in 15 of their 81 patients Bowyer and McCall[5] diagnosed erythrasma caused by *Corynebacterium minutissimum,* which was confirmed by culture and Wood's light examination. Their patients responded to a 10-day course of erythromycin. In other cases a mixed bacterial infection was responsible for the pruritus. Silverman and colleagues,[6] investigating a fecal bacterial cause of pruritus ani, found no qualitative or quantitative differences in the fecal microflora of controls versus patients with pruritus ani.

Gonococcal infections most commonly seen in homosexual men can produce intense erythema, swelling, and maceration of the skin. Syphilitic chancres, while nonpruritic, are often surrounded by macerated local skin folds. Treatment of both of these sexually transmitted diseases leads to improvement, but the patient should receive counseling to avoid recurrence.

Fungal infections are perhaps the most common cause of infectious pruritus ani. Diabetes, recent antibiotic usage, immunocompromised defenses, and poor local hygiene predispose to fungal infections. Dodi and colleagues[7] studied the mycotic floras in controls and patients with pruritus ani. As expected, they found *Candida albicans* to be the most common pathogen associated with pruritus ani, although its presence was associated with pruritus in only 27.4% of their patients. Dermatophytic infections with *Trichophyton mentagrophytes* and *Trichophyton rubrum* were found in fewer patients, but their presence was always associated with pruritic symptoms.[7] Candidiasis and other fungal infections are diagnosed by mixing scrapings with 10% potassium hydroxide solution, warming it, and examining the mixture microscopically.

Parasitic infections should be included in the differential diagnosis of pruritus ani. A history of travel to endemic areas, animals at home, or exposure to children should be clues to this possibility. *Enterobius vermicularis* (pinworms) is the classic parasite to cause rectal itching. The worms tend to migrate at night and produce nocturnal or early morning pruritus. A crawling sensation associated with itching has been reported. The eggs are detected by having the patient press transparent adhesive tape to the anal area on awakening and then examining the tape on a glass slide microscopically.

Pediculosis pubis can cause pruritus ani along with its more characteristic pubic pruritus. Pediculosis pubis is diagnosed when the lice or nits are found on examination. *Sarcoptes scabiei* has been incriminated as a cause of pruritus, although it is usually associated with a more widespread itching. We have also seen a nonspecific colitis associated with this infection. Scabies often causes a characteristic erythematous rash between the fingers and on the volar surfaces of the wrist.

Viral infections can cause pruritus. Sexual promiscuity and anal receptive activity are associated with the development of infections with condyloma acuminatum, molluscum contagiosum, and herpes simplex virus. Characteristic verruciform or ulcerated lesions can lead to their diagnosis. Herpes simplex virus may be associated with buttock pain and bladder difficulties. Rectal mucosal involvement may be found on anoscopy or sigmoidoscopy in these infections.

OTHER IRRITANTS

Diet has been incriminated as causing both increased soiling and creating an irritating feces. Excess liquids in general and coffee, tea, cola, and beer, in particular, have been incriminated. Certain foods including tomatoes, citrus fruits, and chocolate are often cited as causing pruritus. Manometric studies have shown reduction in anal pressures after coffee ingestion.[8]

Certain drugs known to cause diarrhea including antibiotics, laxatives, mineral oil, quinidine, lactulose and colchicine have been incriminated in causing pruritus ani.

Local irritants including soap, toilet paper, feminine hygiene products, and topical ointments have been incriminated as causing pruritus ani. Soaps liberally applied and inadequately removed can be both chemical and allergic offenders. Toilet paper, when used abrasively or when perfumed, can cause mechanical or allergic irritation. Paradoxically, locally applied medications including talcs and steroids, when used repeatedly, have been incriminated as offending agents.

MISCELLANEOUS

Generalized dermatologic problems including psoriasis, seborrheic dermatitis, neurodermatitis, lichen planus, lichen sclerosus et atrophicus, and lichen simplex chronicus have presented with localized anal itching. A careful physical examination should reveal other afflicted areas.

Systemic illnesses associated with itching include renal failure, primary biliary cirrhosis, lymphoma, pellagra, and vitamin A and D deficiencies. As mentioned previously, conditions predisposing to infections such as diabetes and immunosuppressive disorders can lead to opportunistic infections, particularly *Candida*.

Neurologic disorders can be associated with pruritus ani. A history of spinal trauma or neurologic disease leading to bowel dysfunction and anal incontinence predisposes to local perirectal irritations. Patients with dementia, mental illnesses, and developmental disorders may develop pruritus ani due to poor hygienic practices.

Finally, it has been hypothesized that psychologic factors may play a role in the cause of pruritus ani. It has been theorized that pruritus ani is an expression of homosexuality, hypochondriasis, emotional stress, depression, anal erotism, or fear of anal pregnancy.[9]

TREATMENT

Effective treatment is dependent on the determination of the cause of the pruritus ani. Isolation of specific bacterial infections should lead to treatment with oral antibiotics effective against the isolated bacteria. Cephalosporins, 1 g daily for 1 week for *Staphylococcus aureus,* and erythromycin, 1 g daily for *Corynebacterium,* are effective. Topical antifungal creams mixed with 1% hydrocortisone are usually effective for *Candida* infections. Rarely in immunocompromised patients, oral antifungal agents such as fluconazole (Diflucan), 200 mg daily, may be needed. Mebendazole, 100 mg as a single dose repeated in 2 weeks, or pyrantel pamoate, 11 mg/kg as a single dose repeated in 2 weeks, is recommended therapy for *Enterobius vermicularis.* Communicable diseases should be treated appropriately as primary venereal disorders.

Inciting drugs, local irritants, or dietary indiscretions should be stopped, and appropriate dietary deficiencies or systemic dermatologic disorders should be treated. Bowel dysfunction should be improved when possible with the use of bulk agents (psyllium agents), stool thickeners (attapulgite [Kaopectate]), or anticholinergics or antidiarrheal medications (diphenoxylate with atropine [Lomotil], loperamide [Imodium], tincture of opiate).

Surgical treatment of rectal disorders can be effective. Removal of rectal polyps or enlarged papillae and effective treatment of hemorrhoidal disease can lead to resolution of pruritus ani,[10] although a clear-cut association of hemorrhoids with pruritus ani has not been proven. Behavioral modification to correct anal sphincter dysfunction can be helpful. The majority of patients require improved local hygienic regimens to cure their pruritus ani. The following regimen is advocated:

1. Clean the perianal area after each bowel movement with moistened toilet paper or commercially premoistened towelettes. Dry the area gently after cleaning. Avoid abrasive rubbing.
2. At night, clean the area gently with water and a small amount of a nonperfumed mild soap. Remove all soap carefully.
3. Wear cotton underwear, avoid synthetic non-breathing and tight undergarments.
4. If excessive sweating or moisture accumulates in the anal area, place baby powder or thin cotton absorbents on or in the perianal area to absorb moisture.

Occasionally, more aggressive measures may be needed. Shaving the perianal area may improve cleaning and diminish moisture accumulation. A course of corticosteroids for local irritation can be used for brief periods only, as they tend to undermine the skin's normal resistance to fungi and yeasts. Cryotherapy with liquid nitrogen spray has been reported to be effective but at potential risk for scar formation.[11] Intracutaneous methylene blue injections have been reported to be effective in recalcitrant patients, but it may cause abscess and ulcer formation.[12] In certain patients counseling, antianxiety medication, and occasionally formal psychiatric treatment may be necessary for the treatment of pruritus ani when there is an underlying psychologic cause.

REFERENCES

1. Sullivan ES, Garnjobst WM. Pruritus ani: a practical approach. *Surg Clin North Am.* 1978;58(3):505–512.
2. Eyers AA, Thompson JPS. Pruritus ani: is anal sphincter dysfunction important in etiology? *Br Med J.* 1979;2:1549–159.

3. Allan A, Ambrose NS, Siverman S, Keighley MR. Physiological study of pruritus ani. *Br J Surg.* 1987;74:576–579.
4. Baral J. Pruritus ani and *Staphylococcus aureus. J Am Acad Dermatol.* Letter. 1963;9(6):962.
5. Bowyer A, McCall I. Erythrasma and pruritus ani. *Acta Derm Venereol (Stockh).* 1971;51:444–447.
6. Silverman SH, Youngs DJ, Allan A, Ambrose NS, Keighley MR. The fecal microflora in pruritus ani. *Dis Colon Rectum.* 1989;32:466–468.
7. Dodi G, Pirone E, Bettin A, et al. The mycotic flora in proctological patients with and without pruritus ani. *Br J Surg.* 1969;72:967–968.
8. Friend WG. The cause and treatment of idiopathic pruritus ani. *Dis Colon Rectum.* 1977;20(1):40–42.
9. Verbov J. Pruritus ani and its management: a study and reappraisal. *Clin Exp Dermatol.* 1984;9:46–52.
10. Muries JA, Sim AJ, Mackenzie I. The importance of pain, pruritus and soiling as symptoms of hemorrhoids and their response to hemorrhoidectomy or rubber band ligation. *Br J Surg.* 1981;68(4):247–249.
11. Detrano SJ. Cryotherapy for nonspecific pruritus ani. *J Dermatol Surg Oncol.* 1984;10(6):483–484.
12. Eusebio EB, Graham J, Mody N. Treatment of intractable pruritus ani. *Dis Colon Rectum.* 1990;33:770–772.

82

Anal Tumors

GERALD A. ISENBERG

Tumors of the anus often create confusion; there are numerous pathologic terms that describe similar uncommon lesions. Patients with these tumors are frequently treated identically despite this distinctive nomenclature. Regardless, accurate and prompt treatment offers some patients an excellent prognosis.

Understanding the anatomic and histologic features of the anal canal allows a clear understanding of the pathophysiology of anal tumors. The anal canal extends from the anal verge to the anorectal ring. Squamous epithelium is located distal to the dentate line. Columnar epithelium is proximal to the dentate line. Immediately proximal to the dentate line, the cloacogenic zone extends for about 1 cm and may contain columnar, cuboidal, transitional, or squamous epithelium. This cellular variety is responsible for the inconsistent pathologic presentation of anal tumors.

Lymphatic drainage depends on the location of the lesion. Generally, distal to the dentate line, drainage is to the inguinal nodes. Proximal to the dentate line, drainage begins at the inferior, middle, or superior rectal vessels and subsequently drains into the internal iliac chain. Of course, larger lesions may involve both lymphatic systems.

The World Health Organization has divided the tumors into two groups based on location: anal canal proximal to the dentate line and anal margin or anal canal distal to the dentate line. The most common tumors for these zones are listed in Table 82–1.

Patients with anal canal neoplasms commonly present with

- Bleeding (50%)
- Pain (40%)
- A mass (25%)
- Pruritus (15%)

Of course these symptoms are the same for most benign anorectal conditions, hence the diagnostic delay in many cases. *A biopsy should be performed on any anal lesion that is thought to be benign and has not responded to conservative therapy for 1 month.*

ANAL MARGIN

Basal cell carcinoma is a rare lesion, seen more frequently in men. Its appearance is similar to basal cell cancers in other areas; however, the perianal location often causes a delay in diagnosis. The lesions are superficial, have a low potential for invasion, and generally do not metastasize. Basal cell carcinomas should be excised locally. About one third recur and should undergo

TABLE 82–1. TUMORS OF THE ANAL CANAL AND THE ANAL MARGIN

Lesions of the Anal Canal	Lesions of the Anal Margin
Squamous cell	Basal cell
Melanoma	Squamous cell
Adenocarcinoma	Bowen's disease
Sarcoma	Paget's disease
	Verrucous cancer
	Kaposi's sarcoma

reexcision. Massive lesions that occur infrequently require an abdominoperineal resection (APR).

Squamous carcinoma of the anal skin must not be confused with anal squamous cell carcinoma (see below). Squamous carcinoma is similar to skin cancers in other locations. The lesion has rolled, everted edges with central ulceration. Patients present with a slow-growing mass that is either polypoid or ulcerated or both. There is often bleeding and itching. Treatment consists of a wide local excision. Metastases occur in the inguinal nodes. Patients with biopsy-proven lymph node metastases should have a lymph node dissection.

Bowen's disease is an intraepidermal squamous cancer. Patients are usually 50 to 60 years old, more often female and present with itching, burning, and bleeding of the perianal skin. The rash is raised and irregular in shape with scaly brownish-red plaques. Some reports indicate up to one third of patients with Bowen's disease develop other cutaneous premalignant and malignant conditions. Recent studies refute the concept of associated internal malignancy, therefore workup is probably unwarranted. Approximately 5% to 10% of patients have an invasive squamous cell cancer with the perianal lesion.

Bowen's disease is treated by wide local excision. Some authors use frozen sections at the periphery to ensure clear margins. The wound is closed primarily when possible; a split-thickness skin graft or flap is used when indicated. These lesions can recur in up to 10% of Bowen's disease cases and therefore require follow-up every 2 to 3 months for at least 2 years. Reexcision should be performed for recurrences, although there are some reports of 5-fluorouracil (5-FU) cream successfully treating small recurrences.

An interesting subgroup are those patients who present with Bowen's disease as an incidental finding in a hemorrhoidectomy specimen. The affected area is rebiopsied, or excised, or both, hence the importance of separating hemorrhoid specimens during routine hemorrhoid surgery.

Perianal Paget's disease is an intraepithelial adenocarcinoma. There is a long preinvasive phase where patients complain primarily of pruritus. Bleeding, weight loss, and mucous discharge may also occur. Symptoms may be present for years prior to diagnosis. There is a slight male predominance with a mean age of 60 to 70 years. The rash is erythematous and eczematous, often with scaling and oozing. The average size is 5 cm; however, one third of patients may have the entire perianal skin involved. Visceral cancers are commonly associated with perianal Paget's disease and affect the colon, skin, prostate, nasopharynx, and neck, in decreasing frequency. A wide local excision is the treatment of choice; skin grafting is used as indicated. Some authors use vital staining techniques (toluidine blue and acetic acid) intraoperatively to identify the margins of the lesion. Metastases (25%) are found in the inguinal nodes, liver, bone, and lung. Local recurrences should be reexcised. Patients with invasive Paget's disease often have a poor prognosis even with an APR because of metastatic disease.

Verrucous cancer may be associated with giant condylomata or Buschke-Löwenstein tumors. They present as very large warts with erosion and extension into adjacent tissues. Local excision is advised unless the sphincters are involved, requiring an APR. Gordon[7] has suggested these lesions be treated with chemoradiation, which would obviate the need for radical resection.

ANAL CANAL

Squamous cell carcinoma (SCC) is the most common anal tumor representing 70% of all anal lesions. The transition zone is the site of origin of these tumors, hence the array of associated pathology. Squamous, cloacogenic, basaloid, epidermoid, and mucoepidermoid variants of SCC are congregated for this discussion because of their common response to therapy. The patient median age is 60 years with a female predominance of 2:3 in some series despite the higher risk subgroup of homosexual or bisexual men. A number of reports suggest an association of either human papillomavirus 16 or smoking with the clinical manifestation of SCC. Lesions are more common in the upper anal canal in women and in the lower anal canal in men.

Bleeding is seen in half the patients with SCC; weight loss, pain, or a mass is also noted. Physical examination must include inguinal lymph nodes because up to 36% of patients demonstrate inguinal lymph node involvement. Liver function tests, hepatic imaging, chest x-ray examination, and colonic surveillance are needed to exclude metastatic disease. Endorectal ultrasound can help determine the depth of tumor invasion. If smooth muscle is involved, about one third of patients have lymph node metastases, and almost twice as many have lymph node disease with extension to the external sphincter. Tumor size also correlates to lymph node metastases; tumors less than 2 cm have 3% metastases, and tumors greater than 2 cm have 30% lymph node metastases. Distant metastasis is seen in 10% at presentation.

Treatment for SCC represents one of the therapeutic triumphs of this century. The poor results associated with local excision or APR along prompted Nigro[9] to develop multimodality therapy using 5-FU, mitomycin C, and radiation. The original protocol used 5-FU (1000 mg/m²/d) continuous intravenous infusion for 4 days, mitomycin C (15 mg/m²) bolus, and radiation 3000 cGy (200 cGy/d). Many variations to this protocol have emerged with most centers increasing the radiation to 4500 cGy. Inguinal nodes should always be included in the radiation field. Toxicity includes stomatitis, diarrhea, mucositis, dermatitis, and mild hematologic suppression. Five-year survival is 85% to 90%.

Some controversy exists regarding the post-treatment approach; Nigro[9] suggests no biopsy of the scar after therapy if the lesion disappears. Patients are followed closely with office visits every 2 to 3 months, and a biopsy is performed for any suspicious area. Patients who present with large lesions or those who demonstrate only partial initial response, undergo a second round of chemoradiation, substituting cisplatin for mitomycin C. If the initial chemoradiation yields no response or tumor remains after the second round of therapy, APR is recommended. Radiation implants can be used for patients who refuse radical surgery. Patients with recurrent disease should first undergo additional chemoradiation (if possible) before surgery is contemplated. Prophylactic lymph node dissection is controversial, but generally not performed, especially if the lymph nodes have been radiated. Patients who present with lymph node involvement generally have a poor prognosis. Although these patients may respond to the chemoradiation, radical lymph node dissection does not improve survival, is associated with significant morbidity, and therefore is not endorsed.

Melanoma represents 1% to 2% of all anal cancers; however, the anus is the third most common site for primary melanoma, following involvement of skin and eyes. Melanoma in other sites of the gastrointestinal tract usually represent metastases. The mean age of presentation is 50 to 60 years, and there is a female predominance. In contradistinction to skin melanoma, anal melanoma is more prevalent in regions with less sunshine. Although the lesion may appear as a deeply pigmented polypoid mass, some authors report one half to two thirds are amelanotic. Patients usually present with bleeding; thus, melanoma is often confused with bleeding hemorrhoids. The prognosis is poor unless the lesion is small (<2 cm) and superficial (<2 mm penetration), which is rare. Most patients have metastases by the time of presentation (perirectal, perianal, mesenteric and inguinal lymph node, liver, and lung). Five-year survival is 10% to 15% regardless of therapy. Local excision is performed for local control, and APR is used for the palliation of large tumors. Chemotherapy and immunomodulation have not been successful thus far.

Adenocarcinoma of the anal canal is rare; low rectal adenocarcinomas are excluded. The cause is unclear but may stem from a gland, duct, or fistulous tract. Patients present with anal pain, bleeding, and a mass. At initial diagnosis about one half have fistulas and 10% have metastatic disease. Most patients are treated with an APR, and according to a survey of the American Society of Colorectal Surgeons, about half of patients with adenocarcinoma receive adjuvant therapy. Sarcoma is rare and radioresistant and should be treated with an APR.

REFERENCES

1. Abel ME, Chiu YSY, Russell TR, Volpe PA. Adenocarcinoma of the anal glands. *Dis Colon Rectum.* 1993; 36(4):383–386.
2. Adams YG, Schuldenfrei JA, Nonas CJ, Alberts WW. Premalignant and malignant anal lesions. *Surgical Rounds.* September 1992:771–781.
3. Beck DE, Fazio VW, Jagelman DG, Lavery IC. Perianal Bowen's disease. *Dis Colon Rectum.* 1988;31(6):419–422.
4. Berardi RS, Lee S, Chen HP. Perianal extramammary Paget's disease. *Surg Gynecol Obstet.* 1988;167:359–366.
5. Cummings BJ, Rotstein L, Stern H. Anal carcinoma. In: Fazio VW, ed. *Current Therapy in Colon and Rectal Surgery.* Philadelphia, Pa: BC Decker Inc; 1990:64–68.
6. McNamara MJ. Melanoma and basal cell carcinoma. In: Fazio VW, ed. *Current Therapy in Colon and Rectal Surgery.* Philadelphia, Pa: BC Decker Inc; 1990:62–64.

7. Gordon PH. Current status: perianal and anal canal neoplasms. *Dis Colon Rectum.* 1990;33(9):799–808.
8. Nivatvongs S. Perianal and anal canal neoplasms. In: Gordon PH, Nivatvongs S. *Principles and Practice of Surgery for the Colon, Rectum and Anus.* St. Louis, Mo: Quality Medical Publishing; 1991:402–417.
9. Nigro ND. The force of change in the management of squamous cell cancer of the anal canal. *Dis Colon Rectum.* 1991;34(6):482–486.
10. Weinstock MA. Epidemiology and prognosis of anorectal melanoma. *Gastroenterology.* 1993;104(1):174–178.

83

Endometriosis: A Gastroenterologist's Perspective

STEPHEN R. SEVERANCE and C. GREGORY ALBERS

Just as the difficult patient with "atypical" chest pain may tax the combined diagnostic resources of the gastroenterologist and cardiologist, the difficult female patient with pelvic or lower abdominal pain not infrequently presents a frustrating diagnostic challenge to the cooperative efforts of the gastroenterologist and gynecologist.

In the case of *acute* abdominopelvic pain, gynecologic conditions such as ectopic pregnancy, pelvic inflammatory disease, or tuboovarian abscess, complications of ovarian cysts, and adnexal torsion must be differentiated from such diverse gastrointestinal conditions as acute appendicitis, Meckel's diverticulum, inflammatory bowel disease, diverticulitis, and other causes of free perforation. Since the correct diagnosis may potentially avert an unnecessary operation, accurate differentiation of these conditions is both urgent and vital.[1]

In the case of *chronic* abdominopelvic pain, the distinction between gynecologic and gastrointestinal disorders may be somewhat less urgent but is no less critical. The magnitude of this problem is underscored by studies suggesting that close to 50% of women attending gynecologic clinics or of those having diagnostic laparoscopy or hysterectomy meet criteria for the diagnosis of irritable bowel syndrome (IBS).[2-5] Conversely, women with IBS have been shown to be more likely to visit gynecologic clinics.[4] In addition, they are more likely to undergo hysterectomy,[2] further confounding the clinician with the addition of adhesive disorder to the differential diagnosis. The clinical significance of these reports is manifest in several attendant observations:

1. The gastrointestinal diagnosis was often overlooked by the gynecologist.
2. A firm gynecologic diagnosis could be established in only 8% of patients with bowel symptoms as opposed to 44% in those without.[3]
3. With treatment in such clinics, resolution of abdominopelvic pain was far less likely in patients with bowel symptoms (35% response) than in those without (68% response).[3]
4. The success rate of hysterectomy performed primarily for pain was significantly lower in patients with bowel symptoms than in those without.[2]

For both the gynecologist and the gastroenterologist, these observations should foster a constant awareness of the treacherous similarity between two of the most common causes of abdominopelvic pain—IBS and endometriosis. Both disorders are extremely common: endometriosis effects about 10% to 15% of all menstruating women—as high as 30% in infertile women.[6] The incidence of irritable bowel syndrome is probably about 15%.[7] The demographics of the two disorders are likewise very similar. Except for a handful of reports in men receiving hormonal therapy for prostate cancer, endometriosis occurs exclusively in women. Although female-to-male ratios of as high as 21:1 have been reported for IBS, a more realistic figure would be higher than 3:1. Less than 5% of laparoscopically diagnosed endometriosis occurs in postmenopausal women, usually among those receiving estrogen replacement.[8] Similarly, IBS is typically a disorder of the relatively young. To add to the potential for diagnostic confusion, a high incidence of gynecologic symptoms have been reported in women with irritable bowel syndrome, over half experiencing dysmenorrhea and 83% of women in one study reporting sexual dysfunction or dyspareunia.[9-11] Conversely, women with endometriosis or primary dysmenorrhea may experience a higher incidence of gastrointestinal symptoms.[12] Worse yet, a significant number of women with endometriosis, unlike those with primary dysmenorrhea, may experience abdominopelvic pain that is noncyclic in nature. Noncyclic symptoms are particularly common in cases of direct gastrointestinal involvement with endometriosis, and in such cases symptoms may also be influenced by gastrointestinal activities such as eating or bowel movements.

For the practicing gastroenterologist whose office population is commonly almost 50% "functional GI disorders,"[13] a basic understanding of endometriosis and its relationship to both abdominal symptoms and gastrointestinal pathophysiology may convert this seemingly esoteric condition into a fairly commonplace diagnosis.

Several excellent reviews on the subject of endometriosis have been published in the past several years,[6,14-19] including two[18,19] addressing its gastrointestinal manifestations. This is, indeed, a common condition, with reported incidences from 1% to 50%, but a realistic range being from 10% to 15%.[6,17] The condition is defined as the presence of endometrial glands or stroma outside of the uterus. This ectopic tissue has been found in almost every organ system including the gastrointestinal tract, genitourinary system, skin, lymph nodes, extremities, thoracic cage and lungs, peripheral nerves, and central nervous system (CNS), with the one noteworthy exception being the spleen.[17] A detailed discussion of the poorly understood pathogenesis of this common condition is beyond the scope of this chapter but may be found in the excellent review by Rock and Markham.[14] Briefly, the abundant hypotheses concerning the cause of endometriosis may be grouped into four general theories:

1. The "transport" theory, involving "retrograde menstruation" and supported by
   a. The presence of blood in the peritoneal fluid in 90% of women who undergo laparoscopy during menses
   b. The presence of endometrial cells, blood, or both in the peritoneal dialysate of a high percentage of menstruating women undergoing peritoneal dialysis
   c. The increased incidence of endometriosis in women with congenitally narrowed genital outflow tracts or in those simply with regular but prolonged menstruation
2. The "metaplasia" theory, hypothesizing transformation of peritoneal mesothelium to endometrial stroma and possibly supported by the occasional occurrence of endometriosis in men (invariably in those receiving estrogen therapy) or in women with agenesis of the uterus.
3. The "immunologic" theory, supported indirectly by the occurrence of endometriosis following immunosuppression of experimental animals and more directly by the observation of a variety of immunologic aberrancies in afflicted patients.
4. The "embryonic" theory, suggesting, without much scientific support to date, that endometriosis develops from "endometrial rests."

Whichever theory, or more likely combination of theories, ultimately proves valid, this condition presents the paradoxic enigma of a "benign" disorder that behaves in a quasimalignant fashion with documented vascular metastases and with 29% of afflicted individuals displaying endometrial tissue in pelvic lymph glands at autopsy.

The "classic" case of endometriosis confined to the pelvis can be fairly easily distinguished from IBS, other gastrointestinal conditions, or for that matter from most gynecologic disorders.[20] First and foremost, the pain is almost invariably cyclic, occurring in the perimenstrual period. It is often described as "deep," commonly lateral, and may be either sharp or dull. The pain is usually constant, unlike the more rhythmic or crampy pain of both IBS and primary dysmenorrhea. The occasional occurrence of this pain at other times during the cycle together with the frequent occurrence of bowel disturbance in the perimenstrual period does make confusion with IBS sufficiently common to result in fairly frequent gastroenterologic or medical consultation for this condition. With an understanding of endometriosis and a careful history alone, symptomatic pelvic endometriosis should seldom trigger a gastrointestinal workup, and the first appropriate test is often a gynecologic referral. This is supported by the fact that two thirds of patients with endometriosis are nulliparous, and multiparity should militate somewhat against this diagnosis. The disorder should not be suspected in postmenopausal women except for rare cases, which are always associated with estrogen therapy. A history of infertility should be highly suggestive but is present in a minority of cases. A history of dyspareunia is helpful, but far from specific, being present in a substantial number of women with IBS. Finally, a family history of endometriosis should be sought, although this too is present in a minority of cases.[21]

When endometriosis directly involves or "invades" some portion of the gastrointestinal tract, its clinical distinction from primary gastrointestinal disorders is more likely to be problematic. A review of more than 7000 cases of endometriosis reported before 1960 suggested gastrointestinal involvement in about 12%.[22] At either laparoscopy or celiotomy in 573 patients with endometriosis, a later report suggested that 5.4% had "macroscopic" involvement of the gastrointestinal tract with 15% of these having "multiple sites of involvement."[18] Finally, a review published in 1989 suggests gastrointestinal involvement in "up to 25 percent" of patients.[17] Although symptoms may be underreported in pathologic or epidemiologic studies and overreported in clinical series, it is safe to guess that about 50% of these patients were asymptomatic, at least with respect to their gastrointestinal involvement.

In keeping with the "transport" or "retrograde menstruation" theory of pathogenesis, those areas of the gastrointestinal tract most contiguous to the uterus are most commonly involved. Various series have shown considerable disparity in reported distribution. Thus, the Ochsner Foundation series of 163 patients with gastrointestinal endometriosis reported in 1987 found involvement in the descending or rectosigmoid colon (60%), rectum (10%), appendix (20%), ileum (7%), and cecum (6%),[23] whereas others have reported an even higher predilection for the rectum and rectosigmoid.[18] Certainly rectal and rectosigmoid diseases are seen most often and probably represent the greatest challenge to the practicing clinician as well. Here, as in other areas of the intestines, the extent and degree of endometrial implantation may vary from very superficial serosal studs to transmural or circumferential involvement, producing actual luminal compromise or narrowing in up to 18% of cases.[24] The chemical irritation of blood and other products of menstrual "slough" may produce a capsule of adhesions and fibrosis reminiscent of that seen with some carcinoid tumors, often precluding etiologic diagnosis of the lesion by gross inspection in the approximately one out of three patients with no apparent concomitant involvement of other pelvic organs. Indeed, in one surgical series of 14 patients with severe rectosigmoid endometriosis, the correct diagnosis was suspected in only six *even* at the time of laparotomy for resection.[25] These transmural or circumferential lesions represent a minority of cases but account for some of the more dramatic clinical presentations. A small number will present with incomplete or rarely complete large bowel obstruction. Actual perforation classically[26] but not always[27] in the peripartum period may infrequently occur. Hematochezia occurring with menses only is a classical but rarely seen symptom.

The more common and less severe case of rectosigmoid endometriosis (RSE) presents with chronic "colon" symptoms often indistinguishable from IBS. In diminishing order of frequency, crampy pain, usually in the left lower quadrant, constipation, diarrhea, constipation alternated with diarrhea, or proctalgia may occur. Less frequently nausea, vomiting, bloating, or diminished stool caliber may occur. A minority report onset of symptoms with menstruation but, surprisingly, the symptoms are noncyclic in the majority. The noncyclic nature of this condition as well as the absence of any gynecologic symptoms in one third of cases may obscure the gynecologic origin of these symptoms. Indeed, in their review of the more than 200 cases of RSE reported since 1970 (which we suspect represents "the tip of the iceberg" for this underdiagnosed condition), Zwas and Lyon[19] found that the diagnosis was delayed on an average of more than 3.5 years from onset of symptoms. Fortunately, gynecologic symptoms of some kind can be elicited from two thirds of patients with RSE, although similar symptoms in a substantial number of IBS patients render them far from specific.[9-11] A history of infertility is present in approximately one third of patients, and well over half describe dysmenorrhea, menometrorrhagia, or, less frequently, dyspareunia. In absence of any known association with IBS, infertility may be the most useful of these symptoms.

Nearly half of patients with RSE have entirely negative findings from physical examinations. In those with positive findings, simple pelvic or lower abdominal tenderness, often localized to the left lower quadrant, was by far the most common finding. There may be a palpable pelvic mass in as many as 25%, nodularity in the cul-de-sac or uterosacral ligaments in 15%, and an extrinsic "mass" on rectal examination in 15%.[19]

The added possibility of RSE does not change the *initial* diagnostic approach to patients with probable IBS. An occasional patient with RSE may have iron deficiency anemia. This is almost invariably due to menorrhagia, but certainly justifies serial hemoccult determinations. With this exception, the complete blood count should be normal in both conditions. Nonspecific indicators of inflammation such as the erythrocyte sedimentation rate (ESR) or C-reactive protein are likewise normal in both, being helpful largely to screen for inflammatory bowel disease. The presence of diarrhea should be pursued with appropriate stool studies. Except for the "air insufflation test,"[28] sigmoidoscopy or colonoscopy results are usually negative in IBS. Less frequently, air insufflation may be provocative in RSE. Moreover, reporting from the Cleveland Clinic on nine patients with surgically confirmed RSE, Bozdech[29] described endoscopic findings of "polyp, mass, or stricture" in all nine. Endoscopic biopsies confirmed endometriosis in five of six patients with cyclic hematochezia, but in *none* of the others. With the exception of this single small series and isolated case reports, the literature is not sanguine as to the specificity of endoscopy in RSE. To be sure, 59% of cases are endoscopically "abnormal," but almost always nonspecifically so, with extrinsic compression, narrowing, or mass—or more commonly simple fixation, deformity, or angulation.[17,19] Indeed, in a female patient with no prior abdominopelvic surgeries, a frustrating and difficult endoscopy similar to that experienced not uncommonly in the previously operated patient, should always suggest this diagnosis. The theoretic potential for endoscopic ultrasound in this largely submucosal or extrinsic process is obvious but not yet reported. Contrast studies may be a bit more sensitive but are no more specific. Citing 11 series with a total of 63 patients, Zwas and Lyons[19] found 61 to have abnormal results from barium enema studies. External bowel compression and intramural or submucosal filling defects were most common (34 of 63). Actual strictures were seen in 10. Far less frequent were total obstruction, "corkscrewing," and polyps.[19] An air contrast study is preferred.

If results from initial tests are negative or suggestive of IBS (i.e., positive results from "air insufflation test"), a trial of therapy for presumed IBS would seem appropriate. If this trial is unsuccessful and symptoms so warrant, or if the initial tests are suggestive albeit nonspecific, further evaluation should be directed more specifically at the possibility of endometriosis.

Pelvic ultrasonography, especially when transvaginal visualization is added to the traditional transabdominal approach, is often useful in the lower abdomen and pelvis, with a sensitivity of more than 90% for adnexal masses.[30] In his ultrasonographic studies of endometriosis, Bernholz[31] found two discrete forms: the more easily seen discrete pelvic mass (endometrioma) and the diffuse form with multiple implants and adhesions. Unfortunately, the latter pattern is much more common and much more difficult to visualize. A subsequent laparoscopically controlled study of ultrasound detected only 4 (10.8%) of 37 cases of endometriosis, but a transvaginal probe was not routinely used.[32] In spite of this disappointing yield, ultrasonography should probably be performed if for no other reason than to screen for other gynecologic disorders. If endometriosis is a consideration, the ultrasonographer should be alerted, since many of the findings in the diffuse form (generalized increased background echogenicity, "diffusely altered echogenicity," accentuated pelvic arterial pulsations, and poor definition of pelvic structures) are nonspecific or inferential and might not be sought or reported.[31] Especially if RSE is suspected, ultrasound should be performed both before and after voiding.[33] The theoretic attractiveness of *endoscopic* ultrasound, as yet untested, is reiterated.

Computed tomography is probably a bit more sensitive than ultrasound for the diffuse form of endometriosis,[30] but because of the attendant obligatory gonadal radiation exposure in these often reproductive-age patients, it should be used only rarely. If it is used and RSE is suspected, the examination should be performed with rectally instilled water-soluble contrast medium.

A number of studies have espoused the use of magnetic resonance imaging (MRI) in this condition.[20] Reported sensitivity and specificity is as high as 71% and 82%, respectively,[34] but this modality is costly and seldom changes subsequent interventions, notably laparoscopy. MRI should be reserved for very atypical cases or for the rare case in which even laparoscopy is considered risky. In addition, it may have a role in monitoring therapy once the diagnosis is established.[35]

Given the lack of sensitivity and frequent nonspecificity of these indirect or noninvasive pelvic imaging studies, not to mention their rising expense in an era of "cost-benefit" considerations, there is a great deal to be said for proceeding directly to diagnostic laparoscopy if RSE is suspected and preliminary results from evaluation as out-lined above are negative. Indeed, at least 5% to 10% of gynecologic laparoscopies are performed for chronic pain.[36] Unfortunately, 90% or more of examination results are negative, underscoring the need for selectivity. As with IBS, there is a very high percentage of abnormal psychologic profiles in those with negative findings, leading to the suggestion by some that psychologic evaluation be used as one criterion for screening.[36] This procedure has an extremely low mortality, with complications reported in about 3%. The "classic" appearance of diffuse endometriosis on this examination is that of multiple "black powderburn" lesions in the pelvis, but recent studies have increasingly emphasized more subtle variations in appearance, including minute "clear" lesions that can be very difficult to discern.[37,38] For this reason, an experienced gynecologist rather than surgeon or gastroenterologist is preferred in this clinical context. Moreover, even in such experienced hands, biopsy specimens of grossly normal peritoneum have revealed microscopic endometriosis in 13% of patients with gross endometriosis elsewhere in the pelvis and in 6% of patients with completely normal gross laparoscopic inspection.[39] This yield was even higher in one report using electron microscopy.[40] These reports evolved from a study of patients with infertility and are therefore difficult to extrapolate to patients with the presumed "gross" involvement implied by rectosigmoid symptoms. Given that one third of women with RSE have no evidence of endometriosis elsewhere in the pelvis, even at laparotomy,[19] random biopsy specimens at the time of a seemingly normal examination would certainly seem logical.

Indeed, it is this significant percentage of cases with endometriosis seemingly localized to the bowel that causes the greatest diagnostic difficulty and may explain why so much of the literature heretofore is surgical in nature. Very promising in general, recent studies suggesting a serologic approach to the diagnosis of this disorder might be particularly germane to this subgroup. The gynecologic tumor marker CA 125 will be greater than 35 U/ml in less than 1.0% of normal individuals and in 42% of patients with endometriosis.[41] This figure rises to 54% in patients with "advanced" disease.[42] Peritoneal fluid CA 125 may be 100 times that of serum in patients with endometriosis, and both peritoneal fluid and serum levels are more sensitive for this condition at the time of menses.[43] The test may even have a role in monitoring therapy.[44] Endometrial antibodies, first discovered as a by-product of research into the pathogenesis of this condition and best detected by passive hemagglutination, are also present in a large percentage.[45,46] A commercially available assay is anxiously awaited.

Occasionally, on the basis of either history or nonspecific findings the diagnosis of RSE may be highly suspect in an "IBS" patient but elude confirmation after exhausting all of the aforementioned modalities. If such a patient remains symptomatic after routine treatment for IBS, including tricyclic antidepressants, psychologic counseling, and a chronic pain program, exploratory laparotomy might be considered. An unconventional alternative for such a case can be inferred from preliminary studies suggesting that gonadotropin-releasing hormone (Gn-RH) analog, an agent commonly used in the treatment of endometriosis, has recently shown promise in the treatment of IBS.[47] Encouraged by preliminary data, some centers, including our own, have undertaken controlled trials. Enrollment in such a study might be presented as an alternative in these difficult cases.

A detailed discussion of the treatment of endometriosis is beyond the scope of this chapter. Briefly, *symptomatic* therapy would differ from that of IBS only by a greater role for prostaglandin inhibition.[48] Published series of more specific medical or surgical therapy have recently been reviewed.[49] Both the multifocal and the often partially microscopic nature of this disorder makes definitive surgery technically difficult and often noncurative, with 3- and 5-year recurrence rates of 13.5% and 40.3%, respectively.[50] These factors may tax all but the most experienced surgeon, and at our center these cases are often relegated to our highly specialized gynecologic-oncologic surgical team. Presacral or uterine nerve ablation have been done alone or coupled with surgery with improved pain relief.[51,52] Laparoscopic surgery is widely used for pelvic endometriosis,[53] but its benefit in the specific context of *gastrointestinal* endometriosis remains untested and seems doubtful. Medical therapy used independently or in conjunction with surgery consists of various hormonal manipulations.[49-56] Side effects, largely endocrine in nature, have improved with newer preparations, but this modality is appropriately relegated to specialists—either gynecologist or gynendocrinologist. Although fairly effective in pelvic endometriosis, the application of hormonal manipulations to *gastrointestinal* endometriosis has yet to be reported.

The rectosigmoid is by far the most common location for gastrointestinal endometriosis. For this reason and because we believe its potential confusion with IBS is underappreciated by clinicians and not well reflected in the literature, the primary focus of this chapter has been on disease in that location. It should not be forgotten, however, that this disorder, in a way reminiscent of Crohn's disease, has protean gastrointestinal manifestations. Indeed, in the small bowel itself, endometriosis may mimic all the common presentations of Crohn's disease,[57] and less than one third of patients appreciated a cyclic pattern to their symptoms. Moreover, one fourth lacked evidence of *pelvic* endometriosis.[19] More unusual manifestations include protein-losing enteropathy.[58] Appendiceal endometriosis, on the other hand, is almost always cyclic in its presentation and should be considered any time appendicitis occurs in the perimenstrual period.[59] About half of patients with appendiceal endometriosis experience recurrent attacks. Endometriosis has also been found in scar tissue, the umbilicus,[60] inguinal canal,[61] cecum, gallbladder, liver, and pancreas and may result in hemorrhagic ascites. These less common presentations are discussed in greater depth in the excellent review by Zwas and Lyon.[19]

REFERENCES

1. Quan M, Johnson R, Rodney M. The diagnosis of acute pelvic pain. *West J Med.* 1983;139:110–113.
2. Longstreth GF, Preskill DB, Youkeles L. Irritable bowel syndrome in women having diagnostic laparoscopy or hysterectomy: relation to gynecologic features and outcome. *Dig Dis Sci.* 1990;35:1285–1290.
3. Prior A, Wilson K, Whorwell PJ, Faragher EB. Irritable bowel syndrome in the gynecologic clinic: survey of 798 new referrals. *Dig Dis Sci.* 1989;34:1820–1824.
4. Prior A, Whorwell PJ. Gynaecological consultation in patients with the irritable bowel syndrome. *Gut.* 1989; 30:996–998.
5. Hogston P. Irritable bowel syndrome as a cause of chronic pain in women attending a gynaecology clinic. *Br Med J.* 1987;294:934–935.
6. Olive DL, Schwartz LB. Endometriosis. *N Engl J Med.* 1993;328:1759–1769.
7. Talley JT, Zinsmeister AR, Van Dyke C, Melton LJ III. Epidemiology of colonic symptoms and the irritable bowel syndrome. *Gastroenterology.* 1991;101:927–934.
8. Punnonen R, Klemi PJ, Nikkanen V. Postmenopausal endometriosis. *Eur J Obstet Gynecol Reprod Biol.* 1980; 11:195–200.
9. Heitkemper MM, Jarrett M. Pattern of gastrointestinal and somatic symptoms across the menstrual cycle. *Gastroenterology.* 1992;102:505–513.
10. Whitehead WE, Cheskin LJ, Heller BR, et al. Evidence for exacerbation of irritable bowel syndrome during menses. *Gastroenterology.* 1990;98:1485–1489.
11. Guthrie E, Creed FH, Whorwell PJ. Severe sexual dysfunction in women with the irritable bowel syndrome: comparison with inflammatory bowel disease and duodenal ulceration. *Br Med J.* 1987;295:577–578.
12. Heitkemper MM, et al. Gastrointestinal symptoms, function, and psychophysiological arousal in dysmenorrheic women. *Nurs Res.* 1991;40:20–25.
13. Mitchell CM, Drossman DA. Survey of the AGA membership relating to functional gastrointestinal disorders. *Gastroenterology.* 1987;92:1283–1284.
14. Rock JA, Markham SM. Pathogenesis of endometriosis. *Lancet.* 1993;340:1264–1267.
15. Shaw RW. Treatment of endometriosis. *Lancet.* 1992; 340:1267–1271.
16. Schenken RS, ed. *Endometriosis: Contemporary Concepts in Clinical Management.* Philadelphia, Pa: JB Lippincott Co; 1989.
17. Markham SM, Carpenter SE, Rock JA. Extrapelvic endometriosis. *Obstet Gynecol Clin North Am.* 1989;16: 193–219.
18. Prystowsky JB, Stryker SJ, Ujiki GT, Poticha SM. Gastrointestinal endometriosis: incidence and indications for resection. *Arch Surg.* 1988;123:855–858.
19. Zwas FR, Lyon DT. Endometriosis: an important condition in clinical gastroenterology. *Dig Dis Sci.* 1991; 36:353–364.
20. Muse KN. Cyclic pelvic pain. *Obstet Gynecol Clin North Am.* 1990;17:427–438.
21. Simpson JL, Elias S, Malinak LR, Buttram VC Jr. Heritable aspects of endometriosis I: genetic studies. *Am J Obstet Gynecol.* 1980;137:327–331.
22. Macafee CHG, Greer HLH. Intestinal endometriosis: a report of 29 cases: a survey of the literature. *J Obstet Gynaecol Br Emp.* 1960;67:539–555.
23. Weed JC, Ray JE. Endometriosis of the bowel. *Obstet Gynecol.* 1974;50:227.
24. Meyers WC, Kelvin FM, Jones RS. Diagnosis and surgical treatment of colonic endometriosis. *Arch Surg.* 1979;114:169–175.
25. McSwain B, Linn RJ, Haley RL, Franklin RH. Endometriosis of the colon: report of 14 patients requiring partial colectomy. *South Med J.* 1974;67:651–658.
26. Floberg K, Backdahl M, Silfersward C. Postpartum perforation of the colon due to endometriosis. *Acta Obstet Gynecol Scand.* 1984;63:183–184.
27. Ledley GS, Shenk IM, Heit HA. Sigmoid colon perforation due to endometriosis not associated with pregnancy. *Am J Gastroenterol.* 1988;83:1424–1426.
28. Kang JY, Gwee KA, Yap I. The colonic air insufflation test indicates a colonic cause of abdominal pain: an aid in the management of irritable bowel syndrome. *J Clin Gastroenterol.* 1994;18:19–22.
29. Bozdech JM. Endoscopic diagnosis of colonic endometriosis. *Gastrointest Endosc.* 1992;38:568–570.

30. Schwartz LB, Seifer DB. Diagnostic imaging of adnexal masses: a review. *J Reprod Med.* 1992;37:63–71.
31. Bernholz JC. Endometriosis and inflammatory disease. *Semin Ultrasound.* 1983;4:184–192.
32. Friedman H, Vogelzang RL, Mendelson EB, Neiman HL, Cohen M. Endometriosis detection by US with laparoscopic correlation. *Radiology.* 1985;157:217–220.
33. Sack RA, Maharry JM. Misdiagnosis in obstetric and gynecologic ultrasound examinations: causes and possible solutions. *Am J Obstet Gynecol.* 1988;158:1260.
34. Zawin M, McCarthy S, Scoutt L, Comite F. Endometriosis: appearance and detection at MR imaging. *Radiology.* 1989;171:693–696.
35. Zawin M, McCarthy S, Scoutt L, et al. Monitoring therapy with a gonadotropin-releasing hormone analog: utility of MR imaging. *Radiology.* 1990;175:503–506.
36. Levitan Z, Eibschitz I, de Vries K, Hakim M, Sharf M. The value of laparoscopy in women with chronic pelvic pain and a normal pelvis. *Int J Gynaecol Obstet.* 1985; 23:71–74.
37. Stripling MC, Martin DC, Chatman DL, Zwaag RV, Poston WM. Subtle appearance of pelvic endometriosis. *Fertil Steril.* 1988;49:427–431.
38. Redwine DB. Age-related evolution in color appearance of endometriosis. *Fertil Steril.* 1987;48:1062–1063.
39. Nisolle M, Paindaveine B, Bourdon A, Berliere M, Casanas-Roux F, Donnez J. Histologic study of peritoneal endometriosis in infertile women. *Fertil Steril.* 1990; 53:984–988.
40. Murphy AA, Green WR, Bobbie D, dela Cruz ZC, Rock JA. Unsuspected endometriosis documented by scanning electron microscopy in visually normal peritoneum. *Fertil Steril.* 1986;46:522–524.
41. Malkasian GD, Podratz KC, Stanhope CR, Ritts RE Jr, Zurawski VR Jr. CA 125 in gynecologic practice. *Am J Obstet Gynecol.* 1986;155:515–518.
42. Barbieri RL, Niloff JN, Bast RC, Schaetzl E, Kistner RW, Knapp RC. Elevated serum concentration of CA-125 in patients with advanced endometriosis. *Fertil Steril.* 1986;45:630–634.
43. Koninckx PR, Riittinen L, Seppala M, Cornillie FJ. CA-125 and placental protein 14 concentrations in plasma and peritoneal fluid of women with deeply infiltrating pelvic endometriosis. *Fertil Steril.* 1993;57:523–530.
44. Kauppila A, Telimaa A, Ronnberg L, Vuori J. Placebo-controlled study on serum concentrations of CA-125 before and after treatment of endometriosis with danazol or high-dose medroxyprogesterone acetate alone or after surgery. *Fertil Steril.* 1988;49:37–41.
45. Badaway SZA, Cuenca V, Freliech H, Stefanu C. Endometrial antibodies in serum and peritoneal fluid of infertile patients with and without endometriosis. *Fertil Steril.* 1990;53:930–932.
46. Wild RA, Shiver CA. Antiendometrial antibodies in patients with endometriosis. *Am J Reprod Immunol Microbiol.* 1985;8:84–86.
47. Mathias JR, Ferguson KL, Clench MH. Debilitating "functional" bowel disease controlled by leuprolide acetate, gonadotropin-releasing hormone (GnRH) analog. *Dig Dis Sci.* 1989;34:761–766.
48. Kauppila A, Ronnberg L, Naproxen sodium in dysmenorrhea secondary to endometriosis. *Obstet Gynecol.* 1985;65:379.
49. Redwine DB. Treatment of endometriosis-associated pain. *Infertil Reprod Med Clin North Am.* 1992;3:697–721.
50. Wheeler JM, Malinak LR. Recurrent endometriosis: incidence, management, and prognosis. *Am J Obstet Gynecol.* 1983;146:247.
51. Tjaden B, Schlaff WD, Kimball A, Rock JA. The efficacy of presacral neurectomy for the relief of midline dysmenorrhea. *Obstet Gynecol.* 1990;76:89.
52. Lichten EM, Bombards J. Surgical treatment of primary dysmenorrhea with laparoscopic uterine nerve ablation. *J Reprod Med.* 1987;32:37–41.
53. Nezhat CH, Kood J, Winer W, Nexhat F, Crowgey SR, Garrison CP. Videolaseroscopy and laser laparoscopy in gynaecology. *Br J Hosp Med.* September 1987:219–224.
54. Telimaa S, Puolakka J, Ronnberg L, Kauppila A. Placebo-controlled comparison of danazol and high-dose medroxyprogesterone acetate in the treatment of endometriosis. *Gynecol Endocrinol.* 1987;1:13–23.
55. Henzl MR, Corson SL, Moghissi K, Buttram VC, Berklqvist C, Jacobson J. Administration of nasal nafarelin as compared with oral danazol for endometriosis: a multicenter double-blind comparative clinical trial. *N Engl J Med.* 1988;318:485–489.
56. The Nafarelin European Endometriosis Trial Group (NEET). Nafarelin for endometriosis: a large-scale, danazol-controlled trial of efficacy and safety, with a 1-year follow-up. *Fertil Steril.* 1992;57:514–522.
57. Minocha A, Davis MS, Wright RA. Small bowel endometriosis masquerading as regional enteritis. *Dig Dis Sci.* 1994;39:1126–1133.
58. Henley JD, Kratzer SS, Seo S, Davis T. Endometriosis of the small intestine presenting as a protein-losing enteropathy. *Am J Gastroenterol.* 1993;88:130–133.
59. Yelon JA, Green JM, Hashmi HF. Endometriosis of the appendix resulting in perforation: a case report. *J Clin Gastroenterol.* 1993;16:355–366.
60. Michowitz M, Baratz M, Stavorovsky M. Endometriosis of the umbilicus. *Dermatologica.* 1983;167:326–330.
61. Sataloff DM, LaVorgna KA, McFarland MM. Extrapelvic endometriosis presenting as a hernia: clinical reports and review of the literature. *Surgery.* 1989;105: 109–112.

84
Pneumatoses Cystoides Intestinalis

CALVIN E. OLSON

Pneumatosis cystoides intestinalis (PCI) is a relatively rare condition characterized by multiple gas-filled cysts or linear streaks of gas within the wall of the intestine. Air collections may be found anywhere within the wall of the intestinal tract from the stomach to the rectum. Sometimes the cysts on the serosal surface burst and a pneumoperitoneum occurs. PCI is often found in association with a variety of gastrointestinal disorders that are usually characterized by breakdown of the mucosa. By itself, PCI is a benign condition that may resolve with minimal intervention. On the other hand, when associated with other life-threatening conditions, PCI may be a harbinger of a very poor clinical outcome. Each clinical situation involving PCI must be approached individually to make appropriate clinical decisions based on the pathophysiology of the disease.

PCI was first recognized in the 18th century. Gas-filled pockets of air in abdominal hollow organs were first described in 1730 by Du Vernoi. The first microscopic description of the features of the cysts was made by Bang in 1876. The first preoperative diagnosis by x-ray examination was made by Reverdin in 1924. PCI has been recognized for centuries and is not the consequence of modern therapeutic techniques.

SYMPTOMS

Symptoms associated with PCI are nonspecific; that is, PCI cannot be identified by characteristic symptoms. The symptoms range from an incidental finding on abdominal x-ray examinations in an asymptomatic patient to marked clinical deterioration. Symptoms associated with benign PCI include constipation, bloody mucoid stools (like "frothy tomato soup"), and mild abdominal pain. In the more seriously ill patients, the symptoms are those of the primary disorder. Rarely, the cysts can be so large that the patient presents with symptoms of bowel obstruction. The age of presentation can range from infancy to adult. PCI in neonates is invariably associated with fulminant necrotizing enterocolitis. Children with PCI may have short bowel syndrome or various serious medical conditions. In adults PCI is often benign unless bowel infarction is present.

DIAGNOSIS

Since there are no specific symptoms associated with PCI, it is usually discovered serendipitously on radiographs or at surgery. Subserosal or submucosal cystic air pockets can be seen in the bowel wall on x-ray examinations or grossly during surgery or endoscopy. The volume of the cysts can range from microscopic to 100 cm^3. When palpated by the surgeon, the affected bowel feels spongy or crepitant. In the lumen, on barium studies and endoscopy, it may appear as a cluster of polypoid masses. When the cysts are punctured, air escapes under pressure with a hissing sound. When PCI involves the rectum, crepitus may be noted on digital rectal examination. The areas of involvement may be localized or diffuse and sometimes will vary over time in the same patient.

Histologically, the mucosa may have mild focal abnormalities to a severe generalized disturbance in mucosal architecture. The cysts are lined by histiocytes. The lamina propria shows increased numbers of lymphocytes and plasma cells, and neutrophils and eosinophils may also be present. Both single and clustered multinucleated giant cells have been identified, as well as well-formed epithelioid granulomas. Abnormal branching of crypts is frequently seen. There may be variable degrees of cystic dilation of individual crypts with a spectrum from cryptitis to crypt abscesses to partial crypt rupture. These inflammatory changes in the mucosa are seen even without clinical evidence of inflammatory bowel disease.

DEVELOPMENT

PCI develops either by escape of air through a break in the mucosa or by bacterial invasion. Both mechanical and bacterial mechanisms have been proposed to explain the development of gas-filled cysts in the bowel wall. The mechanical theory suggests that gas is forced into the bowel by one or more of several routes:

1. Mucosal breaks in the epithelium
2. Direct trauma
3. Anastomotic leaks
4. Obstruction
5. Increased intraluminal pressure
6. Increased peristalsis
7. Breakdown in pulmonary acini

Mucosal breaks in the epithelium, such as those that occur in ulcerative lesions in the intestine, may permit entry of intraluminal gas, which can then be carried distally along lymphatic channels by peristalsis. Histologic descriptions of the involved colonic mucosa in patients with PCI, without inflammatory bowel disease, show local inflammatory changes and alteration of crypt architecture with cysts oriented toward these abnormal areas. Air pockets are also seen in lymphoid aggregates near mucosal breaks, suggesting that the gut is reacting to the invasion of air or other foreign material. In the face of mechanical obstruction associated with ulceration, increased peristalsis and pressure may drive intraluminal gas through mucosal defects that are too small to allow passage of intestinal contents. Pressures up to 90 mm Hg have been recorded in the intestine; these pressures may drive luminal gas through mucosal defects.

The bacterial mechanism is not mutually exclusive of the mechanical mechanism. Although organisms have not been cultured from the cysts or peritoneal fluid, experimental evidence strongly supports bacterial involvement. The following evidence supports this theory:

1. Cysts have high concentrations of H_2 that can only be produced by bacteria in humans.
2. Patients with PCI have increased fasting breath hydrogen compared with controls with inflammatory bowel disease, irritable bowel syndrome, and postvagotomy diarrhea.
3. Injection of *Clostridium tertium* and *Clostridium perfringens* in pure culture into the peritoneum of germ-free rats causes PCI.

Furthermore, *C. perfringens* is lethal when injected into a closed loop of strangulated bowel. Although *C. perfringens* occurs normally in the intestinal lumen, a functional break in the mucosa with penetration of bacteria in the submucosa might be involved in the cause of PCI.

CONDITIONS PREDISPOSING TO PCI

Several conditions may predispose to PCI. PCI may be classified as either idiopathic (15%) or secondary (85%). Idiopathic PCI is generally unsuspected and has mild symptoms described above. The conditions associated with secondary PCI (Table 84–1) can be predicted from the pathophysiologic mechanisms described above. Fulminant PCI is often associated with *intestinal ischemia or infarction* and *pseudomembranous colitis* in adults and *necrotizing enterocolitis* in neonates or immunocompromised children. PCI has been described in association with obstructing lesions in the intestine including *peptic ulcer disease with pyloric stenosis, esophageal obstruction, gastric carcinoma,* and *obstructing pancreatic carcinoma.*

Mechanical disruption of the mucosa may lead to PCI in *ulcerative colitis, Crohn's disease, tuberculous enteritis, blunt abdominal trauma,* after *gastrointestinal endoscopy,* and postoperatively after *intestinal anastomosis* or *jejunal feeding catheter placement.* PCI has been reported with *collagen-vascular disorders,* particularly *progressive systemic sclerosis,* in which there may be a combination of altered intestinal motility and mucosal breakdown from bacterial overgrowth in the small intestine. PCI has been associated with *steroid therapy* and *immunotherapy.* These

TABLE 84–1. CONDITIONS ASSOCIATED WITH PNEUMATOSIS CYSTOIDES INTESTINALIS (PCI)

Intestinal ischemia or infarction
Necrotizing enterocolitis
Peptic ulcer disease with pyloric stenosis
Intestinal obstruction or ileus
Enteritis or colitis
Blunt abdominal trauma
Gastrointestinal endoscopy
Postsurgical bowel anastomosis or jejunal catheter placement
Collagen disorders, especially progressive systemic sclerosis
Immunotherapy or chemotherapy
Chronic obstructive pulmonary disease
Cystic fibrosis
Trichloroethylene exposure
Lactulose treatment

agents cause depletion of submucosal lymphoid tissues, and the denuded Peyer's patches may produce a localized defect, permitting gas to enter the bowel wall. PCI has been reported after renal, liver, cardiac, and bone marrow transplantation, which is probably due to the associated immunotherapy. Some chemotherapeutic agents are known to cause mucosal breakdown and PCI, the most important of which are *methotrexate, daunorubicin, cytosine arabinoside, 5-fluorouracil,* and *methyl-GAG* (mitoguazone).

Chronic obstructive pulmonary disease has been frequently associated with PCI. It is postulated that air is forced under pressure into the interstitium by coughing or artificial insufflation and then dissects and tracks down to the intestine along the great vessels along the perivascular space through the mesentery to the intestinal wall. This mechanism was demonstrated experimentally in animals and unembalmed cadavers several years ago. However, there have been no reports of pneumomediastinum in association with PCI, leaving this mechanism open to question. Patients with *cystic fibrosis* may develop PCI, particularly after they develop obstructive pulmonary disease. Some authors suggest that idiopathic PCI may be explained by unrecognized chronic obstructive pulmonary disease.

Recently, the Japanese have reported several cases of PCI in workers who use *trichloroethylene* as a degreasing agent. The mechanism is unknown. *Lactulose therapy* has been associated with PCI.

TREATMENT

Supportive care may be sufficient. In adults, PCI is often an incidental finding. If the patient is asymptomatic or has very mild symptoms, no treatment is necessary (Table 84–2). If there is an offending agent, as listed above, it should be removed. Patients usually demonstrate resolution of air on abdominal films within a few weeks. Even patients who may have a severe underlying condition such as bone marrow or renal transplant do well if they are asymptomatic and followed expectantly.

In mild to moderately symptomatic patients, such as those who present with bloody stools or abdominal pain, supportive intervention, including clear liquid diet or nasogastric suction and intravenous hydration, may be necessary. An elemental diet fed for 2 weeks has been used successfully in some patients. The elemental diet

TABLE 84–2. TREATMENT OPTIONS IN PNEUMATOSIS CYSTOIDES INTESTINALIS (PCI)

Observation
Removal of the offending agent
Supportive care: intravenous hydration and nasogastric suction
Elemental diet
Oxygen therapy
Antibiotics
Sclerotherapy?
Surgery

is completely absorbed before reaching the colon, so no carbohydrates are available to gas-forming bacteria. The gas in the cysts then diffuse out into the bloodstream. PCI may recur after discontinuation of the elemental diet, but it can be reinstituted successfully. Nonetheless, an elemental diet may aggravate PCI in patients with small bowel overgrowth, when gas-forming bacteria are present in the small bowel lumen. Empiric antibiotics may be helpful. Metronidazole is a reasonable first choice. Before antibiotic therapy is initiated, a stool sample should be evaluated for the presence of *Clostridium difficile* toxin, and the patient should be treated appropriately if pseudomembranous colitis is suspected.

OXYGEN

Oxygen therapy is particularly helpful if administered cautiously. To hasten the shrinkage of gas-filled cysts, high-concentration oxygen therapy has proven successful. Oxygen may be administered by non-rebreather facemask at 50% to 70% for up to 7 to 10 days with therapy continuing at least 48 hours after radiologic resolution of the ectopic air. A rapid decrease in cyst size may be seen. During treatment, arterial oxygen tension is between 200 and 300 mm Hg and results in a partial pressure gradient of N_2 in the end-capillary and venous blood. The gradient draws the N_2 out of the cyst, and the N_2 is eliminated. The N_2 in the cyst is replaced by O_2, which is metabolized by the tissue, and the cyst collapses. Several investigators have shown the efficacy of oxygen therapy, although the gas cysts may recur after treatment is stopped.

Oxygen therapy, however, is limited by its potential for pulmonary toxicity. Toxicity is dependent on the oxygen concentration and duration of therapy. A decrease in pulmonary vital capacity is a reliable early indicator of oxygen toxicity.

Hyperbaric oxygen successfully treats PCI and avoids oxygen toxicity. Hyperbaric oxygen treatment is maintained at 2.5 atm for 2.5 hours for 2 or 3 consecutive days. As with high-flow oxygen, recurrences have been reported with hyperbaric oxygen treatment. Furthermore, hyperbaric oxygen is not readily available in most centers.

COMPLICATIONS

Pneumoperitoneum and bowel obstruction can complicate the clinical decision making. PCI is the only condition reported that causes pneumoperitoneum without peritonitis. It is critical to look carefully for evidence of PCI when a patient presents with pneumoperitoneum without abdominal symptoms. Recognizing that this is a benign condition avoids the risk of unnecessary surgery. On the other hand, if the patient presents with signs and symptoms of an acute abdomen, the abdomen must be explored for a perforated viscus, since benign PCI rarely presents with severe abdominal pain.

Endoscopic examination of the colon may diagnose benign conditions and surgery can be avoided. Although endoscopic trauma rarely induces PCI, endoscopy has been used for diagnosis without reported complications. Most benign cases of PCI are found in the left colon, whereas more serious forms are found in the small intestine and right colon. Benign PCI may rarely present with signs and symptoms of low colonic obstruction simulating a malignant rectal carcinoma. Sigmoidoscopic examination may be critical to identify the characteristic luminal grape-like projections that pop when biopsied, and unnecessary surgery can be avoided. Endoscopic sclerotherapy has been used to successfully treat a case of recurrent segmental sigmoid obstruction by PCI. Sigmoidoscopic examination may be very useful in identifying patients with pseudomembranous colitis with secondary PCI.

INDICATIONS FOR SURGERY

Since PCI may be a sign of bowel necrosis, consideration for surgical exploration should be undertaken in seriously ill patients (Table 84–3). Patients who have peritoneal signs, acidosis (pH

TABLE 84–3. INDICATIONS FOR SURGERY IN PNEUMATOSIS CYSTOIDES INTESTINALIS (PCI)

Peritoneal signs
Acidosis (pH <7.3 or HCO_3 <20)
Air in the portal vein
Volvulus
Obstruction with clinical deterioration

<7.3 or HCO_3 <20), air in the portal vein, volvulus, or bowel obstruction with deteriorating clinical signs should have surgical exploration for possible resection of nonviable bowel or relief of the obstruction. Exploration is also indicated in seriously ill infants with PCI who likely have necrotizing enterocolitis. Mortality is high even with surgery when the patient has bowel infarction or necrotizing enterocolitis, and the prognosis is better in patients with obstruction from causes other than bowel infarction. As noted above, pneumoperitoneum by itself is not an indication for surgery.

In seriously ill patients with PCI in whom an exploratory operation is being considered, an abdominal computed tomography (CT) scan can identify the underlying cause before exploration is undertaken. The abdominal CT scan is sensitive and specific for detection of air in the bowel wall. Furthermore, a CT scan can demonstrate coexisting abdominal pathology, such as the cause of a bowel obstruction or signs of intestinal infarction. The findings characteristic of PCI on CT scan are bubbly, cystic, linear, or curvilinear gas collections in the periphery of distended, partly fluid-filled loops of bowel. PCI can be distinguished from normal gas in the bowel lumen by identifying air in the dependent aspect of a cross-sectional cut of bowel. The true extent of PCI can be enhanced by using lung settings rather than abdominal settings on the scanner. Coexisting bowel pathology, such as thickening of the bowel wall or air in the portal venous system, alerts the clinician to a high probability of bowel infarction requiring surgery.

REFERENCES

1. Connor R, Jones B, Fishman EK, Siegelman SS. Pneumatosis intestinalis: role of computed tomography in diagnosis and management. *J Comput Assist Tomogr.* 1984; 8(2):269–275.

2. Galandiuk S, Fazio VW. Pneumatosis cystoides intestinalis: a review of the literature. *Dis Colon Rectum.* 1986; 29:358–363.
3. Knechtle S, Davidoff AM, Rice RP. Pneumatosis intestinalis: surgical management and clinical outcome. *Ann Surg.* 1990;212:160–165.
4. Sequeira W. Pneumatosis cystoides intestinalis in systemic sclerosis and other diseases. *Semin Arthritis Rheum.* 1990; 19(5):269–277.
5. West KW, Rescorla FJ, Grosfeld JL, Vane DW. Pneumatosis intestinalis in children beyond the neonatal period. *J Ped Surg.* 1989;24(8):818–822.
6. Yale CE, Balish E, Wu JP. The bacterial etiology of pneumatosis cystoides intestinalis. *Arch Surg.* 1974;109:89–94.
7. Yamaguchi K, Shirai T, Shimakura K, et al. Pneumatosis cystoides intestinalis and trichloroethylene exposure. *Am J Gastroenterol.* 1985;80(10):753–757.

85
Solitary Ulcers of the Colon and Rectum
ROBIN D. ROTHSTEIN and ANN OUYANG

SOLITARY RECTAL ULCERS

Solitary rectal ulcer syndrome was first described over 150 years ago but remains an incompletely and poorly understood entity.[1] The terminology *solitary rectal ulcer syndrome* is confusing, as it is a misnomer. There may be multiple ulcers instead of a solitary ulcer, or in some cases there may not be an ulcer present but instead a flat or polypoid lesion.[2]

CLINICAL FEATURES

Patients may present at any age, but generally the condition afflicts young people, usually in the second and third decades, with a slight female predominance.[3] In a study of 80 patients, the mean age was 49 years with a wide range of ages between 14 to 76 years.[4] Some patients have a long history of straining with defecation and may have required manual assistance for defecation. Patients may be asymptomatic or may present with bleeding, mucus discharge, constipation, alteration of bowel habits, or pain of abdominal, suprapubic, or rectal location.[5,6] Fecal incontinence is not uncommon. A sense of incomplete evacuation is noted by some patients and may be related to the coexistence of rectal prolapse.

Physical findings are uncommon, but patients may have abdominal tenderness, especially in the left lower quadrant. On rectal examination, sphincter tone may be lax or there may be thickening of the anterior rectal wall. Patients may have mild iron deficiency anemia secondary to recurrent, albeit generally mild, rectal bleeding. Other laboratory abnormalities are distinctly atypical. Serious complications are rare in patients with solitary rectal ulcer syndrome, but infrequently, massive bleeding may occur.

Extraintestinal manifestations are occasionally associated with solitary rectal ulcer syndrome, suggesting that perhaps in some patients, the syndrome is part of a systemic process. Erythema nodosa, recurrent oral ulcerations, and sacroiliitis have been reported. In one study of patients with solitary rectal ulcer syndrome, radiologic evidence of sacroiliitis and HLA-B27 positivity occurred in 6 of 19 patients and 4 of twenty patients, respectively.[7]

DIAGNOSTIC STUDIES

Barium radiography of the colon may demonstrate a rectal ulcer. However, the most common, albeit nonspecific, finding is nodularity of the rectal mucosa or thickening of Houston's valves (Fig. 85–1).[8] Other features, including mucosal granularity, spasm, or strictures, may also be seen.[9] A solitary rectal ulcer may not be apparent or an erroneous radiologic diagnosis, including rectal carcinoma or inflammatory bowel dis-

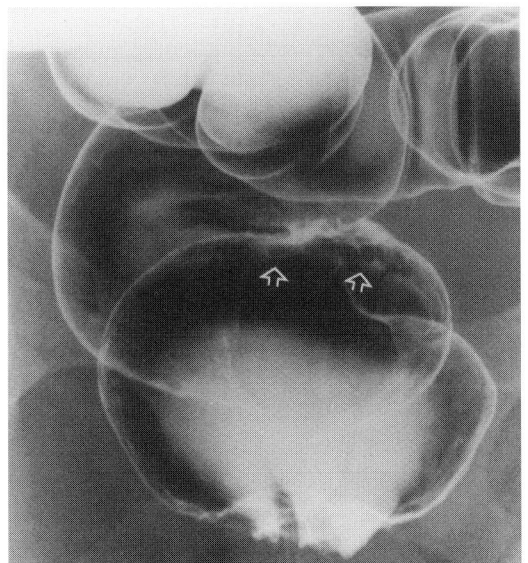

FIGURE 85-1. Focal nodularity is noted of the rectal mucosa. (Courtesy of Stephen E. Rubesin, MD.)

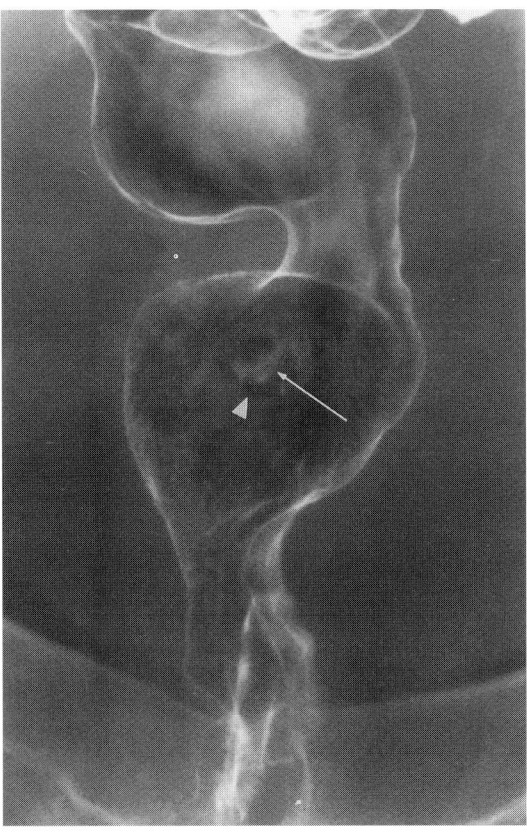

FIGURE 85-2. A solitary rectal ulcer is demonstrated in the rectal ampulla by a focal barium collection *(long arrow)* with a radiolucent halo *(arrow head)* with mild granularity of the distal rectal mucosa. (Courtesy of Stephen E. Rubesin, MD.)

ease, may be contemplated. One or more ulcers may be noted (Fig. 85–2). Less commonly, intussusception or rectal prolapse may be noted.[10] Intussusception is considered to be rectal wall infolding with downward descent into the anal canal with straining. Rectal prolapse is a more severe condition when the intussusceptum protrudes through the anal opening.

Defecography may demonstrate pelvic floor spasm.[11] A high incidence of rectal prolapse or intussusception has been noted on defecograms in patients with solitary rectal ulcer syndrome.[12,13] There may be failure of the puborectalis muscle to relax during defecation or abnormal perineal descent. Dysfunction of the puborectalis muscle may compromise the ability to expel the rectal contents. Balloon proctogram may demonstrate an increased rectoanal angle, which may remain unchanged with squeezing.[14]

Information derived from defecography can be misleading. Some findings on defecography that have been considered abnormal have been noted in normal, healthy subjects. In a comparison study of 32 controls and 32 patients with constipation or incontinence, there was no difference between the anorectal angle or anorectal junction at rest and during squeezing or straining maneuvers.[15] Despite these similarities, there are abnormalities that are more often seen in patients than controls, including intussusception, spasm of the pelvic floor, and prolapse. However, in one study mucosal prolapse was observed more frequently in control subjects than patients.[15]

A classic solitary linear or round ulcer may be found at sigmoidoscopy. Alternatively, multiple ulcers can be seen. In cases where ulceration is not noted, there may be mucosa granularity, erythema, nodules, or polyps.[16] In a review of 51 cases of solitary rectal ulcer syndrome, multiple ulcers were seen in 22%, broad-based lesions in 25%, and granularity or erythema in 18% of patients.[2]

Most ulcers are located on the anterior abdominal wall, within 5 to 10 cm from the anal verge and are 1 to 2 cm in size.[17,18] In a study of 29 total ulcers, 19 were located on the anterior or anterolateral wall of the rectum, and only 10 were located on the posterior or posterolateral wall.[7]

Histopathology

Histology has been instrumental in establishing the diagnosis of solitary rectal ulcer. In general, three criteria are used for diagnosis: fibrous obliteration of the lamina propria, hypertrophy of the muscularis mucosa with muscular fiber extension into the lamina propria, and regenerative changes of crypt epithelium.

A helpful differentiating pathologic finding is the appearance of diffuse excess mucosal collagen deposition, which is characteristic of solitary rectal ulcers and is absent in controls and patients with inflammatory bowel disease.[19] Additional pathologic findings include dilated or cystic mucosal glands, acute or chronic inflammatory infiltration, presence of granulation tissue, and mucosal ulceration. Similar histopathologic findings are noted in colonic intussusception and colitis cystica profunda, which suggests a common underlying pathophysiology.[20]

There may be an evolution of changes in solitary rectal ulcer syndrome with an initial nonulcer phase. The earliest pathologic abnormalities are believed to be fibromuscular obliteration of the lamina propria and hypertrophy of the muscularis mucosa with crypt hyperplasia. Secondary pathologic changes then ensue that result in surface erosion with ongoing, continued damage and subsequent ulcer formation. Fibrosis and hemorrhage are associated with ulcer formation, with cystic changes as part of epithelial repair.[21]

The solitary rectal ulcer syndrome must be considered in the differential diagnosis of inflammatory conditions of the rectum. Crohn's disease, ulcerative proctitis, lymphogranuloma venereum, and infectious colitis may cause similar endoscopic changes but do not cause fibro-obliterative changes of the lamina propria. Alternatively, solitary ulcer syndrome may be confused with rectal carcinoma despite the young age of patients.[22] As the entity of solitary rectal ulcer syndrome is relatively uncommon, it is probably underdiagnosed.[23]

Pathophysiology

The pathophysiology for the solitary rectal syndrome is poorly understood, and several theories have been generated to explain its origin. A basic understanding of the normal anatomy of the anorectum area and the defecation reflex is crucial. The rectum, especially in adults, follows the contour of the sacrum and then turns sharply backward below the coccyx into the anal canal. The pelvic floor provides muscular support at the level of the lower rectum and is composed of the levator ani, which forms a sling of muscle around the rectum. The function of this muscular sling is crucial to the maintenance of continence as the levators elevate the pelvic diaphragm, rectum, and anus and decrease the anal-rectal angle with defecation. The sacral plexus (S-2, S-3, S-4) innervates the levators, except for the puborectalis muscle, which is supplied by the pudendal nerve.

The anal sphincters are divided into internal (smooth muscle) and external (striated muscle) portions. The internal anal sphincter is the distal continuation of thickened circular muscle layer of the rectum. The external anal sphincter fuses with the puborectalis muscle at its superior margin, attaches to the coccyx posteriorly, and connects to the perineal body at its anterior border.

The urge to defecate is associated with internal sphincter relaxation and passage of stool into the anal canal. With sitting, the anal canal is straightened and the stool mass is pushed against the puborectalis sling. The internal anal sphincter relaxes, and the abdominal wall muscles are forcefully contracted, increasing intra-abdominal pressure. The external sphincter relaxes, and stool is passed.

Patients with solitary rectal ulcer syndrome are believed to have abnormalities of anorectal function contributing to the pathophysiology of disease. The puborectalis muscle may not relax with defecation or may paradoxically contract as documented by electromyogram and anal manometry. This abnormal muscle function is probably not sufficient to cause solitary rectal ulcer formation, as it may occur in patients with idiopathic perineal pain and patients with longstanding constipation.[24,25] Pudendal neuropathy has been considered to be an etiologic factor in puborectalis muscle dysfunction. Dysfunction of the pudendal nerve has been documented in some patients with solitary rectal ulcer syndrome, using digitally directed nerve stimulation and single-fiber electromyography.[26]

Anal manometry studies of patients with solitary rectal ulcer syndrome have demonstrated decreased resting tone and squeeze pressures, similar to findings in patients with mucosal prolapse.[27] Reduced rectal sensation and impaired internal anal sphincter relaxation also occur in some patients, despite the presence of normal ganglia on biopsy.[5] Repetitive contractions of the puborectalis muscle may be noted. The maximal intrarectal balloon volume that is tolerated is lower in patients than in controls.

There is a strong association of solitary rectal ulceration with rectal prolapse. In a study of nine patients with solitary rectal ulcer syndrome, rectal prolapse was noted in eight.[28,29] Patients may present with symptoms of the prolapse only, including local pain, incontinence, bleeding, and a sensation of incomplete evacuation. Identical anal manometry findings may occur in both patients with solitary rectal ulcer syndrome and rectal prolapse.

Rectal prolapse or intussusception may be present without the association of the solitary rectal ulcer syndrome. Thus, other factors besides rectal wall defects are important in the development of solitary rectal ulcer syndrome.[30]

Ischemia either due to prolapse or other reasons may contribute to solitary rectal ulceration. Ischemia in the presence of prolapse may cause traction of submucosal vessels or pressure necrosis of the prolapsed mucosa.[17] Bulging of the anterior rectal wall occurs with rectal prolapse and may result in erosions or ulcerations. In turn, these erosive changes may result in destruction of the muscularis mucosa followed by fibrosis and regeneration of the epithelial layer. Pseudoinvasion may follow from regenerating epithelium invading into the submucosa.[31]

Trauma has also been implicated as the cause of solitary rectal ulcer syndrome in some patients. Straining, associated with labor, may lead to trauma and damage to the anterior rectal wall.[16] Alternatively, self-digitation or repeated trauma from introduction of foreign bodies into the rectum has been described in some patients.[32]

Medications may induce solitary rectal ulcers. Ergotamine tartrate–containing suppositories, used for treatment of migraine headaches, have been implicated in the formation of solitary rectal ulcers.[33] Local vasoconstriction occurs with ergotamine, causing mucosal ischemia and ulceration of the rectum. It remains unclear if medication-induced ulcers are part of the solitary rectal ulcer syndrome, or if they represent a completely different entity.

Tuberculosis is a rare cause of solitary rectal ulcers.[34]

THERAPY

Treatment is often based on dietetic changes, including a high-fiber diet and the addition of a fiber supplement.[2] If response to fiber is inadequate, which is often the case, a trial of medication is warranted in the symptomatic patient. Sucralfate enemas have been shown to be helpful in reducing or eliminating symptoms associated with solitary rectal ulcers. Endoscopic reduction in ulcer size has been documented, although complete healing may not ensue.[35] Even in cases of complete macroscopic healing, full histologic improvement has not always occurred.[36]

Therapy with antibiotics, including metronidazole, and other medications, for example, sulfasalazine or corticosteroids, has also been used but with limited success.[37] One exception is HLA-B27–positive patients with sacroiliitis, who have a better response rate to sulfasalazine.[2] Local treatment by sclerosis or coagulation has not met with success.[16]

Persistent symptoms despite medical therapy may lead the patient to surgical intervention. Simple excision of the ulcer is not effective.[28] Rectopexy may reduce symptoms and is primarily used in patients without prolapse.[38,39] More aggressive approaches, including formation of a diverting colostomy, have been performed in patients with solitary rectal ulcer syndrome, but lack of consistent success warrants careful evaluation of this type of approach.[40]

Patients with associated complete rectal prolapse usually derive relief from surgical repair of the prolapse. Surgical intervention for rectal prolapse includes the anterior (Ripstein procedure) or posterior (Wells procedure) sling rectopexy via an abdominal approach.[41,42] For patients who are less than ideal surgical candidates, a perineal procedure may be better tolerated as the operative and anesthesia time is less. Perineal approaches include the Miles rectosigmoidectomy or Deloreme's rectal mucosectomy with plication.[43,44]

Associated with every form of medical or surgical therapy is recurrence or continuation of symptoms. Persistent abnormalities on postoperative defecography closely correlate to the recurrence of problems.[45] Thirty percent of patients continue to have symptoms 5 years after diagnosis.[46] In a study of 52 patients, there was minimal change (either improvement or worsening) of symptoms over 8 years.[16]

Therefore, although solitary rectal ulcer syndrome is considered a benign condition, the difficulty in eradicating symptoms, combined with the difficulty in obtaining histologic and macroscopic resolution, creates frustration on both the part of the patient and physician.

NONSPECIFIC ULCERS OF THE COLON

Nonspecific ulcers of the colon are rare. They are most frequently located in the cecum and the ascending colon, followed by the sigmoid as the second most common site.[47] The cause remains obscure.

CLINICAL FEATURES

Colonic ulcers occur in all age groups, with the greatest percentage occurring in the fifth to seventh decade.[48]

Similar to solitary rectal ulcers, nonspecific ulcers of the colon may cause pain and result in bleeding. In contrast, symptoms are often more acute, and perforation is more common, occurring in 19% of patients.[48] Patients with cecal ulcers may present with acute right lower quadrant pain, fever, and leukocytosis, which may lead to the erroneous diagnosis of appendicitis.[49] An abdominal mass may be palpable in the right lower quadrant.

DIAGNOSTIC STUDIES

Malignancy, inflammatory conditions, including ulcerative colitis and Crohn's disease, and infections, for example, *Entamoeba histolytica,* must be excluded in the evaluation of a patient with a colonic ulcer.

Differentiation of a nonspecific ulcer from a malignant ulcer may be difficult. Radiologic studies and colonoscopy with biopsy are crucial in the identification of a nonspecific ulcer. Although barium contrast studies may be helpful, nonspecific ulcers of the colon may resemble malignancies, including annular carcinomas.[50] Colonoscopy often demonstrates the ulcer, which is generally discrete and well circumscribed. However, surgical intervention may be necessary if the diagnosis cannot be firmly established.

HISTOPATHOLOGY

Nonspecific ulcers of the colon are often solitary, but several may be noted.[51] The lesions are usually located on the antimesenteric wall and, if cecal in location, are often within 2 cm of the ileocecal valve.[52]

Pathologically, the ulcer is nonspecific. Typical changes are seen with a necrotic base of granulation tissue and evidence of surrounding regenerative mucosa.

PATHOPHYSIOLOGY

The cause of nonspecific ulcers of the colon is unclear. Although there are reports of colonic ulcers occurring in association with some medications, including oral contraceptives, the majority of reported cases occur in patients who are not receiving drug therapy.[53]

Colonic ulceration may be the result of diverticulitis. However, diverticuli usually are located on the antimesenteric wall, opposite to the typical location of nonspecific colonic ulcers.

Alternatively, stasis has been implicated in the role of ulcer formation. The cecum is a region of stasis, thus, the reason why the majority of colonic ulcers occur in this area. Alternatively, ischemia has been considered to be a possible mechanism for colonic ulcers, as thrombi and vascular abnormalities have been noted in pathologic specimens.[54] However, colonic ulcers do not occur in the typical distribution for complications of ischemia nor do they occur more frequently in patients at risk for bowel ischemia.

THERAPY

In general, ulcers complicated by peritonitis, perforation, and uncontrollable bleeding require surgical intervention. Local excision has been performed with good results.[55,56] Hemicolectomy has also been used.[52]

The management of more benign colonic ulcers is less clear. Conservative management may be appropriate in some patients in whom the diagnosis is well established.[48] Follow-up has been limited, but spontaneous resolution does appear to occur.[51]

REFERENCES

1. Cruveilhier J. Ulcère chronique du rectum. In: *Anatomie pathologique du corps humain, II, Libre 25. Maladies du rectum.* Paris: Bailliere; 1830:4.
2. Martin CJ, Parks TG, Biggart JD. Solitary rectal ulcer syndrome in Northern Ireland 1971–1980. *Br J Surg.* 1981;68:744.
3. Womach NR, Williams NS, Mist JH, Morrison JF. Anorectal function in the solitary rectal ulcer syndrome. *Dis Colon Rectum.* 1987;30:319.
4. Tjandra JJ, Fazio VW, Church JM, Lavery IC, Oakley JR, Milsom JW. Clinical conundrum of solitary rectal ulcer. *Dis Colon Rectum.* 1992;35:227.
5. Keighley MRB, Shouler P. Clinical and manometric features of the solitary rectal ulcer syndrome. *Dis Colon Rectum.* 1984;27:507.
6. Niv Y, Bat L. Solitary rectal ulcer syndrome: clinical, endoscopic and histological spectrum. *Am J Gastroenterol.* 1986;81:486.

7. Tandon RK, Atmakuri SP, Mehra NK, Malaviya AN, Tandon HD, Chopra P. Is solitary rectal ulcer a manifestation of a systemic disease? *J Clin Gastroenterol.* 1990;12:286–290.
8. Levine MS, Piccolello ML, Sollenberger LC, Laufer I, Saul SH. Solitary rectal ulcer syndrome: a radiologic diagnosis? *Gastrointest Radiol.* 1986;11:187–193.
9. Millward SF, Bayjoo P, Dixon MF, Williams NS, Simpkins KC. The barium enema appearances in solitary rectal ulcer syndrome. *Clin Radiol.* 1985;36:185–189.
10. Goei R, Baeten C, Arends JS. Solitary rectal ulcer syndrome: findings at barium enema study and defecography. *Radiology.* 1988;168:303.
11. Kuijpers HC, Schreve RH, Hoedemakers HTC. Diagnosis of functional disorders of defecation causing the solitary rectal ulcer syndrome. *Dis Colon Rectum.* 1986;29:126.
12. Womack NR, Williams NS, Holmfield JHM, Morrison JFB. Pressure and prolapse: the cause of solitary rectal ulceration. *Gut.* 1987;28:1228.
13. Mahieu PH. Barium enema and defecography in the diagnosis and evaluation of the solitary rectal ulcer syndrome. 1986;1:85.
14. Pescatori M, Maria G, Mattama C, Vulpio C, Vecchio F. Clinical picture and pelvic floor physiology in the solitary rectal ulcer syndrome. *Dis Colon Rectum.* 1985;28:862.
15. Goei R. Anorectal function in patients with defecation disorders and asymptomatic subjects: evaluation with defecography. *Radiology.* 1990;174:121.
16. Madigan MR, Morson BC. Solitary ulcer of the rectum. *Gut.* 1969;10:871.
17. Rutter KR, Riddell RH. The solitary ulcer syndrome of the rectum. *Clin Gastroenterol.* 1975;4:505–530.
18. Schneider A, Fritze C, Bosseckert H, Machnik G. Primary clinical, endoscopic and histologic findings in solitary rectal ulcer. *Dtsch Z Verdau Stoffwechselkr.* 1988;48:183–189.
19. Levine DS, Surazicz CM, Ajer TN, Dean PJ, Rubin CE. Diffuse excess mucosal collagen in rectal biopsies facilitates differential diagnosis of solitary rectal ulcer syndrome from other inflammatory bowel diseases. *Dig Dis Sci.* 1988;33:1345.
20. Levine DS. "Solitary" rectal ulcer syndrome: are "solitary" rectal ulcer syndrome and "localized" colitis cystica profunda analogous syndromes cause by rectal prolapse? *Gastroenterology.* 1987;92:243.
21. Bogomoletz WV. Solitary rectal ulcer syndrome: mucosal prolapse syndrome.
22. Thomson G, Clark A, Handysider J, Gillespie G. Solitary ulcer of the rectum—or is it? A report of 6 cases. *Br J Surg.* 1981;68:21.
23. Saul SH, Sollenberger LC. *Am J Surg Pathol.* 1985;9:411–421.
24. Mackle EJ, Parks TG. The pathogenesis and pathophysiology of rectal prolapse and solitary rectal ulcer syndrome. *Clin Gastroenterol.* 1986;15:985.
25. Jones PN, Lubowshi DZ, Swash M, Henry MM. Is paradoxical contraction of puborectalis muscle of functional importance? *Dis Colon Rectum.* 1987;30:667.
26. Snooks SJ, Nicholls RJ, Henry MM, et al. Electrophysiological and manometric assessment of the pelvic floor in the solitary rectal ulcer syndrome. *Br J Surg.* 1985;72:131–133.
27. Sun WM, Read NW, Donnelly TC, Bannister JJ, Shorthouse AJ. A common pathophysiology for full thickness rectal prolapse, anterior mucosal prolapse and solitary rectal ulcer. *Br J Surg.* 1989;76:290.
28. Ford MJ, Anderson JR, Gilmour HM, et al. Clinical spectrum of "solitary rectal ulcer" of the rectum. *Gastroenterology.* 1984;84:1533.
29. Lowry AC, Goldberg SM. Internal and overt rectal procidentia. *Gastroenterol Clin North Am.* 1987;16:47.
30. Shovron P, Stevenson GW, McHugh •, Somers S. Defecography: a study of normal volunteers. *Radiology.* 1987;165:428. Abstract.
31. Yamagiwa H. Protruded variants in solitary ulcer syndrome of the rectum. *Acta Pathol Jpn.* 1988;38:471.
32. Kuijpers HC, Schreve RH, Hoedemakers HC. Diagnosis of functional disorders of defecation causing the solitary rectal ulcer syndrome. *Dis Colon Rectum.* 1986;29:126.
33. Shpilberg O, Ehrenfeld M, Abramowich C, Samra Y, Bat L. Ergotamine-induced solitary rectal ulcer. *Postgrad Med J.* 1990;66:483.
34. Menezes N, Waingankar VS. Solitary rectal ulcer of tuberculous origin (a case report). *J Postgrad Med.* 1989;35:118–119.
35. Kochhar R, Mehta SK, Aggarwal R, Dhar A, Patel F. Sucralfate enemas in ulcerative rectosigmoid lesions. *Dis Colon Rectum.* 1990;33:49.
36. Zargar SA, Khuroo MS, Mahajan R. Sucralfate retention enemas in solitary rectal ulcer. *Dis Colon Rectum.* 1991;34:454.
37. White CM, Findlay JM, Price JJ. The occult rectal prolapse syndrome. *Br J Surg.* 1980;67:528–530.
38. Nicholls RJ, Simson JNL. Anteroposterior rectopexy in the treatment of solitary rectal ulcer syndrome without overt rectal prolapse. *Br J Surg.* 1986;73:222.
39. McCue JL, Thomson JPS. Rectopexy for internal rectal intussusception. *Br J Surg.* 1990;77:632.
40. Delancy H, Hitch WS. Solitary rectal ulcer: a cause of life-threatening haemorrhage. *Surgery.* 1974;76:830–832.
41. Launer DP, Fazio VW, Weakley FL, et al. The Ripstein procedure: a 16-year experience. *Dis Colon Rectum.* 1982;25:41.
42. Notaeres MJ. The use of mersilene mesh in rectal prolapse repair. *Proc R Soc Med.* 1973;66:686.
43. Miles WE. Rectosigmoidectomy as a method of treatment for procidentia recti. *Proc R Soc Med.* 1933;26:1445.
44. Christianson J, Kirkegaard P. Deloreme's resection for complete rectal prolapse. *Dis Colon Rectum.* 1985;28:721.
45. Goei R, Baeten C. Rectal intussusception and rectal prolapse: detection and postoperative evaluation with defecography. *Radiology.* 1990;174:124.
46. Britto E, Borges AM, Path MRC, Swaroop VS, Jagannath P, DeSouza LJ. Solitary rectal ulcer syndrome: twenty cases seen at an oncology center. *Dis Colon Rectum.* 1987;30:381.
47. Mahoney TJ, Burbick MP, Hitchcock CR. Nonspecific ulcers of the colon. *Dis Colon Rectum.* 1978;21:623.
48. Ona FV, Allende HD, Vivenzio R, Zaky DA, Nadaraja N. Diagnosis and management of nonspecific ulcer. *Arch Surg.* 1982;117:888–894.
49. Bruheim I, Rosseland AR, Holme BF, Solhaug JH. Nonspecific ulcer of the caecum. *Acta Chir Scand.* 1986;152:71–72.
50. Gardiner GA, Bird CR. Nonspecific ulcers of the colon resembling annular carcinoma: subject review. *Radiology.* 1980;137:331–334.
51. Blundell CR, Earnest DL. Idiopathic cecal ulcer. *Dig Dis Sci.* 1980;25:494–503.
52. Cameron JR. Simple non-specific ulcer of the cecum. *Br J Surg.* 1939;26:526–530.

53. Bernardino ME, Lawson TL. Discrete colonic ulcers associated with oral contraceptives. *Am J Dig Dis.* 1976;21:503–506.
54. Butsh JL, Dockerty MB, McGill DB, Judd ES. "Solitary" non-specific ulcers of the colon. *Arch Surg.* 1969;98:171–174.
55. Iuchtman M, Heldemberg D, Auslaender L. Perforated nonspecific ulcer of the colon in children. *Eur J Pediatr Surg.* 1991;1:372–373.
56. Haraguchi M, Matsushima S, Fujie Y, Sugimachi K. Nonspecific giant ulcer of the sigmoid colon: a case report. *Jpn J Surg.* 1991;21:216–219.

86

Diversion Colitis

PAUL J. DeMARTINO and ANTHONY J. DiMARINO, JR.

Diversion colitis may be defined as mucosal inflammation occurring in an excluded colorectal segment. Its pathogenesis has not yet been fully elucidated. Often unrecognized because of its asymptomatic nature, diversion colitis is usually identified by a gastroenterologist or surgeon at endoscopy prior to intestinal reanastomosis or at the time of surgery. The major clinical significance of diversion colitis rests in the fact that some patients are denied an appropriate reanastomosis procedure because of a concern that the mucosal inflammation, identified endoscopically or histologically, may lead to clinically significant disease postoperatively. Diversion colitis was initially described by Morson and Dawson[1] in 1971. Glotzer and colleagues[2] in 1981, reported 10 patients without prior inflammatory bowel disease who developed a form of nonspecific colitis or proctitis that occurred in portions of the colorectum that were devoid of the fecal stream. Glotzer and colleagues were the first to speculate that the mucosal inflammation seen in their patients after a colostomy or ileostomy was causally related to diversion of the fecal stream and therefore coined the term *diversion colitis*.

Since the majority of patients with diversion colitis are asymptomatic, the reported prevalence of this entity is probably grossly underestimated. Orsay and colleagues[3] reported a 74% incidence in asymptomatic patients who were scheduled for colostomy closure. They concluded that diversion colitis occurs frequently in patients with a defunctionalized segment of colon with the major risk factor being the time the intestinal segment is devoid of a normal fecal stream. The clinical significance of diversion colitis remains misrecognition of its benign nature, rather than its clinical symptoms, which are only seen in the minority of patients. This lack of recognition of the benign nature of this entity may inappropriately delay or prevent closure of a temporary colostomy or ileostomy. This misunderstanding may also lead to unnecessary medical therapy for presumed more significant conditions such as ulcerative colitis, Crohn's disease, pseudomembranous enterocolitis, or ischemic colitis.

PATHOGENESIS

The exact pathogenesis of diversion colitis is unknown. However, there are several postulated mechanisms, including prolonged contact of the affected mucosa with toxic luminal contents, alteration in luminal bacterial flora, or deprivation of essential luminal nutrients. The presence of a pathogenic bacterial strain as a result of stagnation of luminal contents has been suggested, but there has been no reproducible pathogen identified to account for the nonspecific changes seen in diversion colitis. Although the pathogenesis of diversion colitis is not fully elucidated, it must not be confused with idiopathic inflammatory bowel disease, since treatment strategies are distinctly different.

Various methods of treatment that have proven to be successful in the management of diversion colitis have provided some insight into the elusive pathogenesis of diversion colitis. Stasis and subsequent bacterial invasion of the mucosa, a theory originally postulated by Morson and Dawson,[1] seems unlikely, since cultures obtained from the diverted colonic segments have failed to reveal a consistent dominant pathogen. In addition, the favorable clinical response often seen with corticosteroids seems incompatible with an infectious cause. A more widely accepted theory, proposed by Glotzer and colleagues,[2] is that fecal diversion deprives the intestinal mucosa of essential nutrients or disrupts the natural bacterial-mucosal relationships that exist in a healthy colon. In support of this theory is the prompt successful resolution of all endoscopic and pathologic changes in the previously defunctionalized colon by restoration of the fecal stream. Roediger[4] demonstrated in vitro that human colonocytes use butyric acid, a short-chain fatty acid (SCFA), as the principal source of fuel for respiration. Anaerobic bacterial flora are solely responsible for the production of SCFAs, which are directly absorbed from the bowel lumen via intact colonocytes. Harig et al[5] concluded that the missing essential nutrients were SCFAs, since local application using SCFA enemas resulted in complete resolution of diversion colitis in all four patients treated. Furthermore, diversion colitis could be kept in remission with repeated instillation of SCFAs, and relapse occurred with withdrawal of SCFAs or when control solutions were instilled via enema form. This eloquent study argues against the presumptive role of bacterial pathogens or of anaerobic bacterial overgrowth in the pathogenesis of diversion colitis and supports the role of SCFAs in prevention of this entity.

CLINICAL PRESENTATION

Most patients with diversion colitis are asymptomatic and the colitis is incidentally discovered during preoperative endoscopic evaluation of the excluded segment prior to colostomy closure. However, the minority of patients (probably less than 20%) may present with a variety of symptoms. Symptoms may include bloody or purulent discharge. If the rectum is involved, which is most often the case, symptoms may include tenesmus, anorectal pain or discomfort at defecation, and rectal bleeding or purulent discharge. The onset of such symptoms may vary from several weeks to 22 years after fecal diversion.[6] Symptomatic patients are generally not debilitated by their symptoms. However, occasionally, severe persistent symptoms may necessitate urgent reestablishment of intestinal continuity if clinically feasible. When symptoms are present, diversion colitis most closely resembles ulcerative colitis and may therefore be misdiagnosed. In addition, the pathologic changes of diversion colitis often include crypt abscesses, which further increases the likelihood of misdiagnosis. It is therefore imperative for the physician to maintain a high index of clinical suspicion of diversion colitis in symptomatic patients who have previously undergone a fecal diversion procedure.

DIFFERENTIAL DIAGNOSIS

The diagnosis of diversion colitis is primarily made by clinical features. However, characteristic endoscopic findings are described. Diversion of the fecal stream may be associated with mucosal abnormalities ranging from mild friability to gross ulcerations. Other endoscopic findings include erythema, mucous plugs, petechiae, edema, friability, mucopurulent exudate, and granularity with occasional nodular inflammatory polyps or aphthous ulcerations.[7-10] Lusk[9] reported two cases of clinically apparent diversion colitis with the occurrence of aphthous ulcerations as the major endoscopic findings. These aphthous ulcers healed after closure of the colostomy. The endoscopic findings are limited to excluded segments of colon and are focal in contrast to the continuous nature of endoscopic findings in ulcerative colitis. Most commonly, the rectum is involved in diversion colitis and the endoscopic appearance is quite similar to that in mild ulcerative colitis. The deep, often serpiginous, ulcerations and cobblestoned appearance of the mucosa in granulomatous colitis are not generally described. The dusky, cyanotic appearance of the mucosa with gross bleeding, often seen in ischemic colitis, is also not generally present in diversion colitis. The lack of pseudomembranes, a frequent history of recent extensive antibiotic use, absence of clinical toxicity and severe diarrhea, and absence of *Clostridium difficile* toxin or byproducts argue against pseudomembranous colitis in the differential diagnosis. The lack of fever, frequent diarrhea, and clinical toxicity generally eliminates an infectious colitis as a consideration.

Radiographic features described in diversion colitis have been relatively nonspecific. Air contrast barium enema may reveal a spectrum of radiographic findings in the defunctionalized segment ranging from isolated inflammatory polyps to diffuse mucosal nodularity, with or without ulcerations.[11] The radiographic appearance of diversion colitis may resemble either ulcerative or granulomatous colitis. Lechner et al[12] suggested the most common air contrast barium enema finding seen in diversion colitis is lymphoid follicular hyperplasia. They demonstrated this finding in excluded segments after colostomy in 12 of 40 patients studied (30%). Regression was demonstrated in eight patients (67%) once reanastomosis was established. The authors note, however, that lymphoid follicular hyperplasia can also be seen in inflammatory bowel disease, sarcoidosis, lower gastrointestinal tract bleeding in children, mononucleosis, lymphoma, familial polyposis coli, colon cancer, and dysgammaglobulinemia or hypogammaglobulinemia. Stein and colleagues[13] suggested the use of radionuclide techniques in helping to diagnose diversion colitis through scans of white blood cells labeled with indium 111. A focal area of prominent radionuclide activity was identified in an excluded segment of colon. This technique is quite sensitive for detecting intestinal inflammation. However, the lack of specificity of the indium 111 technique makes it of minimal value in the diagnosis of diversion colitis.

In view of the low specificity of radiographic and radionuclide techniques for the diagnosis of diversion colitis, endoscopy, histopathologic review of biopsy material, and the presence of a high clinical index of suspicion remain the main methods of diagnosis for diversion colitis.

PATHOLOGY

The histopathologic findings seen in diversion colitis may vary across a spectrum from mild to severe acute or chronic mucosal inflammation. The pathologist must make an attempt to distinguish the changes seen in segments of excluded colon from those that are typical for idiopathic inflammatory bowel disease, especially ulcerative colitis. The main pathologic finding by Murray et al[14] was an inflammatory process (confined to the mucosa) that involved the entire length of the diverted colon and rectum. The most striking finding on gross examination of the resected bowel was a diffuse nodularity involving the entire mucosa. This nodularity correlated with elevations of mucosa of normal thickness and architecture, associated with prominence and hyperplasia of lymphoid nodules throughout the specimen. This so-called nodular lymphoid hyperplasia was the most distinctive pathologic feature noted.

A variety of histologic features have previously been described and a consistent pattern has only recently emerged. Geraghty and Talbot[15] felt the most common pattern in their review of resected specimens from 15 patients with diversion colitis is a diffuse nonspecific chronic proctitis or colitis, with or without mild crypt architectural abnormalities, crypt abscesses, or follicular lymphoid hyperplasia. The presence of crypt abscesses may further confuse the uninitiated pathologist or clinician and suggest a diagnosis of idiopathic ulcerative colitis. Therefore, diversion colitis must be a well-recognized entity by both clinicians and pathologists because a mistaken diagnosis of inflammatory bowel disease can result in inappropriate treatment and unnecessary delay in anastomotic closure.

TREATMENT

Despite a variety of medical treatments for diversion colitis, the mainstay of therapy remains a reanastomosis of the excluded segment. Almost all patients demonstrate prompt reversal of the nonspecific colitis once the fecal stream is restored. Mucosal changes return to normal within 2 weeks after reanastomosis in the majority of cases. Some surgeons and clinicians have been reluctant to proceed with reanastomosis in the presence of inflammatory changes identified by previous endoscopy or radiography. These physicians have attempted to find an effective medical therapy for diversion colitis. Corticosteroids for the treatment of diversion colitis was originally suggested by Glotzer and colleagues[2]; however, Tripodi and colleagues[16] were unable to document a consistent favorable response to treatment with topical corticosteroids, and they treated their patients with 5-aminosalicylic acid (5-ASA) enemas. The authors concluded that 5-ASA enemas are a safe and effective treatment of diversion colitis via two possible mechanisms. First, the well-known antiinflammatory effects of 5-ASA enemas may be operative; interference with the formation of prostaglandins or leukotrienes by these compounds may be the mode of action. Alternatively, 5-ASA enemas also contain potassium acetate, which is a SCFA and may act as a colonic fuel source.

The most interesting form of treatment for diversion colitis is enemas containing SCFAs, which are thought to supply the essential luminal nutrients for colonocytes. Harig et al[5] noted that the instillation of enemas containing SCFAs twice daily resulted in the amelioration of symptoms and the resolution of inflammatory changes noted at endoscopy in five patients over a period of 4 to 6 weeks. Remission was maintained for up to 14 months by daily to twice weekly administered SCFAs. However, a double-blind prospective study by Guillemot et al[17] demonstrated no detectable improvement in endoscopic or histologic changes after SCFA irrigation, as compared with isotonic sodium chloride. The Guillemot study, however, differs from the Harig study, since the duration of treatment

TABLE 86–1. DIFFERENTIAL DIAGNOSIS OF DIVERSION COLITIS

Clinical Entity	Age at Onset	Symptoms	Pathology	Endoscopic Appearance	Comments
Diversion colitis	Variable	Generally asymptomatic Rectal bleeding or discharge, tenesmus, anorectal pain (~25% of patients)	Confined to mucosa Nodular lymphoid hyperplasia	Focal involvement Mild friability to gross ulcerations	Prior surgical diversion of colon Only involves excluded segment Reversed by restoring bowel continuity
Ulcerative colitis	Bimodal: 3rd–5th decades	Chronic bloody or mucopurulent diarrhea Lower abdominal cramping, fever, weight loss, tenesmus	Diffuse inflammation Crypt abscesses Distorted crypt architecture	Continuous involvement Friability, hyperemia, and granularity	Rectosigmoid colon is involved in >90% of cases Extraintestinal manifestations Increased risk of malignancy
Granulomatous colitis (Crohn's disease)	15–30 y	Diarrhea Abdominal pain Fever Weight loss	Transmural or focal inflammation Granulomas, ulcerations, fissures, fistulas	"Cobblestone" appearance Skip areas Mild edema and erythema with serpiginous ulcerations	May involve entire gastrointestinal tract (mouth to anus) Distal ileum and colon are most common sites Perianal disease Extraintestinal manifestations Smaller risk of malignancy than in ulcerative colitis
Pseudomembranous colitis	Variable	Diarrhea Abdominal pain Fever	"Summit" lesion* Adherent fibrinopurulent exudate Preservation of crypt architecture	Pseudomembranes (yellowish-white plaques)	Prior antibiotic use or chemotherapy Usually self-limited Positive *Clostridium difficile* toxin in >95% of cases
Infectious colitis	Variable	Bloody mucoid diarrhea Abdominal pain Fever	Neutrophils within 24–72 h, then plasma cells	Proctocolitis in up to 80% of patients Fecal leukocytes	Positive results from stool cultures
Ischemic colitis	Middle-aged or elderly	Abdominal pain Bloody diarrhea	Hemosiderin deposition Hemorrhagic necrosis	"Dusky" appearance Edematous, hemorrhagic, friable, and ulcerated	Prior history of ischemic heart disease or peripheral vascular disease Mild peripheral leukocytosis Watershed areas Thumbprinting on radiographs
Radiation colitis (XRT)	Variable	Bloody diarrhea Tenesmus	Vascular wall thickening	Acute: resembles acute ischemia Chronic: scarring and telangiectasias	Unpredictable time of clinical onset after XRT (months to years)

*An outpouring of fibrin, mucus, and inflammatory cells from a microulceration of the surface epithelium.

was shorter (2 weeks as compared with 6 weeks), and the concentration of SCFAs was less than the Harig study. Clearly, more studies are needed to further elucidate the role of SCFAs in the treatment of diversion colitis.

Fortunately, the majority of patients with diversion colitis are not symptomatic and clinical confusion with other forms of inflammatory bowel disease is unlikely. In such cases, if surgical reanastomosis is appropriate, it should proceed without attempts at medical therapy for diversion colitis. However, if symptoms are present, one should evaluate the patient with endoscopy and biopsy with radiographic studies performed, if clinically indicated. If, after these studies, confusion exists as to the presence of an alternative diagnosis, the clinician caring for the patient with mucosal inflammation in a diverted segment of the colon could consider an empiric trial of primary therapy for diversion colitis in the form of either topical corticosteroids, 5-ASA enemas, or SCFAs, directly instilled into the diverted segment. Alternatively, the clinician may need to consider the rare but possible presence of a complicating form of colitis in patients who have previously had the fecal stream diverted from a colonic segment. The most common differential diagnosis in such patients would include idiopathic ulcerative colitis, granulomatous colitis, pseudomembranous enterocolitis, infectious colitis, radiation colitis, or ischemic colitis (Table 86–1). Appropriate therapy for these entities may obviously differ from the therapy for diversion colitis. Fortunately, most patients with mucosal disease in an excluded segment of colon respond to either primary therapy for diversion colitis or, preferentially, to intestinal reanastomosis.

REFERENCES

1. Morson BC, Dawson IMP. *Gastrointestinal Pathology.* Boston, Mass: Blackwell Scientific Publications Inc; 1972:485.
2. Glotzer DJ, Glick ME, Goldman H. Proctitis and colitis following diversion of the fecal stream. *Gastroenterology.* 1981;80:438–441.
3. Orsay CP, Kim DO, Pearl RK, Abcarian H. Diversion colitis in patients scheduled for colostomy closure. *Dis Colon Rectum.* 1993;36:366–367.
4. Roediger WE. The starved colon-diminished mucosal nutrition, diminished absorption, and colitis. *Dis Colon Rectum.* 1990;33:858–862.
5. Harig JM, Soergal KH, Komorowski RA, Wood CM. Treatment of diversion colitis with short-chain fatty acid irrigation. *N Engl J Med.* 1989;320:23–28.
6. Ona FV, Boger JN. Rectal bleeding due to diversion colitis. *Am J Gastroenterol.* 1985;80:40–41.
7. Korelitz BI, Cheskin LJ, Sohn N, Sommers SC. The fate of the rectal segment after diversion of the fecal stream in Crohn's disease: its implications for surgical management. *J Clin Gastroenterol.* 1985;7:37–43.
8. Bosshardt RT, Abel ME. Proctitis following fecal diversion. *Dis Colon Rectum.* 1984;27:605–607.
9. Lusk LB, Reichen J, Levine JS. Aphthous ulceration in diversion colitis: clinical implications. *Gastroenterology.* 1984;87:1171–1173.
10. Korelitz BI, Cheskin LJ, Sohn N, Sommers SC. Proctitis after fecal diversion in Crohn's disease and its elimination with reanastomosis: implications for surgical management. *Gastroenterology.* 1984;87:710–713.
11. Scott RL, Pinstein ML. Diversion colitis demonstrated by double-contrast barium enema. *AJR.* 1984;143:767–768.
12. Lechner GL, Frank W, Jantsch H, et al. Lymphoid follicular hyperplasia in excluded colonic segment: a radiologic sign of diversion colitis. *Radiology.* 1990;176:135–136.
13. Stein DT, Paldi JH, Goodwin DA. In-111 leukocyte scan in "diversion" colitis. *Clin Nucl Med.* 1983;8:1–2.
14. Murray FE, O'Brien MJ, Birkett DH, et al. Diversion colitis: pathologic findings in a resected sigmoid colon and rectum. *Gastroenterology.* 1987;93:1404–1408.
15. Geraghty JM, Talbot IC. Diversion colitis: histological features in the colon and rectum after defunctioning colostomy. *Gut.* 1991;32(9):1020–1023.
16. Tripodi J, Garcey S, Burakoff R. A case of diversion colitis treated with 5-aminosalicylic acid enemas. *Am J Gastroenterol.* 1992;87(5):645–647.
17. Guillemot F, Colombel JF, Neut C, et al. Treatment of diversion colitis by short-chain fatty acids: prospective and double-blind study. *Dis Colon Rectum.* 1991;34:861–864.

87
Collagenous and Lymphocytic Colitis
FRANK K. FRIEDENBERG and GARY M. LEVINE

Collagenous colitis and *lymphocytic colitis* are terms used to describe two distinct pathologic entities that are often difficult to distinguish on clinical grounds. Both syndromes are characterized by chronic watery diarrhea and crampy abdominal pain. Patients with these conditions usually have a normal endoscopic appearance to the colon, but histologic examination of patients with either condition reveals infiltration of the lamina propria with lymphocytes and plasma cells. Collagenous colitis differs from lymphocytic colitis only on histologic grounds. In addition to epithelial inflammation, a prominent bandlike collagen deposit is present under the surface epithelium on biopsy.[9] Important differences in epidemiology also exist and are discussed at the end of this chapter. Lymphocytic colitis was formerly known as *microscopic colitis;* however this is a vague, poorly descriptive term, and the current literature suggests that it should be abandoned.

COLLAGENOUS COLITIS

Collagenous colitis was first described in 1976. In this initial description an elderly woman with crampy abdominal pain and chronic watery diarrhea eventually underwent rectal biopsy of apparently normal mucosa, which on microscopy showed a subepithelial collagen layer.[7] Since then, over 320 cases have been reported in the literature.[4]

Clinical Features of Collagenous Colitis

Patients with collagenous colitis characteristically are women in their fifth to sixth decade of life. Women are affected tenfold more often than men, although one relatively large study reported an equivalent sex ratio.[9] Although the typical patient with collagenous colitis is approximately 60 years of age, a very wide age range has been reported. Case reports of children with collagenous colitis have appeared in the literature.[9]

The predominant presenting symptom is chronic, watery diarrhea, which may be admixed with mucus.[2,7,9] Although the stool specimen may test positive for occult blood, gross hematochezia is not seen.[7] Stool white cells are not present. The number of bowel movements per day can total as many as 20, but usually averages around 5 to 10. Stool volume can range from 500 to 2000 cm^3/d (with normal being less than 150 cm^3/d). Fasting often leads to a reduction in stool volume.[2] The duration of diarrhea is often measured in years with reports of up to 20 years of diarrhea preceding the diagnosis.[9]

Another common presenting symptom is diffuse abdominal pain. As mentioned, the pain is often crampy in nature and may be associated with nausea, distension, vomiting, and flatulence.[7] In addition, mild weight loss can occur, and intestinal neoplasm is often appropriately a consideration in the initial differential diagnosis. Because of the abdominal pain, patients are often initially labeled as having irritable bowel syndrome. As discussed later in this chapter, there are important features of collagenous colitis that can be used to distinguish these conditions.[9]

Laboratory Features

There are no characteristic or pathognomonic laboratory findings in these colitides. Routine stool sample examination results for bacterial and parasitic pathogens are negative. Mild steatorrhea (7 to 10 g/d) may be present, but marked steatorrhea is distinctly unusual. For this reason Sudan black B fat stain results for fecal fat are usually negative. Collagenous colitis does not produce nutrient malabsorption so that results from other common tests for malabsorption such as serum carotene level, D-xylose absorption, and the Schilling test are usually normal.[7,9]

On occasion, patients may have an elevated erythrocyte sedimentation rate. These elevations are usually no more than two times the upper limit of normal. Mild eosinophilia, in the range of 5% to 9% of the total white blood cell count, may be present. An associated normochromic, normocytic anemia has been reported in a small number of cases. Rarely, an elevation in titers of antinuclear antibody or rheumatoid factor has been seen.[2] One recent study showed the presence of antineutrophilic cytoplasmic antibodies in collagenous colitis. Elevations in the serum immunoglobulin G level may be seen on protein electrophoresis.[4]

Associated Disorders (Table 87-1)

Histologically, collagenous colitis resembles celiac sprue (also known as gluten-sensitive enteropathy), a disease that typically affects the proximal small bowel. These conditions are similar in that both have a marked inflammatory infiltrate in the lamina propria. Submucosal collagen deposition, the hallmark of collagenous colitis, is also encountered in severe long-standing celiac sprue. Several case reports have appeared in which patients have had both collagenous colitis and sprue. In some cases, collagenous colitis improved with a gluten-free diet, the standard therapy for sprue. Rarely, patients with known celiac sprue have developed Collagenous colitis while maintaining a gluten-free diet. Currently, no dietary allergen or antigen has been implicated in the pathogenesis of collagenous colitis.

Collagenous colitis is frequently associated with autoimmune diseases. Many patients with this condition have abnormalities of thyroid function. Both hypothyroidism and hyperthyroidism are encountered in these patients, and antithyroid antibodies are often demonstrated.[9] Case reports associating collagenous colitis and diseases such as primary biliary cirrhosis, autoimmune hepatitis, rheumatoid arthritis, and scleroderma have been published.[9]

Several investigators have linked a characteristic type of arthritis with collagenous colitis. The estimated incidence is 5% to 10%. The arthritis may be monarticular or polyarticular and is characteristically nondestructive. No association between rheumatoid factor status and the presence of arthritis has been made.[4] Finally, in case-control studies, an association between the chronic use of nonsteroidal antiinflammatory drugs and collagenous colitis has been made. The association is fairly convincing, although no plausible mechanism has been elucidated.[8]

Radiology

In the investigation of patients with chronic diarrhea, radiographic studies are often obtained. Barium contrast studies of both the small and large bowel are usually normal in collagenous colitis. Rare, nonspecific findings such as loss of haustral markings and diverticulosis can be seen, but these are common findings in the elderly. In one patient with collagenous colitis, a benign stricture of the ascending colon has been reported.[7,9]

Endoscopic Findings

At colonoscopy, patients with collagenous colitis usually have a normal mucosa, and the diagnosis is not discernible to the naked eye. Occasionally, patients may have focal areas of mucosal edema, hyperemia, or friability. However, these findings are nonspecific, and their interpretation by different observers is inconsistent. Therefore, it is essential that a physician evaluating a patient with chronic, unexplained diarrhea realize that collagenous colitis and lymphocytic colitis can only be diagnosed if adequate biopsy material is obtained. In many cases, the diagnosis is not initially considered and is never made or is made after a long delay when a repeat colonoscopy and biopsy are performed.

Pathology

As mentioned, the diagnosis of collagenous colitis is made based on the clinical picture in association with characteristic pathologic material. The histologic hallmark is linear, subepithelial fibrous thickening because of collagen deposition. The collagen band is often discontinuous and may be evident only on some biopsy speci-

---

TABLE 87-1. ILLNESSES ASSOCIATED WITH COLLAGENOUS COLITIS

Celiac sprue
Autoimmune thyroid disease
Seronegative arthritis
Chronic nonsteroidal antiinflammatory drug use
Other collagen, vascular, and autoimmune disorders (e.g., autoimmune hepatitis, scleroderma)

mens from a given area. It is important to examine biopsy specimens that are well oriented, since the collagen band may be missed on poorly oriented specimens. Interestingly, the collagen found in this condition is usually type III, which is the type deposited in response to many kinds of inflammation or injury.[9] Another important histologic feature of collagenous colitis is the presence of an inflammatory cell infiltrate within the epithelium. The infiltrate consists of plasma cells, lymphocytes, mast cells, and eosinophils. In some areas of the colon, the dense inflammatory infiltrate is present without collagen deposition. In other areas, only mild inflammation is encountered, but an obvious band of collagen is present. Unlike Crohn's disease, granulomas are not found in collagenous colitis.[9] Resolution of these histologic abnormalities usually parallels improvement of the clinical condition but not always. In addition, the inflammatory infiltrate can appear prior to collagen deposition, raising the question as to whether lymphocytic and collagenous colitis simply represent a continuum of the same disease.[9]

DIFFERENTIAL DIAGNOSIS (Table 87–2)

Based on histologic appearance, at least seven other conditions can be distinguished from collagenous colitis: lymphocytic colitis, idiopathic inflammatory bowel disease (ulcerative colitis, Crohn's disease), ischemic colitis, radiation colitis, amyloidosis, scleroderma, and acute infectious colitis. The pathologist must be aware of the clinical history and endoscopic findings so as to maximize his ability to find the characteristic pathologic changes.

As previously mentioned, collagenous colitis and lymphocytic colitis are histologically distinct, although their clinical presentations and treatment are similar. Idiopathic inflammatory bowel disease is frequently suspected in patients who actually have collagenous or lymphocytic colitis. Ulcerative colitis and Crohn's disease of the colon (Crohn's colitis) are differentiated from collagenous colitis because the former usually have prominent constitutional symptoms, such as abdominal pain, fever, anorexia, and weight loss. In addition, inflammatory bowel disease is frequently associated with extraintestinal symptoms of the joints, eyes, and skin. The characteristics of the diarrhea in inflammatory bowel disease differ from collagenous colitis in that mucopurulent bloody stools are common, whereas watery diarrhea is distinctly uncommon in inflammatory bowel disease compared to collagenous colitis. Results from x-ray examination of the bowel are abnormal in ulcerative colitis and Crohn's colitis but are usually normal in collagenous colitis. Endoscopically, inflammatory bowel disease is characterized by obvious mucosal abnormalities ranging from small aphthous ulcers through a spectrum of ulceration ranging to large, undermined ulcers. Ulcerative colitis is suspected when mucosal edema, erythema, and oozing of blood from a velvety mucosa are found beginning in the rectum and extending proximally for a variable distance.

The irritable bowel syndrome is probably the most difficult condition to differentiate from collagenous colitis because both conditions are marked by diarrhea. However, the irritable bowel syndrome is different in many ways. The irritable bowel syndrome often presents with alternating constipation and diarrhea. Bowel movements often relieve abdominal distress, and weight loss is distinctly uncommon. Patients with irritable bowel syndrome often have a history of symptoms dating back to adolescence or young adulthood and rarely develop this condition in mid- to later life.

Infectious causes of diarrhea are usually self-limited and do not progress to chronicity. However, when a patient with a relatively short history of diarrhea presents, it is important to rule out infectious causes by obtaining stool specimens for ova and parasite examination, particularly for *Giardia* and *Cryptosporidium,* as well as obtaining a stool *Giardia* antigen and a *Clostridium difficile* toxin determination.

Various causes of malabsorption produce diarrhea but usually have associated clinical and laboratory evidence to differentiate them from collagenous colitis. Causes of malabsorption, such as celiac sprue, chronic pancreatitis, and Crohn's disease, should be considered in all patients with chronic diarrhea and weight loss. To

TABLE 87–2. CONDITIONS RESEMBLING COLLAGENOUS COLITIS

HISTOLOGICALLY	CLINICALLY
Ulcerative colitis	Inflammatory bowel disease
Lymphocytic colitis	Irritable bowel syndrome
Ischemic colitis	Giardiasis
Radiation colitis	Malabsorptive disorders
Amyloidosis	Laxative abuse
Scleroderma	Villous adenoma
Infectious colitis	Vipoma
	Gastrinoma
	Carcinoid syndrome

do so, quantitative fecal fat determinations, measurement of serum carotene concentration, and D-xylose absorption tests can confirm the presence or absence of malabsorption. Other blood tests that suggest the presence of malabsorption include evaluations for hypocalcemia, depressed serum iron, folate or vitamin B_{12} concentrations, and an elevated prothrombin time. Occasionally, it is necessary to perform a small bowel biopsy to determine the presence or absence of conditions such as celiac sprue, Whipple's disease, giardiasis, and cryptosporidiosis. Another common cause of malabsorption that should be considered, especially in elderly patients and in patients who have had prior gastrointestinal surgery, is the bacterial overgrowth syndrome. The presence or absence of bacterial overgrowth can be established by obtaining a small bowel aspirate for bacteriologic culture and performing a variety of breath tests that rely on bacterial metabolism of ingested substrates.

Several unusual types of tumors cause hormonal diarrhea, which can produce symptoms similar to that seen in collagenous or lymphocytic colitis. Elevated serum gastrin, vasoactive intestinal polypeptide (VIP), and urinary 5-hydroxyindoleacetic acid levels (5-HIAA) indicate a neuroendocrine tumor. Another cause of chronic watery diarrhea, albeit with abundant mucus production, is a villous adenoma of the distal colon. These tumors may be responsible for chronic diarrhea but should be easily seen on colonoscopic examination. Finally, in some patients with chronic unexplained diarrhea, there may be a factitious cause. Patients should be assessed for chronic laxative abuse by collecting a urine or stool sample for treatment with alkali. The most common cause of laxative use is surreptitious ingestion of phenolphthalein. This drug is excreted in the urine and stool and rapidly turns samples pink to red when alkali is added.

Pathogenesis

Three major hypotheses have been advanced as to the pathogenesis of collagenous colitis. The first holds that collagenous colitis arises from a prior inflammatory event such as an infection or ischemia. This idea is supported by the fact that an acute colitis is reported to occur in some patients prior to the eventual diagnosis of collagenous colitis. In addition, the response of patients with collagenous colitis to antiinflammatory agents such as sulfasalazine supports this hypothesis. Some investigators feel that the cause of inflammation is local mucosal ischemia, as no infectious precipitant has been found. Similarly, the lack of demonstrable deposition of antigen-antibody complexes or immunoglobulins argues against an immune-mediated inflammatory process.[7,9]

The second hypothesis is that collagen deposition occurs because of abnormal collagen synthesis by subepithelial fibroblasts. It is unknown what the inciting event leading to enhanced collagen synthesis or decreased collagen degradation is. This concept postulates that mature collagen-producing cells are not appropriately replaced by immature cells (which initially do not make collagen). This hypothesis fails to explain why most of the collagen is type III rather than the usual type IV. The presence of type III collagen lends more credence to the postinflammatory hypothesis.[7,9]

The third hypothesis holds that a defect in intestinal permeability allows plasma proteins such as fibrinogen to leak out of epithelial capillaries. Fibrinogen is converted to fibrin and the fibrin deposits are slowly replaced by collagen, analogous to the pathogenesis of hyaline arteriosclerosis seen in long-standing hypertension. Although minimal support for this hypothesis is currently available, it is worthy of further study.[7,9]

Cause of Diarrhea

The volume of diarrhea in patients with collagenous colitis is unrelated to the subepithelial collagen layer. No correlations have been established between the thickness and the extent of collagen deposition and clinical symptoms. The diarrhea in collagenous colitis is most probably secretory. Whatever the inciting event, inflammation leads to the release of many mediators such as prostaglandins, prostacyclins, and leukotrienes that produce active secretion of chloride across the chronic epithelium. Sodium and water passively follow the chloride ion, producing an isotonic electrolyte solution.

Several lines of evidence support secretion. First, diarrhea often continues despite fasting, although fasting ameliorates the volume of diarrhea to some degree. Second, fecal electrolyte measurements show that most of the osmolarity of the stool is accounted for by the presence of electrolytes in the diarrheal stool. Twice the sum of the sodium and potassium concentrations usually accounts for most of the osmolarity. The presence of a secretory diarrhea rules out malabsorption or bacterial overgrowth, both of which cause osmotic "gaps."

TREATMENT

The treatment of collagenous colitis requires a high degree of security in the certainty of the diagnosis, since the proposed treatments are not without potential toxicity. In addition, since spontaneous remissions occur in collagenous colitis, the benefits of treatment may be difficult to assess. Most authorities suggest a trial of sulfasalazine at a dosage of 2 to 3 g/d. It is recommended that it be used for 3 to 6 months with an assessment of efficacy made after that time period. Monitoring for leukopenia and sulfa allergy is necessary. Prednisone in dosages of 10 to 20 mg/d may be used in refractory cases.[2] Because there may be no change in histologic findings despite symptomatic improvement from these therapies, the role of repeat colonoscopy after treatment is unclear.[2]

LYMPHOCYTIC COLITIS

Lymphocytic colitis, formerly called microscopic colitis, is very similar to collagenous colitis and need not be discussed in extensive detail, since most information has been highlighted in the discussion of collagenous colitis. Lymphocytic colitis is a chronic secretory diarrhea. Patients often complain of crampy abdominal pain and usually have normal results from radiographic studies. In lymphocytic colitis, an array of associated diseases occurs, as discussed for collagenous colitis, including celiac disease and thyroid abnormalities.[9] In addition, lymphocytic colitis has a normal appearance on x-ray examination and to the naked eye during colonoscopy.

Histologic examination reveals a dense chronic inflammatory infiltrate in the submucosa, but no collagen deposition is seen. Lymphocytic colitis differs from collagenous colitis in two important ways. First, lymphocytic colitis is found as commonly in women as in men, whereas collagenous colitis is more commonly found in women. Second, biopsy specimens show epithelial inflammation similar to collagenous colitis with no evidence of collagen deposition. Many investigators feel that lymphocytic colitis and collagenous colitis represent a spectrum of the same disease. The literature documents cases where colonoscopy showed only epithelial inflammation, but the patient later developed collagen deposition.[9] The same treatments used for collagenous colitis are proposed for lymphocytic colitis. In one study 13 of 16 patients showed improvement when treated with either sulfasalazine or oral corticosteroids. As with collagenous colitis, patients show improvement when treated with antidiarrheal agents such as loperamide or diphenoxylate. In many instances, improvement occurs despite or without treatment.

In summary, collagenous and lymphocytic colitis are difficult problems to manage. Hopefully, as these conditions are more frequently recognized we will learn more about their natural history and pathogenesis, allowing more rational and effective treatment.

REFERENCES

1. Bo-Linn GW, Vendrell DD, Lee E, Fordtran JS. An evaluation of the significance of microscopic colitis in patients with chronic diarrhea. *J Clin Invest.* 1985;75:1559–1569.
2. Giardiello FM, Bayless TM, Jesserun J, et al. Collagenous colitis: physiologic and histopathologic studies in seven patients. *Ann Intern Med.* 1987;106:46–49.
3. Giardiello FM, Lazenky AJ, Bayless TM, et al. Lymphocytic (microscopic) colitis: clinicopathologic study of 18 patients and comparison to collagenous colitis. *Dig Dis Sci.* 1989;34:1730–1738.
4. Giardiello FM. A review of atypical colitides: collagenous and lymphocytic colitis. *Prog Inflammatory Bowel Dis.* 1993;14:1–4.
5. Kingham JGC. Microscopic colitis. *Gut.* 1991;32:234–235.
6. Mills LR, Schuman BM, Thompson WO. Lymphocytic colitis: a definable clinical and histological diagnosis. *Dig Dis Sci.* 1993;38:1147–1151.
7. Ramo H, Rogers AI, Ghandur-Mnaymneh L. Collagenous colitis. *Ann Intern Med.* 1987;106:108–113.
8. Riddele RH, Tanaha M, Mazzoleni G. Non-steroidal anti-inflammatory drugs as a possible cause of collagenous colitis: a case-control study. *Gut.* 1992;33:683–686.
9. Stampfl DA, Friedman LS. Collagenous colitis: pathophysiologic considerations. *Dig Dis Sci.* 1991;36:705–711.
10. Sylwestroiwicz T, Kelly JK, Hwany WS, et al. Collagenous colitis and microscopic colitis: the watery diarrhea-colitis syndrome. *Am J Gastroenterol.* 1989;84:763–768.

88

Infectious Proctitis in the Immunocompetent

RICHARD W. TOBIN and CHRISTINA M. SURAWICZ

A wide variety of infectious organisms can cause inflammation of the rectal mucosa. This can be classified as either proctitis or proctocolitis. Proctitis is characterized by symptoms that are localized to the anorectal area, including anorectal discomfort or pain, tenesmus, constipation, and mucopurulent discharge. These symptoms are due to inflammation of the distal 15 cm of colon and anal canal. Most venereal causes of anorectal disease are limited to the anus or distal rectum and are associated with anal intercourse or oral-anal contact. Proctocolitis, or inflammation of the intestinal mucosa extending proximal to 15 cm from the anal verge, is due to other infectious organisms. These organisms not only produce the symptoms of proctitis but can also cause bloody or watery diarrhea, abdominal cramps, and bloating. Table 88–1 lists the common sexually transmitted diseases (STDs) responsible for anorectal disease. Table 88–2 lists the symptoms and common infectious causes of proctitis and proctocolitis. Acute onset of symptoms is characteristic in infectious proctitis and proctocolitis. Most of the syndromes are self-limited and resolve spontaneously over several days. This chapter briefly reviews the specific causes of proctitis and proctocolitis, discusses the appropriate evaluation of patients with these symptoms, and outlines the empiric and specific treatments available.

SPECIFIC CAUSES OF PROCTITIS

GONORRHEA

Neisseria gonorrhoeae, a gram-negative intracellular diplococcus, is one of the most common STD pathogens in the world. From 28% to 55% of homosexual men at screening STD clinics have positive cultures for *N. gonorrhoeae,*[1] and the rectum is the only site infected in up to 50% of these cases.[2] Transmission is felt to be due to anal-receptive intercourse. In women, the vast majority of patients have concomitant cervical or urethral infection, and transmission is felt more often to be due to autoinoculation into the lower rectum. Isolated anorectal gonorrhea in women occurs only in 0% to 20% of patients, most often less than 10%.[1,3] Most cases are asymptomatic.[4,5] Minimal symptoms such as anal itching and irritation, sensation of rectal fullness, constipation, or mucoid discharge are less common. More acute symptoms include severe rectal burning, tenesmus, hematochezia, mucopurulent drainage, or ischiorectal abscess and account for only approximately 5% of cases.[6] Disseminated disease, which can include perihepatitis, meningitis, endocarditis, pericarditis, and gonococcal arthritis, occurs rarely. The most frequent finding at anoscopy is mucus or mucopus in the anal canal. By applying gentle external pressure during anoscopy, mucopus can often be expressed from the anal crypts under direct visualization and obtained for culture. The proctoscopic appearance is usually normal. Inflammation, if present, causes erythema with localized areas of friability and superficial erosion, confined to the distal 10 cm of the rectum and usually most prominent just above the dentate line. Biopsy is nonspecific, showing patchy disorganization and derangement of the columnar mucus-secreting cells and a mild increase in lymphocytes, plasma cells, and neutrophils in the lamina propria.[7] Diagnosis is best made by culture, since a Gram stain of rectal exudate has been reported as only 58% sensitive.[8] Specimens for culture are best obtained under direct visualization through an anoscope; however, excellent results can be obtained by blindly placing a sterile cotton swab 2 cm into the anal canal, rotating the swab from side to side, and allowing several

TABLE 88–1. SEXUALLY TRANSMITTED DISEASE PATHOGENS CAUSING ANORECTAL DISEASE

Bacteria
Campylobacter sp.
Chlamydia trachomatis
Neisseria gonorrhoeae
Shigella sp.
Treponema pallidum

Parasites
Entamoeba histolytica

Viruses
Herpes simplex virus
Cytomegalovirus
Human papillomavirus

---

seconds for absorption of organisms.[9] Swabs should be discarded if fecal material is obtained, and the test repeated. Specimens for culture should be obtained from other sites, including urethral and pharyngeal cultures in men and women and endocervical cultures in women. Best results are achieved if the specimen is immediately inoculated onto a Thayer-Martin media. A fluorescent antibody technique can be used when gonorrhea is suspected. Isolation of gonorrhea in a homosexual man does not prove gonococcus is responsible for the patient's symptoms, as there is a high prevalence of asymptomatic anorectal gonorrhea, and mixed infections are common in this population. As many nondiagnostic Gram's stains are false-negatives, a high index of suspicion warrants empiric treatment pending culture results.[10] Treatment consists of ceftriaxone, 125 mg intramuscularly, followed by doxycycline, 100 mg orally twice daily for 7 days (to cover possible concomitant chlamydial infection), should be given. As with any STD, all sexual contacts should be treated, and the patient should refrain from sexual contact until cure is proven. Rare complications of untreated anorectal gonorrheal infection include rectal stricture, anal fistulas, fissures, perianal abscesses, and rectovaginal fistulas[1] (Table 88–3).

SYPHILIS

The spirochete *Treponema pallidum* may cause anorectal infection. In homosexual men the prevalence rates are as high as 5% to 10%.[11] Transmission is felt to result from anal intercourse following an incubation period of 9 to 90 days, but primary syphilis usually occurs about 3 weeks after exposure.[12] The patient is often asymptomatic but may have symptoms similar to gonorrheal anorectal infections with prominent perianal pain. The initial chancre is classically at the anal margin or canal. This lesion may be missed, as it can mimic a rectal fissure, fistula, idiopathic rectal ulcer, or even a colonic polyp or carcinoma.[13] In the absence of ulceration or other focal lesion, diffuse distal proctitis has been reported.[13] Inguinal lymphadenopathy is often seen and should aid in making the diag-

TABLE 88–2. COMMON SIGNS, SYMPTOMS, AND PATHOGENS CAUSING PROCTITIS OR PROCTOCOLITIS IN HOMOSEXUAL MEN

SYNDROME	SYMPTOMS	SIGMOIDOSCOPY	PATHOGEN
Proctitis	Anal discharge Anal pain Tenesmus Constipation Mucopurulent discharge	Abnormal distally Below 15 cm in the rectum	Neisseria gonorrhoeae Treponema pallidum Chlamydia trachomatis (Non-lymphogranuloma venereum) Herpes simplex virus Human papillomavirus
Proctocolitis	Anorectal symptoms plus watery or blood diarrhea Abdominal cramps Bloating	Abnormal proximal to 15 cm from anal verge	Shigella sp. Entamoeba histolytica Campylobacter sp. C. trachomatis (lymphogranuloma venereum) Clostridium difficile Escherichia coli Salmonella sp. Yersinia Cytomegalovirus Cryptosporidium

TABLE 88-3. CORRELATION OF SYMPTOMS AND PHYSICAL FINDINGS WITH PATHOGENS CAUSING PROCTITIS OR PROCTOCOLITIS

ORGANISM	CHARACTERISTIC SYMPTOM	ANOSCOPY OR SIGMOIDOSCOPY	LABORATORY DIAGNOSIS	TREATMENT
Neisseria gonorrhoeae	Anal discharge	Proctitis, mucopurulent discharage	Thayer-Martin culture of discharge	Ceftriaxone 125 mg IM + doxycycline 100 mg PO b.i.d. × 7 d
Treponema pallidum	Rectal pain	Anal ulcer or condyloma lata	Dark field examination of fresh scraping; serology	Penicillin G benzathine, 2.4 million units IM (see text)
Chlamydia	Tenesmus	Friable, often ulcerated rectal mucosa; occasional rectal mass	Culture of infected material Immunofluorescent antibody and ELISA tests	Tetracycline, 500 mg, or doxycycline, 100 mg, PO q.i.d. × 7–14 d for non-LGV and 21 d for LGV
Herpes simplex virus	Anorectal pain, occasional urinary retention, impotence dysesthesias	Perianal erythema, vesicles, ulcers; diffusely inflamed, friable rectal mucosa	Viral culture of vesicular fluid, cytologic examination of scrapings	Acyclovir (see text)
Human papillomavirus	Pruritus	Condyloma acuminata	Biopsy (if needed)	Podophyllotoxin, CO_2, laser therapy, cryosurgery
Shigella sp. Enteroinvasive *Escherichia coli* *Yersinia* *Salmonella* sp.	Abdominal cramps, fever, tenesmus, bloody diarrhea	Erythema, edema, and grayish white ulcerations of rectal mucosa	Stool culture	Supportive (fluoroquinolone antibiotic if needed)
Campylobacter	Diarrhea, cramps, bloating	Same as above	Stool culture with selective media	Supportive (fluoroquinolone antibiotic if needed)
Enterohemorrhagic *Escherichia coli*	Abdominal cramps, bloody diarrhea, hemolytic-uremic syndrome, thrombocytopenic thrombotic purpura	Same as above	Stool culture with serotyping	Supportive
Cytomegalovirus	Fever, anorectal pain	Mucosal friability and ulcerations	Culture of biopsy	Supportive (ganciclovir if immunocompromised)
Clostridium difficile	Diarrhea, crampy abdominal pain, tenesmus	Pseudomembranes	*Clostridium difficile* culture and toxin of stool	Metronidazole, 250 mg PO t.i.d. × 10 d, or vancomycin, 125–500 mg PO q.i.d. × 10 d

Adapted with permission from Wexner SD. Sexually transmitted diseases of the colon, rectum, and anus. *Dis Colon Rectum*. 1990;33:1048–1062.

nosis. Rectal syphilis with lymphadenopathy can be mistaken for lymphoma.[14] Secondary anal syphilis occurs approximately 6 to 8 weeks after the primary chancre has healed. The classic finding is condyloma latum, a pale-brown or pink flat verrucous lesion or mucocutaneous rash. This lesion often secretes mucus and is sometimes associated with a foul-smelling odor and pruritus ani. Although extremely rare in Western countries, tertiary syphilis involving the anorectal area can occur. Tabes dorsalis can produce anal sphincter paralysis and severe perianal pain, and syphilitic rectal gumma can be mistaken for malignant growths.[10] Biopsy of infected tissue can reveal an intense infiltrate of plasma cells. Granulomas may sometimes be present. A silver stain may reveal spirochetes in the tissue, but nontreponemal spirochetes also stain positive. The diagnosis is usually made with dark field microscopy of scrapings from the base of a chancre or from condyloma latum, revealing corkscrew-shaped, motile, fluorescent yellowish-green organisms. However, the nonpathogenic spirochetes often present in normal bowel[15] may complicate dark field examination interpretation. Results from the fluorescent treponemal antibody absorption (FTA-ABS) test usually become positive about 4 to 6 weeks after infection. Results from the rapid plasma reagin (RPR) test and Venereal Disease Research Laboratory (VDRL) test become positive after the FTA-ABS test, with a positive VDRL in about 75% of untreated primary syphilis cases and approaching 100% in secondary syphilis.[10] Treatment is penicillin G benzathine 2.4 million units intramuscularly. If long-standing disease is present, this dose may need to be repeated once a week for 3 weeks. Penicillin-allergic patients can be treated with tetracycline or erythromycin, 500 mg four times daily for 15 to 30 days. Again, it is important that all sexual contacts be sought out and treated. Follow-up VDRL or RPR testing should be done at 3-month intervals for 1 year to document a decrease in titer. Patients and contacts should abstain from sexual contact until proven noninfectious by low titers.

CHLAMYDIA

Chlamydia trachomatis, an obligate intracellular pathogen, is a common STD in the United States. *C. trachomatis* has been isolated from the rectum in 4% to 8% of homosexual men attending STD clinics.[5] Transmission is thought to occur via anal-receptive or oral-anal intercourse, and chlamydial proctitis often coexists with other rectal STDs, especially gonorrhea. Chlamydial serotypes D–K are responsible for proctitis, whereas the lymphogranuloma venereum (LGV) serotypes L1, L2, and L3 cause lymphogranula venereum. Non-LGV serotypes can cause a proctitis similar to gonorrhea and syphilis. Severe proctocolitis, often associated with fever and bloody diarrhea, is more characteristic of LGV serotypes. Furthermore, painful anal or perianal ulcerations, strictures, and fistula formation are usually associated with the LGV serotypes.[16,17] Inguinal adenopathy (buboes) occurs with the LGV serotypes.[18] Endoscopic findings include mucosal erythema, friability, and ulceration. Biopsy specimens containing non-LGV serotypes usually reveal only scattered polymorphonuclear cells in the lamina propria. In contrast, biopsy specimens from LGV infected tissue may reveal crypt abscesses, granulomas, and giant cells, findings similar to those in Crohn's disease.[17,19] Confirmation of clinical diagnosis can be difficult. Culture of infected discharge or biopsy material remains the gold standard with an estimated 80% to 90% sensitivity.[20] Fluorescent monoclonal antibody and enzyme-linked immunosorbent assay (ELISA) tests are also available for more rapid diagnosis with reported sensitivity from 81% to 100% and specificity from 82% to 100% versus culture.[20] Antichlamydial antibody titers as determined by complement fixation rise to a level of >1:80 usually 1 month or more after infection[10] but are species specific. Treatment is tetracycline, 500 mg orally four times daily, doxycycline, 100 mg twice daily, or erythromycin, 500 mg four times daily, for 10 to 14 days for non-LGV or for 21 days for LGV strains. Ideally, cultures should be obtained after treatment to verify success. Residual rectal strictures can be a complication of chronic *C. trachomatis* infection. Other more common causes for rectal strictures, including inflammatory bowel disease and ischemia should be ruled out. If the stricture is asymptomatic in an adequately treated patient, no further therapy is needed. For symptomatic strictures, treatment with a 3-week course of tetracycline, doxycycline, or erythromycin should be undertaken; but if unsuccessful, surgery may be required.[10]

HERPES SIMPLEX VIRUS TYPE 2

Herpes simplex virus type 2 (HSV-2) is a common cause of anorectal infection. Six percent to 30% of homosexual men with rectal symptoms are found to have HSV. In one third of these cases HSV is associated with other pathogenic organisms.[21-23] HSV-2 is by far the most common cause, but HSV-1 anorectal infection can occur.[21] Transmission occurs by direct inoculation via anal-receptive intercourse, with symptoms usually beginning 4 to 21 days after exposure. Nonspecific anorectal symptoms such as itching, tenesmus, constipation, or hematochezia may occur, but severe pain is particularly characteristic of herpes simplex infection.[22] Some patients present with urinary retention, impotence, or dysesthesias consistent with a lumbosacral radiculopathy involving the L-4, L-5, and S-1 nerve roots.[24] The symptoms of this radiculopathy often outlive the active clinical infection. On examination, small vesicles to aphthous coalesced ulcers are often evident in the anal canal or perianal area. Inguinal adenopathy is present in about two thirds of cases.[11] Sigmoidoscopy can reveal vesicular or pustular rectal lesions and diffuse friability and ulceration of the distal rectum. Viral culture of vesicular fluid is 90% sensitive, and several antigen detection techniques such as direct immunofluorescence test, immunoperoxidase staining, and ELISA are available. These are generally less expensive and more available than viral culture techniques. Most studies suggest a sensitivity of 70% to 90% compared to viral culture.[25] Cytologic scrapings or biopsies of an ulcer are less sensitive but can reveal the typical intranuclear inclusion bodies, perivascular cuffing of lymphocytes, and multinucleated giant cells. Symptoms usually resolve within 2 weeks, but viral shedding can occur over an additional 2 weeks. Thereafter, patients follow one of three courses: (1) asymptomatic, culture negative; (2) recurrent episodes of a milder nature; or (3) asymptomatic, but continue to shed virus for long periods.[26] Sitz baths, lidocaine ointment, and oral analgesics may be helpful for symptomatic relief. Treatment of first-episode rectal herpes with acyclovir, 400 mg orally 5 times a day for 5 to 10 days, has been shown to produce significant decreases in the duration of viral shedding, presence of the lesions themselves, and length of symptoms.[27] Topical acyclovir is less effective. Intravenous acyclovir at a dosage of 5 mg/kg every 8 hours for 5 to 7 days may be appropriate for patients with severe anorectal herpes or for immunocompromised patients. Recurrent herpes episodes tend to be less severe and heal more quickly. Oral acyclovir is probably modestly effective.[25] Topical acyclovir is ineffective for recurrent herpes. Immunosuppressed patients may benefit from suppressive therapy, and patients with acyclovir-resistant herpes may be candidates for foscarnet or vidarabine.[28,29]

Condyloma Acuminatum

Although they usually do not cause a true proctitis, condyloma acuminata (venereal warts) are a significant cause of anorectal pathology. Human papillomavirus (HPV), the infectious cause of venereal warts, is transmitted via anal intercourse. Up to 50% of homosexual men presenting for proctoscopic examination have evidence of venereal warts, with about 10% of these visible only on anoscopic examination.[30] The warts are usually asymptomatic unless they obstruct passage of stool, but they can be associated with pruritus, bleeding, or odor. On examination, condyloma acuminata are pink to brown papules, usually occurring in clusters and occasionally in large cauliflowerlike masses. Condyloma lata of secondary syphilis, in distinction, tend to be moist, flat papules that have positive results on dark field microscopy. Initial treatment is application of podophyllotoxin; however, if this is unsuccessful, carbon dioxide laser therapy or cryosurgery can be used to ablate the lesions. All forms of therapy carry a high recurrence rate.

SPECIFIC CAUSES OF PROCTOCOLITIS

Shigellosis

Shigella flexneri and *Shigella sonnei* are well-known gastrointestinal pathogens that can cause enteritis or proctocolitis. Transmission is very efficient; as few as 10 organisms can cause infection via a fecal-oral route.[10] Sexual transmission can be via direct or indirect fecal-oral contamination; this is a common method of transmission, as 30% to 50% of patients with *Shigella* are homosexual men.[31,32] Symptoms classically include abrupt onset of crampy abdominal pain, fever, and watery or bloody diarrhea, but asymptomatic carriage can occur. Sigmoidoscopic examination may reveal nonspecific changes consistent with colitis, including patchy hyperemia, petechiae, exudate, and friable mucosa. Gram's stain of rectal discharge often shows white blood cells, and culture is diagnostic. Supportive therapy with hydration and avoidance of antidiarrheal drugs (which can exacerbate cramps, potentiate toxic megacolon, and prolong shedding of the organism) are the mainstays of treatment. Antimicrobial therapy is generally not needed, but if used, choice should be based on sensitivity studies. Treatment with a quinolone antibiotic or trimethoprim-sulfamethoxazole double-strength tablets, one orally twice daily for 7 days, is often successful. It is generally accepted that three consecutive stool specimens negative for *Shigella* indicate resolution of infection.

Amebiasis

Entamoeba histolytica is a protozoan that can exist in a cyst or trophozoite form in the human intestine and cause proctocolitis. Transmission usually occurs via the fecal-oral route, and venereal transmission can occur via oroanal intercourse. Prevalence studies of North American homosexuals screened in STD clinics showed 20% to 32% were passing amebic cysts.[33] Some individuals harbor *E. histolytica* in their stools but do not have intestinal symptoms. This presentation is especially common in homosexual men. It is likely that these amebas have different characteristics and are less pathogenic than those causing symptomatic disease. Symptoms including abdominal pain, diarrhea with or without blood, fever, malaise, and tenesmus can occur. Toxic megacolon and perforation have been reported.[34] Sigmoidoscopy may reveal a nonspecific colitis or the more characteristic picture of punched-out "hourglass" ulcers that contain the trophozoites.[35] Colonoscopy may be necessary to make the diagnosis, as the ulcers are most common in the cecum and ileum. Diagnosis can be made by the analysis of a fresh stool sample for ova and parasites. Ninety percent of stools from symptomatic patients contain amebic trophozoites.[36] If multiple stool collections for ova and parasites are negative and colonoscopic biopsy fails to reveal the diagnosis, amebic indirect hemagglutination titer may establish the diagnosis. Treatment for patients thought to be asymptomatic carriers is controversial. In endemic areas, it may not be worthwhile to treat the patient, as likelihood of reinfection is very high. However, asymptomatic carriers in nonendemic areas should be treated with iodoquinol (Diiodohydroxyquin), 650 mg orally three times daily for 3 weeks. For proctitis or dysentery, oral metronidazole, 750 mg orally three times daily for 10 days, is given. For severe cases oral iodoquinol (Diiodohydroxyquin) is given subsequent to the metronidazole. An alternate to metronidazole for the treatment of amebic colitis is paromomycin sulfate, 25 to 35 mg/kg/d in three divided doses daily for 1 week. Other amebic species that infect the gastrointestinal tract, including *Entamoeba coli*, *Entamoeba hartmanni*, and *Endolimax nana*, are not associated with known human intestinal disease.

CAMPYLOBACTER

Campylobacter sp. including *C. jejuni*, *C. fetus*, and *C. hyointestinalis* cause acute diarrhea in humans, and *C. cinaedi* and *C. fennelliae* have also been associated with acute proctitis in homosexual men.[5,37] Transmission is acquired through ingestion of contaminated milk, water, or food or through close contact with an infected animal or person. Venereal transmission likely occurs, as *Campylobacter* is seen more frequently in homosexual men than in matched heterosexual controls.[10] Approximately 6% of symptomatic and 3% of asymptomatic homosexual men have positive stool cultures for *Campylobacter*.[38] Symptoms include watery diarrhea sometimes mixed with blood, abdominal cramps, and bloating. Arthralgias, fever, and tender hepatosplenomegaly have been reported.[39] Involvement of the small intestine, colon, and rectum may occur. Sigmoidoscopic findings are similar to those in *Shigella* infection and may extend proximally at least to the descending colon. Rectal biopsy specimens may show acute nonspecific inflammation with crypt abscesses and numerous polymorphonuclear neutrophil leukocytes (PMNs). No classic granulomas are seen, but microgranulomas can be present. Gram's stain of rectal discharge will usually reveal PMNs. Culture of the organism on selective media in a microaerophilic atmosphere is diagnostic. Treatment is mainly supportive, as most cases resolve spontaneously over several days. In severe cases or in an attempt to decrease the period of infective shedding, antibiotics may be used. Fluoroquinolone antibiotics or erythromycin, 500 mg orally four times daily for 7 days, is effective.

OTHER ENTERIC PATHOGENS

Although usually involving the more proximal gastrointestinal tract, nontyphoidal *Salmonella* sp., *Escherichia coli*, and *Yersinia enterocolitica* may cause proctocolitis. Nontyphoidal *Salmonella* sp. can cause diarrhea with mucus and pus and cause significant tenesmus, fever, and chills. Food-borne and fecal-oral transmission commonly may occur and cause an idiopathic colitis that may be difficult to distinguish from inflammatory bowel disease.[40] White blood cells are often seen on Gram's stain of the stool, and diagnosis is confirmed by culture. Antibiotics usually are not used and can prolong intestinal carriage. Antibiotics are indicated for complicated infections.

Enteroinvasive *E. coli* (EIEC) can cause bloody diarrhea, fevers, chills, and tenesmus in a syndrome that can be indistinguishable for shigellosis. Transmission is usually via contaminated food. Ulceration and inflammation of the rectal and colonic mucosa reflect the invasion of colonic epithelium by the organism. Stool evaluation with deoxyribonucleic acid (DNA) probes and ELISA techniques are now available for diagnosis. Enterohemorrhagic *E. coli* (EHEC) caused by *E. coli* 0157:H7 can also cause bloody diarrhea and symptoms similar to EIEC but rarely with high fever. EHEC has been associated with hemolytic-uremic syndrome (HUS) and thrombocytopenic thrombotic purpura (TTP).[41] *E. coli* 0157:H7 ferments sorbitol slowly and appears negative on a MacConkey-sorbitol agar. Antigen-specific antisera can be used to specifically identify colonies of *E. coli* 0157:H7.[42] Antibiotics have been advocated for EIEC, but most authors feel antibiotics for EHEC are not currently justified, as they neither shorten the course, eliminate carriage, nor prevent the complications of *E. coli* 0157:H7.[41,43]

Yersinia organisms are gram-negative coccobacilli that can cause a proctocolitis. Fecal-oral and person-to-person transmission can occur. Symptoms usually include tenesmus, watery blood-streaked diarrhea, low-grade fever, and constitutional symptoms. Sigmoidoscopic findings are similar to shigellosis, and as with most enteric pathogens, white blood cells are seen on Gram's stain. Diagnosis can be made by both bacteriologic and serologic means, but specific laboratory techniques may need to be requested for culture. Antibiotics are recommended only for complicated infections.

CLOSTRIDIUM DIFFICILE

Clostridium difficile has been implicated as a cause of proctocolitis, usually associated with recent antibiotic use. Symptoms include diarrhea and crampy lower abdominal pain with occasional tenesmus, vomiting, and fever. Fecal leukocytes are usually present. Sigmoidoscopy reveals the characteristic yellow-white raised plaques scattered over the colonic mucosa, but in about 38% of cases the lesions may spare the rectum and appear only higher in the colon.[44] These pseudomembranes can become confluent, giving the appearance of a shaggy white or yellowish membrane.[45] Diagnosis is usually confirmed by detection of cytotoxin B in the stool. Biopsy specimens of pseudomembranes reveal an outpouring of fibrin, mucus, and inflammatory cells from a microulceration of the surface epithelium. Fulminant colitis can occur secondary to *C. difficile* infection. Treatment is metronidazole, 250 mg orally three times daily for 10 days, or vancomycin, 125 to 500 mg orally four times daily for 10 days.

CYTOMEGALOVIRUS

Cytomegalovirus (CMV) infection can occur in the nonimmunocompromised patient causing perianal ulcers and proctitis. Symptoms of anorectal pain, hematochezia, and fever have been reported.[46] Sigmoidoscopy can reveal friability and ulcerations. Rectal biopsy specimens can reveal diagnostic CMV inclusion bodies within the lamina propria and crypt cells.[46] Diagnosis can be confirmed by culture. The infection is self-limited in the nonimmunocompromised patient and does not usually require treatment. However, in immunosuppressed patients, this infection frequently involves the colon more diffusely, is more severe in nature, and requires treatment with ganciclovir.

CRYPTOSPORIDIUM

Usually a small intestinal pathogen, *Cryptosporidium* organisms can induce a self-limited colitis in immunocompetent patients, producing a profuse mucoid diarrhea.[47] Diagnosis can be established by stool examination or by biopsy of normal-appearing rectal mucosa, which may reveal the characteristic oocysts. Therapy is supportive in the immunocompetent.

RARE CAUSES OF PROCTITIS AND PROCTOCOLITIS

Rarer causes of proctitis and proctocolitis include tuberculosis, fungal infections, schistosomiasis, balantidiases,[48] *Aeromonas* sp, and possibly *Blastocystis hominis*.

EVALUATION AND EMPIRIC THERAPY

By taking a careful patient history, an attempt should be made to determine whether a patient has proctitis or proctocolitis. History of sexual practices, recent antibiotic use, travel, and possible known contact with pathogens should be sought. Perform a physical examination of the oropharynx, abdomen, genitalia, and inguinal nodes. Carefully examine the perianal area, perform a digital rectal examination, and inspect the anal canal with anoscopy in all patients. In patients with probable sexually transmitted proctitis, obtain a culture for *N. gonorrhoeae* and a blood sample for serologic testing for syphilis. If anoscopy reveals mucopus, perform a Gram's stain, culture for *N. gonorrhoeae,* and treat presumptively. If perianal or anal lesions consistent with syphilis are found, collect dark field and serology specimens and treat presumptively for syphilis. Similarly, HSV proctitis can usually be

INFECTIOUS PROCTITIS IN THE IMMUNOCOMPETENT 607

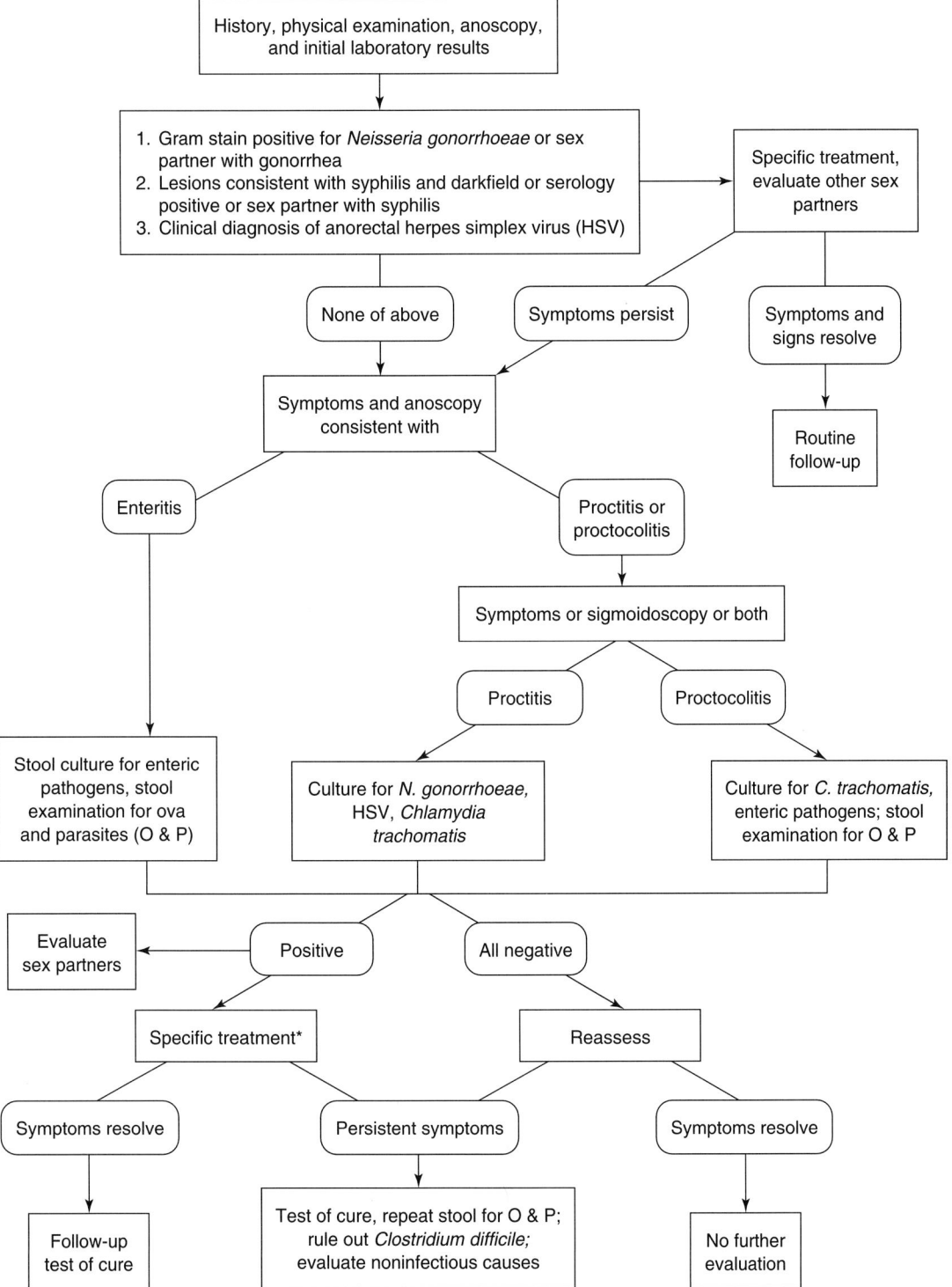

FIGURE 88–1. Algorithm for management of anorectal or intestinal symptoms or both in homosexually active men. Anoscopy, culture for *Neisseria gonorrhoeae,* and a serologic test for syphilis should be performed in all cases. The *asterisk* indicates that specific antiviral therapy for herpes simplex virus proctitis is currently under study. Empiric therapy for enteritis and proctitis can be given pending results of microbiologic studies as discussed in the text. (From Quinn TC, Stamm WE, Goodell SE, et al. The polymicrobial origin of intestinal infections in homosexual men. *N Engl J Med.* 1983;309:576–582. With permission.)

diagnosed by history and anoscopy, and empiric acyclovir can be given. If a history of recent antibiotic use and symptoms consistent with a proctocolitis are present, collect stool for *C. difficile* culture and toxin. Suggested evaluation and therapeutic strategies are outlined in Figure 88–1.

If symptoms are consistent with proctocolitis, if there are no diagnostic abnormalities on anoscopy, or if symptoms persist after treatment, perform sigmoidoscopy. If normal mucosa is seen on sigmoidoscopy, and the patient's symptoms are more characteristic of a generalized enteritis, obtain cultures for enteric bacterial pathogens and examine stool specimens for *E. histolytica* and *Giardia lamblia*. If proctitis is present, collect cultures for *N. gonorrhoeae*, HSV, and *C. trachomatis*. If proctocolitis is present (inflammation >15 cm from the anal verge), culture for *C. trachomatis* and the enteric pathogens and examine any pus for ameba. Characteristic pseudomembranes may also be helpful in the diagnosis of *C. difficile* colitis. Thus, flexible sigmoidoscopy is useful if physical examination and anoscopy do not yield a specific diagnosis or when a pathogen has been treated without response.

Rectal biopsy in patients with acute proctitis or proctocolitis is not usually needed to make the diagnosis, as symptoms due to an infection often resolve spontaneously. Rectal biopsy can be very helpful in patients whose symptoms linger, who do not respond to empiric therapy, or who are severely ill and require prompt diagnosis. In these settings histologic evaluation is often effective in distinguishing acute self-limited colitis (ASLC) from idiopathic inflammatory bowel disease.[50] Furthermore, biopsy can be useful if typical viral inclusions of HSV or CMV infection are found, if specific parasites (such as ameba, *Schistosoma*, or *Cryptococcus*) are seen, or if granulomas are identified. Suggestive of *C. trachomatis* or *T. pallidum* infection, granulomas may also be found in tuberculosis, schistosomiasis, histoplasmosis, and *Yersinia* infections.[49]

REFERENCES

1. Klein EJ, Fisher LS, Chow AW, et al. Anorectal gonococcal infection. *Ann Intern Med.* 1977;86:340–346.
2. Judson FN, Penley KA, Robinson ME, et al. Prevalence and site pathogen studies of *Neisseria meningitidis* and *Neisseria gonorrhoeae* in homosexual men. *Am J Epidemiol.* 1980;112:836–843.
3. Stansfield VA. Diagnosis and management of anorectal gonorrhea in women. *Br J Vener Dis.* 1980;56:319–321.
4. Owen RL, Hill JL. Rectal and pharyngeal gonorrhea in homosexual men. *JAMA.* 1972;220:1315–1318.
5. McMillan A. Bacterial infections. In: Adler MW, ed. *Diseases of the Homosexual Male.* London: Springer-Verlag; 1988:15–39.
6. Catterall RD. Anorectal gonorrhea. *Proc R Soc Med.* 1962;55:871–873.
7. McMillan A, McNeillage G, Gilmour H, et al. Histology of rectal gonorrhea in men with a note on anorectal infection with *Neisseria meningitidis*. *J Clin Pathol.* 1983;36:511–514.
8. McMillan A, Young H. Gonorrhea in the homosexual man: frequency of infection by culture site. *Sex Transm Dis.* 1978;5:146–150.
9. Deherogada P. Diagnosis of rectal gonorrhea by blind anorectal swabs compared with direct vision swabs taken via proctoscope. *Br J Vener Dis.* 1977;53:311–313.
10. Wexner SD. Sexually transmitted diseases of the colon, rectum, and anus. *Dis Colon Rectum.* 1990;33:1048–1062.
11. Peppercorn MA. Enteric infections in homosexual men with and without AIDS. *Contemp Gastroenterol.* 1989;2:23–32.
12. Bingham JS. Syphilis. In: Adler MW, ed. *Diseases in the Homosexual Male.* London: Springer-Verlag; 1988:111–128.
13. Akdamar K, Martin RJ, Ichinose H. Syphilitic proctitis. *Am J Dig Dis.* 1977;22:701–704.
14. Drusin LM, Singer C, Valenti AJ, et al. Infectious syphilis mimicking neoplastic disease. *Arch Intern Med.* 1977;137:156–160.
15. Surawicz CM, Roberts PL, Rompalo A, et al. Intestinal spirochetosis in homosexual men. *Am J Med.* 1987;82:587–592.
16. Bolan RK, Sands M, Schachter J, et al. Lymphogranuloma venereum and acute ulcerative proctitis. *Am J Med.* 1982;72:703–706.
17. Quinn TC, Goodell SE, Mkrtichian E. *Chlamydia trachomatis* proctitis. *N Engl J Med.* 1981;305:195–200.
18. Klotz SA, Drutz DJ, Tam MR. Hemorrhagic proctitis due to lymphogranuloma venereum serogroup 12: diagnosis by fluorescent monoclonal antibody. *N Engl J Med.* 1983;308:1563–1565.
19. Levine JS, Smith PD, Brugge WR. Chronic proctitis in male homosexuals due to lymphogranuloma venereum. *Gastroenterology.* 1980;79:563–565.
20. Lisby SM, Nahata C. Recognition and treatment of chlamydial infections. *Clin Pharm.* 1987;6:25–36.
21. Quinn TC, Corey L, Chaffee RG, et al. The etiology of anorectal infections in homosexual men. *Am J Med.* 1981;71:395–406.
22. Goodell SE, Quinn TC, Mkritchian EE, et al. Herpes simplex virus proctitis in homosexual men. *N Engl J Med.* 1983;308:868–871.
23. Goldmeier D. Proctitis and herpes simplex virus in homosexual men. *Br J Vener Dis.* 1980:111–114.
24. Samarasinghe PL, Oates JK, Maclellan IPB. Herpetic proctitis and sacral radiculomyopathy: a hazard for homosexual men. *Br Med J.* 1979;2:365–366.
25. Mertz GJ. Genital herpes simplex virus infections. *Med Clin North Am.* 1990;74:1433–1446.
26. Artnak EJ, Cerda JJ. The gay bowel syndrome, 1: classic pathogens. *Curr Concepts Gastroenterol.* 1983;6–13.
27. Rompalo AM, Mertz GJ, Davis LG, et al. Oral acyclovir for treatment of first-episode herpes simplex virus proctitis. *JAMA.* 1988;259:2879–2881.

28. Erlich KS, Mills J, Chatis P, et al. Acyclovir-resistant herpes simplex virus infections in patients with the acquired immunodeficiency syndrome. *N Engl J Med.* 1989;320:293–296.
29. Chatis PA, Miller CH, Schrager LE, et al. Successful treatment with foscarnet of an acyclovir-resistant mucocutaneous infection with herpes simplex virus in a patient with acquired immunodeficiency syndrome. *N Engl J Med.* 1989;320:297–300.
30. Sohn N, Robilotti JG. The gay bowel syndrome. *Am J Gastroenterol.* 1977;67:478–484.
31. Bader M, Pederson AHB, Williams R, et al. Venereal transmission of shigellosis in Seattle-King County. *Sex Transm Dis.* 1977;4:89–91.
32. William DC, Felman YM, Marr JS, et al. Sexually transmitted enteric pathogens in male homosexual populations. *NY State J Med.* 1977;77:2050–2052.
33. Allason-Jones E. Protozoal infections. In: Adler MW, ed. *Diseases in the Homosexual Male.* London: Springer-Verlag; 1988:59–75.
34. Ellyson JH, Bezmalinovic Z, Parks SN, et al. Necrotizing amebic colitis: a frequently fatal complication. *Am J Surg.* 1986;152:21–26.
35. Pittman FE, El-Hashimi WK, Pittman JC. Studies of human amebiasis, I: clinical and laboratory findings of eight cases of acute amebic colitis. *Gastroenterology.* 1973;65:581–587.
36. Wiliams DC. The sexual transmission of parasitic infection in gay men. *J Homosex.* 1980;5:291–294.
37. Quinn TC, Goodell SE, Fennell C, et al. Infections with *Campylobacter jejuni* and *Campylobacter*-like organisms in homosexual men. *Ann Intern Med.* 1984;101:187–192.
38. Quinn TC, Stamm WE, Goodell SE, et al. The polymicrobial origin of intestinal infections in homosexual men. *N Engl J Med.* 1983;309:576–582.
39. Guerrant RL, Lahita RG, Winn WC, et al. Campylobacteriosis in man: pathogenic mechanisms and review of 91 blood-stream infections. *Am J Med.* 1978;65:584–592.
40. Miranda AG, Dupont HC. Small intestine: infections with common bacterial and viral pathogens. In: Yamada T, ed. *Textbook of Gastroenterology.* Philadelphia, Pa: JB Lippincott Co; 1991:1447–1472.
41. Griffin PM, et al. Illness associated with *Escherichia coli* 0157:H7 infections: a broad clinical spectrum. *Ann Intern Med.* 1988;109:705–711.
42. Karmali MA, Petric M, Lim C, et al. The association between idiopathic hemolytic uremic syndrome and infection by verotoxin-producing *Escherichia coli*. *J Infect Dis.* 1985;151:775–782.
43. Riley LW, Remis RS, Helgerson SD, et al. Hemorrhagic colitis associated with a rare *Escherichia coli* serotype. *N Engl J Med.* 1983;308:681–685.
44. Tedesco FJ, Corless JK, Brownstein RE. Rectal sparing in antibiotic-associated pseudomembranous colitis: a prospective study. *Gastroenterology.* 1982;83:1259–1260.
45. Price AB, Davies DR. Pseudomembranous colitis. *J Clin Pathol.* 1977;30:1–12.
46. Surawicz CM, Myerson D. Self-limited cytomegalovirus colitis in immunocompetent individuals. *Gastroenterology.* 1988;94:194–199.
47. Quinn TC. Gastrointestinal manifestations of AIDS. *Pract Gastroenterol.* 1985;9:23–34.
48. Marshall JB, Butt JH. Proctitis: approach to diagnosis, causes, and treatment. *J Clin Gastroenterol.* 1982;4:431–444.
49. Surawicz CM. The role of rectal biopsy in infectious colitis. *Am J Surg Pathol.* 1988;12(suppl 1):82–88.

SECTION V

PANCREAS

89
Hereditary Pancreatitis

IVOR D. HILL and EMANUEL LEBENTHAL

Hereditary pancreatitis (HP) is a relatively rare cause of chronic or recurrent pancreatitis. It is distinct from other inherited disorders that may be associated with pancreatitis as a complication, such as cystic fibrosis, hyperparathyroidism, hyperlipoproteinemia (types I, IV, and V), familial hyperchylomicronemia, homocystinuria, and a-1-antitrypsin deficiency. Symptoms due to HP are more common during childhood and early adulthood, and the disorder is often chronic with substantial long-term morbidity.

DEFINITION

Hereditary pancreatitis is defined as an inflammatory condition of the pancreas, which is usually recurrent in nature, and occurs in blood-related individuals over two or more generations.[1] It is inherited as an autosomal dominant trait with apparently complete penetrance but variable expressivity.[2] Onset of symptoms may occur at any age, but most cases first present in childhood.[1]

INCIDENCE

HP was first described in a white American kindred by Comfort and Steinberg in 1952.[3] Subsequently, more than 400 cases and 95 kindreds have been reported from over 20 countries around the world. Most reports have come from the United States and Europe, but patients have now been identified in Brazil, Australia, China, Chile, India, Japan, New Zealand, Pakistan, and South Africa.[4–13] The precise incidence of the condition remains unknown, but in two separate reports it accounted for 5% to 10% of all patients with pancreatitis.[1,14] The number of reported cases in all age groups has increased fourfold over the past two decades. This most probably is indicative of greater awareness of the condition rather than a true increase in incidence. In infants and children, HP is the second most common cause of chronic or recurrent pancreatitis after the pancreatitis that is associated with prolonged protein energy malnutrition.[15]

ETIOLOGY

HP is inherited as an autosomal dominant condition (Fig. 89–1). The precise mechanism causing the pancreatitis remains unknown, and no specific chromosomal abnormality has yet been described. Examination of the pancreatic ducts during pancreatography has shown they may be normal, dilated, or irregularly dilated and constricted,[16–18] and in a number of cases hypertrophy of the sphincter of Oddi has also been identified.[19] These morphologic abnormalities led to speculation that the primary problem is an inherited anatomic defect causing obstruction to the flow of pancreatic secretions. However, it is equally possible that the anatomic abnormalities detected are secondary to the inflammatory process and not the primary event per se.

Increased urinary levels of certain amino acids such as cystine, lysine, and arginine have been documented in some patients with HP, raising the possibility that an inborn error of metabolism is involved in the pathogenesis of the condition.[20–24] Subsequent studies have shown these initial findings to be a nonspecific response to pancreatitis, making a metabolic defect unlikely as the primary causative factor.[2]

An inherited defect in the production of a "stone protein" may be the underlying abnormality in patients with HP.[1] This protein, which inhibits precipitation of insoluble calcium salts within the pancreatic ducts, is a phosphoprotein (MW 14030) secreted by the pancreatic acinar cells.[25,26] Decreased concentrations of "stone protein" have been identified in some patients with nonhereditary pancreatitis (non-HP) and

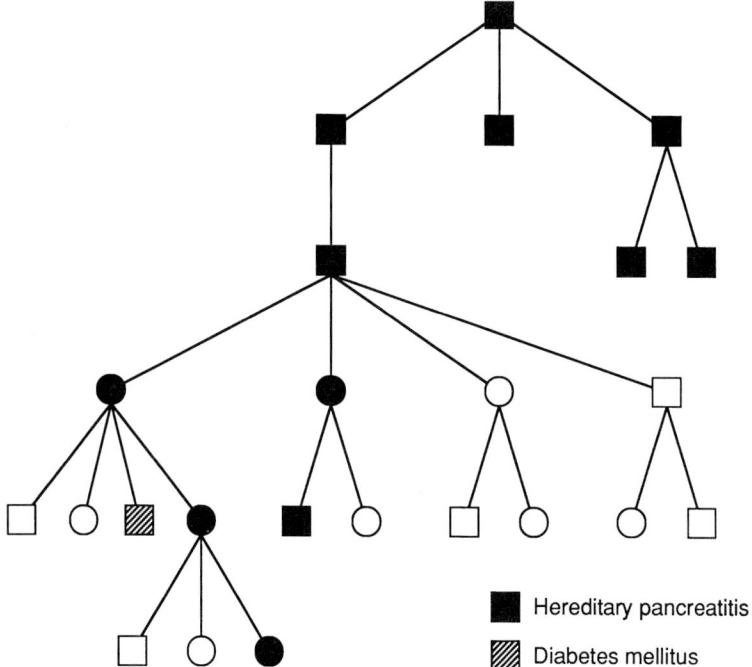

FIGURE 89–1. Family tree showing autosomal dominant inheritance pattern of hereditary pancreatitis. (Courtesy Dr. Y. Elitsur.)

are thought to play a role in the pathogenesis of the condition in these cases.[26,27] Whether this abnormality is also a feature of patients with HP remains to be seen.

ASSOCIATED ABNORMALITIES

A number of developmental abnormalities have been associated with HP. These include strabismus, nystagmus, cerebral palsy, mental retardation, spina bifida occulta, and brachydactyly. Biochemical and serologic changes associated with HP include hypercalcemia,[28] hyperlipidemia,[29,30] raised serum immunoglobulin levels,[31–33] and an increased frequency of HLA types B12, B13, and Bw40.[34–36] In none of these is the relationship strong enough to be considered significant.

PATHOLOGY

HP has no known pathognomonic pathologic features. Knowledge of the early histologic changes in the pancreas of patients with HP is lacking owing to the practical difficulties of obtaining biopsy specimens from this organ. Tissue samples from necropsy specimens or from patients with chronic disease undergoing surgery reveal pancreatic induration, dilation of major and minor ducts, and pancreatic calculi. On histologic examination there is interstitial fibrosis with near-total loss of acinar tissue and partial preservation of normal-appearing islets. These features are indistinguishable from those due to other causes of chronic pancreatitis.[37]

CLINICAL MANIFESTATIONS

Male and female individuals are affected equally.[24] This is in contrast to the male predominance in alcohol-induced pancreatitis and the female predominance in pancreatitis associated with gallstones. Typically, symptoms start during childhood, and the first attack of pancreatitis usually occurs between 1 and 13 years of age. The mean age at first presentation in a large series of patients was 10 years,[24,37] and by 20 years of age up to 75% of patients are symptomatic.[38]

Severe upper abdominal pain due to acute pancreatitis is the most common initial symptom. The character of the pain is no different from that due to any other cause of pancreatitis, and it is usually accompanied by nausea and vomiting. The pain is usually prolonged and of

TABLE 89–1. PHYSICAL SIGNS OF ACUTE PANCREATITIS
Localized epigastric tenderness
Abdominal wall guarding
Rebound tenderness
Abdominal distension
Decreased or absent bowel sounds
Circulatory collapse and hypotension
Oliguria or anuria
Low-grade fever
Grey Turner's sign
Cullen's sign
Ascites and pleural effusion

such severity that it causes the patient to double over. It is frequently localized to the epigastrium but may radiate through to the back or occasionally progress to involve the entire abdominal wall. Symptoms gradually subside, and providing there are no complications, recovery can be expected in 4 to 7 days. Severe hemorrhagic pancreatitis is rare,[38–40] and if it occurs, is more likely to do so during the first or second acute attack.[38] Initially attacks of pain may occur as often as once or twice every 6 months.[1,39] There are currently no known precipitating factors for the attacks. Large fatty meals, alcohol, and stress have been implicated as causes for symptoms, but the evidence for this is weak. With increasing age of the patient the attacks tend to become less severe and less frequent.[20,41,42] Between episodes the patients are usually completely well. In contrast to the usual presentation, the initial attacks in about 5% of cases may be very mild or even painless.[1]

The important physical findings, as listed in Table 89–1, are no different from those found in patients with pancreatitis due to other causes. Epigastric tenderness is the most frequent finding and is often accompanied by decreased bowel sounds. Abdominal distension may occur in up to one third of cases, and guarding and rebound tenderness is usually confined to the upper abdomen or epigastrium. Circulatory shock with hypotension is uncommon and is indicative of severe pancreatitis. The Grey Turner sign (bluish discoloration of the flanks) and the Cullen sign (bluish discoloration of the periumbilical region) are also uncommon and are due to ecchymosis with entrance of blood into the fascial planes. When present, these signs indicate the presence of hemorrhagic pancreatitis. All other signs listed in Table 89–1 are infrequently found with pancreatitis and not specific to the condition.

DIAGNOSIS

Onset of symptoms in childhood in the absence of precipitating factors, such as trauma, alcohol, gallstones, chronic malnutrition or mumps infection, is highly suggestive of HP. When attacks of pancreatitis are accompanied by a history of similar episodes in genetically related individuals spanning a number of generations, the diagnosis of HP can be made with confidence. Without the positive family history, the diagnosis must remain in doubt and may only become apparent with the passage of time.

Acute attacks of pancreatitis are recognized on the basis of the typical history and physical features, together with supportive laboratory findings. Serum pancreatic amylase and lipase levels are elevated and the amylase creatinine clearance ratio is increased. Plain abdominal x-ray examination may show an increase in the gastrocolic separation, sentinel loops of distended bowel in the left upper quadrant, or compression of the duodenal sweep. Edema of the pancreas can be shown with ultrasonography, and this has now become the investigation of choice for diagnosing pancreatitis during the acute phase.

Abdominal ultrasound is also a useful investigation during the chronic stage of the disease. Calcification within the pancreas (Fig. 89–2) is readily detected, and large stones within the major pancreatic ducts are common.[9,16,20,41,43] The characteristics of the stone formation on abdominal x-ray examination may help to distinguish HP from non-HP, as those calculi with central translucency giving an "iris" or "bull's-eye" appearance are suggestive of HP.[1] Conversely, demonstration of concomitant gallstones make the diagnosis of HP less likely. Endoscopic retrograde cholangiopancreatography (ERCP) may show dilation of the duct of Wirsung (Fig. 89–2), but this is not a constant finding.[44–47] Ductular dilation in HP is very variable, and the diameter of the ducts can vary widely over a period of weeks depending on the degree of active inflammation.[1]

COMPLICATIONS

Complications described with HP are the same as those found in patients with non-HP (Table 89–2). Calcification is the most common complication and occurs in 33% to 50% of patients.[1,9,22,48] It is believed to be more common in those with HP as opposed to non-HP. The stones consist of calcium carbonate concretions

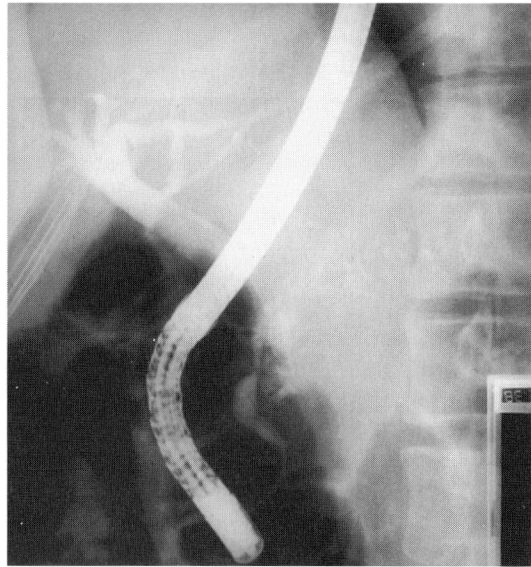

FIGURE 89-2. Endoscopic retrograde cholangiopancreatography showing pancreatic ductular irregularity and extensive calcification. (Courtesy of Dr. S. Glick.)

TABLE 89-2. COMPLICATIONS OF HEREDITARY PANCREATITIS

COMPLICATION	INCIDENCE
Pancreatic calcification	33%–50%
Diabetes mellitus	8%–30%
Exocrine pancreatic insufficiency	5%–50%
Pancreatic pseudocyst (symptomatic)	5%–10%
Pancreatic carcinoma	3%–6%
Portal or splenic vein thrombosis	±4%
Pancreatic ascites	(Rare)
Pleural effusions	(Rare)

and are often very large.[1] They may be deposited in the parenchyma[18,49] but are more often found in the ducts, where they cause obstruction to the flow of pancreatic secretions.[9,16,48,50,51]

The incidence of diabetes in patients with HP varies between 8.5% and 30%.[1,20,37,38,48] This may be an underestimate, as an abnormal glucose tolerance test occurs in a high proportion of asymptomatic cases.[37,38,48] In general, glucose intolerance is a late complication due to progressive pancreatic destruction and is seldom encountered as a clinical problem in the younger patient. With progressive pancreatic destruction some patients develop pancreatic exocrine insufficiency and clinical steatorrhea. The precise incidence of steatorrhea with HP is difficult to determine, as it is not mentioned in a number of reports. Overall estimates have placed the incidence at between 5% and 20%,[1,20,48] but there are reports of this complication occurring in as many as 50% of patients.[37,38]

Symptomatic pancreatic pseudocysts are relatively uncommon and occur in 5% to 10% of patients with HP.[16,20,24,52] With the advent of ultrasound and computed tomography (Figs. 89-3 and 89-4), pseudocysts have been increasingly diagnosed in association with HP and are almost certainly more common than previously recognized.[40,53] The exact incidence has yet to be determined, but it is probably the same as that for pancreatitis from any other cause.

Carcinoma of the pancreas is a well-described late complication of HP. It is said to affect 3% to 6% of cases,[1,24,37,41,49,51,54,55] but in a collective series involving 21 kindreds, it occurred in approximately 20%.[37] Coexistence of chronic inflammation and calcification may predispose to development of duct metaplasia and ultimately pancreatic malignancy.[56] For this reason patients with HP may be at greater risk for developing pancreatic carcinoma than those with non-HP.[2]

Less common complications of HP include portal and splenic vein thrombosis, leading to portal hypertension and gastrointestinal bleeding,[1,9,20,42,48,57] and transient jaundice due to biliary tract obstruction during the acute attack.[1] Prolonged or persistent jaundice should prompt a search for pancreatic carcinoma. Pancreatic ascites from disruption of the pancreatic ductal system with leakage of secretions into the peritoneal cavity is a rare event,[58] as are pleural effusions in association with acute pancreatitis.

MANAGEMENT

Management of the patient with HP during an acute attack of pancreatitis is no different from that of patients with pancreatitis due to other causes.[59–62] Initial treatment is largely symptomatic and supportive and designed to relieve pain, maintain fluid and electrolyte balance, and reduce pancreatic secretions. Pain is often severe and requires strong analgesia. In this regard, meperidine is preferred over codeine or morphine, as the latter causes contraction of the sphincter of Oddi, which can further aggravate pain by obstructing outflow of pancreatic secretions. Reduction of pancreatic secretions is best achieved by stopping all enteral nutrient intake and limiting the passage of gastric secretions into the duodenum by means of continuous nasogastric drainage with suction. H_2-receptor

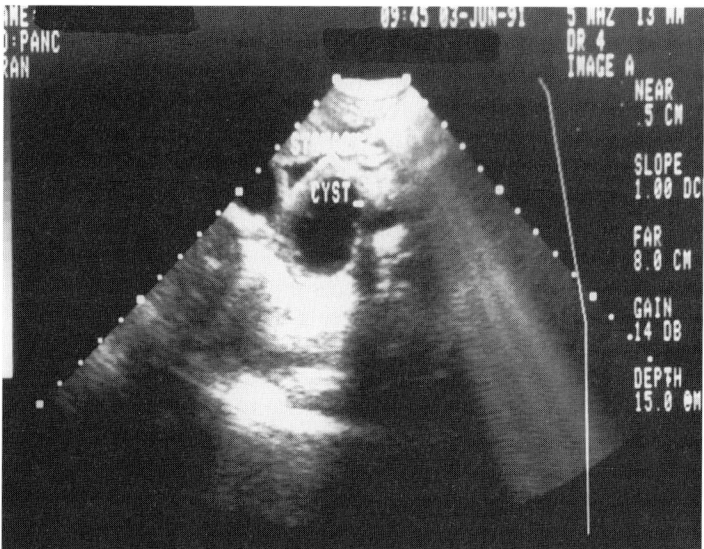

FIGURE 89-3. Abdominal ultrasound demonstrating a pancreatic pseudocyst in the lesser sac. (Courtesy of Dr. Y. Elitsur.)

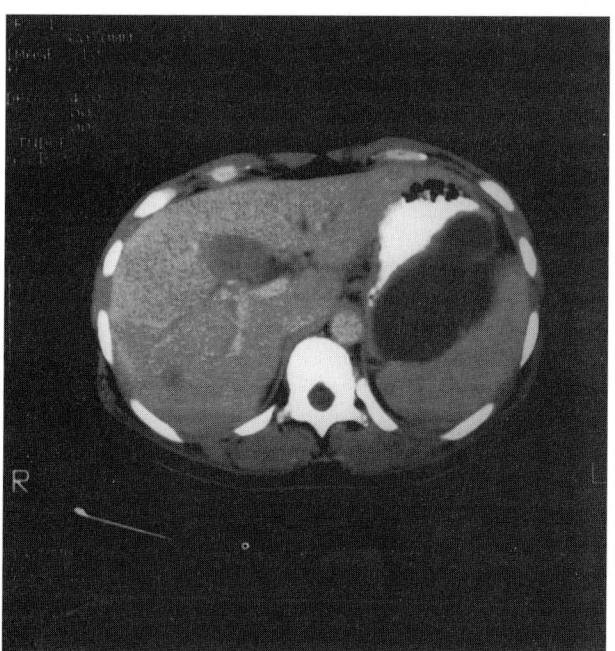

FIGURE 89-4. Computed tomography scan of the abdomen demonstrating a large pancreatic pseudocyst in the lesser sac compressing the stomach, which is filled with contrast material.

antagonists, anticholinergic agents, and trypsin inhibitors have been used as additional modalities during the acute phase but do not appear to be of any benefit. Somatostatin has been employed to decrease pancreatic secretions with variable reported success.[63-66]

Nutritional support is a consideration in patients with prolonged attacks or complicated courses. Early introduction of parenteral nutrition may be of benefit in these cases.[67] Peripheral vein infusion of parenteral nutrients can be used in cases where feeding via the enteral route is likely to be resumed within 7 to 10 days. If enteral feedings are to be withheld for longer periods, a central line should be placed to optimize delivery of sufficient nutrients. Reintroduction of enteral feedings should be considered only after all clinical and biochemical parameters of acute inflammation have resolved.

Antibiotics are frequently prescribed for patients who are febrile during the acute attack or when there is a suspicion of abscess formation.

In some instances antibiotics have been prescribed prophylactically but under such circumstances have not been of proven benefit.[68,69]

Management during the chronic stages of the disease is also similar to that for patients with non-HP. Patients manifesting glucose intolerance require treatment involving dietary manipulation and either oral antidiabetic agents or insulin. Those with exocrine pancreatic insufficiency and steatorrhea should receive pancreatic enzyme supplements with all meals. Pancreatic enzyme supplements have been used prophylactically in an effort to prevent further attacks of pancreatitis, but there is little evidence to show that they are beneficial for this purpose.

The role of surgery in patients with HP is controversial.[1,20,37,70] Pancreatic abscesses are an absolute indication for surgery and always require drainage. In contrast, pseudocysts are no longer considered to need surgical drainage in all cases. Serial ultrasound provides a noninvasive means of monitoring the progression of pseudocysts, and these often resolve completely over a period of months.[1,53] Surgery is now reserved for those pseudocysts that show progressive enlargement on serial ultrasound examination.[1]

Other surgical procedures that have been undertaken include removal of stones, sphincterotomy,[19] ductal dilation,[40] and total or partial pancreatectomy with pancreaticointestinal anastomosis.[70,71] Overall, the results have done little to alter the course of the disease and are of questionable benefit. In many cases sphincterotomy and stone removal can now be achieved with ERCP, rendering surgery unnecessary. Because of the generally disappointing results with surgical procedures[72] and given the tendency for attacks of pancreatitis to decrease in frequency and severity with age, every effort should be made to avoid operative intervention in the young patient. There is always the chance that patients with HP will eventually enter a long phase of clinical remission.

REFERENCES

1. Gross JB. Hereditary pancreatitis. In: Go VLW, ed. *The Exocrine Pancreas: Biology, Pathobiology, and Diseases.* New York, NY: Raven Press Publishers; 1986:829–839.
2. Riccardi VM, Shih VE, Holmes LB, Nardi GL. Hereditary pancreatitis: nonspecificity of aminoaciduria and diagnosis of occult disease. *Arch Intern Med.* 1975;135:822–825.
3. Comfort MW, Steinberg AG. Pedigree of a family with hereditary chronic relapsing pancreatitis. *Gastroenterology.* 1952;21:54–63.
4. Henderson J, Ingram D, House T. Acute pancreatitis in identical twins. *Med J Aust.* 1982;1:432–434.
5. Dani R, Penna FJ, Nogueira CE. Etiology of chronic calcifying pancreatitis in Brazil: a report of 329 consecutive cases. *Int J Pancreatol.* 1986;1:399–406.
6. Lin JT. Hereditary pancreatitis in a Chinese family. *J Clin Gastroenterol.* 1990;12:81.
7. Choudry VP, Srivastava RN, Ghai OP. Familial pancreatitis: a case report. *Indian Pediatr.* 1971;8:466–468.
8. Geevarghese PJ, Pillai VK, Joseph MP, Pitchumoni CS. The diagnosis of pancreatogenous diabetes mellitus: a clinicopathological study of one hundred cases of pancreatic calculi associated with diabetes mellitus. *J Assoc Physicians India.* 1962;10:173–180.
9. Sato T, Saitoh Y. Familial chronic pancreatitis associated with pancreatic lithiasis. *Am J Surg.* 1974;127:511–517.
10. Jones CT, Troughton D, Lindop R. Hereditary pancreatitis: a clinical and biochemical study of a large family with this disorder. In: *Recent Advances in Gastroenterology.* Tokyo: The Third World Congress of Gastroenterology; 1967;4:406–408.
11. Mian TA, Zuberi SJ. Familial pancreatitis with lithiasis. *JPMA.* 1980;30:275–278.
12. Marks IN, Bank S, du Toit A, et al. Genetic and nutritional factors in calcific pancreatitis. In: Riis P, Anthonisen P, Baden H, eds. *Advance Abstracts.* Copenhagen: Danish Gastroenterological Association; 1970:220.
13. Bank S, Marks IN, Novis B. Sweat electrolytes in chronic pancreatitis. *Am J Dig Dis.* 1978;23:178–181.
14. Copenhagen Pancreatitis Study Group. Copenhagen pancreatitis study: an interim report from a prospective epidemiological multicentre study. *Scand J Gastroenterol.* 1981;16:305–312.
15. Pitchumoni CS. Juvenile tropical pancreatitis. In: Walker WA, et al, eds. *Pediatric Gastrointestinal Disease.* Philadelphia, Pa: BC Decker Inc; 1991:1236–1244.
16. Perrault J, Gross JB, King JE. Endoscopic retrograde cholangiopancreatography in familial pancreatitis. *Gastroenterol.* 1976;71:138–141.
17. Stafford RJ, Grand RJ. Hereditary disease of the exocrine pancreas. *Clin Gastroenterol.* 1982;11:141–170.
18. Hardy M, Cornet E, Dupon H, Gordeef A. Chronic pancreatitis associated with familial dilatation of the pancreatic ducts: 6 operated cases. *Bibl Gastroenterol.* 1965;7:189–216.
19. Robechek PJ. Hereditary chronic relapsing pancreatitis: a clue to pancreatitis in general? *Am J Surg.* 1967;113:819–824.
20. Gross JB. Hereditary pancreatitis. In: Gambill EE, ed. *Pancreatitis.* St. Louis, Mo: The CV Mosby Co; 1973:109–114.
21. Gross JB, Ulrich JA, Jones JD. Urinary excretion of amino acids in a kindred with hereditary pancreatitis and aminoaciduria. *Gastroenterology.* 1964;47:41–48.
22. Gross JB, Ulrich JA, Jones JD, Maher FT. Endogenous renal clearances of 12 individual amino acids in four apparently healthy subjects and in four aminoaciduric persons of a kindred with hereditary pancreatitis. *J Lab Clin Med.* 1964;63:933–944.
23. Bergström K, Hellström K, Kallner M, Lundh G. Familial pancreatitis associated with hyperglycinuria. *Scand J Gastroenterol.* 1973;8:217–223.
24. Gross JB, Jones JD. Hereditary pancreatitis: analysis of

experience to May 1969. In: Beck IT, Sinclair DG, eds. *The Exocrine Pancreas*. London: J & A Churchill; 1971: 247–272.
25. Multigner L, De Caro A, Campese D, Lombardo D, Sarles H. Measurement of stone protein in human pancreatic juice during the course of chronic calcific pancreatitis. *Gastroenterology*. 1983;84:1255. Abstract.
26. Multigner L, De Caro A, Lombardo D, Campese D, Sarles H. Pancreatic stone protein, a phosphoprotein which inhibits calcium carbonate precipitation from human pancreatic juice. *Biochem Biophys Res Commun*. 1983;110:69–74.
27. Sarles H, De Caro A, Multigner L, Martin E. Giant pancreatic stones in teetotal women due to absence of the "stone protein"? *Lancet*. 1982;2:714–715.
28. Carey MC, Fitzgerald O. Hyperparathyroidism associated with chronic pancreatitis in a family. *Gut*. 1968;9: 700–703.
29. Brunzell JD, Schrott HG. The interaction of familial and secondary causes of hypertriglyceridemia: role in pancreatitis. *Trans Assoc Am Physicians*. 1973;86:245–254.
30. Cox DW, Breckenridge WC, Little JA. Inheritance of apolipoprotein C-II deficiency with hypertriglyceridemia and pancreatitis. *N Engl J Med*. 1978;299:1421–1424.
31. Bank S, Novis BH, Petersen E, Dowdle E, Marks IN. Serum immunoglobulins in calcific pancreatitis. *Gut*. 1973;14:723–725.
32. Dani R, Antunes LJ, Ribeiro JEF, Nogueira CED, Ribeiro T. Immunological participation in chronic calcifying pancreatitis. *Digestion*. 1974;11:333–337.
33. Malik SA, Van Kley H, Knight WA Jr. Inherited defect in hereditary pancreatitis. *Am J Dig Dis*. 1977;22:999–1004.
34. Gullo L, Tabacchi PL, Corazza GR, Calanca F, Campione O, Labo G. HLA-B13 and chronic calcific pancreatitis. *Dig Dis Sci*. 1982;27:214–216.
35. Gosselin M, Fauchet R, Genetet B, Gastard J. Les antigènes HLA dans la pancréatite chronique alcoolique. *Gastroenterol Clin Biol*. 1978;2:883–886.
36. Angelini G, Boro P, Merigo F, et al. Morphological and functional findings and HLA antigens of three juvenile brothers with chronic pancreatitis. *Digestion*. 1986;35:4.
37. Kattwinkel J, Lapey A, di Sant' Agnese PA, Edwards WA, Hufty MP. Hereditary pancreatitis: three new kindreds and a critical review of the literature. *Pediatrics*. 1973;51:55–69.
38. Durie PR. Pancreatitis. In: Walker WA, et al, eds. *Pediatric Gastrointestinal Disease*. Philadelphia, Pa: BC Decker Inc; 1991:1209–1236.
39. Perrault J, Bartholomew LG. Hereditary and familial pancreatitis. In: Berk JE, Haubrich WS, Kalser MH, Roth JLA, Schaffner F, eds. *Bockus Gastroenterology*. 4th ed. Philadelphia, Pa: WB Saunders Co; 1985:4050–4054.
40. Elliott DW. Familial pancreatitis. In: Howard JM, Jordan GL, Reber HA, eds. *Surgical Diseases of the Pancreas*. Philadelphia, Pa: Lea & Febiger;1987:316–321.
41. Sibert JR. A British family with hereditary pancreatitis. *Gut*. 1975;16:81–88.
42. McElroy R, Christiansen PA. Hereditary pancreatitis in a kinship associated with portal vein thrombosis. *Am J Med*. 1972;52:228–241.
43. Rohrmann CA, Surawicz CM, Hutchison D, Silverstein FE, White TT, Marchioro TL. The diagnosis of hereditary pancreatitis by pancreatography. *Gastrointest Endosc*. 1981;27:168–173.
44. Cotton PB. Progress report: cannulation of the papilla of Vater by endoscopy and retrograde cholangiopancreatography (ERCP). *Gut*. 1972;13:1014–1025.
45. Katon RM, Lee TG, Parent JA, Bilboa MK, Smith FW. Endoscopic retrograde cholangiopancreatography (ERCP): experience with 100 cases. *Am J Dig Dis*. 1974; 19:295–306.
46. Gainsford WD. Endoscopic cannulation of the papilla of Vater. *Arch Surg*. 1974;108:519–525.
47. Pergela K, Cachin M. La pancréato-cholangiographie duodenoscopique per catheritisme de la papille. *Ann Med Interne*. 1972;123:1059–1063.
48. Sibert JR. Hereditary pancreatitis in England and Wales. *J Med Genet*. 1978;15:189–201.
49. Davidson P, Costanza D, Swieconek JA, Harris JB. Hereditary pancreatitis: a kindred without gross aminoaciduria. *Ann Intern Med*. 1968;68:88–96.
50. Gerber BC. Hereditary pancreatitis: the role of surgical intervention. *Arch Surg*. 1963;87:70–80.
51. Logan A Jr, Schlicke CP, Manning GB. Familial pancreatitis. *Am J Surg*. 1968;115:112–117.
52. Freed J, Poley JR, Altman A, Riley HD Jr. Pancreatitis in children. *J Okla State Med Assoc*. 1975;68:153–160.
53. Fried AM, Selke AC. Pseudocyst formation in hereditary pancreatitis. *J Pediatr*. 1978;93:950–953.
54. Gross JB, Comfort MW. Hereditary pancreatitis: report on two additional families. *Gastroenterology*. 1957;32: 829–854.
55. Foster GS, Galdabini JJ. Recurrent abdominal pain and pancreatic calcification with recent jaundice. *N Engl J Med*. 1972;286:1353–1359.
56. Paulino-Netto A, Dreiling DA, Baronofsky ID. The relationship between pancreatic calcification and cancer of the pancreas. *Ann Surg*. 1960;151:530–532.
57. Bartholomew LG, Comfort MW. Chronic pancreatitis without pain. *Proc Staff Meet Mayo Clin*. 1957;32:361–364.
58. Rao SSC, Riley SA, Foster PN, Losowski MS, Stone WD. Hereditary pancreatitis presenting with ascites. *Postgrad Med J*. 1986;62:873–875.
59. Pellegrini CA. The treatment of acute pancreatitis: a continuing challenge. *N Engl J Med*. 1985;312:436–438.
60. Regat PT. Medical treatment of acute pancreatitis. *Mayo Clin Proc*. 1979;54:432–434.
61. Lerner A. Acute pancreatitis in children and adolescents. In: Lebenthal E, ed. *Textbook of Gastroenterology and Nutrition in Infancy*. 2nd ed. New York, NY: Raven Press Publishers; 1989:897–906.
62. Creutzfeldt W, Lankisch PG. Intensive medical treatment of severe acute pancreatitis. *World J Surg*. 1981;5: 341–350.
63. Usadel KH, Uberla KK, Leuschner U. Treatment of acute pancreatitis with somatostatin: results of the multicenter double blind trial (APTS-study). *Dig Dis Sci*. 1985;312:436–438.
64. D'amico D, Favia G, Biasiato R, et al. The use of somatostatin in acute pancreatitis: results of a multicentre trial. *Hepatogastroenterology*. 1990;37:92–98.
65. Choi TK, Mok F, Zhan WH, Fon ST, Lai EC, Wang J. Somatostatin in the treatment of acute pancreatitis: a prospective randomised controlled trial. *Gut*. 1989;30: 223–227.
66. Gislason H, Ga:inbech GE, S:reide O. Pancreatic ascites: treatment by continuous somatostatin infusion. *Am J Gastroenterol*. 1991;86:519–521.
67. Kirby DF, Craig RM. The value of intensive nutritional support in pancreatitis. *JPEN*. 1985;9:353–357.
68. Bradley EL. Antibiotics in acute pancreatitis: current

status and future directions. *Am J Surg.* 1989;158:472–477.
69. Byrne JJ, Treadwell TL. Treatment of pancreatitis: when do antibiotics have a role? *Postgrad Med.* 1989;85:333–334.
70. Williams RA, Caldwell BF, Wilson SE. Idiopathic hereditary pancreatitis: experience with surgical treatment. *Arch Surg.* 1982;117:408–412.
71. Scott HW, Neblett WW, O'Neil JA, Sawyers JL, Avant GS, Starnes VA. Longitudinal pancreaticojejunostomy in chronic relapsing pancreatitis with onset in childhood. *Ann Surg.* 1984;199:610–622.
72. Appel MF. Hereditary pancreatitis: review and presentation of an additional kindred. *Arch Surg.* 1974;108:63–65.

90

Acute Pancreatitis

RUSSELL D. YANG and JORGE E. VALENZUELA

The management of patients with acute pancreatitis is a challenge to any clinician for several reasons. First, acute pancreatitis represents the final common pathway for many diverse etiologic factors. Second, the diagnosis of acute pancreatitis depends heavily on clinical findings, since there is no single laboratory test that is specific for acute pancreatitis. Third, acute pancreatitis represents a wide range of clinical features and pathologic changes from self-limited disease to an acute fulminant course. Fourth, prediction of the clinical course and development of complications is inexact and dependent on nonspecific criteria. Fifth, since we lack an in-depth understanding of the pathogenesis of acute pancreatitis, the treatment and prevention of complications are limited to supportive therapy. This review focuses on the complications of acute pancreatitis and recent developments in the management of those complications.

DIAGNOSIS

The diagnosis of acute pancreatitis is usually made on the basis of clinical features, laboratory findings, and radiographic images. Abdominal pain (a boring sensation located in the epigastrium) is the most frequent clinical symptom. Nausea and vomiting are also common. Since symptoms are nonspecific, elevated levels of circulating pancreatic enzymes, i.e., amylase or lipase (defined as at least three times the upper limits of normal), combined with abdominal pain make the clinical diagnosis of pancreatitis. Other laboratory indexes such as leukocytosis, hyperglycemia, hypertriglyceridemia, transaminasemia, or elevated alkaline phosphatase do not have diagnostic utility. In patients with an unclear clinical picture, imaging studies (ultrasonography or computed tomography [CT] scans) are useful in documenting the presence of pancreatic inflammation and edema with distortion and enlargement of the pancreatic contour. The differential diagnosis of acute pancreatitis should include cholelithiasis or choledocholithiasis, perforation of the gut (i.e., perforated peptic ulcer), and intestinal ischemia or obstruction.

INITIAL TREATMENT

The initial step in the treatment of patients with acute pancreatitis is to remove the offending cause. Thus, a careful history of alcohol usage, medications, recent surgery, or abdominal trauma should be obtained. In addition, the presence of gallstones or peptic ulcer disease should be identified. Finally, metabolic factors such as hypercalcemia or hyperlipidemia should be ruled out.

Once any possible offending cause has been removed, the severity of pancreatitis should be estimated to predict which patients are more likely to develop complications. The clinician should optimize the therapeutic resources and

TABLE 90–1. PROGNOSTIC FACTORS IN ACUTE PANCREATITIS (RANSON'S CRITERIA)

At Admission
Age >55 y
White blood cell count >16,000/mm³
Blood glucose >200 mg/dl
Lactate dehydrogenase >350 IU/L
Aspartate aminotransferase (AST; SGOT) >250 IU/L

Within 48 Hours
Hematocrit fall >10%
PaO$_2$ <60 mm HG
Base deficit >4 mmol/L
BUN rise >5 mg/dl
Fluid sequestration >6 L

---

admit the patient to an intensive care unit when there is any doubt about the patient's clinical stability. Although no single test or observation at the onset of an episode of pancreatitis reliably predicts a patient's subsequent clinical course, several criteria have been established that are useful to determine the severity of an attack. Classically, Ranson's criteria have been used (Table 90–1). Morbidity and mortality increases as more criteria are fulfilled: those patients with two or more criteria are considered to have severe acute pancreatitis, and those patients with three or more criteria carry a greater than 60% mortality.[1] For gallstone pancreatitis, five or more criteria (particularly if the arterial blood gases are worsening) mandate prompt active intervention (see below).[2,3]

A major problem in applying Ranson's criteria is the delay of 48 hours (which may be required to fully assess a patient), since this is often the critical period of resuscitation. Nevertheless, attempts at modification and refinement of Ranson's criteria have not significantly improved prognostication.[4] More recently, Balthazar[5] has used early CT scanning of the pancreas to predict the severity of inflammation in five grades:

- Grade A: normal pancreas
- Grade B: focal or diffuse enlargement of the pancreas with no evidence of peripancreatic disease
- Grade C: intrinsic pancreatic abnormalities and inflammatory changes in the peripancreatic fat
- Grade D: presence of a single inflammatory mass or phlegmon
- Grade E: two or more phlegmonous areas.

The higher grades were associated with increased risk of abscess formation, longer hospital stay, and greater morbidity and mortality.[5] The Balthazar criteria, which identify local complications of pancreatitis, complement Ranson's prognostic signs, which reflect systemic complications.[5] Thus, several investigators have recommended early CT scanning in all patients with two or more Ranson's risk factors and serial scans for patients with grade D and E.[6,7] The search for a single test that will assist in the assessment of early prognosis of acute pancreatitis continues. Newer tests such as determination of urinary trypsin-activated peptide (TAP) are currently being developed.[8]

GENERAL MANAGEMENT OPTIONS

The initial treatment of acute pancreatitis should combine efforts to determine the cause and to assess the severity of an attack with pain relief. Analgesics such as acetaminophen and anticholinergic agents do not give adequate relief, and narcotic administration with meperidine (Demerol) may be necessary. Severe pain itself can induce a shocklike state.

Since the mortality and morbidity of pancreatitis is related to the development of complications, supportive therapy and measures to prevent complications should be initiated. Supportive medical therapy includes nothing by mouth, careful but aggressive volume repletion, and correction of electrolyte disorders. In severe cases of acute pancreatitis, prevention of stress-related gastroduodenal mucosal damage using H$_2$-receptor antagonists or sucralfate may be undertaken.[9] The concept of "putting the pancreas to rest" is still valid. However, efforts to reduce pancreatic secretion have been disproven in several controlled clinical trials.[10,11] Thus, inhibition of pancreatic secretion (i.e., somatostatin, glucagon, calcitonin, anticholinergic agents, prostaglandins), reduction of pancreatic enzyme activity (i.e., aprotinin, inhibition of phospholipase A$_2$), inhibition of gastrointestinal secretion (i.e., H$_2$-receptor antagonists [unless used to prevent stress-related mucosal damage]), inhibition of the inflammatory responses (i.e., corticosteroids), or administration of prostaglandins is obsolete.[10,11]

Although nasogastric suction should not be routinely used in chronic alcoholic patients with acute episodes of pain to "rest the pancreas," it may be useful in patients with gallstone or idiopathic pancreatitis to decrease nausea and vomiting, decompress an ileus, or detect early gastrointestinal tract bleeding. Nasogastric tube placement is usually necessary in the more severe episodes of pancreatitis.

Prophylactic antibiotics play no role in mild-to-moderate cases of acute pancreatitis.[12] However, antibiotics may reduce mortality in severe cases.[13] The lack of beneficial effect may be due to an inadequate selection of antibiotics. More recent studies suggest that newer antibiotics (ciprofloxacin, ofloxacin, and imipenem) achieve higher pancreatic parenchymal tissue levels.[14] Thus, the prophylactic utility of these antibiotics may be beneficial in severe acute pancreatitis. Since acute pancreatitis does induce a hypermetabolic state, total parenteral nutrition should be considered in protracted (>2 weeks) or in complicated cases (i.e., pancreatic fistula).[15,16] However, line sepsis is increased in acute pancreatitis.[17]

There is no consensus on the utility of peritoneal lavage. It can remove vasoactive agents, activated enzymes, and toxic substances associated with the peripancreatic fluid that may accumulate during the course of acute pancreatitis. Although mixed results have been reported, peritoneal lavage does improve cardiopulmonary function and results in pain relief.[18] Apparently, peritoneal lavage is most effective in alcohol-related pancreatitis.[18,19] However, peritoneal lavage does not decrease overall mortality, since necrosis and infection continue to develop.[18,19] Unanswered questions include the completeness of lavage (i.e., does the fluid reach all the compartments of pancreatic fluid?) and length of lavage. Preliminary observations suggest that a 7-day lavage protocol reduces septic complications, whereas a 2- to 4-day lavage does not.[20] Thus, further studies are necessary to determine the optimal number of days for lavage. At present, if peritoneal lavage is contemplated, it should be used early in severe alcoholic pancreatitis and extended for at least 7 days.[20]

Another new therapy for acute pancreatitis is thoracic duct drainage[21] to remove from systemic circulation any activated pancreatic enzymes and toxic substances that may enter the lymphatic system. In combination with peritoneal lavage, this technique may be beneficial in the early phases of severe acute pancreatitis. However, the ability of lymphatic drainage to reduce "late" mortality has not yet been proved.[11]

Surgery is usually avoided in acute pancreatitis. Surgery may be contemplated for the patient with severe pancreatitis and multiorgan failure or gastrointestinal tract bleeding unresponsive to medical therapy.[22] In these patients with an extensive amount of necrotic infected pancreatic tissue, surgical exploration and débridement may increase long-term survival.[23] In more mild cases of pancreatitis, the benefits of surgery are doubtful.[23]

Although endoscopic retrograde cholangio-pancreatography (ERCP) is not routinely performed in acute pancreatitis, urgent intervention by ERCP in the setting of severe biliary pancreatitis can reduce morbidity, mortality, and length of hospital stay.[24] It is generally recommended that patients with mild biliary pancreatitis receive supportive therapy and a cholecystectomy be performed when serum enzyme concentrations have normalized and symptoms have totally abated. However, in severe episodes of biliary pancreatitis (more than three Ranson's criteria), early (within the first 48 hours from the onset of symptoms) intervention with ERCP, endoscopic sphincterotomy, and stone extraction should be undertaken.[24,25] For the elderly or very frail patient, this may be considered definitive surgery. However, once the episode of pancreatitis resolves, consideration of removal of the in situ gallbladder should be undertaken.

COMPLICATIONS OF ACUTE PANCREATITIS

The overall mortality for acute pancreatitis is approximately 10% and rises as complications (either systemic or local) of acute pancreatitis occur. In general, early mortality (<1 week) follows the development of systemic complications, while late mortality is due to local complications. Thus, management of patients with acute pancreatitis is aimed at the prevention, early recognition, and treatment of these complications.

HEMODYNAMIC COMPLICATIONS

A common and early systemic complication of acute pancreatitis is hypovolemia and hemodynamic instability. Hypovolemia arises from the release of vasoactive substances (e.g., kallikreins and other acute phase proteins) that cause increased capillary permeability and subsequent "third spacing" of fluid. *Third spacing of fluid* refers to the sequestration of fluids into the extracellular compartment (i.e., exudation of plasma into the retroperitoneum or peritoneal cavity or collection of fluid in a hollow viscous related to development of an ileus). In addition, actual intravascular volume depletion occurs. Fluid losses from vomiting, nasogastric suctioning, and gastrointestinal tract and retroperitoneal hemorrhage cause further intravascular volume depletion. The resulting hypovolemia of acute pancreatitis may be worsened by concomitant decreased peripheral resistance. Biochemically, this may be manifested initially by a hypokalemic, metabolic alkalosis but metabolic acidosis soon develops as tissue perfusion falls below critical values. In addition, the pancreas gland is susceptible to ischemia, and persistent hypotension can worsen the course of pancreatitis. Clinically, hypovolemia is manifested by tachycardia, hypotension, decreased urinary output, and in severe cases shock. Failure to properly replenish fluids and electrolytes leads to increased early morbidity from pancreatitis.

Circulatory compromise in acute pancreatitis can also occur in the face of adequate circulatory volume. In these instances, a circulating mediator, myocardial depressant factor, may be released[26] or other acute phase mediators may decrease cardiac output.[27]

Fluid repletion should be carefully monitored with serial orthostatic changes and urine output. In more complex cases, placement of a central venous pressure line may be helpful. Crystalloid fluids are appropriate to replace volume unless serial hematocrits suggest the need for blood products. Use of intravenous albumin or other colloids to maintain plasma oncotic pressure has not proven more effective than the use of crystalloids alone. Low-volume infusions of fresh-frozen plasma may be beneficial.[28] Swan-Ganz catheterization is indicated when hypotension persists despite adequate fluid administration if the patient suffers from concomitant heart or lung disease or with adult respiratory distress syndrome (ARDS).

ACUTE RENAL INSUFFICIENCY

Acute renal insufficiency is a relatively common and severe complication of acute pancreatitis.[29] The renal injury that accompanies pancreatitis arises from hypotension and ischemia. In addition, decreased renal perfusion may be caused by selective renovasoconstriction mediated by circulating acute phase mediators (i.e., phospholipase A_2).[30] Furthermore, deposition of fibrin thrombi in the glomeruli related to changes in coagulation induced by acute pancreatitis has also been found.[31] Thus, a spectrum of renal findings from reversible prerenal azotemia to frank acute tubular necrosis can be observed. Clinically, this may be manifested by oliguria (urine output <30 ml/h), rising blood urea nitrogen (BUN) and creatinine levels, and an elevated amylase-creatinine clearance. Furthermore, a diuretic phase of renal failure may evolve if patients fail to concentrate the filtered urine, and loss of excessive amounts of fluids and electrolytes ensues.

Acute renal insufficiency can be prevented by careful fluid and electrolyte management. In addition, restriction of dietary protein may be beneficial. In severe cases, dialysis may be required. More recently, investigators have favored peritoneal dialysis over hemodialysis, since the former also lavages the peritoneal cavity. If dialysis is required during an episode of acute pancreatitis, then mortality may approach 50%.[33]

RESPIRATORY FAILURE

Hypoxemia is common in acute pancreatitis and most often patients are asymptomatic. Usually, the hypoxemia is transient and improves as the course of pancreatitis resolves. In these mild cases, abnormal findings are usually not observed on chest x-ray films. However, if the pancreatitis is severe, hypoxemia and respiratory insufficiency can be quite dramatic. The pathogenesis of pulmonary insufficiency in acute pancreatitis has not been clearly defined but is likely due to the release of elastases, lipases, and other mediators that cause pulmonary edema. Intrapulmonary ventilation-perfusion mismatches caused by microthrombi related to a subclinical state of disseminated intravascular coagulation further exacerbate the respiratory insufficiency.[35] Although the mechanism is poorly understood, hypertriglyceridemia tends to worsen pulmonary symptoms. In addition, the associated abdominal pain and infradiaphragmatic inflammation may cause splinting and atelectasis. The development of a pancreatitis-related pulmonary effusion also contributes to pulmonary difficulties. Pleural effusions are usually left-sided and occur early in the course of acute pancreatitis. Persistence of a pulmonary effusion with high-amylase content suggests the formation of a pancreaticopleural fistula.[36] Hypoalbuminemia and fluid overload during the resuscitation period may worsen symptoms. If the respiratory insufficiency progresses, ARDS can develop. ARDS associated with acute pancreatitis reflects an increased permeability of the pulmonary capillary endothelium caused by inflammatory mediators and is often associated with formation of a pancreatic abscess.

Clinically, respiratory insufficiency begins insidiously and is manifested by tachypnea, agitation, and mental confusion. However, as the pancreatitis progresses and respiratory insufficiency worsens, mechanical ventilation may be necessary. Respiratory failure portends a dismal prognosis (up to 60% mortality).

As mentioned earlier, hypoxemia is common in acute pancreatitis. Usually, the hypoxemia is transient and can easily be treated with supplemental oxygen. However, because respiratory failure can develop insidiously, serial blood gases in the first 24 to 48 hours should be obtained. Chest radiographs are relatively insensitive to changes in pulmonary status. In severe cases, intubation and mechanical ventilation may be required.[37] Avoidance of fluid overload during resuscitation helps to reduce pulmonary complications. Development of ARDS may require the addition of positive end-expiratory pressure.[38]

HYPOCALCEMIA

Hypocalcemia (<8 g/dl) is a poor prognostic indicator in acute pancreatitis and occurs in approximately one third of patients.[1] Possible mechanisms include hypoalbuminemia (low total calcium but normal ionized calcium values), hypomagnesemia, sequestration in areas of fat necrosis, hyperglucagonemia (increased glucagon release can stimulate calcitonin release and thus inhibit bone resorption), or an altered parathyroid hormone axis. Alterations in the parathyroid hormone axis include decreased secretion or end-organ resistance with impaired mobilization of calcium from bone in response to parathyroid hormone.[39]

Clinically, hypocalcemia is only rarely symptomatic. Tetany, Chvostek's sign, and cardiac arrhythmias occur with very low calcium levels but are uncommon in acute pancreatitis. In these extreme cases, calcium replacement may be necessary.

HYPERGLYCEMIA

Blood glucose levels of greater than 200 mg/dl are a common finding in acute pancreatitis and are a poor prognostic indicator. Possible mechanisms include increased release of glucagon or increased responsiveness to glucagon. In addition, there may be a relative insulin deficiency. Hyperglycemia associated with acute pancreatitis is usually transient and does not require specific therapy. However, when diabetic ketoacidosis occurs in a setting of well-demonstrated acute pancreatitis, small doses of regular insulin administration are necessary. Pancreatitis-associated ketoacidosis portends a worse prognosis, and close monitoring of the patient is necessary.[41]

HYPERLIPIDEMIA

Hyperlipidemia is observed in as many as 20% of patients suffering from acute pancreatitis.[42] It is unclear whether hyperlipidemia is a cause of or results from changes induced by acute pancreatitis. Excessive alcohol intake often causes hyperlipidemia. Although there is usually not a preceding history of hyperlipidemias, frequent lipid abnormalities have been observed in patients following their acute attack and include persistent hypertriglyceridemia and abnormal responses to lipid-loading challenges.[42,43] Type IV or V hyperlipidemias associated with extremely high levels of triglycerides (>1000 mg/dl) are often observed in lipid-related pancreatitis.[42,43] Conversely, hypertriglyceridemia induced by pancreatitis is usually <500 mg/dl and gradually resolves as the course of pancreatitis improves.

Clinically, hyperlipidemia is usually silent. However, even though lipid abnormalities are not a poor prognostic indicator, hypertriglyceridemia is associated with a higher incidence of pancreatitis-related ARDS.[44] In addition, it is important to realize that serum amylase levels may be normal in the face of hyperlipidemia because of interference with the amylase assay.[45] In these instances, imaging studies or serum lipase or urinary amylase measurement should be used to help confirm the clinical diagnosis of pancreatitis. Because of the transient nature of hyperlipidemia during the course of acute pancreatitis, specific therapy is usually not necessary. However, if the hyperlipidemia persists once the episode of acute pancreatitis resolves, then chronic therapy should be instituted.

OTHER METABOLIC COMPLICATIONS

Subcutaneous fat necrosis is a rare complication in acute pancreatitis and may mimic erythema nodosum. However, the lesions are usually more diffuse and may be associated with medullary bone lesions and polyarthritis.[46]

Metabolic acidosis can also complicate severe acute pancreatitis. Possible causes include lactic acidosis (due to hypoperfusion or respiratory failure), renal failure, or alcoholic ketoacidosis.

COAGULATION ABNORMALITIES

Severe acute pancreatitis can be complicated by a "hypercoagulable" state due to increased formation of fibrin from fibrinogen related to elevated levels of activated trypsin.[35,47] In addition, there may be increased consumption of antiproteases associated with coagulation by pancreatic proteases.[48] Clinically, this is manifested by disseminated intravascular coagulation (DIC) or to isolated vascular thrombosis.[35,50] As mentioned earlier, end-organ damage with fibrin thrombi in the renal microvasculature may lead to renal insufficiency or in the lungs may lead to increased right-to-left shunting. However, heparin therapy is of no proven benefit in these situations.[50]

GASTROINTESTINAL TRACT BLEEDING

Gastrointestinal tract bleeding occurs in approximately 5% of patients suffering from acute pancreatitis. The most common causes include inflammation of the adjacent gut mucosa (i.e., gastritis or duodenitis) to the area of inflamed pancreas, stress-related mucosal damage (in severe, complicated cases), and peptic ulcer disease. Variceal bleeding in acute pancreatitis could be the result of a alcoholic cirrhosis (with predominantly esophageal varices) or of the development of isolated gastric varices due to splenic vein thrombosis.

Other sources of bleeding are less common. Erosion of a pancreatic inflammatory process (e.g., pseudocyst) into adjacent intestine or a major artery ("pseudoaneurysm") may cause bleeding into the intestine via the pancreatic duct (i.e., hemosuccus pancreaticus). Hemosuccus pancreaticus occasionally can present with a picture of obstructive jaundice if the blood obstructs both the pancreatic and common bile ducts mimicking choledocholithiasis.[51] Intrapseudocyst bleeding may be a cause of rapid blood loss without apparent gastrointestinal tract bleeding.

Because bleeding can rapidly lead to an emergent situation, gastrointestinal tract bleeding in acute pancreatitis should be pursued aggressively with endoscopy and if negative, with imaging (i.e., interventional angiography), which may serve as a diagnostic and therapeutic approach.

NEUROLOGIC COMPLICATIONS

Neurologic complications of acute pancreatitis are rare. Pancreatic encephalopathy can occur in both alcoholic and nonalcoholic pancreatitis. Although the pathogenesis is poorly understood, diffuse demyelination has been observed in these patients.[52] Clinically, it may be difficult to distinguish alcoholic encephalopathy from alcohol withdrawal or delirium tremens or other metabolic encephalopathy. Sudden blindness (Purtscher's angiopathic retinopathy) has also been reported in acute pancreatitis and may be related to the granulocyte plugs in the retinal microvasculature.[53]

PHLEGMON

A pancreatic phlegmon is a solid mass of indurated pancreas and adjacent retroperitoneal tissue–containing edema, inflammatory cells, and limited necrotic tissue. Clinically, a phlegmon may present as a mass (palpable in 20% of cases) with abdominal pain or tenderness and mild fever (usually less than 101°F). A phlegmon can be visualized by either ultrasonography or CT scanning. Phlegmons usually resolve spontaneously in approximately 2 weeks. Possible complications include infection (with evolution into a pancreatic abscess) or pseudocyst formation.[54,55] Thus, phlegmons, once detected, should be monitored to identify these complications.[55]

PERIPANCREATIC FLUID COLLECTIONS, PSEUDOCYSTS, AND ASCITES

Peripancreatic fluid collections (defined as sterile sympathetic effusions of fluid and inflammatory exudate within the pancreatic parenchyma or in surrounding tissues) are common during the initial phases of acute pancreatitis.[56] Peripancreatic fluid collections may resolve spontaneously or evolve into pancreatic pseudocyst(s) or collections of fluid surrounded by a capsule. The fluid contained within the pseudocyst is composed of cellular debris, blood, exudate, and pancreatic enzymes. The capsule may be composed of granulation or fibrous tissue depending on the age of the pseudocyst. Since the capsule lacks a true epithelial lining, it is called a pseudocyst.[57] Pseudocysts complicate up to 15% of cases of acute pancreatitis.[54] Pseudocysts may involve any part of the pancreas but are most commonly seen in the body. In addition, pseudocysts can involve adjacent organs and surrounding structures such as the lesser omental sac, retroperitoneum, and perirenal spaces. In addition, pseudocysts have been reported in remote locations such as the pelvis or mediastinum. Most pseudocysts are unilocular (85%) but may be multilocular or contain several septa.[58]

The pathogenesis of pseudocysts is not exactly known but appears to involve ductal disruption and leakage of fluid into a closed space. However, pseudocysts associated with acute pancreatitis are probably due to tissue destruction and intraparenchymal release of activated pancreatic enzymes, so-called "necrotic pseudocysts."[58] In chronic pancreatitis, pseudocysts more often appear to be secondary to ductal obstruction and retention of fluid containing inactivated enzymes, so-called "obstructive pseudocysts."[58–60]

Classically, pseudocysts usually present following a severe attack of pancreatitis. In addition, prolonged acute pancreatitis lasting more than 1 week or prolonged serum amylase elevation may suggest the formation of a pseudocyst. Less commonly, a pseudocyst may present as a complication (e.g., hemorrhage, infection, rupture) or as an obstruction of an adjacent structure. Pseudocysts may be asymptomatic or accompanied by anorexia, nausea, vomiting, fever, weight loss, abdominal tenderness, vomiting (i.e., obstruction of an adjacent viscus), or jaundice (i.e., compression of the common bile duct). The latter situation is more often observed in chronic alcoholism with chronic pancreatic changes (i.e., obstructive pseudocysts).

Diagnosis of pseudocysts can be made by either abdominal ultrasonography (US) or CT. US is inexpensive and readily available. However, optimal imaging of the pancreas is dependent on the body habitus of the patient and the operator. In addition, complete visualization may not be possible if there is overlying intestinal gas (i.e., an ileus associated with acute pancreatitis).[61] CT scanning is the most reliable technique to visualize the pancreas and yields more additional information regarding the functioning of the pancreas if contrast is injected during the imaging process.[5,6]

Up to 50% of untreated pseudocysts may be complicated by bleeding, infection, or rupture or may cause obstruction of an adjacent structure.[62] Although the natural history of pseudocysts has not been precisely defined, it has been classically taught that pseudocysts that are large (>5 to 6 cm) or persist greater than 6 weeks are more prone to develop complications.[62,63] However, more recent studies suggest that even large pseudocysts may resolve with time and are not associated with an increased complication rate.[64,65] Apparently, pseudocysts associated with acute pancreatitis ("necrotic" pseudocysts) are more likely to resolve spontaneously than those associated with chronic pancreatitis ("obstructive pseudocysts").[60]

Pseudocyst hemorrhage carries a high mortality[66] and may occur by several routes. Bleeding from the wall of the pseudocyst may lead to enlargement of the pseudocyst. An expanding pseudocyst may then rupture into the peritoneal cavity, bleed into the pancreatic duct (i.e., hemosuccus pancreaticus), or erode directly into the stomach or adjacent intestine. If the pseudocyst erodes into a major artery (i.e., pseudoaneurysm), the bleeding can be massive. Clinically, patients may present with signs and symptoms of gastrointestinal tract bleeding. Alternatively, bleeding patients may have a falling hematocrit without gross evidence of gastrointestinal tract blood loss or may suddenly develop an abdominal pain with a mass or obstructive jaundice. Diagnostic evaluation should be carried out promptly and includes upper endoscopy, CT scanning, or angiography. Embolization should be undertaken if technically possible, although definitive surgery is often necessary.[67]

Obstruction of an adjacent organ by a pseudocyst is uncommon. Compression of the duodenum is the most frequent site of obstruction. Obstruction of the common bile duct by a pseudocyst may be further complicated by distal stricture formation in the setting of chronic pancreatitis.[68] Other less common sites include the colon, ureters, and portal vein. Obstruction of an adjacent organ or structure is an indication for drainage. If the common bile duct is obstructed, ERCP should be performed to distinguish between extrinsic compression of the common bile duct by the pseudocyst, a distal common bile stricture related to the surrounding inflammation, and the presence of choledocholithiasis.[69]

Rupture of a pseudocyst can occur into the peritoneal cavity, an adjacent organ, or any adjacent hollow viscus. Classically, rupture into an adjacent intestine occurs suddenly with disappearance of the abdominal mass and massive diarrhea. Free rupture into the peritoneal cavity can cause a severe peritonitis associated with a high morbidity and mortality. Rupture with bleeding or into a solid organ can also be catastrophic, and emergent surgical intervention may be necessary.

Pseudocysts are usually sterile but can become infected. An infected pseudocyst should be suspected in a patient with increasing abdominal pain, fever, chills, and leukocytosis. If an infected pseudocyst is suspected, then US- or CT-guided needle aspiration should be performed diagnostically. Antibiotics and drainage should be undertaken emergently.[70,71] Antibiotics should cover enteric organisms (i.e., combination therapy with ampicillin, gentamicin, and metronidazole). As noted earlier, newer agents such as third-generation cephalosporins, ciprofloxacin, or imipenem may be useful.[14] Classically, internal surgical drainage (into stomach, small intestine, or Roux-en-Y loop) is preferred since external drainages are complicated by infections and fistulization.[72] Recently, percutaneous drainage has gained widespread acceptance, and success rates of greater than 90% have been reported.[70,71] Success rates are greater when the pseudocyst is a single cavity and in a location that is easily drained. Percutaneous drainage may fail in pseudocysts with multiple septa or when they are multiloculated or contain thickened cyst fluid. At present, there are no randomized trials directly comparing surgical drainage to the percutaneous approach.

Pseudocysts that rupture into an adjacent intestine may not require further therapy. However, rupture of a pseudocyst into the free peritoneal cavity or rupture with bleeding often requires surgical intervention.

Pancreatic ascites can be small in volume if associated with acute severe hemorrhagic pancreatitis, but in the setting of chronic pancreatitis it may become massive.[73] In this last instance pancreatic ascites develops from pancreatic ductal disruption with a leakage of pancreatic fluid into the peritoneal cavity. Similarly, acute rupture of the pancreatic duct system following traumatic pancreatitis may cause ascites. In addition, a chronically leaking pseudocyst can also lead to ascites.[74] Clinically, ascites is manifested by increasing abdominal girth, weight loss, and abdominal pain. The patient may appear chronically ill. Paracentesis of the ascitic fluid reveals a high-protein fluid with elevated amylase levels. Pleural effusions may develop in the setting of pancreatic ascites and suggest development of a pancreaticopleural fistula. Since pancreatic ascites usually occurs in the setting of chronic pancreatitis, signs and symptoms of active inflammation may not be present (i.e., pain, fever). Thus, pancreatic ascites should be considered in a chronic alcoholic with an indolent intra-abdominal fluid accumulation.

When pancreatic ascites fails to resolve, a persistent ductular rupture should be identified. Thus, ERCP should be performed in deciding optimal therapy. Similarly, pancreatic fistula should also be visualized, particularly before operative intervention is undertaken. Medical therapy with total parenteral hyperalimentation and somatostatin may be effective in closing fistulas.[75,76] However, if a persistent ductular leak is identified, endoscopic stent placement or surgery is necessary.[77]

ABSCESS

Extensive pancreatic necrotic tissue may become infected and lead to the development of an abscess. Thus, pancreatic abscess usually complicates the more severe episodes of pancreatitis. In particular, patients with postoperative pancreatitis are at higher risk for developing a pancreatic abscess. Since the contaminating bacteria are usually the same as enteric flora, the bacteria are felt to cross the intestinal wall, which is made more permeable to bacteria by the adjacent pancreatic inflammation. Classically, a pancreatic abscess presents as an episode of severe pancreatitis, which seems to improve initially followed by "late" (>2 weeks) clinical deterioration after an episode of pancreatitis. Patients appear to be toxic with fever, abdominal pain, tenderness, nausea, and vomiting. A mass may be palpable, and marked leukocytosis is usually present. CT scanning yields the most accurate imaging of an abscess and may reveal pancreatic edema, fluid within the pancreas, or gas bubbles in the pancreatic bed.[32] CT scanning during rapid bolus injection of contrast (i.e., dynamic imaging) has gained acceptance, since it yields information regarding the extent of necrotic tissue that appears as hypoperfused areas.[6] If an abscess is suspected during pancreatic imaging, needle aspiration should be performed to document the presence of infection.[70,78,79] Other biochemical tests such as serum ribonuclease, phospholipase A_2, C-reactive protein. a-1-antitrypsin, or a-2-macroglobulin levels have not proved to improve the accuracy of diagnosis of pancreatic abscess.[34,40] If untreated or unrecognized, pancreatic abscesses are invariably fatal.

Pancreatic abscess and infected areas of phlegmon, pseudocyst, and necrotic tissue form the spectrum of infectious complications of acute pancreatitis. Since the majority of deaths in the "late" phases of acute pancreatitis are due to abscess formation, diagnosis and therapy should be aggressive. Once CT-guided needle aspiration with Gram's stain and culture has been performed, antibiotic therapy and surgical débridement of the infected necrotic tissue with removal of purulent material and construction of adequate drainage is undertaken. Surgical intervention lowers mortality from 88% to 100% in untreated cases to 25% to 50% postoperatively.[49] Alternatively, percutaneous drainage may be considered. Percutaneous drainage usually is of limited value if the necrotic area is not liquefied enough to allow easy passage of the abscess contents through the drainage catheter or if the abscess is compartmentalized (septated), which would preclude adequate drainage.[79,80] In most instances, well-timed surgical intervention may be superior to percutaneous aspirations.

REFERENCES

1. Ranson JHC, Rifkind KM, Turner JW. Prognostic signs and nonoperative peritoneal lavage in acute pancreatitis. *Surg Gynecol Obstet.* 1976;143:209–219.
2. Ranson JHC. The timing of biliary surgery in acute pancreatitis. *Ann Surg.* 1979;189:654–663.
3. Osborne DH, Imrie CW, Carter DC. Biliary surgery in the same admission for gallstone-associated acute pancreatitis. *Br J Surg.* 1981;68:758–761.
4. Larvin M, McMahon MJ. APACHE-II score for assessment and monitoring of acute pancreatitis. *Lancet.* 1989;2:201–205.
5. Balthazar EJ. CT diagnosis and staging of acute pancreatitis. *Radiol Clin North Am.* 1989;27:19–37.
6. Bradley EL, Murphy F, Ferguson C. Prediction of pancreatic necrosis by dynamic pancreatography. *Ann Surg.* 1989;211:708–718.
7. Balthazar EJ, Robinson DL, Megibow AJ, Ranson JHC. Acute pancreatitis: value of CT in establishing prognosis. *Radiology.* 1990;179:331–336.
8. Gudgeon AM, Heath DI, Hurley P, et al. Trypsinogen activation peptides assay in the early prediction of severity of acute pancreatitis. *Lancet.* 1990;1:4–8.
9. Cook DJ, Witt LG, Cook PJ, Guyatt GH. Stress ulcer prophylaxis in the critically ill: a meta-analysis. *Am J Med.* 1991;91:519–527.
10. Steinberg WM, Schesselman SE. Treatment of acute pancreatitis: comparison of animal and human studies. *Gastroenterology.* 1987;93:1420–1427.
11. Raynaert MS, Dugernier T, Kestens PJ. Current therapeutic strategies in severe acute pancreatitis. *Intensive Care Med.* 1990;16:352–362.
12. Finch WT, Sawyers JL, Schenker S. A prospective study to determine the efficacy of antibiotics on acute pancreatitis. *Ann Surg.* 1976;183:667–671.
13. Beger HG, Bittner R, Bloch S, Buchler M. Bacterial contamination of pancreatic necrosis: a prospective clinical study. *Gastroenterology.* 1986;91:433–438.
14. Buchler M, Malfertheiner P, Frieb H, et al. Human pancreatic tissue concentration of bactericidal antibiotics. *Gastroenterology.* 1992;103:1902–1908.
15. Latifi R, McIntosh JK, Dudrick SJ. Nutritional management of acute and chronic pancreatitis. *Surg Clin North Am.* 1991;71:579–595.
16. Bivins BA, Bell RM, Rapp RP, Toedebusch WH. Pancreatic exocrine response to parenteral nutrition. *J Parenter Enteral Nutr.* 1984;8:34–36.
17. Sax HC, Warner BW, Tolamini MA, et al. Early total parenteral nutrition in acute pancreatitis: lack of beneficial effects. *Am J Surg.* 1987;153:117–124.
18. Stone HH, Fabian TC. Peritoneal dialysis in the treatment of acute alcoholic pancreatitis. *Surg Gynecol Obstet.* 1980;150:878–882.
19. McMahon MJ, Lankisch PG. Peritoneal lavage and dialysis for the treatment of acute pancreatitis. In: Beger HG, Buchler M, eds. *Acute Pancreatitis.* New York, NY: Springer-Verlag New York Inc; 1987:278–284.
20. Ranson JHC, Berman RC. Long peritoneal lavage decreases pancreatic sepsis in acute pancreatitis. *Ann Surg.* 1990;211:708–718.
21. Dugernier T, Reynaert M, Deby-Dupont G. Prospective evaluation of thoracic-duct drainage in the treatment of respiratory failure complicating severe acute pancreatitis. *Intensive Care Med.* 1989;15:372–378.
22. Waltman AC, Luers PR, Athanasoulis CA, Warshaw AL. Massive arterial hemorrhage in patients with pancreatitis: complementary roles of surgery and transcatheter occlusive techniques. *Arch Surg.* 1986;121:439–443.
23. Rattner DW, Warshaw AL. Surgical intervention in acute pancreatitis. *Crit Care Med.* 1988;16:89–95.
24. Neoptolemos JP, Carr-Lock DL, London NJ, Bailey IA, James J, Fossard DP. Controlled trial of urgent endoscopic retrograde cholangiopancreatography and endoscopic sphincterotomy versus conservative treatment for acute pancreatitis due to gallstones. *Lancet.* 1988;2:979–983.
25. Fan ST, Lai ECS, Mok FPT, Lo CM, Zheng SS, Wong J. Early treatment of acute biliary pancreatitis by endoscopic papillotomy. *N Engl J Med.* 1993;328:228–232.
26. Lefer AM, Spatri JA. Pancreatic hypoperfusion and the production of a myocardial depressant factor in hemorrhagic shock. *Ann Surg.* 1974;179:868–876.
27. Beger HG, Bittner R, Buchler M, Hess W, Schmitz JE. Hemodynamic data pattern in patients with acute pancreatitis. *Gastroenterology.* 1986;90:74–79.
28. Leese T, Holliday M, Heath D, Hall AW, Bell PNF. Multicenter clinical trial of low volume fresh frozen plasma therapy in acute pancreatitis. *Br J Surg.* 1987;74:907–911.
29. Goldstein DA, Llach F, Massry SG. Acute renal failure in patients with acute pancreatitis. *Arch Intern Med.* 1976;136:1363–1365.
30. Werner MH, Hayes DF, Lucas CE, Rosenberg IK. Renal vasoconstriction in association with acute pancreatitis. *Am J Surg.* 1974;127:185–190.
31. Gupta RK. Immunohistochemical study of glomerular lesions in acute pancreatitis. *Arch Pathol Lab Med.* 1971;92:267–272.
32. Federle MP, Jeffrey RB, Crass RA, Van Dalsem V. Computed tomography of pancreatic abscesses. *Am J Roentgenol.* 1981;136:879–882.
33. Frey CF. Pathogenesis of nitrogen retention in pancreatitis. *Am J Surg.* 1965;109:747–755.
34. Moosa AR. Diagnostic tests and procedures in acute pancreatitis. *N Engl J Med.* 1984;311:639–642.
35. Ranson JH, Lackner H, Berman IR, Schinella R. The relationship of coagulation factors to clinical complications of acute pancreatitis. *Surgery* 1977;81:502–511.
36. Light RW. Exudative pleural effusions secondary to gastrointestinal disease. *Clin Chest Med.* 1985;6:103–111.
37. Basran GS, Ramasubramanian R, Verma R. Intrathoracic complications of acute pancreatitis. *Br J Dis Chest.* 1987;1:326–331.
38. Warshaw AL, Lesser PB, Rie M, Cullen DJ. The pathogenesis of pulmonary edema in acute pancreatitis. *Ann Surg.* 1975;182:505–510.
39. Weir GC, Lesser PB, Drop LJ, Fisher JE, Warshaw AL. The hypocalcemia of acute pancreatitis. *Ann Intern Med.* 1975;83:185–189.
40. Wilson C, Heads A, Shenkin A, Imrie CW. C-reactive

40. protein, antiproteases and complement factors as objective markers of severity in acute pancreatitis. *Br J Surg.* 1989;76:177–181.
41. Pierce S, Sloane R, Valenzuela JE. Diabetic ketoacidosis (DKA) and elevated pancreatic enzymes: passive bystander or predictor of severe outcome? *Am J Gastroenterol.* 1992;87:1291. Abstract.
42. Guzman S, Nervi F, Llanos O, Leon P, Valdivieso V. Impaired lipid clearance on patients with previous acute pancreatitis. *Gut.* 1985;26:888–891.
43. Cameron JL, Capuzzi DM, Zuidema GD, Margolis S. Acute pancreatitis with hyperlipemia: evidence for a persistent defect in lipid metabolism. *Am J Med.* 1974;56:482–487.
44. Lesser PB, Warshaw AL. Diagnosis of pancreatitis masked by hyperlipemia. *Ann Intern Med.* 1975;82:794–798.
45. Reber HA, Valenzuela JE, Cohen H. Clinical presentation of acute pancreatitis. In: Valenzuela JE, Reber HA, Ribet H, eds. *Medical and Surgical Diseases of the Pancreas.* New York, NY: Igaku-Shoin Medical Publishing; 1991:47–56.
46. Sorensen EV. Subcutaneous fat necrosis: a pancreatic disease. *J Clin Gastroenterol.* 1988;10:71–75.
47. Schmidt A, Svend-Hansen H, Gormsen J. Fibrinogen related antigens in acute pancreatitis. *Acta Chir Scand.* 1976;142:327–328.
48. Lasson A, Ohlsson K. Dissimilated intravascular coagulation and antiprotease activity in acute human pancreatitis. *Scand J Gastroenterol.* 1986;21(suppl 126):35–39.
49. Rattner DW, Warshaw AL. Surgical intervention in acute pancreatitis. *Crit Care Med.* 1988;16:89–95.
50. Ranson JHC, Lackner H. Coagulopathies. In: Bradley EL, ed. *Complications of Pancreatitis.* Philadelphia, Pa: WB Saunders Co; 1982:154–175.
51. Yokoyama I, Hashmi MA, Srinivas D, et al. Wirsungorrhagia or hemoductal pancreatitis: report of a case and review of the literature. *Am J Gastroenterol.* 1984;79:764–768.
52. Estrada RV, Moreno J, Martinez E, Hernandez MC, Gilsanz G, Gilsanz V. Pancreatic encephalopathy. *Acta Neurol Scand.* 1979;59:135–139.
53. Jacob HS, Goldstein IM, Shapiro I, Craddock PR, Hammerschmidt DE, Weissmann G. Sudden blindness in acute pancreatitis: possible role of complement-induced retinal leukoembolization. *Arch Intern Med.* 1981;141:134–136.
54. London NJM, Neoptolemos JP, Lavelle J, Bailey I, James D. Serial computed tomography scanning in acute pancreatitis: a prospective study. *Gut.* 1989;30:397–403.
55. Kourtesis G, Wilson SE, Williams RA. The clinical significance of fluid collections in acute pancreatitis. *Am Surg.* 1990;56:796–799.
56. Siegelman SS, Copeland BE, Sakin GP, Cameron JL, Sanders RC, Zehouni BA. CT of fluid collections associated with pancreatitis. *Am J Roentgenol.* 1980;134:1121–1132.
57. Winship D, moderator. Pancreatitis: pancreatic pseudocysts and their complications. *Gastroenterology.* 1977;73:593–603.
58. Bourliere M, Sarles H. Pancreatic cysts and pseudocysts associated with acute and chronic pancreatitis. *Dig Dis Sci.* 1989;34:343–348.
59. Crass RA, Way LW. Acute and chronic pancreatic pseudocysts are different. *Am J Surg.* 1985;142:660–663.
60. Imrie CL, Buist LJ, Shearer MG. Importance of cause in the outcome of pancreatic pseudocysts. *Am J Surg.* 1988;156:159–162.
61. Silverstein W, Isikoff MB, Hill MC, Barlin J. Diagnostic therapy of acute pancreatitis: prospective study comparing CT and sonography. *Am J Radiol.* 1981;137:497–501.
62. Sankaran S, Walt AJ. The natural and unnatural history of pancreatic pseudocysts. *Br J Surg.* 1975;62:37–44.
63. Bradley EL, Clements JL, Gonzalez AC. The natural history of pancreatic pseudocysts: a unified concept of management. *Am J Surg.* 1979;137:135–141.
64. Yeo CJ, Bastides JA, Lynch-Nyhan A, Fishman EK, Zinner MJ, Cameron JL. The natural history of pancreatic pseudocysts documented by computed tomography. *Surg Gynecol Obstet.* 1990;170:411–417.
65. Vitas GJ, Sarr MG. Selected management of pancreatic pseudocysts: operative versus expectant management. *Surgery.* 1992;111:123–130.
66. Wolsteinholme JT. Major gastrointestinal hemorrhage associated with pancreatic disease. *Am J Surg.* 1974;127:377–381.
67. Stabile BE, Wilson SE, Debas HT. Reduced mortality from bleeding pseudocysts and pseudoaneurysms caused by pancreatitis. *Arch Surg.* 1983;118:45–51.
68. Rohrmann CA, Baron RL. Biliary complications of pancreatitis. *Radiol Clin North Am.* 1989;27:93–104.
69. O'Connor M, Kolars J, Ansel H, Silvis S, Vennes J. Preoperative endoscopic retrograde cholangiopancreatography in the surgical management of pancreatic pseudocysts. *Am J Surg.* 1986;151:18–24.
70. van Sonnenberg E, Wittich GR, Casola G, et al. Percutaneous drainage of infected and noninfected pancreatic pseudocysts: experience in 101 cases. *Radiology.* 1989;170:757–761.
71. Jones SN. The drainage of pancreatic fluid collections. *Clin Radiol.* 1991;43:153–155.
72. Martin EW, Catalan P, Cooperman M, Hecht C, Carey LC. Surgical decision-making in the treatment of pancreatic pseudocysts: Internal versus external drainage. *Am J Surg.* 1979;138:821–825.
73. Mann SK, Mann NS. Pancreatic ascites. *Am J Gastroenterol.* 1979;71:186–192.
74. Sankaran S, Walt AJ. Pancreatic ascites: recognition and management. *Arch Surg.* 1976;111:430–434.
75. Rochey DC, Cello JP. Pancreatopleural fistula: report of 7 patients and a review of the literature. *Medicine.* 1990;69:332–344.
76. Prinz RA, Pickleman J, Hoffman JP. Treatment of pancreatic cutaneous fistulas with a somatostatin analog. *Am J Surg.* 1988;155:36–42.
77. Kozarek RA, Patterson DJ, Ball TJ, Traverso LW. Endoscopic placement of pancreatic stents and drains in the management of pancreatitis. *Ann Surg.* 1989;209:261–266.
78. Ranson JHC, Balthazar E, Caccavale R, Cooper M. Computed tomography and the prediction of pancreatic abscess in acute pancreatitis. *Ann Surg.* 1985;201:656–665.
79. Gerzof SG, Banks PA, Robbins AH, et al. Early diagnosis of pancreatic infection by computed tomography-guided aspiration. *Gastroenterology.* 1987;93:315–320.
80. Steiner E, Mueller PR, Hahn PF, et al. Complicated pancreatic diseases: problems in interventional management. *Radiology.* 1988;187:493–496.

91
Chronic Pancreatitis
CHRIS E. FORSMARK and PHILLIP P. TOSKES

Patients with chronic pancreatitis seek medical attention primarily for abdominal pain or the consequences of pancreatic exocrine insufficiency (steatorrhea, weight loss, or malnutrition). The abdominal pain is quite variable, ranging from a severe acute flare to chronic, persistent pain. A substantial proportion of patients (15% to 25%) do not develop pain and present instead with maldigestion. Chronic pancreatitis is a progressive disease that may evolve over many years, and the process is usually irreversible. Despite this, medical and surgical treatment can often produce substantial improvement in the major complications of abdominal pain and maldigestion.

ETIOLOGY AND PATHOPHYSIOLOGY

In westernized societies, alcohol abuse accounts for 70% of chronic pancreatitis. The mechanism by which alcohol produces pancreatic injury is unknown, but the result is usually substantial damage to the main pancreatic duct and acinar tissue. This damage is characterized by a dilated and strictured main pancreatic duct, usually with associated pancreatic calcifications. At its most extreme, the "chain of lakes" appearance of the pancreatic duct is quite characteristic. This type of disease of the main pancreatic duct ("big duct" disease) is usually easily documented by radiographic imaging, using plain abdominal films in far advanced cases or computed tomography (CT) or endoscopic retrograde pancreatography (ERP) in less advanced cases.

Long-standing obstruction of the main pancreatic duct by stones, strictures, pancreatic duct stents, or tumors may damage the upstream acinar tissue and produce chronic pancreatitis and is likewise characterized by easily demonstrable abnormalities of the main pancreatic duct. Other forms of chronic pancreatitis (idiopathic, hyperlipidemic) appear to damage the acinar tissue and small ducts with relative sparing of the main pancreatic duct. In this case, there is generally no easily visualized abnormality of the main pancreatic duct and little or no pancreatic calcifications. The diagnosis of chronic pancreatitis of this form is therefore more difficult and often requires tests of both pancreatic structure and function. This form of "small duct" or "minimal change" chronic pancreatitis is underdiagnosed and underappreciated by many clinicians.

The specific pathophysiology by which any of these associated conditions produce pancreatic injury and abdominal pain is unknown. Abdominal pain may be produced by a variety of processes in these patients including the following:

1. Inflammation within the pancreas or surrounding tissues
2. Elevated pressure within the pancreatic tissue or pancreatic ducts
3. Associated complications (pseudocyst, duodenal or bile duct obstruction)
4. Hyperstimulation of the pancreas due to a disordered negative feedback–control system

The cause of pain may be different in different patients and may change in any individual patient over time. In some patients, the pain may "burn out" after years of disease.

Maldigestion is not produced until 90% of the exocrine capacity of the pancreas has been lost, making steatorrhea a complication of more advanced chronic pancreatitis. Maldigestion is produced by inadequate delivery of both digestive enzymes and bicarbonate to the small bowel. Malnutrition may occur as a consequence, often promoted by the avoidance of food because of abdominal pain and inadequate intake in individuals with chronic alcoholism.

Endocrine insufficiency (diabetes mellitus) is less common, since the islet cells are more resistant to damage than the acinar cells. Despite this, up to 70% of patients develop glucose intolerance or frank diabetes in far advanced disease characterized by diffuse pancreatic calcifications. The diabetes is characterized by rare ketosis and frequent treatment–associated hypoglycemia. Complications such as nephropathy and retinopathy occur as commonly as in other forms of diabetes if statistics are corrected for disease duration.

DIAGNOSIS

The diagnosis of chronic pancreatitis is usually suggested by the presence of abdominal pain or steatorrhea. There is no pathognomonic pain; the condition varies tremendously in location, radiation, precipitating and alleviating factors, severity, and frequency. Chronic pancreatitis should therefore be included in the differential diagnosis of patients with unexplained abdominal pain. In highly advanced disease, the presence of diffuse pancreatic calcifications may be easily documented by plain abdominal radiography. Unfortunately, these calcifications are not present in many patients with chronic pancreatitis, and more expensive or invasive diagnostic tests must be used to confirm the diagnosis. Various tests of pancreatic structure and function are available to document chronic pancreatitis, and some understanding of these tests and a rational strategy for their use are important in the evaluation of these patients.

Tests of pancreatic structure rely on the presence of ductal dilation, pancreatic calcifications, and pancreatic atrophy to document chronic pancreatitis. In general, more expensive and invasive tests have the greatest sensitivity (such as ERP or CT) and are used only after less expensive and invasive tests have failed to document chronic pancreatitis. The most invasive test, ERP, has a reported sensitivity of 80% to 90%. This is probably an overestimate, since ERP misses those patients who do not have significant abnormalities of the main pancreatic duct (patients with "small duct" disease). In addition, a variety of clinical conditions other than chronic pancreatitis may produce similar changes in the pancreatic duct, including pancreatic carcinoma, acute pancreatitis, pancreatic duct stenting, and even normal aging. Given its expense, need for significant expertise, and risk (approximately 10% complication rate), ERP is used late in the evaluation process. ERP is useful in developing a therapeutic plan. Surgical duct decompression can only be accomplished if the pancreatic duct is adequately dilated; this is best documented by ERP.

Tests of pancreatic function are used in conjunction with tests of structure. The simplest test that carries reasonable accuracy is serum trypsinogen; levels below 20 ng/ml are virtually specific for chronic pancreatitis. More involved evaluations of pancreatic function fall into two categories: indirect and direct tests. The most frequently used indirect test is the bentiromide or nitroblue tetrazolium (NBT)–paraaminobenzoic acid (PABA) test. This test uses a synthetic peptide that is cleaved by pancreatic chymotrypsin, which liberates PABA. This is cleared by the kidney, and a metabolite of PABA is measured in a 6-hour urine collection; the amount collected reflects the level of chymotrypsin in the gut. This test is somewhat more sensitive than serum trypsinogen, but it too is only reliable in highly advanced disease. Like ERP, this test misses patients with less advanced chronic pancreatitis. Direct tests of pancreatic function involve the stimulation of the pancreas with a hormone (secretin or secretin plus cholecystokinin) and collection of the pancreatic secretion by a tube placed in the duodenum. This test is more accurate than any other test for chronic pancreatitis and is able to diagnose patients with less advanced disease. Despite this, it is only performed at a few centers and is unavailable to many clinicians.

TREATMENT

STEATORRHEA

Steatorrhea does not occur until 90% of the excretory capacity of the pancreas has been lost. Fat malabsorption is the most common abnormality, although protein and carbohydrate malabsorption may also occur. The therapy of steatorrhea is directed at delivering adequate amounts of exogenous pancreatic enzymes to the gut lumen. The lipase content of pancreatic enzyme preparations is the most important factor determining efficacy. In most patients, approximately 30,000 U of lipase must be delivered with each meal to the gut lumen for adequate digestion. These enzyme preparations are produced in both conventional (non-enteric-coated) and enteric-coated formulations (Table 91–1). The conventional forms release their contents rapidly after being ingested; the enteric-coated forms do not release their contents until the pH rises above 5.5. The enteric-coated forms there-

TABLE 91–1. PANCREATIC ENZYME FORMULATIONS

Brand Name	Units of Lipase per Pill	Dosage
Viokase*	8,000	8 tablets each time
Cotazym*	8,000	6 capsules each time
Creon†	10,000	3 capsules each time
Pancrease MT10	10,000	3 capsules each time
or MT16†	16,000	2 capsules each time

*Conventional preparation.
†Enteric-coated preparation.
Adjuvant therapy (sodium bicarbonate, H_2-receptor antagonists, or omeprazole) should be given with conventional formulations.

fore are released in the small bowel, whereas the conventional formulations are released in both the stomach and duodenum. The lipase content ranges from 4000 to 20,000 U of lipase per pill, so 2 to 8 pills must be taken with each meal for adequate digestion.

Steatorrhea can rarely be completely corrected, but despite this, the appropriate use of these enzyme preparations results in weight gain and control of diarrhea. The most common reason for failure of enzyme therapy is patient noncompliance with the medication regimen. Another common reason for failure of therapy is inactivation of lipase by gastric acid. This may be corrected by maintaining the gastric pH above 4.0 with the use of sodium bicarbonate, H_2-receptor antagonists, or omeprazole. Alternatively, an enteric-coated preparation may be used.

Dietary manipulation may be useful in selected patients. The diet should generally be high in protein (24%) with moderate fat (30%) and low in carbohydrates (40%). Specific vitamin or trace element deficiencies are rare and are usually a consequence of inadequate intake rather than malabsorption, especially in chronic alcoholism.

PAIN

The management of pain is challenging and often unsatisfactory. Pain is due to a variety of different causes, and hence, no single therapy is effective. Abstinence from alcohol is quite important and often produces significant pain relief. The removal of any other potentially injurious agent (e.g., the use of lipid-lowering agents and diet in patients with hyperlipidemic pancre-

atitis) is also required. Analgesics are often required; nonnarcotic agents or the least potent narcotic agent (e.g., propoxyphene napsylate with acetaminophen [Darvocet N-100]) should be used first. Narcotic addiction is a not infrequent occurrence, particularly in patients with previous substance abuse and little social support. Complications of chronic pancreatitis may also produce pain and are generally amenable to specific therapy; these include duodenal obstruction, bile duct obstruction, or pseudocyst. These should be looked for in any patient with substantial pain or a pain pattern that appears to be worsening.

Exogenous pancreatic enzymes may produce pain relief in a subset of patients. The protease content of the formulation appears to be the active agent that produces pain relief, and these proteases must be released in the duodenum to produce pain relief. For that reason, conventional enzyme formulations must be used. This therapy is most effective in patients with mild-to-moderate disease (no steatorrhea) and with only minor abnormalities of the main pancreatic duct ("small duct" disease). In this subgroup of patients, up to 75% of patients may respond favorably. Eight tablets of a potent conventional enzyme preparation (Viokase or Ku-Zyme HP) should be used at meals and at bedtime. To prevent the breakdown of enzymes by gastric acid, adjuvant therapy with sodium bicarbonate, H_2-receptor antagonists, or omeprazole is usually required. In patients with more advanced disease (steatorrhea or main pancreatic duct abnormalities) this therapy is generally ineffective. Figure 91–1 indicates our approach to the management of abdominal pain in patients with chronic pancreatitis.

Surgical treatment of the pain can be quite effective in some patients with chronic pancreatitis. Surgical therapy may be directed at a complication of chronic pancreatitis or at the pancreas itself. Surgical decompression of the main pancreatic duct by a longitudinal pancreaticojejunostomy (modified Peustow procedure) leads to immediate pain relief in up to 75% of patients and to long-term control of pain in 50%. This therapy is only feasible if the main pancreatic duct is dilated to 7 to 8 mm or more ("big duct" disease), which is best documented by ERP. The performance of a Peustow procedure may also slow the progression of chronic pancreatitis. Subtotal pancreatectomy is generally avoided because of the high incidence of subsequent diabetes mellitus.

In attempts to control the pain of chronic

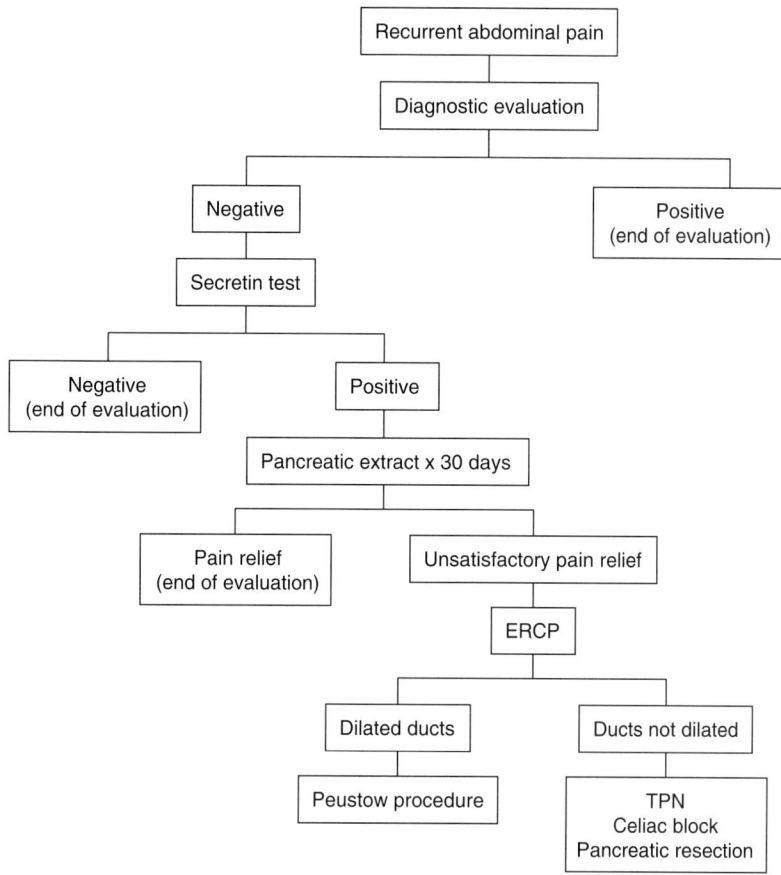

FIGURE 91–1. Management of abdominal pain in patients with chronic pancreatitis. *ERCP* = endoscopic retrograde cholangiopancreatography, *TPN* = total parenteral nutrition. (Modified from Rowell WG, Toskes PP. Pain of chronic pancreatitis: what are the management options? In: Barkin J, Rogers A, eds. *Difficult Decisions in Digestive Diseases.* Chicago, Ill: Year Book Medical Publishers Inc; 1989:192–197.)

pancreatitis, various endoscopic approaches have been used, including pancreatic duct stenting, pancreatic ductal stone removal, dilation of strictures, sphincterotomy of the major or minor papilla, pseudocyst drainage, and biliary decompression. No randomized trials have been performed, and in many reports the response rate is no greater than that seen with placebo. In addition, long-term pancreatic duct stenting appears to produce chronic pancreatitis. With the exception of biliary decompression for cholangitis, these techniques should generally be reserved for clinical trials.

Injection of the celiac axis with an anesthetic or alcohol under CT guidance is generally ineffective in chronic pancreatitis, although it may be quite effective in pancreatic carcinoma, perhaps because of the short survival of those with cancer and the chronicity of chronic pancreatitis. The use of octreotide appears promising, with reported response rates of up to 75%, although further studies are required before this therapy can be widely used.

COMPLICATIONS

PSEUDOCYST

Pseudocysts that occur in the setting of chronic pancreatitis are usually associated with downstream obstruction of the pancreatic duct with upstream development of a pseudocyst. Many patients with pseudocysts remain asymptomatic, with several recent studies suggesting that only 10% to 20% ultimately develop a complication.

This is particularly true in patients with relatively small pseudocysts (<6 cm), which usually are asymptomatic and only rarely produce a complication.

Patients with a pancreatic pseudocyst in the setting of chronic pancreatitis may experience an abrupt complication (bleeding, infection, obstruction of a surrounding structure, or rupture) but may also experience more subtle symptoms such as a worsening of abdominal pain or progressive weight loss. The development of the more severe complications usually requires urgent therapy. Percutaneous aspiration and drainage of an infected pseudocyst is usually successful when coupled with intravenous antibiotics. Surgical therapy is also effective for pseudocyst infection and in addition is usually required for pseudocyst bleeding, rupture, or obstruction of the biliary tree or duodenum.

Pseudocysts that have not produced an abrupt complication can also be treated either percutaneously or surgically. Percutaneous tube drainage has been reported to be successful in over 90% of patients, although many of the pseudocysts reform after the tube is removed. Despite the recurrence, many patients remain asymptomatic. Surgical cystenterostomy is more definitive and, in addition, allows the differentiation of pseudocysts from cystic neoplasms.

OTHER COMPLICATIONS

Splenic vein thrombosis may complicate chronic pancreatitis, producing a segmental portal hypertension characterized by large gastric varices in the absence of significant esophageal varices. Persons with splenic vein thrombosis usually present with gastrointestinal tract bleeding, and the diagnosis is usually established by ultrasound or CT. Endoscopic sclerotherapy or variceal banding may stop bleeding acutely but is generally not effective over the long term; splenectomy is usually curative.

Obstruction of the bile duct may occur as a consequence of a pseudocyst or may be due to fibrosis within the pancreas. Therapy is reserved for those patients with biliary symptoms or signs (jaundice, cholangitis) and for patients with cholestatic liver chemistries. Endoscopic therapy is useful for cholangitis and as a bridge to more definitive surgical biliary bypass.

SUMMARY

Most patients with chronic pancreatitis present with abdominal pain, maldigestion, or both. Steatorrhea is often easy to effectively treat. The treatment of pain is less satisfactory but includes abstinence from alcohol and appropriate analgesia. High-dose, conventional enzyme preparations are useful in a subset of patients with "small duct" disease of moderate severity. Surgical duct decompression is effective for refractory pain if the pancreatic duct is adequately dilated and also is useful for the treatment of associated complications.

REFERENCES

1. Forsmark CE, Grendell JH. Complications of pancreatitis. *Semin Gastrointest Dis.* 1991;2:165–176.
2. Hayakawa T, Kondo T, Shibata T, et al. Relationship between pancreatic exocrine function and histologic changes in chronic pancreatitis. *Am J Gastroenterol.* 1992;87:1170–1174.
3. Jacobson DG, Currington C, Connery K, et al. Trypsin-like immunoreactivity as a test for pancreatic insufficiency. *N Engl J Med.* 1984;310:307–309.
4. Mulvihill SJ, Debas HT. Surgical treatment of pancreatitis and its complications. *Semin Gastrointest Dis.* 1991;2:194–202.
5. Neiderau C, Grendell JH. Diagnosis of chronic pancreatitis. *Gastroenterology.* 1985;88:1973–1995.
6. Slaff J, Jacobson DG, Tillman CR, et al. Protease-specific suppression of pancreatic exocrine secretion. *Gastroenterology.* 1984;87:44–52.
7. Toskes PP. Medical therapy of chronic pancreatitis. *Semin Gastrointest Dis.* 1991;2:188–193.
8. van Sonnenberg E, Casola G, Varney RR, et al. Imaging and interventional radiology for pancreatitis and its complications. *Radiol Clin North Am.* 1989;27:65–72.
9. Vitas GJ, Sarr MG. Selected management of pancreatic pseudocysts: operative versus expectant management. *Surgery.* 1992;111:123–130.
10. Walsh TN, Rode J, This BA, et al. Minimal change chronic pancreatitis. *Gut.* 1992;33:1566–1571.

92

Cancer of the Pancreas

IRVING WAXMAN, STEVEN D. FREEDMAN, and MICHAEL L. STEER

PATHOLOGY AND EPIDEMIOLOGY

Approximately 25,000 Americans develop cancer of the pancreas each year, and more than 95% of these individuals die of their disease within 5 years of its diagnosis. Pancreatic carcinoma is, therefore, the fourth most frequent cause of death from cancer, exceeded only by cancer of the lung, colorectum, and breast. It is the tenth most common form of cancer.

Malignant tumors of the pancreas may arise from its exocrine, endocrine, or supportive elements. Sarcomas and lymphomas of the pancreas are rare. Neuroendocrine tumors, which may or may not be functional, are slow growing and associated with a relatively favorable prognosis. This chapter focuses on carcinomas of the exocrine pancreas, which account for more than 90% of all pancreatic malignancies.

Carcinoma of the exocrine pancreas is more commonly found in the head than in the body or tail of the gland. This predilection has suggested that malignant transformation may involve exposure to carcinogenic agents that reflux into the pancreatic ductal system from either the duodenum or biliary tract. Malignant cystic tumors of the pancreas, although uncommon, represent a clinically important subset because they may be confused with other cystic lesions (e.g., retention cysts, pseudocysts) or benign cystic tumors (i.e., cystadenomas) and because, even in their malignant form, these tumors are slow growing, late to metastasize, and associated with a favorable prognosis if resected.

Pancreatic cancers frequently metastasize via lymphatics and grow, by direct extension, out of the gland into adjacent structures. Most frequent sites for distant metastases include the liver, lung, and peritoneum. In contrast to other malignant tumors, ductal cancers of the pancreas have a predilection for perineural growth and spread within nerve sheaths.

Pancreatic cancer is most common among men and blacks. Several risk factors have been identified. Cigarette smoking is believed to increase the risk of developing pancreatic cancer by 50%. The incidence of pancreatic cancer is also increased among individuals consuming diets that are rich in fat or protein and decreased in those whose diets are rich in fruits and vegetables. Diabetes mellitus and chronic pancreatitis also increase the risk of developing pancreatic cancer. On the other hand, it is currently believed that coffee consumption does not increase the risk of developing cancer of the pancreas.

CLINICAL PRESENTATION

The clinical manifestations of pancreatic cancer are dependent on the location of the tumor within the gland. Cancers of the body and tail of the gland are usually silent until they metastasize, and as a result, many patients with tumors in the body or tail of the gland present with malignant ascites, bowel obstruction, or symptomatic liver metastases. Some present with back pain, which may reflect either nerve compression or pancreatic duct obstruction by the tumor.

Others present with unexplained weight loss, which may be the result of either tumor-associated anorexia or malabsorption from steatorrhea caused by duct obstruction. In contrast to patients with tumors in the body or tail of the pancreas, those with cancers of the head or uncinate process of the pancreas typically develop obstructive jaundice relatively early. Other presenting symptoms may include steatorrhea from pancreatic duct obstruction or gastric outlet obstruction from invasion or obstruction of the duodenum.

Physical examination may reveal a palpable abdominal mass or ascites. In the presence of painless jaundice, a palpable gallbladder is indicative of malignant biliary obstruction (i.e.,

Courvoisier's gallbladder). Supraclavicular adenopathy, Blumer's shelf, or a palpable subumbilical node (Sister Mary Joseph node) indicates widespread metastases. Laboratory studies, in most patients, merely confirm the presence of obstructive jaundice, diabetes, or steatorrhea.

IMAGING STUDIES

Frequently, patients present with jaundice, and thus imaging of the liver should be one of the initial studies performed.

Ultrasound is simple and inexpensive and can determine if there are dilated bile or pancreatic ducts, hepatic metastases, or a pancreatic mass. However, the dependence of ultrasound on body habitus and the frequent difficulty in visualizing the pancreas because of overlying bowel gas limit this technique. The principal advantage of ultrasonography is that it can determine intrahepatic verses extrahepatic causes of jaundice.

Abdominal computed tomography (CT) is generally superior to ultrasonography in the imaging of the pancreas and has a 90% sensitivity and specificity in the detection of pancreatic carcinoma. In a patient with suspected pancreatic tumor, dynamic CT, in which a continuous bolus of contrast is given intravenously, provides the highest resolution images. In conjunction with 5-mm thin cuts through the pancreas, lesions 1 cm or greater can be detected with this method. A mass in the head of the pancreas in conjunction with dilation of the common bile duct should suggest pancreatic neoplasm. Masses may be homogeneous or in some cases cystic. Although the latter may represent a cystic neoplasm, this appearance can be secondary to central necrosis of an adenocarcinoma. An advantage of CT is that dynamic scanning may show vessel encasement and visualize metastases that were not seen by ultrasonography. It should be emphasized that a mass seen on these radiologic studies may overestimate the true size of the actual tumor. Pancreatic adenocarcinoma is frequently surrounded by pancreatic inflammation and fibrosis, making it difficult in certain circumstances to differentiate pancreatitis from carcinoma.

Magnetic resonance imaging (MRI) has only recently been assessed in pancreatic neoplasms. Although early studies did not show an advantage over CT, one recent report suggests MRI is superior to CT in detecting small intrapancreatic tumors and parapancreatic extension. Whether MR angiography can replace conventional angiography for the assessment of vascular involvement by tumor is currently under investigation.

In patients in whom the above radiologic studies are inconclusive, *endoscopic retrograde cholangiopancreatography (ERCP)* is the next test of choice. This modality has the advantage of not only providing diagnostic information but can also be used as a therapeutic tool. At the time of ERCP the following findings may be noted: duodenal invasion along the medial wall due to pancreatic tumor, ampullary neoplasms, choledocholithiasis, and pancreatic and biliary duct strictures. Since 95% of pancreatic adenocarcinomas arise from ductal elements, ERCP frequently demonstrates an abnormal pancreatogram. Occasionally, the "double duct sign" is seen secondary to obstruction of the distal pancreatic and bile duct from a carcinoma in the head of the pancreas. The overall sensitivity of ERCP is between 80% and 90% with false-positives approaching 5%. The difficulty in interpreting pancreatograms arises in the distinction between chronic pancreatitis and carcinoma of the pancreas. Irregular pancreatic strictures longer than 10 mm are more indicative of pancreatic cancer.

Angiography is less helpful in determining the diagnosis. The main utility of this technique is the demonstration of vascular encasement, which makes these hypovascular lesions generally unresectable. Since there is significant variability in pancreatic vascular anatomy, some surgeons also prefer to have an angiogram to guide the surgery.

SERUM MARKERS

A number of markers for pancreatic carcinoma have been examined, although none are sufficient for widespread screening. *The most commonly used marker is the CA 19-9.* The higher the value, the greater the specificity. The CA 19-9 has an overall sensitivity of 80% and specificity of 90%. At levels greater than 1000 U/ml (normal: up to 37 U/ml), the specificity for pancreatic carcinoma rises to 99%. Although the carcinoembryonic antigen (CEA) alone has a low sensitivity and is elevated in many different types of malignancy, the specificity increases to 99% in cases where there is a modest elevation of the CA 19-9 (i.e., <600 U/ml) if the CEA is greater than 5 ng/ml. Of note, elevated CA 19-9 levels are also seen in other adenocarcinomas, especially those that involve the stomach, colon, and bile ducts. There are two conditions where false-positive values for the CA 19-9 are seen in the absence of malignancy. The first is in cirrhosis where it may be elevated in the low hundreds.

The second is in cholangitis where values greater than 1000 U/ml may be found. The CA 19-9 can also be used as a prognostic factor before and after surgery. If the CA 19-9 is elevated prior to resection of pancreatic carcinoma, normalization after surgery suggests a favorable prognosis. Similar to the use of CEA in screening for recurrence of colon cancer after surgery, an increase in the CA 19-9 after surgical resection signifies recurrent tumor.

BIOPSY

If a patient is to undergo surgery, there is no role for obtaining a tissue diagnosis preoperatively. However, in patients with inoperable disease, one may wish to confirm the diagnosis of pancreatic carcinoma by obtaining tissue. If ERCP is performed for palliation, then brushings can be obtained for cytologic analysis. On average, sensitivity approaches 70%. There was initial enthusiasm for aspiration of pancreatic juice at the time of pancreatic duct cannulation to determine if malignant cells were shed. However, this has not been reproducibly found to be a sensitive assay for tumor.

Fine needle aspiration biopsy of the pancreas can be performed using CT guidance. This has a sensitivity of 57% to 90%, depending on the study. However, there are now reports of seeding along the needle tract and perhaps intraperitoneal spread. It is for this reason that this technique should be reserved for nonoperative candidates. Tissue diagnosis should be attempted in these patients, since lymphoma and other tumors may be at least partially cured with chemotherapy.

In addition to abdominal CT and angiography, staging can be approached using laparoscopy with peritoneal washings. In one study, 40% of patients with disease confined to the pancreas by CT were found to have 1- to 2-mm nodules studding the peritoneal and omental surfaces. A similar percentage had malignant cells in peritoneal washings. These findings correlate with resectability, but whether this approach at staging and selecting patients for resection translates into improvement in survival must still be determined.

POTENTIALLY CURATIVE THERAPY

The only potentially curative treatment for carcinoma of the pancreas is radical surgical resection. Rarely, cancers of the body or tail of the gland may be resectable at the time of diagnosis, and in those instances resection involves distal (left) subtotal pancreatectomy and splenectomy. For cancers of the head of the pancreas, resection usually consists of radical pancreaticoduodenectomy (Whipple procedure). Some surgeons perform a pylorus-preserving Whipple procedure in hope of avoiding the unwanted side effects of a distal gastrectomy, but at least on theoretic grounds, this approach may compromise the margins of cancer clearance.

Until relatively recently, the morbidity and mortality associated with the Whipple procedure were extremely high, and perioperative death rates in some series reached 40%. Many groups have now reported perioperative death rates of less than 5%. As a result, most surgeons currently recommend radical resection for appropriate patients who can be resected with the hope of cure, and some surgeons have even suggested that the Whipple procedure might be performed for palliation of symptoms of pancreatic cancer.

The evaluation of patients for surgical therapy of pancreatic cancer has been the subject of considerable controversy. Since pancreatic cancer is resectable in only 20% of patients at the time of diagnosis and the 5-year cure rate of those undergoing resection in various series has ranged from 5% to 30%, at best only 5% to 6% of those diagnosed with pancreatic cancer can be cured by surgical means.

Pancreatic cancer is rare before the age of 40 years, and approximately 80% of all patients are between the ages of 60 to 80 years. As a result, many patients with pancreatic cancer have associated or comorbid diseases that make them poor candidates for a major pancreatic resection. Those individuals should not be considered candidates for surgical resection. On the other hand, some patients present with symptoms of gastric outlet obstruction as a result of duodenal invasion or encasement by tumor. Currently, these patients' symptoms cannot be palliated by nonsurgical methods; since these patients must undergo operation in any case, the question of resectability can be determined at the time of laparotomy.

The remaining patients are neither too infirm to undergo radical resection nor suffering from obstructive symptoms. For the most part, these individuals have already had a CT scan or an ultrasound examination or both that demonstrate a pancreatic mass. If these studies show evidence of metastatic disease such as liver metastases, extrapancreatic adenopathy, or peritoneal nodules, these patients should not be considered as candidates for radical resection. After eliminating these groups from further consideration, there remains a significant number of patients who are acceptable surgical candidates and whose disease appears to be limited to the pancreas, at least on the basis of CT or ultrasound and physical examination. Some of these individuals may, in fact, have only a benign disease such as chronic pancreatitis and be identifiable by performance of an ERCP, which might reveal either no ductal stricture or a stricture longer than 10 mm. However, in practice, the clinical presentation including the history is the major factor used in identifying those individuals with either benign disease or a malignant process. Some patients with benign disease may undergo radical resection in the mistaken belief that they have cancer. It has been our practice to recommend an attempt at resection for acceptable-risk patients believed to have resectable cancer localized to the pancreas and to avoid further attempts at preoperative diagnosis or staging. The only exceptions to this rule are the occasional patients with a lesion at the body or tail of the pancreas or tumors of the head of the pancreas that on CT appear to involve the mesenteric or portal vessels. A visceral arteriogram may be useful in that setting, since obstruction or encasement of major vessels by the tumor would indicate that the cancer is not resectable for cure. Other surgeons, however, have recommended that all potential candidates for radical resection undergo laparoscopy and visceral arteriography, but the potential advantages of this approach have not been established. Recent reports have suggested that endoscopic ultrasound may be a sensitive method of establishing resectability and staging patients with pancreatic cancer. This technology, however, is extremely operator-dependent, and its general applicability remains to be established.

PALLIATIVE THERAPY

Because of significant advancements in pancreatic imaging over the last decade, resectability for pancreatic cancer is currently reported to be about 20%. Nevertheless, 80% of patients are unsuitable for resection and require some form of palliative procedure aimed at relieving obstructive jaundice and pain, which are the most common presenting symptoms in patients with pancreatic carcinoma. Duodenal obstruction, on the other hand, mainly presents in the latter stages of the disease.

OBSTRUCTIVE JAUNDICE

More than 70% of patients with pancreatic cancer develop jaundice in the course of their disease. When prolonged, jaundice impairs liver function and can lead to liver failure. In addition, it is associated with pruritus in 20% of the cases, cholangitis in about 25% of cases, and malabsorption and anorexia, which can lead to malnutrition. Since the 1980s, percutaneous transhepatic stenting (PTS) and endoscopic transpapillary stenting (ETS) have become established methods for the palliation of obstructive jaundice, in addition to surgical biliary bypass. The advantages of PTS and ETS over surgical bypass may reside in their lower mortality and more rapid recovery. In experienced hands, both nonoperative methods can achieve about 90% success in providing biliary drainage. Therefore, ETS is now generally accepted as the first choice for nonsurgical palliation. A combined percutaneous and endoscopic technique has been described for patients who have failed endoscopic drainage procedures and are not surgical candidates; although it has shown an 80% success rate, the combined procedure was associated with significant morbidity and disease-related mortality.

Recent prospective trials have tried to clarify the question of endoscopic versus surgical palliation. It is apparent from these studies that although there is no difference in the long-term survival of the patients, irrespective of treatment, there is a reduction in procedural mortality. The benefit of shorter initial hospital stay for the group that received nonoperative treatment is counterbalanced by frequent readmission for stent changes. Regarding the optimal surgical biliary bypass, it seems that choledochojejunostomy is superior to cholecystojejunostomy. Both procedures carry similar mortality, but recurrence of jaundice or cholangitis seem to be more common after cholecystojejunostomy.

DUODENAL OBSTRUCTION

Although nausea and vomiting are common presenting symptoms of pancreatic cancer and can be seen in 30% to 45% of cases, actual outlet obstruction is present in about 5% of the cases at the time of diagnosis. Tumors in the head of the gland usually obstruct the second part of the duodenum, whereas lesions of the body and tail of the gland can cause obstruction of the distal duodenum at the ligament of Treitz. In addition, a motility disorder may play a role in some of these patients, mimicking gastroparesis or delayed gastric emptying in patients that have undergone gastroenterostomy. Whether this is secondary to a paraneoplastic syndrome mediated by the tumor or due to neural infiltration resulting in autonomic denervation is unknown. Surgical bypass is the only treatment available at the present time. In our opinion, a prophylactic gastrojejunostomy should be performed at the time of the biliary bypass. This is supported by the fact that multiple studies have shown no increase in operative mortality when a gastrojejunostomy is added to a biliary diversion and the fact that up to 25% of patients require a reoperation after the initial biliary bypass. Although we have listed duodenal obstruction as a late complication of pancreatic cancer, we strongly advise a gastroenterostomy combined with a biliary bypass if tumor compression or infiltration of the duodenum is observed during the initial ERCP.

Pain Relief

Abdominal and back pain is a presenting symptom in 70% to 90% of patients with pancreatic cancer. Its cause is unclear. Some believe that pancreatic or bile duct obstruction produces ductal hypertension, and this causes pain. Others suggest that perineural invasion with parapancreatic nerve infiltration may be the explanation. Contrary to jaundice, which does not carry prognostic significance, pain seems to be related to the stage of the disease, being present more often in patients unsuitable for operation. Narcotic analgesics is usually the first line of therapy followed by either percutaneous or intraoperative chemical splanchnicectomy. Series reporting up to an 80% pain reduction are available for both modalities. Another method available for palliation of pain is radiation therapy. Studies using precision high-dose (PHD) external radiation report good results in about 50% to 60% of patients. Intraoperative radiotherapy seems to be more effective but a much more cumbersome alternative. Control studies looking at the effects of stenting an obstructed pancreatic duct to relieve pain are not available yet.

ADJUVANT THERAPY IN UNRESECTABLE PANCREATIC CARCINOMA

When evaluating adjuvant therapy in patients with metastatic pancreatic cancer, one should always keep in mind that the median survival time for these patients is about 3 months. Therefore, quality of life and minimizing iatrogenic side effects is of paramount importance. At best, survival appears to be only marginally increased by adjuvant therapy. Regarding radiotherapy, PHD therapy with adjuvant 5-fluorouracil as a radiosensitizer has shown a median survival time of about 1 year as compared to external beam radiotherapy alone, making it the most attractive regimen currently available. Intraoperative radiotherapy enhances control of local disease and is an effective means of pain control in 50% to 93% of the patients but has not been shown to significantly improve survival. More importantly, however, combination chemotherapy with radiotherapy has a role as an adjuvant therapy for patients who undergo curative resection as shown by the Gastrointestinal Tumor Study Group (GITSG). In the GITSG study median survival rates reached 20 months as compared to 11 months in the control group. A role for hormonal therapy has been suggested by experimental studies that have shown an effect between estrogens and androgens in pancreatic cell function, as well as the finding of receptors for estrogen, progesterone, and androgen in human pancreatic carcinoma. Currently, clinical trials with tamoxifen have shown no clear benefit, but it is clear that much more research is needed in this area.

REFERENCES

1. Arbuck SG. Overview of chemotherapy for pancreatic cancer. *Int J Pancreatol.* 1990;7:209–222.
2. Freeny PC, Marks WM, Ryan JA, Traverso LW. Pancreatic ductal adenocarcinoma: diagnosis and staging with dynamic CT. *Radiology.* 1988;166:125–133.
3. Gastrointestinal Tumor Study Group. Further evidence of effective adjuvant combined radiation and chemotherapy following curative resection of pancreatic cancer. *Cancer.* 1987;59:2006–2010.
4. Huibregtse K. Non-operative palliation for pancreatic cancer. In: Neoptolemos JP, ed. *Bailliere's Clinical Gastroenterology.* London: Bailliere Tindall. 1990;4:995–1004.
5. Steinberg W. The clinical utility of the CA 19-9 tumor associated antigen. *Am J Gastroenterol.* 1990;85:350–355.
6. Warshaw AL, Fernandez del Castillo C. Pancreatic carcinoma. *N Engl J Med.* 1992;326:455–465.
7. Warshaw AL, Zhuo-yun GU, Wittenberg J, Waltman AC. Preoperative staging and assessment of resectability of pancreatic cancer. *Arch Surg.* 1990;125:230–233.
8. Watanapa P, Williamson RCN. Surgical palliation for pancreatic cancer: developments during past two decades. *Br J Surg.* 1992;79:8–20.

SECTION VI

HEPATOBILIARY TRACT

93

Drug- and Toxin-induced Liver Injury

CAROLYN J. HOLESKI and LAURIE D. DeLEVE

The liver is the main drug-metabolizing organ in the body and is therefore a frequent target for toxicity induced by the resulting metabolites. Since drug-induced hepatotoxicity is common and can mimic almost any form of acute or chronic liver disease, it is important to understand the causative mechanisms and to recognize the most common features. This chapter presents an overview of the mechanisms of injury and the clinical patterns by which injury is manifested. This is followed by a discussion of some specific examples of hepatotoxins to illustrate the mechanisms involved in drug- and toxin-induced liver disease.

MECHANISMS OF INJURY

The hepatocyte contains drug metabolizing enzymes, which are responsible for the biotransformation of drugs and toxins. The first step in the metabolism of a drug is usually through a so-called phase I reaction that is carried out by a family of enzymes referred to as the cytochrome P-450 enzymes (by the new convention the word *cytochrome* is omitted and this convention is adhered to throughout the rest of the chapter). In the reactions catalyzed by P-450, a single molecular oxygen is introduced into the drug, usually as a hydroxyl group. This often leads to an unstable compound that rapidly degrades, resulting in the loss of, for example, a carbon atom, so that the net result of the P-450 reaction is a demethylation. Thus, in addition to hydroxylation reactions, the P-450s may catalyze deacylation, oxidation, or reduction reactions. The metabolites that are formed are polar intermediates, which can undergo a phase II conjugation reaction that makes the drug more easily excreted. Drug-induced toxicity is most commonly due to reactive metabolites produced by so-called phase I reactions that react with cellular constituents before conjugation catalyzed by a phase II enzyme can take place (see Fig. 93–1).

Interindividual variation exists in the biotransformation of drugs and toxins and is determined by both genetic and environmental factors. Genetic differences may be due to altered catalytic activity of a specific isozyme or variability in the inducibility of an isozyme. An example of genetic variability of the catalytic activity of an enzyme is the hereditary defect in hydroxylation of debrisoquin, an antihypertensive medication. Ten percent of the population metabolizes this drug poorly, and this appears to be due to at least three separate defects in the genes coding for the P-450 subfamily.[1] Genetic differences in induction have not been well studied in man, but in animals the genetic difference in inducibility of arylhydrocarbon hydroxylase has been well described. Environmental factors such as disease, diet, and exposure to environmental toxins may alter cofactor availability or enzyme induction. The toxic intermediates formed by the P-450s may undergo covalent binding to cellular macromolecules or may oxidize cellular constituents. These actions may impair essential cell functions required for cell viability by inactivating enzymes, disrupting calcium homeostasis, or causing loss of plasma membrane integrity.

The phase II reactions are commonly conjugation reactions with glutathione, glucuronide, sulfate, or acyl groups. Genetic and environmental factors also determine interindividual variation in these conjugation pathways. Increased toxicity in a given individual may therefore be a result of either enhanced phase I formation of toxic metabolites or diminished phase II protection. A genetic anomaly that may predispose to acetaminophen toxicity is uridine diphosphate–glucuronyl transferase deficiency (the enzyme responsible for glucuronide conjugation). An example of an environmental influence that exacerbates toxicity is the increased sensitivity of alcoholics to acetaminophen. This increased sensitivity is due to both induced P-450 activity and diminished glutathione detoxification. Alcohol and acetaminophen share the same P-450 iso-

643

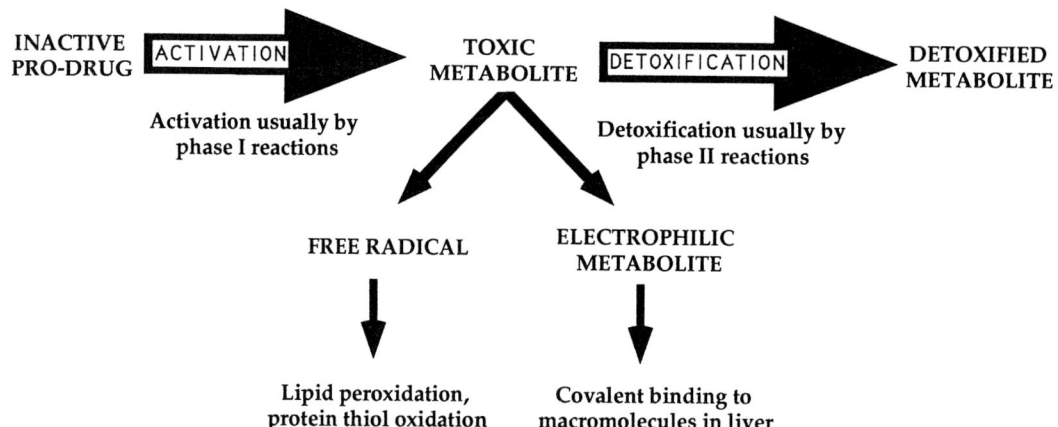

FIGURE 93–1. Imbalance in the equilibrium of the activation and detoxification pathways can allow toxic intermediates to react with cellular macromolecules.

zyme, P-450 IIE1. This isozyme is induced by alcohol, so that activation of acetaminophen to the toxic metabolite may be increased in alcoholics. Long-term alcohol intake may result in a depletion of hepatic glutathione,[2] which is important in the detoxification of the toxic metabolite. Thus, alcoholics may develop hepatotoxicity within the therapeutic range.[2,3,4]

The liver is particularly susceptible to drug- and toxin-induced injury for several reasons. First, the hepatocyte is quite rich in P-450 and is therefore more likely than many other organs in the body to form potentially toxic metabolites. Second, the rich blood supply to the liver ensures intense exposure of the liver to drugs and toxins in the blood; virtually all compounds absorbed from the gastrointestinal tract must pass through the portal vein into the liver. Furthermore, the liver receives approximately 25% of the cardiac output so that parenterally administered drugs (and orally administered drugs that escaped the liver on the first pass) enter the hepatic circulation soon after the drugs enter the bloodstream. A third factor relates to a unique histologic feature of the liver. The endothelium that separates the hepatocyte from the sinusoidal blood is fenestrated, which allows protein-bound drugs direct exposure to the cellular membrane of the hepatocyte.

Hepatotoxins can be classified into two major categories of drug reaction: (1) intrinsic or dose-dependent toxicity and (2) idiosyncratic or host-dependent toxicity (see Fig. 93–2). Intrinsic toxins cause hepatotoxicity at predictable plasma concentrations of the drug. It is reproducible in various species and produces a high incidence in exposed animals. Intrinsic toxicity may be non-specific. An example of this is the formation of highly reactive intermediates that damage membrane lipids of the plasma membrane and organelles indiscriminately. This is exemplified by carbon tetrachloride, which causes lipid peroxidation. Alternatively, an intrinsic toxin may affect a particular metabolic pathway or transport process selectively. This is exemplified by tetracycline, which produces steatosis by interfering with lipid transport from the liver.[5]

In contrast to intrinsic toxins, idiosyncratic toxins produce toxicity in an unpredictable, dose-independent fashion. Although idiosyncratic reactions only occur in a relatively small number of individuals, these adverse reactions are the most common cause of drug- and toxin-induced hepatotoxicity.[6] Idiosyncratic reactions can be divided into reactions due to unusual metabolism of the drug and reactions due to hypersensitivity responses. Metabolic idiosyncrasy may be due to abnormally low levels of detoxifying enzyme or increased activation of the compound. Increased activation may be the result of unusually high levels of activating enzyme or a mutant isozyme that is more active than the normal enzyme. Hypersensitivity reactions are due to toxins that alter endogenous macromolecules. Modifications are due to (1) covalent binding of a toxin to the molecule, (2) alteration of the structure of the protein by mutation of the gene that codes for the protein or by inducing a post-translational modification, or (3) oxidative modification of the macromolecule leading to abnormal disulfide linkages or oxidized residues. The modification of the macromolecule may elicit an immune response against a hapten, a new antigenic determinant or an autoantigen. Haptens

FIGURE 93–2. Hepatotoxins may be categorized as intrinsic or idiosyncratic toxins.

- INTRINSIC: dose-dependent, host-independent
- IDIOSYNCRATIC: dose-independent, host-dependent
  - metabolic: increased activating enzyme or mutant isozyme decreased detoxifying capacity
  - hypersensitivity
    - anti-hapten
    - anti-new antigenic determinant
    - anti-autoantigen

are formed when an immune response is elicited by part or all of the reactive drug bound covalently to a macromolecule. An example of toxicity due to hapten is halothane hepatitis. This injury seems to be due to covalent binding of the trifluoroacetyl chloride metabolite, which forms a trifluoroacetyl hapten. New antigenic determinants can be the result of covalent modification of the macromolecule. Finally, autoantigens are sites that may elicit an immune response due to similarity to previous covalent modifications of the macromolecule.[6]

PATTERNS OF HEPATOTOXICITY

Drug-induced hepatotoxicity can be divided into acute and chronic forms: this describes the clinical presentation and does not necessarily reflect the length of time the patient has been exposed to the drug. Chronic hepatotoxicity may be due to either prolonged exposure to a drug or may be a sequel to acute injury.

ACUTE HEPATOTOXICITY
(see Fig. 93–3)

Acute Parenchymal Toxicity

Parenchymal Necrosis

Drugs that cause acute hepatocellular necrosis usually follow a consistent pattern. For example, zonal necrosis may be related to metabolic differences within the lobule, such as the relatively high P-450 activity or low glutathione availability within the centrizonal portion of the lobule. On the other hand, drugs that cause necrosis of hepatocytes diffusely throughout the lobule are more likely to be dose independent and may be related to genetic variation. Drug-induced hepatocellular necrosis mimics viral hepatitis clinically and histopathologically. Thus, patients may present with fatigue, anorexia, nausea, jaundice, and, in severe cases, with ascites and coagulopathy also. Laboratory studies will show high elevations of aminotransferases and moderate elevations of alkaline phosphatase. Increases of prothrombin time and

HISTOLOGY	LIVER TESTS		CLINICAL PICTURE RESEMBLES
	aminotransferases	alk. phosphatase	
Hepatocellular			
necrosis	↑↑↑	↑	viral hepatitis
steatosis	↑↑	↑	Reye's syndrome
Cholestasis			
hepatocanalicular	Nl-↑↑	↑↑	obstructive jaundice
canalicular	Nl-↑	↑	obstructive jaundice
Mixed	↑↑	↑↑	hepatitis or obstructive jaundice

FIGURE 93–3. Histologic and clinical patterns of acute drug-induced hepatotoxicity.

bilirubin will mirror the severity of necrosis. The most important drugs that cause fulminant hepatic failure are acetaminophen, *Amanita phalloides* toxin (from a poisonous mushroom), phenytoin, halothane, and carbon tetrachloride. Therapy usually consists of supportive medical management for liver failure and coma and hemodialysis for renal failure. In severe cases, orthotopic liver transplantation has become a therapeutic option.

For a small number of agents, specific therapy is based on the metabolism of the drug. The use of hyperbaric oxygen in the management of carbon tetrachloride hepatotoxicity is based on knowledge of the first step of its metabolism, which is a reduction reaction that is inhibited by oxygen.[7,8] Other therapeutic approaches to carbon tetrachloride poisoning have been directed toward scavenging the free-radical intermediates with vitamin E or *N*-acetylcysteine (NAC).[9] Another example of a specific therapy is the use of NAC for acetaminophen intoxication, which is discussed later in this chapter.

Steatosis

Microvesicular steatosis (small fat droplets within the hepatocyte) due to drugs presents with the same clinical and histologic picture as fatty liver of pregnancy or Reye's syndrome. Clinically, patients with microvesicular steatosis present with nausea, vomiting, abdominal pain, renal injury, and progressive neurologic deterioration. The fatality rate in recognized cases is high. Laboratory tests show elevation of aminotransferases, moderate elevation of bilirubin, slight or no elevation of alkaline phosphatase, prolonged prothrombin time, and hypoglycemia. In contrast, patients with macrovesicular steatosis (accumulation of large droplets of fat in the hepatocyte) are often symptom free or may complain of right upper quadrant heaviness and discomfort that worsens with movement. Aminotransferases are usually only moderately elevated. Methotrexate is an example of a drug that can cause macrovesicular steatosis and a clinical picture similar to alcohol-induced fatty change. Therapy for liver injury secondary to steatosis consists of the withdrawal of the offending agent, which frequently results in rapid improvement. For injury that has resulted in fulminant hepatic failure, therapy is primarily supportive with orthotopic liver transplantation as a potential option.

Phospholipidosis

A third form of acute hepatocellular hepatotoxicity is the acute form of phospholipidosis. This is the acute equivalent of nonalcoholic steatonecrosis, which is described later in this chapter under Chronic Hepatotoxicity.

Acute Cholestasis

The second form of acute hepatotoxicity is cholestatic in nature (i.e., arrested bile flow with bilirubin casts in the canaliculi and jaundice). The two main types are hepatocanalicular and canalicular. The two differ in that the hepatocanalicular form is accompanied by a minor degree of parenchymal injury. The clinical picture of drug-induced acute cholestatic hepatotoxicity is similar to extrahepatic biliary tree obstruction with jaundice and itching. Both forms of cholestatic disease show moderate elevations of aminotransferases, but the hepatocanalicular form is accompanied by higher levels of alkaline phosphatase than the canalicular form. Cholesterol may also be elevated in hepatocanalicular cholestasis. Management of acute liver injury due to cholestasis consists of withdrawal of the toxic agent, which often results in gradual improvement of liver function.

CHRONIC HEPATOTOXICITY

Chronic hepatotoxicity can target the hepatocytes leading to chronic hepatocellular injury or can disrupt bile flow, analogous to the changes discussed in acute hepatotoxicity. Additionally, toxicity can be manifested by the formation of granulomas, benign or malignant tumors, or disruption of the hepatic circulation.

Chronic Parenchymal Toxicity

Parenchymal injury can present as chronic active hepatitis, macrovesicular steatosis, or nonalcoholic steatonecrosis; these parenchymal forms of toxicity can potentially progress to fibrosis or cirrhosis.

Chronic Active Hepatitis

Chronic active hepatitis produced by drugs such as alpha-methyldopa is clinically and histologically similar to autoimmune chronic active hepatitis. There is a striking preponderance of female patients, and most patients have the laboratory abnormalities considered typical autoimmune markers, namely antinuclear antibodies, smooth muscle antibodies, and anti-single-stranded DNA. Frequently, there is also hypergammaglobulinemia. Successful management of this adverse reaction depends on timely recognition of the cause followed by withdrawal of the responsible drug. However if the cause is not recognized and the drug is continued, cirrhosis and eventual hepatic failure may develop.

Steatosis

Chronic hepatotoxicity with accumulation of hepatocellular fat is mostly in the macrovesicular pattern. Glucocorticoid-induced steatosis does not appear to lead to any further disease, but methotrexate steatosis may lead to cirrhosis.

The screening process for methotrexate-induced disease is discussed later in this chapter under Specific Examples.

Nonalcoholic Steatonecrosis

Nonalcoholic steatonecrosis has been described with amiodarone. In the acute stage, patients most commonly present with abnormal liver tests, whereas the chronic stage is accompanied by fatigue, wasting, abdominal swelling, hepatomegaly, and jaundice. Biochemical changes consist of twofold to fourfold elevations of aminotransferase levels. Histologic changes in this disorder resemble the findings with acute alcoholic hepatitis.[10] The incidence of mildly increased aminotransferase levels in patients receiving amiodarone has been reported to be between 15% and 50%.[11] In most instances there is no clinical evidence of liver injury, and aminotransferases normalize with continuation of therapy. The incidence of severe hepatotoxicity with amiodarone is 0.3% with 11 reported deaths.

Chronic Cholestasis

Chronic intrahepatic cholestasis can lead clinically to a picture resembling primary biliary cirrhosis. As in primary biliary cirrhosis, there is pruritus, but in drug-induced chronic cholestasis, jaundice occurs early in the course of the disease. Histologically, there is little portal inflammation or granuloma formation and less loss of ducts than in primary biliary cirrhosis. The prognosis for recovery is excellent after discontinuation of the drug responsible for the injury.

Biliary sclerosis occurs in approximately 20% of patients who receive 5-fluorouracil deoxyribonucleoside (FUDR) infused into the hepatic artery. This causes a picture similar to sclerosing cholangitis, with intrahepatic and extrahepatic stricture and possible progression to biliary cirrhosis. Clinical features include upper abdominal aching, anorexia, weight loss, and jaundice.

Vascular Disease

Hepatic vein thrombosis or the Budd-Chiari syndrome has been reported in patients taking oral contraceptives. Clinically, patients present with abdominal pain, hepatomegaly, and ascites. The severity of symptoms depends on the speed of occlusion and the extent of vein involved. In the most severe cases, patients can present with fulminant hepatic failure, whereas a patient with gradual onset of occlusion presents with chronic hepatocellular disease. Portosystemic shunt is a potential therapeutic option, and angioplasty has been proposed for suitable cases.

Hepatic venoocclusive disease, peliosis hepatis, nodular regenerative hyperplasia (discussed later in this chapter under Benign Tumors), and sinusoidal dilation are liver diseases that may be caused by drugs. There are many reports in which a combination of these disorders has been described in the same patient. It has been postulated that all three disorders are manifestations of sinusoidal endothelial damage.[12]

Hepatic venoocclusive disease was originally described as a complication of pyrrolizidine alkaloids present in Jamaican herbal teas ("bush teas"). In the United States it is most commonly seen as a complication of chemotherapeutic drugs, particularly in patients treated with intensive cytoreductive therapy in preparation for bone marrow transplantation. It presents clinically with a syndrome similar to hepatic vein thrombosis (i.e., ascites and painful hepatomegaly preceding the decline in liver function). In this disease, blood flow through the liver is disrupted at the level of the centrizonal sinusoid or the intrahepatic veins or both, followed by parenchymal necrosis. Mortality in patients who develop hepatic venoocclusive disease in bone marrow transplantation units is approximately 50%.[13,14] Clinical trials are currently under way to explore the benefit of thrombolytic therapy with tissue plasminogen activator. Another proposed option is the use of transjugular intrahepatic portosystemic stent shunt (TIPSS) to manage the portal hypertension, but this still requires clinical testing to prove its effectiveness.

Peliosis hepatis consists of large blood-filled cavities without sinusoidal lining. Pronounced sinusoidal dilation may accompany peliosis hepatis, often in parts of the liver remote from the lesion. This is a highly lethal disorder complicated by hemorrhage, cholestasis, portal hypertension, liver failure, and hepatorenal syndrome. The most common compounds associated with this disorder are anabolic steroids, but other causes include tamoxifen, azathioprine, and hypervitaminosis A. Treatment options are hepatic dearterialization and orthotopic liver transplantation.

Granulomatous Hepatitis

Drug-induced granulomatous hepatitis has been reported with many drugs including phenylbutazone, allopurinol, hydralazine, phenytoin, and procainamide. Granulomatous hepatitis due to drugs is usually of the noncaseating type, periportal in location, and associated with tissue and peripheral eosinophilia.[15,16] Common presenting symptoms are fever, hepatomegaly, elevated alkaline phosphatase, and mildly elevated aminotransferases. Granulomatous hepatitis must always be included in the differential diagnosis of fever of unknown cause. Since approximately 50% of cases of granulomatous hepatitis are due to sarcoidosis and tuberculosis, it is essential to exclude these causes in patients receiving drugs that might account for the disease.

Neoplasms

Benign Tumors

Hepatic adenomas are rare benign tumors that have been associated with prolonged oral contraceptive use. Oral contraceptive use for more than 5 years has been estimated to increase the incidence of hepatic adenomas by fivefold to tenfold over the general population.[17] Oral contraceptive use is also associated with larger size of adenomas and greater risk of hemorrhage.[18] Hepatic adenomas may undergo malignant transformation to hepatocellular carcinoma.[19,20] Because of the significant risk of rupture with intraabdominal hemorrhage and the risk of malignant transformation, it has been recommended that these hepatic adenomas be surgically resected.[18]

Nodular regenerative hyperplasia is a lesion characterized by diffuse occurrence of regenerative nodules within the liver parenchyma. Wanless and associates[21] have proposed that the occurrence of nodular regenerative hyperplasia may be due to atrophy and regenerative nodule formation in response to the interruption of portal blood flow. Azathioprine has been implicated as an etiologic factor in some cases of nodular regenerative hyperplasia.[22,23] Azathioprine may damage endothelial cells of the liver, leading to hypoperfusion of portions of the liver. The consequent disruption of blood flow would be consistent with the etiology of nodular regenerative hyperplasia proposed by Wanless. It is estimated that liver abnormalities may occur in approximately 3% to 10% of patients receiving chronic azathioprine therapy.[23] Nodular regenerative hyperplasia is usually asymptomatic and is not detected until portal hypertension has developed. Management of this disease consists of the standard therapeutic options for portal hypertension.

Malignancies

Hepatocellular carcinoma is a malignant tumor arising from hepatocytes. It is a complication of cirrhosis secondary to various types of chronic liver disease, such as hepatitis B, hepatitis C, alcoholic liver disease, and hemochromatosis. This tumor has also been reported in patients exposed to androgenic and estrogenic steroids and thorium oxide. A toxin that is well known for its hepatocarcinogenic potential is aflatoxin B_1. Aflatoxin B_1 is a toxin produced by a fungus, *Aspergillus flavus*. This fungus may contaminate peanut and corn products that have been stored in warm, humid conditions. The toxin is easily detected by its blue luminescence under ultraviolet light. Hepatocellular carcinoma may present with abdominal pain, weight loss, and anorexia. Elevated levels of serum alphafetoprotein, alkaline phosphatase, and bilirubin may be present. Diagnosis may be made by abdominal ultrasound or computed tomography (CT) scan. Very small tumors may be successfully resected, but in general the prognosis is poor.

Angiosarcoma is a rare malignant lesion with a poor prognosis. Chemicals that have been implicated as etiologic factors in the development of hepatic angiosarcoma are vinyl chloride, inorganic arsenicals, thorium dioxide (an x-ray contrast medium), and anabolic and estrogenic steroids.

Cholangiocarcinoma is a malignancy of biliary epithelium. It has been reported to occur in patients exposed to the x-ray contrast medium, thorium dioxide.[24] Patients may present with obstructive jaundice, weight loss, and hepatomegaly. Diagnosis may be made by ultrasound or CT scan imaging and confirmed with endoscopic retrograde cholangiography with brushings for cytologic examination. Prognosis is poor.

SPECIFIC EXAMPLES

ACETAMINOPHEN

One of the best-studied hepatotoxic drugs is acetaminophen, a widely used analgesic and antipyretic agent. Although acetaminophen is considered to be a very safe drug at therapeutic doses, serious hepatotoxicity occurs at high serum concentrations of acetaminophen.

In normal individuals, approximately 90% of a therapeutic dose of acetaminophen is metabolized through two major pathways, glucuronidation and sulfation. Approximately 2% to 3% is excreted unchanged, and approximately 6% to 8% is oxidized by the P-450 enzymes to a more toxic intermediate, N-acetyl-p-benzoquinone imine (NAPQI).[25] This toxic intermediate is detoxified by conjugation with glutathione to form a mercapturate, which is subsequently excreted in the urine. In cases of acetaminophen overdose, the hepatic pools of glutathione become exhausted. The toxic intermediate is then available to either covalently bind to critical cellular proteins or oxidize critical protein sulfhydryl groups, and it eventually causes lethal hepatocellular injury. The therapy for acetaminophen intoxication is administration of NAC, a precursor for glutathione. The mechanism of protection by NAC is not straightforward but may be partially related to its ability to enhance detoxification by hepatic glutathione.

Factors that influence the metabolism and hepatotoxicity of acetaminophen include age, genetic factors, and interactions with other drugs. Cases of acetaminophen overdose in young children are usually associated with a lower incidence of hepatotoxicity than in adults.[26] Although studies on the mechanism of this difference in toxicity in young patients are still under way, it is thought to be due to either increased clearance via sulfation or possibly by increased rates of reduced glutathione (GSH) synthesis.

An important drug interaction that can increase the susceptibility to acetaminophen occurs with chronic alcohol abuse. Alcohol is an inducer of the activating enzyme P-450 IIE1, which enhances the formation of the toxic intermediate, NAPQI.[25] This is compounded by the depletion of hepatic glutathione, which occurs after chronic alcohol administration.[11,12] Toxicity has been described in alcoholics after intake of between 2.6 and 16.5 g of acetaminophen over a 24-hour period.[3,4] This overlaps the upper limit of the therapeutic range, 2.6 g/d.

Patients who have ingested an overdose of acetaminophen may have no symptoms or may experience minor symptoms such as nausea, vomiting, or weakness in the first 24 hours. This is considered stage I of the clinical presentation of acetaminophen toxicity. In stage II the patient usually notes general improvement but may experience right upper quadrant pain; prothrombin time is prolonged, and bilirubin and aminotransferase levels are elevated. Stage III usually occurs 3 to 5 days after the drug ingestion, when bilirubin and prothrombin time reach their peak levels. Stage IV is associated with clinical improvement and normalization of liver tests.[25]

The conventional approach has been to treat only patients who presented with a history of acetaminophen overdose within the last 15 hours. For patients who do present within 15 hours of ingestion the need for therapy may be determined by measuring plasma levels and using the Rumack-Matthew nomogram.[27] However, it has been reported that NAC may improve survival of patients who are treated up to 36 hours after overdose of the drug.[28,29]

NAC is given orally as a loading dose of 140 mg/kg, followed with 70 mg/kg every 4 hours for 18 total doses, or until the acetaminophen level is zero.[14] Activated charcoal should not be given concurrently with NAC, as it will adsorb the NAC and render it ineffective. If charcoal must be used because of ingestion of multiple drugs, then it should be removed by gastric lavage before the administration of NAC. Liver tests (aspartate transaminase [AST], alanine aminotransferase [ALT], bilirubin, and prothrombin time) and plasma acetaminophen levels should be monitored until all tests normalize. With prompt recognition and treatment of acetaminophen toxicity, patients generally recover completely.

ISONIAZID

Isoniazid (INH) is a frequently used antituberculous agent that has been associated with two types of liver injury. The most common form of liver injury associated with isoniazid is a mild, nonspecific focal hepatotoxicity, which has been documented to occur in as many as 10% of all patients taking isoniazid.[30] This mild hepatotoxicity is characterized by modest elevations in serum aminotransferases occurring during the first few months of therapy and is usually asymptomatic. In most cases, the elevated serum aminotransferases appear to be transient and often resolve even if the drug is continued.

A less common form of isoniazid-induced hepatic injury is the more severe, symptomatic and sometimes fatal form seen in approximately 1% of all patients taking isoniazid.[30] There appears to be an increased incidence of this form of isoniazid-induced liver injury in adults compared with children, with an incidence estimated at 2% in persons over 50 years of age. Black women and Asian men appear to be more commonly affected. Approximately half of the cases of isoniazid-induced hepatic injury occur in the first 2 months of therapy, although some cases have occurred up to 12 months after initiation of therapy. The syndrome resembles viral hepatitis and can fall anywhere within the spectrum of mild acute, severe fulminant, or subacute disease. Alternatively, the disease may present as chronic active hepatitis. Rashes and arthritis are very rare findings. Treatment of isoniazid-induced liver failure is supportive.

PHENYTOIN

Phenytoin is classified as an idiosyncratic hepatotoxin, since chronic use may be associated with a dose-independent, hepatitislike injury in a small number of patients. It is metabolized in the liver by the P-450 system to a presumed epoxide intermediate, which in turn is metabolized by epoxide hydrolase to a dihydrodiol. The toxicity is thought to be mediated by covalent binding of the epoxide intermediate to cellular macromolecules.[31] There is evidence to suggest that the hepatotoxicity and aplastic anemia due to phenytoin, carbamazepine, or phenobarbital may be a heritable defect.[32,33] Spielberg and coworkers[32,33] examined lymphocytes from patients with hepatotoxicity or aplastic anemia due to one of these antiepileptics. They demonstrated that when lymphocytes are exposed in vitro in the presence of a microsomal activating system to the drug or drugs that cause in vivo toxicity, the cells show enhanced toxicity. The enhanced response may be to one, two, or all three compounds and can be reproduced in family members who have no prior exposure to the drugs. These findings indicate that the defect may be a hereditary defect in detoxification and that patients who develop hepatotoxicity to one of these antiepileptic agents may be at risk for recurrent injury if exposed to one of the other drugs.

Symptoms of phenytoin-induced toxicity usually develop after 4 to 6 weeks of drug therapy or after rechallenge with the drug. The injury may result in fever, fatigue, lymphadenopathy, rash, vague abdominal pain, hepatomegaly, splenomegaly, jaundice, leukocytosis, and peripheral eosinophilia. Liver test results resemble viral hepatitis with moderate-to-marked increases in serum aminotransferases, alkaline phosphatase, increased serum bilirubin levels, and prolonged prothrombin time. Histologic evidence of focal hepatocellular necrosis with a predominantly centrilobular pattern and increased number of eosinophils may be seen. A granulomatous reaction has also been identified in cases of phenytoin-induced liver injury. Treatment is primarily supportive. There are no specific therapeutic measures, and steroid administration has been tried anecdotally with mixed results.[5]

ESTROGENS

Estrogens rarely induce liver injury; there appears to be tremendous variation in individual susceptibility with increased incidence noted among Scandinavians. Estrogenic steroids may cause a cholestatic pattern of liver injury that usually occurs within the first 2 months of therapy. This manifestation of toxicity may be related to the decreased bile flow and decreased biliary secretion of bile acids and organic anions that have been reported experimentally.[34]

Symptoms of the cholestatic injury include jaundice, pruritus, malaise, vague abdominal complaints, and bilirubinuria. Fever, rashes, and arthritis occur rarely. Moderate increases in serum aminotransferases, alkaline phosphatase, and serum conjugated bilirubin levels occur, but prothrombin time usually remains normal. Histologic evidence of bile stasis is seen within the canaliculi and within the hepatocytes and is predominantly centrizonal. Treatment consists of discontinuing the estrogenic agent, usually resulting in prompt return of normal liver function and resolution of the symptoms and histologic findings of cholestasis.[34]

Estrogens are also associated with increased incidence of hepatic adenomas, focal nodular hyperplasia, hepatocellular carcinoma, and endothelial hemangioendothelioma. The tumors associated with estrogen use are usually vascular, and hemorrhage into the tumor is associated with all of these neoplasms.[19]

ANDROGENIC STEROIDS

Androgenic steroids with a 17-carbon substitution, such as methyltestosterone and norethandrolone, have been shown to produce a clinical syndrome nearly identical to the estrogen-induced cholestatic liver injury. As with estrogen-induced cholestasis, the cholestasis appears to be mild and reversible. Treatment consists of discontinuing the androgenic agent, resulting in rapid return of normal liver function.

Androgenic steroids have also been associated with hepatic adenomas, hepatocellular carcinoma, and hepatic angiosarcoma.[34] Androgen-associated disorders have become more prevalent with the increased use of steroids by ath-

METHOTREXATE

Methotrexate induces macrovesicular steatosis in certain individuals. Chronic methotrexate therapy with large cumulative doses has been associated with hepatic fibrosis and cirrhosis.[35] It has proved difficult to develop recommendations for monitoring patients receiving long-term therapy with methotrexate to detect early onset of hepatotoxicity. Investigations into the use of liver biopsy as a monitoring tool were confounded by the patient population used. Most of the studies involved patients treated for psoriatic arthritis. It later became evident that many patients with psoriatic arthritis had evidence of liver abnormalities before methotrexate administration occurred. Furthermore, patients with psoriatic arthritis were more susceptible to develop methotrexate-induced hepatotoxicity than patients with other rheumatologic disorders (e.g., rheumatoid arthritis).[36,37] Concurrent use of alcohol is the main risk factor for developing hepatotoxicity from methotrexate therapy,[36,37] and continued use of alcohol is considered a relative contraindication to methotrexate therapy.

It is now generally accepted that in patients without known risk factors (diabetes, obesity, impaired renal function, alcohol abuse) or suspected liver disease, there is no need for pretreatment liver biopsy. An exception to this may be patients with psoriatic arthritis, who need more intense follow-up. The issue of routine liver biopsy to diagnose early signs of hepatotoxicity is somewhat controversial. In a meta-analysis of methotrexate-induced histologic liver abnormalities, the incidence of one grade change in the liver biopsy was 20%, and 3% of all patients demonstrated advanced changes in liver histology.[37] Based on their findings the authors recommended that liver biopsies should be done in most patients after every 4 g of methotrexate. In patients with persistently elevated liver enzymes, liver biopsy should be done more frequently.

COCAINE

Rhabdomyolysis and central nervous system and cardiovascular toxicity are well-known complications of illicit recreational use of cocaine. Recent reports have recognized that acute and chronic use of cocaine can also result in hepatotoxicity. Although cocaine hepatotoxicity has been well described in animals, few cases of cocaine hepatotoxicity in humans have been reported in the literature until recently. Perino and coworkers[38] and Silva et al[39] were among the first investigators to report on the histologic patterns seen in cocaine hepatotoxicity in humans. They observed marked elevations in aminotransferases, acute renal failure, and disseminated intravascular coagulation in the most severe cases. Histologic examination via liver biopsy or autopsy specimen showed marked coagulative necrosis and microvesicular and macrovesicular steatosis with variations noted in the zonation of the injury.[38,39,40] The current treatment of cocaine-induced hepatotoxicity is supportive.

REFERENCES

1. Gonzalez FJ, Skoda RC, Kimura S, et al. Characterization of the common genetic defect in humans deficient in debrisoquin metabolism. *Nature.* 1988;331(4):442–446.
2. Lauterburg BH, Velez ME. Glutathione deficiency in alcoholics: risk factor for Paracetamol hepatotoxicity. *Gut.* 1988;29:1153–1157.
3. McClain CJ, Kromhout JP, Peterson FJ, Holtzman JL. Potentiation of acetaminophen hepatotoxicity by alcohol. *JAMA.* 1980;244(3):251–253.
4. Seeff LB, Cuccherini BA, Zimmerman HJ, Adler E, Benjamin SB. Acetaminophen hepatotoxicity in alcoholics: a therapeutic misadventure. *Ann Intern Med.* 1986;104:399–404.
5. Schenker S, Breen KJ, Heimberg M, et al. Pathogenesis of tetracycline-induced fatty liver. In: Gerok W, Sickinger K, eds. *Drugs and the Liver.* Stuttgart: FK Schattaeur-Verlag; 1975:269–289.
6. Pohl LR. Drug-induced allergic hepatitis. *Semin Liver Dis.* 1990;10:305–315.
7. Burk RF, Reiter R, Lane JM. Hyperbaric oxygen protection against carbon tetrachloride hepatotoxicity in the rat: association with altered metabolism. *Gastroenterology.* 1986;90:812–818.
8. Truss CD, Killenberg PG. Treatment of carbon tetrachloride poisoning with hyperbaric oxygen. *Gastroenterology.* 1982;82:767–769.
9. Williams AT, Burk RF. Carbon tetrachloride hepatotoxicity: an example of free radical-mediated injury. *Semin Liver Dis.* 1990;10(4):279–284.
10. Simon JB, Manley PN, Brien JF, Armstrong PW. Amiodarone hepatotoxicity simulating alcoholic liver disease. *N Engl J Med.* 1984;311(3):167–172.
11. Robinson K, Mulrow JP, Rowland E, McKenna WJ. Long-term effects of amiodarone on hepatic function. *Am J Cardiol.* 1989;64:95–96.
12. Haboubi NY, Ali HH, Whitwell HL, Ackrill P. Role of endothelial cell injury in the spectrum of azathioprine-induced liver disease after renal transplant: light microscopy and ultrastructural observations. *Am J Gastroenterol.* 1988;83:256–261.
13. McDonald GB, Shulman HM, Wolford JL, Spencer GD. Liver disease after human marrow transplantation. *Semin Liver Dis.* 1987;7:210–229.
14. Jones RJ, Lee KSK, Beschorner WE, et al. Veno-occlusive disease of the liver following bone marrow transplantation. *Transplantation.* 1987;44:778–783.

15. McMaster KR, Hennigar GR. Drug-induced granulomatous hepatitis. *Lab Invest.* 1981;44(1):61–73.
16. Harrington PT, Gutiérrez JJ, Ramirez-Ronda CH, Quiñones-Soto R, Bermúdez RH, Chaffey J. Granulomatous hepatitis. *Rev Infect Dis.* 1982;4(3):638–655.
17. Rosenberg L. The risk of liver neoplasia in relation to combined oral contraceptive use. *Contraception.* 1991; 43(6):643–652.
18. Shortell CK, Schwartz SI. Hepatic adenoma and focal nodular hyperplasia. *Surg Gynecol Obstet.* 1991;173: 426–431.
19. Gordon SC, Reddy KR, Livingstone AS, Jeffers LJ, Schiff ER. Resolution of a contraceptive-steroid-induced hepatic adenoma with subsequent evolution into hepatocellular carcinoma. *Ann Intern Med.* 1986;105(4): 547–549.
20. Gyorffy EJ, Bredfeldt JE, Black WC. Transformation of hepatic cell adenoma to hepatocellular carcinoma due to oral contraceptive use. *Ann Intern Med.* 1989;110:489–490.
21. Wanless IR, Godwin TA, Allen F, Feder A. Nodular regenerative hyperplasia of the liver in hematologic disorders: a possible response to obliterative portal venopathy. A morphometric study of nine cases with an hypothesis on the pathogenesis. *Medicine.* 1980;59:367–379.
22. Sterneck M, Wiesner R, Ascher N, et al. Azathioprine hepatotoxicity after liver transplantation. *Hepatology.* 1991;14:806–810.
23. Mion F, Napoleon B, Berger F, Chevallier M, Bonvoisin S, Descos L. Azathioprine induced liver disease: nodular regenerative hyperplasia of the liver and perivenous fibrosis in a patient treated for multiple sclerosis. *Gut.* 1991;32:715–717.
24. Ito Y, Kojiro M, Nakashima T, Mori T. Pathomorphologic characteristics of 102 cases of Thorotrast-related hepatocellular carcinoma, cholangiocarcinoma, and hepatic angiosarcoma. *Cancer.* 1988;62:1153–1162.
25. Nelson SD. Molecular mechanisms of the hepatotoxicity caused by acetaminophen. *Semin Liver Dis.* 1990;10(4): 267–277.
26. Briant RH, Dorrington RE, Cleal J, Williams FM. The rate of acetaminophen metabolism in the elderly and the young. *J Am Geriatr Soc.* 1976;24(8):359–361.
27. Rumack BH. Acetaminophen overdose. *Am J Med.* 1983;75(suppl 1):104–115.
28. Harrison PM, Wendon JA, Gimson AE, Alexander GJ, Williams R. Improvement by acetylcysteine of hemodynamics and oxygen transport in fulminant hepatic failure. *N Engl J Med.* 1991;324:1852–1857.
29. Harrison PM, Keays R, Bray GP, Alexander GJM, Williams R. Improved outcome of Paracetamol-induced fulminant hepatic failure by late administration of acetylcysteine. *Lancet.* 1990;335:1572–1573.
30. Black M. Isoniazid-associated hepatitis in 114 cases. *Gastroenterology.* 1975;69:289–294.
31. Watkins PB. Role of cytochrome P-450 in drug metabolism and hepatotoxicity. *Semin Liver Dis.* 1990;10(4): 235–250.
32. Spielberg SP, Gordon GB, Blake DA, Mellits ED, Bross DS. Anticonvulsant toxicity in vitro: possible role of arene oxides. *J Pharmacol Exp Ther.* 1981;217(2):386–389.
33. Spielberg SP, Gordon GB, Blake DA, Goldstein DA, Herlong HF. Predisposition to phenytoin hepatotoxicity assessed in vitro. *N Engl J Med.* 1981;305:722–727.
34. King PD, Blitzer BL. Drug-induced cholestasis: pathogenesis and clinical features. *Semin Liver Dis.* 1990;10(4): 316–321.
35. Scull CJ, Anderson CJ, Cannon GW. Long-term methotrexate therapy for rheumatoid arthritis. *Semin Arthritis Rheum.* 1991;20(5):317–331.
36. Lewis JH, Schiff E. Methotrexate-induced chronic liver injury: guidelines for detection and prevention. *Am J Gastroenterol.* 1988;88(12):1337–1345.
37. Whiting-O'Keefe QE, Fye KH, Sack KD. Methotrexate and histologic hepatic abnormalities: a meta-analysis. *Am J Med.* 1991;90(6):711–716.
38. Perino LE, Warren GH, Levine JS. Cocaine-induced hepatotoxicity in humans. *Gastroenterology.* 1987;93: 176–180.
39. Silva MO, Roth D, Reddy KR, Fernandez JA, Albores-Saavedra J, Schiff ER. Hepatic dysfunction accompanying acute cocaine intoxication. *J Hepatol.* 1991;12:312–315.
40. Wanless IR, Dore S, Gopinath N, et al. Histopathology of cocaine hepatotoxicity: report of four patients. *Gastroenterology.* 1990;98:497–501.

94
Hepatic Encephalopathy

EMMET B. KEEFFE

Hepatic encephalopathy, also called portosystemic encephalopathy, is a neuropsychiatric syndrome occurring in patients with acute or chronic liver failure.[1-3] The term *portosystemic encephalopathy* stresses the role of diversion of portal blood from the liver; however, *hepatic encephalopathy* is a more commonly employed term, since this syndrome occurs regularly in cirrhotic patients without major shunting of portal blood flow. The reversible nature of hepatic encephalopathy and absence of major neuropathologic findings suggest that hepatic encephalopathy is a metabolic syndrome.

Hepatic encephalopathy is often classified into acute hepatic encephalopathy associated with fulminant hepatic failure and the more common chronic hepatic encephalopathy associated with cirrhosis or portosystemic shunts.[1-3] Acute hepatic encephalopathy is a distinct clinical entity that responds poorly to the usual therapy of hepatic encephalopathy and is associated with cerebral edema. The focus of this chapter is the management of chronic hepatic encephalopathy associated with advanced cirrhosis and liver failure.

DEFINITION AND CLINICAL MANIFESTATIONS

A precise definition of hepatic encephalopathy is impossible because there are no uniformly accepted criteria for its diagnosis. A general working definition is that hepatic encephalopathy is a spectrum of neuropsychiatric abnormalities that arise in patients with advanced liver disease.[1-3] The degree of impairment of cerebral function is highly variable, ranging from subclinical changes to the irreversible neurologic syndrome of hepatocerebral degeneration (Table 94–1). When the defect in consciousness is severe and associated with obtundation, the term *hepatic coma* is employed.

Subclinical hepatic encephalopathy is diagnosed on the basis of abnormal scores on psychomotor tests in patients with no overt behavioral, neurologic, or electroencephalographic (EEG) changes.[4] Approximately two thirds of cirrhotic patients have subclinical hepatic encephalopathy as detected by a battery of psychometric tests. These test abnormalities are reversible with conventional treatment of hepatic encephalopathy, and patients may note improved functioning in their daily activities. The recognition of subclinical hepatic encephalopathy emphasizes how frequently encephalopathy is underdiagnosed. Hepatic encephalopathy may also be manifest as a recurrent syndrome related to reversible precipitating events. Between attacks, patients are normal or have subclinical encephalopathy. Chronic hepatic encephalopathy that cannot be fully controlled with dietary modifications or lactulose occurs in patients with far-advanced cirrhosis. Hepatocerebral degeneration, an irreversible neurologic syndrome characterized by ataxia, dementia, and parkinsonian features, is fortunately rare.

Hepatic encephalopathy can be graded into four stages based on mental state and neurologic findings (Table 94–2). The earliest abnormalities of stage 1 are of a psychiatric and cognitive nature and include such signs as personality changes, euphoria, irritability, apathy, slowness, and inverted sleep pattern. In stage 2, asterixis is regularly present, and the patient has obvious personality changes, inappropriate behavior,

---

TABLE 94–1. MANIFESTATIONS OF HEPATIC ENCEPHALOPATHY

Subclinical hepatic encephalopathy
Recurrent hepatic encephalopathy
Chronic hepatic encephalopathy
Hepatocerebral degeneration

TABLE 94–2. CLINICAL STAGES OF HEPATIC ENCEPHALOPATHY

STAGE	MENTAL STATE	NEUROLOGIC SIGNS
1	Mild confusion, euphoria, or depression; decreased attention; slowed ability to perform mental tasks; irritability; inverted sleep pattern	Mild incoordination; slight tremor; impaired handwriting
2	Drowsiness; lethargy; gross deficits in analytic ability; obvious personality changes; inappropriate behavior; intermittent disorientation	Asterixis; ataxia; dysarthria
3	Somnolent but can be aroused; unable to perform mental tasks; disorientation with respect to time or place; marked confusion; amnesia; fits of rage; slurred speech	Hyperreflexia; muscle rigidity; fasciculations; Babinski's sign
4	Coma	Oculovestibular responses lost; response to painful stimuli lost; decerebrate rigidity

drowsiness, lethargy, and gross defects in analytic ability. In stage 3, the patient is somnolent but can be aroused and is disoriented with respect to time or place or both. In stage 4, the patient is comatose with loss of oculovestibular responses and response to painful stimuli and develops decerebrate rigidity while in deep coma.

An abnormal EEG is a classic feature of hepatic encephalopathy, although the changes are nonspecific. There is an initial decrease in wave frequency and increase in amplitude, followed in more advanced stages of encephalopathy by the appearance of triphasic waves and 2 to 3 waves per second. The EEG, as well as other techniques (visual evoked potentials or brain imaging by computed tomography and magnetic resonance), is not routinely employed in the diagnosis of hepatic encephalopathy and appears to offer little beyond clinical diagnosis.

PATHOGENESIS

The precise mechanisms responsible for the development of hepatic encephalopathy have yet to be identified.[1-3] There are a number of metabolic abnormalities that accompany advanced cirrhosis, and it has been difficult to discern which of these abnormalities might be pathogenic in the development of hepatic encephalopathy. It seems likely that there is more than one metabolic factor contributing to the pathogenesis of hepatic encephalopathy. The normal liver detoxifies a number of nitrogenous metabolites from gut metabolism, and failure of hepatocyte function or the formation of portosystemic collaterals allows entry of these neuroactive metabolites into the systemic circulation. Changes in the plasma concentrations of amino acids, free fatty acids, and a number of other toxic metabolites have been noted in liver failure, but the current consensus is that hepatic encephalopathy is primarily related to abnormalities of ammonia metabolism and overactivity of the major inhibitory neurotransmitter, c-aminobutyric acid (GABA).

Multiple studies using variable experimental approaches have demonstrated that ammonia is neurotoxic. The precise mechanism of this neurotoxicity is uncertain but may involve a number of actions of ammonia on nervous tissue, including interference with cellular transport and neurotransmission. Further support for the role of ammonia in the development of encephalopathy is that the concentration of glutamine, a byproduct of brain detoxification of ammonia, correlates well with the degree of severity of hepatic encephalopathy.

There is also accumulating evidence for an increase in central nervous system GABAergic tone in hepatic encephalopathy, and it has been suggested that the neural inhibition of hepatic encephalopathy is mediated at least in part by overactivity of the inhibitory GABA system. The original GABA hypothesis suggested that plasma-derived GABA crossed an abnormally permeable blood-brain barrier and bound to an increased number of receptors, which also serve as the site of action of benzodiazepines. The focus has now switched to the possible role of endogenous benzodiazepines in the pathogenesis of hepatic encephalopathy. Support for this concept is based on the fact that patients with cirrhosis are abnormally susceptible to the effects of benzodiazepines. In addition, preliminary studies suggest a beneficial effect of flumazenil, a benzodiazepine-receptor antagonist, in patients with hepatic encephalopathy. More treatment trials are needed to better define the role of flumazenil in the management of hepatic encephalopathy.

THERAPY

The basic treatment of patients suspected to have hepatic encephalopathy has not changed in recent years. The general approach involves detection and treatment of precipitating factors and initial treatment with a low-protein diet and lactulose. Later, patients are encouraged to eat an adequate diet (including standard daily protein requirements) and to use lactulose as needed to prevent recurrent encephalopathy. In the initial approach to a cirrhotic patient with a change in mental status, it should be emphasized that consideration should always be given to other causes of neurologic dysfunction such as subdural hematoma or meningitis. Some general principles of treatment of hepatic encephalopathy are elucidated first, followed by more detailed discussion of specific therapies.

GENERAL PRINCIPLES

The majority of patients presenting with hepatic encephalopathy have precipitating factors (Table 94–3). Identification and correction of these precipitating factors is the initial step in the management of all patients with hepatic encephalopathy. Conditions that should be sought and corrected include gastrointestinal tract bleeding; excessive dietary protein intake; constipation; infections, particularly spontaneous bacterial peritonitis and pneumonia; volume depletion, which is often associated with diuretic therapy, diarrhea, or vomiting; azotemia, which may be spontaneous or induced by drugs or contrast agents; hypokalemia; use of analgesic or sedative drugs; development of a hepatocellular carcinoma; hepatic injury from alcohol or drugs; and surgery with anesthesia. Another important potential precipitating factor to identify is noncompliance with lactulose therapy. Sepsis is the most challenging precipitating factor to identify, since patients often lack the classic features of infection such as fever, leukocytosis, or localizing signs. Thus, urine, blood, sputum, and ascites must be routinely cultured, and suspected or proven infection must be treated promptly.

SPECIFIC THERAPY

In the following section, the standard therapy and some newer therapies for hepatic encephalopathy are reviewed. The treatment of hepatic encephalopathy is summarized in Table 94–4.

DIET

Dietary protein is a major nutrient that precipitates hepatic encephalopathy. The dilemma in managing cirrhotic patients with encephalopathy is that protein restriction improves hepatic encephalopathy but does not allow long-term prevention or treatment of protein-calorie malnutrition. In patients presenting with severe hepatic encephalopathy, all dietary protein intake is typically stopped for a brief period of time. As hepatic encephalopathy improves, patients should be provided adequate caloric intake (30 to 35 kcal/kg/d), including standard daily protein requirements (1 to 1.5 g/kg/d).[5] This may be provided in the form of oral diet or given as a nasoenteric or parenteral feeding in patients who are anorectic or otherwise unable to eat.

In patients requiring parenteral feeding, standard synthetic amino acid preparations can be used and have only rarely been incriminated as a factor in precipitating hepatic encephalopathy.[5] A practical approach is to provide supplementary intravenous feedings via a peripheral vein to supplement inadequate oral intake. A decrease in the plasma concentration of branched chain amino acids (BCAA) and increase in aromatic amino acids (AAA) have been noted in cirrhotic

---

TABLE 94–3. FACTORS PRECIPITATING HEPATIC ENCEPHALOPATHY

Gastrointestinal bleeding
Excessive dietary protein
Constipation
Infections
   Spontaneous bacterial peritonitis
   Pneumonia
Volume depletion
   Diuretic therapy
   Diarrhea
   Vomiting
Azotemia
   Spontaneous
   Drug-induced
Hypokalemia
Use of analgesic or sedative drugs
Hepatocellular carcinoma
Hepatic injury (e.g., alcohol, drugs)
Surgery with anesthesia
Noncompliance with lactulose therapy

TABLE 94–4. TREATMENT OF HEPATIC ENCEPHALOPATHY

Diet or Drug	Dosage	Potential Problems
Standard Therapies		
Diet	Mild HE: adequate calories (30–35 kcal/kg/d), and protein (1–1.5 g/kg/d)	
	Severe HE: initially no protein intake, then gradual introduction; BCAA-enriched formulas, when standard therapy of HE fails	Cost of BCAA-enriched formulas
Lactulose	Mild HE: 30 ml (20 g) b.i.d. or t.i.d., adjust to 2 or 3 stools/d	Excessive diarrhea and flatulence; sweet taste; cost
	Severe HE: 30 ml q2h (PO or via nasogastric tube) until diarrhea ensues; or enemas (300 ml lactulose and 700 ml tap water) q6–8h	
Metronidazole	250 mg t.i.d. or q.i.d.	Neurotoxicity with long-term therapy
Neomycin	1 g q.i.d. (dosage range, 2–6 g/d)	Nephrotoxicity (rare); ototoxicity (rare)
Alternative or Experimental Therapies		
Sodium benzoate	5 g dissolved in 30 ml of water b.i.d.	Dyspepsia; modest hypernatremia
Zinc acetate or sulfate	200 mg t.i.d.	
Flumazenil	Variable dosages (e.g., 2 mg in 20-ml solution over 5 min)	

BCAA = branched chain amino acids, HE = hepatic encephalopathy.

patients and postulated to be important factors in the pathogenesis of hepatic encephalopathy. A logical development from this hypothesis was the development of BCAA-enriched nutritional formulas for parenteral and oral feeding. These high-BCAA formulations are substantially more expensive than standard formulas. In spite of a large number of studies of the role of parenteral BCAA-enriched formulations in the treatment of hepatic encephalopathy, no consensus has been reached on whether these formulas are effective. However, some studies suggest that oral BCAA-enriched dietary preparations are useful in the management of chronic hepatic encephalopathy. Since BCAA-enriched formulations have been associated with improvement in encephalopathy in some patients, a reasonable recommendation is to reserve this dietary treatment for the minority of patients who fail standard measures to prevent or treat hepatic encephalopathy.

There also are studies suggesting that a diet emphasizing vegetable proteins is associated with improvement in mental functioning and lower blood ammonia levels in patients with chronic hepatic encephalopathy.[6] It appears that meat sources of dietary protein are more likely to induce encephalopathy than are vegetable sources of protein. These vegetable protein sources are postulated to be effective because of their lower AAA and methionine content, a higher fiber content with cathartic action, and their ability to acidify the colon and increase fecal nitrogen content.

LACTULOSE

The standard treatment of hepatic encephalopathy is lactulose administered in divided daily doses ranging from 30 to 120 ml/d (average dosage, 60 to 90 ml/d). Lactulose may be administered orally or by nasogastric tube feeding. The desired result of lactulose therapy is 2 to 3 semisoft stools per day. In the patient with severe hepatic encephalopathy and ileus, lactulose enemas (300 ml of lactulose and 700 ml of water) can be administered every 6 to 8 hours. Although lactulose remains the primary therapy for hepatic encephalopathy, potential problems include excessive diarrhea, excoriation of the buttocks, volume depletion, flatulence, electrolyte imbalance, and high cost.

Lactulose is a synthetic disaccharide composed of galactose and fructose. It is not absorbed or metabolized in the upper gastrointestinal tract and passes into the colon, where it is degraded by anaerobic bacteria and produces several organic acids. The effectiveness of lactulose in hepatic encephalopathy may be explained by a number of potential mechanisms including a cathartic effect, colonic acidification with reduced ammonia absorption, and altered colonic nitrogen metabolism with increased nitrogen excretion.

The effects of lactulose in patients with hepatic encephalopathy are not specific and may be duplicated by lactitol, sorbitol, dietary lactose in lactase-deficient subjects, and possibly even dietary fiber. Lactitol, like lactulose, is a synthetic disaccharide that is malabsorbed by the small intestine.[7] Its effectiveness appears to be equivalent to lactulose; its advantages include its lack of a sweet taste (which may enhance compliance) and its probable lack of certain side effects (particularly flatulence).[7] Lactitol, which is administered in divided dosages of 30 to 50 g/d, is not currently available in the United States.

ANTIBIOTICS

The rationale for the use of antibiotics in hepatic encephalopathy is to reduce the gastrointestinal tract absorption of ammonia and other nitrogenous toxins of bacterial origin. Antibiotics, specifically neomycin, were for many years the primary treatment of hepatic encephalopathy; however, a small amount of neomycin is absorbed, and the potential of significant ototoxicity and neurotoxicity has resulted in lactulose's replacing neomycin as the primary therapy of hepatic encephalopathy. The usual dosage of neomycin is 1 g four times daily, with a range of dosages from 2 to 6 g/d; neomycin is usually administered for 1 to 2 weeks.

In recent years antibiotics have been employed in the treatment of hepatic encephalopathy refractory to lactulose alone, and other antibiotics that reduce intestinal flora have been used more commonly than neomycin. It appears that the combination of lactulose and neomycin is effective for cases of hepatic encephalopathy resistant to lactulose alone, in spite of the concern that neomycin might inhibit the action of lactulose. Vancomycin has been shown to be effective in the management of resistant hepatic encephalopathy, but its expense is prohibitive. Based on a trial demonstrating that metronidazole is as effective as neomycin in the treatment of hepatic encephalopathy, metronidazole has become the oral antibiotic of choice.[8] However, this drug also has a potential for toxicity; it is cleared by the liver, accumulates in patients with chronic liver disease, and may be complicated by peripheral neuropathy and carcinogenic with long-term use. The usual dosage of metronidazole in the treatment of hepatic encephalopathy is 250 mg three times or four times daily, and therapy is usually limited to 1 to 2 weeks.

MISCELLANEOUS

Bowel cleansing with 4 L of a standard colonic lavage preparation may accelerate the resolution of acute episodes of hepatic encephalopathy, particularly when gastrointestinal tract bleeding has been a precipitating factor. Other laxatives such as magnesium citrate may be equally efficacious. However, these regimens are not commonly used, and lactulose alone appears to be adequate for bowel cleansing, particularly when used in initial higher doses to induce diarrhea. Repeated tap water enemas of 1 L may also be used to the end point of a clear return, but this form of therapy is cumbersome and seldom employed.

Sodium benzoate, a commonly used food preservative that also enhances nitrogen excretion and decreases blood ammonia levels, was recently shown to be effective in the treatment of hepatic encephalopathy in a double-blind, controlled trial.[9] Sodium benzoate was compared with lactulose in the treatment of acute episodes of encephalopathy occurring in patients with cirrhosis; 80% and 81% of patients, respectively, recovered with these two forms of therapy. Side effects of sodium benzoate include dyspepsia (which may require therapy with an H_2-receptor antagonist) and modest elevation of serum sodium. The dose of sodium benzoate is 5 g dissolved in 30 ml of tap water administered twice daily. This therapy is up to 30 times cheaper than lactulose.

Zinc deficiency is common in patients with advanced cirrhosis, and zinc deficiency has been postulated to play a contributory role in the pathogenesis of hepatic encephalopathy. Two controlled trials evaluating the effect of short-term oral zinc supplementation showed mixed results in terms of improving hepatic encephalopathy.[10,11] Both studies documented low blood zinc levels that improved with zinc supplementation. Zinc replacement can be accomplished with zinc acetate or zinc sulfate, both of which are well absorbed, at a dose of 200 mg three times daily. Further studies are needed to better define the role of zinc deficiency in the pathogenesis of hepatic encephalopathy and settle the issue of whether zinc supplementation is efficacious.

The logical consequence of the hypothesis implicating increased GABAergic tone in the pathogenesis of hepatic encephalopathy is the use of antagonists of the GABA-benzodiazepine receptor.[12] Benzodiazepine antagonists have induced transient improvement in hepatic encephalopathy in animals with acute liver failure. In a number of small studies, approximately 40% to 60% of patients treated for chronic hepatic encephalopathy with the benzodiazepine antagonist flumazenil have shown improvement, sometimes dramatically within minutes after intravenous administration. Until the results of further trials are reported, it is premature to use flumazenil for the treatment of hepatic encephalopathy. On the other hand, this novel approach to therapy is interesting and shows promise.

Levodopa, amantadine, and bromocriptine have been utilized on the principle of enhancing dopaminergic neurotransmission, which is postulated to be decreased in patients with hepatic encephalopathy. Although bromocriptine appeared to be effective in selected patients with hepatic encephalopathy, a controlled trial showed no benefit.

SURGERY

The most important operation for chronic and intractable hepatic encephalopathy is liver transplantation. Liver transplantation should be considered early in patients with chronic hepatic encephalopathy that is only partially controlled with lactulose and also in patients with encephalopathy that recurs frequently. Other operations play an insignificant role in the management of hepatic encephalopathy. Colonic bypass operations were used briefly but have now been abandoned.

In patients undergoing portosystemic shunt surgery, the distal splenorenal shunt is preferred to a standard portacaval shunt because it better maintains portal perfusion and is associated with less hepatic encephalopathy, particularly in patients with nonalcoholic cirrhosis. Preservation of hepatic portal perfusion, which is also a feature of portacaval H graft and mesocaval shunts, appears to be important in reducing postoperative encephalopathy. If severe and intractable hepatic encephalopathy occurs after the creation of a portosystemic shunt, the shunt may need to be closed, either surgically or radiologically. In the small percentage of patients (approximately 5%) with refractory hepatic encephalopathy following placement of a transjugular intrahepatic portosystemic shunt (TIPS), the stent can be occluded radiologically and will lead to reversal of hepatic encephalopathy. The counterbalancing risk in these circumstances, obviously, is recurrent portal hypertensive bleeding, which is the usual indication leading to shunt surgery or the placement of a TIPS.

REFERENCES

1. Basile AS, Jones EA, Skolnick P. The pathogenesis and treatment of hepatic encephalopathy: evidence for the involvement of benzodiazepine receptor ligands. *Pharmacol Rev.* 1991;43:27.
2. Mullen KD. Hepatic encephalopathy. In: Rector WG, ed. *Complications of Chronic Liver Disease*. St. Louis, Mo: Mosby–Year Book Inc; 1992:127.
3. Marsano L, McClain C. How to manage both acute and chronic hepatic encephalopathy: five hypotheses offer clues to the way toxins affect the brain. *J Crit Illness.* 1993;8:579.
4. Gitlin N. Subclinical portal-systemic encephalopathy. *Am J Gastroenterol.* 1988;83:8.
5. Nompleggi DJ, Bonkovsky HL. Nutritional supplementation in chronic liver disease: an analytical review. *Hepatology.* 1994;19:518.
6. Bianchi GP, Marchesini G, Fabbri A, et al. Vegetable versus animal protein diet in cirrhotic patients with chronic encephalopathy: a randomized crossover comparison. *J Intern Med.* 1993;233:385.
7. Cammà C, Fiorello F, Tinè F, et al. Lactitol in treatment of chronic hepatic encephalopathy: a meta-analysis. *Dig Dis Sci.* 1993;38:916.
8. Morgan MH, Read AE, Speller DCE. Treatment of hepatic encephalopathy with metronidazole. *Gut.* 1992;23:1.
9. Sushma S, Dasarathy S, Tandon RK, et al. Sodium benzoate in the treatment of acute hepatic encephalopathy: a double-blind randomized trial. *Hepatology.* 1992;16:138.
10. Reding P, Duchateau J, Bataille C. Oral zinc supplementation improves hepatic encephalopathy: results of a randomised controlled trial. *Lancet.* 1984;2:493.
11. Riggio O, Ariosto F, Merli M, et al. Short-term oral zinc supplementation does not improve chronic hepatic encephalopathy: results of a double-blind crossover trial. *Dig Dis Sci.* 1991;36:1204.
12. Pomier-Layrargues G, Giguère JF, Lavoie J, et al. Flumazenil in cirrhotic patients in hepatic coma: a randomized double-blind placebo-controlled crossover trial. *Hepatology.* 1994;19:32.

95
Acute Hepatitis
ALBERT J. CZAJA

Acute hepatitis is an inflammation of the liver of less than 6 months' duration. Typically, serum aspartate and alanine aminotransferase abnormalities are the predominant biochemical findings. "Cholestatic" features (predominant serum alkaline phosphatase and c-glutamyltransferase abnormalities) are less frequently encountered (acute hepatitis A virus infection, certain drug toxicities). Hyperbilirubinemia, reflected as jaundice, can be an important feature, and the presence or absence of this finding allows subclassification of patients into "icteric" or "anicteric" categories. Extreme hyperbilirubinemia (serum bilirubin levels greater than 30 mg/dl) suggests concurrent hemolysis and possible renal insufficiency. Persistent and severe (greater than 5 seconds beyond control) hypoprothrombinemia is an indication of disease severity and an important prognostic index.

CLINICAL FEATURES

Patients with acute hepatitis lack cutaneous stigmata of chronic liver disease (spider angiomas, palmar and malar erythema), laboratory features that reflect prolonged suppression of hepatic synthetic function (hypoalbuminemia, low serum pseudocholinesterase levels), and features of portal hypertension (ascites, hypersplenism, esophageal varices), although there are exceptions to every rule. Certainly, hypoalbuminemia, hypergammaglobulinemia, and ascites do not preclude the diagnosis.

Extrahepatic manifestations ("serum sickness prodrome") have been ascribed to circulating immune complexes that develop during acute viral infection. Synovitis involving distal joints, fever, and an erythematous or urticarial eruption typify the prodrome of acute hepatitis B. A polyarteritis syndrome with pancreatitis, membranous glomerulonephritis, and pericarditis is possible, and an aplastic anemia has been described. Urticaria, purpura, synovitis, and aplastic anemia may also complicate the course of acute hepatitis C, and a mixed cryoglobulinemia has been associated with hepatitis B and C virus infections. Fever, headache, myalgias, nausea, vomiting, right upper quadrant discomfort, and an evolving cholestasis with pruritus suggest acute hepatitis A, and this infection has also been associated with aplastic anemia. Lymphadenopathy, pharyngitis, fever, and splenomegaly characterize infections with the Epstein-Barr virus or cytomegalovirus.

In its early stages, acute viral hepatitis may have a leukopenia. Granulocytes are reduced in number, and there may be a relative lymphocytosis with large "atypical" lymphocytes. Leukocytosis is unusual.

HISTOLOGIC FINDINGS

Rarely, liver biopsy assessment is necessary to differentiate acute from chronic hepatitis or to refine the etiologic diagnosis. The histologic findings of acute hepatitis include disruption of liver cell plates (lobular disarray), accumulations of mononuclear cells within the sinusoids and throughout the lobule, Kupffer's cell hyperplasia, acidophilic bodies ("Councilman's bodies") within sinusoids, mixed mononuclear cell infiltrates within expanded portal tracts, and piecemeal necrosis with destruction of the limiting plate of the portal tract. When the necroinflammatory reaction connects recognizable anatomic structures (portal tract to portal tract or portal tract to terminal hepatic venule), bridging necrosis is present. When contiguous lobules are destroyed, confluent necrosis is present. Bile plugs may be evident in canaliculi or in ductules, and with intracanalicular cholestasis there may be bilirubin pigment in hepatocytes and Kupffer's cells. Predominance of these features connotes a cholestatic hepatitis. Cholestasis may be associated with polymorphonuclear leukocytes and ballooning degeneration of contiguous hepatocytes.

Unfortunately, the patterns of necroinflammation are not sufficiently specific to provide a confident etiologic diagnosis, but the demonstration of certain features, such as fat or centrilobular (zone 3) necrosis, can be helpful in the differential diagnosis. The features of lobular hepatitis can be produced by any of several viruses (hepatitis A, B, and C viruses) and drugs (halothane, isoniazid, methyldopa). Similarly, cholestatic changes may be impossible to differentiate from a drug reaction (chlorpromazine, erythromycin estolate, anabolic or contraceptive steroids) or a virus infection (hepatitis A virus). Importantly, bland cholestasis usually connotes drug toxicity.

Fat is unusual in acute hepatitis unless it is associated with alcohol, hepatitis C virus infection, Reye's syndrome, acute fatty liver of pregnancy, or certain drugs (tetracycline, perhexiline maleate, valproate sodium). Centrilobular necrosis connotes ischemia, relative or absolute hypoxemia, or toxic damage, and in the absence of an inflammatory component it does not warrant the designation of hepatitis.

DIFFERENTIAL DIAGNOSIS

The differential diagnosis of an abrupt hepatocellular injury is limited. Viral infection, drug toxicity, ischemic or hypoxic injury, and toxic damage are the main considerations. The diagnosis of hepatitis implies an inflammatory reaction, and therefore diagnoses that connote acute direct tissue injury without an inflammatory component are misclassified as such. Patients with an indolent chronic liver disease may present with an acute decompensation, as in autoimmune hepatitis and Wilson's disease; it is essential to exclude these diagnoses, as they have specific and effective therapies. Rarely, acute cholecystitis, acute choledocholithiasis, or metastatic liver disease may mimic an acute hepatitis.

Ischemic and hypoxic injuries usually occur in the context of congestive heart failure, hypotension, or hypoxemia. A dramatic and rapid resolution of the serum aminotransferase abnormalities after restoration of hemodynamic stability and tissue oxygenation characterizes this type of injury and secures the diagnosis. Similarly, direct hepatotoxins such as carbon tetrachloride and yellow phosphorus are agents of tissue destruction rather than hepatitis.

DIAGNOSTIC CRITERIA

The minimal requirements for the diagnosis of acute hepatitis are (1) a comprehensive clinical history focusing on the nature and duration of symptoms (≤6 months), risk factors for virus infection (blood transfusion, needle use, contacts, homosexual contact), alcohol ingestion, exposure to hepatotoxic medications or chemicals, and family history of liver disease; (2) a complete physical examination evaluating stigmata of chronic liver disease (cutaneous changes, ascites), features of hepatic decompensation (asterixis, encephalopathy, gastrointestinal tract bleeding), and clues to origin (fever, hemodynamic instability, congestive heart failure, dyspnea, rash, pharyngitis, adenopathy, splenomegaly, Kayser-Fleischer rings, vasculitis, synovitis); (3) serologic tests for infections with hepatitis A virus (immunoglobulin M antibodies to hepatitis A virus), hepatitis B virus (hepatitis B surface antigen [HBsAg], antibodies to hepatitis B core antigen [HBcAg], immunoglobulin M antibodies to HBcAg), and hepatitis C virus (antibodies to hepatitis C virus); (4) hemoglobin, leukocyte, and platelet levels with peripheral blood smear to assess atypical lymphocytes; and (5) determinations of serum aspartate and alanine aminotransferase activity, prothrombin time, serum bilirubin level, and serum protein electrophoresis for assessments of albumin and c-globulin concentrations. Additional studies should be obtained as indicated, including other virologic assays (Epstein-Barr virus, cytomegalovirus, herpes simplex virus, adenovirus), drug levels (alcohol, acetaminophen), tests for hemolysis (plasma hemoglobin, haptoglobin, urinary hemosiderin), assays for Wilson's disease (blood ceruloplasmin and copper levels, urinary copper excretion, slit lamp examination for Kayser-Fleischer rings), immunoserologic markers (antinuclear antibodies, smooth muscle antibodies, antibodies to liver-kidney microsome type 1), plasma ammonia levels, cryoglobulins, and coagulation studies. Hepatic ultrasonography is warranted if there is liver tenderness, hepatomegaly, or concerns about hepatic malignancy, steatosis, patency of hepatic vessels, or the presence of ascites. Assessments for the presence of hepatitis B virus DNA and hepatitis C virus RNA in serum by polymerase chain reaction are more sensitive and specific for the diagnosis of acute hepatitis B and C virus infection than the conventional serologic immunoassays for antibodies. Indeed, in acute hepatitis C, antibodies

TABLE 95–1. SEROLOGIC DIAGNOSIS OF ACUTE VIRAL HEPATITIS

DIAGNOSIS	SEROLOGIC FINDINGS	
Hepatitis A virus	Anti-HAV	+
Acute infection	IgM only anti-HAV	+
Past infection/immunity	IgM and IgG anti-HAV	+
	IgM only anti-HAV	−
Hepatitis B virus	HBsAg and anti-HBc	+
Acute infection	IgM only anti-HBc	+
Chronic infection (proliferative stage)	IgM anti-HBc	−
	HBeAg or HBV DNA or both	+
Chronic infection (integrative stage)	IgM anti-HBc and HBeAg	−
	Anti-HBe	+
	HBV DNA	−
Hepatitis C virus	Anti-HCV	+
Acute infection (early stage)	Anti-HCV	−
	HCV RNA	+
Acute or chronic infection	Anti-HCV and HCV RNA	+
False-positive results	Anti-HCV	+
	Recombinant immunoblot assay or HCV RNA or both	−
Hepatitis D virus	HBsAg and anti-HD	+
Acute infection	IgM anti-HD	+
Coincidental with hepatitis B	IgM anti-HBc	+
Superimposed on hepatitis B	IgM anti-HBc	−
Chronic infection	IgM anti-HD	−
Epstein-Barr virus ("mono")		
Acute infection	IgM viral capsid antigen	≥1:5
	Early antigen	≥1:40
	Nuclear antigen	≥1:5

Anti-HAV = antibody to hepatitis A virus, anti-HBc = antibody to hepatitis B core antigen, anti-HBe = antibody to hepatitis B e antigen (HBeAg), anti-HCV = antibody to hepatitis C virus, anti-HD = antibody to delta virus, DNA = deoxyribonucleic acid, HBsAg = hepatitis B surface antigen, IgM = immunoglobulin M, RNA = ribonucleic acid.

to the virus are commonly absent. The serologic findings that establish the diagnosis of the most common forms of acute viral hepatitis are shown in Table 95–1.

ETIOLOGIC FACTORS

Hepatitis A virus is a 27-nm RNA virus (picornavirus) that is most commonly transmitted from person to person by fecal-oral mechanisms (direct contact, food, water, shellfish). The incubation period is short (15 to 49 days), and the virus is present in stool and blood through the latter part of the incubation period until jaundice and peak aminotransferase abnormality ensue. Transmission is mainly during the preicteric phase of the disease, and since viremia is short, transmission by blood inoculation is rare. Asymptomatic disease is common, as only 5% of individuals with serologic evidence of infection have a clinical history of hepatitis. Children are commonly asymptomatic, while in adults the infection has more severe manifestations. Symptoms usually begin abruptly as an influenza-like illness; splenomegaly, lymphadenopathy, and hepatomegaly may be present in icteric patients. Spontaneous resolution occurs in all patients, but the duration of disease may vary from 2 weeks to 6 months or longer. The mean duration of jaundice in patients under 15 years of age is 10.5 days (median, 7 days). Adults may have a more protracted course, and the cholestatic form of the disease may last for 6 months or more. Fulminant hepatitis occurs in less than 1% of patients; but of those with fulminant hepatitis, hepatitis A virus infection accounts for at least 14%. The epidemiology of hepatitis A virus infection is changing, as infection rates have declined in children, presumably because of improvements in sanitation. The number of susceptible adults, therefore, has increased, and these individuals are at high risk for severe disease. Fortunately, there is no chronic carrier state for the virus, and infection does not result in chronic hepatitis.

Hepatitis B virus is a 42-nm DNA virus (hepadnavirus) that is transmitted mainly by blood inoculation or sexual contact. Perinatal transmission is an important mechanism in geographic regions where the virus is endemic. The incubation period ranges from 50 to 180 days (mean, 70 days), and the disease is typically insidious in onset. Viremia is present before, during, and after the clinical illness, and infectivity is not precluded by clinical recovery. Urticaria and synovitis may occur during the prodrome. HBsAg typically disappears from 1 to 13 weeks after the onset of illness, but in 4% to 10% of patients it may persist beyond 6 months. An asymptomatic chronic carrier state is well established, and chronic hepatitis, cirrhosis, portal hypertension, liver failure, and hepatocellular cancer are potential consequences of the infection. Fulminant hepatitis develops in 1% to 2% of acutely infected individuals.

Hepatitis C virus is a single-stranded RNA virus (flavivirus) that is also transmitted by blood inoculation. Transmission by sexual contact or perinatal mechanisms is possible but less well established. Sporadic disease within communities is well recognized, and the existence of an asymptomatic chronic carrier state undoubtedly contributes to an unrecognized reservoir of virus. The incubation period ranges from 15 to 180 days (range, 60 days), and spontaneous resolution usually occurs within 12 weeks. Viremia develops quickly after inoculation, and it may persist indefinitely despite resolution of clinical manifestations. Enzyme immunoassay results for antibodies to hepatitis C virus may be negative during the acute illness, and serial determinations are warranted through the period of convalescence to establish (or exclude) the diagnosis. Chronic hepatitis develops in up to 60% of patients, and serum aminotransferase levels may fluctuate widely during the infection. Intervals of biochemical normality may last up to 18 months before spontaneous exacerbation. Individuals with chronic hepatitis C are at risk for cirrhosis, liver failure, and hepatocellular cancer. Importantly, longitudinal studies in patients with posttransfusion hepatitis have indicated that these consequences are unusual within 18 years of follow-up. Hepatitis C virus has been difficult to detect in patients with fulminant hepatitis, but recent studies have indicated that it is a factor in some geographic regions.

Hepatitis non-A, non-B, non-C is an entity whose existence has been deduced by epidemiologic surveys that have failed to place 20% of patients with viral illness into a confident diagnostic category. The entity has been best described in the community setting where 25% of individuals with this diagnosis lack risk factors for viral infection. Parenteral exposure, sexual or household contact, and low socioeconomic level characterize the remaining 75%. Individuals with community-acquired acute non-A, non-B, non-C ("indeterminate") hepatitis are older, have lower serum aminotransferase elevations, and a lower frequency of chronic hepatitis (29% versus 62%) than counterparts with chronic hepatitis C.

Hepatitis delta virus is a unique virus ("viroid") that requires the hepatitis B virus for expression. It has a single-stranded, circular RNA core and HBsAg coat. Hepatitis delta virus has a direct cytotoxicity; consequently, it produces an aggressive hepatocellular injury. It may infect an individual coincidentally with hepatitis B virus or be superimposed on a chronic hepatitis B virus infection. Coincidental infections are usually self-limited and similar in behavior to acute hepatitis B, although a fulminant presentation is possible. Superimposed infection can result in clinical deterioration and rapid progression to cirrhosis. Some of these patients may be mistakenly diagnosed as having fulminant hepatitis B. Transmission is mainly by parenteral inoculation, and the disease is most common among intravenous drug users, patients receiving hemodialysis, and patients with hemophilia.

Hepatitis E virus is a 27- to 34-nm single-stranded RNA virus (calicivirus) that is transmitted by fecal-oral mechanisms. It is the leading cause of acute viral hepatitis in young to middle-aged adults in developing countries (Pakistan, India, Nepal, Russia, Burma, Borneo, Somalia, Sudan, Algeria, Ivory Coast, Mexico) where epidemics have been described. Sporadic cases of acute hepatitis E do occur in these endemic areas, but they are rare in Western countries. The virus produces a self-limited infection, and chronic hepatitis has not been recognized. Unfortunately, hepatitis E infection has a high mortality (20%) in pregnant women.

Drugs and alcohol are common causes of acute hepatitis, and they must always be excluded even if a viral cause is established. Superimposed or concurrent insults are possible, and they may intensify the manifestations of the primary disease. Viral infection, especially that ascribed to hepatitis C virus, can worsen the prognosis of chronic alcoholic liver disease, and alcohol can potentiate the hepatotoxicity of drugs, such as acetaminophen. Drugs can produce acute hepatitic and cholestatic forms of hepatitis, as well as result in a fulminant presentation, chronic

TABLE 95–2. COMMON DRUGS IMPLICATED AS CAUSES OF ACUTE HEPATITIS

HEPATITIC (LOBULAR) REACTION	CHOLESTATIC REACTION
Aminosalicylic acid	Acetohexamide
Aspirin	Azathioprine
Carbenicillin	Chlorpromazine
Dantrolene sodium	Erythromycin
Disulfiram	Ethinyl estradiol
Isoniazid	Fluoxymesterone
Methyldopa	Flurazepam
Nicotinic acid	Griseofulvin
Nitrofurantoin	Imipramine
Penicillin G	Indomethacin
Propylthiouracil	Meprobamate
	Methandrostenolone
	Phenytoin sodium
	Propoxyphene
	Rifampin
	Sulfonamides
	Tolbutamide

hepatitis, and cirrhosis. Importantly, drugs do not produce a self-perpetuating injury, and discontinuation of the medication typically is followed by resolution of inflammatory activity. Improvement can be anticipated within 1 month of drug withdrawal, although cholestatic forms of alcohol- and drug-induced liver disease may take 2 to 3 months to resolve. The medications most commonly incriminated are shown in Table 95–2.

TREATMENT

There are no therapies of established efficacy in the management of acute hepatitis other than identification and avoidance of injurious substances. Withdrawal of hepatotoxic medication, abstinence from alcohol, and avoidance of toxic substances are standard approaches. Bed rest has not proved to be beneficial, although restriction of strenuous activities is frequently warranted by diminished stamina. The diet should be balanced and nutritious, equalling 1 g of protein and 30 kcal/kg of ideal body weight per day in frequent small feedings.

The intravenous administration of recombinant interferon beta clears serum hepatitis C virus RNA and resolves aminotransferase abnormalities in 91% of patients with acute hepatitis C, whereas only 21% of untreated control patients respond similarly. Such therapy has promise as a means of preventing the progression of acute hepatitis C to chronic hepatitis, but additional studies are necessary to corroborate these preliminary findings and extend the observations to interferon alfa, which can be administered subcutaneously.

Corticosteroids are not effective in patients with acute viral hepatitis, and they may increase the virus burden. Such therapy, however, may be beneficial in selected patients with protracted cholestatic acute hepatitis A and incapacitating symptoms, such as pruritus and diarrhea. Similarly, corticosteroids should be considered in selected patients with severe, potentially life-threatening, alcoholic hepatitis.

The management of fulminant hepatitis is based on the anticipation of spontaneous hepatic regeneration and the prevention of life-threatening complications. Hepatic encephalopathy, cerebral edema, renal failure, bacterial infection, gastrointestinal tract hemorrhage, hypoglycemia, acid-base and electrolyte disturbances, and cardiovascular collapse must be managed aggressively. Cerebral edema is a frequent lethal complication, and patients with advanced hepatic encephalopathy are candidates for direct intracranial pressure monitoring. Intravenous boluses of 20% mannitol (1 g/kg body weight) are effective in reducing intracranial pressure, and they are preferred to corticosteroids or controlled hyperventilation. Thiopental infusion can also be considered if therapy with mannitol is ineffective. Liver transplantation is indicated when prognostic indexes suggest a dismal outcome. The overall 1-year survival of patients undergoing liver transplantation for fulminant hepatitis exceeds 60%. Only 10% of patients with acute liver failure, however, receive a liver graft.

CLINICAL COURSE

The majority of patients have a self-limited clinical course with resolution of the disease within 12 weeks. These patients typically have normal hepatic architecture, and in cases of hepatitis A and B, they develop a homologous immunity to repeat infection. Protracted cholestatic forms of hepatitis or slowly resolving or "relapsing" hepatitis A and C virus infections may require 6 months before resolution. Persistence of inflammatory activity beyond 6 months connotes chronicity. The diagnosis of chronic hepatitis, however, requires features of portal or periportal hepatitis. *Protracted acute hepatitis A infection, impaired regeneration syndrome*, and *slowly resolving acute viral hepatitis* may satisfy temporal criteria for chronicity but not those for chronic hepatitis.

Persistence of inflammatory activity for 6 months or longer in conjunction with histologic features of portal or periportal hepatitis connotes *chronic hepatitis*. The designation implies an unresolving hepatocellular inflammation that has the potential to progress to cirrhosis, liver failure, hepatocellular cancer, and premature death. It is typically a consequence of acute viral infection, occurring in 10% (acute hepatitis B) to 60% (acute hepatitis C) of patients.

The development of hepatic encephalopathy within 8 weeks of illness connotes *fulminant hepatitis*. Mortality relates to patient age and disease origin, but it averages 80%. Survival rates may be as high as 67% for hepatitis A, 53% for acetaminophen toxicity, and 39% for hepatitis B in specialized liver units. In contrast, life expectancies range from 0% to 20% for acute Wilson's disease, halothane hepatitis, and non-A, non-B hepatitis. In these latter instances, orthotopic liver transplantation has been associated with a 54% to 74% survival, and it has become an appropriate treatment option. Auxiliary liver transplantation has the promise of supporting life until the native liver recovers fully from a self-limited and reversible insult. In patients with viral hepatitis and drug reactions, age of less than 11 years or more than 40 years, 7 days or more of jaundice before encephalopathy, serum bilirubin level greater than 17.5 mg/dl (300 1mol/L), and severe hypoprothrombinemia indicate a poor prognosis. In patients with acetaminophen poisoning, an arterial pH of less than 7.3 or a serum creatinine level of greater than 3.4 mg/dl and severe hypoprothrombinemia indicate a dismal outcome.

The development of hepatic encephalopathy more than 8 weeks and up to 24 weeks after the onset of illness connotes *late onset hepatic failure*. These patients resemble those with fulminant hepatitis, and their overall mortality is 81%. A viral cause may be difficult to establish, and patients with late onset hepatic failure are commonly classified as having acute non-A, non-B hepatitis. Corticosteroid therapy is ineffective, and liver transplantation may be necessary.

PREVENTION

Enteric isolation is warranted for patients with acute hepatitis A or E. A private room should be authorized; gowns and gloves should be worn during direct patient contact or exposure to feces; and hand washing should be scrupulous. Blood and body fluid isolation is justified for patients with acute hepatitis B, C, and non-A, non-B, non-C. Precautions are similar to those of enteric isolation except that special care is necessary in the handling and disposal of blood and body fluids.

Immune globulin (0.02 ml/kg body weight intramuscularly) should be given to all close contacts (household members) of patients with acute hepatitis A within 7 days of exposure. Patients who have had a blood inoculation from individuals with acute indeterminate hepatitis can be treated similarly, although the efficacy of this strategy is unestablished. In these instances, the immune globulin (0.06 ml/kg body weight) should be administered intramuscularly within 72 hours of exposure and no later than 7 days.

Hepatitis B immune globulin (HBIG) should be given to susceptible individuals who have been exposed to HBsAg-positive individuals by needle stick, open wounds, blood contact with mucous membranes, and sexual contact. Neonates of HBsAg-positive mothers should be treated immediately at birth. Susceptibility to infection implies absence of previous infection with hepatitis B virus (seronegativity for antibodies to HBcAg) or lack of established immunity (seronegativity for antibodies to HBsAg). Donor seronegativity for hepatitis B e antigen (anti-HBe) or hepatitis B virus DNA should not dissuade the administration of HBIG. The recommended dose in adults is 0.06 ml/kg body weight delivered intramuscularly within 48 hours of exposure (no later than 7 days) and again at 30 days. The recombinant hepatitis B vaccine should be given in conjunction with HBIG to exposed neonates, and it should be encouraged in exposed adults. If exposed individuals receive hepatitis B vaccine in conjunction with HBIG, the second dose of HBIG at 30 days is unnecessary.

The recombinant hepatitis B vaccine is safe and effective. It should be administered to all individuals at risk for exposure to the hepatitis B virus (health care providers, institutionalized individuals, close contacts and newborns of chronic carriers, intravenous drug users, homosexuals, and recipients of multiple transfusions). Universal vaccination is the ultimate goal, and the administration of vaccine to all infants and children has been endorsed. Protective antibodies (antibodies to HBsAg) develop in over 90% of adults who receive 1 ml of vaccine intramuscularly (deltoid) at 0, 1, and 6 months. Immunogenicity should be documented after the course of vaccination. Antibody titers decline with time, but the anamnestic response is well preserved.

Live attenuated and inactivated hepatitis A virus vaccines have been developed and tested in humans. The vaccines seem safe and effective, and FDA approval has recently been obtained for the inactivated vaccine. The formalin-inactivated whole-virus vaccine requires multiple doses, is more expensive, and induces a shorter duration of immunity than the live, attenuated vaccine, but it has better stability and a greater safety margin. Testing and licensing have been hampered because (1) the number of vaccine and placebo recipients required to establish efficacy is prohibitively large; (2) studies in children are ethically difficult to conduct; (3) infection in children is commonly subclinical and inapparent; (4) there are no assays that distinguish natural infection from vaccination; and (5) identification of the appropriate target population for the vaccine has been difficult.

REFERENCES

1. Alter MJ, Margolis HS, Krawczynski K, et al. The natural history of community-acquired hepatitis C in the United States. *N Engl J Med.* 1992;327:1899–1905.
2. Canalese J, Gimson AES, Davis C, et al. Controlled trial of dexamethasone and mannitol for the cerebral oedema of fulminant hepatic failure. *Gut.* 1982;23:625–629.
3. Czaja AJ. Serologic markers of hepatitis A and B in acute and chronic liver disease. *Mayo Clin Proc.* 1979;54:721–732.
4. Gimson AES, O'Grady J, Ede RJ, Portmann B, Williams R. Late onset hepatic failure: clinical, serological and histological features. *Hepatology.* 1986;6:288–294.
5. Houghton M, Weiner A, Han J, Kuo G, Choo Q-L. Molecular biology of the hepatitis C viruses: implications for diagnosis, development and control of viral disease. *Hepatology.* 1991;14:381–388.
6. Lee WM. Acute liver failure. *N Engl J Med.* 1993;329:1862–1871.
7. Ludwig J. Drug effects on the liver: a tabular compilation of drugs and drug-related hepatic diseases. *Dig Dis Sci.* 1979;24:785–796.
8. O'Grady JG, Alexander GJM, Hayllar KM, Williams R. Early indicators of prognosis in fulminant hepatic failure. *Gastroenterology.* 1989;97:439–445.
9. Rizzetto M. The delta agent. *Hepatology.* 1983;3:729–737.
10. Seeff LB, Buskell-Bales Z, Wright EC, et al. Long-term mortality after transfusion-associated non-A, non-B hepatitis. *N Engl J Med.* 1992;327:1906–1911.

96

Interferon Therapy for Chronic Viral Hepatitis B and C

PETER F. MALET

The treatment of chronic hepatitis due to hepatitis B and C viruses has been revolutionized since the mid-1980s by the introduction of therapy with interferon alfa. Interferon alfa-2b has been approved in the United States for treatment of chronic hepatitis B and C/non-A, non-B. Prior to the demonstration of the efficacy of interferon, there were no consistently effective drug therapies for the eradication of chronic hepatitis B and C. While interferon therapy is not effective in nearly all cases and relapses do occur after a course of treatment, its use represents a major breakthrough in the treatment of these types of chronic hepatitis.

Not every patient with chronic hepatitis B or C is a candidate for treatment with interferon, and the choice of which patients to treat involves both objective and also subjective criteria and clinical judgment. The use of interferon continues to be investigated in terms of achieving higher remission and lower relapse rates. Other antiviral therapies for chronic hepatitis B and C are also being explored. This chapter concentrates on the use of interferon alfa for chronic hepatitis B and C, focusing on the diagnosis of chronic hepatitis B and C, indications for therapy, expected response rates, and side effects with interferon administration.

DEFINITION OF CHRONIC HEPATITIS

The term *hepatitis* implies that the liver disease is mainly one involving hepatocellular necrosis; although there may also be a component of cholestasis or steatosis, these are not the primary features. Chronic hepatitis typically is characterized by elevation of serum aminotransferases to a much greater degree than serum alkaline phosphatase. Conversely, chronic cholestatic diseases, such as primary biliary cirrhosis and sclerosing cholangitis, typically exhibit the opposite pattern, in which serum alkaline phosphatase is elevated to a greater extent than serum transaminases.

There are instances in which it may be difficult to readily categorize a particular liver disease as either hepatocellular or cholestatic based solely on the serum liver enzymes. Usually, though, more sophisticated blood and radiologic tests and, ultimately, liver biopsy provide a clearer insight into whether the liver disease is primarily hepatocellular or cholestatic or whether it is truly a mixed picture.

Authorities differ somewhat in their opinions regarding how long hepatitis need be ongoing before applying the term *chronic,* but a reasonable consensus of opinion would be 6 months. The use of at least 6 months' duration as a criterion allows many cases of slowly resolving acute viral or other type of hepatitis to resolve completely. Unnecessary treatment with interferon or other agents can thus be avoided.

DIFFERENTIAL DIAGNOSIS OF CHRONIC HEPATITIS

Viral Causes

The two major causes of chronic viral hepatitis are hepatitis B and C viruses.[1] Prior to 1989, the term *non-A, non-B (NANB) chronic hepatitis* was used to denote those cases of chronic hepatitis thought to be due to a virus or viruses other than hepatitis B virus (HBV); (chronic hepatitis does not result from hepatitis A virus [HAV]). In 1989, the genome of the NANB virus responsible for the majority of chronic NANB hepatitis was elucidated using a recombinant complementary deoxyribonucleic acid (cDNA) technique, and this virus is now termed *hepatitis C virus*.[2,3] Hepatitis C virus (HCV) appears to account for 60% to 90% of NANB hepatitis.[4,5]

It appears likely that there are other NANB viruses; these have not yet been well characterized, though. There is some information regarding hepatitis E, which is a virus that has been found in India and Central and South America and can cause acute hepatitis. Hepatitis E virus (HEV) does not appear to be a cause of chronic hepatitis. Other, as yet unidentified, NANB viruses may result in chronic hepatitis, but if so, they appear to be responsible for only a small proportion of cases of chronic viral hepatitis.

Nonviral Causes

There are a number of other nonviral causes for chronic liver disease (not necessarily strictly hepatocellular in type) including Wilson's disease, α-1-antitrypsin deficiency, autoimmune and drug-induced hepatitis, fatty liver, alcoholic and nonalcoholic steatohepatitis (steatonecrosis), and hemochromatosis. All these conditions must be considered in the differential diagnosis in patients with persistently elevated serum transaminases (Table 96–1).

HEPATITIS C

The HCV is a positive sense, single-stranded ribonucleic acid (RNA) lipid-enveloped virus 50

TABLE 96–1. LABORATORY EVALUATION OF PATIENTS WITH ELEVATED SERUM TRANSAMINASES FOR 6 MONTHS OR MORE

Diagnosis	Findings
Hepatitis B virus	Hepatitis B surface antigen and antibody (if HBsAg positive, obtain hepatitis B e antigen and antibody)
	Hepatitis B core antibody
	Hepatitis B virus deoxyribonucleic acid
Hepatitis C virus	Hepatitis C antibody
Autoimmune hepatitis	Anti-smooth-muscle antibody, antinuclear antibody, liver-kidney microsome antibodies (in selected cases)
Wilson's disease	Serum ceruloplasmin
Hemochromatosis	Serum ferritin, iron, total iron-binding capacity (transferrin)
α-1-Antitrypsin deficiency	Serum α-1-antitrypsin

to 60-nm in diameter with a genome consisting of approximately 9400 nucleotides.[5,6] HCV is responsible for 90% or more of posttransfusional hepatitis worldwide and for 60% to 90% of cases of NANB hepatitis overall.[4,5] HCV has also been associated epidemiologically with hepatocellular carcinoma.[7]

While most cases of hepatitis C are transmitted via the parenteral route (mostly blood transfusions, sharing needles during intravenous drug abuse, and also accidental needle sticks), other cases occur sporadically with no such identifiable risk factors. The risk of chronicity after an episode of posttransfusional acute hepatitis C (which is usually either subclinical or asymptomatic) is at least 50%, possibly even higher.[1,4,5,8,9] Of those with chronic infection, approximately half have active hepatitis on liver biopsy. A significant proportion of cases (estimated to be at least 20%) of chronic hepatitis C eventuate in the development of cirrhosis after a number of years. Although some patients may develop cirrhosis within several years, it is not unusual for up to 20 years or more to elapse between the original infection with HCV and the development of cirrhosis. HCV is suspected to be directly cytopathic to hepatocytes in contrast to HBV, which results in hepatocellular damage through an immunologic mechanism.

HISTOPATHOLOGY OF CHRONIC HEPATITIS C

Patients with chronic hepatitis C may have a variety of histologic findings on liver biopsy ranging from virtually normal to active cirrhosis.[10,11] The histologic progression of hepatitis C from early chronic hepatitis with relatively normal liver architecture and no fibrosis to fully developed cirrhosis is not well understood. In particular, the prognostic significance of minimal changes on liver biopsy in chronic hepatitis C is uncertain. The course of active inflammation that is found in about half of all patients with chronic hepatitis C appears to be one of progressive disease. It is now recommended that the terms *chronic persistent* and *chronic active hepatitis,* which have been used in the past to describe histologic changes associated with chronic hepatitis, no longer be applied in describing chronic hepatitis C[12] or other types of chronic hepatitis. Most experts now favor the use of more specific descriptors, including the activity, grade, and stage of the liver disease, as well as the etiology if known.

There is no single histologic feature or set of histologic features that is diagnostic for hepatitis C. Scheuer et al[10] have found that a common histologic pattern in many patients with chronic hepatitis C is that of mild chronic hepatitis with lymphoid aggregates in the portal tracts with lobular activity, including acidophilic bodies and fatty change. Findings such as this are helpful when combined with a positive serologic test for HCV antibody but absolute diagnostic certainty of chronic hepatitis C on liver biopsy is not currently possible. Efforts to identify the presence of the HCV genome in liver tissue samples, which would further aid in securing the diagnosis, are ongoing.

HEPATITIS C SEROLOGY

The current serologic tests available for HCV represent a major advance over the state of testing up until 1989 when no direct tests were available. Even so, the currently available tests for HCV antibodies or for HCV RNA, although clinically extremely useful, are not 100% sensitive or specific.[13–16] The characterization of the HCV genome is quite complex and far from complete; also the virus exhibits multiple genotypes.[5,6] Newer serologic tests are in a continual state of development and evaluation, and the evolution of serologic tests for HCV will continue.

Prior to 1989, when there were no serologic assays for HCV antibodies, surrogate markers for HCV infection, such as anti-HBc antibody and serum alanine aminotransferase (ALT), were used with some effectiveness for screening donated blood but were not completely adequate. The single most significant breakthrough occurred in 1989 when Choo et al[2] reported the isolation of a cDNA close derived from the plasma of chimpanzees infected by NANB virus. This clone, termed *recombinant 5-1-1,* consisted of 155 base pairs. The discovery of this part of the HCV genome allowed for the development of the first serologic test for HCV antibodies.[3]

ELISA Assays for HCV Antibodies

The first HCV serologic test licensed by the Food and Drug Administration (FDA) was an enzyme-linked immunosorbent assay (ELISA) that used the recombinant antigen c100-3 (Table 96–2). The polypeptide c100 consists of the original clone discovered by Choo et al[2] and two adjacent clones. This type of "first-generation" ELISA assay had significant false-positive and false-negative rates.[15–16]

"Second-generation" ELISA assays and, in-

TABLE 96–2. TYPES OF ASSAYS COMMONLY USED FOR DETECTION OF HCV ANTIBODIES OR HCV RNA IN SERUM

For HCV Antibodies
Enzyme-Linked Immunosorbent Assay (ELISA)
Detects antibodies to recombinant HCV antigens
Second- and third-generation assays

Recombinant Immunoblot Assay (RIBA)
Detects antibodies to recombinant HCV antigens
Second- and third-generation assays

For HCV RNA
Polymerase Chain Reaction (PCR)
Using primers specific for HCV genome, detects cDNA that has been reverse-transcribed from HCV
Does not detect antibodies
May be used in serum or in liver tissue
Increased sensitivity compared to serum HCV antibody detection assays

cDNA = complementary deoxyribonucleic acid, HCV = hepatitis C virus, RNA = ribonucleic acid.

creasingly, "third-generation" ones are now the most widely available tests for HCV antibodies. These assays use, in addition to the c100-3 antigen, other antigens from the HCV genome from both the core and nonstructural regions. These assays are much more sensitive and specific than the first-generation ELISA assay in detecting HCV antibodies, and investigation continues into further refinement of ELISA-type assays.

RIBA Assays for HCV Antibodies

Development of more refined assays for HCV antibodies has also centered around the use of recombinant immunoblot techniques.[14] The first recombinant immunoblot assay (RIBA) detected antibodies to HCV using three antigens: (1) the c100-3 antigen, (2) the 5-1-1 antigen, and (3) superoxide dismutase (SOD).

The second-generation RIBA (termed *RIBA II*) uses five antigens: the same three (two HCV antigens and SOD) as the first-generation RIBA assay plus the c22-3 antigen (which is a structural polypeptide encoded in the core region of HCV) and the c33c antigen (which is a nonstructural polypeptide encoded in the protease [NS_2] region). Interpreting the assay itself is somewhat complex, but basically if there is reactivity to any two or more of the four HCV antigens, the test results are interpreted as reactive (positive). If there is reactivity to only one of the antigens (with or without reactivity to the SOD), the test results are read as indeterminate. If only the SOD band is reactive, the test results are termed *negative*. The RIBA II method has enhanced sensitivity compared to the RIBA I and has been used as a confirmatory test for sera that is positive using the ELISA II assay. Third-generation RIBA assays are being used increasingly.

Polymerase Chain Reaction Assay for HCV RNA

The currently available serologic tests detect only the presence of antibodies to HCV. They provide no insight into the replication of HCV or about the time course of the infection. Test results often do not read as positive until several weeks to months after the acute infection. Detection of actual HCV RNA in the serum provides better elucidation of these points.

HCV RNA generally circulates in extremely low titers in the serum of patients with chronic hepatitis and is not detectable by standard assays, such as northern blot technique, that are used to detect other viral infections such as human immunodeficiency virus (HIV). Polymerase chain reaction (PCR) techniques are currently the most sensitive method of detecting HCV RNA.[17,18] The use of PCR assay amplifies reverse-transcribed cDNA and permits detection of minute quantities of viral RNA either in the serum or in liver biopsy specimens. It appears that primers from highly conserved areas of the HCV genome, such as the 5'-noncoding region, are most useful because of the genetic variability of other areas of the HCV genome. The actual false-positive and false-negative rates for PCR-based assays have not yet been determined. At this time, detection of HCV RNA by PCR techniques is considered the gold standard, although more work is needed to fully elucidate the clinical utility of the test.

CHRONIC HEPATITIS C AND AUTOIMMUNE HEPATITIS

There is occasionally uncertainty in differentiating autoimmune hepatitis from chronic hepatitis C.[19–21] This uncertainty arises because the current serologic tests for HCV can exhibit false-positive and false-negative results and also because not all patients with autoimmune hepatitis have positive results from serologic tests (anti-smooth-muscle antibodies [ASMA] or antinuclear antibodies [ANA]). There is also the question whether HCV may be implicated in the pathogenesis of some cases of autoimmune hepatitis.

In particular, type II autoimmune hepatitis in which only antibodies to liver-kidney microsomes (LKM) are present may present diagnostic difficulties, since the test for anti-LKM is not widely available. There have been reports of worsening of liver disease in some patients with suspected chronic NANB hepatitis with or without positive anti-HCV with type II autoimmune hepatitis treated with interferon. There have also been questions raised whether interferon therapy could induce autoimmune hepatitis in certain patients.

Bach et al[11] have attempted to distinguish the hepatic histologic findings of chronic hepatitis C from that of autoimmune hepatitis. Compared to autoimmune hepatitis, features more commonly observed in hepatitis C were bile duct damage (91% versus 40%), bile duct loss (91% versus 20%), fatty change (72% versus 19%), and lymphoid aggregates with the portal tracts (49% versus 10%). Features seen more often with autoimmune hepatitis than with hepatitis C were piecemeal necrosis (81% versus 10%), severe lobular necrosis and inflammation (76% versus 38%), and broad areas of parenchymal collapse (76% versus 6%). None of these features are diagnostic for hepatitis C, but similar to the findings of Scheuer et al[10] certain combinations of features are more typical of hepatitis C.

Clinical judgment is paramount in deciding about treatment in uncertain cases.[22,23] Autoimmune hepatitis usually responds fairly readily to prednisone alone or combined with azathioprine. In cases where autoimmune hepatitis is suspected but chronic hepatitis C (or NANB hepatitis) is also a consideration, a trial of immunosuppressive therapy seems warranted. Such therapy does not have a deleterious effect on the short-term course of chronic hepatitis C. If the patient fails to respond, as measured by improving symptoms and serum aminotransferases after 2 to 3 months, consideration can then be given to initiating interferon therapy.

MECHANISM OF ACTION OF INTERFERON IN CHRONIC HEPATITIS B AND C

Interferons such as interferon alfa-2b have a variety of effects that can be generally termed *antiviral, immunomodulatory,* and *antiproliferative.*[24–26] Interferon can promote the activity of cytokines and stimulate immune effector cell populations such as macrophages, natural killer cells, and cytotoxic T cells. The enhancement of cytotoxic T lymphocytes may be particularly important in the clearance of hepatocytes infected with HBV. It also enhances target antigen recognition by increasing exposure of various cell surface proteins (HLA class I antigens) that are important in the immune response. For example, it has been shown to enhance the expression of hepatitis B surface antigen (HBsAg) and pre-S2. Among the antiviral effects is the induction by interferon of intracellular proteins such as $2',5'$-oligoadenylate synthetase ($2',5'$ OAS), which enhances cleaving of viral RNA. This effect may be particularly important in clearing HCV. Evidence also suggests that interferon can directly inhibit HCV replication.

Considerations in Initiating Interferon Therapy in Chronic Hepatitis B and C

Although exceptions may exist on a case-by-case basis, interferon therapy is generally not advisable for patients with the following conditions: decompensated liver disease, autoimmune liver disease, and severe psychiatric conditions, particularly depression. The risk of treating patients with decompensated liver disease is increased particularly in those with hepatitis B because of the potential for a flare of the disease during treatment. Careful judgment must be exercised in using interferon, especially at higher doses, in patients with preexisting debilitating medical conditions, coagulation disorders (such as idiopathic thrombocytopenic purpura [ITP]), or severe myelosuppression. Those with preexisting thyroid dysfunction should be carefully monitored during therapy (Table 96–3).

The most important, and often difficult, aspect of treating chronic hepatitis C is deciding which patients to treat. Although there are many cases in which the decision to treat is fairly straightforward, such as those patients with symptomatic progressing disease, there are other cases in which the decision is much more difficult, such as those who are asymptomatic with minimal disease activity on liver biopsy. It should be noted that interferon therapy is approved for chronic NANB hepatitis (that is, whether or not serum HCV antibodies are present). Therefore, although the term *chronic hepatitis C* is used in the following discussion, the information regarding interferon treatment applies to chronic NANB hepatitis as well.

Among the more subjective factors that must be considered in this decision-making process are whether the patient will comply with inter-

TABLE 96–3. INTERFERON TREATMENT FOR HEPATITIS B AND C

Treatment of Hepatitis B with Interferon

Indications
Chronic hepatitis B

Typical Laboratory Findings
Elevation of serum transaminases for >6 mo
Positive HBsAg, anti-HBc, negative anti-HBs
Usually positive HBeAg
Positive serum HBV DNA

Standard Dosage
5 million units SQ daily for 4–6 mo

Laboratory Parameters to Follow During Therapy
Serum transaminases
Hemoglobin, white blood cell count, and platelets
HBsAg, anti-HBs
HBeAg, anti-HBe
Serum HBV DNA
Serum thyroid-stimulating hormone (TSH)

Treatment of Hepatitis C with Interferon

Indications
Chronic hepatitis C
Chronic non-A, non-B hepatitis

Typical Laboratory Findings
Elevation of serum transaminases for >6 mo
Positive anti-HCV antibody (for chronic hepatitis C)
Positive hepatitis C RNA in serum (for chronic hepatitis C)

Standard Dosage
3 million units SQ three times weekly for 6 mo

Laboratory Parameters to Follow During Therapy
Serum transaminases
Hemoglobin, white blood cell count, and platelets
HCV RNA
Serum TSH

anti-HBc = antibody to hepatitis B core antigen, anti-HBe = antibody to hepatitis B e antigen, anti-HBs = antibody to hepatitis B surface antigen, HBeAg = hepatitis B e antigen, HBsAg = hepatitis B surface antigen, HBV DNA = hepatitis B virus deoxyribonucleic acid, HCV RNA = hepatitis C virus, ribonucleic acid.

---

feron administration and whether other diseases the patient might have will significantly shorten the patient's expected life span.

Factored into the decision-making process is the relative lack of knowledge about the long-term prognosis of patients with minimal disease activity on liver biopsy. Whether such patients are at low, medium, or high risk for the development of progressive disease and cirrhosis or hepatocellular carcinoma is not clearly known. Observation is usually the alternative to initiating interferon therapy in those with mild disease activity.

Also incompletely known is whether it is easier to eradicate HCV in the first few years after the patient acquired it or whether the duration of viral infection is not a factor in viral clearance. Clearly, if the former is the case, the trend will be toward treatment as soon as feasible after chronic HCV infection is diagnosed.

Administration of Interferon for Chronic Hepatitis C

The currently recommended regimen for hepatitis C is 3 million units of interferon alfa-2b subcutaneously or intramuscularly three times a week for 6 months (Table 96–2).[27] The use of higher doses of interferon in an attempt to induce higher remission and lower relapse rates is under investigation.[28,29] If the patient has not responded in terms of serum ALT decrease after 4 months, it is unlikely that continuation of therapy will result in improvement; consideration should be given to the accuracy of the diagnosis and to whether therapy should be continued or not.[30] The effect of higher doses and a more prolonged course of interferon in such nonresponders is not yet known but is currently being studied.

Results of Interferon Alfa-2b Therapy for Chronic Hepatitis C

Approximately 40% of patients with chronic hepatitis C respond to a 6-month course of therapy in terms of normalization of serum transaminases.[30–34] Significantly, about 80% to 90% of eventual responders (after a total of 6 months' therapy) achieve a biochemical response within 4 months.

Of the responders after a 6-month course, approximately 50% relapse after discontinuation of interferon. Some patients exhibit rises in serum aminotransferases after discontinuation of interferon that are self-limited, resolving without medical treatment. The majority of first-time relapsers with a sustained elevation of serum ALT in whom interferon is reinitiated at a dose of 3 million units three times a week again achieve a biochemical response. The response is usually seen within a few weeks after restarting therapy. The optimal length of time to continue therapy after a relapse is not known. Questions regarding treatment of relapses, including whether lower dose maintenance therapy is useful in maintaining a remission, are currently being investigated. As yet unknown is whether interferon therapy has any effect on decreasing mortality secondary to chronic hepatitis C or on the future development of hepatoma.

During interferon therapy for chronic hepatitis C, serum anti-HCV antibodies remain positive in patients regardless of the outcome of treatment.[35] Therefore, following anti-HCV antibodies is not helpful in assessing the response to interferon therapy. The effect of interferon therapy on serum HCV RNA (detected by PCR assay) has been reported by Hagiwara et al.[36] In their study HCV RNA became undetectable in all patients whose serum ALT levels fell to normal during interferon treatment; HCV RNA disappeared before serum ALT levels became normal. HCV RNA remained undetectable in those patients who remained in complete remission 6 months after discontinuation of interferon but rose again in patients who had a relapse, based on rising serum ALT levels. In the latter patients, HCV RNA rose within 4 weeks, usually before serum ALT levels. In patients whose serum ALT levels did not normalize during interferon therapy, serum HCV RNA did not disappear during or after therapy. Thus, HCV RNA shows promise as a means of following the response to interferon therapy and for detecting relapses early.

Similar findings have been reported by Shindo et al.[37,38] Thus, although long-term response, in terms of normal serum ALT and HCV RNA, can be achieved after interferon therapy, loss of HCV RNA during therapy cannot be used to predict a favorable long-term response.

A number of other therapies (antiviral and immunomodulatory agents) for chronic hepatitis C are being investigated, and the results of such trials will be forthcoming over the next several years.

Interferon Therapy of Chronic Hepatitis B

Generally, the decision whether to treat a patient with chronic hepatitis B is somewhat more straightforward than is the case for hepatitis C.[39] The serologic tests available for hepatitis B are more readily understood and the viral replicative status of the patient can be better ascertained than with hepatitis C. In addition, the risk of hepatoma development with hepatitis B is a major point favoring an attempt at virus eradication independent of the histologic status of the liver disease. Thus, even in those patients with chronic hepatitis B who are asymptomatic with minimal disease activity on liver biopsy, there is still an indication to consider antiviral therapy. Although a number of more subjective factors still must be considered in the decision to initiate interferon therapy, the impetus to initiate therapy generally is stronger than in those with hepatitis C.

As a useful starting point, albeit somewhat of an overgeneralization, in understanding the response of hepatitis B to antiviral therapy, chronic hepatitis B has been categorized into 2 phases: replicative and nonreplicative. When hepatitis B e antigen (HBeAg) or HBV DNA, or both, are present in the serum, the disease is considered to be in the replicative phase. When these markers are absent, the disease is in the nonreplicative phase. Interferon therapy is most effective in those patients with hepatitis B in the replicative phase.

Some authorities[1] propose that chronic hepatitis B may be better viewed as having three phases:

1. An early high replicative phase
2. A low replicative phase characterized by loss of serologic markers of HBV replication except HBV DNA
3. A nonreplicative phase characterized by loss of all markers of HBV replication, including HBV DNA

These types of classifications are clinically useful in deciding whether interferon therapy is potentially worthwhile, although not all patients can be easily categorized into one phase. For example, children with chronic hepatitis B can often have minimal liver inflammation and minimal or no elevation in serum aminotransferases, yet have high levels of HBV DNA in the serum. They generally do not respond as well to interferon therapy. Other combinations of serologic findings are encountered that may be difficult to readily categorize into high or low replicative phases, and clinical judgment is necessary in deciding whether to proceed with interferon therapy in such cases.

Using these concepts about replication as a framework, the most suitable candidates for interferon therapy are those with serum HBsAg, HBeAg or HBV DNA, and elevated serum aminotransferases. The aim of therapy ideally is to achieve loss of HBV DNA, seroconversion from HBeAg to anti-HBe, and ultimately, seroconversion from HBsAg to anti-HBs. The latter, if it occurs at all, may only occur months or even years after a course of interferon therapy is finished. Accompanying these serologic changes are a normalization of serum transaminases and resolution of liver inflammation.

In clinical trials,[40,41] factors that have been shown to favor a positive response to interferon therapy are:

1. Initial high levels of serum transaminases (>100 units/ml)
2. Initial lower levels of serum HBV DNA (<100 pg/ml)

3. Active liver inflammation on liver biopsy
4. Female gender
5. Acquisition of disease in adulthood
6. Short duration of disease

Factors 1 to 3 are probably interrelated in that they are indicative of a preexisting immune response to HBV by host defenses. Factors 5 and 6 are probably related to lack of progression of HBV disease to a low or nonreplicative phase.

Clinical features that have been shown to favor an unsatisfactory response to interferon therapy are:

1. Initial normal or only mildly elevated levels of serum transaminases
2. Initial high levels of HBV DNA
3. Minimal or no liver inflammation on liver biopsy
4. Chinese ethnicity
5. HIV infection
6. Concomitant HDV infection
7. Acquisition of disease at birth or in childhood
8. Immunosuppressed patients

The use of a short tapering course of corticosteroids prior to initiation of interferon therapy has been suggested as a means of potentially increasing the viral replicative rate and, hence, the subsequent response to interferon. A significant concern, though, has been that the withdrawal of steroids after a short course can lead to a flare in hepatitis activity, which can sometimes be quite severe, particularly in those with advanced liver disease. Studies using this approach have yielded mixed results. It appears that steroid pretreatment most benefits patients who initially have low or normal levels of serum aminotransferases, that is, those in whom the immune system was not already active against HBV-infected hepatocytes. There remains considerable controversy about the role, if any, of steroids before initiation of interferon therapy. For patients with active liver inflammation, this regimen is not necessary. For those without active inflammation, most authorities would not favor pretreatment with steroids.

Administration of Interferon for Chronic Hepatitis B

The recommended regimen for hepatitis B is 5 million units of interferon alfa-2b subcutaneously or intramuscularly daily. Some authorities favor the use of 10 million units three times a week. The duration of treatment varies from 4 to 6 months, depending on whether seroconversion occurs.

Results of Interferon Alfa-2b Therapy for Chronic Hepatitis B

Approximately 40% of patients with chronic hepatitis B achieve a response to interferon therapy. Patients in the typical replicative phase of the disease may achieve a somewhat higher response rate.

The benefits of interferon therapy for chronic hepatitis B were definitively demonstrated in a large, multicenter study in the United States reported in 1988.[41] In this study 169 patients with compensated chronic hepatitis B with at least some elevation of serum ALT were randomized to one of four groups:

1. Prednisone for 6 weeks followed by 5 million units interferon alfa-2b for 16 weeks
2. Placebo followed by 5 million units interferon alfa-2b for 16 weeks
3. Placebo followed by 1 million units interferon alfa-2b for 16 weeks
4. No treatment

Of the group who received 5 million units interferon alone, 37% achieved a loss of HBeAg and HBV DNA versus only 17% of those receiving 1 million units interferon (not different from control subjects) and 7% of untreated control subjects. In the group receiving pretreatment with prednisone, 36% cleared HBeAg and HBV DNA. In the majority of responders serum transaminase levels were normal, and approximately 30% lost serum HBsAg early on. A significant number of patients may lose serum HBsAg over the subsequent several years following a course of interferon therapy.[42,43]

Relapses are not as common after interferon therapy for hepatitis B as for hepatitis C; approximately 5% to 10% of patients may exhibit a relapse.

Side Effects of Interferon Therapy

Side effects of interferon therapy[44] are frequent, although generally mild to moderate in severity. Severe side effects, those requiring discontinuation of therapy, occur in less than 5% of patients. Side effects are generally dose related but not always. The great majority of side effects respond to a decrease in the dosage of the drug, although it is actually not necessary to decrease the dose in the majority of patients experiencing adverse effects. Empiric symptomatic therapy can ameliorate many of the side effects.

The most common side effects of interferon therapy are generally described as "flulike" and include malaise, fatigue, fever, headache, arthralgias, and myalgias. Almost all patients experience one or more of these symptoms. The severity varies from patient to patient, ranging from quite mild to severely debilitating, sometimes necessitating time off from work. The symptoms usually respond to treatment with analgesics such as acetaminophen. These flulike symptoms are most noticeable at the start of therapy, and most patients gradually develop a tolerance to these side effects within 2 to 4 weeks. In those patients who experience severe constitutional symptoms that are not responsive to symptomatic therapy, the dose may have to be decreased temporarily until the symptoms remit, at which time an attempt can be made to increase the drug dosage.

Gastrointestinal side effects include diarrhea, anorexia, and nausea. Some patients experience a burning, itching, or an inflammatory reaction at the site of injection of the drug; this can be empirically treated with topical hydrocortisone cream and by alternating sites of injection. Another side effect is alopecia, which usually becomes apparent after several months of therapy. The alopecia may resolve after discontinuation of therapy, but there have been reports of progression of male pattern baldness that has not resolved after discontinuation of therapy.

Various troublesome neuro-psychiatric side effects can occur that will necessitate lowering the dose or even discontinuing the drug entirely: depression, impaired orientation or concentration, irritability, somnolence, insomnia, and anxiety. Patients complaining of such symptoms during therapy should be monitored more closely than usual, and if the symptoms are interfering with their lifestyle, the dosage must be decreased.

Among the potentially more serious side effects are cytopenias due to interferon's myelosuppressive effects; anemia, leukopenia, or thrombocytopenia can be seen. Generally, the myelosuppression is mild, although occasionally it may be severe enough to warrant a decrease in dosage or even discontinuation of the drug. Neutropenia is the most frequently experienced of the cytopenias and is seen in approximately 35% of patients. Bacterial infections, particularly sinusitis, bronchitis, and urinary tract infections, but also more serious ones, infrequently occur in patients treated with interferon. Anemia is seen in approximately 15% of patients, and thrombocytopenia in about 10%. Clinically overt bleeding, such as epistaxis or gingival bleeding, occurs very uncommonly (approximately 2% incidence). Patients must be monitored with a complete blood count and platelet count periodically during treatment, particularly during the first several weeks after starting therapy. Cell counts return to baseline within a short time after discontinuing treatment.

In about 1% of patients, thyroid dysfunction can occur in association with interferon therapy.[45] Either hyperthyroidism or hypothyroidism may develop. The precise mechanism is unknown, although an autoimmune mechanism has been implicated in some cases. It appears judicious to monitor thyroid-stimulating hormone levels every 3 months or so during interferon therapy.

As noted earlier, patients with presumed hepatitis C who experience an exacerbation of liver disease during treatment with interferon should undergo a careful examination for autoimmune hepatitis.

REFERENCES

1. Davis GL. Chronic hepatitis. In: Kaplowitz N, ed. *Liver and Biliary Diseases.* Baltimore, Md: Williams & Wilkins; 1992:289–299.
2. Choo QL, Kuo G, Weiner AJ, Overby LR, Bradley DW, Houghton M. Isolation of a cDNA clone derived from a blood-borne non-A, non-B viral hepatitis genome. *Science.* 1989;244:359–362.
3. Kuo G, Choo QL, Alter HJ, et al. An assay of circulating antibodies to a major etiologic virus of human non-A, non-B hepatitis. *Science.* 1989;244:362–364.
4. Weiland O, Schvarcz R. Hepatitis C: virology, epidemiology, clinical course, and treatment. *Scand J Gastroenterol.* 1992;27:337–342.
5. Esteban JI, Genesca J, Alter HJ. Hepatitis C: molecular biology, pathogenesis, epidemiology, clinical features, and prevention. In: Boyer JL, Ockner RK, eds. *Progress in Liver Diseases, X.* Philadelphia, Pa: WB Saunders Co; 1992:253–282.
6. Houghton M, Weiner A, Han J, Kuo G, Choo QL. Molecular biology of the hepatitis C virus: implications for diagnosis, development and control of viral disease. *Hepatology.* 1991;14:381–388.
7. Resnick RH, Koff R. Hepatitis C–related hepatocellular carcinoma: prevalence and significance. *Arch Intern Med.* 1993;153:1672–1677.
8. Jeffers LJ, Hasan F, De Medina M, et al. Prevalence of antibodies to hepatitis C virus among patients with cryptogenic chronic hepatitis and cirrhosis. *Hepatology.* 1992;15:187–190.
9. DiBisceglie AM, Goodman ZD, Ishak KG, Hoofnagle JH, Melpolder JJ, Alter HJ. Long-term clinical and histopathological follow-up of chronic posttransfusion hepatitis. *Hepatology.* 1992;14:969–974.
10. Scheuer PJ, Ashrafzadeh P, Sherlock S, Brown D, Dusheiko GM. The pathology of hepatitis C. *Hepatology.* 1992;15:567–571.
11. Bach N, Thung SN, Schaffner F. The histologic features of chronic hepatitis C and autoimmune chronic hepatitis: a comparative analysis. *Hepatology.* 1992;15:572–577.
12. Czaja AJ. Chronic active hepatitis: the challenge for a new nomenclature. *Ann Intern Med.* 1993;119:510–517.
13. Sugitani M, Inchaupse G, Shindo M, Prince AM. Sensitivity of serological assays to identify blood donors with hepatitis C viraemia. *Lancet.* 1992;339:1018–1019.

14. Van Der Poel CL, Cuypers HTM, Reesink HW, et al. Confirmation of hepatitis C virus infection by new four-antigen recombinant immunoblot assay. *Lancet.* 1991; 337:317–319.
15. Alter HJ. New kit on the block: evaluation of second-generation assays for detection of antibody to hepatitis C virus. *Hepatology.* 1992;15:350–353.
16. Aach RD, Stevens CE, Hollinger FB, et al. Hepatitis C virus infection in post-transfusion hepatitis: an analysis with first- and second-generation assays. *N Engl J Med.* 1991;325:1325–1329.
17. Kato N, Yokosuka O, Hosoda K, Ito Y, Ohto M, Omata M. Quantification of hepatitis C virus by competitive reverse transcription-polymerase chain reaction: increase of the virus in advanced liver disease. *Hepatology.* 1993; 18:16–20.
18. Cristiano K, DiBesceglie AM, Hoofnagle JH, Feinstone SM. Hepatitis C viral RNA in serum of patients with chronic non-A, non-B hepatitis: detection by the polymerase chain reaction using multiple primer sets. *Hepatology.* 1991;14:51–55.
19. Czaja AJ, Taswell HF, Rakela J, Schimek CM. Frequency and significance of antibody to hepatitis C virus in severe corticosteroid-treated autoimmune chronic active hepatitis. *Mayo Clin Proc.* 1991;66:572–582.
20. Mitchel LS, Jeffers LJ, Reddy KR, et al. Detection of hepatitis C virus antibody by first and second generation assays and polymerase chain reaction in patients with autoimmune chronic active hepatitis types I, II, and III. *Am J Gastroenterol.* 1993;88:1027–1034.
21. Nishiguchi S, Kuroki T, Ueda T, et al. Detection of hepatitis C virus antibody in the absence of viral RNA in patients with autoimmune hepatitis. *Ann Intern Med.* 1992;116:21–25.
22. Davis GL. Hepatitis C antibody in patients with chronic autoimmune hepatitis: pitfalls in diagnosis and implications for treatment. *Mayo Clin Proc.* 1991;66:647–650.
23. Black M. Alpha-interferon treatment of chronic hepatitis C: need for accurate diagnosis in selecting patients. *Ann Intern Med.* 1992;116:86–87.
24. Katkov WN, Dienstag JL. Prevention and therapy of viral hepatitis. *Semin Liver Dis.* 1991;11:165–174.
25. Perillo RP. Antiviral agents in the treatment of chronic viral hepatitis. In: Boyer JL, Ockner RK, eds. *Progress in Liver Diseases, X.* Philadelphia, Pa: WB Saunders Co; 1992:283–309.
26. Peters M. Mechanisms of action of interferons. *Semin Liver Dis.* 1989;9:235–239.
27. Iino S, Hino K, Kuroki T, Suzuki H, Yamamoto S. Treatment of chronic hepatitis C with high-dose interferon a-2b. *Dig Dis Sci.* 1993;38(4):612–618.
28. Bosch O, Tapia L, Quiroga JA, Carreno V. An escalating dose regimen of recombinant interferon-alpha 2A in the treatment of chronic hepatitis C. *J Hepatol.* 1993;17: 146–149.
29. Alberti A, Chemello L, Diodati G, et al. Treatment of chronic hepatitis C with different regimens of interferon alpha-2. *Hepatology.* 1992;16(?):75A. Abstract.
30. Davis GL, Balart LA, Schiff ER, et al. Treatment of chronic hepatitis C with recombinant interferon alfa: a multicenter randomized controlled trial. *N Engl J Med.* 1989;321:1501–1506.
31. Douglas DD, Rakela J, Ju Lin H, et al. Randomized controlled trial of recombinant alpha-2a-interferon for chronic hepatitis C. *Dig Dis Sci.* 1993;38(4):601–607.
32. Di Besceglie AM, Martin P, Kassianides C, et al. Recombinant interferon alfa therapy for chronic hepatitis C: a randomized, double-blind, placebo-controlled trial. *N Engl J Med.* 1989;321(22):1506–1510.
33. Marcellin P, Boyer N, Giostra E, et al. Recombinant human a-interferon in patients with chronic non-A, non-B hepatitis: a multicenter randomized controlled trial from France. *Hepatology.* 1991;13:393–397.
34. Tine F, Magrin S, Craxi A, Pagliaro L. Interferon for non-A, non-B chronic hepatitis: a meta-analysis of randomised clinical trials. *J Hepatol.* 1991;13:192–199.
35. Magrin S, Craxi A, Fabiano C, et al. Serum hepatitis C virus (HCV)-RNA and response to alpha-interferon in anti-HCV positive chronic hepatitis. *J Med Virol.* 1992; 38:200–206.
36. Hagiwara H, Hayashi N, Mita E, et al. Quantitative analysis of hepatitis C virus RNA in serum during interferon alpha therapy. *Gastroenterology.* 1993;104:877–883.
37. Shindo M, DiBisceglie AM, Hoofnagle JH. Long-term follow-up of patients with chronic hepatitis C treated with a-interferon. *Hepatology.* 1992;15(6):1013–1016.
38. Shindo M, DiBisceglie AM, Cheung L, et al. Decrease in serum hepatitis C viral RNA during alpha-interferon therapy for chronic hepatitis C. *Ann Intern Med.* 1991; 115:700–704.
39. Hoofnagle JH. a-Interferon therapy of chronic hepatitis B: current status and recommendations. *J Hepatol.* 1990; 11:S100–107.
40. Hoofnagle JH, Peters M, Mullen KD, et al. Randomized, controlled trial of recombinant human a-interferon in patients with chronic hepatitis B. *Gastroenterology.* 1988;95:1318–1325.
41. Perillo RP, Schiff ER, Davis GL, et al. A randomized, controlled trial of interferon alfa-2b alone and after prednisone withdrawal in the treatment of chronic hepatitis B. *N Engl J Med.* 1990;323:295–301.
42. Korenman J, Baker B, Waggoner J, Everhart JE, DiBisceglie AM, Hoofnagle JH. Long term remission of chronic hepatitis B after alpha-interferon therapy. *Ann Intern Med.* 1991;114:629–634.
43. Perillo RP, Brunt EM. Hepatic histologic and immunochemical changes in chronic hepatitis B after prolonged clearance of hepatitis B e antigen and hepatitis B surface antigen. *Ann Intern Med.* 1991;115:113–115.
44. Renault PF, Hoofnagle JH. Side effects of alpha interferon. *Semin Liver Dis.* 1989;9:273–277.
45. Lisker-Melamn M, DiBesceglie AM, Usala SJ, Weintraub B, Murray LM, Hoofnagle JH. Development of thyroid disease during therapy of chronic viral hepatitis with interferon alfa. *Gastroenterology.* 1992;102:2155–2160.

97
Fulminant Hepatic Failure

GERALD Y. MINUK and PERRY R. GRAY

Fulminant hepatic failure (FHF) is a medical emergency that requires an extensive understanding of hepatic physiology and pathophysiology. Although patients with FHF are appropriately managed in an intensive care unit by intensivists, the responsibility often falls to the consulting gastroenterologist or hepatologist to direct the investigations and management of these cases. It is also often the responsibility of the gastroenterologist or hepatologist to determine which patients are candidates for liver transplantation and when that procedure should be offered. This chapter reviews various aspects of managing FHF patients and the factors to be considered in making decisions regarding transplantation.

DEFINITION

The classic definition of FHF describes *reversible hepatic failure occurring in the absence of preexisting liver disease, complicated by encephalopathy or coma of stage 3 or 4 severity within 8 weeks of the clinical onset of acute hepatitis.* Although this definition has been useful for many years, recent revelations challenge the validity of certain aspects of it and in so doing establish the need to develop a more accurate definition of the condition as we presently understand it. For example, the classic definition stipulates that hepatic encephalopathy or coma be present. Yet recent data indicate that many FHF patients with decreased levels of consciousness may have cerebral edema rather than hepatic encephalopathy or coma or perhaps a combination of the two. Another problem concerns the issue of underlying liver disease. We now know that all components of the syndrome can occur in patients with preexisting liver disease. Moreover, the natural history of FHF in patients with preexisting liver disease is similar to that in patients without preexisting liver disease. A useful distinguishing feature of patients with chronic liver disease who develop superimposed FHF from patients with chronic liver disease who are undergoing rapid deteriorations in their underlying disorder is the presence or absence of cerebral edema, often being present in the former and absent in the latter group of patients. Finally, the classic definition invokes a time constraint that is unnecessarily rigid. Many patients will not manifest the neurologic abnormalities associated with FHF for 8 to 12 weeks following the onset of acute hepatitis. As a result of these concerns, it would be appropriate to broaden the definition of FHF to read *acute reversible hepatic failure associated with hepatic encephalopathy (coma) or cerebral edema or both in a patient without preexisting liver disease or cerebral edema in a patient with preexisting liver disease.* No time constraints need be applied.

ETIOLOGY

More than 30 distinct causes of FHF have been described in the medical literature (Table 97–1). For diagnostic purposes these causes can be subdivided into infectious agents, drug or toxin exposure, vascular, immunologic, neoplastic, and miscellaneous. From a prevalence point of view, viral hepatitis and acetaminophen overdoses are the most common causes worldwide. Although such classifications are useful for diagnostic and epidemiologic purposes, from a management point of view, causes of FHF are best divided into those in which specific treatment can be offered and those in which only nonspecific management is available. Unfortunately, the former list is relatively short. It consists of acetaminophen toxicity, mushroom poisoning, fatty liver of pregnancy, passive congestion of the liver, Wilson's disease, autoimmune chronic active hepatitis, and perhaps herpes simplex virus infections of the liver. Because specific antidotes are not available for drug-induced FHF, this entity has not been included. However, withdrawal

TABLE 97–1. CAUSES OF FULMINANT HEPATIC FAILURE

Infectious Causes
Common Causes
Viral hepatitis A, B, D, E
Non-A, non-B (?C) hepatitis

Rare Causes
Cytomegalovirus
Epstein-Barr virus
Herpes simplex virus
Paramyxovirus (syncytial giant cell hepatitis)

Metabolic Causes
Acute fatty liver of pregnancy
Reye's syndrome

Drugs or Chemical Exposure
Carbon tetrachloride
Amanita phalloides mushroom poisoning
Acetaminophen overdose
Tetracycline
Halothane
Valproate sodium
Isoniazid
Methyldopa
Monoamine oxidase inhibitors
Yellow phosphorus
Nonsteroidal antiinflammatory drugs

Ischemic or Hypoxic Causes
Hepatic arterial or venous occlusion
Shock
Hyperthermia
Primary graft nonfunction following liver transplantation

Disorders Presenting as Fulminant Hepatic Failure with Histologic Evidence of Chronic Liver Disease
Wilson's disease
Massive malignant infiltration of the liver
Liver failure following jejunoileal bypass
Chronic active hepatitis
Chronic hepatitis B with reactivation or delta superinfection
Erythropoietic protoporphyria

TABLE 97–2. CLINICAL STAGES OF ALTERED LEVELS OF CONSCIOUSNESS

Stage 1	Confused; altered mood or behavior; psychometric defects
Stage 2	Drowsy; inappropriate behavior
Stage 3	Stuporous but speaking and obeying simple commands; inarticulate speech; marked confusion
Stage 4	Coma

On physical examination, diastolic hypotension, tachycardia, tachypnea, fever, jaundice, and occasionally a reduced liver span are evident. By definition, hepatic encephalopathy or coma must be present, but as mentioned earlier, in some patients cerebral edema is of more pathophysiologic importance. Thus, the central neurologic findings should be described as altered levels of consciousness without ascribing an underlying mechanism. The principal components of the various stages of altered levels of consciousness are listed in Table 97–2.

Laboratory results commonly reveal elevated white blood cell counts, serum aminotransferase values, and total and direct bilirubin levels, prolonged prothrombin times, and normal albumin levels. Hypoglycemia and an initial respiratory alkalosis that gives way to metabolic acidosis are also present. In more protracted cases, ascites and renal failure exist.

VIRAL HEPATITIS

With the possible exception of North American variants of the hepatitis C virus (HCV), all hepatotropic viruses have been implicated in causing FHF. The incidence of viral-induced FHF varies from virus to virus. For hepatitis A virus (HAV), 0.1% to 0.4% of infections result in FHF, with the elderly being at highest risk. For hepatitis B virus (HBV), 1% to 3% of acute HBV infections progress to FHF. However, this figure is likely an overestimate in that in certain parts of the world as many as one third of cases represent coinfections or superinfections with HDV. In addition, exacerbations of chronic HBV and acute infection with mutant forms of HBV also contribute to the figure previously ascribed to the wild virus. HEV, HGV (a recently described paramyxolike virus), cytomegalovirus (CMV), Epstein-Barr virus (EBV), and herpes simplex virus (HSV) 1, 2, and 6 rarely cause FHF in the immune competent or nonpregnant host. For

of all nonessential drugs, particularly in FHF patients with rash, fever, and eosinophilia, is mandatory.

CLINICAL FEATURES AND DIAGNOSES

GENERAL

The most common presentation of FHF is that of a perfectly healthy individual who over the course of 1 to 2 weeks develops nausea and general malaise followed by progressive jaundice, a change in the level of consciousness, and finally coma. Drug overdoses and septicemia are often considered in the initial differential diagnosis.

reasons that remain unclear, HEV infections in pregnant women may result in mortality as high as 20%.

A history of sexual promiscuity, parenteral drug abuse, recent return from developing nations, or epidemics of hepatitis within the community are suggestive of viral hepatitis. However, the diagnosis cannot be established with confidence in the absence of serologic testing. For HAV, positive immunoglobulin M (IgM) anti-HAV test results are required. An IgM antibody to hepatitis B core antigen (anti-HBc) is the test of choice for HBV, as the hepatitis B surface antigen (HBsAg) has already cleared in 10% to 50% of FHF cases by the time of onset of neurologic features. Similarly, HBV DNA testing by slot-blot or solubilization assays can be misleading, as the majority of patients have negative results at the time of presentation, presumably because of prompt clearance by the immune system of the invading virus. Because many apparent HBV-induced cases of FHF are associated with concurrent HDV infections, anti-HDV serology should be obtained in all IgM anti-HBc or HBsAg-positive FHF patients. Presently, for FHF patients outside North America, HCV RNA testing (if available) or positive anti-HCV serology test results (present in a minority of cases) help to establish a diagnosis of HCV-induced FHF. Serologic testing for antibody to HEV (anti-HEV) is available in a limited number of centers and should be obtained in undiagnosed FHF patients who have recently returned from trips to developing nations. Specific serologic tests for HGV have not yet been developed, but the diagnosis is suggested by the presence of peripheral eosinophilia, multinucleated giant cells on liver biopsy, and paramyxo-like viral particles on electron microscopy of the liver.

ACETAMINOPHEN-INDUCED HEPATITIS

Acetaminophen is an antipyretic analgesic metabolized by the cytochrome P-450 system of the liver to N-acetyl-p-benzoquinoneimine, which is an unstable toxic metabolite that is quickly conjugated by hepatic glutathione stores and thereby rendered nontoxic. When acetaminophen is taken in excess ($>$10 g/d) or in smaller amounts ($>$6 g/d) but in the presence of cytochrome P-450 inducers such as phenobarbital, phenytoin (Dilantin), rifampin, or alcohol or during periods of starvation, glutathione stores are rapidly depleted and cytoxicity ensues. The diagnosis of acetaminophen toxicity is usually apparent after the history or blood acetaminophen level becomes available. Acetaminophen is also nephrotoxic, and therefore early renal failure in a patient presenting with FHF should increase the index of suspicion for this diagnosis.

MUSHROOM POISONING

Amanita phalloides is a wild mushroom found in Europe and parts of North America that produces a toxin with potent muscarinic properties resulting in excessive sweating, vomiting, and diarrhea. These effects frequently lead to questioning about recent field trips and wild mushroom ingestion, which helps to establish the diagnosis. A bioassay for the toxin is available but difficult to obtain within the time frame of FHF.

FATTY LIVER OF PREGNANCY

Fatty liver of pregnancy, which may result from a fatty acid oxidation defect in the fetus, typically occurs in the third trimester and is often associated with nausea, vomiting, fever, epigastric pain, and features of preeclampsia or eclampsia. Hemolysis and thrombocytopenia may also be present. An ultrasound or computed tomographic (CT) scan of the liver usually confirms the presence of fatty infiltration and occasionally demonstrates hepatic infarcts.

PASSIVE CONGESTION

Passive vascular congestion of the liver from pulmonary, cardiac, or vascular causes results in increased hepatic lobar pressures and decreased arterial perfusion of the liver. Ischemic necrosis ensues. Patients with passive congestion of the liver present with right upper quadrant pain, hepatomegaly, tenderness, and if presentation is delayed, ascites. Features of the underlying disorder (cor pulmonale, pericardial tamponade, tricuspid insufficiency) are also evident. A past or family history of hypercoagulable states, use of hormonal therapy, and radiologic evidence of tumor in the right upper quadrant or retroperitoneal area are frequent findings in patients with hepatic vein thrombosis.

WILSON'S DISEASE

Wilson's disease is a congenital disorder in which copper excretion by hepatocytes into the biliary system is impaired. Free intracellular copper accumulates to levels at which vital organelles are damaged. With hepatocyte death, free copper is released into the systemic circulation causing intravascular hemolysis.

The clinical features suggestive of FHF from Wilson's disease include the young age of the patient, evidence of hemolysis, and disproportionately low serum alkaline phosphatase levels. When present, a history of well-controlled Wilson's disease in a patient who has stopped taking his medications or a family history of Wilson's disease or consanguity is useful. Central nervous system involvement with Wilson's disease, being a late feature of the disease, is uncommon in young FHF patients, and therefore Kayser-Fleischer rings may not be present. Serum ceruloplasmin levels are helpful diagnostic indicators if low or normal but can be elevated as an acute phase reactant. Urine and tissue copper levels ultimately establish the diagnosis.

AUTOIMMUNE CHRONIC ACTIVE HEPATITIS

Autoimmune chronic active hepatitis is an immunologically mediated disorder resembling systemic lupus erythematosus. Hence, the majority of patients are young women with a past history of connective tissue problems such as rashes, arthritis, and Raynaud's phenomenon. Leukopenia, thrombocytopenia, hypergammaglobulinemia, hypocomplementemia, and the presence of high titered autoantibodies are also present.

HSV-INDUCED HEPATITIS

Patients with HSV-induced FHF are frequently immunocompromised, pregnant, or elderly. The hepatitis is often one component of a disseminated infection, but it can occur when only the primary source or no source is evident. Therefore, particularly in undiagnosed cases, a complete physical examination including pelvic examination in women with FHF should be performed. Positive viral serologic test results are frequent findings in the general population and can be misleading. Biopsy specimens and scrapings of skin lesions help to support the diagnosis when present. Liver biopsy specimens reveal fatty infiltration, coagulative necrosis, Cowdry type I inclusion bodies, and positive immunoperoxidase staining.

MANAGEMENT

GENERAL MEASURES

The success or failure of managing a patient with FHF depends on the clinician's attention to detail and ability to anticipate hepatic and extrahepatic events. Those responsibilities are more likely to be met if the clinician considers a simple rule of sevens: seven nondiagnostic medical orders to be entered into the chart and seven lines, tubes, and catheters to be inserted into the patient.

Medical Record

Admittance to the Intensive Care Unit

A practical rule of thumb suggests that FHF patients with stage 1 altered level of consciousness be admitted to the hospital. Stage 2 patients should be admitted to the intensive care unit. Stage 3 patients should be prepared (including evacuation if necessary) for transplantation, and stage 4 patients should be managed in the intensive care unit but not prepared for transplantation.

Vital Signs

Vital signs should be monitored every 1 to 4 hours, depending on the patient's general status. Monitoring should include blood pressure, pulse, respiratory rate, temperature, and mental status. Intakes and outputs should also be recorded on a regular basis because of the increased risk of fluid overload. Elevation of the head of the bed to 20 degrees is suggested to limit increases in intracranial pressure and decrease the risk of reflux aspiration.

Minimum Physical Examinations

Tactile stimuli increase intracranial pressure. As a result, following the initial complete evaluation, physical examinations should be limited to those staff directly involved in the patient's care.

Baseline Assessments (Hepatic and Neurologic)

In isolation, liver enzyme tests (alanine and aspartate aminotransferases, alkaline phosphatase, and c-glutamyl transpeptidase) are not necessarily indicative of an improvement or deterioration of liver status. However, in the presence of unassisted (nontransfusion-related), stable, or improving liver function tests (bilirubins and prothrombin times), a decline in liver enzyme test results often reflects hepatic recovery. On the other hand, in the presence of deteriorating liver function test results, a decline in liver enzyme test results often reflects a complete loss of viable hepatic tissue. Both liver enzyme and function tests need not be repeated more than once or twice daily.

Once the FHF patient is stabilized, an image

of the patient's hepatobiliary system should be obtained by either ultrasound (with Doppler flow studies of all three major vessels: portal vein, hepatic artery, and hepatic vein) or CT scan. Neurologic status should be documented by number connection tests (stages 1 or 2), electroencephalogram (EEG), and CT scan.

Metabolic Studies (Glucose, Electrolytes, and Acid-Base Status)

Approximately 40% of FHF patients become hypoglycemic because of a combination of decreased hepatic glycogenolysis or gluconeogenesis and increased circulating insulin levels. Electrolyte abnormalities are also common, particularly hypokalemia and hyponatremia. The latter, if it developed rapidly, can lead to central pontine myelinolysis. The initial acid-base disturbance is a respiratory alkalosis that gives way to a lactic acid-induced metabolic acidosis. Glucose, electrolyte, and acid-base status should be checked every 2 to 12 hours.

Sepsis Surveillance

All patients should undergo a complete "septic workup" on admission to the intensive care unit. Both bacterial and fungal infections occur in the majority of FHF patients and should be suspected when the patient's status suddenly deteriorates. The clinical, hemodynamic, and hematologic features of sepsis are similar to those that occur in FHF, and therefore a high index of suspicion is required. Blood cultures for fungi are particularly important when serum creatinine levels rise for no apparent reason. Daily blood cultures for bacteria and fungi are mandatory. Additional cultures or radiologic studies or both should be performed if a focus of infection is suspected or if the patient is being evaluated for liver transplantation.

Medications

The only standing order for medication should be antacids. H_2-receptor antagonists, or proton pump inhibitors in sufficient doses and frequency to ensure that gastric pH remains above 5, thereby decreasing the risk of gastrointestinal tract bleeding.

Lines, Tubes, and Catheters

Intravenous Catheters

The initial intravenous solution should be 10% dextrose in water with supplemental KCl given as a constant infusion not to exceed 3 L/d. If the patient's clinical status or blood glucose monitoring indicates hypoglycemia (less than 3.5 mmol/L), 50 ml of 50% dextrose in water should be administered immediately and the rate of the 10% dextrose in water infusion increased thereafter. Constant infusions of high-glucose-containing solutions in the absence of hypoglycemia should be avoided, as they may interfere with hepatic regenerative activity.

Nasogastric Tube

Nasogastric tubes are inserted to decrease the risk of aspiration and monitor gastric acid pH levels.

Urinary Catheter

A urinary catheter is required for monitoring daily outputs.

Arterial Lines

Although there is a risk of continued bleeding at the site, the important information derived from arterial lines outweighs that risk, and these lines should be inserted.

Endotracheal Tubes

When required, endotracheal tubes are inserted to provide ventilatory assistance and to decrease the risk of aspiration.

Central Venous Catheter or Swan-Ganz Catheter

Central pressures are especially useful in FHF patients with cardiac or renal failure or signs of cerebral edema.

Intracranial Pressure Monitors

Under plasma or platelet coverage, epidural or subdural transducers can be safely inserted into patients with severe coagulopathies. The important diagnostic and prognostic data they provide have led to their frequent use in patients with stage 3 or 4 altered levels of consciousness.

SPECIFIC MEASURES

The following are treatment guidelines for causes of FHF in which specific therapy directed toward the underlying cause is available and should be applied.

Acetaminophen-Induced Liver Failure

N-acetylcysteine should be administered by intravenous infusion at a dose of 150 mg/kg body weight in 200 ml of 5% dextrose over 15 minutes, followed by 50 mg/kg in 1 L over 16 hours and continued until the patient is mentally alert. Although the drug is most effective when given within the first 12 to 18 hours of the overdose, it should still be administered when patients present at later time periods.

Mushroom Poisoning

Early hemoperfusion to remove the toxin is indicated. Various antidotes including thioctic acid (a-lipoic acid), penicillin, and silibinin have also been advocated.

Fatty Liver of Pregnancy

Spontaneous or induced delivery of the fetus by the vaginal route, if the mother and fetus are stable, or by cesarean section, if otherwise, is recommended.

Passive Congestion

Uncontrolled trials in small numbers of patients with acute hepatic vein thrombosis suggest that early thrombolytic therapy or portal-systemic shunts and treatment of the underlying hypercoagulable state may avert the need for liver transplantation.

Wilson's Disease

As a temporizing measure until a liver transplant can be arranged or until the patient clinically recovers, penicillamine (1 to 2 g daily), hemodialysis, and two-volume plasmapheresis should be offered. Responders require long-term maintenance penicillamine therapy.

Chronic Active Hepatitis

Chronic active hepatitis should be treated with the equivalent of 60 mg of prednisone daily by intravenous infusion. In patients who continue to deteriorate, the corticosteroids should be discontinued while awaiting a liver transplant. In those who stabilize or show signs of improvement, the steroids should be continued until the patient is mentally alert. Responders who do not undergo transplantation require long-term maintenance immunosuppressive therapy.

Herpes Hepatitis

When the diagnosis is established or considered probable, acyclovir (30 mg/kg/d) by intravenous infusion should be administered.

CYTOPROTECTION

There are four aspects of cytoprotective therapy for FHF:

1. Protect hepatocytes from further injury related to the underlying cause
2. Protect hepatocytes from the complications of FHF
3. Avoid iatrogenic-induced liver injury
4. Maintain hepatocyte structural and functional integrity

The underlying cause of hepatic injury is still active in many FHF patients at the time of hospitalization. Thus, the initial step is to identify and remove or negate that cause where possible (see causes of FHF for specific therapy available).

Hypotension, hypoxemia, and hypoglycemia are complications of FHF that jeopardize hepatocyte survival. As a result, mean arterial pressures should be maintained at levels compatible with optimal hepatic perfusion (100 mm Hg). Arterial oxygen content should be checked and corrected if low. Hemoglobin levels, reflecting the blood's oxygen-carrying capacity, should be normalized with packed cells as required. Finally, hypoglycemia should be avoided and treated promptly when present.

Because the kinetics of many drugs are altered and the ability to withstand even minor hepatic insults is limited in FHF, it is imperative to avoid iatrogenic-induced injury by closely monitoring drug levels and limiting the use of drugs to only those that are essential for patient care. Similarly, the use of blood or blood product transfusions (which could serve as vectors for viral agents or precipitate hypotensive reactions) should be used only when required to maintain normal hemoglobin levels or for hemostasis prior to invasive procedures.

Cytoprotective therapy designed to prevent the release or effect of proinflammatory cytokines such as leukotrienes, procoagulants, tumor necrosis factor, and oxygen free radicals is an area of active research. Preliminary data suggest that the cytoprotective properties of N-acetylcysteine justify its use in the treatment of patients with acetaminophen-induced and non-acetaminophen-induced FHF. However, it should be noted that N-acetylcysteine also increases cardiac output, arterial perfusion pressures, and hepatic oxygen delivery and consumption. Although one controlled clinical trial suggests that patient outcome is improved with such treatment, confirmation of these encouraging results is required.

Based on animal data followed by uncontrolled trials in humans. 16,16-dimethyl prostaglandin E_2 and prostaglandin E_1, respectively, were considered to be promising therapeutic agents for FHF because of their ability to attenuate the effect of cytokines, inhibit platelet aggregation, and perhaps maintain small vessel patency. Unfortunately, recent controlled clinical trials in humans failed to document beneficial effects with these agents unless given very early in the course of FHF. The dosage of prostaglandin E_1 is 0.2 to 0.6 lg/kg/h, administered as a peripheral or central intravenous infusion.

Although the cytoprotective or other properties of corticosteroids have been reported to be effective in animal models of FHF, the results in humans have been discouraging. As a result, corticosteroids are not advocated for use in patients with nonimmunologically mediated forms of FHF.

Regeneration

Most FHF fatalities occur between the period of maximal hepatic injury and restitution of sufficient liver mass to sustain life. The latter process, termed *hepatic regeneration,* has been the subject of extensive research designed to identify mechanisms whereby the liver could be stimulated to regenerate earlier and at a more rapid rate. What has been gleaned from such studies suggests that regenerative activity is impaired in patients with FHF largely because of increased concentrations of circulating growth inhibitors rather than a depletion of growth promotors. Indeed, serum and tissue levels or messenger ribonucleic acid (mRNA) expression of essentially all growth promotors (including hepatocyte growth factor, hepatic stimulator substance, hepatopoietins A and B, and perhaps epidermal growth factor) are significantly increased in FHF, implying that the exogenous administration of these agents is unlikely to be of therapeutic benefit. Early results of studies using these agents (as well as insulin, glucagon, and insulinlike growth factor-II) in animal models of FHF tend to support this pessimistic prediction. To date, much less effort has been expended identifying and designing methods to lower the levels of agents responsible for inhibition of hepatic regeneration. Although transforming growth factor-beta, interleukins 1 and 6, and hepatocyte proliferation inhibitor are presumably some of those inhibitory factors, methods have not yet been developed to limit their production or effect. Fortunately, that is not the case with ammonia, mercaptans, fatty acids, and c-aminobutyric acid (GABA), which also inhibit hepatic regenerative activity and are present in high concentrations in FHF. Treatment with bowel cleansing agents and the use of enterically active antimicrobials decrease the concentrations of these inhibitors and may thereby enhance regenerative activity. Given their relative safety, the use of bowel cleansing agents and enterically active antimicrobials should be considered in all FHF patients regardless of whether encephalopathy is present.

It is important to note that a critical mass (perhaps 10% to 20%) of hepatocytes must survive for regeneration to proceed. Where that is not the case, transplantation presently represents the only opportunity for survival. Unfortunately, with the possible exception of liver histology obtained by the transjugular route, no test or assay is available that documents whether that critical mass of hepatocytes exists.

SUPPORT SYSTEMS

Despite the obvious importance of developing a system (artificial or otherwise) that would sustain patients with FHF until hepatic regeneration was adequate or transplantation could be performed, progress in this area had been lethally slow. Early attempts at developing support systems included exchange transfusions, cross circulations, plasmapheresis and ultrafiltration, hemodialysis, charcoal and serial resin hemoperfusions with and without prostaglandins, and extracorporeal pig liver perfusions. For various reasons these attempts failed or were found to be ineffective in controlled clinical trials. More recent approaches, yet untested in human trials, include the use of infusions of auxiliary partial heterotopic liver transplants, extracorporeal human allografts (designed as a temporizing measure when the graft is not suitable), liver microsomal enzymes bound to biocompatible carriers, transplantation of hepatocytes by collagen-coated microcarriers, and bioartificial liver support devices. The latter are intriguing devices wherein viable, freshly isolated, or cryopreserved hepatocytes (matrix anchored to allow for greater cell differentiation and function) are placed outside or within hollow, readily perfused cartridges and linked in circuit to the subject's systemic circulation. The cartridges serve to clear both toxins and perform hepatic synthetic functions. Early results in dogs and a limited number of humans suggest that these devices may lower plasma ammonia and bilirubin levels, decrease blood transfusion requirements, improve the level of consciousness, decrease intracranial pressure, enhance renal function, and contribute to normoglycemia. Unlike other extracorporeal devices, they have not been associated with hemolysis, thrombocytopenia, a need for heparinization, and in the case of cryopreserved hepatocytes, maintenance of animal colonies. Whether they decrease mortality or the need for transplantation remains to be determined.

ASSOCIATED CONDITIONS

NUTRITIONAL DEFICIENCIES

The most common initial form of nutritional support provided to patients with FHF is the provision of intravenous dextrose to prevent or treat hypoglycemia. As mentioned earlier, impaired gluconeogenesis, decreased glycogenolysis, and a 10- to 20-fold elevation of insulin levels are the mechanisms proposed for this complication. Mild cases can usually be managed using a 10% dextrose solution (initial flow rates 75 to 100 ml/h), which can be safely administered into a peripheral vein. Blood glucose levels should be checked every hour until stable, then the frequency may be decreased. Any deterioration in mental status should include the possibility of hypoglycemia. A blood sample for glucose determination should be obtained, and a 50-ml bolus of a 50% dextrose solution should be administered intravenously. Dextrose should not be withheld pending laboratory analysis. Asymptomatic patients whose blood glucose level is less than 3.5 mmol/L should receive a 50-ml bolus of 50% dextrose immediately, followed by an increase in the hourly flow rate of the dextrose solution, and blood glucose levels should be measured every hour. Patients with moderate-to-severe FHF frequently require massive doses of intravenous dextrose to maintain euglycemia. Use of a 10% dextrose solutions in these patients could result in flow rates up to 500 ml/h. To avoid problems associated with massive administration of water, a 50% or 70% dextrose solution administered via a central venous catheter titrating the flow rate to maintain blood glucose at 6 to 10 mmol/L can be employed.

High-dose carbohydrate infusions can rapidly deplete thiamine stores, creating an acute thiamine-deficient state with resultant lactic acidosis and distributive (high cardiac output, low systemic vascular resistance) shock. To avoid this complication, thiamine (100 mg intravenously daily for 3 days) should be routinely administered to patients with FHF who have any clinical or biochemical evidence of malnutrition.

Plasma amino acid profiles of patients with FHF differ from those of patients with hepatic encephalopathy and cirrhosis. In FHF all amino acids in plasma are elevated except the branched-chain amino acids (leucine, isoleucine, and valine). In hepatic encephalopathy and cirrhosis, branched-chain amino acids are depressed, but not all the remaining amino acids are elevated. Although aromatic amino acids (phenylalanine, tyrosine, and tryptophan) are elevated in both disorders, the magnitude of elevation is much greater in patients with FHF. Therefore conclusions based on nutritional studies of patients with cirrhosis who are acutely encephalopathic cannot necessarily be applied to patients with FHF.

In forming a nutritional plan for patients with FHF, the route of feeding (enteral versus parenteral), total calories, and relative proportions of proteins, carbohydrates, and lipids are considered. Patients with mild FHF (stage 1 altered level of consciousness) can usually be fed enterally. Concern regarding the possibility of aspiration, reluctance to insert a nasojejunal feeding tube in the presence of coagulopathy, theoretic possibility of toxic metabolite production by intestinal bacteria of enteral protein, and ileus are the most common reasons stated for the preference of the parenteral route in patients with moderate-to-severe FHF (stages 2, 3, and 4). Indirect calorimetry has recently been used to measure energy expenditure in fasting patients with FHF resulting in a mean value of 1.2 kcal/min/1.73 m^2. This figure does not include nutrient-induced thermogenesis or physical activity. In the absence of such data, it would be reasonable to add 10% to 15% to the above-mentioned figure. In patients with severe FHF, massive doses of carbohydrates to maintain euglycemia may exceed calculated energy requirements. In these patients carbohydrate, protein, or lipid administration should not be restricted in an attempt to avoid overfeeding. The input of amino acids into plasma from endogenous protein breakdown in patients with FHF is 12 times greater than normal input from dietary protein. Therefore suppressing catabolism is more important than dietary restriction. Patients with FHF should initially receive 40 to 60 g (0.6 to 0.8 g/kg) of a standard amino acid solution daily. In patients with stage 1 to 3 altered levels of consciousness, the amount of protein is increased every 48 to 72 hours, if the level of consciousness remains stable. Protein intake is not increased in patients with stage 4 disease. Recommendations for the use of branched-chain amino acids in FHF are based on anecdotal case reports of reversing encephalopathy, increased branched-chain amino acid loss in patients requiring frequent dialysis, and suppression of endogenous protein catabolism. Most authors have concluded that the superiority of branched-chain amino acids in FHF remains unproven. As previously stated carbohydrate requirements are titrated to maintain euglycemia; however, a minimal recommended dose for all FHF patients is 300 g/d of dextrose to suppress endogenous protein catabolism. Intravenous lipid preparations are almost exclusively metabolized extrahepatically, and clearance has been shown to be normal in patients with severe liver disease. As a general rule one third of the nonprotein calories should be lipid. This is not advisable in patients requiring massive doses of carbohydrates to maintain euglycemia. In these patients total calories should be calculated from the previously mentioned formula. Calculate the nonprotein calories required and administer one third as lipid; (do not decrease carbohydrate infusion based on this calculation unless blood glucose analysis permits). Critically ill patients with FHF may develop complications that would impair triglyceride clearance. Daily monitoring of triglyceride levels is indicated to ensure clearance. The reference range provided by most laboratories is based on fasting subjects. A single value outside the reference range obtained during continuous lipid infusion is difficult to interpret unless greater than 9 mmol/L, which is associated with a risk of triglyceride-induced pancreatitis. Triglyceride levels less than 9 mmol/L but increasing daily indicate accumulation, and the amount of intravenous lipid infused should be decreased.

CEREBRAL EDEMA

Cerebral edema is the leading cause of death in patients with FHF. The cause of cerebral edema in FHF is unknown. Clinical differentiation from hepatic encephalopathy is virtually impossible. Both disorders may present with a decreased level of consciousness, abnormal posturing (decorticate and decerebrate), and no response to painful stimuli. Papilloedema is rarely observed in patients with FHF and cerebral edema. Patients with decreased levels of consciousness should undergo a CT scan of the head to rule out structural causes (such as intracerebral bleeding). CT scans cannot estimate intracranial pressures. Direct intracranial pressure (ICP) monitoring is the most reliable method available to diagnose cerebral edema.

Although it has yet to be demonstrated that ICP monitors reduce mortality in patients with FHF, studies have reported that the use of ICP monitors is associated with prolonged survival, which is an important factor in patients with FHF who are candidates for liver transplantation. There are various types of ICP monitors: epidural transducers, subdural bolts, intraventricular catheters, and pressure transducers placed in direct contact with brain parenchyma. A recent survey of North American transplant centers demonstrated that the epidural transducer was most commonly used and had the lowest complication rate: 1 infection and 5 hemorrhages (2 fatal) in 160 cases.

The current recommendation regarding the timing of insertion of an ICP monitor is when the patient has reached a stage 3 altered level of consciousness. Prior to insertion, infusion of fresh-frozen plasma, with or without plasmapheresis, to maintain the prothrombin time (PT) within 5 seconds of control value is mandatory. If plasmapheresis is required, measurement of the PT should be delayed until 2 to 4 hours after the procedure because of the anticoagulant effect of citrate in fresh-frozen plasma. Intravenous cryoprecipitate is required in patients with persistently low fibrinogen levels (<100 mg/dl). Platelet transfusion is indicated if the platelet count is less than 75,000/1l.

Measurement of mean arterial pressure (MAP) and ICP allow calculation of cerebral perfusion pressure (CPP) (CPP = MAP − ICP). The goal is to maintain CPP greater than 60 mm Hg and ICP less than 20 mm Hg. Mechanisms to elevate MAP are discussed later in this chapter (see *Cardiorespiratory Complications*). Tactile stimulation, isometric muscle contractions, shivering, coughing, sneezing, psychomotor agitation, and Valsalva's maneuver are factors that can increase intracranial pressure. Treatment of such elevations may require the use of benzodiazepines, narcotics, and if necessary neuromuscular blocking agents, which can be given safely to FHF patients with ICP monitors. Fevers are often unresponsive to antipyretic agents, necessitating the use of cooling blankets. In the patient with severe peripheral vasoconstriction, cooling blankets and other external measures may be ineffective. Irrigation of nasogastric tubes and urinary catheters with cool saline solutions is an effective method of internal cooling. Head elevation of 20 to 30 degrees has been standard medical therapy of cerebral edema in FHF for years. It has recently been reported that elevation of the head more than 20 degrees may increase ICP and lower CPP in some patients with FHF. In patients using an ICP monitor, the effect of head elevation on ICP and CPP can be observed and titrated accordingly. There is no reason to prophylactically hyperventilate or administer mannitol to patients with FHF and a normal ICP. The approach to the patient with an elevated ICP should include the following:

1. Ensuring adequate oxygenation
2. Identification and treatment of hypercapnia
3. Administration of appropriate treatment of hypertension and hypotension
4. Identification and treatment of hypoglycemia
5. Assessment of factors related to sedation and neuromuscular blockers (previously mentioned)
6. Identification and treatment of hyperthermia
7. Ensuring the ICP monitor is properly leveled and functional.

If all these measures fail, then hyperventilation titrated to a P_{CO_2} of 25 to 30 mm Hg should be instituted. Excessive hyperventilation (P_{CO_2} less than 25 mm Hg) may lead to cerebral vasoconstriction and reduced cerebral blood flow. Persistent ICP greater than 20 mm Hg and serum osmolality less than 320 mm/kg should be treated with mannitol (0.3 to 1 g/kg intravenous bolus). Repeated doses of mannitol may be required. Rising serum osmolality or widening of the osmotic gap (>20 mmol/kg) indicates accumulation of mannitol, necessitating dosage reduction or discontinuation. Mannitol does not appear to be as effective in patients with FHF with ICP greater than 80 mm Hg. Mannitol administration was associated with an increase in ICP in 60% of such cases. Mannitol is contraindicated in oliguric renal failure, unless given in combination with hemodialysis (usually 30 minutes prior to dialysis). Mannitol may be given to patients receiving continuous arteriovenous hemofiltration (CAVH) or continuous venoveno hemofiltration (CVVH). Corticosteroids are not effective prophylactic or therapeutic agents in cerebral edema secondary to FHF. Patients failing to respond to mannitol should undergo a CT scan of the head to rule out structural complications. Pentobarbital (3 to 5 mg/kg IV over 15 to 30 minutes, followed by a continuous infusion of 1 to 3 mg/kg/h) is indicated for patients with FHF who are unresponsive to mannitol. Barbiturate therapy is titrated to obtain burst suppression on EEG. Patients receiving barbiturate therapy require continuous arterial pressure monitoring to detect and treat hypotension and ICP monitoring to ensure a CPP greater than 60 mm Hg. It is impossible to clinically distinguish between barbiturate coma and brain death. Complete absence of cerebral circulation on four-vessel cerebral angiography is an absolute confirmation of brain death. A CPP of less than 40 mm Hg for greater than 2 hours is considered a contraindication to transplantation in some centers. In a single patient, cerebral edema has been temporarily controlled using an extracorporeal bioartificial liver support system with porcine hepatocytes until a donor liver was found.

Hepatic Encephalopathy

With the realization that many FHF patients have cerebral edema despite the absence of typical neurologic findings and normal CT scans of the brain, much of what was previously ascribed to hepatic encephalopathy must now be reassessed. For example, it is often stated that in FHF, patients with hepatic encephalopathy may present with signs of increased rather than decreased neurologic activity, including delirium, mania, restlessness, violence, and seizures. Whether such presentations are truly the result of hepatic encephalopathy or manifestations of occult cerebral edema or a combination of the two is now unclear. Similarly, it is now unclear whether the minority of patients who develop "hepatic encephalopathy" prior to the onset of jaundice are truly encephalopathic or have unrecognized cerebral edema that might explain the exceptionally poor outcomes in this subgroup. Nonetheless, what is generally considered to be hepatic encephalopathy (i.e., a progressive decrease in mentation associated with fetor hepaticus or asterixis and hyperammonemia) is found in isolation or combination with cerebral edema in over 70% of patients with FHF. Moreover, the extent of encephalopathy correlates with outcome in that patients with mild encephalopathy have survival rates in excess of 80%, whereas those with severe encephalopathy have survival rates of only 20% to 50%.

The cause of hepatic encephalopathy in FHF remains unclear. Theories that are not mutually exclusive have implicated hyperammonemia, aromatic amino acid–generated false neurotransmitters, mercaptans, fatty acids, GABA, and most recently endogenous benzodiazepines that potentiate GABAergic activity.

Regardless of the cause, treatment of hepatic encephalopathy consists of (1) establishing the diagnosis, (2) searching for and correcting precipitating causes, and (3) generic management of the encephalopathy.

Conditions that can mimic hepatic encephalopathy in the setting of FHF include cerebral edema, intracerebral bleeding, encephalitis, hypoglycemia, hypoxemia, Wilson's disease, and Reye's syndrome. An EEG combined with a plasma ammonia level usually helps to distinguish hepatic encephalopathy from these other conditions, but their possible coexistence must also be considered.

The most common precipitating causes of hepatic encephalopathy are as follows:

1. Prerenal azotemia
2. Injudicious use of sedatives, hypnotics, or centrally acting analgesics
3. Electrolyte abnormalities (hyponatremia, hypokalemia)
4. Infection
5. Gastrointestinal tract bleeding
6. Acid-base disturbances
7. Excess dietary protein

If sedatives are required for agitated patients, a small dose of intravenous midazolam should be used but only when necessary and not as a standing order. The benzodiazepine antagonist, flumazenil, should be readily available if coma is inadvertently precipitated by the midazolam.

Treatment of the encephalopathy is confined to withdrawal of dietary protein and administration of lactulose (oral or via nasogastric tube) at an initial dosage of 30 ml every 8 hours, then titrated to result in two loose bowel movements per day. Rectal administration of lactulose may be associated with an increased risk of lower gastrointestinal tract bleeding, increases in ICP (due to agitation), and less efficacy and is rarely accepted with enthusiasm by the intensive care unit staff. Neomycin should be avoided because of the increased risk of nephrotoxicity and ototoxicity. Alternative antimicrobials for bowel decontamination are one of the fluoroquinolone antibiotics (e.g., ciprofloxacin, 250 to 500 mg twice daily) or metronidazole (200 mg four times daily).

Like many other therapeutic interventions for FHF, flumazenil treatment of nonbenzodiazepine-induced hepatic encephalopathy was associated with early promising results that were not supported in subsequent studies. If flumazenil does have a therapeutic role other than reversing the effects of exogenous benzodiazepines, it is in the treatment of patients with early encephalopathy without cerebral edema. The drug can be given intravenously by repeated 0.2- to 2-mg boluses every 3 to 5 minutes, but beneficial results are transient.

CARDIORESPIRATORY COMPLICATIONS

The pattern of respiratory complications in FHF correlates with the severity of the liver failure. Patients with mild FHF often develop tachypnea. Arterial blood gas analysis usually reveals a respiratory alkalosis with or without a metabolic acidosis. In the patient without preexisting respiratory disease, hypoxemia is mild or absent. As the disease progresses, the level of consciousness deteriorates, and the patient becomes susceptible to aspiration. Aspiration of gastric contents may result in pneumonitis, pneumonia, or the adult respiratory distress syndrome (ARDS). ARDS may also develop in patients with severe FHF without aspiration. Administration of large volumes of 10% dextrose, plasma, and sodium bicarbonate to patients with severe FHF and renal failure can result in high-pressure pulmonary edema. Intrapulmonary hemorrhage occasionally occurs in the presence of a severe coagulopathy in FHF. Pneumonitis, pneumonia, ARDS, high-pressure pulmonary edema, and intrapulmonary hemorrhage may result in hypoxemic respiratory failure. A deep comatose state may lead to respiratory depression, resulting in hypercapnic respiratory failure.

Cardiovascular and hemodynamic complications are frequent in severe FHF. Bradydysrhythmias indicate the terminal phase of FHF or increased ICP. Supraventricular tachycardia, premature ventricular contractions, or atrioventricular conduction defects have also been reported. Significant ST segment elevation without myocardial injury has been reported in a patient with FHF and cerebral edema. The hemodynamic pattern of FHF is identical to septic shock: high cardiac output, low systemic vascular resistance, and arterial hypotension (distributive shock).

The timing of intubation is an important issue in patients with FHF. Indications for intubation are respiratory failure (hypoxemic or hypercapnic), controlled hyperventilation for the management of increased ICP and airway protection (with or without tracheal toilet). Hypoxemia exacerbates cerebral edema and delays hepatic recovery. Arterial PO_2 less than 70 mm Hg on maximal face mask supplementation is an indication for intubation. As previously stated, patients with FHF typically hyperventilate. The presence of a normal PCO_2 level or an acidemic pH level in a somnolent patient with FHF is an ominous sign and should prompt immediate intubation. The benefit of hyperventilation in increased intracranial pressure remains controversial, but the detrimental effect of hypoventilation is undisputed. There are risks and benefits to intubation for airway protection in patients with FHF. The placement of an endotracheal tube provides a continuous noxious stimulus to an encephalopathic patient necessitating sedation, which impairs the neurologic assessment and may delay appropriate treatment. In contrast, failure to place an endotracheal tube, resulting in aspiration pneumonia and uncontrolled sepsis, eliminates the option of a life-saving liver transplant. The presence of an intact gag reflex does not guarantee protection of the airway. If stimulation of the gag reflex completely awakens the somnolent patient, intubation for airway protection is not indicated. Intubation is required for unresponsive or incompletely responsive patients.

The goal of ventilatory management of patients with FHF is to provide adequate oxygenation and carbon dioxide excretion using the least amount of positive pressure. Spontaneously breathing patients have a negative intrathoracic pressure during inspiration and passive expiration, which facilitates venous return from the cerebral and hepatic circulation. Intermittent positive pressure ventilation, continuous positive airway pressure (CPAP), and positive end-expiratory pressure (PEEP) have the opposite effect: elevating ICP and theoretically impairing hepatic circulation. A T-piece circuit allows patients to breathe spontaneously and receive inspired oxygen concentrations of nearly 100%. The principal disadvantage of the T-piece circuit is the lack of ventilatory assistance. Patients must have an intact respiratory drive and be able to maintain their minute ventilation. Patients with high minute ventilatory requirements (>15 L/min) or noncompliant lungs (i.e., ARDS, intrapulmonary hemorrhage, or high-pressure pulmonary edema) may induce anaerobic glycolysis in the respiratory muscles, resulting in lactate production, which is poorly tolerated in FHF. Pressure support ventilation (PSV) assists the respiratory muscles while minimizing the mean positive airway pressure. Respiratory depression, respiratory muscle fatigue, or the requirement of neuromuscular blocking agents are contraindications to PSV. These patients require controlled mandatory ventilation (CMV). For the reasons previously mentioned, the routine use of PEEP should be avoided in patients with FHF. PEEP is indicated in hypoxemia unresponsive to high inspired oxygen concentrations. Inverse ratio ventilation (IRV) and jet ventilators (JETS) are often advocated in patients with hypoxemia unresponsive to 100% oxygen and PEEP. The principal disadvantage of IRV and JETS is the accumulation of carbon dioxide.

Distributive shock usually precedes the development of arrhythmias in patients with FHF. Despite the presence of a high cardiac output, cardiac contractility is depressed in distributive shock. Negative inotropic agents should not be used in the treatment of arrhythmias unless all other therapies have failed and the benefit of terminating the arrhythmia outweighs the risk of further cardiac depression. Pulmonary artery catheterization is indicated in hypotensive patients with FHF to enable titration of fluid administration, inotropic agents, and vasopressors. The goals of hemodynamic therapy in FHF are as follows:

1. Cerebral perfusion pressure (CPP) greater than 60 mm Hg
2. Cardiac index greater than 3 L/min/m^2
3. Pulmonary capillary wedge pressure (PCWP) of 8 to 12 mm Hg

Hypotension is often unresponsive to fluid administration and minimally responsive to dopamine. Most patients with FHF require a norepinephrine infusion to maintain an adequate arterial pressure and CPP. Patients with FHF usually maintain a cardiac index greater than 3 L/min/m^2. Excessive doses of vasoconstricting agents produce arterial hypertension and a low cardiac index that is easily recognized and treated. Arterial hypotension and a low cardiac index are usually preterminal events in these patients unless a reversible cause can be identified (i.e., pneumothorax, cardiac tamponade, retroperitoneal bleeding secondary to coagulopathy). An epinephrine (Adrenalin) infusion may temporarily improve the cardiac index.

GASTROINTESTINAL TRACT BLEEDING

H_2-receptor antagonists are the most commonly used agents for prophylaxis of gastrointestinal tract bleeding in FHF. Cimetidine may be administered as an intravenous bolus (150 mg when required) or a continuous infusion (30 to 50 mg/h). Ranitidine has theoretic advantages because of its lower inhibitory effect on the hepatic cytochrome P-450 system. It too may be administered as an intravenous bolus (50 mg every 8 hours) or a continuous infusion (6 mg/h). Dosage should be adjusted in renal failure, and platelet counts should be monitored. Regardless of the agent or dosing regimen, the goal is to maintain gastric pH greater than 5 at all times.

An anecdotal case of FHF associated with the use of the proton pump inhibitor, omeprazole, has been reported.

The most common cause of gastrointestinal tract bleeding in FHF is superficial gastric erosions. Bleeding from esophageal varices is rare. The initial management of gastrointestinal tract bleeding in FHF includes assessment of vital signs, establishing two large-bore intravenous lines and initiating normal saline infusion, grouping and cross-matching at least 4 U of packed red blood cells, and obtaining readings for hemoglobin, platelets, PT, partial thromboplastin time (PTT), and fibrinogen. After appropriate fluid resuscitation, the most important therapy is correction of the coagulopathy. Infusion of fresh-frozen plasma with or without plasmapheresis to normalize the PT, platelet transfusions if the platelet count is less than 75,000/1l, and cryoprecipitate in patients with low fibrinogen levels (<100 mg/dl) may be required. Minor gastrointestinal tract bleeding in the presence of local trauma (i.e., nasogastric tubes) that resolves with correction of the coagulopathy does not require urgent gastroscopy. Gastroscopy is indicated in more severe or ongoing gastrointestinal tract bleeding and may be therapeutic if a lesion amenable to local injection, banding, or cautery is present.

RENAL FAILURE

Mechanisms of renal failure in FHF include prerenal, hepatorenal, acute tubular necrosis (ATN), and direct nephrotoxicity. Frequent determination of serum and urinary creatinine, urinary sodium, and urinary osmolarity and hourly determination of urinary output is necessary to assess renal function in FHF. Serum urea levels are unreliable owing to impaired hepatic synthesis in FHF. Early insertion of a pulmonary artery catheter is required to ensure optimal intravascular filling pressures and an acceptable cardiac index.

Hemodynamically stable patients with FHF but without cerebral edema in renal failure can be safely treated with conventional hemodialysis. Elevation of ICP and decreased MAP commonly occur during hemodialysis in FHF. Cerebral edema or hemodynamic instability are indications for CAVH or CVVH. In general CAVH causes a mild decrease in MAP and does not affect ICP. Intracranial hypertension after initiation of CAVH has been reported in patients with FHF and intravascular volume depletion. Intravascular repletion is required before ultrafiltration is initiated. Standard doses of heparin are often recommended in patients with FHF with or without coagulopathy. Low levels of antithrombin III in patients with FHF minimize the systemic effects of heparin. At high concentrations (greater than 0.3 U/ml) the anticoagulant effect of heparin is independent of antithrombin III. Higher concentrations of heparin within the circuit may inhibit coagulation.

COAGULOPATHY

In FHF the coagulopathy is secondary to decreased synthesis of the majority of clotting factors with or without thrombocytopenia. Enhanced fibrinolysis has been implicated but remains unproved. In the absence of vitamin K deficiency, the one-stage PT test expressed in seconds or international normalized ratio (INR) is the most widely used method to assess coagulopathy and hepatic synthetic capacity in FHF. Factor V and VII levels may be useful in assessing prognosis but are not required to manage the coagulopathy. All patients with FHF require daily monitoring of hemoglobin, PT or INR, and platelet count. A falling hemoglobin level should alert the physician to the possibility of occult blood loss (i.e., retroperitoneal bleeding). Patients who have FHF and are bleeding require measurements of fibrinogen levels and fibrin degradation products (FDP). Monitoring PT or INR, platelet counts, and fibrinogen levels enables appropriate administration of fresh-frozen plasma (with or without plasmapheresis), platelet transfusion, and cryoprecipitate, respectively (see above *Gastrointestinal Tract Bleeding*). Transfusion of 2 to 4 U of fresh-frozen plasma every 3 hours may be required to improve coagulation and control bleeding. Marked elevation of FDP indicates the development of disseminated intravascular coagulation (DIC) in patients with FHF.

Treatment of the coagulopathy is indicated in the presence of active bleeding or prior to performing invasive procedures (see above *Cerebral Edema*). Treatment is not indicated for asymptomatic patients with mild-to-moderate coagulopathy (INR less than 7). Some authors recommend prophylactic fresh-frozen plasma if the INR is greater than 7. Other authorities argue that the benefits of prophylactic administration of fresh-frozen plasma remain unproved. Vitamin K, 10 mg intravenously daily for 3 days, should be given to patients with FHF to ensure adequate stores.

Sepsis

In one series of 50 patients with FHF, 80% developed a bacterial infection, and 32% were also infected with fungi. *Staphylococcus aureus, staphylococcus epidermidis,* streptococci, coliform, and candidal organisms were found most often, and the respiratory and urinary tracts were the most common sites of infection. Bacteremias occurred within 72 hours of hospital admission in 26% of patients and correlated strongly with the development of renal failure.

In the absence of positive cultures or a classic infiltrate on chest radiograph, the diagnosis of sepsis in the patient with FHF is virtually impossible. Fever and leukocytosis can be a feature of hepatic necrosis. One third of septic patients with FHF have a normal white cell count and body temperature. The hemodynamic pattern of FHF is identical to septic shock. Therefore patients with moderate-to-severe FHF (stages 2 to 4) should receive prophylactic antimicrobials (e.g., cefuroxime 1.5 g intravenously every 8 hours), and daily blood, urine, and sputum cultures should be obtained. The efficacy of systemic antimicrobial prophylaxis is not improved by the addition of enteral antimicrobial regimens. Antibiotic therapy should be adjusted on the basis of positive cultures and documented sensitivities. Foley catheters should be removed in anuric patients. This approach has reduced infection rates but not mortality in patients with FHF. However, uncontrolled sepsis is a contraindication to liver transplantation.

Metabolic

Glucagon levels are inconsistent but usually elevated in patients with FHF. Glucagon increases blood glucose levels by increasing glycogenolysis and gluconeogenesis. Given the underlying pathophysiology of FHF, there is no role for the use of glucagon in the treatment of hypoglycemia in these patients.

Renal failure, massive chloride administration, and accumulation of lactate are common causes of metabolic acidosis in FHF. Sodium bicarbonate is therapeutic in hyperchloremic metabolic acidosis and may temporarily improve the pH in renal failure. Repeated administration of sodium bicarbonate to anuric patients may precipitate pulmonary edema and hypernatremia. Sodium bicarbonate is not indicated in patients with FHF and lactic acidosis. Dialysis lowers lactate levels and reverses the acidosis but does not correct the underlying defect.

PROGNOSIS

Survival figures for patients with FHF have more than doubled since the early 1970s when rates of 20% were reported. Although increased access to liver transplant programs and improvements in the transplant procedure may result in even higher survival figures, they may also claim the lives of patients with FHF that might have otherwise survived.

Presently, there are six possible outcomes for the patient with FHF admitted to the intensive care unit:

1. Survival without transplantation
2. Survival with transplantation in a patient requiring a transplant
3. Survival with transplantation in a patient not requiring a transplant
4. Death in a patient in whom a transplant was required and was obtained
5. Death in a patient in whom a transplant was required but not obtained
6. Death in a patient in whom a transplant was not required but was obtained

Adverse outcomes 3, 5, and 6 are potentially avoidable if the proper prognosis is assigned and correctly adjusted during the patient's hospital stay.

A useful method for assigning prognosis but one that is often overlooked is frequent clinical evaluation of the patient. Rapidly deteriorating levels of consciousness, a shrinking liver, ascites, decerebrate rigidity, and loss of oculovestibular reflexes are ominous signs.

Also useful for prognostic purposes is monitoring of certain laboratory results. Factor V levels in particular may correlate with outcome. In nonacetaminophen cases, values less than 20% in the young and less than 30% in the elderly or rapidly falling levels in any age group have been associated with a poor prognosis. Serum alpha-fetoprotein levels have also been advocated by some as a prognostic variable in that high levels are assumed to reflect active regenerative activity. However, this test is only useful beyond 5 days after admission to the hospital when most decisions regarding liver transplantation have already been made. Moreover, the test may not be accurate in non–hepatitis B virus (HBV) cases.

Perhaps the most widely used approach to determining prognosis is that identified by the King's College Hospital group, which incorporates various clinical and laboratory parameters including underlying cause, age, interval be-

TABLE 97–3. CRITERIA ADOPTED IN KING'S COLLEGE HOSPITAL FOR LIVER TRANSPLANTATION IN FULMINANT HEPATIC FAILURE

Acetaminophen Patients
pH <7.30 (regardless of grade of encephalopathy)
OR
Prothrombin time >100 s and serum creatinine >300 1mol/L in patients with grade III or IV encephalopathy

Nonacetaminophen Patients
Prothrombin time >100 s (regardless of grade of encephalopathy)
OR
Any three of the following variables (regardless of grade of encephalopathy):
  Age <10 or >40 y
  Etiology: non-A, non-B hepatitis, halothane-induced hepatitis, idiosyncratic drug reactions
  Duration of jaundice before onset of encephalopathy >7 d
  Prothrombin time >50 s
  Serum bilirubin >300 1mol/L

tween jaundice and evidence of encephalopathy in nonacetaminophen cases, total bilirubin values, PT and serum creatinine for acetaminophen cases, and pH levels (Table 97–3). A more accurate but complicated formula has recently been developed by Japanese investigators who by incorporating age, coexisting disease, white blood cell counts, alanine aminotransferase values, bilirubin (total and direct) levels, and PT were able to achieve high positive and negative predictive values, predictive accuracy, and sensitivity and specificity values in retrospective and prospective generated data. The major drawback of the Japanese, King's College, and other equations for predicting FHF outcome is their etiologic specificity. For example, although the Japanese equation works well for patients with HBV-related FHF, it must be modified for non-A, non-B cases and cannot be applied to drug or halothane-induced FHF.

Two less cumbersome and more generic approaches to establishing a prognosis have come through the analysis of liver tissue findings and CPP monitoring. The former involves determining the extent of hepatocyte necrosis on transjugular liver biopsy with greater than 70% necrosis being associated with a poor outcome. The latter consists of monitoring ICP and CPP. Patients with ICPs greater than 40 mm Hg that are refractory to pressure lowering techniques and those with CPPs less than 40 mm Hg for more than 2 hours are considered to have advanced disease and a low probability of surviving transplantation.

LIVER TRANSPLANTATION

Decisions that lead to liver transplantation begin at the time of the patient's presentation to the hospital. Those with acute hepatitis and signs of hepatic decompensation (jaundice, ascites, gastrointestinal tract bleeding, or encephalopathy) or those unable to maintain adequate caloric intake should be hospitalized. Patients who develop stage 2 decreased levels of consciousness should be admitted to the intensive care unit, and the closest available liver transplant unit should be notified. If stage 3 is reached, a decision must be made as to whether to list or evacuate the patient for transplantation. Contraindications to transplantation for FHF include the presence of decerebration, advanced cerebral edema, impaired pupillary or brainstem reflexes, ICP and CPP described above, positive serologic results for human immunodeficiency virus, active bacterial infections, extrahepatic malignancy, refractory hypotension, severe chronic cardiovascular or respiratory disease, active substance abuse, or mental instability. On the other hand, transplantation should be pursued when contraindications are not present and the patient's liver or renal function continues to deteriorate (i.e., rising bilirubin, PT, and serum creatinine levels or falling factor V levels) or liver biopsy findings reveal extensive necrosis. The importance of not procrastinating or awaiting the response to an unproven therapeutic intervention cannot be overemphasized. By doing so, the chances of a successful transplant may be greatly diminished. Simply stated, liver transplantation should dictate the timing of experimental therapy and not vice versa. ABO incompatibility does not preclude transplantation, as retransplantation with a more compatible donor liver is an option in the 50% of patients who subsequently develop liver failure or primary allograft nonfunction.

The results of liver transplantation for FHF vary. Recent data from eight international centers revealed survival rates from 33% to 71%, presumably reflecting in part different thresholds for listing patients in the different sites. Although the procedure itself is technically less difficult (patients with FHF tend to be relatively young and without adhesions or varices), survival figures remain lower than for patients with chronic liver disease. The short time frame available to locate donor livers and the need to use suboptimal grafts are the major reasons why survival figures are not higher. Finally, it must be noted that despite reports of improved survival rates for patients with FHF with liver transplantation, controlled studies comparing transplantation with optimal medical management have yet to be reported.

REFERENCES

1. Blei AT, Olafsson S, Webster S, Levy R. Complications of intracranial pressure monitoring in fulminant hepatic failure. *Lancet.* 1993;341:157–158.
2. Donaldson BW, Gopinath R, Wanless IR, et al. The role of transjugular biopsy in fulminant liver failure: relation to other prognostic indicators. *Hepatology.* 1993;18:1370–1374.
3. Fingerote RJ, Bain VG. Fulminant hepatic failure. *Am J Gastroenterol.* 1993;88(7):1000.
4. Fischer JE, Rosen HM, Ebeid AM, et al. The effect of normalization of plasma amino acids on hepatic encephalopathy in man. *Surgery.* 1976;80:77–91.
5. Keays R, Harrison PM, Wendon JA, et al. Intravenous acetylcysteine in paracetamol-induced fulminant hepatic failure: a prospective controlled trial. *Br Med J.* 1991;303:1026–1029.
6. Lee WM. Acute liver failure. *N Engl J Med.* 1993;329:1862–1872.
7. Lidofsky SD, Bass NM, Prager MC, et al. Intracranial pressure monitoring and liver transplantation for fulminant hepatic failure. *Hepatology.* 1992;16:1–7.
8. Munoz SJ. Difficult management problems in fulminant hepatic failure. *Hepatology.* 1993;17:196–201.
9. O'Grady JG, Alexander GJM, Hayllar KM, Williams R. Early indicators of prognosis in fulminant hepatic failure. *Gastroenterology.* 1989;97:439–445.
10. Rolando N, Gimson A, Wade J, et al. Prospective controlled trial of selective parenteral and enteral antimicrobial regimen in fulminant liver failure. *Hepatology.* 1993;17:196–201.
11. Sherlock S. Fulminant hepatic failure. *Adv Intern Med.* 1993;38:245–265.

98

Ischemic Hepatitis

MICHAEL W. FRIED

DEFINITION

Hypoperfusion of any viscera may result in ischemic damage. *Ischemic hepatitis* can be defined as hepatocellular necrosis associated with a decrease of hepatic perfusion. The cause of ischemic hepatitis is most often related to cardiovascular insufficiency, although any condition that results in severe intravascular volume depletion, and thus hypoperfusion, may precipitate ischemic injury to the liver. The clinical manifestations of ischemic hepatitis may vary from mild biochemical abnormalities to frank jaundice and fulminant hepatic failure. The prognosis is largely dependent on the outcome of the underlying disease process.

HEPATIC CIRCULATION

The liver receives approximately 25% of cardiac output. Blood flow via the hepatic artery is well-oxygenated and accounts for approximately one third of the total hepatic blood flow. The remainder is derived from the portal vein that supplies the liver with less well-oxygenated blood, which is rich in nutrients absorbed from the gastrointestinal tract.[1]

A fall in cardiac output is reflected as a decrease in hepatic perfusion. The liver is able to compensate for changes in hepatic blood flow via vasoactive mechanisms and by increasing oxygen extraction during periods of decreased hepatic perfusion. However, when a critical level of hypoperfusion is reached, the compensatory mechanisms are overwhelmed and hepatic injury may result.

Blood enters the hepatic lobule via branches of the hepatic artery and portal vein in the periportal area. The blood in the periportal area has the highest level of oxygen. As it passes through the hepatic sinusoids toward the terminal hepatic (central) vein, oxygen is extracted so that hepatocytes in the centrilobular area are perfused by blood that is the least well oxygenated.[1] It is in this area where the histologic changes of ischemic hepatitis become manifest.

HEPATIC HISTOLOGIC FINDINGS

Histologic studies of ischemic hepatitis are limited. Patients in whom a diagnosis of this syndrome is being considered are usually critically ill, often with multiorgan failure, making a liver biopsy impractical. Nevertheless, the hallmark of ischemic hepatitis is centrilobular necrosis in the absence of an inflammatory infiltrate.[2] Gibson and Dudley[3] studied 17 patients diagnosed with ischemic hepatitis based on these characteristic histologic findings and concluded that a diagnosis of ischemic hepatitis could be made without a liver biopsy in patients with the appropriate clinical setting (patients who had a potential cause for a fall in cardiac output) and a rapid rise in levels of serum aminotransferases and lactate dehydrogenase (LDH). Acute viral and toxic injury was excluded by appropriate serologic tests and medical history.

DIAGNOSIS

Several studies have looked at the clinical features of ischemic hepatitis.[3-5] The criteria that were used in these studies to define this syndrome varied greatly and ranged from purely clinical observations to liver biopsy diagnosis of centrilobular necrosis. Despite these limitations, it is still possible to ascertain a general picture of the clinical and biochemical characteristics of ischemic hepatitis.

The diagnosis of ischemic hepatitis should be considered in any patient with elevations of liver enzymes (aspartate aminotransferase [AST], alanine aminotransferase [ALT], LDH) in the setting of systemic hypotension. Hypotension resulting in hepatic hypoperfusion may be very brief, and documented episodes of hypotension may be absent in as many as 70% of patients who otherwise fulfill the criteria for ischemic hepatitis.[3] Cardiogenic shock from any cause is the most commonly reported risk factor for the development of ischemic hepatitis. Transient decreases in cardiac output that occur with arrhythmia or valvular heart disease may also result in hepatic injury. Other causes for ischemic hepatitis include hypovolemic shock from hemorrhage or dehydration and septic shock. Rare episodes of ischemic hepatitis have been reported in patients who ingest vasoactive medications (ergotamine overdose) and after protracted seizures in children.[6,7]

The incidence of ischemic hepatitis is difficult to determine. In two studies that retrospectively analyzed cases of ischemic hepatitis over a defined 20-month time frame, a total of 26 patients with ischemic hepatitis were identified.[3,4] Unfortunately, neither study attempted to provide a denominator against which to judge the frequency of the event. In another study that retrospectively identified patients with ischemic hepatitis based on marked elevation in serum AST activity, 29 patients, or 0.2% of the 18,000 hospital admissions that were reviewed over a 6-month period, were diagnosed with ischemic hepatitis.[5] In a group of 130 cirrhotic patients with gastrointestinal tract bleeding, only two patients (1.5%) developed ischemic hepatitis. This rate of ischemic hepatitis is quite low considering that these patients were at high risk for developing hemorrhagic shock and their total hepatic blood flow was already compromised due to their underlying cirrhosis.[8]

Ischemic hepatitis can affect any age group, although it is most frequently reported in older populations. This probably reflects the increased risk for underlying cardiovascular disease associated with increasing age. In the two studies that reported demographic data,[3,4] the mean age for patients with ischemic hepatitis was 50 and 64 years (range 24 to 80 years). Ischemic hepatitis has also been reported in children, however, often in association with congenital heart disease or overwhelming sepsis that results in hepatic hypoperfusion.[9] In the latter, ischemic hepatitis developed in 0.7% of children admitted to the intensive care unit over a 4-year study period. Their mean age was 26 months (range 2 days to 14 years).

BIOCHEMICAL CHANGES

The biochemical changes of ischemic hepatitis have been well described, and a distinct pattern

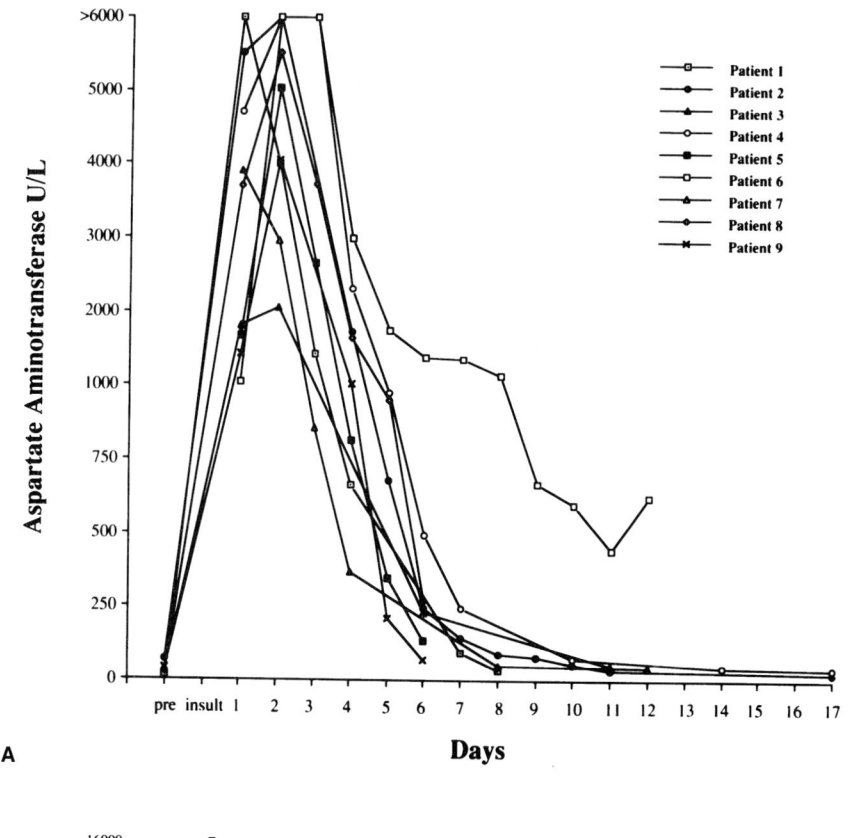

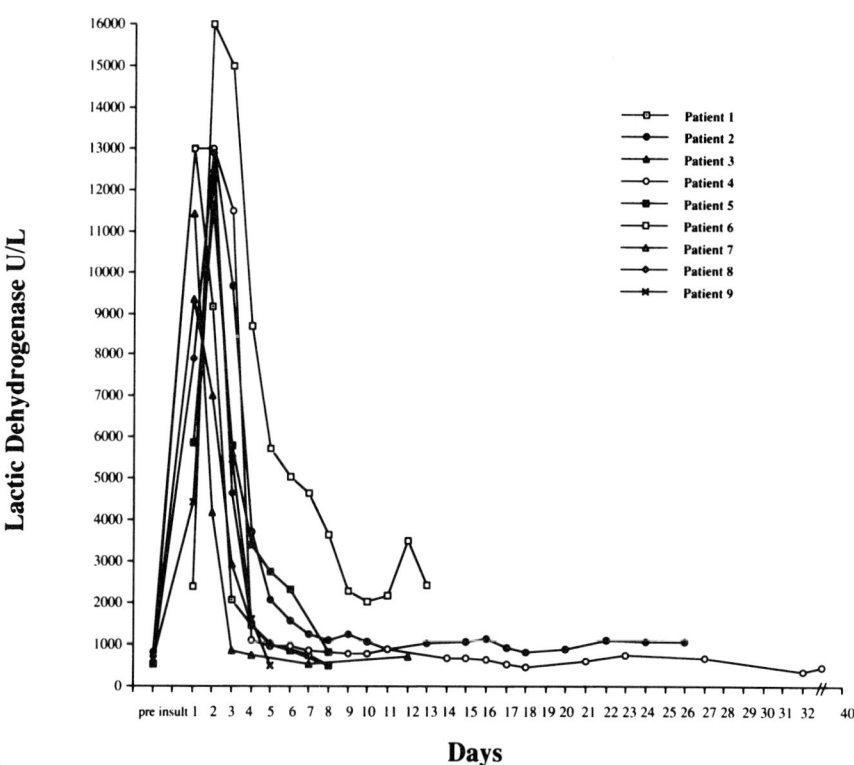

FIGURE 98–1. A, Serial changes in serum aspartate aminotransferase (AST) activity in nine patients with ischemic hepatitis. Note the rapid peak and resolution of enzyme abnormalities. **B,** Serial changes in serum lactate dehydrogenase (LDH) activity in nine patients with ischemic hepatitis. These changes follow the same pattern as serum aminotransferases. (From Gitlin N, Serio KM. Ischemic hepatitis: widening horizons. *Am J Gastroenterol.* 1992;87:831–836. Reprinted with permission.)

of liver enzyme abnormalities is characteristic of this disorder. Serum aminotransferases rise rapidly after an ischemic episode and peak within 1 to 3 days. With improvement in hepatic blood flow through treatment of the underlying illness, serum aminotransferases return to near normal usually within 7 to 10 days of the initial insult. Persistent elevation of serum aminotransferases beyond this period implies a poor prognosis because of continued hepatic hypoperfusion.

Serum ALT and AST activity is strikingly elevated and may exceed 200 times the upper limits of normal (Fig. 98-1A). Less marked elevations (<500 U/L) have also been reported in biopsy-proven ischemic hepatitis.[3] Serum LDH activity is also markedly elevated in patients with ischemic hepatitis. When fractionated, serum LDH activity is mostly of hepatic origin.[3] The level of LDH may rise to 30 times the upper limits of normal and parallels the pattern of aminotransferase activity with a brisk rise and rapid resolution (Fig. 98-1B). Of note, the serum LDH is usually only slightly elevated in patients with acute viral hepatitis.

Elevation of alkaline phosphatase or serum bilirubin is not a usual feature of ischemic hepatitis, and cholestasis has not been demonstrated by liver biopsy specimens of these patients. Mild elevations of serum bilirubin may be seen, but it rarely exceeds four times the upper limit of normal.[3] In contrast, chronic congestion of the liver in patients with heart failure commonly results in hyperbilirubinemia and increased alkaline phosphatase levels.

Gitlin and Serio[4] noted several other biochemical features in their series of patients with ischemic hepatitis. All patients had transient abnormalities of serum creatinine and blood urea nitrogen (BUN). These changes were sometimes marked, consistent with acute renal failure, but resolved over 7 to 10 days. They speculated that the same hypotensive insult to the liver had similar adverse effects on the kidneys. In this series, two thirds of patients with ischemic hepatitis had new onset hyperglycemia that occurred within 48 hours of their illness. All patients eventually became normoglycemic within 2 weeks, but insulin therapy was required transiently in three patients.

DIFFERENTIAL DIAGNOSIS

Few primary liver diseases besides ischemic hepatitis give such marked elevations of serum aminotransferases followed by rapid resolution. The diagnosis of ischemic hepatitis can be made readily in a patient in the intensive care unit with a rapid and striking increase of serum aminotransferase and LDH activities who has recently suffered a documented, acute hypotensive episode that required pressor support. The clinical picture is dominated by the cardiovascular, septic, or hemorrhagic illness that precipitated the hepatic hypoperfusion.

Acute viral hepatitis, particularly hepatitis A, may on occasion mimic the clinical picture seen with ischemic hepatitis. Acute viral hepatitis is usually accompanied by a symptomatic prodrome or a history of exposure that can be ascertained in the medical history. Viral serologic assays and screenings for hepatitis A-IgM, hepatitis B surface antigen and core antibody-IgM, and anti-hepatitis C virus antibody help to exclude a viral cause. Patients with acute viral hepatitis more commonly are jaundiced at the time of presentation, and serum aminotransferases fall to normal much more slowly. Serum LDH activity is only mildly elevated. In patients who have only modest elevations in serum aminotransferases, chronic hepatitis B and hepatitis C should be excluded by history and appropriate serologic assays. Attempts to locate previous liver enzyme results prior to the current illness may be invaluable in distinguishing the acute illness from chronic viral hepatitis.

Special care should be taken to identify all medications that had been used by the patient prior to admission, as well as those that were started since hospitalization. Drug hepatotoxicity is associated with striking elevations of serum aminotransferases and LDH. Acetaminophen toxicity should be considered in patients with marked elevations of serum aminotransferases and renal insufficiency. Idiosyncratic reactions to therapeutic doses of certain drugs, such as isoniazid, may also present in this manner. Discontinuing the offending medication is crucial to recovery (Table 98-1).

Other causes of marked, acute elevations of serum AST activity include rhabdomyolysis, acute myocardial infarction, hepatic trauma, and hepatic infarction, all of which should be distinguishable from ischemic hepatitis by history and additional laboratory investigation.

TREATMENT AND PROGNOSIS

The treatment of ischemic hepatitis is directed at the underlying illness. Therapy to improve cardiac output with inotropic agents and pressors will improve hepatic perfusion and result in res-

TABLE 98-1. CLINICAL FEATURES OF ISCHEMIC HEPATITIS VERSUS ACUTE VIRAL HEPATITIS OR DRUG HEPATOTOXICITY

FEATURE	ISCHEMIC HEPATITIS	ACUTE VIRAL HEPATITIS	DRUG TOXICITY
Symptomatic prodrome	No	Yes	Possible
Intensive care unit setting	Usual	Rare	Rare
AST and ALT >20 times normal	Yes	Yes	Possible
Rapid rise to peak	Yes	Possible	Unlikely
Resolution <10 d	Yes	Unlikely	Possible
Marked LDH elevation	Yes	Unusual	Yes
Jaundice	Unlikely	Often	Possible
Renal failure	Frequent	Only late in course	No (acetaminophen)
Fulminant hepatic failure	Unusual	Rare (<<1%)	Possible

ALT = alanine aminotransferase, AST = aspartate aminotransferase, LDH = lactate dehydrogenase.

olution of ischemic hepatitis. Similarly, volume resuscitation for patients with hemorrhagic shock and appropriate treatment for septic shock indirectly improve cardiac output and hepatic perfusion.

Special consideration should be given to prescribing medications in patients with circulatory failure and ischemic hepatitis. The metabolism of certain drugs, such as lidocaine and calcium channel blockers, is dependent on hepatic blood flow, and therefore clearance of these medications is greatly diminished in this setting. Indeed, an association has been reported between the use of calcium channel blockers and antiarrhythmic agents and increased mortality in patients with ischemic hepatitis, although it was not clear from that study if the worse prognosis was merely related to the presence of more severe cardiac disease.[10] Opiates and analgesics that are often prescribed for these critically ill patients also have the potential to accumulate and cause neurologic and respiratory depression.

The prognosis of ischemic hepatitis is largely dependent on the prognosis of the underlying illness. Mortality has been reported as high as 50% in patients with ischemic hepatitis. However, despite the massive hepatic necrosis that may occur, deaths due to hepatic failure are extremely rare, and the cause of death is usually a result of poor cardiac reserve.[5]

The level of AST elevation does not correlate with survival. When stratified according to peak AST activity, the survival for patients with AST less than 2000 was 43% compared to 41% for patients with a peak AST activity above this cutoff. The pattern of AST activity, however, does seem to have some prognostic value. In patients with ischemic hepatitis who died, the level of serum AST did not drop appreciably from peak values, whereas in those who survived, with effective treatment of their underlying disease, AST rapidly returned toward normal.[5]

REFERENCES

1. Lautt WW, Greenway CV. Conceptual review of the hepatic vascular bed. *Hepatology.* 1987;7:952–963.
2. Bynum TE, Boitnott JK, Maddrey WC. Ischemic hepatitis. *Dig Dis Sci.* 1979;24:129–135.
3. Gibson PR, Dudley FJ. Ischemic hepatitis: clinical features, diagnosis, and prognosis. *Aust N Z J Med.* 1984;14:822–825.
4. Gitlin N, Serio KM. Ischemic hepatitis: widening horizons. *Am J Gastroenterol.* 1992;87:831–836.
5. Hickman PE, Potter JM. Mortality associated with ischemic hepatitis. *Aust N Z J Med.* 1990;20:32–34.
6. Deviere J, Reuse C, Askenasi R. Ischemic pancreatitis and hepatitis secondary to ergotamine poisoning. *J Clin Gastroenterol.* 1987;9:350–352.
7. Ussery XT, Henar EL, Black DD, Berger S, Whitington PF. Acute liver injury after protracted seizures in children. *J Pediatr Gastroenterol Nutr.* 1989;421–425.
8. Henrion J, Colin L, Schmitz A, Schapira M, Heller FR. Ischemic hepatitis in cirrhosis. *J Clin Gastroenterol.* 1993;16:35–39.
9. Garland JS, Werlin SL, Rice TB. Ischemic hepatitis in children: diagnosis and clinical course. *Crit-Care Med.* 1988;16:1209–1212.
10. Potter JM, Hickman PE. Cardiodepressant drugs and the high mortality rate associated with ischemic hepatitis. *Crit Care Med.* 1992;20:474–478.

99

Hepatorenal Syndrome

JACOB GREEN

The hepatorenal syndrome (HRS) is a unique form of acute renal failure occurring in patients with liver disease for which a specific cause cannot be elucidated. Despite the severe derangement of renal function and ominous prognosis when renal failure develops, minimal and inconsistent pathologic abnormalities of the kidneys are found at autopsy. Furthermore, the kidneys, if transplanted, are capable of normal function, which supports the concept that the renal failure is functional and potentially reversible. In contrast to patients with classic acute tubular necrosis (ATN), patients with HRS manifest characteristic alterations of renal function that mimic prerenal azotemia (i.e., hyperosmolar urine and very low urinary sodium concentration). The past several years have witnessed newer insights into both the pathophysiology and the therapeutics of this syndrome. For example, the characterization of endothelin and the nitric oxide-arginine pathway and their roles in biology and medicine has provided additional new insights into the mechanisms of peripheral vasodilation, hyperdynamic circulation, and decreased renal perfusion, all of which constitute the clinical picture of HRS. Finally, recently initiated therapeutic approaches lend a note of optimism to the future management of a syndrome that is so often incompatible with recovery. These include the acceptance of orthotopic liver transplantation as definitive treatment for patients with end-stage liver disease and attempts to improve renal function by countervailing the decrease in systemic vascular resistance while minimizing concomitant increments in renal vascular resistance.

The purpose of this chapter is to summarize current concepts with regard to the pathophysiology of HRS and to survey newer modalities that have been recently added to the therapeutic armamentarium of this disorder.

DIFFERENTIAL DIAGNOSIS

Although HRS is the most dreaded renal complication in patients suffering from liver disease, clinicians should be discouraged from equating decreased renal function with HRS. There are many other conditions, some of which are more common than HRS, that can involve both the liver and the kidneys. For didactic purposes one must consider seven categories of clinical conditions that may be confused with HRS.

1. Simultaneous injury can occur to both the liver and the kidneys ("pseudohepatorenal" syndrome).
   a. Infections (sepsis, leptospirosis, Reye's syndrome, cytomegalovirus [CMV], and others)
   b. Circulatory problems (shock, heart failure)
   c. Genetic disorders (e.g., polycystic disease)
   d. Collagen vascular diseases (systemic lupus erythematosus [SLE], polyarteritis nodosa [PAN])
   e. Toxins (e.g., CCl_4, tetracyclines)
   f. Neoplasms (metastatic or nonmetastatic renal cell carcinoma)
2. Immune complex glomerulonephritis can be associated with hepatitis B disease.
3. Glomerulopathies can be associated with chronic liver disease (e.g., immunoglobulin A [IgA] nephropathy with alcoholic cirrhosis).
4. Disseminated intravascular coagulation (DIC) in association with acute liver disease may damage the kidney.
5. ATN can be secondary to hypotension, nephrotoxic drugs, sepsis, gastrointestinal tract bleeding, coagulopathies, and bilirubinemia (obstructive jaundice). Renal failure occurring in patients with liver disease is more commonly ATN than the HRS.

6. Prerenal azotemia is a likely occurrence in patients who are actively forming ascites, especially if their intake of solute and fluid is meager and there are associated losses of body fluids because of vomiting, diarrhea, and forced diuresis. Distinguishing between prerenal azotemia and HRS is one of the big challenges facing the clinician treating patients with combined liver-kidney dysfunction (see below).
7. With the introduction of liver transplantation as a therapeutic option for decompensated liver disease, the spectrum of combined liver-kidney dysfunction has been expanded. Various forms of liver transplant–related renal dysfunction are currently recognized. These are mainly related to severe volume deficit during the operation, preexisting renal disease, cyclosporine nephrotoxicity, and de novo HRS secondary to the liver graft dysfunction.

In view of the broad spectrum for combined liver-kidney disease it is prudent to meticulously search for the precise cause of renal failure before making a diagnosis of HRS.

An additional cause for concern during evaluation of patients with liver-kidney disease is the potential pitfalls in the assessment of glomerular filtration rate (GFR) in the presence of liver disease. First, interference by bilirubin with the measurement of serum creatinine performed by means of automated chemical analytic techniques has been reported.[1] The magnitude of the error (a lower creatinine reading) is variable but may be as great as a 57% decrement with some commonly used automated analyzers. This interference may mask a true elevation of serum creatinine in a markedly jaundiced patient or result in the erroneous assumption that a decrease in serum creatinine level represents a real improvement in renal function. It has been suggested, however, that the end point Jaffee method can overcome the interference by bilirubin.

Second, a number of medications such as spironolactone, triamterene, amiloride, cimetidine, and trimethoprim that are commonly used in patients with liver disease inhibit the tubular secretion of creatinine resulting in a variable rise in serum creatinine and a decline in the calculated creatinine clearance (Ccr).

Third, because of poor nutrition, severe muscular wasting, and hepatic disease or failure, many adult cirrhotic patients have more severe renal dysfunction than that suggested by the level of their measured serum creatinine.[2] This is a situation resembling the relatively low creatinine levels observed in small children or elderly patients, because of their relatively small muscle mass and low body creatinine pools. Thus, a serum creatinine concentration "within the range of normal" may actually represent important renal dysfunction in some cirrhotic patients.

Papadakis and Arieff[2] have stressed the unpredictability of the use of serum creatinine levels and Ccr values in estimating the degree of renal dysfunction in patients with liver disease, particularly those with HRS. In a recent prospective study, they reported that the serum creatinine level frequently failed to rise above the usually accepted "normal" level even when the GFR was very low (less than 25 ml/min) and that Ccr overestimated inulin clearance by a factor of two in patients with HRS. They further stated that many patients with cirrhosis and ascites have a GFR less than 60 ml/min but a normal serum creatinine level.

DEFINITION

HRS is defined as renal failure occurring in patients with liver disease in the absence of clinical, laboratory, or anatomic evidence of other known causes.[3]

HRS is characterized by marked variability in both clinical presentation and course. It usually occurs in alcoholic patients with cirrhosis, although cirrhosis is not necessary for its development. HRS may also complicate other liver diseases, including acute hepatitis, fulminant hepatic failure, and hepatic malignancy. The fact that HRS often follows events that reduce effective blood volume, including abdominal paracentesis, vigorous diuretic therapy, and gastrointestinal tract bleeding, has been well documented. However, HRS can also occur in the absence of an apparent precipitating event. In this context, several observers have noted that patients with HRS seldom arrive at the hospital with preexisting renal failure; rather, renal failure seems to develop while the patient is in the hospital, suggesting that events or procedures in the hospital may precipitate the occurrence of this syndrome.

Virtually all patients with HRS have ascites (often tense) and clinical signs of portal hypertension. The degree of jaundice is extremely variable; occasionally, renal failure may develop even while the serum bilirubin concentration is decreasing. The majority of patients have a modest decrease in systemic blood pressure with significant hypotension usually occurring as a terminal event. Most of the patients die within 3 weeks of the onset of azotemia.

In his series of 200 patients, Papper[4] observed only two patients who recovered spontaneously. Even though other investigators have reported a higher incidence of recovery from HRS,[5] a careful analysis of these cases revealed that some of the patients suffered from prerenal azotemia rather than from HRS. Also, the carefully documented recoveries have appeared to follow a rapid improvement in the condition of the liver.

It is a remarkable fact that 130 years after the original description of the essential features of HRS,[6] the pathogenesis of this condition still remains an enigma. A substantial body of evidence suggests that the renal failure in patients with HRS is functional. Despite a severe derangement of renal function, renal pathologic abnormalities are minimal and are not consistently present.[3] Furthermore, the functional integrity of the renal tubules is maintained during the renal failure, as manifested by relatively normal capacity for both sodium reabsorption and urine concentration. In these patients, the biochemical characteristics of the urine are the same as in patients with hypovolemia, which underscores the importance of considering hypovolemia in any diagnostic evaluation of azotemia in liver disease.

The most direct evidence for the functional nature of HRS is derived from the demonstration that the kidneys transplanted from patients with HRS are capable of resuming normal function in the recipient[7] and from the return of renal function when a patient with HRS successfully receives a liver transplant.[8]

In spite of the elusive nature of the pathogenesis of HRS, it is now well established that renal hypoperfusion with preferential renal cortical ischemia underlies the renal failure in this condition. Renal angiographic studies performed in a group of cirrhotic patients with kidney failure[9] disclosed marked beading and tortuosity of the interlobar and proximal arcuate arteries and an absence of distinct cortical nephrograms and vascular filling of the cortical vessels. Postmortem angiography performed on the kidneys of five patients (who had been studied during life) disclosed a striking reversal of all the vascular abnormalities in the kidneys (Fig. 99–1). These findings lend further support to the functional basis of the renal failure in HRS operating through an active renal vasoconstriction.

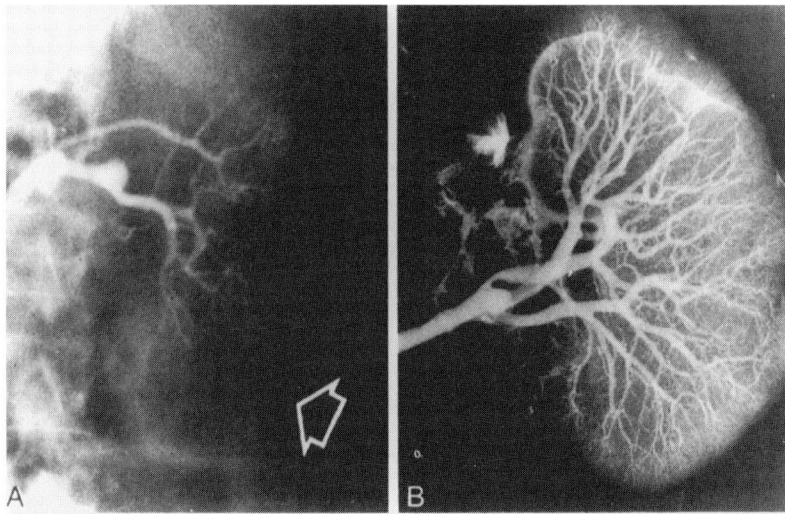

FIGURE 99–1. **A,** Selective renal arteriogram in patient with hepatorenal syndrome. Primary intrarenal and interlobular arteries are tenuous and tortuous; cortical vessels are not filled. **B,** Postmortem arteriogram of same kidney. Intrarenal arterial system appears normal, with good filling of cortical vessels. Vessels are histologically normal. (Reproduced with permission from Epstein M, Berk D, Hollenberg N, et al. Renal failure in the patient with cirrhosis. *Am J Med.* 1970;49:175–184.)

POSTULATED CONTRIBUTING MECHANISMS

Although the hallmark of HRS is a "de novo" severe renal vasoconstriction, it is postulated that certain abnormalities occurring in patients with liver disease can contribute toward this extreme reduction in renal blood flow. These abnormalities involve the cardiovascular system and the volume status of cirrhotic patients, and they are subgrouped as "afferent" events and "efferent" events.

"AFFERENT EVENTS"

Low "Effective Blood Volume"

Traditionally, cirrhotic patients are characterized as having "diminished effective blood volume." The concept of "effective blood volume" (EBV) is not always easy to understand, but in simplistic terms it refers to that part of the circulating volume that appears to stimulate volume receptors (high-pressure sinoaortic and low-pressure cardiopulmonary baroreceptors). In normal circumstances, EBV correlates with total extracellular fluid (ECF) volume. However, in chronic liver disease (as in other edematous states) EBV does *not* correlate with total ECF volume. Despite massive retention of salt and water, EBV remains functionally contracted. Patients with chronic liver disease may suffer from low EBV because of the following:

- Disturbance in Starling forces leading to pooling of ECF in the splanchnic circulation
- Peripheral vasodilation
- Impaired cardiac function

Altered Starling Forces

It has been classically proposed that because of destruction of the architecture of the liver parenchyma there is blockage of hepatic venous outflow with subsequent sinusoidal hypertension. The resulting imbalance of Starling forces in the hepatic sinusoids and splanchnic capillaries causes an excessive amount of lymph formation, exceeding the capacity of the thoracic duct to return this excessive lymph to the circulation.[4,10] Consequently, excess lymph accumulates in the peritoneal space as ascites with a subsequent contraction of circulating plasma volume (see further discussion in Chapter 102). The diminution of plasma volume in turn constitutes an afferent signal, causing a secondary augmentation of renal sodium and water reabsorption. Thus, despite a progressive increase in total ECF volume, most of the excess volume is sequestered in the splanchnic fluid compartment (because of the prevailing Starling forces) without normalizing EBV. It appears therefore that the imbalance of Starling forces in the splanchnic circulation is responsible for two abnormalities seen in cirrhotic patients:

1. Expansion of total ECF (by stimulating renal salt and water reabsorption)
2. Impaired kidney perfusion (due to redistribution of the plasma volume)

Cardiovascular Response in Chronic Liver Disease

Cirrhosis is often complicated by altered cardiovascular homeostasis characterized by a reduction in total peripheral resistance, an increase in cardiac output, and a tendency toward systemic hypotension at rest.[11] These changes are accompanied by increased activity of the sympathetic nervous system, as reflected by elevations in plasma concentrations of norepinephrine and by urinary excretion of norepinephrine.[12] The perturbed peripheral hemodynamics in the face of augmented sympathetic activity have been traditionally ascribed to the presence of anatomic arteriovenous shunts. It has also been proposed that several circulating vasodilators that accumulate in this condition could play a role in diminishing the "fullness" of the arteriovenous tree. These vasodilators include bradykinin, substance P, vasoactive intestinal polypeptide, glucagon, prostacycline, and atrial natriuretic peptide. However, there is no clear evidence of substantial involvement of any of these agents. Recently, attention has also focused on nitric oxide as a mediator of peripheral vasodilation in cirrhosis. Nitric oxide, a vasodilator synthesized from L-arginine, accounts for the biologic activity of endothelium-derived relaxant factor (EDRF). The synthesis of nitric oxide in both endothelium and vascular smooth muscle can be induced by lipopolysaccharide (endotoxin) and various cytokines.[13] Based on these findings and given the fact that circulating endotoxins can be detected in the circulation of many cirrhotic patients, Vallance and Moncada[13] have postulated that the endotoxemia in cirrhosis may induce the synthesis of nitric oxide, which in turn causes peripheral vasodilation in these patients. Indeed, in a preliminary communication, these investigators reported that serum nitrite and nitrate concentrations, indexes of nitric oxide production, were elevated in a group of patients with cirrhosis.[14] Furthermore, there was a direct correlation between serum nitrite and nitrate concentrations and endotoxemia.

Aside from circulating vasodilators, both experimental and clinical evidence suggest that in liver disease there might be an inherent disorder within the vascular wall that renders the wall refractory to vasoactive agents.[15,16] One of the first descriptions of loss of vascular responsiveness to norepinephrine in cirrhotic patients was made by Morandini and Spanedda.[17] Subsequent studies by Lunzer and his colleagues[16] in 1973 and 1975 confirmed the findings that the vasculature of cirrhotic patients was refractory to endogenous and exogenous norepinephrine. However, diminished end-organ responsiveness to norepinephrine is not a consistent finding in all of the clinical studies. Thus, early studies by Laragh et al[18] found that while the vasculature is refractory to angiotensin II, the reactivity to norepinephrine is normal. Furthermore, recently, Lenz et al[19] reported that the pressor response to norepinephrine in 11 patients with hepatic encephalopathy (nine of which had chronic liver disease) was enhanced.

Cardiac Function in Liver Disease

Cirrhotic patients have been classically described as having "hyperkinetic circulation" characterized by tachycardia, cardiac enlargement, and high cardiac output.[11] However, more extensive cross-sectional studies have shown that patients with advanced liver disease can have either an increased, normal, or depressed cardiac output.[20] Of interest is the observation that in these patients renal blood flow does not correlate with the level of cardiac output. Comparable reductions in total renal blood flow and cortical flow were observed in the low- and high-output groups.[20] This finding is compatible with the notion of "primary" renal vasoconstriction's being responsible for renal dysfunction in patients with liver disease.

Studies of global left ventricular function in cirrhosis should be interpreted with caution, since peripheral vasodilation and reduced left ventricular afterload (often found in cirrhosis as described above) can mask latent left ventricular disease. In fact, correction of hypotension with vasopressors, thereby increasing the afterload of the heart, may precipitate pulmonary edema in cirrhotic patients.[21] Similarly, an overzealous administration of colloid solutions to cirrhotic patients may also precipitate pulmonary edema if not properly monitored. Gould et al[22] performed cardiac catheterization in 10 patients with cirrhosis who had a presystolic gallop. When exercising, all 10 patients showed an average increase in left ventricular end-diastolic pressure from 6 to 19 mm Hg (an increase of 216%). A striking increase also was noted in pulmonary artery pressure (24 to 47 mm Hg; +96%). This observation is another indication for the fact that by "stressing" the cardiovascular system, one may unmask latent cardiac dysfunction in cirrhotic patients.

The reasons for impaired heart function in liver disease could be multifactorial. Diminished venous return due to tense ascites, alcoholic myopathy, malnutrition, and electrolyte derangements accompanying liver disease (hypomagnesemia, hypophosphatemia, hypocalcemia, alkalosis) can interfere with myocardial performance. There may be also an inherent defect related to the cirrhotic milieu. This may be suggested by the observation that heart muscles taken from dogs with severe liver disease (the CBDL model) show a blunted contractile response to isoproterenol.[23] Also, in vivo studies in patients and experimental animals with cirrhosis have demonstrated attenuated positive inotropic and chronotropic responsiveness to catecholamines and desensitization of myocardial b-adrenergic receptors.[24]

In conclusion, chronic liver disease may lead to diminished effective blood volume because of pooling of ECF in certain compartments and because of disturbed cardiovascular function. These abnormalities act in concert to diminish the relative "fullness" of the arteriovenous tree despite an increase in total plasma volume. This in turn activates the various "efferent" mechanisms promoting a decrease in renal perfusion and GFR.

"EFFERENT" EVENTS

As outlined in the previous section, it is postulated that "afferent" events activate certain effectors (i.e., "efferent" factors), which in turn bring about certain changes that eventuate in renal ischemia and a decrease in GFR. The postulated mechanisms that may play a role in the pathogenesis of renal failure of liver disease have to do with an imbalance between humoral and intrarenal vasoconstrictors and vasodilators.

Among the agents that have been implicated in the pathogenesis of the renal vasoconstriction characterizing HRS are the renin-angiotensin system,[25,26] renal prostaglandins,[27-30] sympathetic nervous system,[12,31] endothelins,[32] and endotoxemia.[33] In addition, blunted vasodilatory response to the kallikrein-kinin system and to atrial peptides may enhance the cortical vasoconstriction encountered in this disease.

Although many hormonal systems are altered in HRS, there is no clear-cut proof to assign a role to any of the hormonal systems' being the sole mediator of HRS. Thus, it is often hard to establish a cause-and-effect relationship between a given hormonal abnormality and the appearance of renal failure. Furthermore, attempts to block pharmacologically the renin-angiotensin system or the sympathetic nervous system in cirrhotic patients have failed to reverse HRS. It is, therefore, possible that altered hormonal status in these patients is an epiphenomenon without having a pathogenetic role in the renal vasoconstriction. Alternatively, renal failure in cirrhotic patients can be attributable to a panoply of hormonal and neural mediators acting in concert, rather than to a single hormonal system.

The role of altered synthesis of renal prostaglandins (PGs) has attracted a great deal of attention because of its clinical relevance. Administration of inhibitors of PG synthesis (e.g., indomethacin) to patients with cirrhosis results in a significant decrement in GFR and renal plasma flow (RPF).[27] This complication is mainly seen in patients who are retaining sodium avidly (i.e., patients with ascites). Since the kidney is a major site for the production of both vasodilatory (e.g., PGE_2, PGI_2) and vasoconstrictor PGs (e.g., thromboxane), it is tempting to speculate that an imbalance between the two groups of PGs underlies the pathogenesis of cortical vasoconstriction in HRS. It is clear that although PGs do not play an important role in modulating renal function in normal subjects, these agents constitute a critical modulator of kidney function and sodium excretion during disease states involving volume contraction. Thus, in the setting of decompensated cirrhosis (i.e., associated with ascites or edema), the ability to enhance PG synthesis in the kidney provides a compensatory or adaptive mechanism inasmuch as the vasodilatory PG (e.g., PGE_2) counterbalances the decrement in GFR and RPF associated with the disease and mitigates sodium retention owing to their natriuretic effect. The corollary of this formulation is that the administration of agents that impair such an adaptation (i.e., PG synthetase inhibitors) might result in a clinically important deterioration of renal function. This occurs primarily in patients who suffer from low EBV and are retaining sodium avidly.

Further support for such a postulate derives from recent observations by Govindarajan et al.[28] They used an immunofluorescence technique to localize and semiquantitate the PG-synthesizing enzymes PGH synthase and PGI_2 synthase obtained in postmortem, biopsy, and nephrectomy specimens from human renal tissue. Medullary collecting tubule PGH synthase–positive staining was graded 4+ or 5+ in kidney samples from patients with ATN or acute tubulointerstitial nephritis and from patients with liver failure without HRS. However, PGH synthase–positive staining was markedly diminished or absent (average 1+) in patients with HRS. The authors interpreted their data to suggest that loss of the medullary PGH synthase is the cause of diminished urinary PGE_2 excretion in HRS.

DIAGNOSTIC CONSIDERATIONS

The abrupt onset of oliguria in a cirrhotic patient does not necessarily imply the presence of HRS. The two most common conditions to consider in addition to HRS are "prerenal azotemia" (due to volume extraction or cardiac pump failure) and ATN. Table 99–1 outlines the biochemical characteristics of HRS, prerenal azotemia, and ATN. Although the laboratory features are helpful in differentiating ATN from HRS, clinicians must acknowledge that often the urinary indexes are confusing and fall in the "grey zone." Furthermore, patients with HRS often develop classic ATN as their condition deteriorates. Therefore, in many cases the natural history appears to be a continuum between the two conditions.

Low $[U_{Na}]$ is considered to be the laboratory hallmark of HRS. However, one needs to be aware of certain deviations from this rule. For example, HRS can be accompanied by elevated $[U_{Na}]$.[34] Conversely, various clinical settings of intrinsic renal damage may be associated with low $[U_{Na}]$. These conditions include oliguric and nonoliguric ATN, urinary tract obstruction, acute glomerulonephritis, contrast nephropathy, and myoglobinuric renal failure.

Clearly, one particular urinary index cannot be expected to reliably discriminate between HRS and other forms of acute renal failure in liver disease. Any set of laboratory data must be interpreted in conjunction with the patient's clinical course and the use of additional urinary and serum tests.

As shown in Table 99–1, HRS and prerenal azotemia share similar urinary indexes. In both conditions, urinary concentrating ability is preserved and $[U_{Na}]$ is low. Therefore, distinction between prerenal azotemia and HRS remains

HEPATORENAL SYNDROME

TABLE 99-1. DIFFERENTIAL URINARY FINDINGS IN ACUTE AZOTEMIA ASSOCIATED WITH LIVER DISEASE

	PRERENAL AZOTEMIA	HEPATORENAL SYNDROME	ACUTE TUBULAR NECROSIS
Urine sodium concentration (mEq/L)	<10	<10	>30
Urine osmolality	At least 100 mOsm > plasma osmolality	At least 100 mOsm > plasma osmolality	Equal to plasma osmolality
Urine sediment	Normal	Unremarkable	Casts, cellular debris

one of the big challenges facing the clinician who provides medical care to a cirrhotic patient with oliguria. For all practical purposes, the diagnosis of HRS can be established only after a diligent search for reversible causes of prerenal azotemia has been made and after the exclusion of ATN and other conditions leading to a combined liver-kidney dysfunction (as outlined in the introduction to the chapter under Differential Diagnosis). A useful algorithm that can assist the clinician in the evaluation and management of acute azotemia in patients with liver disease is described in Figure 99-2.

MANAGEMENT AND TREATMENT

Realistically, the management of HRS is frustrating. This grim outlook is understandable if one considers the fact that HRS usually appears in a setting of a terminal decompensated liver disease. Therefore, several therapeutic approaches that have been employed through the years had only limited success. At the present, liver transplantation is the only definitive treatment that can be offered to these patients (see below). Because therapy of established HRS is so cumbersome, the importance of prevention of the syndrome cannot be overemphasized.

PREVENTIVE MEASURES

Avoidance of Volume Contraction

Avoidance of volume contraction can be achieved by avoiding unnecessary use of loop diuretics and the use of therapeutic abdominal paracentesis (unless for tense ascites with respiratory distress). Any other obvious volume loss such as gastrointestinal tract bleeding, vomiting, or diarrhea should be promptly corrected. One

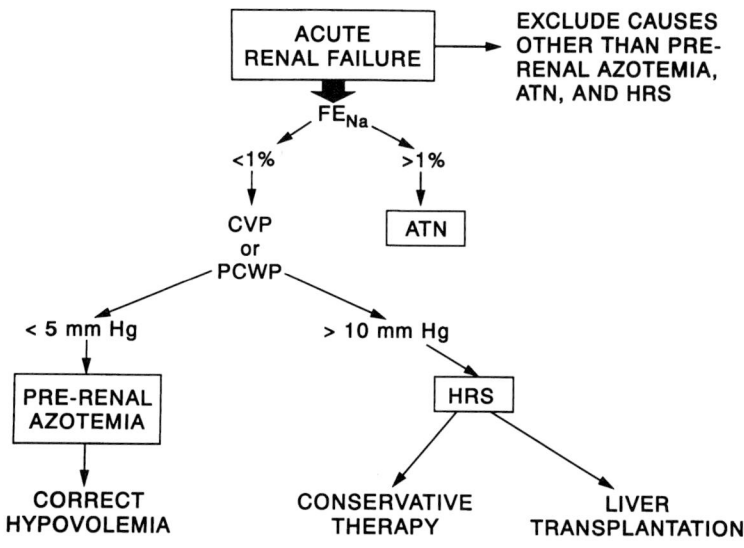

FIGURE 99-2. Algorithm for the evaluation and management of a cirrhotic patient with renal dysfunction. ATN = acute tubular necrosis, CVP = central venous pressure, FE_{Na} = excreted fraction of filtered sodium, HRS = hepatorenal syndrome, PCWP = pulmonary capillary wedge pressure.

cannot stress enough the importance of looking diligently for correctable causes of azotemia (e.g., volume contraction, heart failure, ATN) before the diagnosis of HRS is made. Since HRS and prerenal azotemia have similar urinary diagnostic indexes, one must often use a functional maneuver (i.e., administration of volume expanders) to differentiate between these two entities. The clinician should realize, however, that because of low peripheral resistance associated with cirrhosis the degree of volume expansion necessary to replenish the cirrhotic patient may at times be marked, occasionally requiring the infusion of massive amounts of colloids. To assist in determining when to discontinue volume expanders (to avoid fluid overload), one must consult the clinical status of the patient (e.g., blood pressure, urine flow rate, creatinine clearance) and monitor central hemodynamic parameters such as central venous pressure (CVP) or data derived from Swan-Ganz catheter.

Avoidance of Nephrotoxic Drugs

It is now well established that nonsteroidal anti-inflammatory drugs that inhibit prostaglandin synthetase activity often adversely influence renal function in patients with liver disease and ascites.[27] Similarly, the broad spectrum antibiotic demeclocycline (often used for hyponatremia due to excess antidiuretic hormone [ADH] activity) may induce acute azotemia in patients with cirrhosis and ascites.[35] Lactulose, which is often used for the treatment of hepatic encephalopathy, can induce profound hypovolemia secondary to diarrhea, thereby resulting in azotemia. Patients with liver disease have been reported to be at increased risk for aminoglycoside nephrotoxicity.[36] The pathogenesis for this link remains unclear. It has been suggested that aminoglycosides might interfere with a vasodilatory PG that may be activated in decompensated cirrhotic patients and that counterbalances the renal vasoconstrictor activity of angiotensin II. An additional explanation relates to the synergism between gentamicin and endotoxin. Zager and Prior[37] have demonstrated an association between gram-negative sepsis and enhanced gentamicin nephrotoxicity. This phenomenon was attributable to the effect of endotoxin and to an enhanced renal cortical uptake of the aminoglycoside. The relevance to decompensated cirrhotic patients, who very often suffer from endotoxemia, is quite obvious. This factor should be kept in mind when treating these patients with aminoglycosides.

THERAPEUTIC MANEUVERS

Several therapeutic modalities have been proposed to alter the relentless course of HRS. All these maneuvers are partially successful at most. Some of them may result in transient improvement in GFR, but survival of the patients is not altered. Moreover, critical analysis of the reports where a "limited" success has been reported reveal that many of the patients did not fit the strict criteria of HRS.

Expansion of Extracellular Volume

Increasing EBV by infusion of colloids, head-out water immersion, and paracentesis with reinfusion of ascites has been almost uniformly disappointing in the management of established HRS. The latter procedure is fraught with serious complications such as bacterial peritonitis, intravascular volume depletion, hepatic encephalopathy, and protein depletion.

Recently, there has been a flurry of enthusiasm for the use of LeVeen peritoneovenous shunt (PVS) in the management of HRS. Since the underlying abnormality in decompensated cirrhosis is not solely an excess of total body fluid but also a maldistribution of ECF with a resultant diminished EBV, a redistribution of body fluids between compartments may be a reasonable approach to reverse many of the abnormalities contributing to renal failure.

In 1974, LeVeen and associates developed the PVS with a one-way valve system activated by the increased intraabdominal pressure. Originally used for the treatment of refractory ascites, several investigators have suggested its use for HRS as well.[38] Unfortunately, although there have been a few well-documented "successes," the majority of reports have been anecdotal with insufficient details to allow critical assessment. Even where sufficient data were available, we must conclude that the majority of putative "successes" occurred in patients who were not clearly documented to have HRS; rather, many patients probably had reversible azotemia secondary to a diminished effective blood volume.

Recently, Linas et al[39] carried out a prospective study comparing PVS ($n=10$) with medical therapy in 20 patients with well-documented HRS associated with alcoholic liver disease. The insertion of a PVS resulted in an increase in pulmonary capillary wedge pressure and in cardiac index, with a concomitant decrease in serum creatinine. Despite improvement in renal function, survival was prolonged significantly in only one patient. In the remainder, survival was 13.8 ± 2.2 days compared to 4.1 ± 0.6 days with medical therapy. The investigators concluded that whereas PV shunting often stabilizes renal function, it does not prolong life in patients with HRS. Additional studies are currently under way to assess the role of PVS in HRS patients with less advanced disease.

The study of Stanley et al (Veterans Administration Cooperative Study)[40] in its preliminary report, indicated that although there were seven long-term survivors in a group of 14 patients with HRS treated with PVS, the results were not statistically different from those of 19 patients with HRS randomized to medical therapy.[40] It is clear that some patients with HRS (particularly those with mild liver disease) exhibit improvement in renal function following PVS implantation, but the benefits must be balanced with the high occurrence of major adverse reactions and mortality. Further controlled prospective randomized studies are necessary to assess the effects of PVS on liver and kidney function, complications, long-term survival, and quality of life obtained.

Pharmacologic Modulation

In view of the prominent role assigned to renal cortical ischemia in the pathogenesis of HRS, it is not altogether surprising that there have been numerous attempts to treat HRS with vasodilators. Pharmacologic modulation of renal vasoconstriction has been tried by intrarenal or systemic infusion of acetylcholine, dopamine, a-adrenergic blockers (phenoxybenzamine, phentolamine), captopril, saralasin, PGs (PGE_1, PGA_1, PGI_2), and thromboxane synthesis inhibitors.[41,42] None of these agents have shown effects that resulted in any sustained improvement of renal function or patients' outcome.

Another investigative approach that merits consideration is the potential role of atrial natriuretic peptide and calcium channel blockers in the setting of HRS. Both agents have been shown to constitute selective renal vasodilatory effect in specific settings of renal ischemia.[43] Thus, if it can be demonstrated that atrial natriuretic peptide and calcium antagonists can be safely administered to patients with decompensated cirrhosis without inducing concomitant hypotension, they may constitute an additional therapeutic approach to the management of HRS.

In addition to the use of vasodilators as an attempt to reduce renal vasoconstriction, a different pharmacologic approach puts more focus on the disturbed *peripheral* hemodynamics observed in HRS patients (i.e., peripheral vasodilation). It was proposed that reversal of the low peripheral resistance redistributes blood to the kidney, thereby ameliorating HRS. Thirty years ago, Gornel et al[44] demonstrated that the administration of the pressor amine metaraminol to cirrhotic patients is often followed by increased GFR, an increase in urine flow, and the elaboration of a more dilute urine. Although the use of metaraminol was fraught with problems, it would appear that the general approach might be valid. Cohn et al[45] demonstrated that a synthetic analog of lysine vasopressin (Octapressin) has the unique property of producing renal vasodilation (small dose) combined with systemic vasoconstriction (larger dose), thereby producing a redistribution of blood flow to the kidney. Based on this finding, Cohn and colleagues proposed a possible role for this agent in the management of HRS. Unfortunately, additional studies were not undertaken.

Recently, there has been renewed interest in the hemodynamic derangements and attempts to improve renal function by countervailing the hyperdynamic state associated with cirrhosis. Lenz et al[46] investigated the effects of the infusion of ornipressin on renal and circulatory function. In a preliminary report, they observed that ornipressin reversed the hyperdynamic state. Concomitantly, there was improvement in renal function, as assessed by a more than 70% increase in creatinine clearance and a doubling in urine flow. These preliminary observations lend support to the concept that the peripheral vasodilation of liver disease contributes importantly to the renal dysfunction. Consequently, maneuvers that counter the vasodilation may possibly prove to be of benefit in improving renal function. In this regard, clinical trials that attempt to reverse the HRS should be undertaken with additional vasoactive agents that selectively increase systemic vascular resistance.

Dialysis

Dialysis, in general, has been reported to be ineffective in the management of HRS.[47] In spite of the dismal prognosis of HRS patients who receive dialysis, there are special circumstances when dialysis is justified. Thus, dialysis may be indicated for correction of fluid and electrolyte and acid-base disturbances and for prevention and treatment of pulmonary edema in patients in need of large volume replacement. Dialysis is also useful in patients who receive parenteral hyperalimentation. Hemodialysis rather than peritoneal dialysis is the therapeutic modality of choice, since the efficiency of peritoneal dialysis may be blunted by the presence of ascites.

The major problem encountered when employing hemodialysis in cirrhotic patients is severe hypotension. This results undoubtedly from the known cardiovascular instability of these patients, itself due to contracted plasma volume, ascites-induced hemodynamic changes, bleeding, and septic shock. Hypotension is difficult to control and frequently limits the usefulness of the dialysis. This problem can be circumvented by using continuous arteriovenous hemofiltration (CAVH). This technique allows successful mobilization of fluids and solutes with hemodynamic stability in a continuous rather than intermittent fashion.

CAVH has recently gained a great deal of popularity because of its simplicity and its ability to be used in most intensive care units. Since this procedure can be used to remove large amounts of fluid, it is the preferred choice of treatment in cirrhotic patients who suffer from volume overload, particularly if the patient manifests hemodynamic instability.

Aside from management of life-threatening complications in HRS, dialysis is indicated for several other conditions that combine liver-kidney failure (Table 99–2). It is, however, clear that the "typical" chronic alcoholic cirrhotic patient who has developed renal failure in the absence of the clinical situations outlined in Table 99–2 and failed to respond to volume expansion is not a candidate for dialytic therapy and almost invariably does not benefit from the procedure.

LIVER TRANSPLANTATION

Liver transplantation (LT) is the only definitive therapeutic modality that can be offered at the present time to patients with end-stage liver disease. In 1973, Iwatsuki et al[8] demonstrated for the first time that HRS can be reversed by orthotopic LT. In that report, two of three patients died in the perioperative period despite normal kidney function. Since then, there have been sporadic reports on long-term survival of these patients. In spite of the remarkable progress made in the technical aspects of LT and the remarkable increase in patients' survival, many of the published LT series do not make specific mention regarding the long-term kidney function in these patients. One study from Children's Hospital in Pittsburgh[48] reported that HRS was

TABLE 99–2. INDICATIONS FOR DIALYSIS THERAPY IN PATIENTS WITH LIVER AND KIDNEY FAILURE

- Acute fulminant liver disease when recovery from liver failure is expected
- While awaiting or undergoing consideration for liver transplantation
- When HRS is not the major cause of acute renal failure (e.g., aminoglycoside nephrotoxicity, contrast nephropathy, sepsis)
- When etiology of acute renal failure is not clear
- When uremia is a major factor in encephalopathy
- When obstructive jaundice is complicated by renal failure

present in 7 of 133 patients (5.3%) who underwent LT. Four of these seven patients recovered renal function 2 to 4 weeks after transplantation. More recent LT series in adult patients[49] found a 10% preoperative incidence of HRS (31 of 300 patients) (Table 99–3). These patients did quite well with a perioperative mortality (first 90 days) comparable to that of the patients without HRS (12.9% versus 9.5%). This was despite worse preoperative status (greater percentage in the intensive care unit) and rockier postoperative course, as evidenced by longer time in the intensive care unit and greater requirement for dialysis. Although the 1- and 2-year survival rates for patients with HRS were numerically less than the rates for patients without HRS, it was not statistically different. Assessment of kidney function (by iothalamate method) over time (2 years) revealed that 24 patients of 31 (77%) recovered sufficient renal function to avoid dialysis. Thus, with aggressive pretransplant and posttransplant management, one can expect excellent results following LT in patients with HRS.

Notwithstanding the comparable perioperative survival and long-term survival between patients with HRS and patients without HRS, there were some major differences between the two groups. Ten percent of patients with HRS developed end-stage renal disease after transplantation compared with 0.8% of patients who did not have HRS. Based on these data, more LT centers would consider a combined liver and kidney transplantation for patients with preoperative HRS. In spite of the low incidence of end-stage renal disease, patients without HRS have a progressive decline in GFR following the transplantation. In the series published by Gonwa et al[49] a preoperative GFR of 97 ml/min was decreased to 47 ml/min 3 years after transplantation. A progressive decline in renal func-

TABLE 99–3. RENAL EFFECTS OF LIVER TRANSPLANTATION IN 300 PATIENTS WITH AND WITHOUT HEPATORENAL SYNDROME (HRS)

	NON-HRS	P VALUE	HRS
Number of patients	263	–	31
Age (y)	44 ± 31	NS	41 ± 1
GFR (ml/min)*			
Preoperative	97 ± 3	<0.001	20 ± 4
(2 mo)	57 ± 2	<0.001	33 ± 3
(1 y)	63 ± 3	<0.05	46 ± 6
(2 y)	58 ± 4	<0.05	38 ± 6
(3 y)	47 ± 7	–	–
Patient survival (%)			
1 y	87	NS	77
2 y	82	NS	77
3 y	80	NS	66
4 y	79	NS	65

Adapted from Gonwa TA, Morris CA, Goldstein RM, et al. Long-term survival and renal function following liver transplantation in patients with and without hepatorenal syndrome: experience in 300 patients. *Transplantation*. 1991;51:428–430.
Results are mean ± SE.
*[135]Iodothalamate technique.
NS = not significant.

tion has also been described in infants and children who have survived liver transplantation.[50] The mechanism for this long-term reduction in kidney function is not absolutely clear. Chronic cyclosporine nephrotoxicity probably plays a major role in this regard.

Renal dysfunction in the immediate post-LT period is not only related to pretransplant HRS but can result from a host of acute insults to the kidney in this setting. In fact, it is the current experience in most transplant centers that virtually all patients (more than 90%) undergoing LT exhibit an elevation of serum creatinine of at least 50% above their baseline value. Important factors that appear to play a role in acute renal dysfunction include hypotension due to blood loss, endotoxemia, suboptimal renal perfusion during the anhepatic stage, drug nephrotoxicity (mainly, cyclosporine), sepsis, and de novo HRS secondary to graft dysfunction. It is possible that preexisting renal disease (albeit, unrecognized clinically) is a predisposing factor for post-LT acute renal failure. Intraoperative needle renal biopsies were performed during LT in 18 patients with nonalcoholic liver disease at the Royal Brisbane Hospital.[51] The authors reported that despite preserved Ccr, all patients had variable glomerular abnormalities. Eight had minor glomerular changes, whereas seven exhibited the classic hepatic glomerulosclerosis associated with cirrhosis. The causal relationship between the presence of these lesions before LT and the development of renal dysfunction after LT is entirely conjectural at this time. In a most recent report, the group at Baylor[52] demonstrated that the use of venovenous bypass during the anhepatic phase protected the systemic and renal hemodynamics during the operation but did not prevent early post-LT renal failure. Intraoperative or long-term postoperative verapamil showed no protective function against post-LT renal dysfunction.

Because of the potential role of cyclosporine in inducing acute renal dysfunction, it is recommended that this immunosuppressive drug be withheld until a post-LT diuresis begins. The nephrologist caring for these patients should also be aware of the fact that patients who have had a LT may receive very large intraoperative fluid replacement (of the order of 10 to 30 L). Therefore, ultrafiltration may be required to control severe fluid overload. Dialysis may be indicated to correct symptoms of renal failure and to treat acid-base and electrolyte abnormalities that may accompany the post-LT renal failure.

SUMMARY

The appearance of HRS in a patient with acute or chronic liver disease is associated with dismal outcome. Thus, management of HRS remains a formidable challenge to the aggressiveness and perseverance of the physician. The best treatment for the HRS remains prevention based on avoidance of circulating volume contraction or the use of nephrotoxic drugs. Treatment for established HRS remains a frustrating experience with recovery being rare. A successful liver transplantation is currently the only definitive treatment that can reverse HRS. As this procedure is being performed with increasing frequency and encouraging results, a new window of hope has been opened for these patients.

REFERENCES

1. Halstead AC, Nanji AA. Artifactual lowering of serum creatinine levels in the presence of hyperbilirubinemia. *JAMA*. 1984;251:38–39.
2. Papadakis MA, Arieff AI. Unpredictability of clinical evaluation of renal function in cirrhosis: prospective study. *Am J Med*. 1987;82:945–952.
3. Epstein M. Hepatorenal syndrome. In: Epstein M, ed. *The Kidney in Liver Disease*. 3rd ed. Baltimore, Md: Williams & Wilkins; 1988:89–118.

4. Papper S. Hepatorenal syndrome. In: Epstein M, ed. *The Kidney in Liver Disease.* 2nd ed. New York, NY: Elsevier Science Publishing Co Inc; 1983:87–106.
5. Goldstein H, Boyle JD. Spontaneous recovery from the hepatorenal syndrome: report of four cases. *N Engl J Med.* 1965;272:895–898.
6. Flint A. Clinical report on hydro-peritoneum, based on an analysis of forty-six cases. *Am J Med Sci.* 1863;45:306–339.
7. Kopple MH, Coburn JW, Mims MM, et al. Transplantation of cadaveric kidneys from patients with hepatorenal syndrome: evidence for the functional nature of renal failure in advanced liver disease. *N Engl J Med.* 1969;280:1367–1371.
8. Iwatsuki S, Popovtzer MM, Corman JL, et al. Recovery from hepatorenal syndrome after orthotopic liver transplantation. *N Engl J Med.* 1973;289:1155–1159.
9. Epstein M, Berk D, Hollenberg N, et al. Renal failure in the patient with cirrhosis. *Am J Med.* 1970;49:175–184.
10. Better OS, Schrier RW. Disturbed volume homeostasis in patients with cirrhosis of the liver. *Kidney Int.* 1983;23:303–311.
11. Kowalski HJ, Abelman WH. The cardiac output at rest in Laennec's cirrhosis. *J Clin Invest.* 1953;32:1025–1033.
12. Ring-Larsen H, Hesse B, Henriksen H, Christensen NJ. Sympathetic nervous activity and renal and systemic hemodynamics in cirrhosis: plasma norepinephrine concentration, hepatic extraction and renal release. *Hepatology.* 1982;2:304–310.
13. Vallance P, Moncada S. Hyperdynamic circulation in cirrhosis: a role for nitric oxide? *Lancet* 1991;337:776–778.
14. Tomas A, Soriano G, Guarner C, et al. Increased serum nitrite and nitrate in cirrhosis: relationship to endotoxemia. *J Hepatol.* 1992;16(suppl 1):4. Abstract.
15. Finberg JPM, Syrop HA, Better OS. Blunted pressor response to angiotensin and sympathomimetic amines in bile-duct ligated dogs. *Clin Sci.* 1981;61:535–539.
16. Lunzer MR, Manghani KK, Newman SP, et al. Impaired cardiovascular responsiveness in liver disease. *Lancet.* 1975;2:382–385.
17. Morandini G, Spanedda M. Contributo allo studio della reattività vascolare periferica all'an-giotensina ed alla noradrenalina in corso di affezioni epatiche. *Minerva Medica.* 1966;57:2175–2180.
18. Laragh JH, Cannon PJ, Bentzel CJ, et al. Angiotensin II, norepinephrine and renal transport of electrolytes and water in normal man and in cirrhosis with ascites. *J Clin Invest.* 1963;42:1179–1192.
19. Lenz K, Hortnagel H, Magometschnigg D, Kleinberger G, Druml W, Langger A. Function of the autonomic nervous system in patients with hepatic encephalopathy. *Hepatology.* 1985;5:831–836.
20. Epstein M, Schneider N, Befeler B. Relationship of systemic and intrarenal hemodynamics in cirrhosis. *J Lab Clin Med.* 1977;89:1175–1187.
21. Limas CJ, Guiha NH, Lekagul O, et al. Impaired left ventricular function in alcoholic cirrhosis with ascites. *Circulation.* 1974;69:755–759.
22. Gould L, Shariff M, Zahir M, et al. Cardiac hemodynamics in alcoholic patients with chronic liver disease and a presystolic gallop. *J Clin Invest.* 1969;48:860–864.
23. Binah O, Bomzon A, Blendis LM, et al. Obstructive jaundice blunts myocardial response to isoproterenol: a clue to the susceptibility of jaundiced patients to shock? *Clin Sci.* 1985;69:647–653.
24. Lee SS, Marty J, Mantz J, Samain E, Braillon A, Lebrec D. Desensitization of myocardial β-adrenergic receptors in cirrhotic rats. *Hepatology.* 1990;12:481–485.
25. Epstein M, Levinson R, Sancho J, et al. Characterization of the renin-aldosterone system in decompensated cirrhosis. *Circ Res.* 1977;41:818–829.
26. Cade R, Wagemaker H, Vogel S, et al. Hepatorenal syndrome: studies of the effect of vascular volume and intraperitoneal pressure on renal and hepatic function. *Am J Med.* 1987;82:427–438.
27. Epstein M, Lifschitz M, Ranachandran M, et al. Characterization of renal PGE responsiveness in decompensated cirrhosis: implications for renal sodium handling. *Clin Sci.* 1982;63:555–563.
28. Govindarajan S, Nast CC, Smith WL. Immunohistochemical distribution of renal prostaglandin endoperoxide synthase and prostacyclin synthase: diminished endoperoxide synthase in the hepatorenal syndrome. *Hepatology.* 1987;7:654–659.
29. Zipser RD, Radvan GH, Kronborg KJ, et al. Urinary thromboxane B_2 and prostaglandin E_2 in the hepatorenal syndrome: evidence for increased vasoconstrictor and decreased vasodilator factors. *Gastroenterology.* 1983;84:697–703.
30. Rimola A, Gines P, Arroyo V, et al. Urinary excretion of 6-keto-prostaglandin F_1 alpha, thromboxane B_2 and prostaglandin E_2 in cirrhosis with ascites: relationship to functional renal failure (hepatorenal syndrome). *Hepatology.* 1986;3:111–117.
31. Bichet DB, Van Putten VJ, Schrier RW. Potential role of increased sympathetic activity in impaired sodium and water excretion in cirrhosis. *N Engl J Med.* 1982;307:1552–1557.
32. Moore K, Wendon J, Frazer M, et al. Plasma endothelin immunoreactivity in liver disease and the hepatorenal syndrome. *N Engl J Med.* 1992;327:1774–1778.
33. Liehr H, Jacob AI. Endotoxin and renal failure in liver disease. In: Epstein M, ed. *The Kidney in Liver Disease.* 2nd ed. New York, NY: Elsevier Science Publishing Co Inc; 1983:535–551.
34. Dudley FJ, Kanel GC, Wood LJ, et al. Hepatorenal syndrome without avid sodium retention. *Hepatology.* 1986;6:248–251.
35. Carrilho F, Bosch J, Arroyo V, et al. Renal failure associated with demeclocycline in cirrhosis. *Ann Intern Med.* 1977;87:195–197.
36. Moore RD, Smith CR, Lietman PS. Increased risk of renal dysfunction due to interaction of liver disease and aminoglycosides. *Am J Med.* 1986;80:1093–1097.
37. Zager RA, Prior RB. Gentamicin and gram negative bacteremia: a synergism for the development of experimental nephrotoxic acute renal failure. *J Clin Invest.* 1986;78:196–204.
38. Epstein M. The peritoneovenous shunt in the management of ascites and the hepatorenal syndrome. *Gastroenterology.* 1982;82:790–799.
39. Linas SL, Schaffer JW, Moore EE, et al. Peritoneovenous shunt in the management of the hepatorenal syndrome. *Kidney Int.* 1986;30:736–740.
40. Stanley MM, Ochi S, Lee KK, et al. Peritoneovenous shunting as compared with medical treatment in patients with alcoholic cirrhosis and massive ascites. *N Engl J Med.* 1989;321:1632–1638.
41. Epstein M, Berk DP, Hollenberg NK, et al. Renal failure in the patient with cirrhosis: the role of active vasoconstriction. *Am J Med.* 1970;49:175–185.
42. Fevery J, Van Cutsem E, Nevens F, et al. Reversal of hepatorenal syndrome in four patients by peroral miso-

43. Loutzenhiser RD, Epstein M. The effects of calcium antagonists on renal hemodynamics (editorial review). *Am J Physiol.* 1985;249:F619–F629.
44. Gornel DL, Lancestremere RG, Papper S, et al. Acute changes in renal excretions of water and solute in patients with Laennec cirrhosis induced by the administration of the pressor amine, metaraminol. *J Clin Invest.* 1962;41:594–603.
45. Cohn JN, Tristani FE, Khatri IM. Systemic vasoconstriction and renal vasodilator effects of PLV-2 (Octapressin) in man. *Circulation.* 1964;38:151–156.
46. Lenz K, Hortnagel H, Druml W, et al. Beneficial effect of 8-ornithin vasopressin on renal dysfunction in decompensated cirrhosis. *Gut.* 1989;30:90–96.
47. Perez GO, Epstein M, Oster JR. Role of dialysis and ultrafiltration in the treatment of the renal complications of liver disease. In: Epstein M, ed. *The Kidney in Liver Disease.* 3rd ed. Baltimore, Md: Williams & Wilkins; 1987:613–624.
48. Wood RP, Ellis D, Starzl TE. The reversal of the hepatorenal syndrome in four pediatric patients following successful orthotopic liver transplantation. *Ann Surg.* 1987; 205:415–419.
49. Gonwa TA, Morris CA, Goldstein RM, et al. Long-term survival and renal function following liver transplantation in patients with and without hepatorenal syndrome: experience in 300 patients. *Transplantation.* 1991; 51:428–430.
50. McDiarmid SV, Ettenger RB, Fine RN, et al. Serial decrease in glomerular filtration rate in long-term pediatric liver transplantation survivors treated with cyclosporine. *Transplantation.* 1989;47:314–318.
51. Crawford DHG, Endre ZH, Axelsen RA, et al. Universal occurrence of glomerular abnormalities in patients receiving liver transplants. *Am J Kidney Dis.* 1992;19:339–344.
52. Gunning TC, Brown MR, Swygert THF, et al. Perioperative renal function in patients undergoing orthotopic liver transplantation: a randomized trial of the effects of verapamil. *Transplantation.* 1991;51:422–427.

100

Alcoholic Liver Disease

FLORENCE WONG and LAURENCE BLENDIS

Alcohol is the single most common cause of chronic liver disease in the Western world. Alcoholic liver disease is defined as the development of liver damage following long-term heavy alcohol consumption. It ranks fourth as a cause of death in adults between the ages of 20 and 70 years in the United States and Canada. In terms of health costs, it equals the treatment of many cancers. This is not yet taking into account the social costs of chronic alcoholism, the silent forerunner of alcoholic liver disease, in terms of loss of productivity and disruption to personal and family lives. Therefore, the development of a treatment strategy toward controlling alcoholism and its medical complications has of necessity become important.

MANAGEMENT OF CHRONIC ALCOHOLISM

Chronic alcoholism is a behavioral disorder that is often unrecognized, especially in the absence of alcoholic liver disease. It is composed of tolerance, physical dependence, impaired control over drinking, craving during abstinence, and continued drinking despite its destructive effects. Diagnosis is often difficult, especially in the silent drinker who maintains an appearance of functional stability. Every effort should be made to identify patients with alcoholism, as continued drinking adversely affects prognosis (Table 100–1). Recent alcohol intake can be detected by alcohol levels in blood, urine, and sweat. For those who abstain on the day of sampling, current research is exploring the development of objective biochemical markers. Acetaldehyde, the first metabolite of alcohol, has been shown to form adducts by binding to a variety of proteins. Adducts are now being investigated as potential markers of drinking, and antibodies are being used to detect their presence in serum.[1] Indeed, various studies have indicated that this approach is showing promise. Similarly, desialylated transferrin or carbohydrate-deficient transferrin is also being developed to identify the drinking pa-

TABLE 100-1. LABORATORY MARKERS OF EXCESSIVE ALCOHOL CONSUMPTION

MARKER	ABNORMAL IN ALCOHOLIC PATIENTS WITH ≥60 G DAILY INTAKE	COMMENTS
γ-glutamyltranspeptidase	70–80%	A sensitive (90%) but nonspecific marker of alcoholism; not reliable in patients receiving enzyme-inducing medications
Aspartate aminotransferase (AST)	30–75%	Indicative of alcoholic liver disease; although high levels suggest severe liver damage, low levels may not correspond to minimal liver injury
Alanine aminotransferase (ALT)	30–45%	Poor marker of alcoholic liver injury
AST-ALT ratio >1	90%	Highly suggestive of alcoholic hepatitis or cirrhosis or both
Mean corpuscular volume	75–90%	Present even in the absence of folate and vitamin B_{12} deficiency because of alcohol's direct action on developing erythrocytes
High-density lipoprotein–cholesterol (HDL-cholesterol)	50–80%	Graded increase with low levels of alcohol consumption; not a reliable index of alcohol abuse; severe liver disease with impaired liver function tends to lower HDL-cholesterol levels
Transferrin	81%	Abnormal only in patients with alcoholic liver disease with normal AST
Uric acid	10%	Levels increase with increasing alcohol consumption

All tests are fairly nonspecific but when combined with other observations contribute to an accurate diagnosis of alcoholism and alcoholic liver disease.
Adapted from Holt S, Skinner HA, Israel Y. Early identification of alcohol abuse: clinical and laboratory indicators. Addiction Research Foundation of Ontario, Canada.

tient. The levels of this protein are elevated in heavy drinking and fall with abstinence.

Once alcoholism is recognized, the physician is obliged to confront the patient and begin intervention. Detailed treatment strategy of chronic alcoholism is beyond the bounds of this review, but the patient must be seen safely through withdrawal, and then appropriate referral must be made to help the patient maintain long-term sobriety, as the best treatment for the dependent alcoholic patient is abstinence.

THE TREATMENT OF ALCOHOL WITHDRAWAL

The benzodiazepines have remained the treatment of choice for acute alcoholic withdrawal. They not only control the sympathetic overactivity associated with withdrawal, but can also prevent seizures and possibly delirium tremens. Benzodiazepines probably act on the inhibitory c-aminobutyric acid (GABA)-benzodiazepine receptor complex. Chlordiazepoxide, a long-acting benzodiazepine, can be given either as a single large bolus or as tapering doses over several days.[2] The optimal dosage should be individualized, as patient response may vary. Since most benzodiazepines are metabolized more slowly in patients with liver disease, a conservative dosage regimen is indicated, as a large bolus may prove to be an overdose. Oxazepam or lorazepam may be preferred, since they are metabolized by glucuronidation, a pathway not affected by liver disease.

Chlormethiazole, a short-acting sedative, is an alternative for the treatment of acute alcoholic withdrawal. It appears to act via mechanisms that differ from those of the benzodiazepines. It does not interact with the GABA- or benzodiazepine-binding sites, and yet it potentiates the inhibitory effects of GABA. The mechanism by which chlormethiazole enhances the inhibitory effects of GABA is not known. Given as frequent tapering doses over several days, chlormethiazole can be used to safely sedate the patient during withdrawal. Once again, the dosage must be individualized, as the drug is extensively metabolized by the liver; bioavailability depends on the functional capacity of the liver.

Attention must also be given to fluid and electrolyte replacement and avoidance of hypoglycemia in the ill patient. Thiamine and other water-soluble vitamins should be administered, as vitamin deficiency is common in these patients.

The safety of unmedicated withdrawal has remained a difficult question. It is true that patients with mild withdrawal symptoms can be managed without medications. However, recent literature suggests that increases in plasma cortisol during withdrawal may be damaging to the hippocampus, an area important for learning and memory. Furthermore, a succession of unmedicated withdrawals may eventually culminate in more severe withdrawal and even seizures. Therefore, withdrawal without medications, although less expensive because it can be done outside the hospital setting, may not be a suitable option for many.

LONG-TERM SOBRIETY MAINTENANCE

During abstinence, craving for alcohol appears unpredictably and often of sufficient intensity to override any serious intention to remain alcohol free. Controlled drinking to overcome this craving has been advocated, but enthusiasm for this treatment option has waned, as it is now recognized that the best goal for the alcoholic patient is total abstinence. This is particularly so in the patient with alcoholic liver disease. Pharmacotherapy, behavioral modification, and psychosocial support have remained the mainstay of treatment for long-term maintenance for sobriety.

Disulfiram produces irreversible inhibition of acetaldehyde dehydrogenase. The accumulation of acetaldehyde contributes to the unpleasant reaction after alcohol ingestion in patients treated with disulfiram. It has been used as a deterrent to alcohol consumption and an aid to the overall management of selected alcoholic patients in an integrated program. However, disulfiram was not found to be superior to placebo in a recent study comparing its effect on total abstinence, although the number of drinking days was reduced.

New pharmacotherapeutic agents are now being developed to attenuate the pathologic craving for alcohol. In particular, newer knowledge gained in the understanding of neuroscience is employed. Opioid antagonists may be useful in the early weeks after withdrawal to reduce craving and the probability of relapse.

Abstinence must be monitored, and early detection of relapse in patients who have been rehabilitated is an important part of therapy. Random blood or urinary alcohol levels and c-glutamyl transpeptidase have been used in the past to identify those who have succumbed to the temptation of alcohol. Now on the horizon are markers, such as acetaldehyde adducts, that will not only allow detection of drinking but also provide an objective means of assessing various treatment modalities, thereby improving the chance for survival for the alcoholic patients.

TREATMENT OF ALCOHOLIC LIVER DISEASE

Three types of histologically detectable alcohol-induced liver damage are recognized: fatty liver, alcoholic hepatitis, and cirrhosis. Fatty liver is usually a benign, reversible condition that disappears on abstinence from alcohol. Alcoholic hepatitis can present acutely with high mortality or be present in a chronic form. It is a condition characterized by liver cell necrosis and inflammatory reaction. It may occur separately or in combination with established cirrhosis. Alcoholic cirrhosis is micronodular. Widespread pericellular fibrosis around hepatocytes is prominent (especially in zone 3 of the liver acinus) and extends to portal areas as the disease progresses. Extensive fibrosis contributes to the development of portal hypertension with its many complications. Therefore, therapy of alcoholic liver disease should aim at reducing hepatic damage and preventing cirrhosis. The pivotal factor in the treatment of alcoholic liver disease is prolonged abstinence from alcohol and good nutritional support, together with specific drug therapies for certain indications. Abstinence alone has been shown to improve clinical status and survival.

FATTY LIVER

Fatty liver occurs commonly after ingestion of moderate amounts of alcohol. Ethanol ingestion leads to increased triglyceride synthesis, decreased lipid oxidation, and impaired secretion by the liver. This results in the accumulation of triglycerides in the hepatocytes within 3 to 7 days. The fat is usually macrovesicular and less often microvesicular. Initially, fat accumulates mostly in zone 3, while in the more severely affected, it becomes diffuse. Alcoholic fatty liver in the ambulatory population is usually asymptomatic. Severe fatty infiltration is associated with malaise, anorexia, nausea, jaundice, and tender hepatomegaly. Portal hypertension with splenomegaly, and occasionally bleeding varices may occur in the most severe cases. The treatment of fatty liver requires recognition of the problem and therapy for alcohol withdrawal, together with an adequate diet. With this regimen, fat disappears from the liver in 4 to 6 weeks.

Acute Alcoholic Hepatitis

Patients with alcoholic hepatitis are usually malnourished. There is a 2- to 3-week prodrome of fatigue, anorexia, nausea, and weight loss. Clinical signs include a mild fever, tender hepatomegaly, and jaundice. In the most severe cases, which usually follow a period of binge drinking, the patient is gravely ill with fever, marked jaundice, ascites, and evidence of a hyperdynamic circulation such as systemic hypotension and tachycardia. Florid spider nevi are usual on the skin. Hepatic decompensation can be precipitated by vomiting, diarrhea, intercurrent infection, or gastrointestinal tract bleeding, leading to encephalopathy and liver failure. The clinical picture may occasionally be confused with fulminant viral hepatitis, especially since viral markers are more common in patients with alcoholic liver disease; however, in acute alcoholic hepatitis there is usually a history of heavy drinking, and evidence of hepatic decompensation is more prominent.

Histologically, alcoholic hepatitis is characterized by a combination of inflammation and necrosis, on a background of hepatocyte enlargement and macrovesicular steatosis. The hepatocyte nucleus is small and hyperchromatic. On hematoxylin and eosin (H & E), alcoholic hyaline or Mallory's bodies are purplish red intracytoplasmic inclusions consisting of randomly orientated intermediate microfilaments. Polymorphs are seen surrounding cells that contain Mallory's bodies and damaged hepatocytes.

Collagen deposition is maximal in the sinusoidal Disse's space and terminal hepatic venular regions and extends in a perisinusoidal pattern to enclose hepatocytes, giving a "chicken wiring" effect. Blood in the liver acinus normally flows from the periportal (zone 1) to the perivenular (zone 3) area, therefore making zone 3 relatively hypoxic with respect to zone 1. The increase in hepatic metabolism due to increased alcohol oxidation renders zone 3 more hypoxic. This in turn is exacerbated by the combination of hepatocyte swelling and collagen deposition, causing sinusoidal compression and portal hypertension. Chronically, this results in the development of shunts, further exacerbating zone 3 hypoxia. Collagen deposition also increases the resistance to flow and reduces sinusoidal perfusion. This renders the normally relatively hypoxic zone 3 to be even more susceptible to hypoxic damage (Table 100–2). Changes in the portal triad are often inconspicuous. When the acute inflammation settles, a varying degree of fibrosis is seen, which may eventually lead to cirrhosis.

TABLE 100–2. CAUSES OF ZONE 3 HYPOXIA IN ALCOHOLIC LIVER DISEASE

Intrahepatic Predisposing Factors
Zone 3 normally hypoxic relative to zone 1
Disse's space expansion due to collagen deposition and capillarization
Defenestration of sinusoidal endothelial membrane
Hepatocyte enlargement compressing sinusoidal lumen
Portosystemic shunts aggravated by sinusoidal compression

Extrahepatic Predisposing Factors
Chronic anemia as a result of chronic blood loss or nutritional deficiency
Chronic obstructive pulmonary disease secondary to smoking

Extrahepatic Precipitating Factors
Acute anemia from hemorrhage that causes systemic hypotension
Sleep apnea with hypoxia
Pneumonia with hypoxia
Anesthetic that causes decreased hepatic perfusion
Alcoholic stupor or coma with hypoxia

Therapy in acute alcoholic hepatitis has been directed toward reducing the severity of the necroinflammatory process and preventing hepatic fibrosis. In addition, attempts to improve the nutritional status of the patient and stimulate hepatic regeneration have also been tried. Clinical trials have reviewed various treatment modalities, and the results are summarized as follows.

Nutritional Supplementation

The severity of protein-calorie malnutrition has been shown to correlate with the severity of liver disease and mortality. Achievement of positive nitrogen balance by oral, enteral, or parenteral route has been suggested to improve survival in hospitalized patients with alcoholic hepatitis. Furthermore, severely ill patients with or without hepatic encephalopathy have an abnormal amino acid pattern characterized by a decrease in the levels of branched-chain amino acids and an increase in aromatic amino acid. Therefore, many trials have been conducted to manipulate various combinations of nutritional supplements in an attempt to improve the well-being of these patients.

Enteral feeding in malnourished alcoholic patients improves digestibility and protein and fat absorption. Several studies assessing the effect of either oral or enteral feeding with branched-chain amino acids have shown improvement in nutritional parameters and liver function tests but not in mortality.[3]

Parenteral amino acid supplementation for 1 month in patients with moderately severe biopsy-proven alcoholic hepatitis resulted in more rapid clinical improvement in one study. There was greater improvement in nitrogen balance and greater resolution of fatty infiltration on histologic examination. However, this early advantage was no longer apparent at the end of 1 month, and survival was not affected. Another study reported that parenteral amino acid supplementation resulted in greater clinical and laboratory improvement and improved survival. In the most recent study conducted by Mezey et al,[4] patients were randomized to receive either amino acids and dextrose or dextrose alone. Five and six patients died in the control and treatment groups, respectively. Parenteral amino acid supplementation improved nutritional status but did not affect 1-month or 2-year follow-up survival.

Despite the lack of effect on survival, patients who were treated with amino acids continued to have improvement in serum bilirubin, prothrombin time, retinol-binding protein, and transferrin even after discharge from the hospital. Quite remarkably, the patients tolerated the amino acid infusions well with no evidence that the infusions promoted the development of hepatic encephalopathy. Many patients maintain an improved nutritional status after completion of their course of amino acid therapy.

Corticosteroids

There have been 12 randomized controlled trials evaluating corticosteroid therapy in patients with alcoholic hepatitis. Possible mechanisms of action include inhibition of hepatic necrosis and secondary inflammation, blunting of immunologic responses that perpetuate liver injury, modification of cytokine production including tumor necrosis factor, reduction of collagen production, and suppression of the acetaldehyde adducts–induced antibody production. It is now generally agreed that corticosteroids are of no benefit in the treatment of patients with mild-to-moderate disease. However, corticosteroids were noted to improve the 1-month survival in a subset of patients with severe illness, manifested by encephalopathy, prolonged prothrombin time, or elevated bilirubin. Similar findings were noted in a study where either prednisolone or placebo was administered to 55 patients for 1 month. Six of 31 patients who received placebo died compared to only 1 of 24 patients who received prednisolone. A discriminant function of greater than 32 emerged as a predictor of poor prognosis and favorable response to corticosteroid therapy.

Discriminant function = 4.6 × (Prothrombin time − Control prothrombin time) (in seconds) + Serum bilirubin (in 1mol/L) ÷ 17.[5]

Subsequent meta-analysis of the various studies confirmed a protective effect of corticosteroids in a subgroup of severely ill patients with encephalopathy.[6] Corticosteroid therapy also resulted in more rapid improvement in serum aspartate aminotransferase (AST), bilirubin, albumin, and prothrombin time. However, there is no clear benefit of corticosteroids in patients with encephalopathy secondary to gastrointestinal tract bleeding. In fact, corticosteroids may actually be detrimental.

Propylthiouracil

Patients with alcohol-induced liver disease often have evidence of hepatic hypermetabolism. The relative hypoxia of zone 3 of the liver acinus makes it more vulnerable to ischemic damage. Therefore, it would seem reasonable to reduce hypermetabolism and oxygen consumption in this area to minimize hypoxic damage. Propylthiouracil was suggested because it reduced the hypoxic damage in the liver in animals with alcohol-induced hypermetabolic state that were exposed to low oxygen tension. Two studies assessing the use of propylthiouracil at a dosage of 300 mg/d in patients with acute alcoholic hepatitis reported an improvement in their clinical state but not survival. Another group of investigators failed to show any short-term benefit of therapy. Subsequently, a much larger randomized controlled study by Orrego et al[7] assessing the long-term effects of propylthiouracil in chronic alcoholic liver disease reported a significantly reduced mortality in the treated group. The patients who benefited most were those with severe disease and who consumed the least alcohol. Those who continued to drink heavily were not protected by therapy. Thus far, there have been no further double-blind controlled trials of long-term propylthiouracil therapy. At present, propylthiouracil is not widely used in patients with chronic alcoholic liver disease, although minimal side effects (except occasional clinical hypothyroidism) have been found.

Anabolic Steroids

Enthusiasm about anabolic steroids waxed and waned over the years. Administration of oxandrolone, 80 mg/d for 1 month, did not affect survival during the time of treatment. However, in those who survived the acute phase, there was a significant improvement in survival in those with moderate but not severe alcoholic hepatitis at 6 months compared to placebo or prednisolone alone. In another study, oxandrolone combined with branched-chain amino acid supplements resulted in an increase in survival in a subgroup of patients with alcoholic hepatitis and moderate protein-calorie malnutrition. No such effect was seen in patients with mild or severe malnutrition. In a multicenter trial of long-term testosterone therapy (200 mg three times daily) from Copenhagen, there was no evidence that testosterone improved survival, liver function, or histologic findings when compared to placebo.[8]

Insulin and Glucagon

A number of hormones have been used to stimulate liver regeneration following necrosis. Insulin and glucagon have been studied in four separate trials to assess their hepatotropic effect. All studies administered daily infusions of either insulin or glucagon or placebo for 3 weeks. Two of these studies reported favorable outcome in terms of improved survival and liver function parameters. The other two, however, did not support the use of insulin or glucagon. Equal numbers of patients died in the treated and placebo groups. Furthermore, there is the added danger of inducing hypoglycemia in patients who are already at risk for hypoglycemic episodes. Therefore, insulin and glucagon should not be used in the treatment of alcoholic hepatitis.

D-Penicillamine

The rationale for using D-penicillamine lies in the fact that it interferes with the cross-linking of collagen molecules, thereby reducing collagen synthesis. Two small trials assessing the use of D-penicillamine in patients with alcoholic hepatitis showed no improvement in survival, although in one of these reports, a second liver biopsy specimen revealed less hepatocellular injury and fibrosis in patients in the treated group.

CIRRHOSIS

Established cirrhosis is usually a disease of middle age after many years of drinking. The onset of cirrhosis is often insidious, and a history of alcoholic hepatitis may not be always present. Advanced cirrhosis can develop in apparently well-nourished, asymptomatic patients. This is particularly so in social drinkers. When symptoms do occur, they often are nonspecific and include fatigue, anorexia, weight loss, nausea, and abdominal discomfort. Occasionally, the patient may present with end-stage liver disease with malnutrition, ascites, encephalopathy, and bleeding tendency. Rapid deterioration should raise the suspicion of a complicating hepatocellular carcinoma.

The treatment for uncomplicated cirrhosis consists of abstinence from alcohol and a balanced nutritious diet that is not restricted in protein but reduced in salt. Multivitamins and folic acid should be given if there is evidence of vitamin deficiency or in those with poor dietary intake. In malnourished anorexic patients, oral or enteral supplements of amino acids or casein as the protein source should be given. Administration of up to 80 g of branched-chain amino acids per day can improve nitrogen balance without worsening of mental status.

Colchicine

Colchicine interferes with the assembly of microtubules and the transcellular movements of collagen and increases the production of collagenase in vitro. In patients with cirrhosis of all causes including alcohol, treatment with colchicine at a dose of 1 mg/d led to an improved 5-year survival in one Mexican study.[9] In addition, liver histologic findings also improved in 18% of the treated patients. However, no clear benefit was seen before 30 months of therapy. It is uncertain how effective colchicine is in patients who continue to drink alcohol. Additional controlled trials are presently ongoing.

Liver Transplantation

Liver transplantation is being increasingly considered as a treatment option for patients with alcoholic cirrhosis who have recognized their alcoholism and achieved sobriety. The 1-year survival rate in patients who required a liver transplant because of alcoholic cirrhosis is similar to that found in patients who required a liver transplant for other conditions.[10] In a recent report from Pittsburgh, 7% of patients who required liver transplants because of alcoholic liver disease returned to alcohol abuse with varying severity of liver damage. With the growing disparity between availability of donor organs and demand, the optimal period of abstinence before transplantation is still the subject of debate. Therefore, liver transplantation cannot be provided for the majority of patients with end-stage alcoholic cirrhosis.

Prognosis of Alcoholic Liver Disease

When fatty liver is not associated with alcoholic hepatitis, the prognosis is excellent. It is completely reversible on cessation of alcohol. It is generally not regarded as a precirrhotic lesion, and the 1-year mortality has been estimated to be 6%.

The prognosis for patients with alcoholic hepatitis is variable and depends on the severity of the acute lesion and the presence or absence of underlying cirrhosis. Bad prognostic indicators are encephalopathy, low serum albumin, elevated serum bilirubin above 340 lmol/L, and a prolonged prothrombin time to more than 8 seconds above control value. Patients with alcoholic hepatitis and encephalopathy have the worse prognosis, with 1-year mortality of 50% reported in one series. Those with hepatitis not complicated by encephalopathy still have a 1-year mortality of 20%. Long-term follow-up of patients with alcoholic hepatitis revealed that almost 40% of these patients develop cirrhosis after a mean period of 3.3 years. Interestingly, 50% of these patients have alcoholic hepatitis without progressing to cirrhosis. Once cirrhosis is superimposed on alcoholic hepatitis, the 5-year survival rate is only 46%, with most of the deaths occurring in the first year after diagnosis.

Inactive cirrhosis without any complications is associated with a favorable prognosis, similar to that of alcoholic steatosis, especially in those who stop drinking alcohol. The 5-year survival rate is reduced from 89% to 68% in those who continue to drink alcohol. Once complications occur, the 5-year survival rate is reduced to 60% in the abstainers and 34% in those who continue to abuse alcohol. Clinical features with bad prognostic significance include encephalopathy, ascites, peripheral edema, and presence of collateral circulation.

THE FUTURE

Better understanding of the pathogenesis of alcoholic liver disease has led to the development of new tools for earlier detection of alcoholism and research into specific therapies for its many complications. Perivenular fibrosis is a predictor of rapid progression to cirrhosis in patients who continue to drink alcohol. Increased serum levels of tissue inhibitor of metalloproteinase have been shown to correlate with the development of cirrhosis and therefore could serve as a screening marker of those individuals who have a greater propensity to develop cirrhosis. Polyunsaturated lecithin has been found to prevent acetaldehyde-mediated increase in collagen accumulation, possibly by increasing collagenase activity. It can therefore potentially be used to prevent the progression from perivenular fibrosis to cirrhosis. Antagonists to cytokines or antibodies to cytokine receptors could block the cytokine-induced hepatocellular necrosis of alcoholic hepatitis. Similarly, prostaglandins, with their cytoprotective properties, have been demonstrated to exert some protection against alcohol-induced mitochondrial injuries in rats and therefore may be beneficial in patients with alcoholic hepatitis. Finally, oxygen free radicals have been shown to mediate hepatic injuries produced by alcohol. Substances, such as allopurinol, that inhibit enzymes involved in the production of oxygen free radicals are now being evaluated. Prospects for more successful medical treatments of alcoholic liver disease are therefore promising in the foreseeable future.

REFERENCES

1. Crabb DW. Biological markers for increased risk of alcoholism and for quantitation of alcohol consumption. *J Clin Invest.* 1990;85:311–315.
2. Romach MK, Sellers EM. Management of alcohol withdrawal syndrome. *Annu Rev Med.* 1991;42:323–340.
3. Mendenhall C, Bongiovanni G, Goldberg S, et al. VA cooperative study on alcoholic hepatitis III: changes in protein-calorie malnutrition associated with 30 days' hospitalization with and without enteral nutrition therapy. *JPEN.* 1985;9:590–596.
4. Mezey E, Caballeria J, Mitchell MC, et al. Effects of parenteral amino acid supplementation on short-term and long-term outcomes in severe alcoholic hepatitis: a randomized controlled trial. *Hepatology.* 1991;14:1090–1096.
5. Ramond MJ, Poynard T, Rueff B. A randomised trial of prednisolone in patients with severe alcoholic hepatitis. *N Engl J Med.* 1992;326:507–512.
6. Reynolds TB, Benhamou JP, Naccarato R, Orrego H. Treatment of acute alcoholic hepatitis. *Gastroenterol Int.* 1989;2:208–216.
7. Orrego H, Blake JE, Blendis LM, Compton KV, Israel Y. Long term treatment of alcoholic liver disease with propylthiouracil. *N Engl J Med.* 1987;317:1421–1427.
8. The Copenhagen Study Group for Liver Diseases. Testosterone treatment of men with alcoholic cirrhosis, a double blind study. *Hepatology.* 1986;6:807–813.
9. Kershenobich D, Vargas F, Garcia-Tsao G, et al. Colchicine in the treatment of cirrhosis of the liver. *N Engl J Med.* 1988;218:1709–1713.
10. Starzl TE, Van Thiel D, Tzakis AG, et al. Orthotopic liver transplantation for alcoholic cirrhosis. *JAMA.* 1988;260:2542–2544.

101
Variceal Bleeding

CHARLES N. BERNSTEIN

Esophageal varices result from portal hypertension. Gastric and intestinal varices may also result from portal hypertension, although gastric varices may arise in the setting of splenic vein thrombosis. Varices in these extraesophageal sites are less common than esophageal varices and are not as frequently diagnosed as the cause of severe upper gastrointestinal tract hemorrhage. Portal hypertension caused by primary extrahepatic obstruction of the portal vein or secondary to noncirrhotic portal fibrosis (seen typically in India and Japan) carries a better prognosis than portal hypertension secondary to cirrhosis. Worldwide the most common cause of portal hypertension is probably schistosomiasis, whereas in the West the most common cause is alcoholic cirrhosis. The origin and severity of the underlying cause of portal hypertension impacts on the morbidity and mortality after variceal bleeding.

Approximately 50% of patients with cirrhosis have esophageal varices, and of these patients, one third eventually experience variceal bleeding. For patients with cirrhosis, each variceal bleeding episode has a mortality of approximately 50%. The rebleeding rate is 25% to 35% within 6 weeks and may be as high as 70% overall. Of patients with esophageal varices who present with an upper gastrointestinal tract bleeding episode, endoscopy reveals that one third have actively bleeding varices, one third have varices that are not bleeding but no other lesion is present, and one third have another nonvariceal source for the bleeding. The challenges to the clinician caring for these patients are to determine the exact cause of bleeding in the patient with varices, stop the acute bleeding, prevent recurrent bleeding after an initial bleeding episode, and determine if any impact can be made on the underlying cirrhosis or portal hypertension to prevent progression. Another strategy is to consider some form of prophylactic therapy to prevent initial variceal bleeding.

INITIAL MANAGEMENT OF ACUTE VARICEAL BLEEDING

The initial management of patients with acute variceal bleeding is resuscitative. This includes adequate volume support with crystalloid and usually blood transfusion. Since patients with cirrhosis are predisposed to hepatic encephalopathy and since these patients are at added risk for encephalopathy when there is a large intestinal protein load like blood, an assessment of the patient's ability to maintain his airway is mandatory. There should be a low threshold to perform endotracheal intubation in patients with cirrhosis whose mental status is altered during upper gastrointestinal tract hemorrhage. Patients require hemodynamic monitoring and are best cared for in an intensive care unit.

A complete blood count and a prothrombin time should be checked and platelets should be transfused if the count is less than 50,000/mm³ or if the patient has a clear history of recent aspirin ingestion. In the setting of recent aspirin ingestion, an alternative approach to improve platelet adhesiveness, albeit unproven, is the use of desmopressin (DDAVP). If the prothrombin time is prolonged, plasma should be transfused, and vitamin K should be administered subcutaneously (although vitamin K does not have a short-term effect). Serial blood counts should be checked to dictate the need for further blood transfusion. The patient should be lavaged with a large-bore orogastric tube (i.e., Ewald tube) to facilitate endoscopy. The endoscopy should be performed as early as possible once the patient's vital signs have been stabilized and the blood parameters are known. If the patient is particularly combative or obtunded, he might require endotracheal intubation for airway protection and for facilitating the endoscopy. Approximately 50% of patients stop bleeding spontaneously, so all therapeutic interventions must be judged accordingly.

ACHIEVING INITIAL HEMOSTASIS

SCLEROTHERAPY

Sclerotherapy has become the primary treatment for bleeding esophageal varices after endoscopic diagnosis is made.[16] In North America, sclerotherapy is typically performed in a freehand fashion through a flexible endoscope and with intravariceal injections. The optimal approach is to begin injecting at or just below the spurting variceal site or at the gastroesophageal junction in the patient who is not acutely bleeding. Approximately 2 ml are injected into each varix at 2 cm intervals along the course of each varix moving from distal to proximal, for at least three injections, or to ensure that the distal 5 to 6 cm of the varices are sclerosed, since this is where variceal bleeding usually occurs. All varices (not just the spurting one) are injected, if possible, during the initial session. In Europe, paravariceal injections are more popular, and some centers advocate a combination of intravariceal and paravariceal injections. It has been shown that up to 40% of attempted intravariceal injections are actually paravariceal, and as much as 40% of what is injected by the intravariceal route is carried away systemically. In North America, combinations of sodium tetradecyl sulphate or morrhuate sodium and alcohol or saline are usually used as the injected solution. In Europe, polidocanol or ethanolamine are often used.

Esophageal sclerotherapy can induce hemostasis in approximately 90% of patients with acute variceal bleeding. Only 30% of patients experience acute rebleeding during hospitalization and require further sclerotherapy or alternate therapy. Ninety percent of these patients achieve hemostasis with a second session of sclerotherapy. In those patients who then embark on a course of long-term sclerotherapy, a clear reduction in rebleeding has been shown; however, no sclerotherapy trials have impacted acute mortality. The most common complication of esophageal variceal sclerotherapy is esophageal stricture formation, which usually can be managed easily medically. Esophageal perforation or inducing bleeding occurs in 3% of cases. Postinjection fever may occur up to 50% of the time and depends on the sclerosing agent, since it is more common with fatty acid–based agents than with water-soluble ones. If fever occurs, it subsides within 48 hours. Bacteremia may occur after sclerotherapy, but antibiotic prophylaxis is not typically recommended unless there are more specific indications (i.e., rheumatic heart disease, prosthetic heart valves, or a history of spontaneous bacterial peritonitis in patients who have ascites). Substernal chest pain is also common after injection sclerotherapy and also subsides within 48 hours. If endoscopic sclerotherapy is not available or fails or early rebleeding occurs, then pharmacologic therapy or balloon tamponade are often considered.

PHARMACOLOGIC THERAPY

Vasopressin is administered intravenously by constant infusion. The literature reveals that the therapeutic efficacy of achieving initial hemostasis is 50% to 70%. Vasopressin, by vasoconstricting the splanchnic circulation and also lowering cardiac output, decreases portal inflow and therefore portal pressure. The side effects are mostly related to its vasoconstricting properties, including coronary ischemia and arrhythmias, mesenteric ischemia, and increased gut motility, causing abdominal pain and peripheral vascular and cerebrovascular ischemia. The dose used is 0.3 to 0.9 U/min, and the use of a bolus dose is of questionable benefit. Nitroglycerin, which is a powerful vasodilator (particularly on the venous circulation), has been added to vasopressin therapy to limit the cardiotoxic effects of vasopressin.[2] Nitroglycerin may also lower portal pressure by reducing portal resistance and by limiting portal flow through systemic venodilation. Nitroglycerin can be administered by constant intravenous infusion adjusted to a systolic blood pressure of at least 90 mm Hg, or by the sublingual or transdermal route. It is crucial to recognize that there is a tolerance to nitrates after 24 to 48 hours of consecutive administration. Because of the questionable benefit of vasopressin compared to controls in randomized studies and because of significant side effects, use of vasopressin has been abandoned in some centers as a therapeutic option. Terlipressin is a vasopressin analog that has been used in Europe with a view that there will be less side effects seen with terlipressin than with vasopressin. Another advantage of terlipressin is that it can be administered in bolus doses every 6 hours. There is a lack of data supporting terlipressin as being a therapeutic advance over vasopressin.

Somatostatin also functions as a mesenteric vasoconstrictor, either through direct effects on the mesenteric vascular smooth muscle or through hormonal effects (i.e., inhibiting glucagon, a smooth muscle relaxant). Somatostatin at a dosage of 250 1g bolus and 250 1g/h infusion over 5 days has been shown to be more effective than placebo at controlling variceal bleeding.[4] The one multicenter US study[17] showing it to be less effective than placebo had a remarkable 83% cessation of bleeding rate on placebo. In that trial 65% of the patients who were given somatostatin stopped bleeding. This rate is compatible with other data collected for somatostatin, including trials that directly compared its use to vasopressin. Somatostatin lacks the side effects of vasopressin, although it is considerably more expensive. It may find a role as a temporizing measure prior to sclerotherapy. No data are available on the use of the long-acting analog octreotide (Sandostatin).

Drugs that increase lower esophageal sphincter pressure may reduce variceal bleeding by compressing the varices and reducing their blood flow. Metoclopramide has been shown to significantly reduce transmural variceal pressure when measured by direct puncture of the varices. Other vasoactive agents that may find a role in the management of variceal bleeding and in reducing portal hypertension include clonidine, a central-acting a-adrenergic agonist, and serotonin antagonists.

Although vasopressin and nitroglycerin or somatostatin may control variceal bleeding, no pharmacologic agent has been shown to impact patient mortality.

Balloon Tamponade

The two main types of balloon devices used for variceal tamponade are the Linton-Nachlas (LN) tube (gastric balloon and two separate ports to aspirate esophageal and gastric contents) and the Sengstaken-Blakemore (SB) tube (gastric balloon, esophageal balloon and a port to aspirate the stomach). A variation on the SB tube is the Minnesota tube, which has a fourth port for aspirating the esophagus. Balloon tamponade provides initial hemostasis in up to 90% of patients. However, up to 40% of these patients rebleed during the initial hospitalization. The main complication from these devices is pulmonary aspiration. Other complications include esophageal and gastric ulceration and perforation. The complication rate may be as high as 10%. Almost invariably patients treated with these devices should have an endotracheal tube in place, and a pair of scissors should be kept at the bedside to cut the tube at the first sign of respiratory compromise. Either tube may be placed through the nose or the mouth, and traction should be kept on the tube via a pulley and a 1-kg weight or by taping the tube to a face guard on a football helmet. The gastric or esophageal balloons should not be inflated for longer than 48 hours.

One trial that directly compared the LN tube to the SB tube found a statistically significant advantage for achieving hemostasis in bleeding esophageal varices using the SB tube.[12] There was an advantage, although not statistically significant, for achieving hemostasis with the LN tube in gastric varices. In a trial of SB tube tamponade compared to vasopressin infusion in patients with Child's classes A and B cirrhosis, the two modalities of therapy achieved similar initial hemostasis rates. Another trial showed similar efficacy of an SB tube compared to a terlipressin and nitroglycerin combination. Sclerotherapy has been shown to have a statistically significant better rate of hemostasis than SB tube therapy in two controlled trials. Thus, if sclerotherapy is not available or fails, balloon tamponade may be useful for achieving hemostasis until more definitive therapy can be performed, such as a second round of sclerotherapy, transjugular intrahepatic portosystemic shunt (TIPS) procedure, or surgery.

Surgery

Portosystemic shunting procedures are the most successful way of achieving hemostasis for bleeding varices with success rates of 95%. However, in the acute bleeding setting mortality may be as high as 50% in the patients who have Child's class C cirrhosis. Esophageal staple transection is also effective at inducing and maintaining hemostasis. Recently the group at the Royal Free Hospital[3] has shown this surgical modality to achieve hemostasis in 90% of patients as a primary therapy (when compared to sclerotherapy in a randomized controlled trial) or as a salvage therapy in those patients who failed to stop bleeding after sclerotherapy. Adding a devascularization procedure to esophageal transection may increase the operative risk and therefore is best reserved for more elective cases. Orthotopic liver transplantation is the most definitive surgery for control of portal hypertension.

Other Therapies

Variceal band ligation is gaining more widespread use, as similar rates of hemostasis have been achieved when this technique has been compared to sclerotherapy.[15] This technique is performed through a flexible endoscope and requires an overtube to be in place, since the band device needs to be reloaded after each band is placed. The bands are placed beginning at the gastroesophageal junction and within 6 cm of the gastroesophageal junction on each varix. Follow-up banding sessions are undertaken similar to sclerotherapy. Injection of cyanoacrylate glues into varices has been advocated in Europe but has only been used experimentally in North America.

Emergency percutaneous transhepatic obliteration of varices relies on selective catheterization of the left and short gastric veins feeding gastroesophageal varices to introduce agents for variceal obliteration or embolization. This procedure has been abandoned in favor of the TIPS procedure. This technique is performed by radiologists who place an expandable, flexible metallic stent intrahepatically. A large early report has come from San Francisco where the investigators found no immediate complications from the procedure, a significant reduction in portal pressure, and excellent early hemostasis rates. They found this therapy to be a useful adjunctive technique, allowing the patients to undergo successful orthotopic liver transplantation.[14] Other investigators subsequently have reported portosystemic encephalopathy rates comparable to those seen from surgical shunts and high rates of TIPS occlusion at 1 year.

PREVENTION OF RECURRENT BLEEDING

Variceal bleeding is likely to recur in at least 70% of patients who are treated medically after an acute esophageal or gastric variceal hemorrhage. The risk of rebleeding rapidly diminishes over the first few days after an episode of variceal bleeding, but the risk of rebleeding returns to baseline within 2 to 3 months. The most crucial management step in reducing variceal rebleeding for patients with alcoholic cirrhosis is to stop all alcohol consumption.

SCLEROTHERAPY

In many centers long-term sclerotherapy is the accepted approach for reducing rebleeding rates.[10,16] However, it will be likely of no benefit in the alcoholic patient who continues to drink alcohol. For sclerotherapy to be effective, it is imperative that sessions are continued within days after the initial hemostasis is achieved, at weekly to biweekly intervals until all varices are obliterated. This usually takes 4 to 6 sessions. A repeat endoscopy should be performed at 6- to 12-month intervals to detect recurrent varices, which should be reinjected if they occur. Approximately 50% of patients enrolled in chronic sclerotherapy rebleed, but this usually occurs before complete eradication is achieved. All trials have shown sclerotherapy to effectively reduce rebleeding rates, but sclerotherapy only impacts mortality if the patients survive the first 3 to 6 months after initial variceal bleeding. A recent series of 1000 consecutive patients treated with sclerotherapy in Japan revealed that after a mean of 4.2 sessions, 78% of patients achieved complete eradication of esophageal varices. Varices recurred at a rate of 22%. Sclerotherapy-related transient esophageal strictures occurred in 137 patients and were uniformly dilated with Maloney dilators.[8]

Other than esophageal strictures, major complications, which are uncommon, include perforation and bleeding from esophageal ulceration. Esophageal ulcers are an expected sequelae of effective sclerotherapy. Both omeprazole and sucralfate have been reported to be useful adjunctive agents in the management of postsclerotherapy ulceration. Chronic esophageal variceal sclerotherapy in the patient with prominent gastric varices is controversial. There is a theoretic risk of increasing gastric variceal pressure if the esophageal channels are obliterated, particularly since it has been shown that portal pressure increases after obliterative sclerotherapy. In patients with gastroesophageal varices, particularly when neither site has stigmata of recent hemorrhage (active bleeding or adherent clot), surgical therapy should be considered. It has been shown that portal hypertensive gastropathy may worsen after esophageal variceal sclerotherapy. Variceal band ligation has been shown to achieve variceal eradication and reduce rebleeding similarly to sclerotherapy. It may be associated with fewer nonbleeding complications, like esophageal stricture, compared to sclerotherapy.

PHARMACOLOGIC THERAPY

Propranolol given twice daily in a dose sufficient to reduce resting heart rate by 25% was shown in a large randomized, controlled French study to prevent recurrent variceal or gastric mucosal bleeding in well-compensated patients with alcoholic cirrhosis.[1] A subsequent study from Scotland later confirmed these results, including a successful reduction of rebleeding in patients with Child's class C cirrhosis. In this later study, there still was a 39% rebleeding rate at 2 years of follow-up in patients with Child's class C cirrhosis.[6] Two other studies confirmed an advantage for b-blocker therapy, but three other randomized controlled trials did not confirm these results. Several of these studies have found an "early" (2 to 6 weeks after acute bleeding) high incidence of rebleeding in the patients treated with propranolol.

Propranolol acts by reducing splanchnic arterial inflow (secondary to a fall in cardiac output and an increased resistance in the splanchnic vessels) and a consequent decrease in portal and portocollateral flow. Propranolol has been shown to reduce portal pressure, although patients who benefit from this drug may not have their hepatic venous pressure gradient (HVPG) reduced to less than 12 mm Hg, the value below which variceal bleeding is not seen. Propranolol may increase portal vascular resistance because it has been shown to reduce portal pressure to a smaller degree than portal vein flow.

Propranolol provided no additional benefit to repeated sclerotherapy in lowering rebleeding rates in one trial. When compared to sclerotherapy as a primary therapy for reducing rebleeding rates, propranolol has been shown to have a comparable benefit. One trial showed that a combination of propranolol plus isosorbide-5-mononitrate lowered HVPG to a greater extent than propranolol alone. However, it remains to be proved whether this combination translates into better clinical efficacy. Propranolol has been shown to lower rebleeding rates in variceal bleeding from noncirrhotic portal hypertension caused by schistosomiasis and bleeding from portal hypertensive gastropathy. Propranolol has been shown to have few adverse effects in patients with cirrhosis, and the fear that patients would be unable to hemodynamically respond should they have a rebleeding episode has not been borne out. The usual contraindications to b-blocker use apply, and, of course, compliance with the drug regimen may be an issue. Calcium channel blockers have also been considered for long-term management.

SURGERY

Portosystemic shunt surgery is the gold standard for reducing rebleeding from varices with success rates as high as 95%. Portacaval and mesocaval shunts were initially advocated, but the more technically demanding distal splenorenal shunt has gained greater acclaim. This shunt is thought to reduce the incidence of encephalopathy following shunt surgery, because more hepatopedal flow is preserved, while being far enough away from the portal bed so as to not interfere with prospective orthotopic liver transplantation. Nonetheless, in the studies directly comparing the selective distal splenorenal shunt to the nonselective shunts, no differences were found in the incidence of encephalopathy after shunt surgery. Preoperatively, it is difficult to predict who will likely suffer from significant postoperative encephalopathy. The group at Emory University has shown that patients with alcoholic cirrhosis may have a lower survival after shunt surgery than patients with nonalcoholic cirrhosis.[9] Portosystemic and distal splenorenal shunts may thrombose over time.

Shunt surgery has not been shown to have any effect on long-term survival, which depends on the evolution of the underlying liver disease. Reported operative mortality ranges from 1% to 20% and varies depending on the severity of the liver disease. The incidence of encephalopathy after shunt placement ranges from 4% to 40% (although disabling encephalopathy is seen in less than 10%).

Shunt surgery has found a firm place in the management of patients who have failed sclerotherapy or in patients with nonesophageal variceal bleeding. The group at Emory University recently reported that particularly alcoholic patients treated with sclerotherapy had an improved mortality compared to patients treated with selective shunt surgery and that rescue shunt surgery was very effective in those patients who rebled after sclerotherapy (35% of the sclerotherapy group).[9] Other studies have not found a survival advantage for either modality but have confirmed the usefulness of surgical rescue in patients who fail sclerotherapy.

Other successful nonshunt surgical interventions have included esophageal transection with and without devascularization and splenectomy. Finally, all patients who experience a variceal bleeding episode should be evaluated for orthotopic liver transplantation, although sclerotherapy, one of the surgical techniques, or possibly the TIPS procedure can certainly buy time for transplantation.

PROPHYLACTIC THERAPY

Since nearly one third of patients with varices bleed and since the mortality associated with each bleed is approximately 50%, there has been a significant interest in treating either the varices specifically or the portal hypertension prophylactically. The key issue that most prophylactic studies have not addressed is selecting the very high-risk patients for inclusion in the studies. One reason for this is that it has been difficult to accurately predict which varices are likely to bleed. The factors that seem to be predictive of variceal bleeding include the following:

1. Size of varices
2. Specific variceal characteristics (red wale markings, cherry red spots or veins on veins)
3. HVPG greater than 12 mm Hg
4. Child-Pugh score
5. Continued alcohol ingestion

Variceal wall tension, a product of the size of the varices and the variceal pressure, is thought to be the major factor determining variceal rupture. One study found size and HVPG to be independent predictors and advocated that determination of HVPG is indicated to predict which patients should be treated.

Pharmacologic Therapy

Groszmann et al[4] studied the effect of propranolol prospectively compared to placebo in patients with cirrhosis and varices who had not yet experienced variceal bleeding. The dose of propranolol chosen for each patient was based on a 25% reduction in HVPG or a decrease in heart rate to less than 55 beats/min after short-term administration of the drug. At 3 months the group receiving propranolol had a significant reduction in the HVPG (by 14%), whereas the placebo group did not. By 12 months both groups showed comparable decreases in HVPG. The improvement in HVPG seen in the propranolol group had no relation to improvement in Child's score, as was seen in the placebo group. None of the patients who achieved a HVPG less than 12 mm Hg bled during follow-up. Although propranolol had a statistically significant effect at reducing the incidence of bleeding, the majority of patients receiving propranolol did not achieve a HVPG less than 12 mm Hg. It remains to be proved that sequential measurement of HVPG positively affects patient management.

Pascal et al[13] showed that propranolol compared to placebo could decrease the incidence of variceal bleeding and improve survival in a large group of mostly alcoholic patients. Since then, a number of trials have confirmed a beneficial effect of propranolol on decreasing the incidence of initial bleeding, including in patients with less severe liver disease.[11] A recently published meta-analysis reported that prophylactic propranolol could decrease bleeding incidence by 40% and decrease mortality by about 25%. The benefit at reducing bleeding is generally accepted; however, the benefit of impacting mortality is still questionable. When used, the usual dosage of propranolol required is approximately 160 mg/d; however, the dosage should be titrated to decrease heart rate by 25%. Nadolol has also been used and may have theoretic advantages over propranolol, since nadolol has less effects on renal blood flow and less central nervous system effects.

Sclerotherapy

Prophylactic sclerotherapy has been shown in some European studies to effectively reduce variceal bleeding. The large US Veterans' Affairs study[12] not only failed to show a reduction in bleeding in the patients treated with sclerotherapy, but also showed that sclerotherapy had a deleterious effect on patient mortality. A recent meta-analysis revealed that prophylactic sclerotherapy reduced the 13-month mortality by 13% and also significantly reduced initial bleeding rates, particularly in patients with alcoholism. Another meta-analysis revealed a positive effect only in those patients with a high risk of variceal bleeding and a negative effect in low-risk patients. Two recent studies have compared sclerotherapy to propranolol and to no therapy as prophylaxis. Neither study showed a beneficial effect of sclerotherapy. The key to prophylactic sclerotherapy is to ensure that all esophageal varices are eradicated, although in general, prophylactic sclerotherapy is not advised.

Surgical Therapy

Four earlier trials, revealed that portal decompressive surgery could reduce bleeding rates in patients with varices, but the technique was associated with unacceptably high mortality in the treated patients. A recent report from Japan using prophylactic portal nondecompressive surgeries, including esophageal transection, devascularization, and selective shunts, revealed a survival advantage for those patients undergoing the procedures.

OTHER CONSIDERATIONS

Acutely bleeding gastric varices may be treated with sclerotherapy or band ligation. Both techniques have been successful for achieving initial hemostasis when performed by skilled endoscopists. Large volumes of sclerosants and subsequent endoscopic treatment sessions are required. However, rebleeding rates are high. In general, bleeding gastric varices are best approached with a portal decompressive shunt or a TIPS procedure, unless they are secondary to splenic vein thrombosis, where a splenectomy is curative. Often gastric balloon tamponade is required to stop gastric variceal bleeding until more elective surgery can be undertaken. Portal decompression surgery or TIPS should also be considered for bleeding from portal hypertensive gastropathy. Use of b-blockers in this setting, although theoretically sound, is as yet unproven.

SUMMARY

After resuscitative measures, the patient with bleeding esophageal varices should undergo urgent upper endoscopy with variceal sclerotherapy or variceal band ligation. If the patient is too unstable for endoscopy, intravenous vasopressin with transdermal, sublingual, or intravenous nitroglycerin should be administered. Alternatively, intravenous somatostatin may be used, or the patient may be treated with balloon tamponade. If the patient fails to stop bleeding after endoscopic therapy, balloon tamponade can buy time until subsequent endoscopic therapy sessions are attempted or until the patient can be taken for urgent TIPS procedure, portal decompressive surgery, or nondecompressive surgery, such as esophageal transection.

If the patient has severe enough liver disease, he should be seriously considered for transplantation. To prevent rebleeding while the patient is awaiting transplantation or if the underlying liver disease is not too advanced, the primary therapy should be obliterative sclerotherapy or obliterative band ligation. As a primary alternative choice or if endoscopic therapy fails, the patient should undergo one of the surgical options or the TIPS procedure. b-Blockers may be substituted for any of these options, but these drugs have not been definitively proven to be of benefit in preventing rebleeding.

For patients who have never bled but who have a high risk of variceal bleeding as determined by the varices' endoscopic characteristics, by the severity of the underlying liver disease, or by the HVPG, prophylactic b-blockers should be used, but sclerotherapy or prophylactic surgery are not advocated.

For patients who drink alcohol, the primary recommendation should be abstinence whether the setting is to prevent recurrent bleeding or primary bleeding.

REFERENCES

1. Andreani T, Poupon RE, Balkav BJ, et al. Preventative therapy of first gastrointestinal bleeding in patients with cirrhosis: Results of a controlled trial comparing propranolol, endoscopic sclerotherapy and placebo. *Hepatology.* 1990;12:1413–1419.
2. Bosch J, Groszmann RJ, Garcia-Pagan JC, et al. Association of transdermal nitroglycerin to vasopressin infusion in the treatment of variceal hemorrhage: a placebo-controlled clinical trial. *Hepatology.* 1989;10:962–968.
3. Burroughs AK, Hamilton G, Phillips A, Mezzanote G, McIntyre N, Hobbs KEF. Comparison of sclerotherapy with staple transection of the esophagus for the emergency control of bleeding from esophageal varices. *N Engl J Med.* 1989;321:857–862.
4. Burroughs AK, McCormick PA, Hughes MD, Sprengers D, D'Heygere F, McIntyre N. Randomized, double-blind, placebo-controlled trial of somatostatin for variceal bleeding. *Gastroenterology.* 1990;99:1388–1395.
5. Conn HO. Prophylactic propranolol: the first big step. *Hepatology.* 1988;8:167–170.
6. Garden OJ, Mills PR, Birnie GG, Murray GD, Carter DC. Propranolol in the prevention of recurrent variceal hemorrhage in cirrhotic patients. *Gastroenterology.* 1990;98:185–190.
7. Groszmann RJ, Bosch J, Grace ND, et al. Hemodynamic events in a prospective randomized trial of propranolol versus placebo in the prevention of a first variceal hemorrhage. *Gastroenterology.* 1990;99:1401–1407.
8. Hashizume M, Kitano S, Koyanagi N, et al. Endoscopic injection sclerotherapy for 1,000 patients with esophageal varices: A nine-year prospective study. *Hepatology.* 1992;15:69–75.
9. Henderson JM, Kutner MH, Millikan WJ, et al. Endoscopic variceal sclerosis compared with distal splenorenal shunt to prevent recurrent variceal bleeding in cirrhosis: a prospective randomized trial. *Ann Intern Med.* 1990;112:262–269.
10. Infante-Rivard C, Esnaola S, Villeneuve JP. Role of endoscopic variceal sclerotherapy in the long-term management of variceal bleeding: a meta-analysis. *Gastroenterology.* 1989;96:1087–1092.
11. Pagliaro L, Burroughs AK, Sorenson TIA, et al. Therapeutic controversies and randomised controlled trials (RCTs): prevention of bleeding and re-bleeding in cirrhosis. *Gastroenterol Int.* 1989;2:71–84.
12. Panes J, Teres J, Bosch J, Rhodes J. Efficacy of balloon tamponade in treatment of bleeding gastric and esophageal varices: results in 151 consecutive episodes. *Dig Dis Sci.* 1988;33:454–459.
13. Pascal JP, Cales P, Multicenter Study Group. Propranolol in the prevention of first upper gastrointestinal tract hemorrhage in patients with cirrhosis of the liver and esophageal varices. *N Engl J Med.* 1987;317:856–861.
14. Ring EJ, Lake JR, Roberts JP, et al. Using transjugular intrahepatic portosystemic shunts to control variceal bleeding before liver transplantation. *Ann Intern Med.* 1992;116:304–309.
15. Stiegmann GV, Goff JS, Sun JH, Davis D, Bozdech J.

Endoscopic variceal ligation: an alternative to sclerotherapy. *Gastrointest Endosc.* 1989;35:431–434.
16. Terblanche J, Burroughs AK, Hobbs KEF. Controversies in the management of bleeding esophageal varices (parts one and two). *N Engl J Med.* 1989;320:1393–1398 and 1469–1475.
17. Valenzuela JE, Schubert T, Fogel MR, et al. A multicenter, randomized, double-blind trial of somatostatin in the management of acute hemorrhage from esophageal varices. *Hepatology.* 1989;10:958–961.
18. The Veterans' Affairs Cooperative Variceal Sclerotherapy Group. Prophylactic sclerotherapy for esophageal varices in men with alcoholic liver disease: a randomized, single-blind, multicenter clinical trial. *N Engl J Med.* 1991;324:1779–1784.

102

Ascites

EDWARD P. TOFFOLON

Ascites is the abnormal accumulation of fluid in the peritoneal cavity. Clinically, this common entity has a broad spectrum of manifestations. Symptoms range from none in early stages to incapacitating in later stages. Similarly, physical findings may be absent initially but dramatically obvious when ascites is tense. Etiologies are numerous and pathophysiology variable. Finally, therapy also ranges from safe and simple to aggressive and invasive. All these aspects are discussed in more detail with particular emphasis on therapeutic options.

SYMPTOMS

Symptoms of ascites are absent when the volume of fluid is small. As the volume increases, vague symptoms of abdominal fullness and bloating are common. When ascites is tense, early satiety and anorexia can lead to malnutrition and loss of lean body mass. Interestingly, weight may not change because loss of tissue mass is balanced by the weight of fluid accumulation. In is final stages, respiratory embarrassment results from elevated diaphragms and severe pain from stretched peritoneal surfaces.

Physical findings are minimal in early stages of ascites accumulation. Interestingly, when ascites is moderate, the classic physical findings of flank dullness, fluid wave, and shifting dullness are accurate only 50% of the time.[1] This is an important fact to remember before performing a paracentesis in a patient suspected of having ascites. When ascites is massive, there is rarely any question that fluid is present in the abdomen. It is at this time that organ size can only be appreciated by the technique of balloting.

ETIOLOGIES

Decompensated cirrhosis is by far the most common cause of ascites, but any cause for portal hypertension may result in ascites (Table 102–1). Hypoalbuminemia is frequently associated with cirrhosis but rarely can be a sole contributor to ascites formation. Other benign causes include disturbances in lymph formation or clearance, inflammatory diseases of the peritoneum, pancreatic ductal disruption, and rare complications of renal failure. Malignant causes for ascites include malignant involvement of peritoneal surfaces, malignant blockage of lymphatic channels, and ovarian neoplasms (Table 102–1).

DIAGNOSIS

The diagnosis of small amounts of ascites is difficult because symptoms are vague and physical findings absent. As the amount of ascites increases, then the classic physical findings of bulging flanks, shifting dullness, and fluid wave begin to appear.

When the diagnosis of ascites is in doubt, an abdominal ultrasound is very helpful. The ultrasound is much more sensitive than either the

TABLE 102–1. ETIOLOGIES OF ASCITES

Benign
1. Portal hypertension
   a. Cirrhosis
   b. Hepatic congestion
      (1) Right ventricular failure
      (2) Constrictive pericarditis
      (3) Inferior vena cava obstruction
      (4) Hepatic vein obstruction (Budd-Chiari syndrome)
   c. Portal vein obstruction
2. Hypoalbuminemia
3. Pancreatic duct disruption
4. Renal failure
5. Urinary bladder or ureteral disruption
6. Chylous ascites
7. Tuberculous peritonitis
8. Myxedema

Malignant
1. Ovarian cancer (Meigs' syndrome)
2. Metastatic disease involving peritoneum
3. Malignant obstruction of inferior vena cava or hepatic vein
4. Lymphoma (obstructing lymphatic flow)

physical examination or a plain radiograph of the abdomen, and it is less expensive and cumbersome than a computed tomography or magnetic resonance image. Once the diagnosis of ascites is secure, a diagnostic paracentesis should be performed. Complications, such as hemorrhage or bowel perforation, would be anticipated in less than 1% of cases if simple guidelines are followed. Choosing a site in the avascular midline or left lower quadrant, avoiding surgical scars and the rectus muscle, and using a fine-bore needle in the presence of a coagulopathy are standard recommendations. Dilated bowel would increase the risk of perforation as would bowel adherent to the abdominal wall.

The analysis of the ascites should always include routine culture and sensitivity, cell count and differential, cytology, glucose and protein, and albumin. A simultaneously obtained serum albumin should also be obtained. Other tests on ascites fluid would be determined by the clinical setting, i.e., lactate dehydrogenase (LDH), amylase, mycobacterial or fungal culture, pH, lactate, triglyceride, and carcinoembryonic antigen (CEA).

The serum-ascites albumin gradient (SAAG) is the best way to distinguish ascites associated with portal hypertension from that due to neoplasm or inflammatory diseases. A gradient of 1.1 g/dl or greater indicates portal hypertensive ascites with an accuracy of greater than 95%.[2] Other gradients, i.e., total protein or LDH, or other absolute values, i.e., ascites total protein, have not been nearly as discriminating.

Perhaps the most important reason to perform a diagnostic paracentesis in a patient who appears to have "routine" cirrhotic ascites is to rule out spontaneous bacterial peritonitis (SBP). It has been well documented that patients with SBP need not have fever, abdominal pain, or tenderness. Neutrocytic ascites (polymorphs >250/ml) should be considered diagnostic of SBP and should trigger therapy with a broad spectrum antibiotic while waiting for culture results.[3] A culture negative for SBP in the face of neutrocytic ascites should be considered a false-negative, and treatment should be continued for 10 days. A second paracentesis should reveal a decreased polymorph count if the diagnosis is accurate and the treatment is effective. Direct inoculation of 5 ml of ascites into blood culture bottles in addition to sending samples for culture and sensitivity has been recommended to improve the yield of ascites culture.

PATHOPHYSIOLOGY

The most common cause of ascites is decompensated cirrhosis. The pathophysiology of ascites formation in cirrhosis is due to excessive hepatic lymph formation. As scarring progresses in the liver, the hydrostatic pressure in the hepatic sinusoid increases. This "driving" pressure causes increased amounts of protein-rich fluid to cross the sinusoidal membrane into the Disse space and then into hepatic lymphatics. The capacity of the hepatic lymphatics is eventually overcome, and lymph "weeps" off the liver into the peritoneal cavity.

The kidney plays an important role in ascites formation by retaining sodium and water despite a normal-to-increased blood volume and cardiac output in cirrhotic patients. There is a redistribution of central blood volume, perhaps explained by splanchnic congestion due to portal hypertension or by decreased systemic vascular resistance due to atrioventricular shunting in the extremities.[4] Increased levels of norepinephrine and antidiuretic hormone (ADH) and decreased levels of atrial natriuretic peptide support the concept of a decreased effective blood volume. Increased plasma renin activity, angiotensin, and aldosterone levels and a redistribution of intrarenal blood flow from cortex to medulla are consistent with the concept of decreased effective renal blood flow. This "underfill" theory is the most attractive explanation for renal sodium and water retention in cirrhotic patients with ascites.

MANAGEMENT

Since cirrhotic ascites is by far the most common form of ascites, we focus primarily on the treatment of this entity. Bed rest, a time-honored and effective modality to mobilize ascites, is too slow and consequently cannot be used as the sole therapy of hospitalized patients, especially in these days of managed care. Sodium restriction is frequently recommended and makes sense, although its importance has been debated in the literature. A 20-mEq sodium-restricted diet makes hospital food unpalatable and is rarely adhered to after discharge from the hospital. The importance of good nutrition should probably take precedence over sodium restriction. Fluid restriction to 1000 ml/d and sodium to 40 mEq/d is consistent with a nutritionally complete diet and is helpful in establishing negative fluid balance.

Spironolactone (Aldactone), an aldosterone inhibitor, is perhaps the safest diuretic for the management of ascites. It works by inhibiting aldosterone's effect on sodium reabsorption in the distal tubule. Its main drawback is delayed onset of action (up to 48 hours). An initial dosage of 100 mg/d is reasonable with slow increases to as high as 600 mg/d. Hyperkalemia may be a serious side effect, and consequently potassium supplementation should never be ordered for more than 24 hours without rechecking the serum potassium level. Although spironolactone has been shown to be effective in up to 75% of patients with ascites, much of that data comes from outpatient studies. More often than not, in hospitalized patients, if effective diuresis is not achieved in several days, a loop diuretic (furosemide or bumetanide) is added to the regimen. These powerful diuretics inhibit sodium reabsorption in the loop of Henle and cause marked increase in the delivery of sodium to the distal tubule at a rate that exceeds its capacity to reabsorb it. When loop diuretics are coupled with spironolactone, the sodium excretion by the kidney may be significantly increased. Ninety percent of patients respond to this combination with significant sodium and water excretion. The dose of furosemide required is between 40 to 120 mg/d. If the blood urea nitrogen (BUN) rises above 25% or 30%, one must weigh the risks of precipitating irreversible renal failure with the desire to rid the patient of ascites fluid.

Rarely, in patients with ascites that is difficult to mobilize, a third diuretic that acts on the proximal renal tubule (thiazide or metolazone) may be added. *Extreme caution* must be used because blocking the proximal tubule, loop of Henle, and distal tubule may result in rapid and profound fluid and electrolyte losses.

The goal of mobilizing ascites must be balanced against the risk of precipitating severe intravascular volume depletion, azotemia, electrolyte disturbances, and hepatic encephalopathy. A good rule of thumb is to limit negative fluid balance to 500 ml (~0.45 kg [1 lb] weight loss) per day in patients with ascites and no edema, or 1000 ml (~1 kg [2 lb] weight loss) per day in patients with ascites and edema. These guidelines are based on the data from the early 1970s,[5] which were redefined more recently. Even when guidelines are followed, frequent checks of BUN, creatinine, and electrolytes must be obtained.

Patients with ascites that is resistant to diuretic therapy or patients who develop significant complications of diuretics may be candidates for more invasive forms of therapy to remove ascites.

Therapeutic paracentesis of 5 L or more per session has recently been shown to be a very safe and effective method for removing ascites. Most physicians avoided "large-volume" paracentesis in the past for fear of precipitating renal underperfusion and the hepatorenal syndrome. Elegant studies from Barcelona have shown that plasma volume can be maintained and renal function preserved during large-volume paracentesis by the simultaneous intravenous administration of 25 to 50 g of albumin.[6] In fact, the Barcelona group makes a cogent argument that large-volume paracentesis for patients with tense ascites may be safer than diuretic therapy.[7] It is only fair to mention that the need for plasma volume expansion at the time of large-volume paracentesis has been debated in the literature. The risks of bleeding, perforation, or ascites leak could be avoided by paying close attention to the techniques and precautions that have been previously described. In this way, patients unresponsive to diuretics alone may be managed by diuretics and periodic large-volume paracentesis.

If reaccumulation of ascites is so rapid that paracentesis must be performed more frequently than every 2 to 3 weeks or if complications of paracentesis make subsequent procedures too uncomfortable or risky, then the transjugular intrahepatic portosystemic shunt (TIPS) may be considered. Recent studies have shown that patients with refractory ascites can now be maintained ascites free with minimal to no diuretic therapy after the TIPS procedure.[8] The risk of immediate complications from the TIPS procedure diminishes with the skill of the interventional radiologist. Significant hepatic encephalopathy occurs in a minority of patients. Patient's portal blood flow velocity is monitored on a regular basis by Doppler portal venography, and shunts may be modified as flow dynamics decrease or ascites reaccumulates.

Hopefully, the need to resort to peritoneovenous shunts can be avoided with our current therapeutic options for treating ascites. Peritoneovenous shunts have been associated with significant complications and do not improve survival when compared to medical management of ascites.[9] Similar comparative studies for TIPS are eagerly awaited.

REFERENCES

1. Callan EL Jr, Benjamin SB, Knuff TE, et al. The accuracy of the physical examination in the diagnosis of suspected ascites. *JAMA.* 1982;247:1164.
2. Runyon BA, Montano AA, Akriviadis EA, et al. The serum-ascites albumin gradient is superior to the exudate-transudate concept in the differential diagnosis of ascites. *Ann Intern Med.* 1992;117:215.
3. Runyon BA, Hoefs JC. Culture negative neutrocytic ascites: a variant of spontaneous bacterial peritonitis. *Hepatology.* 1984;4:1209.
4. Fernandez-Rodriguez CM, Prieto J, Zozaya JM, et al. Arteriovenous shunting, hemodynamic changes, and renal sodium retention in liver cirrhosis. *Gastroenterology.* 1993;104:1139.
5. Shear L, Chang S, Gabuzda GJ. Compartmentalization of ascites and edema in patients with hepatic cirrhosis. *N Engl J Med.* 1970;282:391.
6. Gines P, Tito LL, Arroyo V, et al. Randomized comparative study of therapeutic paracentesis with and without intravenous albumin in cirrhosis. *Gastroenterology.* 1988;94:1493.
7. Gines P, Arroyo V, Quintero E, et al. Comparison between paracentesis and diuretics in the treatment of cirrhosis with tense ascites. *Gastroenterology.* 1987;93:234.
8. Somberg KA, Lake JR, Tomlanovich SJ, et al. Transjugular intrahepatic portosystemic shunt for refractory ascites: assessment of clinical and humoral response and renal function. *Gastroenterology.* 1993;104:A998.
9. Stanley MM, Ochi S, Lee KK, et al. Peritoneovenous shunting as compared with medical treatment in patients with alcoholic cirrhosis and massive ascites. *N Engl J Med.* 1989;321:1632.

103
Spontaneous Bacterial Peritonitis

J. EILEEN HAY

Spontaneous bacterial peritonitis (SBP) is infection of ascitic fluid that occurs in the absence of a local source of infection. It is a common, frequently recurrent complication that, together with its variants, occurs in 10% to 30% of patients hospitalized with cirrhotic ascites.[1] The clinical presentation of SBP may be subtle and its recognition missed unless clinical suspicion is high. Yet once considered, the diagnosis can easily be made by diagnostic abdominal paracentesis to allow treatment with appropriate antibiotics.

SBP is defined by ascites, usually cirrhotic, with the following characteristics:

1. Ascitic fluid culture positive for pathogenic bacteria
2. Presence in the ascites of an increased polymorphonuclear neutrophil leukocyte (PMN) count
3. No intraabdominal source of infection.

In patients with the last two characteristics but a culture negative for bacteria, a diagnosis of culture-negative neutrocytic ascites (CNNA) is made. Since patients with CNNA behave in an identical manner clinically and biochemically to those with microbiologically confirmed SBP, they are assumed to represent cases missed by present culture techniques[2]; clinically such cases are considered a variant of SBP. The other variant, bacteriascites, is an ascitic fluid culture positive for bacteria without an increased PMN count and is usually the transient residence of bacteria in ascites.

PATHOGENESIS

CAUSAL ORGANISMS

The most frequently isolated bacteria in SBP are normal flora of the gastrointestinal tract; about 70% of cases are due to gram-negative bacilli, especially *Escherichia coli* (responsible for about half of all cases of SBP) and *Klebsiella* spp. Aerobic gram-positive cocci are the next most frequent etiologic agents with streptococci (in particular, *Streptococcus pneumoniae*) accounting for about 20% of cases and enterococci for 5%. Anaerobes rarely cause SBP (about 5% of cases), perhaps because the oxygen tension in ascites is too high to sustain their growth. Most infections are monomicrobial with only 10% polymicrobial.

PATHOGENETIC MECHANISMS

The frequent isolation of enteric bacteria in SBP suggests that most causal organisms originate from the gastrointestinal tract, a hypothesis supported by the success of selective bowel decontamination in preventing SBP due to susceptible organisms. Spontaneous bacteremias are also more common in cirrhotic patients, and now most experimental data support seeding of ascites, not directly through the bowel wall but from bacteremia. The mechanism(s) by which bacteria reach the bloodstream in cirrhotic patients is unknown, although bacterial translocation exacerbated by congestion and edema of the bowel wall because of portal hypertension may play a role; an additional factor may be shunting of portal blood away from the influence of the hepatic reticuloendothelial system.

Bacteremia in the cirrhotic patient may then be perpetuated by reduced phagocytic activity, impaired bactericidal activity of Kupffer's cells, and impaired peripheral destruction of bacteria and yeasts by neutrophils, the latter due to several defects including low serum complement levels, defective neutrophil chemotaxis and bactericidal immunoglobulin M (IgM) antibody activity, and decreased intracellular destruction of phagocytosed bacteria. The net result of the above defects is that bacteremia of whatever source persists longer in the cirrhotic patient and may be followed by colonization of ascites.

After seeding of ascites, whether SBP develops depends on the antibacterial effect of the ascites. The ascitic fluid of cirrhotic patients has been shown to have low complement levels, low opsonic activity, and reduced bactericidal activity, which therefore allows proliferation of bacteria and the production of infection.

PREDISPOSING FACTORS

Early recognition of SBP was almost exclusively in alcoholic cirrhosis; although SBP is most common in patients with alcoholism, it is now well established that SBP can occur in any type of cirrhotic ascites and occasionally in patients with Budd-Chiari syndrome and severe acute liver disease with ascites, e.g., viral or alcoholic hepatitis. Since ascites is a prerequisite for its development, SBP occurs only in the setting of decompensated liver disease, and patients who develop SBP generally have more severe liver disease than those who do not develop SBP. Patients with ascites and SBP have been shown to have lower ascitic complement levels and reduced opsonic activity, these parameters correlating very closely with the total protein concentration of the ascitic fluid.

It has now been well established by prospective studies that a major risk factor for the development of SBP is a low protein concentration of the ascitic fluid, with SBP occurring in about 20% of patients with ascitic fluid protein of less than 1 g/dl and in only 2% of those with protein levels greater than 1 g/dl.[1] Other predisposing factors are the occurrence of gastrointestinal tract hemorrhage and use of indwelling urinary catheters; whether endoscopy or sclerotherapy increases the risk is not firmly established, although case reports have demonstrated the temporal relationship between SBP and these procedures.

Patients who have already experienced an episode of SBP are very likely to have a further episode, and the recurrence rate at 1 year is at least 50% and as high as 70% in some series.

CLINICAL FEATURES

The typical patient with SBP is one hospitalized with advanced, decompensated liver disease; but even within this group of patients, the clinical spectrum of SBP is broad, ranging from a silent, asymptomatic state to a severe, rapidly fatal illness. Earlier reports describe the "typical" patient with sudden onset of fever, abdominal pain, general deterioration, large-volume ascites, and rebound tenderness. The onset, however, is often more insidious and can be asymptomatic in 10% of patients. Single elements of the typical presentation occur more frequently, with fever and abdominal pain being the most common presenting complaints, each occurring in about 60% of patients. Other common manifestations are encephalopathy, rebound tenderness, and decreased bowel sounds, with less frequent features being hypothermia, hypotension, diarrhea, renal dysfunction, and refractoriness to diuretic therapy. Although ascites is essential for SBP, in a small number of cases the ascites may not be clinically detectable.

Patients with SBP usually have a prompt response to antibiotic therapy, although this may be masked by other, often life-threatening complications of their liver disease. Although patients with CNNA are indistinguishable clinically (including response to antibiotics), biochemically, and by the Child-Pugh score from those with SBP, recent data have shown patients with CNNA have a lower PMN count and lower mortality than patients with SBP, suggesting that this may represent a less severe variant.[2] Patients with bacteriascites have less severe liver disease than patients in the other two categories.

The diagnosis of SBP and its variants cannot be made with certainty clinically and may well be obscured by other complications of the chronic liver disease. Diagnostic paracentesis is essential whenever there is any suspicion of infection. However, because the clinical presentation of SBP can be subtle and easily missed clinically, diagnostic paracentesis is also recommended in the following situations:

1. All patients who present with new onset ascites
2. All cirrhotic patients who are hospitalized for ascites
3. All patients with ascites who develop any compatible symptoms (e.g., fever, abdominal pain, encephalopathy, diarrhea, leukocytosis)
4. Any patient with stable ascites who deteriorates suddenly

It should be remembered that SBP not infrequently develops during hospitalization, necessitating consideration of a second paracentesis or more during the hospital stay.

Recent clinical factors predictive of the first episode of SBP have been sought. Univariate analysis has found poor nutritional status, increased serum bilirubin or aspartate aminotransferase (AST) level, reduced prothrombin activity, and reduced total protein concentration in the ascitic fluid to be predictive; multivariate analysis established the latter to be the most important predictor for a first episode of SBP.

DIAGNOSIS

DIAGNOSTIC CRITERIA FOR SBP, CNNA, AND BACTERIASCITES
(Fig. 103–1)

A presumptive diagnosis of SBP is made with the finding of neutrocytic ascites, i.e., greater than 250 PMN per milliliter of ascitic fluid, in a patient with cirrhosis and no secondary source of infection (see below). The ascites PMN count has been shown to be the main laboratory indicator for the presence of SBP with a diagnostic accuracy of about 90% and is used to establish the presumptive diagnosis until bacterial culture results are available. Confirmation is by ascitic fluid culture positive for bacteria. If the ascitic fluid culture is negative for bacteria in a patient who has received antibiotics, a presumed diagnosis of SBP is made, since it is rarely possible to isolate an organism from ascites in the presence of antibiotic therapy. If there has been no recent antibiotic therapy and there is no evidence for any other cause of neutrocytic ascites (e.g., cholecystitis, pancreatitis, intraperitoneal hemorrhage, or carcinomatosis), a diagnosis of CNNA is made. Because of their clinical similarities, it is likely that most, if not all, patients with CNNA are cases of SBP missed by present culture techniques.[2]

Bacteriascites is defined by an ascitic fluid count of less than 250/ml and a culture positive for bacteria, and it is usually the transient residence of bacteria in the ascitic fluid. Patients with bacteriascites generally have less severe liver disease than those with SBP, and usually it will clear spontaneously without antibiotic therapy[1,3]; indeed, in asymptomatic patients with bacteriascites, SBP rarely develops and signs and symptoms of infection are the best indicator of progression to SBP.[3] It does seem prudent, however, to repeat diagnostic paracentesis at the time of culture positivity; if at that time, neutrocytic ascites is present, the diagnosis of SBP can now be made. Where cultures are positive for non-

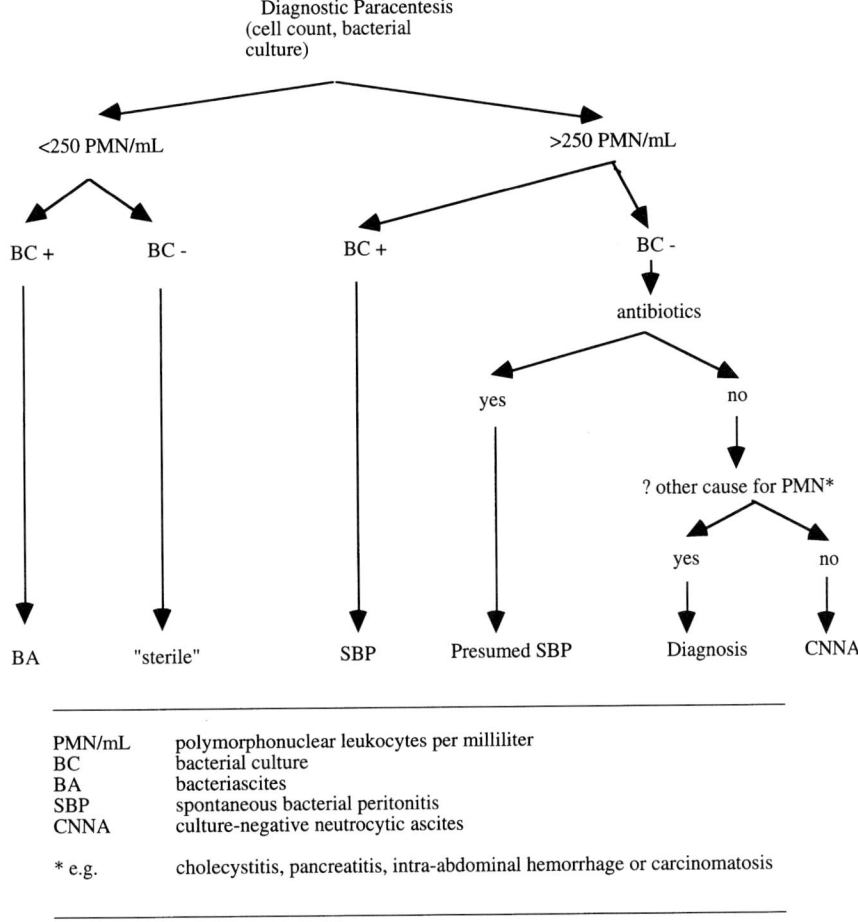

FIGURE 103–1. Algorithm for the diagnosis of spontaneous bacterial peritonitis. PMN/ml = polymorphonuclear neutrophil leukocytes per milliliter, BC = bacterial culture, BA = bacteriascites, SBP = spontaneous bacterial peritonitis, CNNA = culture-negative neutrocytic ascites.

pathogenic bacteria such as diphtheroids, *Bacillus,* and *Staphylococcus epidermidis* and the patient has neither symptoms nor neutrocytic ascites, contamination of the cultures has probably occurred.

DIAGNOSTIC PARACENTESIS

Ascitic fluid analysis is essential for the diagnosis of SBP and for appropriate antibiotic therapy. Abdominal paracentesis is an easy, safe procedure with a very low complication rate even in the presence of coagulopathy. The clinical indications for pursuing diagnostic paracentesis are given in the previous section.

Because the concentration of causal organisms in ascitic fluid is typically very low (one organism per milliliter), conventional laboratory culture techniques have historically yielded poor results. Microbiologic studies have now clearly established the greatly increased sensitivity of bedside (as opposed to laboratory) inoculation of larger volumes of ascites into media that provides enrichment for a small number of organisms[4] rather than selection of organisms. Bedside inoculation of blood culture bottles (e.g., tryptic soy broth), each with at least 10 ml of ascites, has greatly improved the sensitivity of culture techniques,[5] although 10% to 20% of cases continued to have negative culture results. In our own institution, conventional methods of culture, using direct laboratory inoculation of specimens onto agar plates and into thioglycollate broth, yielded very poor results with positive cultures in only 20% of patients; conversion to bedside blood culture techniques has increased this sensitivity to greater than 80%. Unfortunately, negative culture results are the rule where the patient has already received even one dose of antibiotics. Despite recent progress, there is still a need for improved culture techniques for SBP, especially in patients who have already received antibiotic therapy prior to the diagnostic paracentesis.

Ascitic fluid analysis should include a cell count (total white blood cells and PMNs), bacterial culture (aerobic and anaerobic), amylase, glucose and lactate dehydrogenase (LDH), the latter two parameters[6] being helpful in differentiating SBP from secondary infection.[6] Other ascitic fluid indexes (e.g., lactate and pH) have generally been found to offer little or no additional clinical information and have not proven as useful as the PMN count for the presumptive diagnosis of SBP. Routine culture for mycobacterial infection is not recommended and is reserved for cases in which there is high clinical suspicion; even in these cases, the sensitivity of ascitic fluid culture is poor, and peritoneoscopy is often necessary.

Blood cultures should also be performed when a diagnosis of SBP or its variants has been made, although positive results are found in only half the cases of SBP.[1]

DIFFERENTIAL DIAGNOSIS

The main differential diagnosis of SBP is secondary bacterial peritonitis, where ascites is infected from a local source, most commonly a perforated viscus (e.g., perforated peptic ulcer, ruptured appendix, or perforated diverticulum) or an abscess, particularly perinephric. Secondary bacterial peritonitis is less common than SBP, occurring in about 15% of cases, but it must be diagnosed to allow appropriate therapy. The operative mortality in cirrhotic patients with infected ascites is about 85%, but it is 100% in secondary cases without surgery.

Clinical features do not allow a reliable differentiation between SBP and secondary cases, and in all patients with infected ascites, surgically treatable sources of infection must be considered before a decision to treat with antibiotics alone is made. At the time of the initial paracentesis, two of the following criteria identify cases of secondary infection with high sensitivity but moderate specificity[6]; ascitic fluid total protein greater than 1 g/dl, glucose less than 50 mg/dl, and LDH greater than the upper limit of normal serum range. It has also been established that, although the ascitic fluid PMN count may rise in some patients after initiation of antibiotic therapy, it will have decreased to below the pretreatment levels in all patients with SBP after 48 hours of appropriate antibiotic therapy. However, about a third of patients with secondary bacterial peritonitis have 48-hour PMN counts above baseline.[6] Virtually all cases of secondary peritonitis have positive culture results, often by multiple organisms, and this culture is often still positive for bacteria after 48 hours of therapy. By contrast, in SBP ascitic fluid becomes sterile in greater than 80% of cases after a single dose of antibiotic.

In summary, factors suggesting secondary infection are a very high white cell count in ascites (>10,000 cells/ml), multiple organisms, unusual organisms (anaerobes or fungi), ascitic fluid glucose less than 50 mg/dl, or LDH greater than the upper limit of normal for serum and an increase in ascitic PMN count with antibiotic therapy.[6]

All patients with bacterial peritonitis should undergo a plain and upright abdominal x-ray examination to detect free air, a urine culture, and chest x-ray examination; with suspicion for secondary bacterial peritonitis, emergency investigations with computed tomography (CT) scan of the abdomen, surgical consultation, and water-soluble contrast studies of the gastrointestinal tract must be considered.

TREATMENT

ANTIBIOTIC THERAPY

Intravenous antibiotics are indicated as soon as a presumptive diagnosis of SBP is made, i.e., when the PMN count of the ascitic fluid is greater than 250/ml or with a typical clinical picture independent of the PMN count. Therapy is continued in all patients subsequently diagnosed with SBP or CNNA. Because more than 90% of cases are due to gram-negative aerobes (predominantly *E. coli* and *Klebsiella* spp.) or gram-positive cocci (predominantly streptococci), cefotaxime, a third-generation cephalosporin, in doses of 1 to 2 g intravenously every 6 to 8 hours is generally the first choice of antibiotic for the empiric treatment of SBP. Few randomized trials have been performed in this group of patients. In one randomized study of 73 patients with cirrhosis, cefotaxime therapy was shown to be effective in 85% of cases, more effective than the combination of ampicillin and an aminoglycoside; in addition, the latter combination was associated with more renal toxicity and superinfection in cirrhotic patients.[7] Ceftriaxone, 2 g/d, has been effective in some patients.

As could have been predicted, aztreonam (a b-lactam antibiotic), although well tolerated, is less effective as empiric treatment because of its lack of activity against gram-positive organisms.[8] Parenteral amoxicillin-clavulanic acid has been found to be clinically useful with an efficacy of 85% and minimal side effects in 27 treated patients; as yet, it has not been tested against cefotaxime.

With organism identification, antibiotic therapy can be adjusted according to sensitivity testing. In CNNA cases, antibiotic therapy should be tailored to the clinical response, and in most cases cefotaxime is effective.

Because SBP rarely develops in the asymptomatic patient with bacteriascites, antibiotic therapy is not required in the asymptomatic patient. If the patient is or becomes symptomatic or if the subsequent paracentesis shows an increasing PMN count, then therapy is instituted.

SUBSEQUENT PARACENTESIS

Diagnostic paracentesis should be repeated after 48 hours of antibiotic therapy to observe the PMN response. If the PMN count is greater than baseline, the patient must be carefully re-examined and tested (retested) for secondary sites of infection (see above). In addition, antibiotic therapy can be adjusted according to sensitivity testing, and antibiotic coverage can be extended if it is considered necessary. In the vast majority of patients with SBP, the PMN count falls after 48 hours of antibiotic therapy.[6]

DURATION OF ANTIBIOTIC THERAPY

Most patients with SBP respond quickly to antibiotic therapy. Whereas it was formerly common practice to continue treatment for 10 to 14 days, a recent randomized study of 90 patients[4] has shown that short-course treatment (5 days) is as efficacious as 10 days of therapy in terms of bacteriologic cure, mortality, and recurrence. Additionally, it has been shown that a PMN count of less than 250/ml, checked at 2- to 3-day intervals, can be used as an index to stop therapy, often again after shorter courses of therapy.[9] Duration of therapy is of economic consequence, both in terms of drug cost and length of hospitalization. In patients with a blood culture positive for bacteria, it seems reasonable to continue therapy for 10 days, although the value of this is unproven.

MORTALITY

Inpatient mortality for cirrhotic patients with SBP has been reported to range between 30% and 50%, although in many cases, death occurs after resolution of the SBP; this reflects not only the SBP itself but the severity of the underlying liver disease in the typical patient who develops SBP, death occurring frequently because of variceal bleeding or liver failure. In more recent years, the published hospital mortality has dropped to less than 30%,[10] presumably reflecting improvement both in diagnosis and management of SBP and other complications of chronic liver disease. A recent study of 213 episodes of SBP treated with cefotaxime with a mortality of 38% showed the following parameters to be indicative of infection resolution and patient survival: blood urea nitrogen level, serum AST level and site (community or hospital) of peritonitis acquisition; patients developing SBP in the hospital have particularly low survival rates.

In terms of mortality, patients with CNNA appear to have less severe disease with better early survival reflected by a 20% 1-month mortality compared to 50% for those with a culture that was positive for disease[2]; in addition, the late mortality at 1 year after diagnosis was 41% for those with CNNA and 75% for those with SBP. Patients with bacteriascites have an even better prognosis, closer to those patients with sterile ascites.

SBP AND LIVER TRANSPLANTATION

Patients who develop SBP have more severe liver disease and poorer prognosis than those without SBP, and their 1-year survival is dismal at less than 40%. In an otherwise suitable patient with chronic liver disease, an episode of SBP, therefore, can be considered an indication for liver transplantation.

PREVENTION

Three groups of patients with cirrhotic ascites are known to be at particularly high risk for development of severe infection including SBP: namely patients who have recovered from the first episode of SBP, patients with gastrointestinal tract hemorrhage, and those with low total protein concentrations in ascitic fluid.

Patients with an episode of SBP have an extremely high recurrence rate of greater than 50% at 1 year after diagnosis, and it is reasonable to consider prophylactic measures in patients who survive the acute illness. Rarely can anything be done to influence the course of the underlying disease, and in only the occasional patient does diuretic therapy clear the ascites. However, increased opsonic activity has been demonstrated in ascites during diuresis, proportional to the increase in protein concentration, giving further rationale for the use of maximal supportive measures for ascites control in these patients. In addition, because most cases of SBP are due to gram-negative bacteria of gut origin, selective bowel decontamination can be used to eliminate gram-negative organisms leaving gram-positive and anaerobic flora unaffected (a maneuver that prevents overgrowth with resistant and fungal organisms). Indeed, in cirrhotic patients, oral norfloxacin has been shown to be associated with disappearance of gram-negative bacilli from the fecal flora without significant changes in gram-positive cocci and anaerobic bacteria.[10] In a randomized trial of 80 cirrhotic patients who had survived an acute episode of SBP, norfloxacin in doses of 400 mg/d reduced the recurrence rate of SBP to 20% in treated patients (only one case was due to a gram-negative bacillus [*E. coli*]) compared to 68% in controls, this difference being due to the great reduction of gram-negative infections in treated patients; only one patient developed side effects (oral and esophageal candidiasis) from the antibiotic therapy, and there was no emergence of antibiotic-resistant bacteria.[10]

Norfloxacin has also been used with success to reduce the incidence of SBP in two groups of hospitalized patients who are known to be at high risk for this complication, namely those with low ascitic fluid total protein levels (<1.5 g/dl) and those with gastrointestinal tract hemorrhage. In 63 noninfected patients hospitalized with ascites and low ascitic fluid protein levels (<1.5 g/dl), norfloxacin significantly lowered the incidence of SBP to 0% in 32 treated patients compared to 22% in 31 control subjects. Similarly, in a randomized, prospective study of 119 patients hospitalized with cirrhotic ascites and gastrointestinal tract hemorrhage, prophylactic norfloxacin reduced the incidence of bacteremia or SBP from 17% in control subjects to 3% in treated patients.

Whether long-term primary prophylaxis would be beneficial in these two groups of patients or in any other group of cirrhotic patients with ascites awaits further controlled studies, and at the present time, the only patients in whom long-term prophylaxis can be recommended are those who have already had an episode of SBP. Even in this latter group of patients, it is not established whether the long-term benefit of antibiotic prophylaxis exceeds the value of early diagnosis and treatment of the individual infective episodes or whether prevention is cost effective. Indeed, it would seem that perhaps the patients who would most benefit from prophylaxis are patients with advanced liver failure, poor nutritional status, poor renal function, or intractable ascites with very low ascitic protein concentration who not only are at high risk of SBP but in very poor condition to withstand the acute infection. During the waiting period for liver transplantation, it would seem reasonable to place such a patient on selective bowel prophylaxis, although the clinical benefit of this has not been studied.

REFERENCES

1. Garcia-Tsao G. Spontaneous bacterial peritonitis. *Gastroenterol Clin North Am.* 1992;21(1):257–275.
2. Pelletier G, Salmon D, Ink O, et al. Culture-negative neutrocytic ascites: a less severe variant of spontaneous bacterial peritonitis. *J Hepatol.* 1990;10:327–331.
3. Runyon BA. Monomicrobial nonneutrocytic bacteriascites: a variant of spontaneous bacterial peritonitis. *Hepatology.* 1990;12(4):710–715.
4. Runyon BA, McHutchison JG, Antillon MR, Akriviadis EA, Montano AA. Short-course versus long-course antibiotic treatment of spontaneous bacterial peritonitis: a randomized, controlled study of 100 patients. *Gastroenterology.* 1991;100:1737–1742.
5. Runyon BA, Canawati HN, Akriviadis EA. Optimization of ascitic fluid culture technique. *Gastroenterology.* 1988;95:1351–1355.
6. Akriviadis EA, Runyon BA. Utility of an algorithm in differentiating spontaneous from secondary bacterial peritonitis. *Gastroenterology.* 1990;98:126–133.
7. Felisart J, Rimola A, Arroyo V, et al. Cefotaxime is more effective than is ampicillin-tobramycin in cirrhotics with severe infections. *Hepatology.* 1985;5(3):456–462.
8. Ariza J, Xiol X, Esteve M, et al. Aztreonam vs. cefotaxime in the treatment of gram-negative spontaneous peritonitis in cirrhotic patients. *Hepatology.* 1991;14:91–98.
9. Fong TL, Akriviadis EA, Runyon BA, Reynolds TB. Polymorphonuclear cell count response and duration of antibiotic therapy in spontaneous bacterial peritonitis. *Hepatology.* 1989;9(3):423–426.
10. Gines P, Rimola A, Planas R, et al. Norfloxacin prevents spontaneous bacterial peritonitis recurrence in cirrhosis: results of a double-blind, placebo-controlled trial. *Hepatology.* 1990;12:716–724.

104
Porphyria
JOSEPH R. BLOOMER and CLAUS A. PIERACH

The porphyrias are metabolic disorders in which there are increased production, accumulation, and excretion of porphyrins and porphyrin precursors.[1,2] These compounds are intermediates of the heme biosynthetic pathway. Thus, the liver and bone marrow are the principal sites of expression of the biochemical abnormality because they are the major sites of heme production. This is the basis for the early classification of the porphyrias as either hepatic or erythropoietic.

There are eight types of porphyria, each of which is associated with an enzyme abnormality in the heme biosynthetic pathway that produces a characteristic pattern of abnormal accumulation and excretion of porphyrins and porphyrin precursors. The diagnosis of a specific porphyria is made by documenting this pattern and in some cases may be confirmed by demonstrating a deficiency of the enzyme activity that underlies the biochemical abnormalities. In recent years, genes that code for the enzymes have been cloned and sequenced, and the diagnosis may be aided in the future by identifying gene defects.

The clinical manifestations of the porphyrias are varied, and patients with these disorders may be seen by many different physicians. The gastroenterologist or hepatologist may be consulted for several clinical situations:

1. Management of abdominal pain in patients with the inducible (acute) types of porphyria
2. Evaluation and management of liver disease in patients with porphyria cutanea tarda
3. Management of liver disease in patients with protoporphyria
4. Evaluation of patients with secondary porphyrinuria.

A characteristic feature of the porphyrias is the relationship between the clinical manifestations and biochemical abnormalities. Porphyrias associated with acute porphyric attacks have increased urinary excretion of the porphyrin precursor ᴅ-aminolevulinic acid (ALA) and also porphobilinogen (PBG), except in the rare disorder ᴅ-aminolevulinic acid dehydrase deficiency (Fig. 104–1 and Table 104–1). Porphyrias associated with tissue damage, either photocutaneous lesions or liver disease, have increased accumulation and excretion of the porphyrin compounds themselves (Fig. 104–1 and Table 104–1). Two of the porphyrias, variegate porphyria and hereditary coproporphyria, have both.

MANAGEMENT OF INDUCIBLE (ACUTE) PORPHYRIAS

Acute intermittent porphyria is the most common type of inducible porphyria in the United States. This autosomal dominant disorder has a prevalence of 5 to 10 affected individuals per 100,000 in the general population. Two other types of porphyria, which are also inherited as autosomal dominant disorders, that cause acute porphyric attacks are variegate porphyria and hereditary coproporphyria. A fourth disorder, caused by a recessive deficiency of ᴅ-aminolevulinic acid dehydrase, is very rare and unlikely to be encountered by most physicians.

ACUTE PORPHYRIC ATTACK

A variety of signs and symptoms occur during an acute porphyric attack, reflecting widespread involvement of the nervous system. The most frequent complaint is abdominal pain, which occurs in more than 90% of patients. Although there is no characteristic pattern to the pain, it is often described as severe, colicky, and localized to the lower quadrants of the abdomen. Pain may occur in any portion of the abdomen, however, and may radiate to the back, thighs, and chest. The abdominal pain is frequently accompanied by nausea and vomiting. Despite the intensity of the pain, physical examination is usu-

732 HEPATOBILIARY TRACT

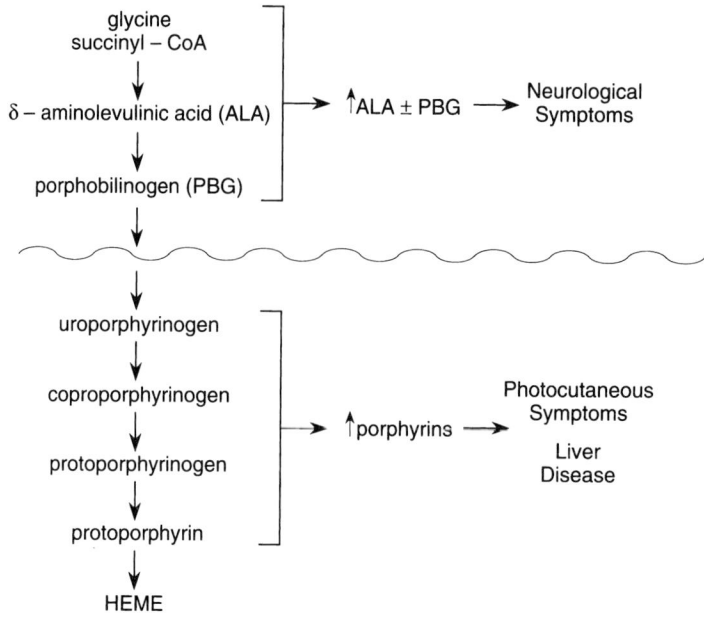

FIGURE 104-1. Relationship between biochemical abnormalities and clinical manifestations in the porphyrias. The porphyrias associated with acute attacks of neurologic dysfunction have increased urinary excretion of δ-aminolevulinic acid with or without porphobilinogen (ALA±PBG), whereas those associated with photocutaneous lesions or liver disease have increased accumulation and excretion of porphyrin compounds.

TABLE 104-1. CLASSIFICATION OF THE PORPHYRIAS ACCORDING TO CLINICAL MANIFESTATIONS

Neurologic symptoms only
   Acute intermittent porphyria
   δ-Aminolevulinic acid dehydrase deficiency
Photocutaneous symptoms only
   Porphyria cutanea tarda
   Protoporphyria*
   Hepatoerythropoietic porphyria
   Congenital erythropoietic porphyria
Both types of symptoms
   Variegate porphyria
   Hereditary coproporphyria

*Neurologic symptoms similar to those in acute porphyric attacks may occur in patients with advanced protoporphyric liver disease.

---

ally unremarkable, specifically noteworthy for the absence of abdominal rigidity and rebound tenderness. Abdominal x-ray films demonstrate the pattern of pseudoobstruction, with segmental dilation and spasm of the intestine. In 10% to 40% of patients, fever and leukocytosis may accompany the abdominal pain, necessitating consideration of an intraabdominal inflammatory process even when the patient is known to have porphyria.

The abdominal pain is caused by autonomic neuropathy. Other features of autonomic neuropathy may also occur, supporting the diagnosis of porphyria as the cause of the abdominal pain. Chief among these is a sinus tachycardia (heart rate >100). Hypertension, constipation, and urinary retention are also common.

Peripheral neuropathy, with both motor and sensory components, may develop as the attack progresses. Peripheral neuropathy in its more severe form can lead to paralysis, and complications of respiratory paralysis have been the leading cause of death during acute attacks. Hypothalamic lesions have been found at postmortem examination and are probably the cause of the inappropriate secretion of antidiuretic hormone during some attacks, leading to hyponatremia. Central nervous system manifestations include an organic brain syndrome, depression, and neuroses. Seizures and coma occur in some cases.

If the diagnosis of porphyria has not been established in the patient, the above-mentioned array of signs and symptoms may be helpful to the physician in considering the diagnosis. Other features of the history that may be helpful in directing the physician toward the diagnosis include the following:

1. An acute attack of porphyria rarely occurs before the age of puberty.
2. The patient's symptoms may have been temporarily related to ingestion of certain drugs or to a period of decreased food intake.
3. In women the attack may be cyclic in nature, regularly occurring a few days before menstruation begins.
4. There may be a history of unexplained abdominal pain in other members of the family.

If the history and physical findings strongly suggest porphyria as the cause of the patient's symptoms, it is nonetheless very important for the physician to establish the diagnosis biochemically. Unfortunately, the quantitative measurement of urinary excretion of ALA and PBG is not rapidly available to many physicians. Nevertheless, two screening tests can be used to show an increased level of PBG in urine. These are the Watson-Schwartz Test and the Hoesch Test, both of which rely on the fact that PBG reacts with Ehrlich's aldehyde reagent in an acidified solution to form a red compound (Fig. 104–2). Positive results indicate that there is at least twice the normal level of PBG in the urine (normal excretion is <4 mg in 24 hours). Urobilinogen in urine also reacts with Ehrlich's aldehyde reagent to form a red compound, so particular care must be used to extract the solution with organic solvents, or false-positive results occur (Fig. 104–2). When allowed to stand in air and light, urine that contains excess PBG may also turn black because of conversion of PBG to porphobilin and other pigments. If the screening test results are positive, quantitative determination of urinary PBG and ALA should be done to confirm the diagnosis. However, it is not necessary to do this before beginning therapy, particularly if the patient is severely ill.

It is also not important to document the specific type of porphyria responsible for the acute attack, since treatment is the same regardless of the type. Therapy of the acute porphyric attack should follow several steps (Fig. 104–3). First, any potential porphyrinogenic drug should be stopped.[1,2] If the attack has been precipitated by an infection, this should be promptly treated. An adequate caloric intake should be maintained, as negative caloric balance may aggravate an attack, and diminished oral intake is recognized as a precipitant of attacks. The daily diet should provide at least 400 g of glucose or another readily metabolized carbohydrate. It has been known for many years, both as a result of experimental and clinical studies, that a high carbohydrate intake is beneficial in the porphyric attack, probably through a suppressive effect of glucose on

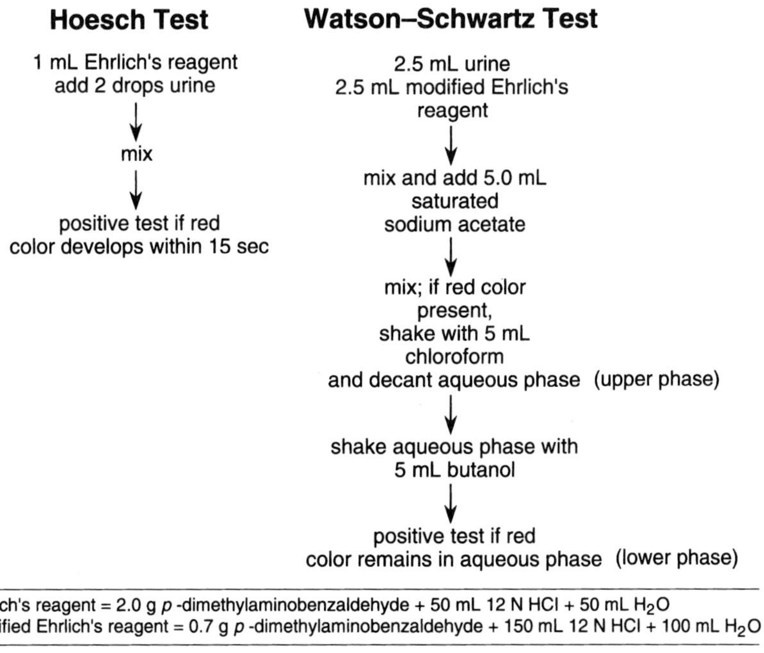

Hoesch Test

1 mL Ehrlich's reagent
add 2 drops urine
↓
mix
↓
positive test if red color develops within 15 sec

Watson–Schwartz Test

2.5 mL urine
2.5 mL modified Ehrlich's reagent
↓
mix and add 5.0 mL saturated sodium acetate
↓
mix; if red color present, shake with 5 mL chloroform and decant aqueous phase (upper phase)
↓
shake aqueous phase with 5 mL butanol
↓
positive test if red color remains in aqueous phase (lower phase)

Ehrlich's reagent = 2.0 g p-dimethylaminobenzaldehyde + 50 mL 12 N HCl + 50 mL H_2O
Modified Ehrlich's reagent = 0.7 g p-dimethylaminobenzaldehyde + 150 mL 12 N HCl + 100 mL H_2O

FIGURE 104–2. Screening tests to detect increased urinary porphobilinogen (PBG) in a patient suspected of having an acute porphyric attack.

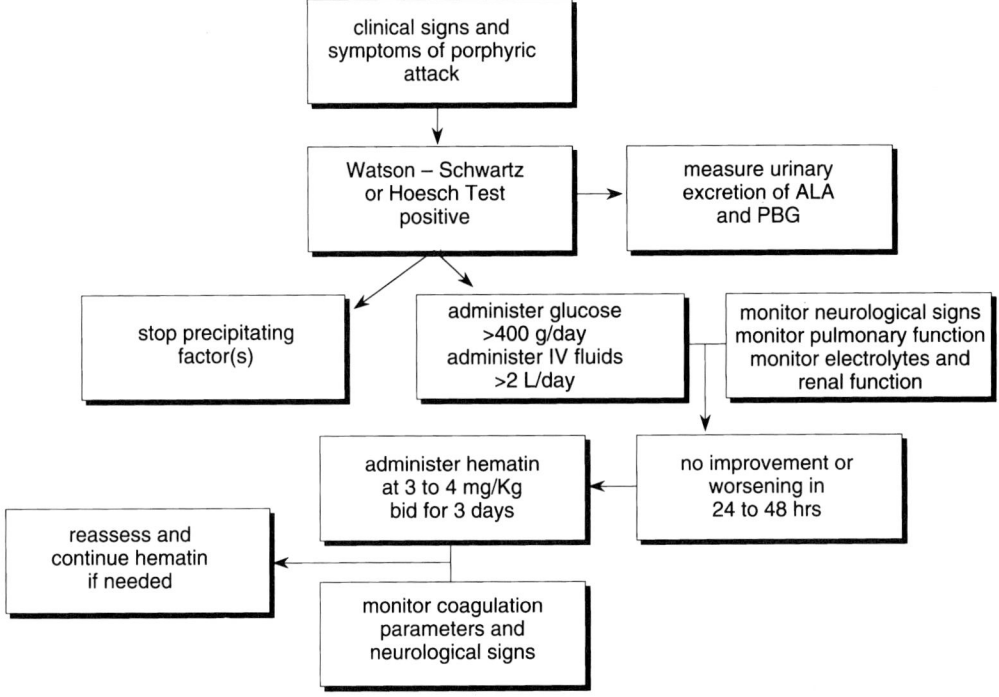

FIGURE 104-3. Scheme for management of the patient with an acute porphyric attack.

ALA synthase, the rate-limiting enzyme in hepatic heme biosynthesis. This is due specifically to carbohydrates and cannot be reproduced through a similar caloric intake with protein or fat. If the patient is unable to take carbohydrates by mouth, they should be given through a nasogastric feeding tube or by intravenous route. Intravenous fluids should be administered to maintain a fluid intake greater than 2 L/d. It is probably best to give this as normal saline to guard against the development of hyponatremia, which occasionally occurs during a porphyric attack because of the inappropriate secretion of antidiuretic hormone.

The patient should be carefully monitored for the development of a neuropathy. Particular attention should be paid to respiratory function. Daily measurements of vital capacity and forced expiratory volume should be done to assess the progress of the attack, and ventilatory support should be provided if respiratory depression occurs.

If the patient does not show improvement within 24 to 48 hours after beginning therapy, hematin should be administered.[3] Hematin (ferriheme hydroxide) is the chemical form of heme in aqueous solution at physiologic pH. Experimental and clinical studies have demonstrated that exogenously administered hematin represses hepatic ALA synthase, the rate-limiting step in the formation of hepatic heme, and thereby reduces the formation of ALA and PBG. Hematin was first administered to patients in the early 1970s and was made commercially available as an orphan drug in 1983. In the United States it may be purchased in the form of a sterile, lyophilized powder (Panhematin). In Europe it is also available as heme arginate (Normosang from Leiras Oy Pharmaceuticals in Helsinki, Finland); this has not yet become available for commercial use in the United States.

Hematin in a dosage of 3 to 4 mg/kg body weight, administered twice daily for 3 days, generally produces a prompt decline in serum and urine levels of ALA and PBG. There is no need to give a larger amount, and renal failure has been precipitated by high doses (12 mg/kg). Despite the impressive effect of hematin administration on urinary ALA and PBG excretion, the clinical effect is less predictable. In fact, there have been no randomized controlled studies that have shown a clinical benefit to the administration of hematin during an acute porphyric attack, although physicians who are experienced with managing such patients widely believe that it is of benefit. It is important to administer hematin before advanced neuronal damage occurs during an attack, as the damage is usually not reversed.

Hematin is well tolerated if given in the proper manner. The most common side effect is thrombophlebitis, which can be prevented by administering the solution slowly over 15 to 30 minutes through a freely flowing intravenous line. A transient coagulopathy is also produced, which is caused by the breakdown products of heme. Thus, hematin should be administered as soon as possible after it is dissolved in aqueous solution. The platelet count and coagulation parameters should be monitored during therapy; however, overt bleeding has been observed only when hematin has been given to a patient who is already receiving anticoagulant therapy. Heme arginate appears to present less problem with thrombophlebitis and coagulopathy than hematin. Dissolving hematin in human serum albumin protects it from degradation, and this solution is as effective as hematin administered alone.[4] More recently tin protoporphyrin, which is an inhibitor of heme oxygenase and thereby prevents the catabolism of heme, has been used in combination with hematin to prolong the biochemical remission.[5] Further studies are needed to determine how this compares to the use of hematin alone.

Measures must also be taken to manage the symptoms and signs of the porphyric attack while glucose administration or hematin administration is being provided. Particular attention should be given to the control of pain, which can be very severe, and narcotics should be administered if necessary (Table 104–2). Anxiety and agitation can be controlled with chlorpromazine, and ondansetron is used to relieve nausea and vomiting. Propranolol in a dosage of 20 to 200 mg/d can be given to control hypertension and tachycardia, although some studies have indicated this should be done cautiously. Seizure activity may be a particularly difficult manifestation of the porphyric attack to treat, as most of the anticonvulsants (particularly the barbiturates and phenytoin) are known to precipitate acute attacks. Bromides are safe, but there is a narrow range between the therapeutic and toxic dose. Clonazepam in low doses, producing levels less than or equal to 6 mg/dl, may also be administered. New drugs such as felbamate and gabapentin are promising, but there is little experience with their use. Status epilepticus can be controlled with diazepam (up to 10 mg intravenously), paraldehyde (8 to 10 ml rectally), or magnesium sulfate (0.5 to 1.0 g/h by intravenous infusion).

Patients With Chronic Pain Syndrome

Many patients with acute porphyria have a limited number of porphyric attacks in their lifetime, and they do well if they avoid precipitating factors such as certain drugs, decreased food intake, excessive alcohol intake, and recurrent infections. However, there are some patients who have recurrent attacks, and they pose a particularly challenging problem to the clinician. As with any other chronic pain syndrome, these patients are prone to narcotic addiction, and pain management becomes a critical feature of their care. A limited number of studies have evaluated the regular administration of hematin to prevent the attacks. Available studies show uncertain benefit, perhaps because hematin cannot be administered frequently enough to suppress the biochemical abnormalities on a continuous basis. Whether the addition of tin porphyrin to the regimen benefits such patients remains to be answered. It is helpful to document the basal urinary excretion of ALA and PBG, since an objective sign that the patient is suffering an attack is a marked increase in the urinary excretion of these compounds.

In some women porphyric attacks are regularly related to the menstrual cycle, beginning a few days prior to the onset of menses and ending after menstruation has begun. Oral contracep-

TABLE 104–2. SAFE DRUGS FOR USE IN THE ACUTE PORPHYRIAS

Pain	Aspirin, acetaminophen, propoxyphene, ibuprofen, naproxen, codeine, methadone, meperidine, morphine
Nausea, vomiting	Phenothiazines, domperidone, ondansetron
Tachycardia, hypertension	Propranolol, atenolol, labetalol, metoprolol, reserpine
Anxiety	Chloral hydrate, chlorpromazine, haloperidol, paraldehyde
Seizures	Bromides, magnesium sulfate, clonazepam (low doses), felbamate (experience limited), diazepam for status epilepticus
Infection	Aminoglycosides, penicillin and derivatives, amphotericin B, tetracyclines
Anesthetics	Procaine, ether, nitrous oxide, succinylcholine, cyclopropane, neostigmine (Prostigmin)

tive therapy has been used in these patients successfully, even though oral contraceptives are known to precipitate acute attacks. Analogs of luteinizing hormone–releasing hormone (LHRH) have also been administered to prevent cyclic attacks related to the menstrual cycle.[6] These agents appear to act by blocking the effect of LHRH on the pituitary, thus preventing the normal cyclic secretion of luteinizing hormone (LH) and follicle-stimulating hormone (FSH).

PREVENTION AND CARRIERS OF THE LATENT GENE DEFECT

The measurement of activity of heme biosynthesis enzymes in individuals who are relatives of patients with acute porphyria has made it possible to identify carriers of the latent gene defect. The future ability to identify gene defects in the porphyrias will enhance this possibility.

In families with acute intermittent porphyria, the measurement of erythrocyte PBG deaminase activity has shown that many carriers of the gene defect are latent. These individuals have no clinical manifestations of the disease, and many have normal levels of urinary ALA and PBG. Although the natural history of the latent state remains unclear, the risk of developing an acute attack appears to be low. However, some individuals have experienced devastating attacks in later life when exposed to precipitating factors (Bloomer and Pierach. Personal observations). Thus, carriers of the gene defect should always be considered to have the potential for developing an acute attack, and they should avoid those factors that have been most incriminated in precipitating attacks (sulfonamides, barbiturates, hydantoins, meprobamate, estrogens, fasting, and excessive use of alcohol).

Erythrocyte PBG deaminase activity should be assessed in all first-degree relatives of patients with acute intermittent porphyria, particularly in children who are approaching puberty. As gene testing becomes more widely available, gene testing may also be used in families in which acute intermittent porphyria or the other types of acute porphyria are present. Patients in whom the enzyme abnormality or gene defect is documented should be managed along the same lines as those outlined above for carriers of the latent gene defect. They should also be counseled regarding the genetics of the acute porphyrias.

Individuals who have suffered porphyric attacks should be instructed to wear a bracelet stating that they have porphyria and giving the phone number of their physician. They should also be instructed to avoid drugs and other factors that have either been demonstrated to precipitate porphyric attacks or have been shown experimentally to be porphyrinogenic.[1,2] Although this is a long list, many safe drugs are available. (Table 104–2).

LIVER DISEASE IN PORPHYRIA CUTANEA TARDA

CLINICAL AND BIOCHEMICAL FEATURES

Porphyria cutanea tarda is the most common type of porphyria in the United States. It is also common in European countries, especially those with sunny climates. Porphyria cutanea tarda is of three types. In some patients the activity of uroporphyrinogen decarboxylase is decreased to approximately 50% of normal in liver and erythrocytes, and approximately half of their first-degree relatives have a similar decrease in activity. These patients have a familial form of the disorder. More commonly there is no family history of the disease, and uroporphyrinogen decarboxylase activity in erythrocytes is normal. These patients have the sporadic form of the disease, which can be precipitated by a variety of factors including alcoholism, use of estrogen compounds, and chronic hemodialysis. Recently, there has been an association with hepatitis C. Finally, there is a toxic form of the disease, which can be caused by the exposure to substances such as haloaromatic compounds. Most notable was the outbreak in Turkey in the 1950s following the ingestion of flour made from seed wheat that had been treated with the fungicide hexachlorobenzene.

The principal clinical manifestation of porphyria cutanea tarda is cutaneous lesions that appear in sun-exposed areas of the body. Patients usually present with vesicles and sores on their hands and complain of increased facial hair on the cheeks and in the periorbital region. The hand lesions result from increased skin fragility caused by porphyrin-induced damage. If untreated, skin lesions may become infected and heal slowly, causing pigment changes. In the most severe form of porphyria cutanea tarda, sclerodermatous changes can occur. Whereas cutaneous symptoms usually prompt the patient to seek medical care, liver disease is also a common feature in the patient with overt porphyria cutanea tarda. Patients frequently have a mild-to-moderate elevation of the serum aminotransferase level. Liver biopsies show abnormalities, which include red fluorescence of unstained tissue when exposed to ultraviolet light, the presence of cytoplasmic needlelike inclusions in hepatocytes, fatty infiltration, and siderosis. The serum iron concentration and transferrin saturation are typically increased in these patients.

In addition to these features, varying degrees of hepatocellular damage are noted, which range from mild portal inflammation to cirrhosis. An increased incidence of hepatocellular carcinoma has also been found in patients with long-standing untreated porphyria cutanea tarda. This has occurred most commonly in European countries, and a high prevalence of exposure to hepatitis B virus has been noted in these patients as compared to the general population. More recently, a prevalence of hepatitis C antibody of 60% to 80% has been found in patients with porphyria cutanea tarda in Spain and Italy, far in excess of that found in control populations. The presence of active viral infection has been documented by polymerase chain reaction for hepatitis C RNA. Liver biopsy specimens from the patients who were positive for hepatitis C antibody demonstrated histologic changes similar to those found in chronic hepatitis C infection alone.

These findings suggest that the cause of liver damage in patients with porphyria cutanea tarda is multifactorial. Alcoholism may contribute to the liver damage when it is the precipitating factor. Experimental studies suggest that the metabolic disorder itself may also cause liver damage because of the formation of activated oxygen species when porphyrinogens are oxidized to porphyrins in the presence of iron. The common finding of hepatitis C virus in these patients, at least in European countries, indicates that viral infection also contributes to the liver damage.

The diagnosis of porphyria cutanea tarda is made by demonstrating a marked increase in the urinary excretion of uroporphyrin in a patient with compatible clinical manifestations. If the history indicates an occurrence of the disorder in other family members, then measurement of uroporphyrinogen decarboxylase activity in erythrocytes may be used to substantiate the diagnosis and provide evidence that the patient has the familial form of the disease. Liver biopsy is not necessary to make a diagnosis, but the presence of red fluorescence in the biopsy specimen, along with the other features mentioned above, is strongly supportive of the diagnosis. Liver biopsy documents the severity of hepatocellular damage and should be considered in the patient who also has hepatitis C infection.

MANAGEMENT

Treatment of porphyria cutanea tarda is mainly directed toward the photocutaneous symptoms (Fig. 104–4).[7] Patients with active skin lesions should be instructed to stop the ingestion of ethanol, and women taking birth control pills should be given some other form of contraceptive. Patients should also stop the ingestion of iron-containing compounds (e.g., multivitamin preparations). Despite discontinuing the precipitating factors, cutaneous manifestations show only slow improvement unless other therapy is initiated. The mainstay of therapy in porphyria cutanea tarda is phlebotomy,[8] based on the observation that hepatic siderosis is common in these patients and that iron probably plays an important role in the pathogenesis of the disease. The liver contains an excess of 2 to 4 g of iron, and the amount of phlebotomy needed is on the order of 4 to 8 L of blood. The usual schedule for phlebotomy is to remove 500 ml of blood every 1 to 3 weeks until the patient becomes anemic or the urinary excretion of uroporphyrin diminishes below 500 lg daily. After completion of phlebotomy, urine levels of uroporphyrin continue to fall toward normal, and more than 90% of treated patients have normal levels after 6 to 12 months. Accompanying the decrease in uroporphyrin excretion is improvement in skin fragility, and patients no longer develop vesicles or erosions. However, hirsutism, hyperpigmentation, and milia may take many months to clear after therapy is terminated, and sclerodermoid changes may not resolve for several years.

Approximately 10% of patients relapse within 1 year after treatment but respond to a second course of phlebotomy therapy. Ingestion of iron-containing compounds has been shown to be a reason for relapse and should be avoided. For patients who are either intolerant of phlebotomy or in whom cutaneous symptoms continue despite an adequate course of phlebotomy, chloroquine or related compounds should be administered. These compounds appear to form a water-soluble complex with uroporphyrin and heptacarboxyl porphyrin, enhancing their removal from tissue sites and their excretion in urine. They should be administered initially in a low dose, starting with 100 mg of hydroxychloroquine or 125 mg of chloroquine three times a week. Larger doses may cause acute hepatic in-

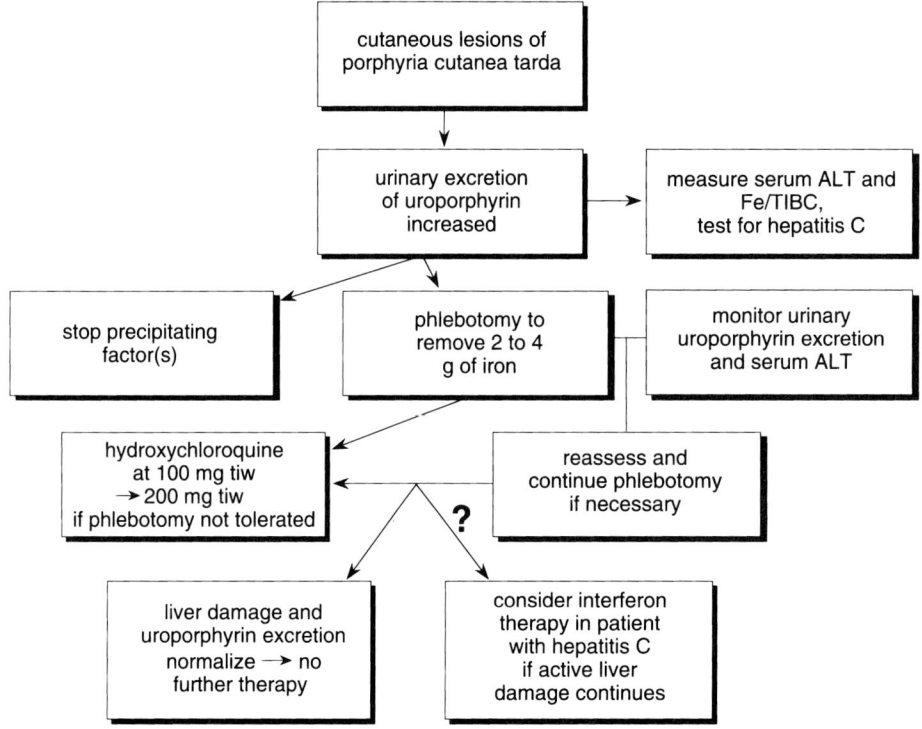

FIGURE 104–4. Scheme for management of the patient with active porphyria cutanea tarda. ALT = alanine aminotransferase, Fe/TIBC = iron/total iron binding capacity ratio.

jury related to the massive removal of uroporphyrin from the liver.

It is not presently known if therapy of hepatitis C infection improves the clinical manifestations of porphyria cutanea tarda as well. Since some studies suggest that interferon therapy is less effective in the patient with hepatitis C who has iron overload, the initial therapy in the patient with porphyria cutanea tarda who has concomitant hepatitis C infection should be phlebotomy anyway. When adequate phlebotomy has been completed, a decision can be made about interferon treatment based on the residual level of serum alanine aminotransferase (ALT) and the findings from a liver biopsy specimen.

For the patient with chronic renal failure who is receiving hemodialysis and develops cutaneous lesions identical to porphyria cutanea tarda, standard phlebotomy is usually contraindicated because of anemia. In such a situation plasmapheresis, deferoxamine infusions (4 g intravenously during each dialysis session), and erythropoietin therapy (150 U/kg body weight intravenously after each dialysis session) accompanied by small-volume phlebotomies have been used in individual patients successfully.

LIVER DISEASE IN PROTOPORPHYRIA

CLINICAL AND BIOCHEMICAL FEATURES

Protoporphyria is also a relatively common type of porphyria, probably second to porphyria cutanea tarda in prevalence. In occurs in all ethnic groups and is inherited as an autosomal dominant trait with variable expression. More complex mechanisms of inheritance have been proposed, but examination of ferrochelatase activity (the enzyme that is deficient in protoporphyria) in tissues of families with the disease indicates that autosomal dominant inheritance is most likely.

The principal clinical manifestation of protoporphyria is photosensitivity. Unlike the other types of porphyria in which photocutaneous symptoms occur, patients with protoporphyria have a direct reaction to sunlight, complaining of burning or pain in sun-exposed areas. Erythema and edema follow in these areas, and vesicles may develop if sun exposure is intense and prolonged. Chronic skin changes of protoporphyria are those of shallow, depressed scars on the nose and hands, as well as thickening and lichenification of the skin.

The photosensitivity is usually present from infancy, although an occasional patient does not exhibit symptoms until adolescence or adulthood. Mothers may note that their children become acutely uncomfortable on exposure to the sun. Window glass does not prevent the photosensitivity, since the wavelength of light that produces reaction (approximately 400 nm) is not filtered by window glass. The dermatologist is usually the first physician consulted, and a diagnosis is made in a patient with compatible cutaneous symptoms by demonstrating an increased level of protoporphyrin in erythrocytes and stool. In contrast to lead poisoning and iron deficiency anemia, in which zinc protoporphyrin levels are increased, the increased protoporphyrin in erythrocytes occurs as free protoporphyrin. In some cases this may be an important distinguishing feature, since approximately 20% to 30% of patients with protoporphyria have mild anemia that is characterized by hypochromic microcytic indexes.

Although photosensitivity is the symptom in protoporphyria for which patients usually seek medical evaluation, the more important clinical manifestation is liver disease. Often this has insidious development, with jaundice being the first manifestation. In early case reports the onset of jaundice was followed by a progressive and rapid downhill course, with only occasional patients recovering. However, those patients had often undergone exploratory laparotomy for evaluation of the jaundice, which probably contributed to their deterioration. More recent studies indicate the course may be drawn out over several months even when the bilirubin level has become elevated.

The livers of patients who have died in hepatic failure have been black in color because of massive deposits of protoporphyrin pigment. When examined by polarization microscopy, these pigment deposits show a diagnostic birefringence due to the presence of crystals. The isolation and characterization of these crystals have shown that they are composed principally of protoporphyrin, and liver disease in protoporphyria is thus considered to be due to the toxic effects of protoporphyrin on the liver. Clinical data have usually indicated that other factors do not contribute to the liver toxicity. However, use of alcohol has been reported to have a synergistic effect and should be avoided in patients in whom liver damage has occurred. Biochemical data have been nonspecific, showing variable degrees of elevation in the serum bilirubin, aminotransferase, and alkaline phosphatase levels. Characteristically, erythrocyte and serum protoporphyrin levels are significantly higher than in the usual patient with protoporphyria, exceeding 2000 µg/dl in red cells and 100 µg/dl in serum.

Fortunately, liver disease in protoporphyria is uncommon, developing in less than 10% of patients. Unfortunately, there is as yet no good means by which to identify those patients who are susceptible to hepatic damage. In patients with high erythrocyte protoporphyrin levels, monitoring of liver chemistries on a periodic basis should be done. Liver biopsy should be carried out in patients with abnormalities in liver chemistries and high erythrocyte protoporphyrin levels.

MANAGEMENT

Usually, the only symptom of protoporphyria that requires therapy is photosensitivity. Most sunscreens do not protect against the photosensitivity because they do not screen the wavelength of light (400 nm) that activates protoporphyrin, but some have broader action (e.g., Photoplex Broad Spectrum Sunscreen) and should be used before sun exposure. There are also films that can be installed on windows to provide protection against light at the 400-nm wavelength. A clear film called CLS-200-X (Madico Co, in Woburn, Mass) blocks 88% of light at 400 nm. Amber films provide better protection (TA-81 from Madico Co), but visibility is altered by these films. Finally, it has been shown that oral administration of betacarotene (Solatene from Roche Dermatologics) in a dosage of 60 to 180 mg daily reduces photosensitivity in over 80% of patients with protoporphyria.[9]

For the patient in whom liver disease has developed, definitive therapy is not available, although a number of therapeutic approaches have been used. These have in common the attempt to diminish the production of excess protoporphyrin, facilitate its transport and secretion into bile, or interrupt its enterohepatic circulation. For reasons not understood, the oral administration of chenodeoxycholic acid has reduced protoporphyrin levels in some patients. Correction of iron deficiency in some has dramatically reduced erythrocyte protoporphyrin levels, although iron therapy must be used cautiously because some patients appear to have a worsening of their protoporphyrin metabolism. Red blood cell transfusions and the administration of hematin have also been successful in diminishing protoporphyrin levels. Oral administration of cholestyramine, or activated charcoal, has been used to interrupt the enterohepatic circulation of protoporphyrin. Administration of vitamin E has been used, on the premise that oxidant-induced damage may be a factor in the pathogenesis of liver disease. Although each of these has a rational basis and does not pose a major risk to the patient, none has been shown in a large group of patients or in controlled studies to be optimal. For the patient with early liver damage a combination of chenodeoxycholic acid (10 to 15 mg/kg/d), cholestyramine (8 to 12 g daily), and vitamin E (100 to 400 IU daily) should at least be given a trial, monitoring liver chemistries and erythrocyte protoporphyrin levels during therapy.

If liver damage progresses despite the above-mentioned treatment, or if liver disease is already advanced at the time the diagnosis is established, there is no therapy to effectively reverse the situation. These patients have often had symptoms of a crisis, showing many of the features that occur during acute attacks of the inducible porphyrias. The symptoms include severe abdominal pain that often radiates into the back, mild degrees of hypertension, tachycardia, and weakness. These symptoms are felt to be caused by the neurotoxic effects of protoporphyrin when blood levels are very high. Limited studies indicate that the condition can be stabilized by hematin administration. This allows the patient to be maintained until liver transplantation can be accomplished. The weekly or twice weekly administration of hematin in a dose of 3 to 4 mg/kg body weight has ameliorated the symptoms of crisis and corrected the biochemical abnormalities toward normal. It is uncertain whether long-term use of this therapy can keep patients in remission, but it is probably impractical to continue the therapy over any extended period of time.

Thus, liver transplantation has become the main option for patients in whom liver disease is advanced.[10] There are now several reports of successful transplantation. During transplantation, the patients are susceptible to a number of unique problems because of their high levels of protoporphyrin in blood and tissue. In particular, the patients are sensitive to photodamage of their skin tissue and abdominal tissue during exposure to fluorescent lights used in operating rooms, and the CLS-200-X filter mentioned above should be used to cover the operating room lights. Their tissues should also be protected from light as much as possible during the operation. Exchange transfusion should not be used just prior to transplantation, as transfused red cells are uniquely sensitive to photohemolysis caused by circulating protoporphyrin. Instead, plasmapheresis should be considered just prior to transplantation.

Unfortunately, liver transplantation does not correct the ferrochelatase deficiency in the bone marrow, and erythrocyte protoporphyrin levels may remain high in patients following transplantation. Their new livers thus remain susceptible to the toxic effects of protoporphyrin, a condition that can be exacerbated by other cholestatic problems that may arise in the posttransplantation period such as rejection and biliary abnormalities. It remains undetermined as to what percent of patients develop significant damage in the new liver.

SECONDARY PORPHYRINURIA

The most common abnormality of porphyrin metabolism encountered by the gastroenterologist or hepatologist is secondary porphyrinuria. This condition is characterized by a mild-to-moderate increase in the urinary excretion of porphyrins, particularly coproporphyrin. It is associated with several different diseases. These include hepatobiliary diseases (acute and chronic hepatitis, alcoholic liver disease, cirrhosis of varying causes, and cholestatic disorders), hematologic diseases (various anemias, leukemias, and Hodgkin's disease), toxic exposures (heavy metal poisoning, toxic exposure to haloalkanes and haloaromatic compounds), and miscellaneous conditions such as diabetes, infections, and starvation. Acute alcoholism may also cause a significant increase in the urinary excretion of coproporphyrin, which begins within a few days of ingestion. Since the bile is an important route for excretion of the porphyrins, the increase in the urinary excretion of porphyrin that occurs in hepatobiliary disorders is explained by the diversion of coproporphyrin from bile to urine. This may be particularly excessive when there is intense cholestasis.

Secondary porphyrinuria is an acquired condition, and it is critical to providing proper treatment for the patient that the clinician avoid making the diagnosis of a genetic porphyria. This may initially be difficult, since some patients with secondary porphyrinuria have symptoms of an acute porphyric attack, including abdominal pain, nausea, and vomiting. Usually a careful history indicates that a genetic type of porphyria is unlikely to be the cause of the excess urinary porphyrin excretion. As an additional means to establish that the patient has secondary porphyrinuria, it is important to remember that the inducible porphyrias associated with acute porphyric attacks have increased urinary excretion of ALA and PBG. This is not the case in those conditions associated with secondary porphyrinuria, except in the situations of lead poisoning and hereditary tyrosinemia, where urinary ALA is increased. The most important time to obtain urine for measurement of these compounds is when the patient is symptomatic. If urinary excretion of ALA and PBG is normal during a symptomatic period, then the diagnosis of a genetic type of porphyria is ruled out.

Management of the secondary porphyrinurias is not directed toward the abnormality in porphyrin metabolism, since by itself it does not cause any symptoms. Management is instead directed toward the underlying abnormality with which the excessive urinary coproporphyrin excretion is associated. The gastroenterologist or hepatologist should be particularly aware of the association of secondary porphyrinuria with hepatobiliary disorders and evaluate the patient appropriately.

REFERENCES

1. Kappas A, Sassa G, Galbraith RA, Nordmann Y. The prophyrias. In: Scriver CR, Beaudet AL, Sly WS, Valle D, eds. *The Metabolic Basis of Inherited Diseases.* 6th ed. New York, NY: McGraw-Hill Book Co; 1989:1305.
2. Bloomer JR, Straka JG, Rank JM. The porphyrias. In: Schiff L, Schiff ER, eds. *Diseases of the Liver.* 7th ed. Philadelphia, Pa: JB Lippincott Co; 1993:1438.
3. Mustajoki P, Tenhunen R, Pierach C, et al. Heme in the treatment of porphyrias and hematological disorders. *Semin Hematol.* 1989;26:1.
4. Bonkovsky HL, Healey JF, Lourie AN, et al. Intravenous heme-albumin in acute intermittent porphyria: evidence for repletion of hepatic hemoproteins and regulatory heme pools. *Am J Gastroenterol.* 1991;86:1050.
5. Dover SB, Moore MR, Fitzsimmons EJ, et al. Tin protoporphyrin prolongs the biochemical remission produced by heme arginate in acute hepatic porphyria. *Gastroenterology.* 1993;105:500.
6. Anderson KE, Spitz IM, Sassa S, et al. Prevention of cyclical attacks of acute intermittent porphyria with a long-acting agonist of luteinizing hormone-releasing hormone. *N Engl J Med.* 1984;311:643.
7. Poh-Fitzpatrick MB. Pathogenesis and treatment of photocutaneous manifestations of the porphyrias. *Semin Liver Dis.* 1982;2(2):164.
8. Epstein JH, Redeker AG. Porphyria cutanea tarda: a study of the effect of phlebotomy. *N Engl J Med.* 1968;279:1301.
9. Matthews-Roth MM, Pathak MA, Fitzpatrick TB, et al. Beta-carotene as an oral photoprotective agent in erythropoietic protoporphyria. *JAMA.* 1974;228:1004.
10. Bloomer JR, Weimer MK, Bossenmaier IC, et al. Liver transplantation in a patient with protoporphyria. *Gastroenterology.* 1989;97:188.

105

Hepatobiliary Complications of Ulcerative Colitis and Crohn's Disease

VIJAYAN BALAN and NICHOLAS F. LaRUSSO

Although hepatobiliary abnormalities occur frequently in patients with inflammatory bowel disease (IBD) (Table 105–1), there are only three associated conditions of major clinical importance: primary sclerosing cholangitis (PSC), autoimmune chronic active hepatitis, and cholelithiasis. In this review, we comment briefly on the latter two diseases but concentrate principally on PSC, since it is the most frequent and clinically important hepatobiliary disorder found in conjunction with IBD.

TABLE 105–1. CONDITIONS INVOLVING THE LIVER ASSOCIATED WITH INFLAMMATORY BOWEL DISEASE (IBD)

Abnormalities on liver biopsy
  Pericholangitis
  Steatosis
  Fibrosis
  Cirrhosis
  Amyloidosis
  Hepatitis
Diseases of the biliary tract
  Cholelithiasis
  Sclerosing cholangitis
  Benign and malignant tumors of biliary tract
Hepatic abscess
Hemosiderosis
Sarcoidosis
Hepatic vascular abnormalities
  Portal vein thrombosis
  Liver infarct
  Hepatic vein occlusion

PRIMARY SCLEROSING CHOLANGITIS

PSC is a chronic, progressive, idiopathic, cholestatic liver disease that principally affects young men and is characterized by diffuse inflammation and fibrosis of the entire biliary tree. The natural history of PSC usually is one of slow progression with eventual development of cirrhosis, portal hypertension with its accompanying complications, and death from liver failure unless liver transplantation is performed.

ETIOLOGY

Currently, the cause of neither PSC nor IBD is known. However, both have a familial predilection and are associated with immunologic disturbances. One study addressing the familial occurrence of PSC and chronic ulcerative colitis (CUC) found that members of three families had both PSC and CUC; in each family, two siblings were affected, with six having PSC and five also having CUC. In this study, approximately 5% of first-degree relatives of patients with PSC (with or without IBD) had PSC, whereas approximately 30% had IBD. In addition, there is an increased frequency of HLA haplotypes HLA-B8, HLA-DR3, HLA-DRw52A, and HLA-DR2 in PSC, supporting a genetic predisposition.

A number of alterations in the immune system of PSC patients have been described. Humoral changes include increased serum immunoglobulin M levels, decreased hepatic clearance of circulating immune complexes, and increased complement activation. Recently, neutrophil cytoplasmic and nuclear antibodies have been described in well over 75% of patients with PSC with or without associated IBD. A colitis-associated antibody has been demonstrated to cross-react with antigens on colonic, skin, and biliary epithelia, suggesting that antibodies against mutual antigens may be involved in the pathogenesis of both PSC and CUC. Cellular abnormalities in the immune system in patients with PSC include inhibition of leukocyte migration by biliary antigens and alterations in T-cell subsets in the blood and liver of patients with PSC. Furthermore, biliary epithelia, which probably represent the target cells for PSC, aberrantly express major histocompatibility complex (MHC) class II antigens in PSC. A viral infection affecting the biliary tree and triggering immunologic bile duct destruction has also been implicated. The search for pathogenetic viruses, including reo type 3, cytomegalovirus, and other viruses, has thus far been unsuccessful.

Thus, the pathogenic relationship of PSC and IBD is unclear but may hold a clue to the cause of at least some types of each disease. Increased permeability of the diseased colonic mucosa to potential hepatotoxic agents, epitheliotropic viruses, abnormal immune responses to mutual antigens, or some combination of these disturbances may be an essential feature of the pathogenesis of these diseases in genetically predisposed individuals.

CLINICAL FEATURES

Although PSC can occur alone, at least 70% of patients with PSC have associated IBD, most commonly CUC. CUC usually precedes the onset of PSC but can be diagnosed simultaneously or subsequent to the diagnosis of PSC. Indeed, a number of patients have developed PSC following proctocolectomy for CUC. In general, CUC associated with PSC is quiescent, and 80% of patients with PSC and CUC are either asymptomatic or mildly symptomatic from CUC at the time PSC is diagnosed. Seventy percent of patients with PSC are male with a mean age of 43 at diagnosis. Typically, patients with PSC present with the gradual onset of pruritus without jaundice; jaundice then develops within 6 months to 2 years. Patients may also present with fatigue, right upper quadrant discomfort, and lethargy. Symptoms of advanced liver disease such as gastrointestinal tract bleeding, as-

TABLE 105-2. SYMPTOMS AND SIGNS AT PRESENTATION OF PRIMARY SCLEROSING CHOLANGITIS (PSC)

SYMPTOMS		SIGNS	
Fatigue	75%	Hyperpigmentation	25%
Pruritus	70%	Hepatomegaly	55%
Jaundice	65%	Splenomegaly	30%
No symptom	4%	Xanthelasma	4%

cites, and encephalopathy usually occur late in the course of the disease. Table 105-2 summarizes the symptoms and their relative frequency in PSC. Clinical cholangitis marked by recurrent fever, right upper quadrant pain, and jaundice occurs most often in patients who have had previous reconstructive biliary surgery or in those patients who develop a dominant stricture of the extrahepatic bile duct.

On physical examination, jaundice and excoriations may be present. Xanthelasma and xanthomas are occasionally seen about the eyes and the extensor surfaces in the later stages of the disease. Hyperpigmentation, especially in the sun-exposed areas, is not uncommon. The liver is usually enlarged and firm, and the spleen may also be palpable. Signs of end-stage liver disease (i.e., ascites, spider angiomas, and evidence of hepatic encephalopathy) appear only in the latter stages of the disease and are rare as presenting features.

The widespread use of automated blood chemistries has resulted in an increasing number of patients being diagnosed at the presymptomatic stage; such patients are usually identified because of an elevated serum alkaline phosphatase level on routine examination.

DIAGNOSIS

Blood Chemistries

The hepatic chemistries usually reveal an elevated alkaline phosphatase (three or four times normal), with mild-to-modest elevations in alanine aminotransferase (ALT) and aspartate aminotransferase (AST). In about half the patients with PSC, serum bilirubin values are modestly increased at the time of diagnosis. Serum albumin level and prothrombin time generally remain normal until late in the course of the disease. Tests related to copper metabolism are virtually always abnormal in both diseases. Total cholesterol levels also increase in PSC with advancing liver disease.

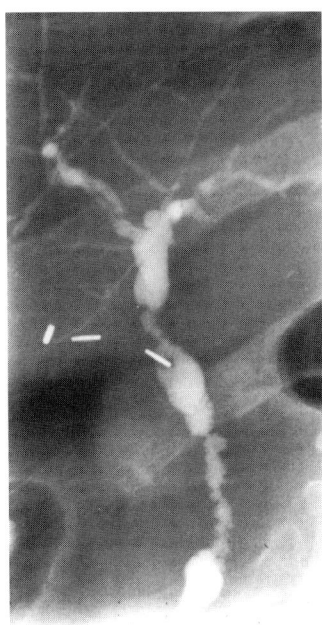

FIGURE 105-1. A retrograde cholangiogram exhibiting classic features of PSC, showing diffuse stricturing and beading of intrahepatic and extrahepatic bile ducts. (Reprinted by permission from LaRusso NF, Wiesner RH, Ludwig J, MacCarty RL. Primary sclerosing cholangitis. *N Engl J Med.* 1984;310:899-903.)

Autoantibodies

Anticolon antibodies, antineutrophil nuclear antibodies, and neutrophil cytoplasmic antibodies are present in the majority of patients with PSC. These antibodies also occur in a high percentage of patients with CUC without evidence of PSC. In contrast, antibodies to mitochondria (AMA), smooth muscle (SMA), and nuclei (ANA) are usually absent.

Evaluation of the Biliary Tree

In PSC, biliary tract visualization by endoscopic or transhepatic cholangiography is diagnostic and cholangiograms usually exhibit diffuse stricturing and beading of the intrahepatic and extrahepatic bile ducts (Fig. 105-1). Most commonly, strictures are short and annular with intermediate segments of slightly dilated bile ducts. Morphologically, these findings represent localized areas of cholangiectasis.

Hepatic Histology

Early in this disease, histologic abnormalities found on liver biopsy are highly characteristic of PSC and include enlargement of portal tracts characterized by edema, increased connective

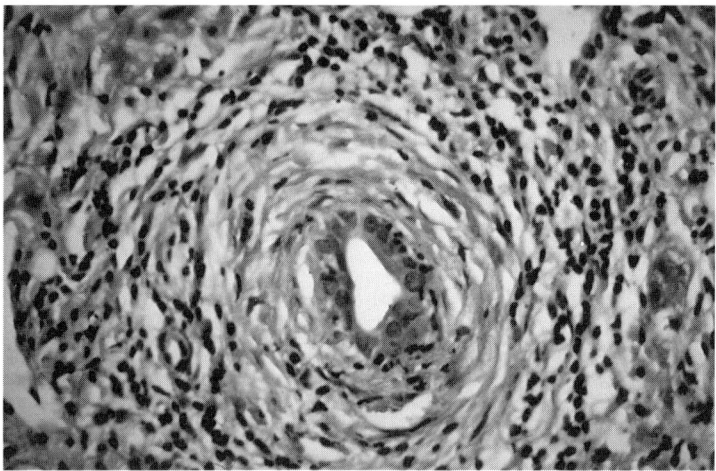

FIGURE 105–2. Fibrous obliterative cholangitis in PSC. The interlobular bile duct shows a typical fibrous collar, and epithelium appears undamaged. (Reprinted by permission from LaRusso NF, Wiesner RH, Ludwig J, MacCarty RL. Primary sclerosing cholangitis. *N Engl J Med.* 1984;310:899–903.)

tissue, and proliferation of interlobular bile ducts. The diagnostic histologic abnormality in PSC is fibrous obliterative cholangitis, which results in replacement of the duct segments by fibrous chords and connective tissue, leading to complete loss of interlobular and adjacent septal bile ducts (Fig. 105–2). The end stage of the disease is marked by histologic findings that include ductopenia and biliary cirrhosis.

PSC has been subdivided into three categories based on the cholangiographic and hepatic histologic findings. Classic or global PSC is the most common variety of the syndrome and involves disturbances of the bile ducts, both inside and outside the liver; both liver biopsy and cholangiogram show typical abnormalities. Small duct PSC (formerly termed *pericholangitis*) represents a stage in the evolution of global PSC at which time the cholangiogram may be normal but the liver biopsy shows evidence of nonsuppurative obliterative cholangitis. The least common variety of PSC is large duct PSC in which the abnormalities of the biliary system are limited largely, if not exclusively, to the extrahepatic and large intrahepatic ducts. The cholangiogram is diagnostic in this condition, although liver biopsy specimens may show minimal or nonspecific changes.

RELATIONSHIP OF PSC TO IBD

IBD is the most important disease associated with PSC, although other diseases (pancreatitis, arthritis, thyroid disease, sarcoid, celiac sprue) occur with increased frequency in association with PSC. Several studies have shown that between 54% and 100% of patients with PSC have associated IBD, with a mean of 77%. In the vast majority (48% to 82%, mean 67%), CUC is the form of IBD associated with PSC. Much less frequently (0% to 13%, mean 8%), Crohn's disease is found in association with PSC. On the other hand, the frequency of PSC in a subgroup of patients with CUC has varied from 2.4% to 5.6%. As discussed earlier, the cause of both PSC and CUC is unclear; however, there is unequivocal evidence of a genetic predisposition to both PSC and CUC supported by familial occurrence of both PSC and CUC together and an increased frequency of certain HLA haplotypes in patients with PSC.

Chronologically, the diagnosis of IBD usually precedes the diagnosis of PSC; however, PSC may precede IBD, PSC may develop after proctocolectomy, and PSC and IBD may be diagnosed simultaneously. IBD associated with PSC is usually symptomatically quiescent or mild; however, some patients with PSC and CUC require colectomy for colitic symptoms. CUC in association with PSC most commonly involves a major portion of the colon and frequently is characterized by rectal sparing. Patients with IBD and PSC are more likely to be male than are patients with IBD but without PSC. Barium enema results may be normal in as many as 50% of patients with PSC and CUC. Unfortunately, patients with PSC are at risk for adenocarcinoma of both the colon, because of their CUC, and the bile duct, because of their PSC (see below). Recent unconfirmed data suggest that patients with PSC and CUC may have an increased risk of colon cancer compared to patients with CUC alone. However, no significant differences have been identified between the two groups of patients (PSC alone versus PSC with IBD) with regard to symptoms and signs, standard biochemical tests, cholangiograms, and hepatic histology. Neutrophil cytoplasmic and nuclear antibodies have been found in 65% to 80% of patients with CUC, PSC, or PSC and CUC, suggesting shared immunopathogenic mechanisms.

When patients with PSC alone are compared to patients with PSC and CUC with regard to cholangiographic abnormalities, no significant differences in the frequency of bandlike strictures, diverticula, or mural irregularities are observed. Similarly, on comparing these two groups of patients (PSC and CUC versus PSC alone) with regard to morphologic abnormalities on liver biopsy, no significant differences were found in the frequency of periductal fibrosis, periductal inflammation, cholestasis, or cirrhosis. In addition, hepatic copper levels, which are universally elevated in PSC because of chronic cholestasis, are elevated to an equal extent in patients with PSC with CUC compared to patients with PSC alone.

Historically, PSC has been considered an extracolonic manifestation of IBD, suggesting that the latter causes the former. Experimentally, animal models of colitis have been demonstrated to have associated liver and biliary tract abnormalities. Clinically, the fact that most patients with PSC have IBD and the fact that at least in one multivariate analysis IBD represented an independent risk factor for survival in PSC have been taken to suggest that IBD indeed does cause PSC. In contrast are the observations that not all patients with PSC have IBD, that patients can develop PSC after a curative proctocolectomy for CUC, that proctocolectomy does not affect the progression of PSC, that PSC and IBD progress independently, and that cholangiograms and liver biopsies are not different in patients with PSC with or without IBD. Thus, it seems that PSC and CUC are diseases that have a common link in their pathogenesis but are distinct diseases without any clear-cut or demonstrable causal relationship.

From a clinical point of view, the implications of the association of PSC and IBD include the aforementioned common pathogenic mechanisms, the morbidity from each disease, the fact that each disease represents a premalignant condition for a distinct organ, and the need to take into account the association of both diseases in developing treatment strategies for either.

NATURAL HISTORY AND COURSE

The understanding of the natural history of PSC continues to evolve. In PSC, although some symptomatic or minimally symptomatic patients do well for many years, the majority experience progression of disease. Analysis at our institution of 174 patients with PSC revealed the following:

1. The median survival from time of diagnosis of PSC was 11.9 years.
2. Both symptomatic and asymptomatic patients had a shorter survival as compared to a US population matched for age, sex, and race.
3. Thirty-one percent of patients died as a result of underlying liver disease or the development of cholangiocarcinoma.
4. An additional 10% were referred for liver transplantation.

Statistical models have been devised to predict the probability of survival for individual patients with PSC. These models are useful in the selection of patients and timing of liver transplantation, designing treatment trials, for stratification of patients entering trials, and developing end points of treatment failure. Models for PSC developed at the Mayo Clinic rely on measures such as age, serum bilirubin, hepatic histologic stage, and the presence of splenomegaly.

COMPLICATIONS

Complications associated with any type of chronic liver disease, such as liver failure, pruritus, ascites, and esophageal varices occur in PSC. Because of the cholestatic nature of the syndrome, patients with PSC are also susceptible to fat-soluble vitamin deficiencies and metabolic bone disease.

Complications *specific for PSC* include recurrent bacterial cholangitis, dominant stricturing of the extrahepatic bile ducts, and cholangiocarcinoma. Recurrent episodes of bacterial cholangitis are unusual initial symptoms in PSC; however, cholangitis is frequent in patients with previous biliary surgery and in those with dominant stricture formation.

Strictures

Dominant strictures of the biliary tree occur in approximately 10% to 15% of patients with PSC during the course of their disease. The strictures occur most often at the hilum, and they can also involve the common bile duct, as well as the right and left hepatic ducts. Dominant strictures are frequently associated with the acute onset of jaundice, pruritus, and bacterial cholangitis with fever and chills.

Adenocarcinoma of Bile Ducts

During the course of their disease, 8% to 15% of PSC patients with or without CUC develop adenocarcinoma of the bile duct. The highest incidence appears to occur in those patients with long-standing CUC and cirrhotic-stage PSC. Hence, PSC can be considered a premalignant condition of the biliary tree just as CUC is considered a premalignant condition of the colon. Because patients with PSC often have long-standing, relatively quiescent colitis, they are at risk for developing both cholangiocarcinoma and colon cancer. Unfortunately, it has been difficult to diagnose bile duct cancer early in patients with PSC, since fine-needle aspiration, brush cytology, and exfoliative cytology have been rather insensitive in detecting cholangiocarcinoma in the presence of PSC. A recent report suggests that the measurement of serum concentrations of the glycoprotein CA-19-9 may be promising for the detection of cholangiocarcinoma that accompanies PSC.

DIFFERENTIAL DIAGNOSIS

The differential diagnosis of PSC should include primary biliary cirrhosis and extrahepatic biliary obstruction due to stones, iatrogenic strictures, and tumors. Although ultrasonography or computed tomography may suggest biliary dilation, cholangiography is the definitive diagnostic study. Drug-induced cholestasis should also be considered in the differential diagnosis.

Autoimmune chronic active hepatitis (AICAH) can sometimes overlap with PSC. During the course of AICAH, patients may develop a cholestatic biochemical profile, and a cholangiogram may show changes consistent with PSC. Therefore, patients with AICAH and associated CUC should have a cholangiogram to exclude PSC.

TREATMENT

Treatment of Complications

The management of symptoms from decompensated liver disease in PSC (e.g., recurrent bleeding from gastroesophageal varices, ascites, or hepatic encephalopathy) is essentially the same as the management of these complications in other forms of liver disease. Sclerotherapy is preferred to shunt surgery for bleeding esophageal varices, as the latter procedure may make future liver transplantation more technically difficult. Transjugular intrahepatic portosystemic shunt (TIPS) placement is also being employed more frequently for bleeding esophageal varices.

Bacterial Cholangitis in PSC

Bacterial cholangitis in PSC should be treated with broad spectrum antibiotics. The effectiveness of prophylactic therapy with antibiotics is not yet clearly established. Ciprofloxacin can be used because of its high biliary concentrations and broad bacterial coverage. The ability of ciprofloxacin to reduce the frequency of bacterial cholangitis in PSC in patients who have a history of recurrent bacterial cholangitis seems impressive; however, controlled data remain unavailable.

Strictures of the Biliary Tree in PSC

Strictures of the biliary tree in PSC and the ensuing biliary obstruction can be alleviated by balloon dilation of dominant strictures by either a transhepatic or endoscopic retrograde approach, depending on the location and available expertise. Dominant strictures developing in patients with PSC can often be successfully treated with percutaneous balloon dilation, and long-term stenting and biliary surgical intervention can generally be avoided. Balloon dilation seems to be most effective in patients who had a recent increase in serum bilirubin levels or a recent onset of bacterial cholangitis; the approach appears less effective in patients with a long-standing jaundice or with a long-standing history of recurrent bouts of bacterial cholangitis.

Medical Therapy

A number of therapies for PSC have been tested in controlled trials. None are totally effective. Specific therapeutic agents that have been tested are summarized in Table 105–3 and include cupruretic, antifibrinogenic, immunosuppressive, and anticholestatic agents.

TABLE 105-3. MEDICAL THERAPY FOR PSC

CUPRURTIC	IMMUNOSUPPRESSIVE	ANTIFIBRINOGENIC	CHOLERETIC
D-Penicillamine*	Corticosteroids Cyclosporin* FK506 Methotrexate* Azathioprine*	Colchicine	Ursodeoxycholic acid*

*Controlled trial performed or under way.

However, two agents, methotrexate and ursodeoxycholic acid (UDCA), may have some place in selected patients with PSC. After 24 months of treatment with methotrexate in a open-labeled trial, patients with PSC showed significant biochemical improvement in alkaline phosphatase but not in other biochemical parameters, liver histologic parameters, or final outcome. Several studies have demonstrated UDCA to significantly improve biochemical abnormalities in patients with PSC; however, none have demonstrated improvement in patient survival. Methotrexate and UDCA may help in precirrhotic patients with PSC, and larger randomized control trials need to be performed.

Surgical Therapy

Reconstructive Biliary Tract Surgery

Choledochoduodenostomy or choledochojejunostomy for PSC are palliative measures to alleviate symptoms. Unfortunately, no good published data exist presenting confident evaluation of surgical procedures for the treatment of PSC. Reconstructive surgery is unlikely to have a beneficial effect on the natural history of PSC, particularly if performed in patients with cirrhotic-stage disease. In addition, bouts of bacterial cholangitis develop postoperatively in more than 60% of patients who undergo such surgical procedures. However, patients with severe hilar or extrahepatic biliary structuring and persistent jaundice or cholangitis but without cirrhosis may benefit from biliary reconstruction, particularly if efforts at endoscopic or transhepatic balloon dilation are unsuccessful.

Proctocolectomy

Some clinicians have suggested that proctocolectomy in patients with PSC and CUC may favorably affect the hepatobiliary disease. However, such surgery is associated with considerable morbidity from the development of peristomal varices after ileostomy. Furthermore, proctocolectomy has not been shown to have a beneficial effect on clinical, biochemical, hepatic histologic, and radiologic features of PSC and on overall survival. Currently, proctocolectomy should not be performed simply to remove the colon in a patient with PSC in anticipation of having a beneficial effect on liver disease. If carcinoma or precancerous lesions develop in the colon, a proctocolectomy is indicated. Patients who require a proctocolectomy and are potential candidates for liver transplantation should undergo an ileoanal anastomosis to avoid the potential formation of peristomal varices and to eliminate the constant threat of bacterial contamination from the ileostomy at the time of liver transplantation.

Liver Transplantation

The treatment of choice for patients with end-stage PSC is liver transplantation. The development and use of prognostic models has shown liver transplantation to be a valuable life-extending therapeutic modality in patients with end-stage PSC. One-year survival after liver transplantation is currently about 80%. Factors that promote consideration for liver transplantation are decreased quality of life, progressive cholestasis (bilirubin >10 mg/dl), deteriorating hepatic synthetic function, or intractable symptoms. Disabling fatigue, pruritus, uncontrolled ascites, hepatic encephalopathy, or variceal bleeding not controlled with sclerotherapy are also indications for liver transplantation. Successful liver transplantation normally results in increased survival and dramatic improvement in the quality of life. Most patients resume normal activities after recovering from the postoperative period.

Patients with PSC seem to have an increased incidence of chronic ductopenic rejection and graft loss from rejection, as well as an increased incidence of biliary structuring. After liver transplantation, there is evidence of recurrence of PSC in a very small number of patients. However, it is difficult to conclusively attribute the biliary stricturing after liver transplantation to recurrent PSC, since these strictures may be attributable to low-grade bacterial cholangitis, which could be related to the Roux-en-Y biliary anastomosis that is routinely performed in PSC patients. In addition, rejection, ischemia, ABO mismatch, prolonged graft preservation prior to transplantation, and possibly cytomegalovirus or other viral infections may contribute to biliary stricturing after liver transplantation.

CHRONIC HEPATITIS

Chronic persistent hepatitis and CAH occur with increased frequency in association with inflammatory bowel disease, usually CUC. In general, these chronic hepatitides are idiopathic or autoimmune in nature. The role of the hepatitis B and C viruses in causing these conditions remains somewhat obscure. The natural history of the underlying hepatitis is independent of progression or lack of progression of IBD and generally similar to patients without IBD. However, response to medical therapy may not be as beneficial. There is a situation in which a patient with CUC may have biochemical and histologic evidence for CAH at one point in time and then subsequently develops biochemical, histologic, and ultimately cholangiographic evidence of PSC, suggesting the existence of an overlap syndrome between CAH and PSC. Thus, it seems reasonable that patients with CAH who have associated IBD should have a cholangiogram to exclude PSC.

CHOLELITHIASIS

Gallstones are known to be increased in frequency (approximately 30%) in Crohn's disease and after ileocolectomy. The stones are predominantly cholesterol in composition and reflect alterations in the enterohepatic circulation of bile acids that result from malabsorption of bile acids by a diseased or absent ileum; a subsequent diminution in the bile acid pool results in an increase in cholesterol saturation of bile. There is no apparent increase in gallstones in association with CUC. Therapy of the gallstones in association with IBD should be the same as in patients with gallstones without associated IBD.

SUMMARY

PSC is the most common and most important hepatobiliary disease seen in association with IBD. Approximately 5% of all patients with CUC have PSC, and most patients with PSC ultimately develop IBD, usually CUC. PSC and CUC appear to be associated diseases; one does not cause the other, but common pathogenic mechanisms are likely involved. PSC alone does not differ from PSC with IBD with regard to clinical, biochemical, cholangiographic, and hepatic histologic features. There is an overlap syndrome of CAH and PSC in patients with CUC, suggesting that patients with CAH and CUC should have a cholangiogram. Colectomy in patients with PSC and CUC does not influence the PSC and, if done for colitic indications, should be accompanied by an ileal pouch-anal anastomosis. Serologic markers frequently found in PSC with or without CUC are being identified, including markers for the dreaded complication of cholangiocarcinoma. Unfortunately, patients with PSC and CUC are doubly at risk for malignancies of the colon and biliary system. Medical therapies that may beneficially affect both PSC and CUC are being assessed, and liver transplantation is life saving for patients with advanced PSC. Although CAH and gallstones are also found in association with IBD, they are much less common and of considerably less clinical importance than PSC associated with IBD.

REFERENCES

1. Chapman RW. Role of immune factors in the pathogenesis of primary sclerosing cholangitis. *Semin Liver Dis.* 1991;11:1–4.
2. Fausa O, Schrumpf E, Elgjo K. Relationship of inflammatory bowel disease and primary sclerosing cholangitis. *Semin Liver Dis.* 1991;11:31–39.
3. LaRusso NF, Wiesner RH, Ludwig J, MacCarty RL. Primary sclerosing cholangitis. *N Engl J Med.* 1984;310:899–903.
4. Quigley EMM, LaRusso NF, Ludwig J, MacSween RNM, Birnie GG, Watkinson G. Familial occurrence of primary sclerosing cholangitis and ulcerative colitis. *Gastroenterology.* 1983;85:1160–1165.
5. Wiesner RH, LaRusso NF, Ludwig J, Dickson ER. Comparison of the clinicopathologic features of primary sclerosing cholangitis and primary biliary cirrhosis. *Gastroenterology.* 1985;88:108–114.

Major Radiologic Abnormalities in PSC
1. Cotton PB, Nickl N. Endoscopic and radiologic approaches to therapy in primary sclerosing cholangitis. *Semin Liver Dis.* 1991;11:40–48.

2. MacCarty RL, LaRusso NF, Wiesner RH, Ludwig J. Primary sclerosing cholangitis: findings on cholangiography and pancreatography. *Radiology.* 1983;149:39–44.

Histologic Abnormalities in PSC

1. Batts KP, Ludwig J. Histopathology of autoimmune chronic active hepatitis, primary biliary cirrhosis, and primary sclerosing cholangitis. In: Krawitt EL, Wiesner RH, eds. *Autoimmune Liver Diseases.* New York, NY: Raven Press Publishers; 1991:75–92.

Bone Disease in PSC

1. Hay JE, Lindor KD, Wiesner RH, Dickson ER, Krom RAF, LaRusso NF. The metabolic bone disease of primary sclerosing cholangitis. *Hepatology.* 1991;14:257–261.

Complications and Treatment

1. Cangemi JR, Wiesner RH, Beaver SJ, et al. Effect of proctocolectomy for chronic ulcerative colitis on the natural history of primary sclerosing cholangitis. *Gastroenterology.* 1989;96:790–794.
2. Dickson ER, Murtaugh PA, Wiesner RH, et al. Primary sclerosing cholangitis: refinement and validation of survival models. *Gastroenterology.* 1993;103:1893–1901.
3. Kaplan MM. Medical approaches to primary sclerosing cholangitis. *Semin Liver Dis.* 1991;11:56–63.
4. Marsh JW Jr, Iwatsuji S, Makowka L, et al. Orthotopic liver transplantation for primary sclerosing cholangitis. *Ann Surg.* 1988;207:21–25.
5. Nichols JC, Gores GH, LaRusso NF, Wiesner RH, Nagorney DM, Ritts RE Jr. Diagnostic role of CA 19-9 for cholangiocarcinoma in primary sclerosing cholangitis. *Hepatology.* 1992;16:62A. Abstract.
6. Rosen CB, Nagorney DM, Wiesner RH, Coffey RJ Jr, LaRusso NF. Cholangiocarcinoma complicating primary sclerosing cholangitis. *Ann Surg.* 1991;213:21–25.

106

Primary Biliary Cirrhosis

VIJAYAN BALAN, E. ROLLAND DICKSON, and KEITH D. LINDOR

Primary biliary cirrhosis (PBC) is a chronic, usually progressive, cholestatic liver disease that primarily affects middle-aged women and is characterized by ongoing destruction of interlobular and septal bile ducts. The name *primary biliary cirrhosis* is commonly used, although it is only descriptive of the last stage of the disease. The more accurate name *chronic nonsuppurative destructive cholangitis* describes the characteristic abnormality seen on the liver biopsy specimen. The natural history of the disease usually is one of slow progression with eventual development of cirrhosis, portal hypertension, with its attendant complications, and death, unless liver transplantation intervenes.

EPIDEMIOLOGY

PBC has been reported from virtually all parts of the world and affects all races. However, most epidemiologic studies are from Europe and North America; based on these studies, the number of patients affected suggest an annual incidence of 4 to 15 per million individuals. The prevalence, or the number of individuals alive at any time with the disease, is estimated to be between 40 to 180 per million. These numbers primarily reflect the symptomatic cases, and the size of the asymptomatic group is not known. Women are more commonly afflicted, with most reported series showing eight to nine times more women than men.

GENETICS

Familial clustering of PBC has been documented, for instance, in sisters, twins, and mothers and daughters, but is uncommon. The prevalence of circulating antibodies is also increased in relatives of patients afflicted with PBC. The class II major histocompatibility complex (MHC) antigens, especially HLA-DRw8, have been demonstrated to be present with increased frequency in patients with PBC. The MHC class

II antigens are the gene products of the D region loci within the MHC on human chromosome 6 and are important in generating the immune response.

Concanavalin A–induced suppression of mitogen-stimulated immunoglobulin production is impaired in patients with PBC and in normal relatives of patients with PBC. This finding suggests that hereditary immunoregulating abnormalities may play a role in the cause of PBC.

ETIOLOGY

Although the cause of PBC remains unknown, many investigators believe that PBC is associated with an immunologic disturbance that is related to the bile duct destruction. PBC's origin as an autoimmune disease is supported by the following features:

1. Frequent association of PBC with other autoimmune diseases
2. Presence of circulating antibodies (Table 106–1)
3. Multiplicity of functional immunologic abnormalities (Table 106–1)
4. Hepatic histologic findings suggesting immunologic bile duct destruction.

However, as of yet, no unifying theory exists to explain how these above findings relate to the pathogenesis of PBC.

CLINICAL FEATURES

SYMPTOMATIC DISEASE

Nine out of ten patients with primary biliary cirrhosis are female, usually in their fourth to sixth decade of life. A typical presentation is one of gradual onset of pruritus without jaundice. In many of these patients, jaundice may develop within 6 months to 2 years after the onset of pruritus. In a smaller number of the patients, jaundice and pruritus start simultaneously. Jaundice that precedes pruritus is unusual but may be the most common presenting complaint in men. Pruritus may begin during pregnancy and therefore be confused with idiopathic cholestatic jaundice of the last trimester.

In addition, patients may present with fatigue, right upper quadrant pain, and lethargy. Symptoms of advanced liver disease such as jaundice, gastrointestinal tract bleeding, ascites, and encephalopathy usually occur late in the course of the disease. Table 106–2 summarizes the symptoms and their relative order of frequency.

On physical examination, the patient often appears well nourished. Hyperpigmentation, especially in the sun-exposed areas, is not uncommon. Jaundice may be present, as well as excoriations from scratching. Xanthelasma and xanthomas are occasionally seen about the eyes and the extensor surfaces in the later stages of the disease. The liver is usually enlarged and firm, and the spleen is also palpable. Signs of end-

TABLE 106–1. AUTOANTIBODIES AND IMMUNOLOGIC ABNORMALITIES ASSOCIATED WITH PRIMARY BILIARY CIRRHOSIS

Incidence of Associated Autoantibodies
Antimitochondrial antibodies	96%
Rheumatoid factor	70%
Smooth muscle antibody	66%
Thyroid-specific antibodies	41%
Extractable nuclear antigen	30%
Antinuclear antibody	23%
Antibody to native DNA	22%

Associated Immunologic Abnormalities in Decreasing Order of Frequency
Autoantibodies
Skin test anergy
Increased serum immunoglobulin G
Increased serum immunoglobulin M
Increased complement activation and turnover
Circulating immune complexlike activity
Suppressor T-lymphocyte dysfunction
Decreased autologous mixed lymphocyte response
Increased autoreactive T lymphocyte
Circulating activated B lymphocytes
Alteration of T-cell subsets
Cytotoxic lymphocyte infiltrating bile duct epithelium
Expression of class II major histocompatibility complex antigens by bile duct epithelium
Decreased Kupffer's cell function

TABLE 106–2. INCIDENCE OF SYMPTOMS AND SIGNS OF BILIARY CIRRHOSIS AT PRESENTATION

Fatigue	70%
Pruritus	69%
Jaundice	30%
No symptom	30%
Hyperpigmentation	55%
Hepatomegaly	50%
Splenomegaly	30%
Xanthelasma	20%

TABLE 106–3. DISEASES ASSOCIATED WITH PRIMARY BILIARY CIRRHOSIS

DISEASE	INCIDENCE (%)
Keratoconjunctivitis sicca	70–90
Arthritis or arthropathy	15–20
Scleroderma and variants	15–20
Scleroderma	3
CREST syndrome	7
Raynaud's phenomenon	8
Thyroid disease	15–20
Cutaneous disorders (lichen planus, discoid lupus erythematosus, bullous pemphigoid)	11
Renal tubular acidosis	60
Breast cancer	Fourfold increase in risk

stage liver disease (i.e., ascites, spider angiomas, and evidence of hepatic encephalopathy) appear only in the latter stages of the disease and are rare as presenting features.

A number of diseases have been reported to be associated with PBC and are summarized in Table 106–3. Many of the diseases found in association with PBC may be related to disturbances in the immune system. These are scleroderma, which may be seen in 3% to 4% of patients, and the CREST syndrome (calcinosis cutis, Raynaud's phenomenon, esophageal dysfunction, sclerodactyly, and telangiectasia) variant of scleroderma. Various components of this combination may be seen in up to a fifth of patients with PBC. Sjögren's syndrome (defined by the presence of dry eyes [keratoconjunctivitis sicca] and dry mouth and by specific testing) may be seen in as many as 75% of patients.

Inflammatory arthritis may be present in one fifth of patients with PBC. Thyroid disease, usually lymphocytic thyroiditis may also be seen in 20% of patients with PBC. Various antithyroid antibodies, such as antimicrosomal or antithyroglobulin antibodies, are present in a large percentage of patients. Renal tubular acidosis, which may be either proximal or distal, is relatively common in PBC and may be found in up to 50% to 60% of patients. The cause of the renal tubular acidosis is unknown but, as in Wilson's disease, may be related to excess copper deposition within the kidney. A threefold to fourfold increased risk of breast cancer has been reported in patients with PBC. The mechanism of this increased risk is unknown, but a regular screening for breast cancer in these patients is warranted.

ASYMPTOMATIC DISEASE

The widespread use of automated blood chemistries has resulted in an increasing number of patients being diagnosed at presymptomatic stage. These patients are usually identified because of an elevated serum alkaline phosphatase level on routine examination or during investigation of a related complaint such as hypercholesterolemia. Other patients may present with symptoms specific for other diseases known to be associated with PBC.

DIAGNOSIS

BLOOD CHEMISTRIES

The hepatic chemistries usually reveal an elevated alkaline phosphatase (three or four times normal), with mild elevations in alanine aminotransferase (ALT) and aspartate aminotransferase (AST). The serum bilirubin values are usually normal initially. Serum albumin level and prothrombin time generally remain normal until late in the course of the disease. Serum immunoglobulin M (IgM) is elevated in 90% of patients.

LIPID PROFILE

Serum cholesterol levels are usually elevated in PBC. In the early stages, the increases in high-density lipoprotein (HDL) cholesterol exceed those of low-density lipoprotein (LDL) and very low density lipoprotein (VLDL). As the disease progresses, the concentration of HDLs decreases, and a marked elevation in LDL occurs. However, the hyperlipidemia associated with PBC does not appear to place these patients at increased risk for atherosclerotic disease.

AUTOANTIBODIES

The circulating antimitochondrial antibodies (AMA) are found in virtually all patients with PBC. AMA are nonorgan and nonspecies specific, usually detected by an ELISA technique, and not specific for PBC. Positive test results for AMA can be seen in a quarter of patients with chronic active hepatitis, 3% of patients with connective tissue diseases, and occasionally with patients with primary sclerosing cholangitis. However, the AMA is nearly always absent in patients with mechanical obstruction to the bile ducts.

Recent work has defined a specific group of antigens in PBC that are located on the inner membrane of mitochondria and antibodies that recognize AMA. The autoantigens, termed *M2*, and the antibodies directed against it, anti-M2, are present in 95% to 98% of patients with PBC. The antigenic targets of anti-M2 have been identified and characterized as immunodominant sites in three vital enzymes of the 2-oxoacid dehydrogenase family, which include pyruvate dehydrogenase, branched-chain 2-oxoacid dehydrogenase, and 2-oxoglutarate dehydrogenase. This discovery is likely to help increase the sensitivity and specificity of the AMA. Other AMA subtypes related to PBC have also been described and react with antigens on the outer mitochondrial membrane. Anti-M4 is present in patients with anti-M2 and with features both of chronic active hepatitis and PBC. Anti-M8 is present in patients with anti-M2 and may be associated with a more rapid course of PBC. Anti-M9 has been seen in patients with and without anti-M2 and may be helpful in the diagnosis of early and asymptomatic PBC.

Evaluation of the Biliary Tree

In the patient who has chronic cholestasis, positive test results for AMA, and liver biopsy results consistent with PBC, an ultrasound examination of the biliary tree is usually adequate to exclude biliary obstruction. However, in a male patient with negative test results for AMA or with atypical features of PBC, an endoscopic retrograde cholangiography or percutaneous cholangiography is recommended to exclude primary sclerosing cholangitis and other causes of biliary obstruction.

HEPATIC PATHOLOGY

Morphologically, the disease progresses through sequential histologic changes, which have been descriptively divided into four stages (Fig. 106–1). The visible chain of events begins with an inflammatory reaction, which presumably is immunologically mediated, involving the interlobular and septal bile ducts. Inflammatory cells accumulate in the portal tracts, which often appear expanded *(portal hepatitis, stage I)*. The epithelium of the interlobular and septal bile ducts degenerates segmentally. This process is accompanied by the formation of a poorly defined, noncaseating epithelioid cell granuloma. The "florid duct lesion" (granulomatous duct

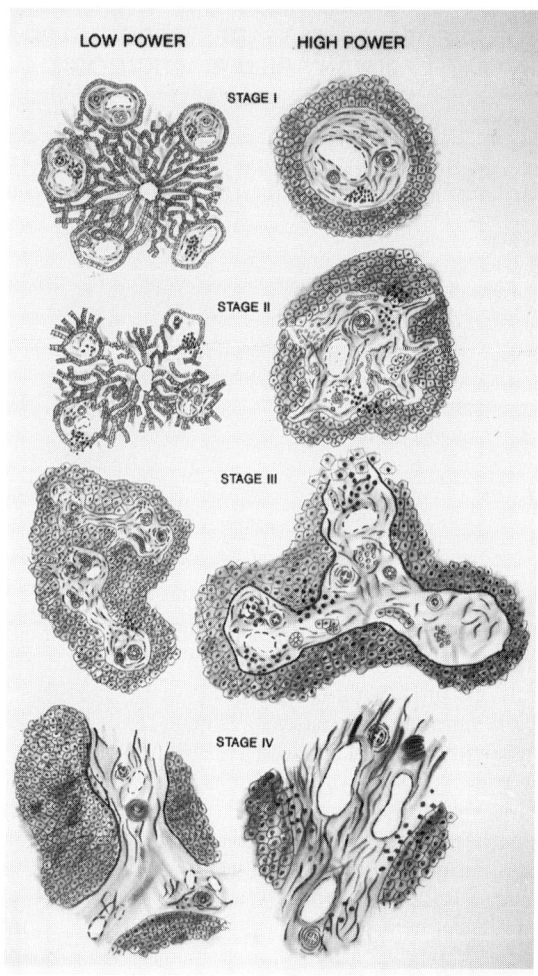

FIGURE 106–1. Histologic stages of primary biliary cirrhosis (PBC) III at low- and high-power magnification. *Stage I*, portal hepatitis; *stage II*, periportal hepatitis; *stage III*, septal stage; *stage IV*, cirrhotic stage. (From Lindor KD, Dickson ER. Primary biliary cirrhosis. In: Kaplowitz N, ed. *Liver and Biliary Diseases.* Baltimore, Md: Williams & Wilkins Co; 1992. © 1992, the Williams & Wilkins Co, Baltimore.)

destruction) is nearly diagnostic of PBC. The only convincing exceptions have occurred in a few patients with sarcoidosis. However, the "florid duct lesion" is infrequently found on single-blind biopsy specimens.

As the disease progresses, the inflammatory infiltrate spills from the portal tracts into the surrounding parenchyma and causes piecemeal necrosis *(periportal hepatitis, stage II)*. Small granulomas outside the bile ducts and in the lobules may appear at this time and may remain until late in the disease. Periportal inflammation may be associated with much ductular (small bile ducts) proliferation, but the presence of these ductules merely represents a futile attempt by the parenchyma to regenerate, as ductules cannot replace ducts. Advancing inflammation, often accompanied by fibrosis, begins to connect portal tracts, and lobules become dissected. Bridging necrosis and septal fibrosis becomes a dominant histologic feature *(septal stage, stage III)*. By this time, segmental granulomatous bile duct destruction becomes inconspicuous because most ducts have already been destroyed and are no longer identifiable. Most patients become symptomatic at this stage. Finally, nodular regeneration begins to appear, ductopenia is prominent, and true biliary cirrhosis develops *(cirrhotic stage, stage IV)*. Histologic progression may occur over many years in the absence of overt symptoms in some patients. In addition, some patients may present with advanced histologic disease (stage III or IV) despite mild-to-modest biochemical alterations and have a benign clinical course for many years.

NATURAL HISTORY AND COURSE

Our understanding of the natural history of PBC is being clarified as more patients are being recognized in the asymptomatic phase of the disease. Initially, it was thought that patients in the asymptomatic phase have a normal life expectancy; however, this has not been the experience of most groups. Presymptomatic patients follow the same course as those with symptoms, except that mortality lags behind by approximately 4 years (Fig. 106–2). In a Mayo Clinic study, 32 of the 44 patients with asymptomatic PBC followed for 4 to 6 years developed increasing bilirubin and decreasing serum albumin. Furthermore, 84% of the patients developed symptoms related to the liver disease and had a fourfold increase in mortality compared to the general population. In any case, in most patients the course of PBC is long and may exceed 10 to 15 years.

Statistical models have been devised to predict the probability of survival for individual patients with PBC. One such model developed at the Mayo Clinic relies on simple noninvasive measures such as serum bilirubin, albumin, prothrombin time, presence or absence of peripheral edema, and patient's age. Other models have also used similar criteria with some variation in the predictive variable used. These models are useful in the selection of patients and timing of liver transplantation. They may also be useful in designing treatment trials, for stratification of patients entering trials, and for developing end points of treatment failure.

COMPLICATIONS

Steatorrhea is a common finding as PBC progresses. Steatorrhea may be due to decreased bile acid micelle concentration in the small intestine, pancreatic exocrine insufficiency, or coexisting celiac sprue. Fat malabsorption may lead to vitamin D and calcium malabsorption, causing osteomalacia, which may contribute to the development of metabolic bone disease in some patients. *Metabolic bone disease* may lead to disabling pathologic fractures and is a serious complication of PBC. Osteoporosis is the major

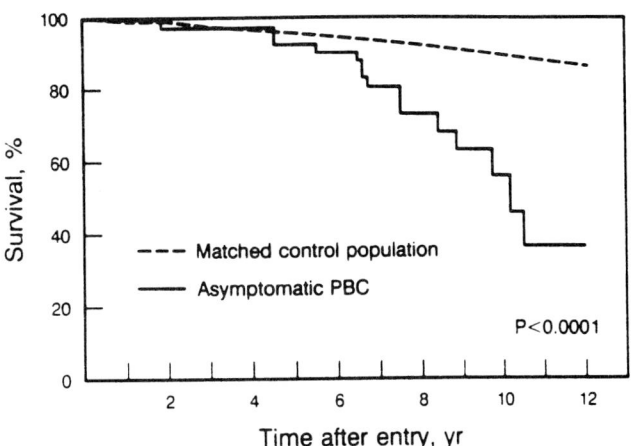

FIGURE 106–2. Survival (Kaplan-Meier estimate) of age-, sex-, and race-matched controls (---) and patients with asymptomatic primary biliary cirrhosis (PBC) (—). (From Balasubramaniam K, Grambsch PM, Wiesner RH, et al. Diminished survival in asymptomatic primary biliary cirrhosis: a prospective study. *Gastroenterology*. 1990;98:1567–1571. By permission of the American Gastroenterological Association.)

component of the bone disease. Although the cause of osteoporosis is uncertain, it has recently been reported that elevated levels of serum bilirubin may inhibit osteoblast proliferation in vitro.

Other fat-soluble vitamins may also be low secondary to steatorrhea. *Vitamin K deficiency* leads to prolonged prothrombin time; *vitamin A deficiency* may lead to difficulty with night vision. *Vitamin E deficiency* on rare occasions can cause a neurologic abnormality primarily affecting the posterior columns and is characterized by areflexia or ataxia and loss of proprioception.

Portal hypertension may develop at any time during the course of the disease and may lead to gastrointestinal tract bleeding from esophageal varices, even in the earlier stages before cirrhosis has developed. The development of esophageal varices in patients with PBC has a more favorable prognosis than in patients with alcoholic cirrhosis (Fig. 106–3). Hence, prophylactic therapy is not indicated for patients with PBC and varices that have not previously bled. Finally in the last stages of the disease, hepatocellular failure leads to death unless liver transplantation intervenes.

DIFFERENTIAL DIAGNOSIS

Other causes of chronic cholestasis such as extrahepatic biliary obstruction due to biliary stones, iatrogenic strictures, and tumors should be considered in the differential diagnosis. In these patients, although ultrasonography or computed tomography may suggest biliary dilation, cholangiography is the definitive diagnostic study. AMA would be absent in most of these patients.

Primary sclerosing cholangitis (PSC) is also in the differential diagnosis of PBC. PSC is more common in patients with inflammatory bowel disease, affects men more often than women, and test results for AMA are negative. Cholangiography is diagnostic in these patients and shows areas of irregular structuring and dilation of the intrahepatic and extrahepatic biliary tree. Liver biopsy specimens may be suggestive but not always adequate to differentiate PBC from PSC.

Drug-induced cholestasis secondary to administration of phenothiazine, estrogens, androgens, and a number of other drugs should also be considered in the differential diagnosis.

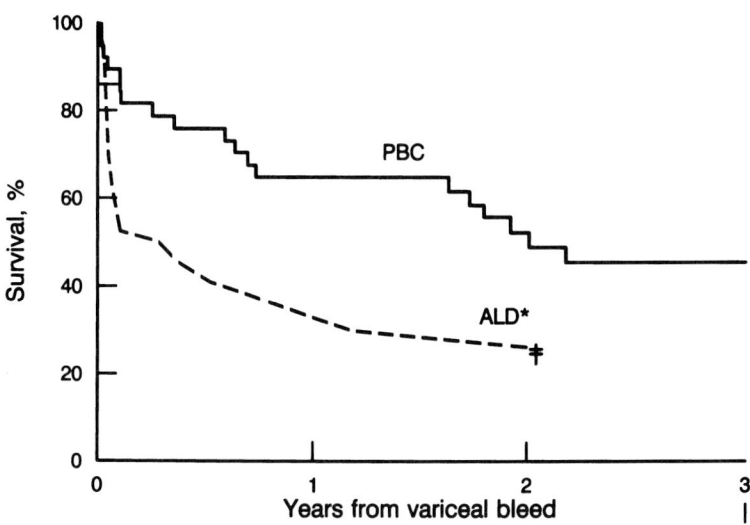

†Smith, JL, Graham DY:Gastroenterology 82:968, 1982
*ALD = Alcoholic Liver Disease

FIGURE 106–3. Comparison of the survival of patients with primary biliary cirrhosis *(PBC)* and alcoholic liver disease *(ALD)* after initial variceal bleed. †Smith JL, Graham DY. *Gastroenterology.* 1982;82:968. (From Smith JL, Graham DY. Variceal hemorrhage: a critical evaluation. *Gastroenterology.* 1982;82:968–973; Graham DY, Smith JL. The course of patients after variceal hemorrhage. *Gastroenterology.* 1981;80:800–809; Gores GJ, Wiesner RH, Dickson ER, et al. Prospective evaluation of esophageal varices in primary biliary cirrhosis: development, natural history, and influence on survival. *Gastroenterology.* 1989;96:1552–1559. By permission of the American Gastroenterological Association.)

Autoimmune chronic active hepatitis (AICAH) can be confused with PBC in some patients. Patients with AICAH may have positive test results for AMA but usually in low titer (<1:40). A liver biopsy specimen may be helpful, as bile duct abnormalities are uncommon in AICAH and characteristic in PBC. AMA subtypes such as anti-M4 may allow differentiation between CAH and PBC when this rare, confusing, overlap situation arises.

TREATMENT

TREATMENT OF SYMPTOMATIC DISEASE

Pruritus

Cholestyramine relieves itching and lowers serum bile acids in patients with cholestasis. Cholestyramine increases intestinal excretion of bile acids by preventing their reabsorption. There is little controversy regarding the dramatic relief of pruritus from cholestyramine in many patients with PBC, but the role of bile acids in the pathogenesis of itching remains unclear. Cholestyramine is given in 4-g doses (mixed with liquids) with meals for a total daily dose of 12 to 16 g. Cholestyramine should be given one and a half hours before or after other medications to avoid nonspecific binding and diminished intestinal absorption. Once the itching remits, the dosage should be reduced to the minimum that maintains relief.

If cholestyramine is ineffective, phenobarbital may be added in a dosage of 120 to 160 mg/d. Rifampin, 300 to 600 mg/d, has also been effective in relieving pruritus. This may be due to P-450 enzyme induction or inhibition of bile acid uptake. Additional experimental approaches include phototherapy and plasmapheresis to remove bile acids.

Osteopenia

The bone disease associated with PBC, as discussed earlier, is often due to osteoporosis and seldom due to osteomalacia. However, if serum levels of vitamin D are low, they can readily be corrected by administering 50,000 U of vitamin D given once or twice per week. Patients with PBC generally do not have difficulties in 25-hydroxylation of vitamin D and hence do not require the expensive 1,25-dihydroxyvitamin D or 25-hydroxyvitamin D replacement therapy. Osteoporosis, however, has no effective therapy in patients with PBC. In postmenopausal osteoporosis, estrogen therapy, especially when instituted soon after menopause, has been associated with slowing of bone loss. In cholestatic patients, estrogen therapy was thought to be contraindicated, as it may further contribute to intrahepatic cholestasis. However, this does not seem to be a problem with a standard estrogen replacement therapy and has been shown to improve osteoporosis in a recent retrospective study. However, it would be prudent to reassess the patient clinically and biochemically within 2 to 3 months after starting estrogen therapy.

Fat-Soluble Vitamin Deficiency

Vitamin A deficiency may cause problems with night vision. Vitamin A level can be readily measured in the blood, and when it is low, oral administration of vitamin A (25,000 to 50,000 U two to three times per week) improves this symptom. Excessive vitamin A intake is associated with hepatotoxicity and should be monitored. Vitamin K deficiency is associated with a prolonged prothrombin time. In patients with vitamin K deficiency a trial of vitamin K (5 to 10 mg) should be given; if the prothrombin time improves, these patients should be maintained on a water-soluble vitamin K replacement, 5 mg/d. In patients with low vitamin E levels, replacement therapy can be instituted with 100 mg twice daily, although replacement is not always effective.

Hypercholesterolemia

Because patients with PBC do not appear to have an increased risk of atherosclerotic disease despite high serum cholesterol, lipid-lowering agents such as mevacor are not usually recommended. In some patients with xanthelasma, cholestyramine may stabilize or even decrease the size of cutaneous lipid deposits.

TREATMENT OF DECOMPENSATED CIRRHOSIS

The management of complications associated with decompensated PBC, such as recurrent bleeding from gastroesophageal varices, ascites, or hepatic encephalopathy, is essentially the same as the management of complications with other end-stage liver diseases. Sclerotherapy rather than shunt surgery is usually preferred for bleeding esophageal varices, as the later procedure may make future liver transplantation more technically difficult. Transjugular intrahepatic portosystemic shunt (TIPS) placement is also being employed more frequently for bleeding esophageal varices; however, its role in PBC is not defined. TIPS can rapidly decompress the portal system and in turn decompress not only the esophageal varices but also gastric varices, which are not accessible to sclerotherapy. TIPS can also reduce ascites quite dramatically. Unfortunately, the incidence of hepatic encephalopathy may increase after TIPS.

SPECIFIC TREATMENT FOR PBC

A number of therapies for PBC have been tested in controlled trials, and none has been proved to be totally effective. Specific therapeutic agents that have been tested are summarized below.

Corticosteroids were the first of the immunosuppressive agents used to treat patients with PBC. Corticosteroids would be expected to be beneficial by reducing the hepatic inflammatory response in PBC. It is also suggested that corticosteroids interfere with antigen processing by macrophages prior to presentation to lymphocytes. In a controlled trial evaluating corticosteroids, patients experienced biochemical and some histologic improvement but at the expense of accelerating bone loss. Currently, corticosteroids have an uncertain role in the treatment of PBC, especially until drugs are available to help stabilize or actually improve the osteopenia.

Azathioprine is a purine analog and acts by competitive enzyme inhibition to block the precursors of purines. The drug has potent antiinflammatory properties and, when used in combination with corticosteroids, has successfully inhibited graft rejection. Recognition of similarities between the graft-versus-host reaction and PBC strengthened the rationale for studying this drug. However, in large, prospective, controlled trials azathioprine has not shown any definite benefits. Currently azathioprine is seldom, if ever, used in the treatment of PBC.

Chlorambucil, commonly used for cancer chemotherapy, has been considered for use in PBC because of its potential antiinflammatory and immunosuppressive effects. A small, prospective clinical trial indicated biochemical and histologic improvement, but bone marrow toxicity occurred in a third of the patients who received chlorambucil, requiring discontinuation of the drug. This major toxicity has hampered further large trials and seems to preclude its use in PBC.

Cyclosporine, a potent immunosuppressive drug widely used in transplantation, has been evaluated in PBC as well. A recent clinical trial from the Mayo Clinic found clinical, biochemical, and histologic improvement with cyclosporine treatment when compared to placebo. Unfortunately, half the patients treated with cyclosporine developed hypertension, and half developed depressed renal function. Because of these side effects, the role of cyclosporine in the treatment of PBC remains indeterminate. However, this study did suggest that immunosuppressive therapy may be of benefit provided that other drugs with less toxicity than cyclosporine are available.

D-*Penicillamine (*D-*PCA)* has been the most extensively tested drug in patients with PBC. D-PCA has a variety of effects including immunosuppressive activity, copper mobilization, and suppression of fibrogenesis, all of which were considered to be important in the development of PBC. Unfortunately, despite these potential beneficial actions, the drug resulted in no clinical, biochemical, histologic, or survival benefit when tested in patients with PBC.

Colchicine, an antifibrogenic drug, has been studied in several placebo-controlled trials in patients with PBC. The drug appears to have minimal toxicity and is generally well tolerated by patients. However, colchicine has minimal effect on clinical symptoms and in slowing the histologic progression of the disease on liver biopsy and has little, if any, effect on survival.

Methotrexate is a folic acid antagonist that directly blocks the synthesis of nucleic acids and indirectly blocks the synthesis of protein. Furthermore, low-dose methotrexate acts as an immunosuppressive agent. Methotrexate has been used extensively as an immunosuppressive drug in rheumatoid arthritis. In a small uncontrolled trial performed at the New England Medical Center, nine patients with symptomatic precirrhotic PBC received methotrexate. All patients became asymptomatic; biochemical tests improved or were normalized but deteriorated in three when methotrexate was stopped. Liver histologic features improved in five patients and remained stable in four.

On rare occasions, methotrexate leads to bone marrow suppression (<1%) and idiosyncratic pulmonary infiltrates, with cough, dyspnea, and hypoxemia. These potential complications require close monitoring. The most concerning toxicity of methotrexate is hepatic fibrosis. The hepatic toxicity of methotrexate is increased with alcohol consumption and cumulative doses. Methotrexate may be efficacious in the treatment of PBC if the side effects of long-term therapy can be controlled.

Ursodeoxycholic acid (UDCA) has been evaluated in randomized, controlled trials for the treatment of PBC. This drug appears to replace endogenous hydrophobic bile acids, some of which may be hepatotoxic, with the hydrophilic nonhepatotoxic UDCA. Alterations in the bile pool may occur by competition for ileal uptake sites or by direct action at the level of the liver. Furthermore, UDCA may reduce class I and class II HLA antigen expression on the hepatocytes and bile duct epithelial cells and may also decrease the number of CD8 cells surrounding bile duct epithelial cells in patients with PBC. Preliminary results reported from clinical trials show that UDCA reduces symptoms, improves liver tests, and may improve some histologic features while having minimal toxicity. Limited information is available on the effects of UDCA on survival, need for liver transplantation, histologic progression to cirrhosis, or development of varices or ascites in patients with PBC. Hence, long-term treatment results are awaited before this drug can be recommended for the treatment of PBC.

LIVER TRANSPLANTATION

Liver transplantation is an excellent therapeutic option for end-stage PBC. The development and use of prognostic models (see Natural History and Course earlier in this chapter) have shown liver transplantation to be a valuable life-extending therapeutic modality in patients with end-stage PBC. One-year survival after liver transplantation is currently about 80% and over 60% at 5 years. Factors that promote consideration for liver transplantation are decreased quality of life, progressive cholestasis (bilirubin >10 mg/dl), deteriorating hepatic synthetic function, or intractable symptoms. Disabling fatigue, pruritus, uncontrolled ascites, hepatic encephalopathy, or variceal bleeding that is not controlled with sclerotherapy are indications for liver transplantation. Successful liver transplantation normally results in increased survival and dramatic improvement in the quality of life. Most patients resume normal activities after recovering from the postoperative period. Positive test results for AMA persist after liver transplantation, and long-term follow-up studies indicate that in up to 7% there is evidence of histologic recurrence of PBC (florid duct lesion) in the grafted liver. However, the presence of an isolated florid duct lesion has thus far not been of clinical significance and should not influence the decision of liver transplantation in PBC patients.

SUMMARY

PBC is a chronic, usually progressive, cholestatic liver disease. It is of presumed autoimmune origin and mainly affects middle-aged women. PBC is nearly always associated with positive test results for AMA and a number of other autoimmune disorders. There is no totally effective medical treatment for PBC, although UDCA appears to be beneficial. Liver transplantation is a proven and effective therapeutic modality for end-stage PBC.

REFERENCES

Clinical Features
1. Dickson ER, Fleming CR, Ludwig J. Primary biliary cirrhosis. In: Popper H, Schaffner F, eds. *Progress in Liver Disease.* Vol. 6. New York, NY: Grune & Stratton Inc; 1979:487.
2. Wiesner RH, LaRusso NF, Ludwig J, et al. Comparison of the clinicopathologic features of primary sclerosing cholangitis and primary biliary cirrhosis. *Gastroenterology.* 1985;88:108–114.

Associated Diseases
1. Culp KS, Fleming CR, Duffy J, Baldus WP, Dickson ER. Autoimmune association in primary biliary cirrhosis. *Mayo Clin Proc.* 1982;57:365–370.
2. Wolke AM, Schaffner F, Kapelman B, et al. Malignancy in primary biliary cirrhosis: high incidence of breast cancer in affected women. *Am J. Med.* 1984;76:1075–1078.

Diagnosis
1. Ludwig J, Dickson ER, McDonald GSA. Staging of chronic non-suppurative destructive cholangitis (syndrome of primary biliary cirrhosis). *Virchows Arch [A]* 1978;379:103–112.
2. Mackay IR, Gershwin ME. Molecular basis of mitochondrial autoreactivity in primary biliary cirrhosis. *Immunol Today.* 1989;10:315–318.
3. Portmann B, Popper H, Neuberger J, Williams R. Sequential and diagnostic features in primary biliary cirrhosis based on serial histologic study in 29 patients. *Gastroenterology.* 1985;88:1777–1790.

Pathogenesis
1. Gores GJ, Moore SB, et al. Primary biliary cirrhosis: associations with class II major histocompatibility complex antigens. *Hepatology.* 1987;7:889–892.
2. Kaplan MM. Primary biliary cirrhosis. *N Engl J Med.* 1987;316:521–528.
3. Miller KB, Schwartz RS. Familial abnormalities of immunoregulation in PBC. *Am J Med.* 1983;75:75–80.

Complications
1. Crippin JS, Lindor KD, Jorgensen R, et al. Hypercholesterolemia and atherosclerosis in primary biliary cirrhosis: what is the risk? *Hepatology.* 1992;15:858–862.
2. Kaplan MM, Elta GH, Furie B, et al. Fat-soluble vitamin nutrition in PBC. *Gastroenterology.* 1988;95:787–792.
3. Maddrey WC. Bone disease in patients with primary biliary cirrhosis. *Prog Liver Dis.* 1990;9:537–554.

Natural History and Prognosis
1. Balasubramaniam K, Grambsch PM, Wiesner RH, et al. Diminished survival in asymptomatic primary biliary cirrhosis: a prospective study. *Gastroenterology.* 1990;98:1567–1571.
2. Beswick DR, Klatskin G, Boyer J. Asymptomatic primary biliary cirrhosis: a progressive report on long-term follow-up and natural history. *Gastroenterology.* 1985;89:270–271.
3. Dickson ER, Grambsch PM, Fleming TR, et al. Prognosis in primary biliary cirrhosis: model for decision making. *Hepatology.* 1989;10:1–7.

Specific Treatment for PBC
1. Dickson ER, Fleming TR, Wiesner RH, et al. Trial of penicillamine in advanced primary biliary cirrhosis. *N Engl J Med.* 1985;312:1011–1015.
2. Hoofnagle JH, Davis GL, Schafer DF, et al. Randomized trial of chlorambucil for primary biliary cirrhosis. *Gastroenterology.* 1986;91:1327–1334.
3. Kaplan MM, Alling DW, Zimmerman HJ, et al. A prospective trial of colchicine for primary biliary cirrhosis. *N Engl J Med.* 1986;315:1448–1454.
4. Markus BH, Dickson ER, Grambsch PM, et al. Efficacy of liver transplantation in patients with primary biliary cirrhosis. *N Engl J Med.* 1989;320:1709–1713.
5. Wiesner RH, Grambsch PM, Lindor KD, et al. Clinical and statistical analyses of new and evolving therapies for primary biliary cirrhosis. *Hepatology.* 1988;8:668–676.

107
Hepatic Granulomas
ROBERTO CHIPRUT

Hepatic granulomas are a frequent manifestation of infectious or noninfectious systemic illnesses.[1-6] The importance of granulomas is not in the hepatic functional disturbance they may cause but as a means of diagnosing the causative condition. Hepatic biopsy specimens can be used to confirm the diagnosis. It is often difficult to establish a conclusion when systemic manifestations are absent or no pathogens are isolated. The treatment is directed at the specific etiologic agents or the systemic process. A therapeutic trial of antituberculous chemotherapy or corticosteroids is indicated when systemic manifestations are of significant severity.

DEFINITION

The granuloma results from an immune reaction to contain and eventually destroy degradable, harmful stimuli. This proliferative inflammatory reaction results in the formation of a granular circumscribed lesion that is clearly distinct from the adjacent uninvolved tissue.[3]

It is a compact organized collection of inflammatory cells predominantly composed of mature mononuclear phagocytes (macrophages), lymphocytes, and fibroblasts. A lesser number of other inflammatory cells may surround the periphery of the granuloma.

Four categories have been described, depending on the type and disposition of the cells.[7,8]

EPITHELIOID GRANULOMA

Epithelioid granuloma is characterized by the presence of large cells with round-to-oval, clear nuclei and an eosinophilic cytoplasm (epithelioid histiocytes). It is surrounded by plasma cells and lymphocytes. These granulomas are located in the parenchyma and the portal tract. They vary in size, sometimes approaching the size of the entire hepatic lobule. When the granulomas acquire considerable size, central necrosis can be present. These granulomas are associated with multinucleated giant cells and can present in two forms: (1) horseshoe configuration along the periphery of the cells, so-called *Langhans' type,* and (2) *foreign body type* in which giant cells contain a considerable number of nuclei arranged in a compact cluster, frequently containing paralyzed foreign material (e.g., silica or talc). Granulomas of foreign body or Langhans' type may contain fungi or mycobacteria. In chronic granulomatous states, a dense fibroblastic reaction involving the portal tracts may occur and may result in presinusoidal portal hypertension (sarcoidosis).

INFLAMMATORY GRANULOMA

Inflammatory granuloma is a cluster of lymphocytes, macrophages, plasma cells and, in some instances, neutrophils and eosinophils. They are poorly delineated, small and located mainly in the parenchyma. Giant cells are uncommon.

LIPOGRANULOMA

Lipogranuloma is a collection of inflammatory cells that react against extracellular fat. In fatty infiltration of the liver, necrosis may occur with phagocytosis of the fat by macrophages. The macrophages contain small fat droplets and are surrounded by a variable number of lymphocytes. These type of granulomas are most frequently seen in diabetic, obese, and alcoholic patients. Chronic exposure to mineral oil used in the food industry has been associated with lipogranulomas.[9]

Gold therapy for rheumatoid arthritis has also been recently associated with lipogranulomas.[10]

HEPATIC FIBRIN RING GRANULOMA

Hepatic fibrin ring granuloma is a thin, well-demarcated granuloma with a rim of fibrin observed in Q fever (43%), visceral leishmaniasis (22%), and boutonneuse fever (9%). These granulomas have also been reported in toxoplasmosis, Hodgkin's disease, allopurinol hypersensitivity, cytomegalovirus infection, and hepatitis A.[11,12]

PATHOGENESIS

The formation of hepatic granulomas results from the cellular immune response of the reticuloendothelial tissue to antigens or a foreign body.[13] In this process, antigens stimulate T lymphocytes to secrete lymphokines; these substances help recruit monocytes and fibroblasts, promoting the formation of giant cells. Suppressor T cells modulate the magnitude of the inflammatory response. The mechanism whereby granulomas form to foreign bodies depends on phagocytosis by either Kupffer's cells or monocytes. The cells stimulate the secretion of a wide variety of substances that initiate the granulomatous reaction. In recent studies, it has been shown that interleukin-1 secreted by Kupffer's cells and macrophages plays a major role in the recruitment of other inflammatory cells and fibroblasts and in the formation of collagen.[14,15] Fibrosis or cirrhosis is an infrequent complication in granulomatous disease. The only exception is schistosomiasis, in which extensive portal fibrosis results in portal hypertension.

ETIOLOGY

Hepatic granulomas are found in 4% to 10% of needle biopsy specimens. They are always part of a generalized disease process. In a significant number of patients, no etiologic diagnosis is established, in spite of classic histologic scrutiny, staining for organisms, and extensive cultures.[16] With the exception of primary biliary cirrhosis, hepatic granulomas do not significantly alter hepatic function. Granulomas represent a clue for the recognition of a systemic disorder. The specific characteristics of the granuloma may enhance the possibility of establishing a diagnosis.[16,17] When granulomas are present, a comprehensive diagnostic approach should be pursued. Even after this is completed, the cause may remain a mystery.

There is definitive geographic variation in the etiologic agents that cause hepatic granulomas. In the United States and in particular southern California, sarcoidosis and tuberculosis are the most common causes, accounting for more than 50% of the cases.[8] Also in patients with acquired immunodeficiency syndrome (AIDS), atypical mycobacteria and mycoses are frequent causes of hepatic granulomas.

The etiologic factors of hepatic granulomas can be divided into two main groups: noninfectious and infectious (Table 107–1). *Noninfectious causes* include sarcoidosis, primary biliary cirrhosis, drug hypersensitivity reactions, and neoplasia.

Infectious causes include tuberculosis and atypical mycobacterial diseases. Although brucellosis, leprosy, Q fever, tuberculosis, and other mycobacteria have increased in prevalence, other causes remain rare and often produce distinctive types of granulomas. Other infectious diseases that rarely result in hepatic granulomas are viral diseases (cytomegalovirus, infectious mononucleosis), secondary syphilis, and mycoses (histoplasmosis and coccidioidomycosis). In patients

TABLE 107-1. ETIOLOGY OF HEPATIC GRANULOMAS

Noninfectious

Systemic Diseases
Idiopathic*
Sarcoidosis*
Hodgkin's disease*
Crohn's disease

Lymphoma
Wegener's granulomatosis
Systemic lupus erythematosus
Periarteritis nodosa

Ulcerative colitis
Hypogammaglobulinemia
Whipple's disease
Carcinoma

Drug Reactions
Sulfonamides*
Methyldopa*
Allopurinol*
Hydantoin*
Penicillin
Cephalosporins
Hydralazine
Quinidine

Halothane
Phenylbutazone*
Chlorpropamide
Diltiazem
Amoxicillin (clavulanic acid)
Chlorpromazine
Procainamide
Carbamazepine

Oral contraceptives
Tocainimide
Methimazole
Gold therapy
Quinine
Clofibrate

Foreign Substances
Starch (parenteral drug abuse)
Beryllium
Copper (vineyard sprayers)
Mineral oil

Cement
Mica dust
Silica

Miscellaneous Causes
Primary biliary cirrhosis*
Jejunoileal bypass

Autoimmune liver diseases
Administration of bacille Calmette-Guérin*

Infectious

Bacterial
Tuberculosis*
Brucellosis*
Leprosy*
Atypical *Mycobacterium** (*Mycobacterium avium-intracellulare*)
Salmonellosis

Tularemia
Yersinia
Melioidosis
Listeriosis

Mycosis
Histoplasmosis*
Coccidioidomycosis*
Aspergillosis

Candidiasis
Blastomycosis
Actinomycosis

Cryptococcosis
Torulosis
Nocardiosis

Viral
Cytomegalovirus*
Mononucleosis
Influenza B

Lymphogranuloma venereum
Psittacosis
Hepatitis A virus

Cat-scratch fever
Chickenpox

Parasitic
Schistosomiasis*
Toxocariasis
Fascioliasis
*Cryptosporidium**

Strongyloidosis
Tongue worm
Toxoplasmosis
Giardiasis

Visceral larva migrans
Ascariasis
Clonorchiasis

Rickettsial
Q fever*

Spirochetal
Secondary syphilis

*Most frequent.
Adapted from Wright LT. Parasitic, bacterial, fungal and granulomatous liver disease. In: Wyngaarden JB, Smith LH, Bennett JC, eds. *Cecil Textbook of Medicine.* 19th ed. Philadelphia, Pa: WB Saunders Co; 1992:778–782.

with AIDS, granulomas can be a manifestation of infection with multiple opportunistic organisms.

There is a group of patients with severe systemic symptoms and hepatic granulomas in which, in spite of extensive evaluation, the cause is not identified. This group has been labeled *idiopathic granulomatous disease of the liver.* In the midwestern United States, this is the most frequent cause of hepatic granulomas.[4]

CLINICAL FEATURES

The symptoms and findings in patients with hepatic granulomas are those of the causative disorder.[1,4,8] Patients may be asymptomatic or present with a transient fever, malaise, weight loss, abdominal pain, night sweats, nausea, or vomiting. Fever of unknown origin may occur. In patients with sarcoidosis, jaundice is common. Erythema nodosum is a nonspecific finding and associated with tuberculosis, sarcoidosis, and secondary syphilis. Hepatomegaly is usually moderate and sometimes associated with splenomegaly. The presence of lymphadenopathy suggests sarcoidosis, tuberculosis, syphilis, and AIDS. Portal hypertension can be a feature of schistosomiasis, sarcoidosis, and primary biliary cirrhosis (Table 107–2).

DIAGNOSTIC EVALUATION

Biochemical tests suggest liver dysfunction or injury. Liver tests frequently demonstrating a disproportionate increase in alkaline phosphatase (greater than five times normal) over aminotransferases. There is moderate elevation of the serum bilirubin, usually less than 3 ng/dl. In some cases of tuberculosis, sarcoidosis, and primary biliary cirrhosis, bilirubin levels may be higher. In patients with autoimmune disorders, hypergammaglobulinemia occurs. Hepatic synthetic function measured by the prothrombin time and albumin usually remains normal.[1,4,6,8] Before an extensive evaluation, it is imperative to note that tuberculosis and sarcoidosis are the most prevalent causes of hepatic granulomas. The standard laboratory evaluation should include a complete blood cell count, liver test, erythrocyte sedimentation rate, chest x-ray examination, and purified protein derivative (PPD) skin test. The microbiologic evaluation consists of cultures and serologic examinations for *Mycobacterium,* fungi, syphilis, and *Brucella.* Following the liver biopsy, culture material should be obtained from liver material and from blood, gastric washings, sputum, and bronchial washings. If suspected, serologic examinations for cytomegalovirus, Epstein-Barr virus, and Q fever should be ordered. Finally, antinuclear antibody, rheumatoid factor, antimitochondrial antibody, and angiotensin-converting enzyme may establish specific diagnoses.[4]

RADIOGRAPHIC STUDIES

Ultrasonography may suggest the presence of hepatic granuloma. Hepatic granulomas appear as multiple echogenic lesions, measuring between 3 and 5 mm, surrounded by a hypogenic halo.[18] A computed tomography (CT) scan of the liver may reveal the presence of multiple low-density areas.[19] Magnetic resonance imaging can also define the presence of granulomas.

MOST FREQUENTLY ASSOCIATED DISORDERS

GRANULOMATOUS HEPATITIS[4,6]

Liver granulomas may reflect an occult systemic disease that may remain undiagnosed. When no cause is evident, hepatic granulomas are often manifested by nonspecific symptoms including fever of unknown origin, malaise, anorexia, and asymptomatic liver function abnormalities. The patient is often a middle-aged or elderly man. Granulomas are not widespread. Pulmonary involvement is unusual. Liver tests are impaired with marked increase in serum alkaline phosphatase and slight elevation in serum aminotransferase and globulins. Serum bilirubin is usually normal.

In the Mayo Clinic series, 50% of the cases were attributed to idiopathic granulomatous hepatitis. Sarcoidosis was the second most frequent cause, and the rest were attributed miscellaneous causes.

The majority of patients with fever of unknown origin due to idiopathic granulomatous hepatitis have a favorable prognosis. Forty percent resolve spontaneously; the remaining respond to a trial of prednisone for 3 to 33 months in a 3-year follow-up. All patients became afebrile and asymptomatic.[20] This entity has often been considered a form of sarcoidosis, but in the Mayo Clinic series, granulomas were absent in other organs.

SARCOIDOSIS

Sarcoidosis, a disease of unknown origin, is characterized by diffuse multiorgan involvement by epithelioid granulomas.[17,21] The most frequent sites of extrahepatic involvement are the skin, eyes, lymph nodes, lung, and neurologic system. This disease is characterized by a wide variety of well-recognized clinical manifestations.[21–23] The hepatic granulomas are usually concentrated in the portal tracts and periportal zones but may also be located within the hepatic lobule. The granulomas frequently coalesce and become segmented by fibrous tissue that is eventually replaced by collagen. When granulomas are located adjacent to the interlobular bile ducts, bile duct lesions may appear almost iden-

TABLE 107-2. DIFFERENTIAL DIAGNOSIS AND TREATMENT OF HEPATIC GRANULOMAS

ETIOLOGY	CLINICAL FEATURES	DIAGNOSTIC EVALUATION	TREATMENT
Idiopathic granulomas	Fever, malaise, weight loss, abdominal pain, hepatomegaly	Extensive evaluation with negative results	Observation or trial of prednisone, 40 mg/d × 4–6 wk, tapered once symptomatic improvement occurs
Sarcoidosis	Diffuse organ involvement (eyes, lungs, heart, liver, intestine, kidneys, skin, lymph nodes, nervous system)	Chest x-ray examination (lymphadenopathy, pulmonary fibrosis), abnormal pulmonary function test, anergy skin test, positive results from Kveim reaction, elevated angiotensin-converting enzyme, positive results from calcium 67 scanning	Prednisone, 40 mg/d, tapered after clinical improvement; long-term maintenance of lowest effective dose may be necessary; treatment does not affect natural course; spontaneous remission
Tuberculosis	Pulmonary symptoms; occasional multiorgan involvement	Positive results from skin test, isolation organism, sputum pulmonary lavage, bone marrow aspirate, urine, liver biopsy	Isoniazid, 5 mg/kg/d, with rifampin 10 mg/kg/d, and pyrazinamide, 20–30 mg/d OR Isoniazid, 5 mg/kg/d, and ethambutol, 15 mg/kg/d, treatment for 6–9 mo
Brucellosis	Occupational history (dairymen, farmers, veterinarians, etc.), ingestion of goat milk cheese; several clinical stages: acute, relapsing, chronic; systemic symptoms: hepatosplenomegaly, lymphadenopathy, occasional neuropsychiatric symptoms	Isolation of organism from blood, bone marrow aspirate, lymph node spinal fluid, positive results from agglutination test (STA), new test ELISA, RIA more sensitive	Doxycycline, 2.5 mg/kg/d, with rifampin, 10 mg/kg/d, treatment for 6 wk
Q fever	Inhalation of aerosols containing organisms; exposure to sheep, cattle, goats, cats; flulike illness with pneumonia, hepatitis, and occasionally endocarditis	Positive complement fixing antibodies OR indirect fluorescent antibody; chest x-ray examination: patchy infiltrate, consolidation	Tetracycline, 25–30 mg/kg/d OR Doxycycline, 2.5 mg/kg/d, for 7–10 d

ELISA = enzyme-linked immunosorbent assay, RIA = radioimmunoassay.

tical to those observed in primary biliary cirrhosis. Epithelioid granulomas of sarcoidosis frequently have multinucleated giant cells and, when they coalesce, may exhibit a central fibrinoid necrosis. Intracytoplasmic inclusions have also been observed (Schaumann's bodies and asteroid bodies).

Several biochemical changes have been observed. The involvement of sarcoid tissue in the reticuloendothelial tissue leads to elevation of the γ-globulins. Characteristically, the liver tests show a predominance of alkaline phosphatase elevation with serum bilirubin levels within normal range. Recent studies have revealed that vitamin D_3 produced by macrophages is involved in systemic calcium metabolism. Stimulated macrophages also produce angiotensin-converting enzyme within the granulomas.[24,25] Serum angiotensin-converting enzyme is usually increased when pulmonary involvement is present.[4] The gallium scan demonstrates positive results in affected organs.[25]

Patients with hepatic sarcoidosis can develop three complications:

1. *Portal hypertension* is usually presinusoidal because of involvement of the portal tract by granulomatous and fibrous tissue. Thrombotic occlusion of the portal and splenic vein can occur. When esophageal variceal bleeding occurs, patients tolerate portosystemic shunt surgery well. Therapy with corticosteroids

TABLE 107–2. DIFFERENTIAL DIAGNOSIS AND TREATMENT OF HEPATIC GRANULOMAS *Continued*

ETIOLOGY	CLINICAL FEATURES	DIAGNOSTIC EVALUATION	TREATMENT
Leprosy	Wide variety of cutaneous lesions: erythema nodosum, nerve damage, leonine facies, saddle nose, endemic area exposure	Positive results from acid-fast bacilli test in skin, lymph node, liver, spleen, bone marrow; positive results from skin and serologic test (questionable values)	Dapsone, 100 mg/d for 5–7 y to life, and rifampin, 600 mg/d for 6 mo; if resistant organism, clofazimine, 50–100 mg is substituted for dapsone
Histoplasmosis	Variety of clinical syndromes: influenzalike to progressive disseminated multiorgan disease, endemic area exposure, bat guano source of infection, prevalence in immunosuppressed patients, adrenal insufficiency	Chest x-ray examination (cavitation, calcifications, adenopathy), presence of complement fixing antibody; RIA to detect antigen; positive results from culture from blood, bone marrow, lymph nodes, liver, skin	Itraconazole, 200–400 mg/d, is drug of choice for 6 mo Amphotericin B (total dose 2–2.5 g) reserved for failure of itraconazole
Coccidioidomycosis	Primary or extrapulmonary dissemination (skin, joint, basilar meninges)	Positive results from culture from lung, liver, spinal fluid, identifications of spherules; presence of complement fixing antibodies in blood and spinal fluid	Amphotericin B, total dose 1–3 g; new triazole drugs are under investigation
Schistosomiasis (Bilharziasis)	Endemic areas depend on the unsanitary disposal of urine and feces; chronic form produces egg granuloma; portal hypertension with normal wedged hepatic pressure (presinusoidal)	Eosinophilia is common; identification of eggs in stool, rectal or liver biopsy specimen, or serologic culture	Praziquantel, 50 mg/kg/d for 30 d

does not ameliorate or prevent portal hypertension.[26]

2. *Budd-Chiari syndrome* can result from extensive granulomatous involvement of the liver and the hepatic vein. It frequently leads to thrombotic occlusion of the main hepatic veins or granulomatous involvement of the hepatic vein radicals.[27]

3. *Cholestasis* due to bile duct involvement is frequently indistinguishable from primary biliary cirrhosis.[28]

Corticosteroid therapy has been shown of benefit in the prevention of certain complications but has little or no effect on the liver biopsy appearance.[22,23]

TUBERCULOSIS

Hepatic granulomas are present in almost all cases of miliary tuberculosis; thus, they occur in 80% of cases of extrapulmonary tuberculosis and in a small proportion of cases of primary pulmonary infection. Aspiration liver biopsy specimens yield positive results in up to 80% of patients with extrapulmonary tuberculosis.[29] Cultures of liver biopsy are positive for tubercle bacilli. Characteristically, the granulomas are epithelioid and are localized in the portal tracts. Granulomas frequently exhibit a central eosinophilic caseation. Langhans' giant cells are usually positive for *Mycobacterium tuberculosis* by acid-fast staining. In chronic tuberculosis, granulomas are less frequent, and giant cell reaction and caseation are usually absent. Distinction between tuberculosis and sarcoidosis may be impossible.[21] Corticosteroids may activate the disease and precipitate caseation.

Recently, two complications have been associated with hepatic tuberculosis. First, obstruction of the biliary tree may occur with extensive tuberculous calcifications.[30] Second, pseudotumor of the liver, characterized by extensive calcified granulomatous lesions may mimic primary or metastatic neoplasia. Patients with immunosuppression and those who have received bacille

Calmette-Guérin (BCG) can develop diffuse granulomatous changes within the liver. Administration of intravesical BCG has been associated with hepatic granulomatosis.[31]

The response to antituberculous therapy may be evident after 1 or 2 weeks but occasionally takes longer. Therapy should be continued for up to 2 months before concluding it is ineffective. After 2 months of unresponsive therapy, idiopathic granulomatous disease of the liver of sarcoidosis should be considered as an alternative diagnosis.

BRUCELLOSIS

In brucellosis, there is usually an occupational history of ingestion of unpasteurized dairy products. Clinically, patients experience a typical fever pattern, extreme malaise, and clinical evidence of hepatosplenomegaly. The diagnosis is confirmed by the presence of positive cultures obtained from blood, bone marrow aspirate, liver biopsy material, or lymph nodes. A rise in titer of agglutinating antibody is very suggestive of disease; however, there is a high incidence of false-negatives.

The cause of brucellosis depends on three different types of *Brucella* species. *Brucella abortus* predominates in the chronic form of the disease. The granulomas are epithelioid and are located within the hepatic lobule rather than within the portal zone. They frequently cannot be distinguished from those of sarcoidosis. Lung granulomas may undergo central necrosis with secondary fibrosis and calcification.[32,33] *Brucella melitensis* is associated with the acute stage of the disease. The granulomas are composed predominantly of Kupffer's cells and macrophages. They are well defined, and the liver parenchyma exhibits intense Kupffer's cell hyperplasia. Focal hepatitis may also occur.[34] *Brucella suis* is more invasive and causes hepatic suppuration, with hepatic abscesses ultimately calcified. A portion of fixed biopsy specimens should be cultured, since they are occasionally positive for *Brucella abortus* or *Brucella melitensis*.

MYCOSES

Histoplasmosis is the most frequent fungal infection that affects the liver. The granulomas are usually epithelioid and large and frequently are histologically identical with those observed in sarcoidosis, except for the presence of the intracellular encapsulated fungus in Kupffer's cells. When the granulomatous lesions enlarge, they often progress to central necrosis. Occasionally, multinucleated giant cells are found. Biopsy sections should be silver stained to identify the *Histoplasma capsulatum*, and a portion of the biopsy specimen should be sent for special cultures.[35] Frequently, histoplasmosis causes extensive hepatic calcification and diffuse fibrosis.[36]

Coccidioidomycosis has increased in incidence in patients with AIDS. A careful history frequently reveals that the patient has either traveled or is a resident of an endemic area. The patients frequently exhibit signs of meningeal infection. Laboratory workup frequently reveals eosinophilia. The diagnosis is confirmed by tissue biopsy culture or a rise in the complement fixation antibody titer.

The granulomas are epithelioid with large, multinucleated giant cells that contain the organisms that appear as spherules. Special silver stains are necessary. Resolution with fibrosis occurs.[37,38]

Q FEVER

A history of raw milk ingestion is usually associated with Q fever, and the pulmonary manifestations are frequent. The hepatic granulomas are predominantly inflammatory; occasionally epithelioid cells and multinucleated giant cells are seen. Characteristic *"doughnut"* granulomas are composed of a clear space surrounded by a ring of fibrin tissue and peripherally surrounded by inflammatory cells, predominantly macrophages. The hepatic lobule in the portal tract contains increased numbers of plasma cells and lymphocytes. The results of liver biopsy cultures frequently are negative.[39,40] These classic fibroid ring granulomas have also been observed with other clinical entities.[11,12]

LEPROSY

Leprosy is endemic in Mexico. Patients frequently exhibit pale, anesthetic, macular or nodular, erythematous lesions involving several body tissues including skin, superficial nerves, nose, pharynx, larynx, eyes, and testicles. The lesions range from 1 to 10 cm in diameter. Extensive neurologic disturbances result from nerve infiltration and thickening. The disease is divided clinically into two different types: *lepromatous* and *tuberculoid leprosy*. In the *lepromatous* type, the course is progressive and malignant. In *lepromatous leprosy*, granulomas are present in 60% to 80% of patients; they are inflammatory, mainly composed of histiocytes (foam cells), and located either in the parenchyma or portal tract. The granulomas frequently contain abundant acid-fast organisms (Fite's stain), but results from biopsy cultures are usually negative.

In *tuberculoid leprosy,* the granulomas are present in 20% of patients. They are epithelioid with multinucleated giant cells and are located mainly in the hepatic parenchyma. Results of staining tests are usually negative for the organisms.[41,42]

SCHISTOSOMIASIS

The patient with schistosomiasis usually has been exposed to *Schistosoma* or resides in an endemic area. Schistosomiasis is one of the leading causes of presinusoidal portal hypertension. The diagnosis is confirmed by the detection of ova in feces or biopsy specimens of rectal mucosa or liver. *Schistosoma mansoni* (South America, Caribbean, and Africa) and *Schistosoma japonicum* (Southeast Asia and Japan) are the causative parasites. During the schistosome life cycle, eggs migrate into the portal space, causing an inflammatory and epithelioid reaction. The eggs are surrounded by inflammatory cells and fibrous tissue, described as having a "pipe stem" appearance. These lesions result in the development of severe portal hypertension.[43]

LYMPHOMA

Hepatic granulomas are present in 12% of patients with Hodgkin's disease[44,45] and in 2% of patients with non-Hodgkin's lymphoma.[46] The granulomas are epithelioid without caseation and occasionally contain giant cells. Some patients with granulomatous hepatitis may have lymphoma also. Peripheral T-cell lymphoma has also been associated with epithelioid granulomas.[47]

PRIMARY BILIARY CIRRHOSIS

In up to 60% of patients with primary biliary cirrhosis, hepatic granulomas appear in the early stages. They are epithelioid in type and are located within the portal tract or throughout the parenchyma. They are associated with interlobular bile duct destruction.[48] The histologic picture frequently resembles sarcoidosis. The presence of granulomas is associated with a favorable prognosis. An overlap syndrome has been described between primary biliary cirrhosis and sarcoidosis.[49] The diagnosis of primary biliary cirrhosis is established with the presence of antimitochondrial antibody, elevated serum immunoglobulin M (IgM), and the characteristic lesions of the interlobular bile ducts. Patients with sarcoidosis have a more favorable response to corticosteroid therapy than do patients with primary biliary cirrhosis.

DRUG-RELATED GRANULOMAS

Multiple drugs have been implicated as causing hypersensitivity reactions and eosinophilia. The granulomas are inflammatory or epithelioid, with no specific location. The most frequent drugs are sulfa, methyldopa, allopurinol, and hydantoin (see Table 107–1). On discontinuation of the medication, there is complete resolution without hepatic sequelae.[50] The presence of granulomas in patients with AIDS should raise the suspicion of drugs in the differential diagnosis.[51]

ACQUIRED IMMUNODEFICIENCY SYNDROME

The spectrum of liver disease in patients with AIDS is multifactorial and is caused by a wide variety of infections, neoplasias, and drug-related reactions (Table 107–3).[50,53] Usually, the clinical and histologic expression is attenuated as a result of impaired immune response. Frequently, the entire hepatobiliary system is affected by more than one process.[51-55] Almost two thirds of unselected patients with AIDS have increased liver enzymes. Granulomas appear in up to 40% of patients and usually are poorly formed, hypocellular, and without central caseation. Multinucleated cells are absent. The portal and periportal inflammation is mild. The presence of eosinophilia suggests a drug re-

TABLE 107–3. HEPATIC GRANULOMAS AND AIDS

Infectious	
Viral	Cytomegalovirus, hepatitis A
Bacterial	*Mycobacterium avium-intracellulare, Mycobacterium tuberculosis*
Mycosis	Histoplasmosis, coccidioidomycosis, aspergillosis
Parasitic	Toxoplasmosis
Noninfectious	
Neoplasia	Hodgkin's and non-Hodgkin's lymphoma
Drugs	Sulfonamide, isoniazid, hydantoin, cephalosporins, amoxicillin

action. *Mycobacterium avium-intracellulare* is the most frequent cause of granuloma. Acid-fast stain is positive for these organisms, which are widely distributed throughout the hepatocytes and Kupffer's cells (Table 107–2).

TREATMENT (Table 107–2)

When the diagnosis of hepatic granulomas is confirmed on clinical and laboratory studies, effective and definitive therapy is instituted. In patients with continuous fever and clinical illness in which after extensive laboratory and radiographic evaluation, the diagnosis remains unknown, a therapeutic trial is recommended.

If tuberculosis is suspected, the combination of isoniazid and ethambutol is preferred. The treatment should be continued for a period of at least 2 weeks. In most of the patients with tuberculosis with fever and clinical illness, the fever will subside. In those patients who remain symptomatic, a trial of corticosteroids is warranted in view of the possibility of sarcoidosis.[4,8]

Demonstration of hepatic involvement in sarcoidosis in association with generalized illness should indicate treatment with corticosteroids.[23] In rare cases of portal hypertension and sarcoidosis, treatment is beneficial. Confirmation of brucellosis by culture should prompt specific treatment with a combination of doxycycline with rifampin. The treatment is continued for 6 weeks. In Q fever, tetracycline is the drug of choice. Frequently, there is rapid resolution in a 10-day treatment period.[56]

Leprosy requires treatment with a combination of dapsone and rifampin. Frequently, therapy for life is required. In leprosy for resistant organisms, clofazimine has proven effective.[56]

Amphotericin B is the drug of choice for mycotic infections.[57] Ketoconazole is also effective.[58] A new group of triazole compounds shows promise in resistant cases. Schistosomiasis has been treated successfully with Praziquantel.[59] In patients with advanced fibrosis, the results are less dramatic.

The patient with AIDS is often a special challenge. Frequently, multidrug therapy is necessary to treat the granulomatous process.

REFERENCES

1. Guckian JC, Perry JE. Granulomatous hepatitis: an analysis of 63 cases and review of literature. *Ann Intern Med*. 1966;65:1081.
2. Fauci AS, Wolf SM. Granulomatous hepatitis. In: Popper H, Schaffner F, eds. *Progress in Liver Diseases*. Vol. 5. New York, NY: Grune & Stratton Inc; 1976:609.
3. Adams DO. The granulomatous inflammatory response: a review. *Am J Pathol*. 1976;84:164.
4. Sartin JS, Walker RC. Granulomatous hepatitis: a retrospective review of 88 cases at the Mayo Clinic. *Mayo Clin Proc*. 1991;66:914.
5. Neville E, Piyasena KHG, James DE. Granulomas of the liver. *Postgrad Med J*. 1975;51:361.
6. Mir-Madjlessi SH, Farmer RC, Hawk WA. Granulomatous hepatitis: a review of 50 cases. *Am J Gastroenterol*. 1973;60:122.
7. Wagoner GP, Anton AT, Gall EA, et al. Needle biopsy of the liver, VIII. Experiences with hepatic granulomas. *Gastroenterology*. 1953;25:487.
8. Reynolds BT, Campra CJ, Peters RL. Hepatic granulomata. In: Zakim D, Boyer TD, eds. *Hepatology: A Textbook of Liver Disease*. 2nd ed. vol 2. Philadelphia, Pa: WB Saunders Co; 1990:1101.
9. Wanless IR, Geddie WR. Mineral oil lipogranulomata in liver and spleen. *Pathol Lab Med*. 1985;109:283.
10. Landas SK, Mitros FA, Furst DE, et al. Lipogranuloma and gold in the liver in rheumatoid arthritis. *Am J Surg Pathol*. 1992;16(2):171.
11. Marazuela M, Moreno A, Yebra M, et al. Hepatic fibrin granulomas: a clinopathologic study of 23 patients. *Human Pathol*. 1991;22:607–613.
12. Ponz E, Garcia Pagian JC, Bruguera M, et al. Hepatic fibrin ring granuloma in hepatitis A. *Gastroenterology*. 1991;10:268.
13. Boros DL. Granulomatous inflammation. *Prog Allergy*. 1978;24:184.
14. Kresina TF. In vitro regulation of *S. japonica* granuloma formation by an IL-2 antagonist. *Parasitology*. 1991;2: 243–249.
15. Dinarrello CA. Interleukin-I. *Rev Infect Dis*. 1984;6:51–60.
16. Scheuer P. *Liver Biopsy Interpretation*. 4th ed. London: Bailliere Tindall; 1988:223.
17. Klastin G. Hepatic granulomata problems in interpretation. *Mt Sinai J Med*. 1977;44:798.
18. Millis P, Saverymuttu S, Fallowfield M, et al. Ultrasound in the diagnosis of granulomatous liver disease. *Clin Radiol*. 1990;41:113.
19. Nakata K, Iwata K, Kojima K, et al. Computed tomography of liver sarcoidosis. *J Comput Assist Tomogr*. 1989; 13:707.
20. Zoutman DE, Ralph ED, Frei JV. Granulomatous hepatitis and fever of unknown origin: an 11-year experience of 23 cases with three years follow-up. *J Clin Gastroenterol*. 1991;13:69.
21. Klastin G, Yesner R. Hepatic manifestation of sarcoidosis and other granulomatous diseases: a study based on histological examination of tissue obtained by needle biopsy of the liver. *Yale J Biol Med*. 1950;23:207–246.
22. James DG, Jones Williams W. *Sarcoidosis and Other Granulomatous Disorders*. Philadelphia, Pa: W.B. Saunders Co; 1985.
23. Maddrey WC, Johns CJ, Boitnott JK, et al. Sarcoidosis and chronic hepatic disease: a clinical and pathological study of 20 patients. *Medicine*. 1970;49:375.
24. Nishimura M, Hara A, Nojima H, et al. Possible role of the hormonal form of vitamin D_3 in the associated-converting enzyme activity. *Sarcoidosis*. 1991;8(2):101.
25. Nojal A, Schleisser LA, Mishkin FS, et al. Angiotensin converting enzyme and gallium scan in non-invasive evaluation of sarcoidosis. *Ann Intern Med*. 1979;90:328.
26. Valla D, Pessegueiro-Miranda H, Degott C, et al. He-

patic sarcoidosis with portal hypertension: a report of 7 cases with a review of the literature. *Q J Med.* 1986; 63:531.
27. Russe EW, Bansky G, Pfaltz M, et al. Budd-Chiari syndrome in sarcoidosis. *Am J Gastroenterol.* 1986;81:71.
28. Maddrey WC. Sarcoidosis and primary biliary cirrhosis associated disorders. *N Engl J Med.* 1983;308:588.
29. Korn RJ, Kellow WF, Heller P, et al. Hepatic involvement in extrapulmonary tuberculosis. *Am J Med.* 1965; 27:60.
30. Maglinte DD, et al. Patterns of calcifications and cholangiographic findings in hepatobiliary tuberculosis. *Gastrointest Radiol.* 1988;13:331–335.
31. Graziano DA, Jacobs D, Lozano RG, et al. A case of granulomatous hepatitis after intravesical bacillus Calmette-Guérin administration. *J Urol.* 1991;146:1118–1119.
32. Cervantes F, Bruguera A, Carbonell J, et al. Liver disease in brucellosis: a clinical and pathological study of 40 patients. *Postgrad Med J.* 1982;58:346.
33. Williams RK, Crossley K. Acute and chronic hepatitis involvement of brucellosis. *Gastroenterology.* 1982;83: 1985.
34. Fogel R, Lewis S. Diagnosis of *Brucella melitensis* infection by percutaneous needle biopsy of the liver. *Ann Intern Med.* 1960;53:204.
35. Sarosi GA, Voth DW, Dahl BA, et al. Disseminated histoplasmosis results of long-term follow-up: a center for disease control cooperative mycosis study. *Ann Intern Med.* 1971;75:511.
36. Okudaira M, Straub M, Schwarz J. The etiology of discrete splenic and hepatic calcifications in an endemic area of histoplasmosis. *Am J Pathol.* 1961;39:599.
37. Coodley EL. Disseminated coccidioidomycosis: diagnosis by liver biopsy. *Gastroenterology.* 1967;53:947.
38. Craig JR, Hilberg RJ, Balchum OJ. Disseminated coccidioidomycosis: diagnosis by needle biopsy of the liver. *West J Med.* 1975;122:171.
39. Hofmann CE, Heaton JW. Q fever hepatitis: clinical manifestations and pathological findings. *Gastroenterology.* 1982;83:474.
40. Bernstein M, Edmondson HA, Barbour BH. The liver lesion in Q fever: clinical and pathologic features. *Arch Intern Med.* 1965;116:491.
41. Karat ABA, Job CK, Rao PSS. Liver in leprosy: histological and biological findings. *Br Med J.* 1971;1:307.
42. Chen TSN, Drutz DJ, Whelan GE. Hepatic granulomas in leprosy: their relation to bacteremia. *Arch Pathol Lab Med.* 1976;100:182.
43. Dunn MD, Kamel R. Hepatic schistosomiasis. *Hepatology.* 1981;1:653–661.
44. Bagley CM Jr, Roth JA, Thomas LB, et al. Liver biopsy in Hodgkin's disease: clinicopathologic correlation in 127 patients. *Ann Intern Med.* 1972;76:219.
45. Kadin ME, Donaldson SS, Durfman RF. Isolated granulomas in Hodgkin's disease. *N Engl J Med.* 1970;283: 859.
46. Braylan RC, Long JC, Jaffe ES, et al. Malignant lymphoma obscured by concomitant extensive epithelioid granulomas: report of 3 cases with similar clinicopathologic features. *Cancer.* 1977;39:1146.
47. Saito K, Nakanuma Y, Ogawa S, et al. Extensive hepatic granulomas associated with peripheral T-cell lymphoma. *Am J Gastroenterol.* 1991;86:1243–1246.
48. Roll J, Boyer JL, Barry D, et al. The prognostic importance of clinical and histologic features in asymptomatic and symptomatic primary biliary cirrhosis. *N Engl J Med.* 1983;308:1.
49. Rudzki •, Ishak KG, Zimmerman HJ. Chronic intrahepatic cholestasis of sarcoidosis. *Am J Med.* 1975; 59:373.
50. McMaster KR, Hennigar GR. Drug-induced granulomatous hepatitis. *Lab Invest.* 1981;44:61–73.
51. Orenstein MS, Tavitian A, Yonk B, et al. Granulomatous involvement of the liver in patients with AIDS. *Gut.* 1985; 26:1220.
52. Lebovics E, Thung SN, Schaffner F, et al. The liver in the acquired immunodeficiency syndrome: a clinical and histologic study. *Hepatology.* 1985;5:293.
53. Schneiderman DJ, Arenson DM, Cello JP, et al. Hepatic disease in patients with the acquired immune deficiency syndrome (AIDS). *Hepatology.* 1987;7:925.
54. Glasgow BJ, Anders K, Layfield LJ, et al. Clinical and pathologic findings of the liver in the acquired immune deficiency syndrome. *Am J Clin Pathol.* 1985;83:582.
55. Schneiderman JD. Hepatobiliary abnormalities of AIDS. *Gastroenterol Clin North Am.* 1988;17(3):615.
56. The choice of antibacterial drugs. *The Medical Letter.* 1992;34(871):49, 56.
57. McKinsey DS, Gupta MR, Riddler SA, et al. Long-term amphotericin B therapy for disseminated histoplasmosis in patients with acquired immunodeficiency syndrome (AIDS). *Ann Intern Med.* 1989;3:655.
58. Dismukes WE, Cloud G, Bowles C, et al. National Institute of Allergy and Infectious Diseases Mycosis Group treatment of blastomycosis and histoplasmosis with ketoconazole: result of a prospective randomized clinical trial. *Ann Intern Med.* 1985;103:861.
59. King CH, Mahmoud AAF. Drugs five years later: praziquantel. *Ann Intern Med.* 1989;110:290.

108
Amebic Abscess
ANTHONY S. TORNAY, JR.

DISEASE

Entamoeba histolytica is a protozoan parasite that infects 10% of the world's population. It is believed that there are pathogenic and nonpathogenic strains, and only 10% of those infected ever exhibit clinical disease. The organism has a simple life cycle with only two forms; the cyst and the trophozoite. Cysts are ingested in contaminated food or water or passed by direct person-to-person contact. Cysts are resistant and can survive dormant for some time. Once in the host intestinal tract, mobile trophozoites can be released. This form is capable of producing tissue invasion in the colon and subsequent spread, usually through the portal system.

There are several different clinical syndromes in those infected. Obviously the most common is that of asymptomatic cyst passage. What factors, such as pathogenicity, host susceptibility, play a role in this phenomenon have yet to be delineated. If followed for a period of time, most or all individuals exhibit clearance of the organism. Those who manifest intestinal disease have three different clinical syndromes: acute amebic dysentery, fulminant amebic colitis, and ameboma.

Extraintestinal amebiasis likewise exhibits a host of different presentations. Because of the portal mode of spread, the majority of the presentations center around the liver. However, there have been isolated reports of retroperitoneal abscess, perforated amebic appendicitis, and isolated lung involvement that may indicate other pathways. Of the patients with clinical disease in an endemic area, 10% present with amebic liver abscess (ALA).

Amebiasis predominates in tropical and subtropical areas of the world and is a major public health problem in parts of Asia, South America, and Africa. The level of public sanitation and personal hygiene is considered the most important factor in the degree of infestation of an area. In the United States the prevalence is much lower, but a statistic of 1% to 4% is often quoted, depending on the area studied and the intensity of investigation. Groups including recent immigrants, homosexuals, and institutionalized persons are most likely to present with disease. Travelers to endemic areas are also at risk. The most difficult problem for physicians in developed countries may be just considering the diagnosis, since one is not often confronted with the differential. Treatment is usually quite easy once the diagnosis is established, and the diagnosis is easy to make when looked for.

PRESENTATION

The typical presentation of ALA is that of a right upper quadrant pain syndrome (80% to 90% of cases). It may occur in any age group but for unexplained reasons occurs in men (ratio 5 to 10:1) between the ages of 20 and 40 most commonly. The onset may be acute with symptoms lasting up to 10 days or less frequently subacute with more indolent symptoms going on for 6 months prior to diagnosis. Diarrhea suggestive of an intestinal disease is present in less than 33%. On physical examination, tenderness in the right upper quadrant, often with hepatomegaly, is associated with the pain. Constitutional symptoms such as fever, chills, sweats, and nausea occur in the majority of patients and may predominate. Findings from routine laboratory workup are abnormal but nonspecific. Elevation of white blood cell count, along with a mild anemia and increase in inflammatory markers, is present in greater than 75% of patients. Slight elevations in liver function test results including bilirubin and all enzymes are likewise common. Jaundice is rare.

In addition to the abdominal symptoms,

pleuropulmonary complaints are present in 20% to 50% and may predominate or occur alone. These likewise may be acute or chronic and consist of cough and pleuritic pain with an associated sympathetic effusion and elevated right hemidiaphragm. In addition, there may be parenchymal consolidation and even abscess formation in the contiguous right lower lobe. The more dramatic presentation is that of empyema or tracheobronchial fistula associated with ALA rupture. Presumably, it is the thin wall characteristic of ALA, along with its propensity to occur in the periphery of each lobe, that leads to abscess rupture.

The direction of rupture dictates the clinical picture in those with complications of ALA. It can be intraperitoneal, intrapericardial, or intrapulmonary. Peritonitis is more often an indolent process associated with a leak, whereas pericardial rupture, although rare, presents with tamponade and shock.

DIAGNOSIS

Prompt therapy and, therefore, response hinges on rapid recognition. Ideally the initiation of therapy should occur within 24 to 48 hours based on a presumptive diagnosis made on immunologic and radiologic criteria and the clinical presentation. As the organism is infrequently seen or cultured from liver material, response to therapy is the final parameter used in clinical studies in establishing the diagnosis of ALA.

Noninvasive radiologic testing has always been very important in the management of ALA. However, the advent of ultrasound has been a dramatic advancement and has improved patient care and outcome. Because of its lack of expense and widespread availability even in underdeveloped areas, it is the most widely used modality. Computed tomography (CT) and magnetic resonance imaging (MRI) are seldom needed, although they can be of value in unusual cases. A sonogram of the right upper quadrant, including the liver, is indicated in most cases of abdominal pain in that area. Typically the abscess is well defined, round, or oval and hypoechogenic with distal sonic enhancement. Sonography demonstrates the presence of an abscess 90% to 95% of the time. The majority of abscesses are located in the right lobe (80% to 85%), with multiple lesions in about 20%. Isolated left lobe lesions occur in less than 5% of cases.

Serologic confirmation of ALA is an essential part of the diagnosis. Fortunately, serologic confirmation is quite easy, although most hospitals send the specimens to reference laboratories. Results should be available within 24 to 48 hours with the assist of a phone call or facsimile transmission. The preferable test in most series is indirect hemagglutination (IHA) based on availability, cost, and sensitivity. IHA test results should be positive 97% to 100% of the time if one keeps in mind that very early on (first 5 to 7 days after exposure) the test results may be negative, with positive titers occurring on subsequent testing 1 to 4 weeks later. The other concern is that in endemic areas a low-level antibody persists for years after any invasive amebic event and can be confusing. A titer of 1:512 would be considered diagnostic, whereas lesser titers down to 1:128 are just suggestive and should be repeated. Numerous other immunologic tests, e.g., complement fixation (CF), immunoelectrophoresis (IEP), counter immunoelectrophoresis (CIEP), enzyme-linked immunosorbent assay (ELISA), and gel diffusion (GD) are available, but none have compelling reasons to replace IHA. Of all the numerous new tests being studied, the one that might prove most useful is the immunologic detection of amebic antigen in the pus of an aspirated abscess. If the test is readily available at the hospital, this would circumvent the fact that trophozoites are infrequently found in aspirate specimens.

Percutaneous aspiration is the final diagnostic tool available in ALA. This is almost always done with ultrasound guidance, which has improved the accuracy and safety of the procedure. Two very important concepts have evolved from numerous studies of this technique. First, it is infrequently needed to establish the diagnosis (therapeutic aspiration is dealt with in the next section of this chapter). Second, it is an extremely easy and safe procedure with no contraindications and should be performed whenever considered necessary. The classic aspirate is the anchovy paste (red-brown) necrotic debris, which is not foul smelling. However, the aspirate can be yellow or creamy white. Active organisms are infrequently identified, the best chance occurring on immediate wet mount study of the final volume removed. It is presumed that this material is coming from the interface of normal liver with expanding abscess where live organisms are actively at work. As noted above, immunologic studies to detect antigen in the pus may become more widely available for rapid diagnosis. Probably the major indication for diagnostic aspiration is to perform a culture and a

Gram stain on pus to rule out the diagnosis of pyogenic abscess.

TREATMENT

The amebicide of choice in the treatment of ALA is metronidazole given in a dosage of 750 mg three times daily for 10 days. The efficacy is reported as greater than 90% in all studies and close to 100% in recent reviews. As in other protozoan infections, even single-dose (2.4 g × 1) therapy has been shown effective, although this is not to be recommended. The side effects of nausea, vomiting, headache, metallic taste, and rash rarely require stopping the drug. Metronidazole can be given intravenously, but oral therapy is effective and the route of choice in almost all patients. Alternative drugs include dehydroemetine, 1.5 mg/kg (maximum dose 90 mg/d) for 10 days, and chloroquine (1 g for two days and then 500 mg every day for 20 days). Most recommend a crossover to chloroquine if metronidazole fails, which is an uncommon event. Therapy should begin as quickly as possible and hopefully within 24 hours of presentation based on a presumptive diagnosis as outlined above. To avoid a diagnostic aspiration, some centers begin empiric therapy for pyogenic abscess with ampicillin combined with gentamicin for 48 hours until the serologic studies confirming the clinical and radiologic impression are available. In typical cases empiric therapy is not needed, and if pyogenic abscess is a serious consideration, a diagnostic aspiration should be done for Gram's stain and culture.

A major debate still exists in the literature over the need for therapeutic aspiration in the treatment of ALA. There have been several prospective studies and even one randomized (not double-blinded) study[7] to look at this issue. In the majority of patients who present with ALA and certainly in those with mild-to-moderate disease, antiamebicidal therapy is all that is needed. The time to clinical improvement and length of hospital stay are the same with and without aspiration. In patients with larger, painful abscesses, there may be some benefit to drainage with quicker clinical improvement. It would appear that in other countries the tendency to more frequent drainage is at least in part due to a different population of patients. In underdeveloped areas the majority of patients are at least moderately or even severely malnourished and often present later for therapy.

Generally accepted criteria for therapeutic aspiration include large abscesses of the left lobe (to prevent pericardial rupture), failure to respond to medical therapy ([?] after 3 to 5 days), or imminent rupture as defined by a tender or painful peripheral abscess. Some consider a "large" abscess (7 to 10 cm) to be an indicator. It is important to remember that there are no contraindications to aspiration, but it may not be needed. Drainage is most often performed with an ultrasound-guided needle aspiration, but some prefer to leave an indwelling catheter or perform daily drainage. Although drainage has not been shown to definitely shorten hospital stay, in more seriously ill patients the trend is to shorten the duration of the illness.

It should be noted that resolution of the abscess cavity has been used as a criteria for selection of therapy. When followed by ultrasound with just amebicidal therapy, scans show a defect (the "amebic cyst") months to years later. The defect usually resolves with a scar and is not clinically significant. When treated with aspiration, particularly with a prolonged indwelling catheter, this defect often resolves immediately. However, this is not a reason to select catheter drainage.

An interesting proposal by Filice et al[2] is to instill intralesional amebicidal therapy when performing therapeutic aspiration. They use metronidazole, 37.5 mg/kg in 5 mg/ml solution, to achieve high intralesional concentration of the drug. This concept has merit and certainly requires study in those patients with an indication for aspiration.

Patients with a complicated amebic abscess must be treated on an individual basis. It is no longer considered a situation that mandates urgent surgery. More commonly today surgery is undertaken for an "acute abdomen," and the diagnosis becomes apparent at that time. In that setting it is appropriate to establish closed suction drainage of any significant localized collection and then proceed with amebicidal drugs. There have been enough reports of nonsurgical treatment of perforated ALA to consider this as established therapy. Whether the leak is intraperitoneal or intrathoracic, establishment of appropriate drainage and amebicidal therapy has proved successful in most cases. The mortality from this type of complication has decreased from up to 50% to less than 5% in most series. Intrapericardial rupture is fortunately quite uncommon, as it is dramatic and still quite dangerous. Open drainage is still the treatment of choice when intrapericardial rupture is recognized.

After the successful treatment of ALA, there is still the issue of whether to treat the patient with a luminal drug, since metronidazole does not effectively eliminate all cysts. The patient may become an asymptomatic cyst passer with the potential for reinfection with either colitic or extracolitic manifestations. Fortunately, this occurs quite infrequently with an incidence of 0.1% to 1% in most series. Most authorities formally recommend treatment with a luminal drug. However, in real practice very few patients are treated. There are two reasonable strategies. The first would be to look for those who become cyst passers and treat only that group. This requires a laboratory experienced at identification and more than a cursory search of one old stool specimen. Fresh specimens and even wet mounts at sigmoidoscopy are needed for accuracy. The second approach would be to simply treat everyone.

There are three luminal drugs available for use. The most widely used in the United States is iodoquinol (Diiodohydroxyquin) in a dosage of 650 mg three times daily for 20 days. It is contraindicated in iodine allergy and liver failure. Diloxanide, 500 mg three times daily for 10 days, has been used successfully worldwide without significant side effects but is available only through the Centers for Disease Control and Prevention. Paromomycin, 500 mg three times daily for 10 days, is the third drug, with less established experience. Diloxanide seems to have gained favor among clinicians in endemic areas who favor treatment.

REFERENCES

1. Donovan AJ, Yellin AE, Ralls PW. Hepatic abscess. *World J Surg.* 1991;15(2):162–169.
2. Filice C, Di Perri G, Strosselli M, et al. Outcome of hepatic amebic abscesses managed with three different therapeutic strategies. *Dig Dis Sci.* 1992;37(2):240–247.
3. Irusen EM, Jackson TF, Simjee AE. Asymptomatic intestinal colonization by pathogenic *Entamoeba histolytica* in amebic liver abscess: prevalence, response to therapy, and pathogenic potential. *Clin Infect Dis.* 1992;14(4):889–893.
4. Nordestgaard AG, Stapleford L, Worthen N, Bongard FS, Klein SR. Contemporary management of amebic liver abscess. *Am Surg.* 1992;58(5):315–320.
5. Reed SL. Amebiasis: an update. *Clin Infect Dis.* 1992;14(2):385–393.
6. Sharma MP, Dasarathv S. Amoebic liver abscess. *Trop Gastroenterol.* 1993;14(1):3–9.
7. Van Allan RJ, Katz MD, Johnson MB, Laine LA, Liu Y, Ralls PW. Uncomplicated amebic liver abscess: prospective evaluation of percutaneous therapeutic aspiration. *Radiology.* 1992;183(3):827–830.
8. Vinayak VK, Shandil RK. Immunological approaches in the diagnosis of amoebiasis. *Trop Gastroenterol.* 1991;12(4):165–175.
9. Widjaya P, Bilic A, Bibic Z, Ljubicic N, Bakula B, Pilas V. Amoebic liver abscess: ultrasonographic characteristics and results of different therapeutic approaches. *Acta Med Iugosl.* 1991;45(1):15–21.

109

Hepatic Tumors

STEVEN D. SEAGREN and ROWEN K. ZETTERMAN

Primary liver tumors comprise a heterogeneous group of benign and malignant lesions. Different cellular populations of the liver including hepatic parenchymal cells, bile duct epithelium, and endothelium may each give rise to tumors with varying characteristics. This chapter addresses the most common malignant tumors, hepatocellular carcinoma, cholangiocarcinoma, and hepatic angiosarcoma, along with the selected benign tumors of hepatic adenoma and focal nodular hyperplasia.

HEPATOCELLULAR CARCINOMA

EPIDEMIOLOGY

The worldwide incidence of hepatocellular carcinoma (HCC) is approximately one million cases annually and is the most common malignancy in portions of Asia and Africa. In the United States, it is the seventh most common malignancy, with an annual incidence of two cases per 100,000 population, and it is identified at autopsy in 1.4% of those with cirrhosis. The male-to-female ratio of HCC in the United States is 2 to 3:1, which is independent of other risk factors.

Multiple lines of evidence point to chronic hepatitis B virus (HBV) infection as a risk factor that is felt to be directly oncogenic. The worldwide geographic variability in HCC occurrence parallels hepatitis B surface antigen (HBsAg) carrier prevalence with an up to 100-fold increased incidence of HCC in HBsAg carriers. Integrated HBV DNA can be found in both normal hepatocytes and HCC tissue of HBsAg carriers. Integration occurs at multiple sites on different chromosomes, unrelated to known oncogenes. In the United States, 10% to 26% of those with HCC are HBsAg positive.

Hepatitis C virus (HCV) is also associated with HCC. It may not be directly hepatocarcinogenic, but rather it promotes HCC by causing cirrhosis. The role of HCV is striking in Japan, where the incidence of HCC doubled from 1966 to 1981 while HBV infections were essentially unchanged. In the United States, where HCV is more common than HBV, up to 58% of patients with HCC have evidence of prior HCV infection.

Cirrhosis of any cause is found in up to 90% of patients with HCC and the incidence of development of HCC in patients with cirrhosis may approach 2% to 5% per year. Adenomatous hyperplasia may be a precursor lesion, representing the link from regenerative nodules to development of HCC. Alcohol seems to confer risk via cirrhosis, rather than as a direct carcinogen. Use of androgenic steroids, aflatoxin ingestion, thorotrast exposure (with a 20-year latency), and hemochromatosis are also risk factors.

HISTOLOGY

HCC may be undifferentiated, macrotrabecular or microtrabecular, acinar, pseudoglandular, adenomatous, or fibrolamellar. Growth patterns are described as expanding, infiltrative, or diffuse (multicentric). Tumor growth rates are variable, with a median doubling time of 4 to 6 months and a range of 1 to 19 months. In Eastern countries, tumors are more often solitary, whereas in the West, they are typically multicentric. Portal vein involvement by HCC is common. Metastases typically reach the lung, regional lymph nodes, pancreas, adrenals, and bone.

Fibrolamellar HCC (FLHCC) carries a better prognosis. It occurs in younger patients, with a mean age of 23 years and a male-to-female ratio of 3:4, and is typically unassociated with cirrhosis. In FLHCC, well-differentiated neoplastic hepatocytes are surrounded by fibrosis, and tumor nodules are well-demarcated from normal tissue. On noninvasive imaging, FLHCC may resemble focal nodular hyperplasia. Tumor markers are negative. Resectability rates are high (50% to 75%), and the 5-year survival in this group is 50% to 60%. If nonresectable, the median survival is 13 months.

CLINICAL PRESENTATION

HCC may cause malaise, abdominal pain, weight loss, or anorexia; however, these usually occur late in the disease course. Often, these symptoms are incorrectly attributed to the underlying cirrhosis. If sudden clinical deterioration occurs in a cirrhotic patient, HCC must be suspected. On physical examination, a rub or bruit may be heard over the liver.

LABORATORY ASSESSMENT

Liver enzymes are inconsistently and nonspecifically abnormal with HCC. Erythrocytosis may be observed in 5% to 10% because of erythropoietin production by tumor. Hypercalcemia and hypoglycemia may develop.

Alpha-fetoprotein (AFP) is the most useful tumor marker, and levels greater than 400 ng/ml (normal <20 ng/ml) are highly suggestive of HCC. In the United States, an elevated AFP level is seen in 30% to 70% of patients at diagnosis, with false-positive tests reported in acute and chronic hepatitis and pregnancy. Germ cell tumors also produce AFP elevation. The size of tumor is positively correlated with AFP levels, indicating that small, resectable tumors are less likely to be identified by AFP alone. Other tumor markers such as carcinoembryonic antigen and des-gamma-carboxy prothrombin have been studied, but none offer better sensitivity or specificity than AFP.

RADIOLOGIC ASSESSMENT

The differential diagnosis of a lesion suggestive of HCC should include regenerative nodules, adenomatous hyperplasia, focal or diffuse fat, metastatic disease, cholangiocarcinoma, hepatic adenoma, focal nodular hyperplasia (FNH), and hemangioma. Ultrasound is usually the first radiologic test chosen and has a sensitivity for small HCC (<3 cm) of 55% to 84% and for vascular thrombosis of 27%. Diffuse tumor and lesions less than 2 cm may be missed by ultrasound. If ultrasound findings are equivocal, a subsequent examination with AFP measurement should be performed at 2 to 4 months. If operation is undertaken, intraoperative ultrasound increases the sensitivity to 95% for lesions less than 2 cm and 67% for vascular thrombosis.

Computed tomography (CT) with conventional contrast has a sensitivity for small HCC essentially equal to ultrasound, although vascular thromboses and intraabdominal metastases are better demonstrated. Lipiodol is an oil-based contrast agent, which when injected intraarterially, is preferentially retained by HCC. A CT scan performed 10 to 14 days after Lipiodol injection can demonstrate small HCC, with up to 67% of lesions less than 5 mm identified in some series. FNH may also take up Lipiodol because of its hypervascular nature, although Lipiodol "washes out" of FNH much more rapidly than HCC.

A tissue diagnosis of small lesions can be obtained by ultrasound- or CT-guided biopsy using thin-gauge (21 to 22) needles or by fine needle aspiration (FNA) for cytologic examination. Guided FNA offers greater safety but has higher false-positive and false-negative rates than does percutaneous biopsy.

Angiography, with or without portography, may assist in determination of tumor resectability or aid in diagnosis. Angiography is 82% to 89% sensitive for tumors less than 5 cm and 61% to 81% for those less than 3 cm.

Percutaneous liver biopsy can be successful because of the multicentric nature of HCC. In addition, laparoscopy with guided biopsy offers direct visualization of the lesion and the remainder of liver surface for micrometastases overlooked by ultrasound or CT.

TREATMENT

Hepatic Resection

Hepatic resection has been felt to be the best hope for cure of HCC when feasible. Patients should be carefully evaluated prior to operation. Exclusion criteria may include multifocal disease, lesions greater than 7 cm in diameter, vascular thrombosis, distant metastases, Child's class 2 or 3 cirrhosis, ascites, and underlying severe cardiac or renal disease. Overall, resectability rates range from 13% to 31% in western countries. Intraoperative ultrasound can aid the surgeon by accurately identifying the site and extent of lesions.

Survival rates following resection are related to tumor size and encapsulation, AFP level, and Child's class. Five-year survival of carefully selected patients are up to 60% for tumors of 4 to 5 cm in diameter, 82% if 2 to 3 cm, and 85% if less than 2 cm. Survival of patients with Child's class 1 cirrhosis is superior to that of patients with Child's class 2 and 3; 57% versus 12% at 3 years after resection in one study.

Depending on the severity of underlying liver disease, patients may develop liver failure, new onset of ascites, and bleeding due to portal hypertension following resection. Operative mortality may approach 28%, although more recent series cite figures of less than 10% to as low as 2%.

Recurrent tumor is common after resection, occurring in 55% to 100% at 5 years. Almost all recurrences are remote from resection margins, suggesting that residual tumor is not the cause and that metachronous HCC that develops in a "preneoplastic" cirrhotic liver is the explanation. Re-resection is an option for some recurrences but only if functioning reserve permits. A 5-year survival of 43% is reported in a select group eligible for a second resection.

Orthotopic Liver Transplantation

Orthotopic liver transplantation (OLT) should be the ideal therapy for HCC when a preoperative evaluation (chest and head CT with bone scan) appears to have ruled out metastases. Unfortunately, recurrence rates after OLT have been disappointingly high, often occurring early with aggressive growth. Early series of OLT reported 5-year survivals as low as 15% and median survivals of only 9 to 18 months due to recurrent tumor in lung or the transplanted liver. Possible reasons for high recurrence of tumor include unnoticed micrometastases, seeding of tumor at the time of OLT, and increased rates of growth with immunosuppression. Patients with bilobar tumor, vascular invasion, or metastasis in regional lymph nodes do worse after OLT, and in almost all patients tumors recur within 1 year. Tumor size also predicts recurrence. Initial tumors over 8 cm in diameter recur in up to 78%, whereas single lesions less than 5 cm recur in less than 5% of cases. One problem is that preoperative radiographic studies tend to underestimate the size and extent of disease. The number of radiographically identified tumors also predicts a high likelihood of recurrence with poor outcome when more than three tumor nodules are present.

Currently, OLT should be reserved for patients with known HCC that is coincidental (or incidental) to the underlying liver disease that requires transplantation or when there are no more than three nodules, each less than 5 cm in diameter. Patients with Child's class 1 cirrhosis and small (<5 cm) tumors can be considered for either OLT or resection. One study suggests neoadjuvant chemotherapy for tumors larger than 5 cm may promote tumor shrinkage and contribute to higher success rates with transplantation.

Ethanol Injection

Percutaneously guided ethanol injection has gained acceptability for treatment of HCC since it was first introduced in 1983 and is considered an alternative to resection in certain patients. Pioneered in Japan, this therapy employs thin-gauge needle injection of ethanol directly into tumor to produce tissue necrosis. Typically, 2 to 8 ml of ethanol is used per session, one or two times per week in the outpatient setting, depending on size and number of lesions. Optimal candidates have fewer than three lesions that are less than 3 cm in diameter, although larger tumor burdens have been treated. Contraindications include massive ascites and uncorrectable coagulopathy. Side effects are usually mild and include fever in up to 50%, abdominal pain, elevated c-glutamyltransferase (GGT), and pleural effusion (2.4%). Portal vein thrombosis and seeding of tumor have been reported.

Ethanol injection was shown to be superior to symptomatic treatment in a randomized trial, with 1- and 3-year survivals of 82% and 53% versus 91% and 13%, respectively. Nonrandomized trials have shown survival equal to that of resection, a result more impressive considering that the patients treated with ethanol often have more advanced liver disease or were not surgical candidates. Recurrence after ethanol injection is common and parallels surgical resection with 87% to 96% recurrence within 5 years. Recurrent lesions may be injected again.

Ethanol injection should be considered for HCC in Child's class 3 disease when the patient is not an OLT candidate. It can also be considered for primary therapy of small (<3 cm) HCC. A randomized trial comparing resection to ethanol injection is needed.

Chemotherapy

Chemotherapy alone is of limited value. Doxorubicin (Adriamycin) is the most effective single agent, producing a partial response in up to 20%. However, numerous studies have demonstrated no survival advantage over placebo for peripherally delivered single agent or combination chemotherapy. To avoid first-pass metabolism and lessen systemic exposure, direct hepatic arterial infusion has been tested, again without survival benefit.

Chemoembolization

Lipiodol or gelfoam pledgets are used as carriers for the chemotherapeutic agent(s) to deliver treatment as selectively as possible to the tumor at angiography. Results depend on the agent used, severity of underlying cirrhosis, presence of metastases, and vascular anatomy. When used alone, chemoembolization seems to offer little or no survival benefit because of residual viable tumor cells in the capsule (which receive some portal blood supply) and incomplete initial necrosis of the tumor. However, chemoembolization may assist in tumor shrinkage prior to OLT or resection, although potential complications such as vasculitis, hepatic artery thrombosis, and tumor abscess may make subsequent surgery more difficult. Portal vein thrombosis is an absolute contraindication to chemoembolization.

Other Therapies

Hormonal therapy has been examined because of the presence of estrogen and androgen receptors on HCC. Antiandrogens such as ketoconazole, cyproterone acetate, and buserelin (a gonadotropin-releasing hormone antagonist) have been studied and appear to be of no benefit. In a randomized trial versus placebo, tamoxifen prolonged median survival from 1 to 5 months in advanced, nonoperative disease. Interferon alfa-2b and interleukin-2 are of no benefit, nor are ferritin and AFP antibodies labeled with iodine 131.

External beam radiation must be limited to 3000 rads because of hepatic sensitivity, and doses below this level are ineffective for tumor control. Although intraoperative radiation can deliver higher, localized doses, randomized trials are lacking. Another form of intraoperative treatment is cryosurgery. This therapy involves ultrasound-guided liquid nitrogen and is useful for lesions felt to be nonresectable. It appears to be safe, but further studies on efficacy are needed.

As the HCC vascular supply is arterial, hepatic artery ligation has been tried. Although tumor necrosis occurs, neovascularization is rapid, benefit is minimal, and the effect of dearterialization on the cirrhotic liver can provoke hepatic failure.

SCREENING

Screening to identify tumors at an earlier stage in high-risk individuals is widely advocated. Those at high risk include all cirrhotic patients (Wilson's disease and primary biliary cirrhosis are of less risk) and HBsAg-positive patients. Screening protocols vary but generally include checking AFP levels every 6 months and annual ultrasound examinations. If universally applied, such screening would be very costly. Although screening in high-risk regions such as China has demonstrated an increase in resectability rates, controlled trials showing survival benefit or cost-effectiveness in the United States are not available. Efforts should be placed on eradication of HBV by universal infant vaccination programs.

CHOLANGIOCARCINOMA

EPIDEMIOLOGY

Cholangiocarcinoma is a primary liver malignancy of bile duct origin with an autopsy incidence in the United States of 0.01% to 0.46%. Peak occurrence is in the seventh decade of life, with a male-to-female ratio of 1.3:1. Risk factors for development of cholangiocarcinoma include gallstones (present in 50% of cases), ulcerative colitis, cystic diseases, toxins, and infections. In ulcerative colitis the incidence of cholangiocarcinoma is elevated to 0.4% to 1.4% (for a relative risk of 22 to 31), where it often presents in the fifth decade, typically after 15 to 20 years of pancolitis and usually in the presence of underlying primary sclerosing cholangitis. Early colectomy does not reduce this risk.

Caroli's disease, congenital liver cysts, and choledochal cysts confer an elevated risk of developing cholangiocarcinoma, also typically in the fourth or fifth decade. The pathogenesis is unclear but may include biliary stasis with chronic inflammation, intraductal stones, and exposure to pancreatic secretions. Other risk factors include thorotrast, hepatolithiasis, and *Opisthorchis sinensis* infection. There are possible associations with isoniazid, a-methyldopa, birth control pills, asbestos, and polychlorinated biphenyl exposure.

HISTOLOGY

Most bile duct tumors are cholangiocarcinomas or adenocarcinomas (90% to 95% of cases), although squamous and mucoepidermoid carcinomas, leiomyosarcomas, rhabdomyosarcomas, and cystadenocarcinomas occur. Hilar cholangiocarcinoma, which includes the common hepatic duct or main left and right hepatic ducts, is also known as a Klatskin's tumor. It offers special difficulties because of its strategic location. Among extrahepatic tumors, 33% to 40% are located in the common bile duct, 30% to 32% in the common hepatic duct, 20% at the bifurcation, and 4% in the cystic duct.

Cholangiocarcinoma expresses three types of growth characteristics. The sclerosing type is most common and coincidentally most difficult to diagnose and treat. Nodular and papillary types also exist, usually in the distal extrahepatic biliary system. Cholangiocarcinoma is slow growing, and blood-borne metastases are unusual, occurring late in the disease course. The tumor typically extends locally with submucosal spread. Cholangiocarcinomas may be multifocal in approximately 10% of cases.

CLINICAL PRESENTATION

Obstructive jaundice is the most common presentation of symptomatic extrahepatic cholangiocarcinoma. Pruritus and abdominal pain are frequent, and weight loss is seen in 50%. Physical examination is usually unremarkable except for jaundice, although hepatomegaly or ascites are occasionally present. Patients may also present with bacterial cholangitis. A diagnosis is often delayed in more proximal tumors, as unilateral bile duct obstruction does not produce jaundice. Determination of alkaline phosphatase and GGT levels are more sensitive, although nonspecific, tests than determination of bilirubin levels and are elevated even with only single duct involvement.

RADIOLOGIC ASSESSMENT

Ultrasound should be the first imaging test employed. Obstruction may be suggested by biliary tree dilation, but a primary tumor mass is seen in only 12% to 20% of cases. CT may be better able to demonstrate a tumor mass (40% to 54% sensitivity) or identify lobar atrophy or hypertrophy, evidence of metastatic disease, and other sources of bile duct obstruction such as pancreatic disorders.

As the differential diagnosis of obstructive jaundice includes benign strictures, intraductal stone disease, gallbladder carcinoma, sclerosing cholangitis, cholangiocarcinoma, and pancreatic disease, the elucidation of the location and extent of biliary obstruction is important. This requires direct imaging of the biliary tree via percutaneous transhepatic cholangiography (PTC) or endoscopic retrograde cholangiopancreatography (ERCP).

ERCP allows direct visualization of the ampulla of Vater, definition of pancreatic duct anatomy, identification of bile duct diseases, duct biopsy or cytologic examination, and therapeutic intervention such as stone extraction or biliary stenting. If the biliary tree, including ducts proximal to an obstruction, cannot be satisfactorily visualized at ERCP, PTC can be used. Because of the risk of bacterial cholangitis, prompt biliary drainage by endoscopic stent or percutaneous drain may be necessary when emptying of contrast from above a stricture is delayed.

Tissue diagnosis may be attempted with bile or brush cytologic examination, FNA, or biopsy of the lesion at ERCP or PTC. Bile cytologic examination and FNA are 33% to 56% and 50% to 77% sensitive, respectively. If surgical resection is contemplated, angiography including portal venography to document vascular anatomy and look for possible tumor encroachment or vascular thrombosis should be considered.

TREATMENT

Resection

Treatment of cholangiocarcinoma focuses on surgical resection, as resection offers the only hope for cure. Operability ranges from 5% to 50% of cases, although hilar cholangiocarcinomas are resectable in only 20%. Untreated, hilar cholangiocarcinoma carries a mean survival of 3 to 6 months. Patients with bilobar arterial or portal vein involvement or patients with unilateral vascular involvement with contralateral intrahepatic duct tumor extension are poor operative candidates. Although main portal vein involvement has been an absolute contraindication to resection, some surgeons are reporting success with vein excision and grafting.

Based on the patient's general medical condition and the results of radiographic studies, only 40% appear to be resectable. Of these, half cannot be resected based on intraoperative findings. Manipulation or biopsy of the tumor at operation may spread the carcinoma and preclude future treatment by OLT.

Surgical options for cholangiocarcinoma are based on the location of the tumor. Peripheral tumors require lobectomy, and 3-year survival rates up to 56% are reported. Extrahepatic bile duct tumors are divided into distal, middle, and proximal by thirds. Distal cholangiocarcinoma has a 47% to 70% resectability rate and includes pancreaticoduodenectomy with 3-year survival rates of up to 36% and 5-year survival rates of 20% reported. Middle tumors are resectable in 32% to 40% of cases, usually requiring both local resection and pancreaticoduodenectomy, although survival rates are poor.

For hilar cholangiocarcinoma surgical options include local resection or a radical excision including segmentectomy with Roux-en-Y hepaticojejunostomy to either the segment III duct (left lobe) or segment V duct (right lobe). If considered, radical excision is favored, as the likelihood of positive margins and early tumor regrowth following local excision is high. There are no randomized trials of local versus radical resection for hilar carcinomas. Unfortunately, because of the infiltrative nature of tumor growth, adequate surgical margins are difficult to assess at laparotomy, and residual microscopic tumor has been reported in up to 100% of those undergoing "curative" resection in some series.

Caudate lobe involvement with hilar cholangiocarcinoma is frequent and often undetectable. Caudate lobe resection had been recommended only if grossly involved by tumor, although a consensus is building for inclusion of caudate resection in all radical excisions. Preoperative cholangioscopy has been used to assess tumor extent. Of 55 patients studied, 53 had caudate involvement, and 46 underwent resection, all but one including segmentectomy and caudate lobectomy. Operative morbidity and mortality compared favorably to published rates, but 3- and 5-year survival rates were striking at 52% and 38%, respectively. Cholangioscopy is not widely employed and requires a 15F transhepatic channel; but despite these limitations, cholangioscopy should be further studied.

Median survival for hilar cholangiocarcinoma after resection varies between 7 to 23 months in large series, most likely reflecting patient selection. Ten-year survival rates of 4% to 14% have been reported for radical resection. Tumor-free surgical margins and lymph nodes confer survival advantage. Preoperative biliary drainage does not offer any additional advantage. "Palliative" resection offers no survival benefit over tumor stenting. Resection morbidity includes sepsis, cholangitis, acute renal failure, bleeding, pancreatic and biliary fistulae, and liver failure. Biliary leaks are common. Morbidity rates are 39% to 56% for radical excision with an attendant mortality of 6% to 27%.

Orthotopic Liver Transplantation

OLT has been used for cholangiocarcinoma with generally poor results. Most centers report 1- and 2-year survivals of less than 33% and 10%, respectively. Almost all patients die of recurrent disease. At present, most clinicians suggest that cholangiocarcinoma be transplanted only under study protocol, usually involving some form of neoadjuvant radiation or chemotherapy. If transplantation is to be considered, prior operative bile duct manipulation and biopsy should be avoided.

Palliation

The majority of cholangiocarcinomas are not resectable. In patients with cholangiocarcinomas, the main goal of palliation should be to effect relief of obstructive jaundice. Unilateral drainage relieves jaundice in 80% of patients with hilar tumors unless the segment drained is atrophic.

The method by which obstruction is bypassed must take into account issues of available expertise, the site of the lesion, patient acceptance and life expectancy, nutritional factors, and long-term bypass patency. Surgical bypass and stenting via endoscopic or percutaneous routes are most commonly employed. One series showed median survival rates for resection, surgical bypass, and stenting to be 23, 6.6, and 3.5 months, respectively; however, direct comparison of treatment efficacy is not valid, as patients were not randomized to different treatment groups.

Endoscopically or percutaneously placed biliary stents are the most frequently chosen palliative procedures. Internal endoscopically placed stents entail little morbidity and a 70% success rate, although the success rate is lower for hilar tumors. Endoprostheses have the advantages of lower rates of cholangitis, lack of an external appliance to care for, and ease of insertion. The major disadvantage is stent obstruction, typically occurring after 3 to 4 months, due to biliary sludge deposition, migration, initial malposition, or tumor overgrowth. Metallic wall stents, with a large inner diameter of 7 to 10 mm, offer improved patency rates. Migration is rare, although tumor overgrowth can occur.

Drainage through a percutaneous stent is also an option, both for initial obstruction relief and long-term palliation, and may be easier to place than endoscopic stents, especially for hilar tumors. This arrangement alone results in high rates of cholangitis (up to 50% to 60%); ongoing fluid, bile salt, and electrolyte loss; and additional care required for an external appliance. Subsequent internalization of these stents is possible and controls most of these problems. Wall stents may be placed percutaneously in a one-step procedure, requiring only a 7F transhepatic route, with stent expansion after it has crossed the stricture. Fully internal endoprostheses can be inserted percutaneously, but they are technically demanding and require prolonged hospitalization.

If at laparotomy a patient is found to have a nonresectable tumor, a surgical bypass may be done. Elective surgical bypass is less commonly performed today, since other modalities are available. Some nonrandomized studies suggest that this type of palliation may offer less chance of cholangitis, longer lasting obstruction relief, and better quality of life.

Other Therapies

Chemotherapy and radiation therapy are considered palliative. Controlled trials of chemotherapy have demonstrated partial responses in a minority of patients but have not shown survival benefit. External beam radiation is not an option because of the radiosensitivity of the liver at doses needed for tumor treatment. Transtumoral placement of iridium 192 or cobalt 60 wires within biliary stents has been used. However, randomized trials of efficacy are lacking.

HEPATIC ANGIOSARCOMA

Hepatic angiosarcoma (HAS) is a rare malignant tumor of mesenchymal origin. It accounts for only 2% of all primary liver tumors, with a male-to-female ratio of 3:1. Patients exposed to known risk factors account for up to 50% of cases. These factors include exposure to thorotrast, a thorium-containing contrast agent used from 1928 to the late 1950s. The first case of HAS linked to thorotrast was reported in 1947. Thorium is radioactive and has a half-life of 200 years, and 70% of a dose is taken up by the liver. There is a 24- to 37-year latency from contrast administration to tumor diagnosis. Polyvinyl chloride exposure is also linked to HAS, with a latency of approximately 19 years.

HAS may exhibit sinusoidal, cavernous, or solid tumor growth patterns. The tumors are poorly circumscribed and are often multiple. Central necrosis and hemorrhage are common. Tumor growth is aggressive, with early metastasis via vascular and lymphatic invasion. Distant metastasis to lung, regional lymph nodes, adrenals, spleen, and other abdominal viscera are present in 60% at diagnosis.

Symptoms are constitutional and nonspecific. Abdominal pain is most common, but fatigue, weakness, and weight loss also occur. Hepatomegaly (58%), ascites (28%), and jaundice (24%) are found on physical examination. A bruit over the liver may be noted. AFP and carcinoembryonic antigen levels are normal. Decreased platelets are seen in 54% to 62%, and frank disseminated intravascular coagulation occurs in up to 5%. Liver enzymes may be nonspecifically elevated in 70% to 85%, with γ-glutamyl transpeptidase (GGTP) being the most sensitive.

HAS can mimic hemangiomas by CT appearance. With contrast, heterogeneous and persistent tumor enhancement is noted. Ultrasound and technetium Tc 99m sulfur colloid scans are nonspecific. Angiography is the most useful test. Classic findings include early edge enhancement, delayed central enhancement, and increasing opacification over 3 to 15 minutes. Percutaneous biopsy specimens are diagnostic in only 25% of cases, and the procedure carries a high morbidity and mortality (18% bleeding rate and 12% death). If HAS is suspected, open biopsy is indicated when tissue diagnosis is required. Overall, two thirds of cases are diagnosed at autopsy.

Prognosis is poor, with a 5.5-month median survival. Only 2% of patients live more than 2 years, with death due to liver failure in half and intraabdominal hemorrhage in one quarter of patients. Most treatment interventions offer little or no benefit. Indeed, screening those at high risk for tumor development has not improved survival. Chemotherapy can afford temporary tumor regression, and in one retrospective series chemotherapy prolonged median survival to 13 months. Chemotherapeutic agents used in other soft tissue sarcomas are employed such as doxorubicin (Adriamycin), 5-fluorouracil, and cyclophosphamide (Cytoxan). Radiation therapy is not useful.

HEPATIC ADENOMA

Hepatic adenoma (HA) is the most common benign liver tumor found in women using oral contraceptives. Glycogenesis types IA and 6, use of androgenic steroids (in men), and pregnancy are also related to an increased risk. A history of estrogen use is present in 89% of patients with HA, and these tumors were in fact rare before the introduction of birth control pills. The risk of HA increases with the dose and duration of estrogen use. At 5 years the relative risk is 2.5%; at 9 years, 7.5%; and at more than 9 years the relative risk approaches 25%. Discontinuation of birth control pills usually decreases HA size.

HAs are typically solitary and surrounded by a pseudocapsule. They are often subcapsular and range from 5 to 30 cm in size. Hepatocytes with vacuolated cytoplasm are arranged in trabeculae, and sinusoids are compressed. Portal veins, bile ducts, and central veins are absent.

Unlike FNH, HA presents due to symptoms in up to 80% of cases, usually as a consequence of mass effect or bleeding. In fact, one third of patients present with an acute abdomen due to intratumoral or intraperitoneal bleeding or infarction. Both the size of the tumor and bleeding potential are increased with use of birth control pills.

Ultrasound and CT appearance are nonspecific, although CT may reveal evidence of hemorrhage. Liver enzymes and AFP are normal. Technetium Tc 99m sulfur colloid scan usually shows decreased uptake, whereas angiography shows a hypervascular mass with peripherally located vessels. Needle biopsy may provoke hemorrhage and is often nondiagnostic. Laparotomy with biopsy is occasionally necessary, but most cases are readily diagnosed by patient characteristics, x-ray studies, and percutaneous biopsy.

If HA is suspected in the absence of bleeding or rupture, birth control pills should be discontinued, and tumor size should be periodically observed by ultrasound. As long as the tumor regresses in size, expectant observation is warranted. However, with increasing size or development in the absence of birth control pills or pregnancy, resection may be required. Mortality from a free intraperitoneal rupture is 5% to 10%, whereas elective resection carries a less than 1% mortality. Cases of malignant transformation of HA to hepatocellular carcinoma have been reported. Pregnancy and oral contraceptive use should be avoided, if possible, following resection, as tumor recurrence in this setting has been described.

FOCAL NODULAR HYPERPLASIA

FNH is a benign liver tumor that affects up to 8% of the population. The female-to-male ratio is 2:1, with a peak incidence in the third to fifth decade. Unlike hepatic adenoma, no firm links have been made between FNH and estrogen use. There appears to have been an increased incidence in the past three decades, but this is likely secondary to improved awareness and imaging.

Discovery of FNH tumors is usually incidental. Only 10% of patients present with symptoms (usually due to mass effect), and bleeding is very rare. If the tumor is pedunculated, torsion may occur with associated pain. Liver enzyme levels are normal, and tumor markers are negative.

Histologically, FNH is composed of normal hepatocytes, sinusoids, bile ducts, and Kupffer's cells. There are, however, no portal triads, as the blood supply is exclusively arterial. The pathogenesis of FNH is unclear. One theory is that a primary arterial anomaly is present with a subsequent hyperplastic cellular response. Another possibility is that normal portal flow is somehow obliterated, which results in an area of tissue receiving only arterial flow, again with resultant hyperplasia.

The appearance of FNH on ultrasound and CT is nonspecific. Most commonly the finding is of an incidentally noted, sharply demarcated focal liver mass. More than 95% of these tumors are less than 10 cm in diameter. CT without contrast may show a slightly hypodense lesion, which becomes isodense with contrast administration. The differential diagnosis in this setting would include HA and HCC. Suggestion of a stellate central scar at CT or magnetic resonance imaging is classic for FNH. Angiography may show a characteristic hypervascular tumor with a central blood supply, spoke-and-wheel arterial arrangement, and a dense capillary blush. This finding is unfortunately neither sensitive nor specific. If FNH is suspected, colloid scintigraphy may be helpful and is recommended by some authors as the next test after ultrasound or CT. Normal or increased uptake of colloid strongly suggests FNH. This finding is due to a normal complement of Kupffer's cells, which HA and HCC lack.

Percutaneous biopsy is generally safe but often nondiagnostic. If focal arteriole wall thickening is demonstrated, the diagnosis may be made. It may be difficult to exclude normal liver, HA, or even HCC (especially FLHCC variant) unless wedge biopsy is performed. Once the diagnosis of FNH is established, it may safely be left in situ if asymptomatic, as the natural history of this lesion is benign.

REFERENCES

1. Belghiti J, Panis Y, Farges O, et al. Intrahepatic recurrence after resection of hepatocellular carcinoma complicating cirrhosis. *Ann Surg.* 1991;214:114–117.
2. Colombo M. Hepatocellular carcinoma. *J Hepatol.* 1992;15:225–236.
3. Hadjis NS, Blenkharn JI, Alexander N, et al. Outcome of radical surgery in hilar cholangiocarcinoma. *Surgery.* 1990;107:597–604.
4. Liang TJ, Jeffers LJ, Reddy R, et al. Viral pathogenesis of hepatocellular carcinoma in the United States. *Hepatology.* 1993;18:1326–1333.
5. Livraghi T, Bolondi L, Lazzaroni S, et al. Percutaneous ethanol injection in the treatment of hepatocellular carcinoma in cirrhosis. *Cancer.* 1992;69:925–929.
6. McLean GK, Burke DR. Role of endoprostheses in the management of malignant biliary obstruction. *Radiology.* 1989;170:961–967.
7. Nimura Y, Hayakawa N, Kamiya J, et al. Hepatic segmentectomy with caudate lobe resection for bile duct carcinoma of the hepatic hilus. *World J Surg.* 1990;14: 535–544.
8. Shortell CK, Schwartz SI. Hepatic adenoma and focal nodular hyperplasia. *Surg Gynecol Obstet.* 1991;173: 426–431.
9. Stain SC, Baer HU, Dennison AR, Blumgart LH. Current management of hilar cholangiocarcinoma. *Surg Gynecol Obstet.* 1992;175:579–588.
10. Van Thiel DH, Carr B, Iwatsuki S, et al. The 11-year Pittsburgh experience with liver transplantation for hepatocellular carcinoma: 1981–1991. *J Surg Oncol.* 1993(suppl 3);78–82.

110
Disorders of Liver Function in Systemic Disease

PETER V. BARRETT

The purpose of this chapter is to offer the reader an approach to the diagnosis and management of disorders of liver function that are commonly seen in the presence of systemic disease. No attempt is made to provide a detailed account of specific disease processes, since this information is available in a number of excellent textbooks, some of which are given as references.[1,2]

LIVER FUNCTION: SPECTATORS AND TARGETS

In the clinical setting, liver function is most commonly described in terms of a panel of "LFTs," or liver function tests, such as those listed in Table 110–1. *Function* must be broadly defined for such tests, since the tests reflect a variety of cellular mechanisms. Nevertheless, clinical usage has demonstrated that this small group of tests can be very helpful in clinical diagnosis if they are properly interpreted. Interpretation requires an appreciation of the origins of a *marker*, such as alkaline phosphatase, and an understanding that these tests, as a group, demonstrate a high sensitivity but low specificity for the diagnosis of liver disease.

It may be helpful to consider systemic diseases with abnormal liver function tests as falling into one of two large groups: clinical settings in which the liver is primarily a "spectator," and settings in which the liver is the major "target" of the disease process. Congestive heart failure is an example of the liver as spectator; effective treatment of the heart disease resolves liver function test abnormalities. Viral hepatitis is a classic example of the latter group; here, eradication of the hepatic infection by the host or by antiviral therapy results in normalization of liver function tests. Thus, one of the clinician's most important roles is to be able to distinguish between these two general categories. An appreciation that liver function falls into the spectator category in a very large number of systemic diseases can prevent diagnostic distractions and many unnecessary tests.

FIVE LIVER FUNCTION TESTS

Clinical testing for diagnosis in medicine has become increasingly more sophisticated and costly in recent years, and it is therefore worthy of emphasis that the bedside history remains the single best diagnostic tool. Evaluations of patients with a variety of disease states from heart disease to jaundice have shown that a careful history provides an accurate diagnosis in three quarters of patients; physical examination and routine clinical laboratory testing (e.g., a liver function test panel) can provide diagnosis for most of the remainder. Invasive and expensive testing is needed in only a small percentage of patients. Therefore, it follows that clinicians should make every effort to glean as much information as possible from the routine but high-yield approaches to patient evaluation. In the same manner, patience and thoughtful interpretation of the five standard tests listed in Table 110–1 are usually sufficient to explain abnormalities of liver function. The individual tests in this table are briefly discussed to serve as a basis for a review of hepatic dysfunction in systemic disease.

ALBUMIN

The serum albumin concentration is widely viewed as a measure of hepatocyte synthetic function, and consequently low values are generally interpreted to indicate diminished synthe-

TABLE 110–1. FIVE COMMON TESTS OF LIVER FUNCTION (SERUM TEST AND NORMAL RANGE)

Albumin (3.5–5.5 g/dl)
Alkaline phosphatase (30–120 IU/L)
Aminotransferases (transaminases)
　Aspartate aminotransferase (0–35 U/L)
　Alanine aminotransferase (0–35 U/L)
Bilirubin (total <1 mg/dl)
Prothrombin time (9–11 s)

sis or nutritional deficiency. Furthermore, because of its relatively long biologic half-life of 20 days, a low value is suggestive of a chronic process, and this information can be useful in distinguishing chronic liver disease in relapse from an acute process. However, there are several common clinical settings that may limit the usefulness of this test. As noted above, nutritional deficiency itself can result in low serum concentrations of albumin; in conditions associated with an expanded extracellular volume (e.g., pregnancy, ascitic cirrhosis), a low serum concentration may be found without a decrease in total body albumin.

ALKALINE PHOSPHATASE

Serum alkaline phosphatase (SALP), a product of the biliary epithelium, has been used in the evaluation of liver function for many years, but interpretation of abnormal serum levels may be difficult at times because the enzyme can also be released from other tissues such as bone and placenta. Liver disease is clearly the most frequent reason for elevated serum concentrations of alkaline phosphatase, and it is usually sufficient to judge the enzyme's source by "the company it keeps"; thus, the liver is the most likely source of the enzyme if other liver function tests are abnormal. However, caution must be exercised in using it as a marker for liver disease in pregnant women and in children during periods of rapid growth, since both of these conditions are associated with increased serum levels of the enzyme. In these clinical settings additional testing with either of two serum enzymes, c-glutamyl transpeptidase or 5′-nucleotidase, is useful in the differential diagnosis, since neither is released from bone.

In patients with liver disease, an elevated SALP has almost become synonymous with *cholestasis,* a term that should be used with care, since it may have different connotations for the pathologist, biochemist, and clinician. Thus, one may encounter the term in a description of bile plugs on liver biopsy or description of a very high SALP, whereas at the bedside the term may be used by a clinician to describe an icteric patient. However, each of the above represents a different consequence of the same primary problem, namely, impaired bile formation or solute excretion, or both. Furthermore, it is important to remember that the impairment can result from either mechanical obstruction or from abnormal function of the bile secretory apparatus.

The absolute level of SALP can be of some help in the differential diagnosis, especially at very high levels. SALP activities greater than 500 IU/L may be seen in intrahepatic or extrahepatic biliary obstruction, granulomatous diseases, and some diseases of bone such as Paget's disease. On the other hand, low-level or moderate elevations of SALP occur in a wide variety of conditions, and they are therefore of little help in identifying specific disease states.

AMINOTRANSFERASES

Alanine aminotransferase (ALT) and aspartate aminotransferase (AST), previously known as transaminases, are two of the most useful tests of liver function. AST is present in a wide variety of tissues, but ALT is primarily found in the liver. The elevated serum levels that occur in a variety of disease processes result not only from hepatocellular necrosis but also from cellular injury, and in general there is a poor correlation between serum levels and the extent of necrosis. Hepatotoxins such as acetaminophen are an exception to this rule, and patients with the greatest elevations of serum aminotransferase (SAT) may be expected to have more serious clinical illness.

The highest levels of SAT occur in patients with viral hepatitis, acute hypoperfusion states, and hepatotoxins; levels are commonly greater than 1000 U/L under these circumstances. Rarely, patients with acute biliary obstruction may have transient elevations of SAT that approach this level.

BILIRUBIN

Measurement of the serum bilirubin concentration was one of the first procedures introduced into clinical chemistry. Eighty years ago van den Bergh and Snapper published the details of a diazo method, which has undergone little modification over the years. These early workers found that color development occurred promptly ("directly") when diazo reagent was added to serum of patients with hepatitis or obstructive jaundice; however, color did not appear immediately after the addition of diazo reagent to serum from newborns or patients with hemolytic anemia unless an accelerator, such as alcohol, was added. This latter type of bile pigment, "indirect bilirubin," is now known to represent unconjugated bilirubin, whereas direct bilirubin represents water-soluble conjugated bilirubin. Precise research methods that are now available have validated the diazo method, especially for measurement of total bilirubin, which includes both indirect and direct bilirubin. However, measurements of direct bilirubin are unreliable if the total bilirubin concentration is less than 5 mg/dl. Thus, in suspected hemolytic disease or other conditions associated with unconjugated hyperbilirubinemia, the disease cannot be excluded if testing fails to reveal an increased indirect bilirubin level.

PROTHROMBIN TIME

The two commonly used tests of liver function that directly reflect synthetic function of the hepatocyte are the albumin concentration and the prothrombin activity, in contrast to other function tests that reflect either cell integrity (SAT), clearance (bilirubin), or production by bile duct epithelial cells (SALP). It may also be helpful to recall that the in vivo half-life of prothrombin is 2 to 5 days, and albumin is 20 days; thus, a loss of prothrombin out of proportion to the albumin value may suggest fulminant liver disease, whereas a decrease in the levels of both albumin and prothrombin suggests a more chronic process.

OTHER LIVER FUNCTION TESTS

One may argue that newer, more specific tests such as the alpha-fetoprotein or hepatitis B surface antigen (HBsAg) should also be thought of as liver function tests, and indeed, under certain circumstances such tests are clearly indicated. However, the "core" of the five simple tests listed above provides sufficient information for the initial phase of evaluation.

THE LIVER AS SPECTATOR

Table 110–2 lists some of the systemic disease processes that affect the liver in an incidental manner, where liver dysfunction usually plays little role in the patient's outcome.

TABLE 110–2. CLINICAL CONDITIONS IN WHICH THE LIVER MAY BE A SPECTATOR IN SYSTEMIC DISEASE

Hypoperfusion states
  Congestive heart failure
  Cardiogenic or hypovolemic shock
Systemic infections
  Sepsis, especially gram-negative type
  Granulomatous disease
Drug-induced disease
Fatty liver
  Ethanol abuse
  Malnutrition
  Obesity
  Corticosteroids
  Diabetes mellitus
  Gastrointestinal tract disease
  Pancreatitic disease
  Intestinal bypass for morbid obesity
  Total parenteral nutrition
Acquired immunodeficiency syndrome
Collagen-vascular disease
Miscellaneous
  Amyloidosis
  Lymphoma (Hodgkin's disease and Non-Hodgkin's lymphoma)
  Nephrogenic hepatic dysfunction syndrome
  Sickle cell anemia

HYPOPERFUSION

A variety of acute and chronic conditions associated with a decreased cardiac output may result in liver function abnormalities. Prior to the advent of potent diuretics and cardiac surgery, many patients with valvular heart disease developed cirrhosis because of long-standing, decompensated congestive heart failure. This entity may still be seen, but it is now much more common to encounter patients with acute or subacute cardiac dysfunction. In patients with chronic hypoperfusion, the abnormalities of liver function are variable, but twofold to threefold elevations of the SAT and a 1- to 2-second prolongation of the prothrombin time are usually the earliest changes to be noted. Although case reports of congestive heart failure that presents as obscure liver disease have been published, for the most part the relationship between heart failure and liver dysfunction is not subtle.

Acute hypoperfusion of the liver may result in abnormalities of some or all of the clinical tests of liver function, and changes in the SAT may be striking. Aminotransferase values may match levels commonly seen in patients with acute viral hepatitis (25- to 50-fold elevation); however, with prompt restoration of perfusion these very high values decline to near-normal levels within a few days, in contrast to a slow decline over several weeks, which is typical of acute viral hepatitis. Uncommonly, patients who have experienced an acute episode of hypoperfusion may develop 1 to 2 weeks later a clinically confusing syndrome that mimics the biochemical pattern of extrahepatic obstruction, with markedly elevated serum concentrations of bilirubin and SALP and only moderate increases in the levels of the SAT.[3] The importance of correct diagnosis cannot be over emphasized, since the syndrome resolves without treatment and since surgery in such patients carries with it a high rate of morbidity and mortality. The cause of this syndrome is unknown but presumably results from prolonged ischemia.

Systemic Infections

Abnormal results from liver function tests occur with great regularity in patients in an intensive care unit, and it is often difficult to attribute the abnormalities to a single factor. Hypoperfusion has been discussed as one of these factors, but the roles of recent surgery or trauma, drugs, malnutrition, and sepsis must also be considered.

The association of jaundice with serious systemic infection has long been recognized, but only in recent decades has it become clear that clinically significant abnormalities in hepatic function can occur without evidence of biliary infection. Jaundice is a frequent accompaniment of serious extrahepatic infection in neonates, and indeed may be the earliest indicator of sepsis. In adults, the incidence of jaundice varies widely in accordance with the severity of the infection and the specific organism involved, but jaundice is generally uncommon. However, as many as one half of such patients have moderately severe abnormalities of other liver function tests.[4]

The association between sepsis and abnormalities of liver function is most commonly encountered in patients with gram-negative infections, especially with *Escherichia coli* bacteremia. However, a large number of organisms have the potential to produce such changes, and common examples include pneumococcal pneumonia and the toxic shock syndrome induced by staphylococci. The pathogenesis of the liver function abnormalities is not well understood, but there is appealing laboratory evidence that endotoxins derived from *E. coli* and *Salmonella enteritidis* can produce a dose-dependent decrease in bile flow; thus, circulating endotoxin could be responsible, at least in infections with these organisms, for the observed clinical picture.

Drug-Induced Disease

Abnormalities of liver function may be observed frequently in the course of management with a variety of drugs. For the most part the abnormalities consist of onefold to twofold elevations of SAT and SALP (which are often transient), and the patient is asymptomatic. Thus, most such reactions fall into the category of spectator abnormalities; however, the unpredictable specter of a devastating reaction, albeit rare, should be always present in the clinician's mind. Prudence suggests that a potential cause-and-effect relationship exists in any clinical setting in which liver function abnormalities occur during drug treatment. Ordinarily, observation alone is sufficient, but withdrawal is sometimes indicated. Especially in critically ill patients who are receiving multiple medications, the clinical decision to withdraw drugs is often a very difficult one in large part because of our poor understanding of the natural history of drug hepatotoxicity.

As an example, isoniazid is well known to produce liver function abnormalities in at least 10% of patients; however, most of these abnormalities resolve in the face of continued treatment, and it is unclear whether this mild "transaminitis" bears any relationship to the fulminant presentation of hepatitis that is seen in fewer than 1% of patients who take the drug. There is little evidence that monitoring has prevented morbidity or mortality. Until better information is available, however, the most reasonable course of action is to proceed in a conservative manner in the management of possible hepatotoxicity related to drug treatment. The reader is referred to the hepatology texts referenced above for a more detailed account of drug hepatotoxicity.

Fatty Liver (Steatosis)

Table 110–2 lists most clinical settings in which fatty liver may be found. For the purposes of general discussion, the liver may again be described as a spectator for most patients who are affected by these disease processes, but it is obvious that on occasion serious disease may result as well.

Of the conditions listed in Table 110–2, ethanol abuse, malnutrition, and obesity are responsible for the greatest number of patients; in fact, many of the remaining entities, such as diabetes mellitus, may be considered "derivative" associations. For example, obesity is probably the process responsible for the development of fatty liver in diabetic patients, rather than diabetes mellitus itself, and malnutrition may account for the fatty liver found in a variety of diseases of the gastrointestinal tract system. Malnutrition may also play a role in the development of fatty liver and liver function abnormalities that occur in some patients who receive total parenteral nutrition; Quigley and colleagues[5] have recently published a helpful review of this complex problem.

Abnormal liver function is commonly observed in patients with disturbances of energy metabolism, but there has been disagreement about causation. The coexistence of other diseases and the increased incidence of gallstone disease in patients who have diabetes mellitus or obesity have made it difficult to identify responsible factors. Nevertheless, in recent years most investigators have concluded that diabetes mellitus, malnutrition, and obesity, singly or in combination, are frequently associated with minor abnormalities of aminotransferases, alkaline phosphatase, albumin and, less commonly, bilirubin.

Kwashiorkor is a dramatic clinical demonstration of abnormalities that result from severe protein-calorie malnutrition. The livers of such patients are enlarged, and microscopic examination reveals the presence of large amounts of fat (triglyceride) in the hepatocytes. Modest abnormalities of liver function may also be present, and cirrhosis has been found in some patients; however, the cirrhosis in kwashiorkor probably results from coexisting disease processes. In general, fatty liver, per se, is not considered to have deleterious long-term effects on hepatic function.

In most instances fatty liver results from an imbalance between rates of delivery of fatty acids to the liver from the periphery and the rate of secretion of very low density lipoproteins by the liver. Ethanol abuse, of course, may produce fatty liver and a panorama of clinical syndromes that relate in part to the duration of abuse and to the amount consumed. A number of studies have convincingly demonstrated that ethanol can produce fatty liver in the absence of associated nutritional deficiencies.

Fasting also produces a fatty liver, ordinarily without changes in alkaline phosphatase or aminotransferase; however, a twofold to threefold increase in serum bilirubin may be expected. The increase in serum bilirubin under fasting conditions passes unnoticed in patients with normal values (<1 mg/dl); however, for those with underlying liver disease or Gilbert syndrome who have baseline bilirubin concentrations greater than 2 mg/dl, a twofold to threefold increase in bilirubin concentration to a level of 4 to 6 mg/dl produces obvious jaundice and generates much diagnostic confusion. The elevated bilirubin concentration probably reflects the decrease in hepatic clearance of organic anions that has been demonstrated under fasting conditions; the elevated bilirubin concentration causes no harmful consequences, provided that the elevation is not taken as an indication for surgery.[6]

ACQUIRED IMMUNODEFICIENCY SYNDROME

A wide array of disease and drug-related processes combine to produce spectator abnormalities of liver function in most patients with acquired immunodeficiency syndrome (AIDS), and on occasion serious hepatobiliary disease requires difficult medical and surgical management decisions. Table 110–3 lists disease processes commonly encountered in patients with AIDS.[7,8]

Autopsy studies do not fairly represent the frequency of disease processes through the full course of an illness, but they are nevertheless helpful in providing insight into the types of processes to be encountered. Livers of patients with AIDS have been found to be abnormal in 80% to 90% of patients at autopsy, and half this number are AIDS-specific processes such as *Mycobacterium avium-intracellulare,* cytomegalovirus, granulomatous disease, Kaposi's sarcoma, and intrahepatic lymphomas. In life, liver function abnormalities are the rule, rather than the exception. Ordinarily, the abnormalities are limited to aminotransferase and alkaline phosphatase, and the latter can be markedly elevated in patients with hepatic granulomas, lymphoma, and sclerosing cholangitis. Liver biopsy is seldom indicated, since the parenchymal liver disease in AIDS patients usually represents a manifestation of previously diagnosed, disseminated disease.

TABLE 110–3. DISEASES AFFECTING THE HEPATOBILIARY SYSTEM IN ACQUIRED IMMUNODEFICIENCY SYNDROME (AIDS)

Viral hepatitis
  Hepatitis A, B, C, D
  Cytomegalovirus
  Epstein-Barr virus
  Herpes simplex virus
  Human immunodeficiency virus
Opportunistic infections
  Mycobacterium avium-intracellulare
  Cryptosporidium
  Pneumocystitis carinii
  Mycobacterium tuberculosis
  Coccidioides immitis
  Candida albicans
  Histoplasma capsulatum
  Cryptococcus neoformans
AIDS cholangiopathy
  Acalculous cholecystitis
  Sclerosing cholangitis
  Papillary stenosis
  Lymphoma of biliary tree
Neoplasms
  Kaposi's sarcoma
  Non-Hodgkin's lymphoma
  Drug-induced hepatitis
Histologic findings
  Steatosis (fatty liver)
  Granulomatous hepatitis
  Portal inflammation
  Sinusoidal dilation
  Peliosis hepatitis

From Reddy KR, Schiff ER. Hepatobiliary manifestations of AIDS. In: Rustgi VK, Van Thiel DH, eds. *The Liver in Systemic Disease.* New York, NY: Raven Press Publishers; 1993.

COLLAGEN-VASCULAR DISEASE

Liver function test abnormalities are common in collagen-vascular disease, but once again the liver usually plays the role of spectator. Mild hepatomegaly may be found in a quarter of patients with rheumatoid arthritis and systemic lupus erythematosus (SLE), usually related to steatosis. Mild elevations in SALP levels may be seen in half of patients with rheumatoid arthritis, and in most instances the SALP is derived from liver rather than bone. Elevations of aminotransferase may also occur in the various collagen-vascular diseases, particularly in patients with SLE. However, in many cases the elevation results from drugs used in treatment, particularly salicylates.

Early investigators who described patients with autoimmune chronic active hepatitis (AICAH) were impressed by clinical and laboratory features that may also be found in SLE such as hyperglobulinemia, arthritis, and a positive "LE cell" test. Therefore, the term *lupoid hepatitis* was introduced to indicate the possible relationship of this form of liver disease to SLE. However, over the years numerous studies have addressed this issue, and it is now clear that AICAH bears no direct relationship to SLE. The term *lupoid hepatitis* should be abandoned. Nevertheless, it should be borne in mind that associations do exist between various collagen-vascular diseases and autoimmune diseases of the liver such as AICAH and primary biliary cirrhosis; furthermore, in patients with persistent abnormalities of liver function, clinical circumstances may warrant additional serologic testing (e.g., antinuclear and antimitochondrial antibodies).

MISCELLANEOUS

Several uncommon disease processes that may be associated with abnormalities of liver function are listed in Table 110–2. The nephrogenic hepatic dysfunction syndrome (Stauffer's syndrome) bears emphasis, since the observed liver function abnormalities may be mistakenly interpreted as indicating metastatic disease. The syndrome is found in 15% to 20% of patients with renal cell carcinoma and is characterized by fever, weight loss, and focal hepatic necrosis without metastasis. Symptoms and abnormalities of liver function may be expected to resolve within 1 or 2 months following resection of the tumor, suggesting that a circulating factor produced by the tumor may be responsible.

Spectator abnormalities of liver function are frequently observed in patients with sickle cell anemia with minor elevations of alkaline phosphatase and aminotransferase enzymes. In past years patients with sickle cell anemia often received transfusions, and liver function abnormalities were often seen as a consequence of transfusion-induced chronic hepatitis from hepatitis B or C viruses (HBV or HCV). However, because transfusions are now used sparingly and serologic testing of donated blood for viral hepatitis has become routine, the frequency of such abnormalities can be expected to diminish in the future. More striking liver function abnormalities may occasionally be seen in patients with hepatic sickle crisis, and the constellation of right upper quadrant pain, fever, leukocytosis, and jaundice may be indistinguishable from acute cholecystitis with choledocholithiasis and ascending cholangitis. The differential diagnosis is especially difficult because of the increased frequency of pigment gallstones in patients with sickle cell anemia. To avoid this dilemma, elective cholecystectomy should be considered for patients known to have gallstones.

GENERAL APPROACH

A frequent clinical problem encountered by the generalist and subspecialists in hepatology is the finding of abnormal aminotransferase and alkaline phosphatase tests on a routine biochemical screening panel in an asymptomatic patient. Many such patients are obese or female and therefore liable for complications of gallstone disease; additionally, they may have obscure complaints and are often receiving multiple medications. The following outlines the best and most cost-effective way to proceed in the evaluation of such patients.

In the absence of significant symptoms or abnormalities on physical examination, a stepwise approach to medical evaluation should be pursued over a period of several months. The patient should be observed on several occasions while important aspects of the history are reviewed and routine liver function tests are repeated. Additional information concerning the use of drugs and alcohol, prior transfusions, and homosexual contacts may be elicited during this time. The ALT for a small proportion of such patients with low-grade abnormalities becomes normal without any form of treatment, and liver function test abnormalities improve or revert to normal in half of obese patients with weight reduction and general conditioning.[9]

However, after following the systematic approach to medical evaluation outlined above, a small but important subset of asymptomatic patients with persistent, unexplained abnormalities of SAT may be identified who have clinically significant liver disease. Hay and colleagues[10] at the Mayo Clinic prospectively studied asymptomatic patients with persistent abnormalities of liver function and found 47 who had elevations of SAT that were threefold or greater for more than 6 months. On biopsy, 34 of the 47 patients were found to have chronic active hepatitis, and among these patients, half were shown to have AICAH.[10] Thus, most of the patients in this study with persistent abnormalities of SAT deserved consideration for treatment of either chronic viral or autoimmune hepatitis.

Despite the clinician's best efforts, some abnormalities of liver function tests cannot be explained. Abnormal liver function tests in asymptomatic individuals pose a frequent diagnostic dilemma, and judgment must be exercised in balancing risks and costs of extensive testing with possible benefits of accurate diagnosis. An algorithm illustrating an approach to the evaluation of abnormal liver function tests in patients with persistently abnormal results is shown in Figure 110–1.

As noted earlier, the highest diagnostic yield for most clinical problems comes from a good history obtained from the patient, family, and old records. An important additional strategy to shed light on asymptomatic liver function abnormalities is the "brown bag maneuver"; in this approach the patient is instructed to bring into the office all medications, vitamins, and health foods from the home. The harvest can be astounding!

A review of Table 110–4 suggests that among patients with these broad categories of disease, intervention has greatest impact on those with gallstone disease. Treatment of patients with various types of hepatitis is in its infancy; the treatment of ethanol-induced liver disease (abstinence) is well known but seldom successful; chemotherapy and surgery for tumors of the liver is discouraging; and the treatment of drug-induced disease depends primarily on the identification and withdrawal of the noxious agent.

Thus, with the exception of gallstone disease, treatment of hepatic disease is often limited to supportive care and withdrawal of alcohol or drug. It behooves the clinician to be thorough in the search for evidence of gallstones and for evidence that the gallstones are in fact producing the patient's symptoms or observed abnormalities of function. The prevalence of gallstones increases throughout life, and at least 20% of women over the age of 60 years may be expected to have cholelithiasis. However, at least two thirds of such patients are asymptomatic, and the rate at which symptoms or complications de-

TABLE 110–4. COMMON CLINICAL CONDITIONS IN WHICH THE LIVER CAN BE CONSIDERED THE TARGET OF THE DISEASE PROCESS

Hepatitis (viral, autoimmune)
Ethanol abuse
Tumor (primary and metastatic)
Drug- and toxin-induced disease
Biliary tract disease (gallstone, autoimmune)

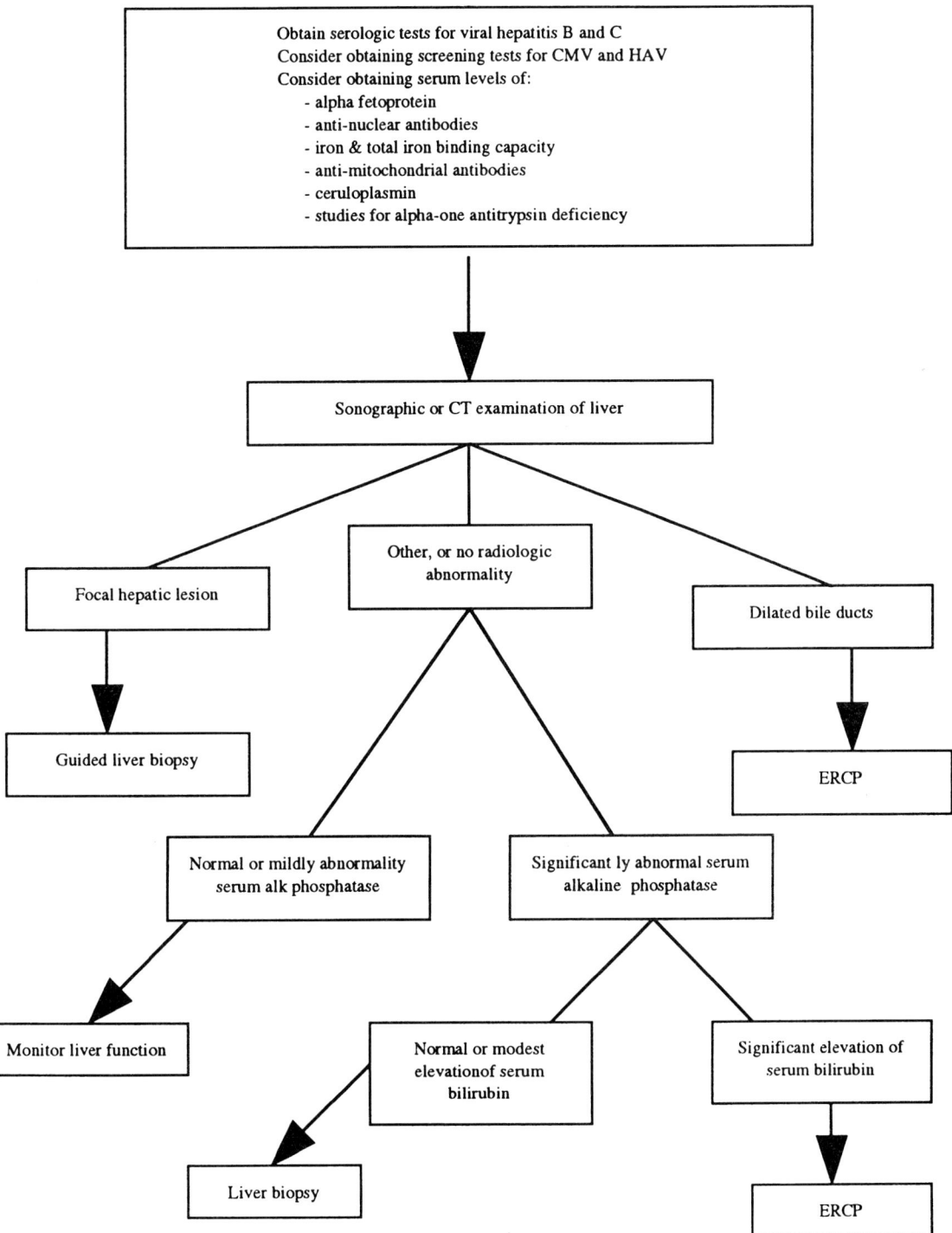

FIGURE 110–1. Algorithm for evaluation of hepatic dysfunction. *Arrow* indicates that one alternative is available in the algorithm; *lines* indicate that multiple choices are available. *CMV* = cytomegalovirus, *CT* = computerized tomographic scan, *ERCP* = endoscopic retrograde cholangiopancreatography, *HAV* = hepatitis A virus. (Adapted from Cappell MS, Hepatobiliary manifestations of the acquired immune syndrome. *Am J Gastroenterol.* 1991;86:1–15.)

velop is very low, probably in the range of 1% per year. This low rate is the basis for recommending observation as the approach to management of asymptomatic gallstones until symptoms or complications occur, which contrasts with the more aggressive, surgical approach that was advocated 25 years ago.[11]

THE LIVER AS TARGET

The liver may be viewed as the major target of a variety of disease processes, the most common of which are listed in Table 110–4. It may be argued that some of the disease processes listed are not "systemic," which is the focus of this chapter. Nevertheless, they must be considered at least to a sufficient degree to allow exclusion; diagnosis in liver disease is, of course, a process of both inclusion and exclusion of various possibilities.

HEPATITIS

The classic clinical manifestations of acute viral hepatitis consist of a prodrome of lassitude and nausea for several weeks, followed by the appearance of jaundice; it is the latter that often brings the patient to the attention of a physician. However, it is important to emphasize that viral hepatitis is one of the "iceberg" diseases with a high frequency of subclinical infection. Furthermore, symptomatic hepatitis may not represent acute disease at all but instead may represent a relapse of chronic hepatitis caused by viral infection (e.g., HBV, HCV), autoimmune hepatitis, drug-induced disease, or metabolic processes (e.g., Wilson's disease). Thus, the physician cannot be completely certain during the first encounter whether such a clinical presentation represents acute disease or a relapse of chronic active disease. A mathematic analogy can be imagined in considering acute and chronic disease. At least two points are necessary to define the slope of a line, and similarly, at least two clinical observations are required over a period of time to allow the clinician to distinguish between acute and chronic disease. Much anxiety is generated and resources are wasted when excessive numbers of tests are ordered on the basis of conclusions drawn from a single office visit. Further history, observation, and confirmation of simple tests often provide sufficient information to distinguish between acute and chronic disease processes.

An approach to the evaluation of abnormal liver function with emphasis on acute and chronic viral hepatitis is shown as an algorithm in Figure 110–2.[12]

ETHANOL ABUSE

The liver may be a spectator in patients with ethanol abuse, as listed in Table 110–2, but a broad spectrum of hepatic involvement clearly exists, and the liver may also serve as a major target of symptomatic disease. A comprehensive discussion of this topic is beyond the scope of this chapter but can be found in the references previously cited.[1,2]

TUMOR

The sensitivity and specificity of standard liver function tests for the detection of metastatic or primary tumors of the liver is poor; however, minor abnormalities (onefold to twofold elevations) of SALP and SAT can often be detected, and clinical evaluation should follow the approaches outlined in Figures 110–1 and 110–2. In addition to the routine tests of liver function, measurement of alpha-fetoprotein can be helpful in the diagnosis of hepatocellular carcinoma; approximately two thirds of patients are found to have abnormal elevations in the serum. In the absence of cirrhosis, synthetic vital functions of the liver are usually well preserved until late in the course of the illness.

A number of bedside clues may be helpful in the diagnosis of hepatic cancer. Auscultation may reveal a rub in the right upper quadrant in up to 10% of patients, and in a smaller number bruits resulting from the development of arteriovenous shunts or arterial impingement by tumor may be detected over the liver. A palpable gallbladder (Courvoisier's gallbladder) is a rare but very helpful physical finding in the diagnosis of pancreatic carcinoma with common duct obstruction. It is easily overlooked because of its superficial location and cystic character.

DRUG- AND TOXIN-INDUCED DISEASE

As with ethanol, a wide spectrum of liver disease may be induced by drugs and toxins. These issues are addressed above.

BILIARY TRACT DISEASE

Although the term *biliary tract disease* encompasses a vast number of disease processes, it is nevertheless useful as a bedside approach to differential diagnosis, since the therapeutic im-

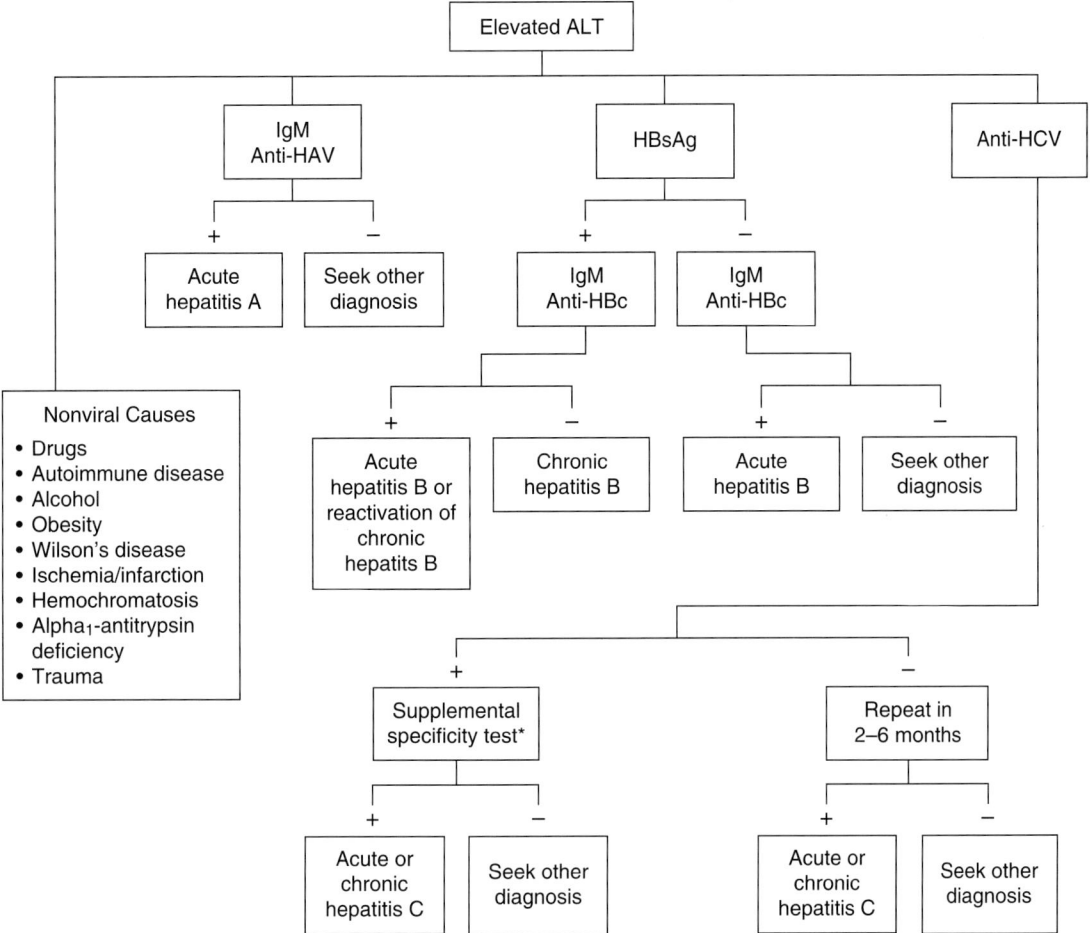

FIGURE 110–2. Algorithm for evaluation of alanine aminotransferase elevation with emphasis on viral hepatitis. *ALT* = alanine aminotransferase, *(−)* = nonreactive, *(+)* = reactive, *anti-HAV* = antibody to hepatitis A virus, *anti-HBc* = antibody to hepatitis B core antigen, *anti-HCV* = antibody to hepatitis C virus, *HBsAg* = hepatitis B surface antigen, *IgM* = immunoglobulin M. (Adapted from Advanced Therapeutic Communications, Secaucus, NJ, 1993.)

plications are vastly different from problems related to viral hepatitis, ethanol, tumor, or drugs.

Cholesterol gallstones account for the vast majority of gallstones and are considered to be of local origin rather than part of a systemic process. However, pigment gallstones and related biliary disease may result from chronic hemolytic conditions, such as sickle cell anemia, or may be associated with parasitic infestations, as seen with *Clonorchis sinensis*. Autoimmune diseases of the biliary tract can more easily be categorized as systemic processes in which hepatic dysfunction plays a prominent role.

Primary biliary cirrhosis (PBC) is a disease of unknown origin, but much evidence exists to suggest that autoimmunity plays a role in the pathogenesis. As a term, *nonsuppurative destructive cholangitis* is a more accurate pathologic description of the disease process and avoids confusion about the role of cirrhosis, since it is clear that cirrhosis does not appear until late in the course of the disease. Nevertheless, common usage has generally favored *PBC* as the term to describe this clinical entity. Evidence for autoimmunity in PBC is found in the form of autoantibodies, notably antimitochondrial antibodies, and associations with a variety of autoimmune diseases such as scleroderma, Sjögren's syndrome, rheumatoid arthritis, and hypothyroidism.

The clinical presentation of PBC commonly mimics that of chronic extrahepatic biliary obstruction with jaundice and pruritus and with a gender ratio greatly favoring women. Because of such similarities, PBC was not clearly identified as a distinct entity until the 1950s when radiographic imaging and liver biopsies allowed more accurate diagnosis. The reason for the clinical similarities becomes clear on review of microscopic sections of liver, which demonstrate a chronic inflammatory process affecting the small and intermediate intrahepatic bile ducts. Eventually, these pathologic changes result in obliteration of ducts, cirrhosis, and liver failure. Diagnosis is based on the clinical picture, an "obstructive" or cholestatic pattern of liver function test abnormalities, the presence of antimitochondrial antibodies, and a compatible liver biopsy. The clinical presentation may also require studies to demonstrate patency of the biliary system, since gallstone disease is relatively common in the middle-aged female group affected by PBC, and both disease processes may coexist.

An elevated SALP is often the earliest abnormality of liver function to be detected, and levels are frequently increased 5- to 10-fold. As noted in an earlier section, if the elevated SALP constitutes an isolated abnormality of liver function the diagnosis is far from secure, and additional testing is required. However, other changes in liver function are also usually present, with twofold to fivefold elevations of SAT and modest elevations of globulins and cholesterol. In the later stages of disease patients may demonstrate a rising serum bilirubin and prolongation of the prothrombin time.

Symptomatic relief of pruritus may be obtained with administration of cholestyramine early in the disease process. The mechanism involved is unclear, but the resin may bind bile acids or the metabolic products responsible for pruritus. A number of approaches to treatment of PBC have been studied, but none have been proven to be effective despite initial enthusiasm. For most patients, the possibility of liver transplantation must eventually be considered.

Primary sclerosing cholangitis (PSC) is another autoimmune process affecting the liver that can produce a chronic cholestatic disease and potential confusion with obstructive gallstone disease. Unlike PBC, PSC is more common among young men and attacks the larger ducts of the biliary tree. The pathologic process consists of an inflammatory fibrosis that frequently results in bile duct obliteration and biliary cirrhosis. As with PBC, satisfactory medical management is lacking, and patients with PSC often become candidates for liver transplantation.

Liver function abnormalities in PSC characteristically consist of minor elevations of SAT and bilirubin and moderate, severalfold elevations of SALP. The striking levels of SALP typically found in PBC are usually not present in PSC. However, as with PBC, hypergammaglobulinemia and a variety of autoantibodies may be found. Recent studies have identified an antineutrophil nuclear antibody that is present in most patients with PSC and may become useful in diagnosis.

The greatest aid to diagnosis of PSC is the knowledge that approximately 70% of patients with PSC have coexisting ulcerative colitis. The basis for this relationship is far from clear, but proposed explanations include portal bacteremia or various immunologic mechanisms. Liver biopsy is of little help in diagnosis, but endoscopic cholangiography usually demonstrates characteristic ductal changes.

CONCLUSION

The evaluation of patients with abnormalities of liver function remains difficult, but our improved understanding of hepatic dysfunction allows earlier and more precise diagnosis. An important part of this advance has resulted from the recognition that it is often possible to distinguish between clinical settings in which the liver is an important target of the disease process and those in which it takes the role of a spectator to the main event.

REFERENCES

1. Schiff L, Schiff ER, eds. *Diseases of the Liver.* 7th ed. Philadelphia, Pa: JB Lippincott Co; 1993.
2. Zakim D, Boyer TD, eds. *Hepatology: A Textbook of Liver Disease.* 2nd ed. Philadelphia, Pa: WB Saunders Co; 1990.
3. Kantrowitz PA, Jones WA, Greenberger NJ, et al. Severe postoperative hyperbilirubinemia simulating obstructive jaundice. *N Engl J Med.* 1967;276:590–598.
4. Sikuler E, Guetta V, Keynan A, et al. Abnormalities in bilirubin and liver enzyme levels in adult patients with bacteremia. *Arch Intern Med.* 1989;149:2246–2248.
5. Quigley EMM, Marsh MN, Shaffer JL, et al. Hepatobiliary complications of total parenteral nutrition. *Gastroenterology.* 1993;104:286–301.

6. Crawford JM, Gollan JL. Bilirubin metabolism and the pathophysiology of jaundice. In: Schiff L, Schiff ER, eds. *Diseases of the Liver.* 7th ed. Philadelphia, Pa: JB Lippincott Co; 1993:42–84.
7. Reddy KR, Schiff ER. Hepatobiliary manifestations of AIDS. In: Rustgi VK, Van Thiel DH, eds. *The Liver in Systemic Disease.* New York, NY: Raven Press Publishers; 1993:321–336.
8. Cappell MS. Hepatobiliary manifestations of the acquired immune syndrome (clinical review). *Am J Gastroenterol.* 1991;86:1–15.
9. Palmer M, Schaffner F. Effect of weight reduction on hepatic abnormalities in overweight patients. *Gastroenterology.* 1990;99:1408–1413.
10. Hay EI, Czaja AJ, Rakela J, et al. The nature of unexplained chronic aminotransferase elevations of a mild to moderate degree in asymptomatic patients. *Hepatology.* 1989;9:193–197.
11. Sama C, Labate AMM, Taroni F, et al. Epidemiology and natural history of gallstone disease. *Semin Liv Dis.* 1990;10:149–158.
12. Advanced Therapeutics Communications, Secaucus, NJ, 1993.

111

Alpha$_1$-Antitrypsin Deficiency

DAVID H. PERLMUTTER

Homozygous PiZZ alpha$_1$-antitrypsin (a_1AT) deficiency affects approximately 1 of every 1600 to 2000 live births in North America[1] and constitutes the most common genetic disorder to cause liver injury in infants and children.[2] a_1AT deficiency is also a common cause of chronic hepatitis, cirrhosis, and hepatocellular carcinoma in adults. Because it is an inhibitor of the destructive protease neutrophil elastase, a_1AT is thought to play an important role in connective tissue turnover, especially that of the elastin-rich tissues of the lung. Inherited deficiencies of a_1AT result in premature development of emphysema, and acquired a_1AT deficiency syndromes may be associated with destructive lung disorders, often referred to as adult respiratory distress syndrome.

Because the clinical manifestations of liver disease associated with a_1AT deficiency are similar to those of many other causes of chronic liver injury, it is difficult to make the diagnosis of this disorder on a purely clinical basis. Nevertheless, the diagnosis can be relatively easily made by subjecting small quantities of serum to isoelectric focusing or lymphocytes to polymerase chain reaction–based diagnostic techniques.

Three key observations have led to greater understanding of the pathogenesis of liver disease associated with a_1AT deficiency. First, a single amino acid substitution is responsible for the synthesis of an abnormal protein that is unable to transverse the secretory pathway and accumulates within the endoplasmic reticulum (ER) of liver cells.[2] Second, experiments in transgenic mice have confirmed previous suspicions that the liver injury results from the hepatotoxic effects of intracellular accumulation of the abnormal a_1AT molecule.[3] This means that the liver disease of a_1AT deficiency is unlikely to respond to protein or gene replacement therapy. Third, follow-up studies of nationwide prospective newborn screening in Sweden have clearly demonstrated that only a subpopulation of individuals with a_1AT deficiency develop significant liver injury.[1,4] This leads to the prediction that unlinked genetic traits or environmental factors predispose, or protect, individuals with a_1AT deficiency from liver injury. In this chapter I review our current knowledge of the clinical manifestations, diagnosis, and pathophysiology of this deficiency and associated liver disease and argue that an understanding of predisposing genetic traits or environmental factors represents our best hope for developing rational, specific long-term therapy.

CLINICAL MANIFESTATIONS

Liver involvement is usually first noticed at 1 to 2 months of age because of persistent jaundice (Table 111–1). Serum transaminases are mild-to-moderately elevated. The liver may be enlarged. Such infants are often first admitted to the hospital with a diagnosis of "neonatal hepatitis syndrome." Many of these infants have minimal clinical liver disease but persistent serum transaminase abnormalities for the first few years of life. Approximately 10% of the population have moderate-to-severe clinical liver disease with complications of liver synthetic dysfunction (bleeding diathesis, ascites, feeding difficulties, poor growth) during the first few years of life. A few infants are recognized initially because of a cholestatic clinical syndrome characterized by pruritus, hypercholesterolemia, and paucity of intrahepatic bile ducts on histopathologic examination.

Liver disease associated with a_1AT deficiency may also be first discovered in late childhood or early adolescence when the affected individual is seen with abdominal distension from hepatosplenomegaly or ascites or has upper intestinal bleeding caused by esophageal variceal hemorrhage (Table 111–1). In some of these cases there is a history of unexplained prolonged obstructive jaundice in the neonatal period. In others there is no evidence of any previous liver injury, even when the neonatal history is carefully reviewed. Although many of these children have progressive hepatic decompensation necessitating liver transplantation, a few lead relatively uncomplicated lives for several years despite moderate-to-severe liver synthetic dysfunction.

Several studies have attempted to define clinical signs of poor prognostic significance in children with liver disease related to a_1AT deficiency.[2] These studies suggested that persistence of hyperbilirubinemia, hard hepatomegaly, early development of splenomegaly, and progressive prolongation of the prothrombin time were indicators of poor prognosis. It was argued that these signs could be used to determine the appropriate time for recommending liver transplantation. However, these are the same type of clinical abnormalities on which we ordinarily rely in assessing the need for liver transplantation in any of the childhood liver disorders. Moreover, in my experience, there are children with a_1AT deficiency who have survived years after developing hepatosplenomegaly and prolongation of the prothrombin time.

a_1AT deficiency should be considered in the differential diagnosis of any adult who presents with chronic hepatitis, cirrhosis, portal hypertensin, or hepatocellular carcinoma of unknown origin. In fact, on a purely clinical basis it may be impossible to distinguish adult patients with autoimmune hepatitis, drug-induced hepatitis, chronic viral hepatitis, and Wilson's disease from those with a_1AT deficiency.

There is very little information about the incidence of liver enzyme abnormalities or liver histologic abnormalities in individuals with a_1AT deficiency and emphysema. Autopsy studies have indicated the presence of cirrhosis or hepatocellular carcinoma in adults who were only known to have emphysema.[5] Further studies of the prevalence of clinical and subclinical liver injury in individuals with a_1AT deficiency and emphysema are needed.

DIAGNOSIS

Diagnosis is established by a serum a_1AT phenotype determination in isoelectric focusing or agarose gel electrophoresis at acid pH (Fig. 111–1). The phenotype should be determined in all cases of neonatal hepatitis or unexplained chronic liver disease in older children, adolescents, and adults. Serum concentrations of a_1AT may be helpful, when used together with the phenotype, to distinguish individuals who are homozygous for the Z allele from SZ compound heterozygotes, both of which may develop liver disease. In some cases, phenotype determinations on parents or other relatives are also necessary to be certain about the distinction between ZZ and SZ allotypes, a distinction which is important for genetic counseling. Serum concentrations of a_1AT are occasionally misleading.

TABLE 111–1. CLINICAL MANIFESTATIONS OF LIVER DISEASE ASSOCIATED WITH α-1-ANTITRYPSIN DEFICIENCY

Infancy	Prolonged obstructive jaundice; mild elevation transaminases; occasionally symptoms of cholestasis
Early childhood	? Mild elevation transaminases; severe liver dysfunction (10%–15%)
Late childhood and adolescence	Portal hypertension; severe liver dysfunction
Adulthood	Chronic active hepatitis; cryptogenic cirrhosis; portal hypertension; hepatocellular carcinoma

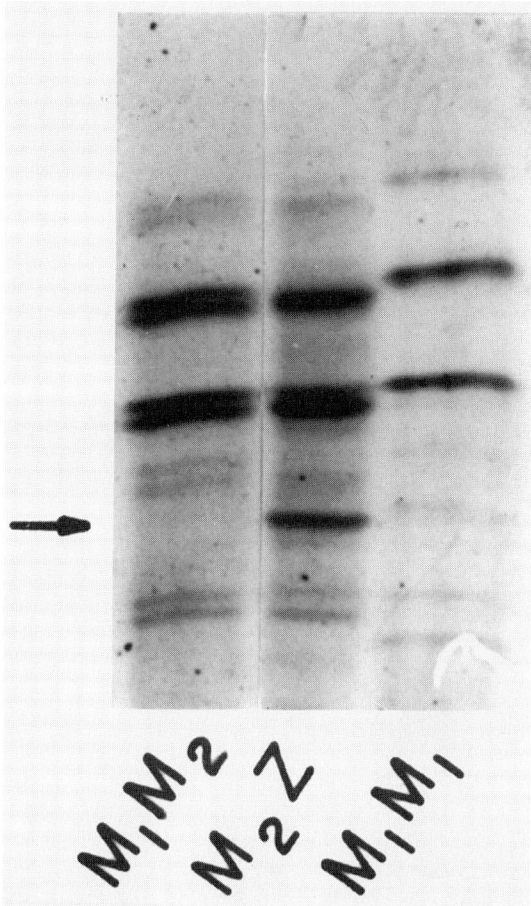

FIGURE 111–1. Isoelectric focusing of human serum samples for diagnosis of α_1AT deficiency. Sera from a normal M_1M_2 individual, an M_2Z heterozygote, and a normal M_1M_1 individual were subjected to isoelectric focusing with the anode at top and cathode at bottom. Migration of the Z allele is indicated by the *arrow*. (Gel courtesy JA Pierce, St. Louis, Mo.)

Siiyama, hepatocyte inclusions without any evidence of parenchymal injury were reported.[9]

It is now also possible to detect specific α_1AT variants by amplification of genomic DNA using the polymerase chain reaction.[10] This is a rapid and sensitive technique and requires only a small amount of cellular material. It should prove useful for confirmation of diagnoses, population screening, prenatal diagnosis, and research studies. Determination of α_1AT serum concentration and phenotype is still necessary for diagnosis in most clinical situations.

The distinctive histologic feature of homozygous PiZZ α_1AT deficiency is periodic acid-Schiff–positive, diastase-resistant globules in the ER of hepatocytes (Fig. 111–2; see also Color Plate IV). According to some observers, these globules are not as easy to detect in the first few months of life as at later ages. The presence of these inclusions should not be interpreted as diagnostic of α_1AT deficiency. Similar structures are occasionally observed in PiMM individuals with other liver diseases.[11] The inclusions are eosinophilic, round to oval, and 1 to 40 µm in diameter. They are most prominent in periportal hepatocytes,[12] but may also be seen in Kupffer's cells and cells with the appearance of bile duct epithelial origin.[13] There may be evidence of variable degrees of hepatocellular necrosis, inflammatory cell infiltration, periportal fibrosis, or cirrhosis. There is often evidence of bile duct epithelial cell destruction and, occasionally, as mentioned above, there is paucity of intrahepatic bile ducts. In several cases, extrahepatic biliary atresia has been reported in Pi ZZ individuals.[14]

PATHOPHYSIOLOGY OF α_1AT DEFICIENCY IN PiZZ INDIVIDUALS

It is now well established from pulse-chase experiments in several cell culture systems, in vitro microsomal translocation assays, and morphologic studies that there is a selective defect in secretion of the PiZ α_1AT gene product and that this protein accumulates in the ER.[2] Only 15% of the newly synthesized α_1AT molecules are able to transverse the secretory pathway to reach the extracellular medium and ultimately the body fluids. The defect is not specific for liver cells; it also affects extrahepatic sites of α_1AT synthesis such as macrophages. It has recently been recognized that the substitution of Glu 342 by Lys 342, the substitution that characterizes PiZ α_1AT, is sufficient to produce this cellular defect.[15–16] Site-directed mutagenesis experiments

For instance, serum α_1AT concentrations may increase during the host response to inflammation, even in homozygous PiZZ individuals, giving a falsely reassuring impression.

It is still not entirely clear whether heterozygous MZ individuals are predisposed to liver injury. Studies that examined the prevalence of the MZ phenotype in adults who had undergone liver biopsy[6] suggest that there is a relationship between heterozygosity and the development of liver disease. Liver dysfunction has also been identified in several individuals with the M Malton and M Duarte allotypes,[7,8] but there are still not enough individuals with these allotypes to determine whether they really predispose to liver injury. In one individual with deficiency allotype

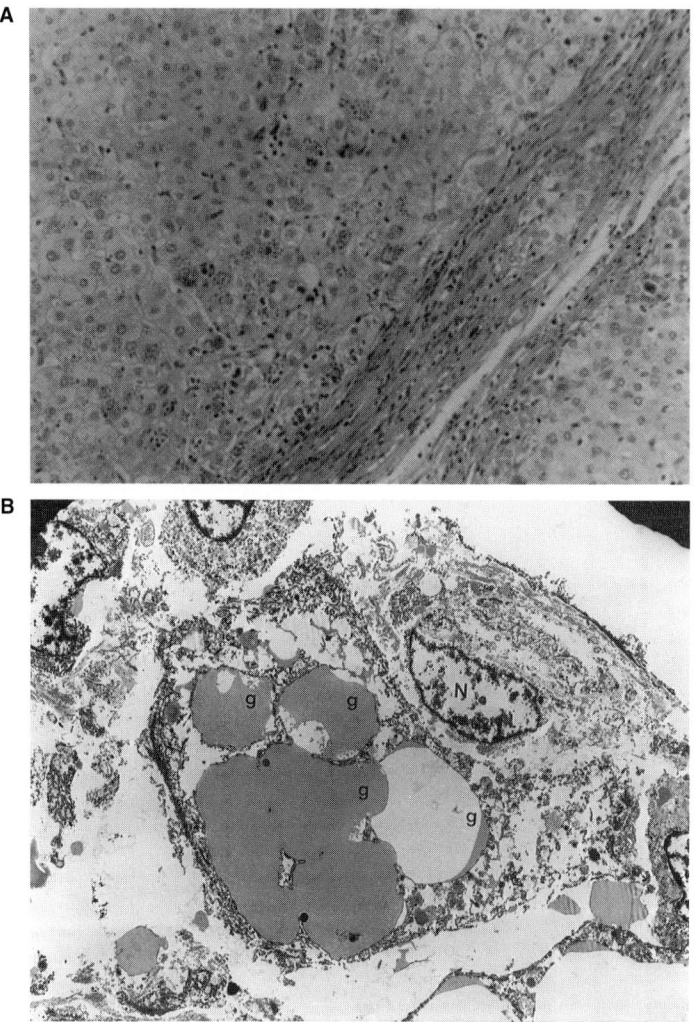

FIGURE 111–2. Liver histology in homozygous PiZZ α_1AT deficiency. **A,** Photomicrograph of a liver biopsy in α_1AT deficiency (periodic acid-Schiff [PAS], diastase stain; magnification ×40) demonstrating PAS-positive, diastase-resistant globules in hepatocytes, especially periportal and adjacent to a broad band of fibrous tissue. (**A** also Color Plate II.) **B,** Electron photomicrograph of the same biopsy demonstrating globules in the endoplasmic reticulum. N = nucleus, g = globules. (Courtesy Dr. C. Coffin, St. Louis, Mo; reproduced with permission from Perlmutter DH. Alpha-1 AT deficiency. In: Suchy FJ, ed. *Liver Disease in Children*. St. Louis, Mo: Mosby–Year Book; 1994:697.)

show that it is the change in charge of this amino acid residue, rather than disruption of a potential salt bridge, that leads to intracellular retention. This molecular abnormality presumably results in a change in the conformation or folding of the nascent α_1AT polypeptide after translocation into the lumen of the ER.

Several recent studies have raised the possibility that the substitution of Glu 342 by Lys 342 reduces the stability of α_1AT in the monomeric form and increases the likelihood that α_1AT polymers are generated.[17,18] This concept was first suggested by studies of the structure of α_1AT and other serpins. These studies show that the native α_1AT molecule is extremely labile. Its reactive center is probably projected onto the external surface of the molecule as an alpha-helical loop, leaving a gap in the conserved A-sheet of 5 beta-helixes (Fig. 111–3 in Color Plate IV). On interaction with an adjacent cognate enzyme, such as neutrophil elastase, or a cleaving enzyme, such as collagenase, there is a dramatic structural rearrangement, often associated with hydrolysis of a reactive site bond and insertion of the reactive site loop into the gap. This interaction results in an extremely stable "complex" or "cleaved" form of α_1AT. In a recent study by Mast et al,[17] it has been shown that during cleavage polymers of α_1AT may be formed by insertion of reactive site loops of some α_1AT molecules into the gap in the A-sheet of other α_1AT molecules. Lomas et al[18] then showed that Z α_1AT may undergo this polymerization to a certain extent spontaneously and to a greater extent during relatively minor perturbations, such as raising the temperature to 37°C. Lomas et al[18] then showed by electron microscopic examination the presence of such polymers in the hepatocytic ER inclusions of α_1AT. This is a potentially important observation. If correct, it would imply that synthetic peptides that could be pharmacologically targeted to the ER of hepatocytes and that could insert into the gap in the A-sheet of the mutant (Z) α_1AT molecule could prevent polymerization and concomitant intracellular accumulation of hepatotoxic mutant protein. However, it must first be shown that polymers of Z α_1AT accumulate to a greater extent or are more toxic to hepatocytes than is monomeric Z α_1AT.

There are several possible ways by which polymerization or alteration of the conformation of monomeric α_1AT might affect secretion. An alteration in folding might preclude the interaction of α_1AT with another protein that ordinarily facilitates its secretion, such as a transport receptor or a key glycosylating enzyme. Despite relatively extensive investigation, however, there is no evidence for a receptor that binds α_1AT in the secretory pathway.[19] Furthermore, fundamental cell biologic experiments have provided evidence that transport of secretory proteins from the ER is controlled by relatively nonspecific factors,[20] whereas retention of secretory proteins within the ER is controlled by specific protein-protein interactions such as ligand-receptor interactions.[21] Thus, it is possible that an alteration in folding of α_1AT, as occurs in the mutant (Z) α_1AT, permits an otherwise sequestered domain to be recognized by another protein in the ER and that the consequent protein-protein interaction is responsible for specific intracellular retention of α_1AT. In fact, several observations suggest that misfolded proteins are selectively retained within the ER by interaction with members of the heat shock–stress protein family. First, two members of the stress protein family, glucose-regulated proteins GRP 78 and GRP 94, are known to be localized to the ER.[22] Second, one of these stress proteins (GRP 78) binds loosely and transiently to secretory proteins until the assembly or folding of these proteins is complete. Once a "translocation-component" conformation is achieved, secretory proteins dissociate from GRP 78 in a reaction dependent on adenosine triphosphate (ATP), calcium, and magnesium to allow for subsequent transport.[21] If a translocation-component conformation is not achieved, as might occur with a genetically altered protein, the secretory protein does not dissociate from GRP 78 and remains within the ER until it is degraded.[21] Third, it has been shown that synthesis of stress proteins (the so-called stress response) is activated by the presence of misfolded or denatured proteins in the cell.[23] Thus, binding of stress proteins to misfolded proteins or decreases in the free pool of heat shock–stress protein mediate feedback induction of new stress protein synthesis, ensuring an excess of these proteins for chaperoning functions, especially during times of cellular stress.

PATHOPHYSIOLOGY OF LIVER INJURY IN INDIVIDUALS WITH PiZZ α_1AT DEFICIENCY

Several theoretic explanations for the pathogenesis of liver injury in individuals with α_1AT deficiency have been discussed in the literature. In one theory, liver damage is thought to be a consequence of diminished serum concentrations of α_1AT, rendering the liver susceptible to proteolytic attack. There has been no experimental or applied clinical evidence to support this theory. In a second theory, liver damage is thought to result from an abnormal immune response to liver antigens.[24] This theory is based on the observation that peripheral blood lymphocytes from PiZZ infants are cytotoxic for isolated hepatocytes. However, this is probably a nonspecific effect of liver injury in that peripheral blood lymphocytes from PiMM infants with a similar degree of neonatal hepatitis syndrome are also cytotoxic for isolated hepatocytes.[24] More recent evidence has indicated an increase in the HLA-DR3-Dw25 haplotype in α_1AT deficient individuals with liver disease.[24] However, there is no difference in the expression of class II major histocompatibility complex (MHC) antigens in the livers of these individuals compared to those of normal controls.[25] Moreover, an increase in the prevalence of a particular HLA-DR haplotype in the affected population does not by itself imply altered immune function. In fact, because of the linkage disequilibrium displayed by genes within the MHC, it is possible that increased susceptibility is caused by the products of unrelated but linked genes. For instance, the MHC contains genes for several heat shock–stress proteins,[26] proteins that play an important role in intracellular translocations. The MHC also encodes genes for proteolytic processing of peptides in the cytoplasm and for translocation of peptides from cytoplasm to the ER.[27]

In the third, more widely accepted, theory, accumulation of α_1AT in the ER of liver cells is thought to be directly related to liver injury.[28] Experiments in transgenic mice carrying the mutant (Z) allele of the human α_1AT gene[5,6] have provided direct experimental support for this "accumulation theory." These mice have periodic acid–Schiff–positive, diastase-resistant intrahepatocytic globules and exhibit neonatal hepatitis and growth failure. Because there are normal levels of α_1AT and presumably other antielastases in these animals, as directed by the endogenous murine genes, liver injury cannot be attributed to diminished serum or tissue levels of α_1AT. It is, therefore, likely that liver injury is related to the intracellular accumulation of the abnormal human α_1AT gene product. It should be noted, however, that high levels of expression of α_1AT in transgenic mouse lineages that carry the normal (M) α_1AT allele were also associated with histologic liver disease. Furthermore, murine hepatitis virus infections that have been noted in transgenic mouse facilities could complicate the analysis. Finally, severe impairment of growth is not necessarily characteristic of neonatal hepatitis in α_1AT deficiency. In fact, many infants with this deficiency do not have evidence of liver injury, as noted above. Thus, some caution must be exercised in drawing conclusions about human disease from results of studies in this animal model.

Any theory for the pathogenesis of liver injury in α_1AT deficiency must take into consideration the fact that only a subpopulation of these individuals develop significant liver injury. This was shown by Sveger,[1] who prospectively screened 200,000 newborn infants in Sweden. One hundred twenty-seven PiZZ infants were identified and have been followed clinically since that time. Fourteen of the 127 PiZZ infants had prolonged obstructive jaundice. Nine of these infants had severe liver disease, and five had mild liver disease by clinical and laboratory criteria. Eight other PiZZ infants had minimal abnormalities in serum bilirubin, serum transaminases, and liver size. Approximately 50% of the remaining infants had abnormal serum transaminases. Sveger[4] has collected data regarding the clinical outcome for these infants at 12 years of age. More than 75% of the 127 prospectively identified PiZZ children have normal serum transaminases and no evidence of liver injury at this age. One issue not addressed by the Sveger study is whether these 12-year-old children with α_1AT deficiency had persistent subclinical histologic abnormalities despite lack of evidence of liver injury by clinical and biochemical criteria and that liver disease tends to become clinically evident during adolescence or adulthood.

With these considerations in mind, we have proposed a conceptual model for the cellular basis of liver injury in α_1AT deficiency (Fig. 111–4).[2] In normal PiMM individuals *(left panel)* with or without liver disease, α_1AT is translocated into the lumen of the ER. It may transiently associate with polypeptide chain–binding proteins, most of which are members of the heat shock/stress protein family, until it has folded into its translocation-component, native conformation, allowing it to transverse the remainder of the secretory pathway. A few newly synthesized α_1AT molecules may ordinarily undergo degradation in the ER. In PiZZ individuals with α_1AT deficiency *(right panel)*, α_1AT is translocated into the lumen of the ER. It also associates with polypeptide chain-binding proteins, but because of its single amino acid substitution, the mutant α_1AT is much less efficient at folding into the translocation-component shape so that only 15% of the newly synthesized molecules dissociate and exit through the secretory pathway. Most newly synthesized α_1AT molecules remain bound and ultimately undergo degradation in the ER or ER salvage compartment. This model also provides a reasonable explanation for the development of significant liver injury in a subpopulation of PiZZ individuals with α_1AT deficiency. Genetic or environmental factors that increase the net balance of abnormally folded α_1AT in the ER would predispose the PiZZ individual to liver disease. These other factors could affect the rate of synthesis of α_1AT *(right panel, 1)*, interaction of α_1AT with polypeptide chain-binding proteins in the ER *(right panel, 2)*, rate of degradation in the ER *(right panel, 3)*, or rate of secretion for the 15% of newly synthesized α_1AT molecules that reach this step *(right panel, 4)*. For instance, a genetic trait that decreases the efficiency of the putative ER degradative system *(right panel, 3)*, would lead to higher steady-state levels of misfolded α_1AT in the ER, a sustained increase in synthesis of stress protein and the cellular pathophysi-

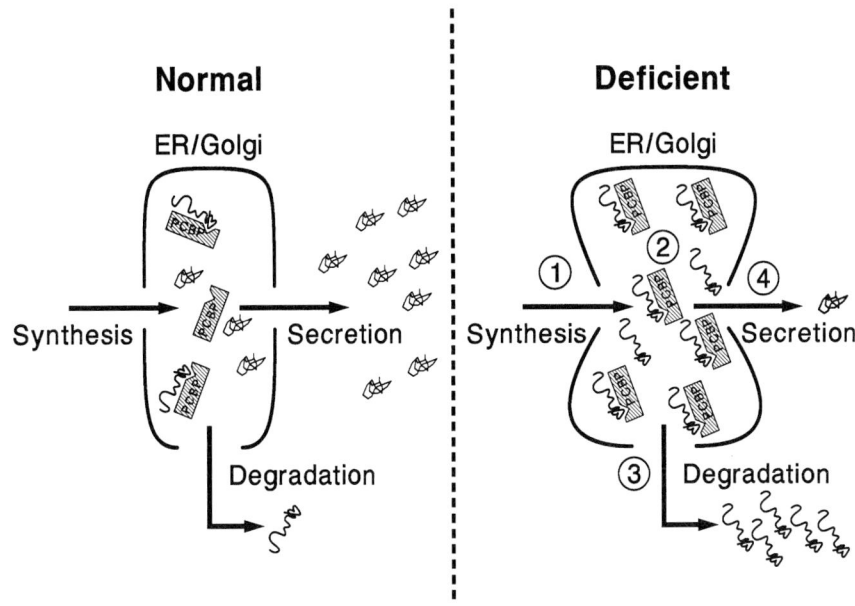

FIGURE 111–4. Conceptual model for liver injury in α_1AT deficiency. See text for description. (From Perlmutter DH. The cellular basis for liver injury in alpha-1-antitrypsin deficiency. *Hepatology.* 1991;13:172–185.)

ologic concomitants of this phenomena. Such a genetic trait would be silent in the general population, which is not exposed to a chronic burden of mutant misfolded secretory protein. In another example, PiZZ individuals exposed to higher or more sustained concentrations of environmental factors that enhance synthesis of α_1AT *(right panel, 1)* would be expected to have higher steady-state levels of abnormally folded α_1AT molecules in the ER if the putative ER degradative system(s) is already operating at maximal efficiency.

This conceptual model is substantiated to a certain extent by our study of heat shock/stress proteins in α_1AT–synthesizing cells of PiZZ individuals.[29] We examined synthesis of several members of this stress protein family in monocytes from normal PiMM and deficient PiZZ individuals. Net synthesis of proteins in the heat shock/stress gene family was increased only in the subset of PiZZ individuals with liver disease. It was not significantly increased in PiZZ individuals with emphysema or in those without apparent tissue injury. There was also an increase in steady-state levels of RNA for several of the heat shock/stress genes in liver from PiZZ individuals compared to PiMM individuals. This "uninduced" or "constitutive" stress response could not be attributed to a nonspecific effect of tissue injury or inflammation: net synthesis of stress proteins was not increased in PiMM individuals with severe liver disease. Net synthesis of stress proteins was not increased in individuals with another variant of the α_1AT gene (PiS α_1AT). Finally, the increase in synthesis of stress proteins in the absence of thermal or chemical stress was confined to α_1AT–synthesizing cells of the affected patients and was exaggerated by regulatory factors that caused greater intracellular accumulation of α_1AT in these patients. It is still possible that the induction of stress proteins in these individuals is only a marker for liver disease. In either case, these data taken together provide evidence for the involvement of a class of polypeptide chain-binding proteins, particularly members of the heat shock/stress gene family, in intracellular accumulation of the mutant (Z) α_1AT molecule and for an exaggeration of the accumulation in a subpopulation of PiZZ individuals with α_1AT deficiency who exhibit liver disease.

The development of liver injury probably involves a sequence of events; only the initial steps are considered in detail by our conceptual model. There is still relatively little information on which to base hypotheses for the subsequent events that lead to liver injury after accumulation of the misfolded α_1AT protein within the secretory pathway. In one report, accumulation of mutant (Z) α_1AT in *Xenopus* oocytes was associated with release of lysosomal enzymes.[30] It is likely that other intracellular metabolic systems are affected by accumulation of abnormal α_1AT molecules, or the cellular response to accumulation, and may contribute to liver cell damage.

This conceptual model predicts several targets for potential pharmacologic intervention. For instance, if the alteration in conformation or polymerization of the mutant (Z) α_1AT protein could be prevented, interaction with polypeptide chain-binding proteins would be transient and the α_1AT molecules released by bulk flow. One relatively reasonable approach is treatment with synthetic peptides, which insert into the gap in the A-sheet and prevent polymerization of the mutant (Z) α_1AT protein. Although it is not yet entirely clear, there is some evidence from studies on the assembly of MHC class I molecules that synthetic peptides may be delivered to the endoplasmic reticulum from the extracellular medium of cultured cells.[31] There is also evidence that certain molecules may be transported retrograde to the endoplasmic reticulum by receptor-mediated endocytosis.[32]

The conceptual model also predicts that a pharmacologic intervention that blocks the upregulating effect of specific environmental factors on synthesis of α_1AT will tend to lower the steady-state level of abnormally folded α_1AT molecules in the ER. This may be enough to protect liver cells from hepatotoxic consequences. With this consideration in mind, we have identified several specific mechanisms by which synthesis of α_1AT is upregulated, including a mechanism mediated by interleukin-6 (IL-6) and a mechanism mediated by endotoxin.[33] We have also shown that synthesis of α_1AT is upregulated by the enzyme it inhibits, neutrophil elastase.[33] Because we believed that this was a dominant mechanism for regulation of α_1AT and a mechanism that could be a target for pharmacologic treatment, we have studied it in great detail. These studies have shown that the effect requires formation of a complex of elastase with endogenous α_1AT or requires an exogenous, preformed α_1AT–elastase complex. Second, the effect can be elicited by synthetic peptides corresponding to a domain of the α_1AT molecule that is only exposed after the structural rearrangement that accompanies complex formation. These synthetic peptides bind specifically and saturably to a single class of receptors on the cell surface of monocytes and hepatoma cells HepG2 (K_d ~40 nmol/L; 4.5×10^5 plasma membrane receptors per cell). We now refer to this class of receptor molecules as serpin-enzyme complex (SEC) receptors because they recognize the same highly conserved domain of other serpin-enzyme complexes AT III–thrombin, α_1 ACT-cathepsin G, and to a lesser extent C1 inhibitor-C1s complexes, as well as that of α_1AT–elastase complexes. In fact, it now appears that a pentapeptide domain in the carboxyl terminal fragment of α_1AT (amino acids 370–374, FVFLM) is sufficient for binding to the SEC receptor.[33] Photoaffinity cross-linking studies and purification by ligand affinity chromatography indicate that the SEC receptor, or at least its ligand-binding subunit, is approximately 76 kDa.[33] The SEC receptor is probably involved in in vivo clearance or catabolism of α_1AT–elastase complexes because it mediates endocytosis and lysosomal degradation of these complexes in tissue culture[33] and because its ligand specificity is similar to that for in vivo clearance of serpin-enzyme complexes in mice.[34] The SEC receptor also mediates the previously described neutrophil chemoattractant properties of α_1AT–elastase complexes,[35] and this biologic activity can be abrogated by desensitization of the SEC receptor.[33] Thus, receptor-mediated recognition of α_1AT–elastase complexes leads to intracellular catabolism of the complex, activation of a signal transduction pathway for upregulation of α_1AT gene expression, and directed migration of neutrophils. When synthesis of α_1AT is upregulated by this mechanism in cells from individuals with homozygous PiZZ α_1AT deficiency, there is a marked increase in the intracellular accumulation of α_1AT[33] and, therein, a proclivity toward hepatotoxicity. Mapping of the receptor-binding domain on α_1AT, purification and characterization of the receptor and its ligand-binding domain, and definition of the mechanism for desensitization of the SEC receptor will allow us to block this receptor as a potential therapeutic intervention in individuals with α_1AT deficiency who are at risk for liver injury.

In contrast to liver injury in which accumulation of the abnormal α_1AT molecule is involved, destructive lung disease in α_1AT deficiency almost certainly results from the deficiency of antielastase activity in the lung. This has led to the elastase-antielastase model for emphysema: any perturbation in the balance of protease and antiprotease, specifically in the balance of neutrophil elastase and α_1AT, in favor of proteolytic activity results in lung injury.[36] According to this theory, an individual is predisposed to lung injury by a decrease in numbers of α_1AT molecules, as might occur in genetic deficiencies of α_1AT, or by a decrease in the function of each α_1AT molecule, as might occur by oxidative inactivation of α_1AT during cigarette smoking.

The incidence and prevalence of emphysema in α_1AT deficiency has not been studied prospectively. Autopsy studies suggest that 60% to 65% of individuals with homozygous PiZZ α_1AT deficiency develop clinically significant lung injury.[36] There are, however, PiZZ individuals who smoke cigarettes but do not have any symptoms of lung disease or evidence of pulmonary function abnormalities or do not develop them until the seventh or eighth decade of life.[36]

TREATMENT

The most important treatment for α_1AT deficiency is avoidance of cigarette smoking. Cigarette smoking markedly accelerates the destructive lung disease associated with α_1AT deficiency, reduces the quality of life, and significantly shortens the longevity of these individuals.[36]

Liver disease associated with α_1AT deficiency has been treated by orthotopic liver transplantation (OLT). In a study of 250 infants and children who underwent OLT and received cyclosporine or prednisone treatment in Pittsburgh from 1980 to 1986, 29 children had α_1AT deficiency. Five of the 29 died during the follow-up period.[37] This represents 75% to 80% survival, slightly higher than the overall 69.2% 5-year survival in children who have undergone OLT. Five of the surviving patients were affected by chronic complications of transplantation at the time of the report. These results did not appear to be affected by the severity of liver disease at the time of OLT because 80% had ascites and 59% had experienced variceal hemorrhage. More recently compilations of survival rates report approximately 80% at 1 year and 70% at 5 years after OLT.[37] Nevertheless, it should be noted that even individuals with α_1AT deficiency and moderate-to-severe liver dysfunction may have relatively low rates of disease progression. A selective group of these patients may, therefore, not require OLT as urgently as do patients with other forms of liver disease. Individuals with α_1AT deficiency and mild liver dysfunction do not necessarily have poor prognoses, as demonstrated by Sveger,[1,4] and, therefore, should not be considered for OLT until there is evidence for progressive deterioration. Because it is not known whether extrahepatic α_1AT synthesis is an important factor in the development of emphysema or whether α_1AT synthesis by Kupffer's cells that repopulate the donor liver is an important factor in the development of liver disease, it is not known whether individuals with α_1AT deficiency who have undergone OLT are susceptible to emphysema or recurrent liver disease.

Most individuals with α_1AT deficiency and liver disease are not candidates for alternative surgical interventions. However, there are rare specific clinical situations in which a portacaval or splenorenal shunt might be considered (e.g., an individual with only mild liver synthetic dysfunction and mild parenchymal liver injury but severe portal hypertension). Several children with severe liver disease and α_1AT deficiency have survived 10 to 15 years after shunt surgery before requiring OLT. Moreover, previous hepatobiliary surgery is not a statistically significant risk factor for poor outcome of subsequent OLT.[37]

There have been trials of pharmacologic therapy for α_1AT deficiency. Patients have been given synthetic androgens danazol or stanozolol because of the dramatic effects of the same agents in individuals with hereditary angioedema (a deficiency of the homologous serine proteinase inhibitor C1 inhibitor) and because danazol was initially found to increase serum levels of α_1AT in PiZZ individuals.[38] However, further evaluation has demonstrated that danazol increases serum levels of α_1AT in only 50% of individuals with α_1AT deficiency, and the magnitude of the effect is small.[39] If the effect of the pharmacologic agent is at the level of synthesis of α_1AT, this type of therapy has the theoretic drawback of causing greater intracellular accumulation of the mutant α_1AT and thereby the potential pathophysiologic consequences of intracellular retention of misfolded protein (see above).

Patients with α_1AT deficiency and emphysema have undergone replacement therapy with purified plasma α_1AT. Twenty-one PiZZ and Pi null individuals were treated for 5 months with weekly infusions of purified α_1AT.[39] There was improvement in serum concentrations of α_1AT and concentrations of α_1AT and neutrophil elastase inhibitory capacity in bronchoalveolar lavage fluid. No significant side effects were seen during these trials. Although this study demonstrates only biochemical efficacy, purified plasma α_1AT has been licensed for use in individuals with α_1AT deficiency and established emphysema because it is thought that data regarding clinical efficacy are virtually impossible to collect. Recent data suggest that it may also be possible to deliver α_1AT by aerosol administration.[40] This therapy is designed for individuals with established and progressive emphysema. Protein replacement therapy is not being considered for individuals with liver disease because there is little information to support the notion that deficient serum levels of α_1AT are mechanistically related to liver injury. There are several potential complications of this form of therapy. These relate to the fact that α_1AT is being infused into a host with high levels of free elastase and, if effective, would be expected to generate high levels of α_1AT–elastase complexes. As mentioned previously, such complexes mediate, through the SEC receptor, increases in synthesis of α_1AT and increases in intracellular retention of α_1AT, constituting therein a potential environmental factor predisposing a given host with α_1AT deficiency to liver injury.

Gene replacement therapy for α_1AT deficiency has been discussed in the literature.[36] Experiments in animals have indicated that somatic gene therapy with recombinant α_1AT is theoretically possible. A retroviral vector bearing the α_1AT coding sequence was transferred into mouse fibroblasts and these fibroblasts were transplanted into the peritoneal cavities of nude mice. The product of the transferred gene, human α_1AT, was detected in sera and bronchial washings for up to 4 weeks. More recently, secretion of α_1AT was directed by lymphocytes into which the retroviral vector had been transferred. Lymphocytes are being used as the cell target for the first experiments in gene replacement therapy for human disease. These provide the advantage of a target cell population that can be expanded in vitro and in vivo by IL-2 administration and of the possible localization to specific tissues on the basis of adhesion-receptor expression. Rosenfeld et al[41] have also shown that a replication-defective adenoviral vector containing the human α_1AT gene could be used to make recombinant adenovirus particles, and these particles could infect respiratory epithelium after tracheal instillation. The infection conferred α_1AT expression to pneumocytes for at least 1 week.

Several other approaches have been used recently to deliver genes to hepatocytes for gene therapy. Chowdhury et al[42] showed that hepatocytes from the Watanabe heritable hyperlipidemic rabbit could be transduced ex vivo with recombinant retroviruses containing low-density lipoprotein receptor (LDLR) complementary DNA (cDNA). The hepatocytes were cultivated from liver tissue that was removed by partial hepatectomy, transduced, and then transplanted into the liver. There was a 30% to 50% reduction in serum cholesterol levels for over 4 months.

Gene therapy may also be mediated by in vivo infection of the liver with recombinant retroviral particles. Ferry et al[43] perfused rat liver with recombinant retroviral particles through the portal vein. The transduced gene was expressed in approximately 5% of hepatocytes for at least 3 months. Wilson et al[44] have demonstrated the reconstitution of hepatic LDLR expression in the Watanabe rabbit by peripheral infusion of the cloned LDLR covalently attached to a ligand for the hepatocyte-specific asialoglycoprotein receptor.

Nevertheless, there are still major issues that must be addressed before gene therapy becomes a realistic alternative therapy. In all the methods described above, the levels of the transferred gene product were low and were sustained for short intervals. Even more important for α_1AT deficiency is the problem of concomitant expression of the endogenous mutant allele, which is potentially hepatotoxic. Moreover, reconstitution of α_1AT in plasma and tissue would lead to enhanced levels of α_1AT–proteinase complexes, feedback upregulation of α_1AT synthesis, increased intracellular accumulation of α_1AT, and, in turn, increased likelihood of liver injury.

Alternative strategies for at least partial correction of this defect may result from a more detailed understanding of the intracellular fate of the abnormal α_1AT molecule. The conceptual model proposed in this article suggests several novel potential treatment approaches. For instance, mapping of the binding domain of α_1AT, which is recognized for intracellular retention, might allow the design of synthetic peptides to saturate the binding reaction and result in release of mutant α_1AT by default. Such an intervention would not only prevent the intracellular accumulation of α_1AT and the consequent pathophysiologic effects but would also provide delivery of functionally active α_1AT to extracellular fluid and tissues. The mutant α_1AT is at least 85% as active as normal α_1AT in inhibition of neutrophil elastase.[45,46] Delivery of synthetic peptides to the ER to insert into the gap in the A-sheet and prevent polymerization of α_1AT, as mentioned above, might have the same effect. Second, elucidation of the biochemical mechanism by which abnormally folded α_1AT undergoes intracellular degradation might allow pharmacologic manipulation of this degradative system in the subpopulation of PiZZ individuals predisposed to liver injury. Third, a competitive antagonist of binding or signal transduction by α_1AT–proteinase complexes at the SEC receptor might prevent increases in intracellular accumulation of α_1AT during augmentation of α_1AT levels with protein replacement or gene replacement therapies.

REFERENCES

1. Sveger T. Liver disease in alpha-1 antitrypsin deficiency detected by screening of 200,000 infants. *N Engl J Med.* 1976;294:1216–1221.
2. Perlmutter DH. The cellular basis for liver injury in alpha-1-antitrypsin deficiency. *Hepatology.* 1991;12:172–185.
3. Dycaico JM, Grant SGN, Felts K, et al. Neonatal hepatitis induced by alpha-1-antitrypsin: a transgenic mouse model. *Science.* 1988;242:1409–1412.
4. Sveger T. The natural history of liver disease in alpha-1-antitrypsin deficient children. *Acta Paediatr Scand.* 1988;77:847–851.
5. Eriksson S, Carlson J, Velez R. Risk of cirrhosis and primary liver cancer in alpha-1-antitrypsin deficiency. *N Engl J Med.* 1986;314:736–739.
6. Hodges JE, Millward-Sadler GH, Barbatis C, Wright R. Heterozygous MZ alpha-1-antitrypsin deficiency in adults with chronic active hepatitis and cryptogenic cirrhosis. *N Engl J Med.* 1981;304:357–360.
7. Curiel DT, Holmes MD, Okayama H, et al. Molecular basis of the liver/lung disease associated with the alpha-1-antitrypsin deficiency allele M malton. *J Biol Chem.* 1989;264:13938–13945.
8. Crowley JJ, Sharp HL, Freier E, Ishak KG, Schow P. Fatal liver disease associated with alpha-1-antitrypsin deficiency PiM/PiM duarte. *Gastroenterology.* 1987;93:242–244.
9. Seyama K, Nukiwa T, Takabe K, Takahashi H, Myake K, Kira S. Siiyama (serine 53 [TCC] to phenylalanine 53 [TTC]): a new alpha-1-antitrypsin deficient variant with mutation on a predicted conserved residue of the serpin backbone. *J Biol Chem.* 1991;266:12627–12632.
10. Petersen KB, Kolvroa S, Bolund L, Braun-Peterson G, Koch J, Gregerson N. Detection of alpha-1-antitrypsin genotypes by analysis of amplified DNA sequences. *Nucleic Acids Res.* 1988;16:352.
11. Qizibash A, Young-Pong O. Alpha-1-antitrypsin liver disease: differential diagnosis of PAS-positive diastase-resistant globules in liver cells. *Am J Clin Pathol.* 1983;79:697–702.
12. Feldmann G, Gignon J, Chabinian P, Degott C, Benhamou J-P. Hepatocyte ultrastructural changes in alpha-1-antitrypsin deficiency. *Gastroenterology.* 1974;67:1214–1224.
13. Yunis EJ, Agostini RM, Glew RH. Fine structural observations of the liver in alpha-1-antitrypsin deficiency. *Am J Clin Pathol.* 1976;82:265–286.
14. Nord KS, Saad S, Joshi VJ, McLoughlin LC. Concurrence of alpha-1 antitrypsin deficiency and biliary atresia. *J Pediatr.* 1987;111:416–418.
15. Wu Y, Foreman RC. The effect of amino acid substitutions at position 342 on the secretion of human alpha-1-antitrypsin from *Xenopus* oocytes. *FEBS Lett.* 1990;268:21–23.
16. McCracken AA, Kruse KB, Valentine J, Roberts C, Yohannes TZ, Brown JL. Construction and expression of alpha-1-protease inhibitor mutants and the effects of these mutations on secretion of the variant inhibitors. *J Biol Chem.* 1991;266:7578–7582.
17. Mast AE, Enghild JJ, Salvesen G. Conformation of the reactive site loop of alpha-1-proteinase inhibitor probed by limited proteolysis. *Biochemistry.* 1992;31:2720–2728.
18. Lomas DA, Evans DL, Finch JJ, Carrell RW. The mechanism of Z alpha-1-antitrypsin accumulation in the liver. *Nature.* 1992;357:605–607.
19. Lodish HF, Kong N, Hirani S, Rasmussen J. A vesicular intermediate in the transport of hepatoma secretory proteins from the rough endoplasmic reticulum to the Golgi complex. *J Cell Biol.* 1987;104:221–230.
20. Weiland F, Gleason ML, Serafini TA, Rothman JE. The rate of bulk flow from the endoplasmic reticulum to the cell surface. *Cell.* 1987;50:289–300.
21. Rothman JE. Polypeptide chain binding proteins: catalysts of protein folding and related processes in cells. *Cell.* 1989;59:591–601.
22. Munro S, Pelham HRB. An HSP 70-like protein in ER: identity with the 78kD glucose-regulated protein and immunoglobulin heavy chain binding protein. *Cell.* 1988;46:291–300.
23. Kozutsumi K, Segal M, Normington K, Gething M-J, Sambrook J. The presence of misfolded proteins in the endoplasmic reticulum signals the induction of glucose regulated proteins. *Nature.* 1988;332:462–464.
24. Povey S. Genetics of alpha-1-antitrypsin deficiency in relation to neonatal liver disease. *Mol Biol Med.* 1990;7:161–162.
25. Lobo-Yeo A, Senaldi G, Portmann R, Mowat AP, Mieli-Vergani G, Vergani D. Class I and class II major histocompatibility complex antigen expression on hepatocytes: a study in children with liver disease. *Hepatology.* 1990;12:224–232.
26. Sargent CA, Dunham I, Trowsdale J, Campbell RD. Human major histocompatibility complex contains genes for the major heat shock protein HSP 70. *Proc Natl Acad Sci USA.* 1989;86:1968–1977.
27. Perlmutter DH. Liver disease in alpha-1-antitrypsin deficiency. In: Ockner RK, Boyer J, eds. *Progress in Liver Disease.* Philadelphia, Pa: WB Saunders Co; 1993;11:139–165.
28. Carrell RW. Alpha-1-antitrypsin molecular pathology, leukocytes and tissue damage. *J Clin Invest.* 1986;77:1427–1431.
29. Perlmutter DH, Schlesinger MJ, Pierce JA, Punsal PI, Schwartz AL. Synthesis of stress proteins is increased in individuals with homozygous PiZZ alpha-1-antitrypsin deficiency and liver disease. *J Clin Invest.* 1988;84:1555–1561.
30. Bathurst IC, Errington DM, Foreman RC, Judah JD, Carrell RW. Human Z alpha-1-antitrypsin accumulates intracellularly and stimulates lysosomal activity when synthesized in the *Xenopus* oocyte. *FEBS Lett.* 1985;183:304–408.
31. Elliott T, Cerundolo V, Elvin J, Townsend A. Peptide-induced conformational change of the class I heavy chain. *Nature.* 1991;351:402–406.
32. Sandvig K, Garred O, Prydz K, Kozlov JV, Hansen SH, van Deurs B. Retrograde transport of endocytosed Shiga toxin to the endoplasmic reticulum. *Nature.* 1992;358:510–512.
33. Perlmutter DH. Alpha-1-antitrypsin: structure, function, physiology. In: Mackiewicz A, Kushner I, Baumann H, eds. *Acute Phase Proteins: Molecular Biology, Biochemistry, Clinical Application.* Miami, Fl: CRC Press Inc; 1993:149–167.
34. Mast AE, Enghild JJ, Pizzo SV, Salvesen G. Analysis of plasma elimination kinetics and conformational stabilities of native, proteinase-complexed and reactive site cleaved serpins: comparison of alpha-1-proteinase in-

hibitor, alpha-1 antichymotrypsin, antithrombin III, alpha-2-antiplasmin, angiotensinogen, and ovalbumin. *Biochemistry.* 1991;30:1723–1730.
35. Banda MJ, Rice AG, Griffin GL, Senior RM. The inhibitory complex of human alpha-1-proteinase inhibitor and human leukocyte elastase is a neutrophil chemoattractant. *J Exp Med.* 1988;167:1608–1615.
36. Crystal RG. Alpha-1-antitrypsin deficiency, emphysema and liver disease: genetic basis and strategies for therapy. *J Clin Invest.* 1990;95:1343–1352.
37. Starzl TE, Demetris AJ, Van Thiel D. Liver transplantation. *N Engl J Med.* 1989;321:1014–1022, 1092–1099.
38. Wewers MD, Gadek JE, Koegh BA, Fells GA, Crystal RG. Evaluation of danazol therapy for patients with PiZZ alpha-1-antitrypsin deficiency. *Am Rev Respir Dis.* 1986;134:476–480.
39. Wewers MD, Casolaro A, Sellers SE, et al. Replacement therapy for alpha-1-antitrypsin deficiency associated with emphysema. *N Engl J Med.* 1987;316:1055–1062.
40. Hubbard RC, McElvaney NG, Sellers SE, Healy JT, Czerski DB, Crystal RG. Recombinant DNA-produced alpha-1-antitrypsin administered by aerosol augments lower respiratory tract antineutrophil elastase defenses in individuals with alpha-1-antitrypsin deficiency. *J Clin Invest.* 1989;84:1349–1354.
41. Rosenfeld MA, Siegfried W, Yoshimura K, et al. Adenovirus-mediated transfer of a recombinant alpha-1-antitrypsin gene to the lung epithelium in vivo. *Science.* 1991;252:431–434.
42. Chowdhury JR, Grossman M, Gupta S, Chowdhury MR, Baker JR, Wilson JM. Long-term improvement of hypercholesterolemia after ex vivo gene therapy in LDLR-deficient rabbits. *Science.* 1991;254:1802–1804.
43. Ferry N, Duplessis O, Houssin D, Danos O, Heard J-M. Retroviral-mediated gene transfer into hepatocytes in vivo. *Proc Natl Acad Sci USA.* 1991;88:8377–8381.
44. Wilson JM, Grossman M, Wu CH, Chowdhury NR, Wu GY, Chowdhury JR. Hepatocyte-directed gene transfer in vivo leads to transient improvement of hypercholesterolemia in low density lipoprotein receptor–deficient rabbits. *J Biol Chem.* 1992;267:963–967.
45. Bathurst IC, Travis J, George PM, Carrell RW. Structural and functional characterization of the abnormal Z alpha-1-antitrypsin isolated from human liver. *FEBS Lett.* 1984;177:179–183.
46. Ogushi F, Fells GA, Hubbard RC, Strauss SD, Crystal RG. Z-type alpha-1-antitrypsin is less competent than M1-type alpha-1-antitrypsin as an inhibitor of neutrophil elastase. *J Clin Invest.* 1987;89:1366–1374.

Acknowledgments

Studies from my laboratory described in this chapter have been supported by grants from the March of Dimes, Arthritis Foundation, an American Heart Association Established Investigator Award and US Public Health Service HL37784. I am grateful to Karen Jaboor for preparing the manuscript.

112

Wilson's Disease

MICHAEL L. SCHILSKY and IRMIN STERNLIEB

Wilson's disease (WD) is an autosomal recessive disorder in which copper accumulates primarily within the liver (as a result of reduced biliary excretion of this metal) and later in the nervous system and other tissues. Unless specific treatment is instituted, copper accumulation is progressive and its toxicity is ultimately fatal. However, timely and appropriate treatment offers patients excellent long-term survival.

The prevalence of the disease in almost all populations is about 1:30,000 individuals, with higher frequencies found in certain ethnic or geographic groups in which the probability of consanguinity is increased. The gene for WD, localized to chromosome 13 (specifically to 13q14-q21), encodes a putative copper transporting P-type ATPase.

DIAGNOSIS

The modes of presentation and clinical signs and symptoms of WD are listed in Table 112–1. To establish the diagnosis of WD combinations of clinical, biochemical, and histochemical criteria are used. These are discussed below and are summarized in Table 112–2. Diagnostic difficulties encountered in the patient presenting with

TABLE 112–1. MODES OF CLINICAL PRESENTATION OF WILSON'S DISEASE

Asymptomatic (with or without transaminasemia)
Liver disease
  Hepatic insufficiency
  Portal hypertension with splenomegaly or hypersplenism
  Clotting abnormalities
  Chronic hepatitis
  Fulminant hepatitis with hemolysis
Neurologic disease
  Tremors
  Rigidity
  Dystonia
  Drooling
  Amimia
  Grimacing
  Posturing of extremities
  Abnormal gait
  Athetosis
Psychiatric disease
  Behavioral abnormalities
  Irritability
  Depression
  Moodiness
  Anxiety
  Sexual preoccupation
  Psychosis
Renal dysfunction
  Proximal tubular dysfunction
  Distal tubular dysfunction
  Calculi
  Nephrocalcinosis

a sudden onset of jaundice with an associated nonimmune hemolytic anemia, so-called Wilsonian fulminant hepatitis, are addressed separately.

KAYSER-FLEISCHER RINGS

Most symptomatic patients with WD display characteristic peripheral corneal, copper deposits within Descemet's membrane that are grossly visible in some patients. The presence of these Kayser-Fleischer rings must be confirmed by slit lamp examination. The rings may be absent in young patients but are invariably present when neurologic or psychiatric manifestations of WD are observed. Although similar rings are rarely found in patients with long-standing cholestasis, the clinical setting and biochemical abnormalities distinguish these patients from patients with WD.

SERUM CERULOPLASMIN

Circulating levels of the blue copper-protein ceruloplasmin are reduced in nearly 95% of patients with WD to less than 20 mg/dl of serum. However, since 20% of heterozygotes for the WD gene display similar abnormal values, this determination alone is not sufficient for a diagnosis. Moreover, because of the physiologic reduction of ceruloplasmin during the first 6 months of life, diagnostic values may not be obtained until later in the first year. In patients with severe hepatic insufficiency, severe protein-losing enteropathies, or nephropathies and in rare patients with familial hypoceruloplasminemia, the concentration of ceruloplasmin in serum may be reduced without any associated pathologic changes.

URINARY COPPER

Urinary copper excretion generally exceeds 100 μg/24 h in symptomatic patients with WD. However, it is often below this diagnostic level in young, asymptomatic patients. By contrast, in patients with advanced non-Wilsonian liver disease, particularly in association with cholestasis, the excretion of urinary copper may be increased. Loss of ceruloplasmin into the urine due to proteinuria is another cause of hypercupriuria.

Urinary copper excretion increases dramati-

TABLE 112–2. DIAGNOSTIC INDEXES FOR WILSON'S DISEASE

	NORMAL VALUES	CHARACTERISTIC FOR WILSON'S DISEASE
Kayser-Fleischer rings	Absent	Present
Hepatic copper concentration	<50 μg/g dry weight	>250 μg/g dry weight
Hepatic histologic findings	Normal	Steatosis; glycogen nuclei; fibrosis; cirrhosis
Rhodanine histochemistry	Negative	Positive throughout certain, but not all, nodules
Serum ceruloplasmin	20–40 mg/dl	<20 mg/dl*
24-hour urinary copper excretion	<50 μg	>100 μg
Radiocopper incorporation into ceruloplasmin	Normal	Very low

*In 95% of patients with Wilson's disease and in 20% of heterozygous carriers.

cally in untreated patients with WD following the administration of chelating agents like penicillamine, trientine, British antilewisite (BAL), or tetrathiomolybdate. Penicillamine, 500 mg given orally, prior to a 24-hour urine collection for copper, may be helpful in diagnosing WD in children without Kayser-Fleischer rings.

Liver Biopsy

The determination of hepatic copper concentration provides critical data for the diagnosis of WD. The normal human liver contains less than 50 1g of copper per gram of dry weight, whereas that of patients with WD typically contains more than 250 1g/g dry tissue. In long-standing cholestatic disorders, such as primary biliary cirrhosis (PBC), sclerosing cholangitis, or childhood cholestatic syndromes, hepatic copper content may reach values encountered in patients with WD. Even higher concentrations, often in excess of 1000 1g/g dry weight are present in the livers of patients with Indian childhood cirrhosis or in the rare non-Indian idiopathic copper toxicosis. The clinical, histologic, biochemical, and serologic features of these disorders are distinctive and therefore it is unlikely that they might be confused with those of WD.

Light and electron microscopic studies of liver specimens may provide supportive evidence for the diagnosis of Wilson's disease. During the early stages of WD, microvesicular or macrovesicular fatty changes are common findings in the hepatocytes, particularly in asymptomatic patients. Glycogen nuclei and vacuolated nuclei containing cytoplasmic invaginations are seen. In the untreated patient, steatosis is typically followed by fibrosis and ultimate progression to cirrhosis. Submassive necrosis and Mallory's bodies are seen in the livers of patients presenting clinically with fulminant hepatitis or chronic active hepatitis, both forms always superimposed on an existing cirrhosis.

The cytochemical demonstration of copper or copper-binding protein in histologic sections treated with rhodanine, rubeanic acid, orcein, or Victoria blue is of diagnostic value only if positive. Even though hepatic copper content is higher during the early stages of WD, this copper may not be stainable because of its diffuse distribution in the cytoplasm. As the evolution toward cirrhosis progresses, copper is concentrated in hepatocellular lysosomes and becomes detectable as stainable granules with the routine histochemical stains. Characteristically in WD, copper staining can be seen throughout certain liver nodules while being absent from neighboring areas. This pattern differs from that encountered in cholestatic disorders in which copper accumulates at the peripheries of most nodules.

Ultrastructural examination of liver tissue is occasionally useful for diagnosis in young patients. Pleomorphic mitochondria with increased matrix density, matrical inclusions, and widened intermembranous and intracristal spaces are unique to WD. They are present during the early stages of fatty infiltration but disappear with progression of the pathologic process toward cirrhosis or with treatment specific for WD.

Radiocopper Loading Tests

Radiocopper loading tests are used mainly for distinguishing WD from other liver or neurologic diseases in patients with *normal* levels of serum ceruloplasmin. Typically, 1 to 2 hours following the administration of an oral dose of radiolabeled copper, radioactivity in the serum reaches a peak and then falls. Normally, the serum concentration of radiocopper rises over the next 24 to 48 hours, corresponding to its incorporation into newly synthesized ceruloplasmin secreted by the liver into the circulation. In patients with WD this secondary rise is absent, thus enabling the differentiation of Wilsonian from non-Wilsonian disorders.

Molecular Genetic Analysis

Identification of the WD gene to a specific region of chromosome 13 enables the molecular identification of family members of affected individuals by haplotype analysis. Specific familial patterns distinguish homozygotes for WD from heterozygotes and nonaffected individuals within families. At present, molecular analysis is limited to screening families of affected individuals, since DNA polymorphisms are too varied among the general population to allow the identification of unrelated individuals and because multiple disease-specific mutations have been identified.

Diagnosis of WD With Fulminant Hepatitis

Patients exhibiting a clinical picture of Wilsonian fulminant hepatitis present unique diagnostic problems because of the urgency of the diagnosis in this rapidly progressive fatal condition. The patients are often so young that they may not exhibit Kayser-Fleischer rings. Moreover, hepatic biopsy may be too hazardous because of the associated coagulopathy. In some patients, serum levels of ceruloplasmin may be elevated to the normal range because of an acute phase response to hepatic inflammation in a patient who may otherwise have diagnostic low levels of this protein. Conversely, occasional patients with non-Wilsonian severe hepatic insufficiency exhibit a temporary reduction of serum levels of ceruloplasmin due to synthetic failure.

Levels of serum copper, specifically non-ceruloplasmin-bound serum copper, and urinary copper excretion are invariably markedly elevated in patients with Wilsonian fulminant hepatitis. Still unexplained are other diagnostic features of Wilsonian fulminant hepatitis, namely the unexpectedly low serum alkaline phosphatase activities and disproportionately modest serum transaminase levels in the presence of profound jaundice and hepatocellular necrosis. The ratio of serum alkaline phosphatase (in IU/L) to total serum bilirubin (mg/dl) was proposed as a diagnostic criterion for Wilsonian fulminant hepatitis. However, recent data have cast doubt on the reliability of this ratio. Nonetheless, if the ratio is less than 2, it is likely that WD is etiologic. However, a ratio greater than or equal to 2 does not exclude this diagnosis.

TREATMENT

Pharmacologic treatment aims at preventing or reversing the toxic effects of copper by reducing its absorption, inducing synthesis of endogenous chelators such as metallothioneine, promoting the excretion of copper in urine or bile, or by a combination of these processes. Correction of the metabolic defect of WD can only be achieved by orthotopic liver transplantation.

Penicillamine (Cuprimine, Depen, Trolovol)

Mode of Action and Indications for Use

D-Penicillamine is a chelating agent that forms soluble metal complexes that are readily excreted by the kidneys. This drug acts by promoting cupriuresis and reducing tissue copper stores. It may also promote the induction of cellular metallothioneine, interfere with fibrogenesis, and modulate the immune system.

Penicillamine is the drug of choice for all modes of presentation of WD. Most patients treated with this drug improve, often dramatically, and live essentially a normal life span.

Dosage

Adult: 1 to 2 g daily, administered in four divided doses about 30 minutes before meals or 2 hours after eating. Once the dosage of 1 g is well tolerated, the dosage of D-penicillamine should be adjusted in accord with the patient's clinical and biochemical responses. A useful index for adequacy of the dose and for compliance is the concentration of non-ceruloplasmin-bound serum copper (see *Monitoring of Pharmacotherapy* below). The dosage should be reduced temporarily to no less than 250 mg/d prior to elective surgery or delivery.

Pediatric: (for children weighing less than 40 kg) 0.02 g/kg body weight (rounded to the nearest 125 mg) administered orally in four divided doses about 30 minutes before meals or 2 hours after eating.

Pyridoxine, 25 mg daily administered orally, should be given to patients taking D-penicillamine as compensation for the drug's weak antipyridoxine action.

Early Side Effects

Sensitivity reactions, almost always reversible, may occur in up to 20% of patients within the first few weeks of D-penicillamine therapy. These include fever; diffuse, erythematous, macular, slightly papular, pruritic rash; lymphadenopathy, most commonly localized to the nodes of the neck; and leukopenia or thrombocytopenia, apart from that due to hypersplenism. The medication should be immediately discontinued if any of these occur.

Neurologic manifestations may worsen temporarily in about 10% of patients who manifest such signs or symptoms prior to treatment. This occurs typically in the first weeks or months following the initiation of therapy. D-Penicillamine should be continued, barring occurrence of other adverse reactions, since the neurologic condition often remits with time. However, in some patients the deterioration is progressive. Unfortunately, there are no prognostic criteria that permit the early identification of such individuals, nor is there evidence that this response does not occur with other regimens.

Late Effects

Renal toxicity is generally heralded by the onset of proteinuria. It occurs in fewer than 5% of penicillamine-treated patients with WD. Proteinuria should be quantitated in a 24-hour urine collection. If proteinuria is less than 0.5 g/d, D-penicillamine may be continued. But if it exceeds 1 g, an alternative medication should be used.

In rare instances patients with WD may develop a lupuslike syndrome, usually preceded by hematuria and proteinuria and often accompanied by arthralgias. Serum titers of antinuclear antibodies are frequently elevated. Corticosteroids and reduction of the D-penicillamine dosage may control this reaction. However the use of alternate medication should be considered. Goodpasture's syndrome, marked by pulmonary and renal hemorrhages, in patients with WD who had received penicillamine in excess of 1 g/d, has not been reported in recent years, possibly because lower doses of D-penicillamine are generally used.

Several types of skin lesions may occur after years of continued D-penicillamine therapy. Most common is the increased wrinkling of the skin, particularly on the neck, giving it a progeric appearance. Unrelated to this effect are the raised, arcuate lesions of elastosis perforans serpiginosa. These appear singly or in groups, most commonly on the axilla, neck, and buttocks but rarely at other sites. No specific treatment exists; however, the lesions may disappear spontaneously whether or not D-penicillamine therapy is discontinued.

Penicillamine dermatopathy, resulting in friability with milia-like lesions, and weakening of subcutaneous tissue due to interference of cross-linking of elastin and collagen, is seen when daily dosages of 3 to 4 g are used for prolonged periods. Pemphigus or pemphigoid lesions, lichen planus, and aphthous stomatitis have also been reported in several patients receiving penicillamine.

Very rare late side effects occurring in patients with WD include anaphylaxis, myasthenia gravis, polymyositis, loss of taste, depression of immunoglobulin A (IgA), and serous retinitis, all of which are reversible.

Desensitization

Early reactions to D-penicillamine (except for severe leukopenia) are managed by stopping the medication, waiting for a few days for the reaction to disappear, and then starting prednisone 30 mg, daily for 3 days prior to administering 125 mg D-penicillamine once daily for 3 days, and progressing slowly to 1 g daily. Prednisone is reduced to 20 mg daily and ultimately tapered if no recurrence of the adverse reaction develops.

Pregnancy

The regular dose of penicillamine should be continued during the first two trimesters of pregnancy. It can be reduced to 500 mg/d during the last trimester. If a cesarean section is contemplated, the dosage should be reduced to 250 mg daily for 6 weeks before and until normal wound healing has occurred. In over 150 pregnancies carried by women with WD, no toxicity of the drug to either mother or fetus was seen.

TRIENTINE (SYPRINE, TRIENTINE HYDROCHLORIDE, TETA)

Mode of Action and Indications for Use

Trientine promotes cupriuresis less effectively than penicillamine, but seems to be clinically as effective as penicillamine as maintenance therapy for patients with WD. Its role as primary treatment for patients presenting with severe liver disease or marked neurologic or psychiatric manifestations remains to be determined.

Dosage

Adult: 1 to 1.5 g orally administered daily in divided doses 30 minutes before meals or 2 hours after eating.

Pediatric: 0.5 to 0.75 g daily in two divided doses.

Side Effects

No hypersensitivity reactions have been reported. In patients with penicillamine-induced lupus, there may be a recurrence with trientine. Few patients have developed a sideroblastic anemia. This is thought to be the result of drug-induced copper deficiency in the erythropoietic stem cells, which inhibits the effective utilization of iron.

Pregnancy

A daily dosage of 1 g of trientine maintained during pregnancy has not resulted in any known complications to date.

ZINC (ZINC SULFATE, ZINC GLUCONATE, ZINC ACETATE)

Mode of Action and Indications for Use

Orally ingested zinc reduces the intestinal absorption of copper by stimulating the synthesis of metallothioneine in enterocytes. This protein sequesters copper in the small intestinal cells, which are subsequently shed into the intestinal lumen and excreted. Zinc may also be hepatoprotective by stimulating metallothioneine synthesis in hepatocytes.

Zinc was shown to be effective maintenance therapy for asymptomatic WD and for patients who have reached a plateau with D-penicillamine or trientine. Its precise role in the schema of treatment of patients presenting with severe liver disease or with neurologic or psychiatric manifestations is not clear.

Dosage

150 to 200 mg of metallic zinc as zinc sulfate, zinc acetate, or zinc gluconate, given in divided doses at least 1 hour before meals, daily.

Side Effects

Gastric irritation, which may be in part dependent on the chemical form of the zinc compound, is most likely to occur with zinc sulfate.

Pregnancy

Zinc therapy during pregnancy has not resulted in known complications to date.

BRITISH ANTILEWISITE (BAL) (DIMERCAPROL, DIMERCAPTOPROPANOL)

Mode of Action and Indications for Use

BAL was the first chelating agent successfully utilized for the treatment of WD. BAL increases the urinary copper excretion and results in clinical improvement in some patients with WD. Its present role is restricted to that of an adjunct to oral therapy for patients with WD with severe neurologic involvement, occasionally with dramatic results. Being an uncharged hydrophobic molecule, BAL is thought to be able to cross the blood-brain barrier, as well as cellular plasma membranes.

Dosage

Three milliliters of 10% BAL in peanut oil is injected intramuscularly daily, in repeated 5-day courses, up to 40 to 60 doses. Because of local pain caused by the injections, not all patients tolerate this treatment. BAL should not be administered in conjunction with medicinal iron because of possible formation of complexes with BAL that are highly nephrotoxic.

Side Effects

Sterile abscesses may develop. These can be avoided by carefully alternating injection sites. Other effects include tachycardia and anaphylaxis, which are probably related to an allergic reaction to the vehicle for BAL and hemolysis in patients with glucose-6-phosphate dehydrogenase deficiency.

TETRATHIOMOLYBDATE

Tetrathiomolybdate, used for decades by farmers and veterinarians for treatment of copper toxicosis in sheep, is being evaluated as an investigational drug for its role as initial treatment for WD in the hope of avoiding the initial clinical deterioration that occurs in some patients treated with D-penicillamine. It is a more effective chelator of copper than D-penicillamine or trientine. Tetrathiomolybdate reduces intestinal copper absorption, and administered parenterally, enhances cupriuresis. Injury to intestinal lining cells was observed in some treated animals. Whether these alterations are due to copper deficiency within enterocytes or to toxic actions of this agent is unclear.

TRANSPLANTATION

Hepatic transplantation plays an important role for the treatment of patients with WD with severe hepatic failure refractory to pharmacologic treatment, for those presenting with Wilsonian fulminant hepatitis with hemolysis, and for patients with hepatic decompensation following noncompliance with the pharmacologic regimen. In a recent survey of the outcome of hepatic transplantation for WD, survival was 79%, comparable to that of other patients with liver disease. The role of liver transplantation for neurologic WD without hepatic insufficiency is uncertain.

HEMOFILTRATION AND PLASMAPHERESIS

Hemofiltration and plasmapheresis have been used in few patients with Wilsonian fulminant hepatitis awaiting suitable donor livers. In none did these treatments stay the need for transplantation.

MONITORING OF PHARMACOTHERAPY

There are three major goals of monitoring pharmacotherapy: (1) determination of the adequacy of therapy; (2) recognition and screening for side effects or intolerance; and (3) determination of therapeutic compliance.

Adequacy of therapy is determined foremost by the patient's clinical response; the normalization of abnormal laboratory tests; the reduction of the concentration of non-ceruloplasmin-bound copper in the serum to less than 10 1g/dl; and by maintaining the 24-hour urinary copper excretion above or close to 0.5 1g/d. Most clinical neurologic abnormalities and biochemical parameters of liver dysfunction improve within 6 months to 1 year after initiation of therapy. However, normalization of the prothrombin time may take longer or may be delayed indefinitely.

Patients should be alerted to look out for fever, rash, or lymphadenopathy. Complete blood counts should be obtained at weekly, then biweekly, intervals, and periodically thereafter. Urine should be routinely tested for protein and cellular sediment.

The importance of monitoring compliance cannot be overstated. The patient's refusal to take the prescribed dosages of medication accounts for lack of improvement occasionally. Discontinuation of therapy after intervals of apparent well-being results in the sudden severe appearance of some noncompliant patients in hepatic insufficiency, requiring liver transplantation. Compliance is best achieved by repeatedly stressing the importance of taking medication regularly; counting pills; periodic slit lamp examinations for documentation of the disappearance of Kayser-Fleischer rings; serum testing for biochemical evidence of liver disease; determinations of the fraction of nonceruloplasmin-bound serum copper; and measurements of urinary copper excretion. Imaging studies (including magnetic resonance imaging), neurophysiologic investigations (visual- and auditory-evoked responses), and serial hepatic copper determinations may be of academic interest but contribute little to a thorough clinical and biochemical examination.

REFERENCES

1. Brewer JB, Yuzbasiyan-Gurkan V. Wilson's disease. *Medicine*. 1992;71:139–163.
2. Martins da Costa C, Baldwin D, Portmann B, Lolin Y, Mowat AP, Mieli-Vergani G. Value of urinary copper excretion after penicillamine challenge in the diagnosis of Wilson's disease. *Hepatology*. 1992;15:609–615.
3. Scheinberg IH, Jaffe ME, Sternlieb I. The use of trientine in preventing the effects of interrupting penicillamine therapy in Wilson's disease. *N Engl J Med*. 1987;317:209–213.
4. Scheinberg IH, Sternlieb I. *Wilson's Disease*. Philadelphia, Pa: WB Saunders Co; 1984.
5. Schilsky ML. Identification of the Wilson's disease gene: clues for disease pathogenesis and the potential for molecular diagnosis. *Hepatology*. 1994;20:529–533.
6. Schilsky ML, Scheinberg IH, Sternlieb, I. Liver transplantation for Wilson's disease: Indications and outcome. *Hepatology*. 1994;19:583–587.
7. Sternlieb I. Perspectives on Wilson's disease. *Hepatology*. 1990:12:1234–1239.
8. Walshe JM, Yealland M. Chelational treatment of neurological Wilson's disease. *QJ Med*. 1993;86:197–204.

113

Hemochromatosis

BRUCE R. BACON

There are several iron overload syndromes that have been described in adults. Classification is based on the cause and the distribution of the increased iron deposition (Table 113–1). Since humans have no excretory pathway for iron, iron overload occurs either as a result of an increase in intestinal iron absorption or from the parenteral administration of iron either as medicinal iron chelates (e.g., iron-dextran) or as iron in hemoglobin in transfused red blood cells.

Hereditary hemochromatosis (HHC) refers to the disorder in which there is homozygous in-

TABLE 113–1. CLASSIFICATION OF IRON OVERLOAD SYNDROMES IN ADULTS

Hereditary Hemochromatosis (HHC)
Primary
Genetic
Idiopathic

Secondary Iron Overload
Anemia due to ineffective erythropoiesis
    β-Thalassemia
    Sideroblastic anemia
    Aplastic anemia
Liver disease
    Alcoholic cirrhosis
    Chronic viral hepatitis
    Following portacaval shunts
    Porphyria cutanea tarda
Increased oral intake of iron
Congenital atransferrinemia

Parenteral Iron Overload
Red blood cell transfusions
Iron-dextran injections
Associated with long-term hemodialysis

African Iron Overload

heritance of the HHC gene. This results in increased iron absorption from the gut with subsequent deposition in parenchymal cells of the liver, heart, pancreas, and other organs. *Secondary iron overload* encompasses a variety of clinical disorders in which there is an underlying condition that results in an increase in intestinal iron absorption. The best examples of secondary iron overload are the various disorders of ineffective erythropoiesis such as β-thalassemia, sideroblastic anemia, or aplastic anemia where anemia is the underlying condition and parenchymal iron overload can occur in the absence of prior red blood cell (RBC) transfusions. Secondary iron overload is also seen in patients with a variety of liver diseases, including alcoholic cirrhosis, viral hepatitis with and without cirrhosis, following portacaval shunts, and in porphyria cutanea tarda (PCT). It is unknown how liver disease results in increased iron deposition. *Parenteral iron overload* refers to the situation in which individuals receive excessive amounts of iron in the form of injectable iron chelates or from chronic RBC transfusion in the absence of blood loss. Most patients with ineffective erythropoiesis have a combination of both secondary and parenteral iron overload, since RBC transfusion is often necessary. In parenteral iron overload, iron is initially deposited in reticuloendothelial cells; but with enough iron loading, redistribution to parenchymal cells occurs. Finally, it has recently been reported that a second form of inherited iron overload, genetically distinct from HLA-linked HHC, occurs in sub-Saharan Africans. Enhanced expression of this genetic form of *African iron overload* occurs with the consumption of traditional home-brewed beer, which is high in iron content, but can also be seen in the absence of dietary iron ingestion. In African iron overload, cellular iron distribution is different from that observed in HHC.

HEREDITARY HEMOCHROMATOSIS

The gene responsible for hereditary hemochromatosis has not yet been precisely localized but is known to be on the short arm of chromosome 6 in close proximity to the HLA-A locus. Pedigree analysis and population screening studies in North America, Australia, and Europe have shown that the gene frequency is approximately 5%, with homozygotes being described in 0.2% to 0.7% and heterozygotes in 8% to 14% of the population. Although the disorder is not sex linked, the disease is more pronounced and presents at an earlier age in male than in female subjects. Excessive iron accumulation in female patients is usually delayed by as much as 10 years when compared to accumulation in male patients, in part because of physiologic losses of iron from menstruation and pregnancy. The main organs that are affected include the liver, heart, pancreas, joints, and pituitary. In homozygotes, coincident alcohol ingestion seems to accelerate the progression of the liver disease; thus, cirrhosis can be found at lower hepatic iron concentrations in those who drink excessive amounts of alcohol compared to those who do not. Approximately 25% of heterozygotes for HHC have minor increases in hepatic iron content with alterations in blood tests of iron status, but progressive tissue damage does not occur.

CLINICAL MANIFESTATIONS OF HHC

Iron absorption is increased throughout the lifetime of patients with HHC, resulting in the gradual accumulation of toxic levels of tissue iron, eventually leading to organ damage. Symptoms typically develop after tissue damage has occurred, which is usually associated with the accumulation of from 10 g to 20 g of storage iron. Although some patients may present with fully expressed clinical disease in their twenties, it is more usual for patients in their forties or fifties to present either with abnormal blood test results or with symptoms. Typical presenting symptoms (Table 113–2) are often nonspecific and include weight loss, fatigue, weakness, apathy, and lack of libido. Other clinical findings (Table 113–2) and symptoms seen in HHC include arthritis, impotence, diabetes, amenorrhea, cirrhosis, and heart failure; these can mimic symptoms and findings seen in other common disorders, and as a result, diagnosis and treatment are frequently delayed. Finally, with the advent of increased awareness of the disease and the introduction of multiphasic screening that includes serum iron levels, many patients are now being detected prior to the development of symptoms.

In most older series of patients with HHC, hepatomegaly and skin pigmentation were found in as many as 80% to 90% of patients. Because the liver is the primary storage organ for iron, it is often damaged early in the course of HHC. The pancreas and heart are other organs that accumulate excess iron and are susceptible to tissue damage, resulting in diabetes and heart failure, but the pancreas and heart are less commonly affected than the liver. More recent studies of patients with HHC have reflected an increased awareness of the disease with earlier diagnosis; fewer patients have had cirrhosis, diabetes, heart disease, or endocrine abnormalities, and many have been asymptomatic. The full clinical expression of HHC is influenced by age, gender, dietary habits, and other unknown factors, and some homozygous patients may live a full life without developing life-threatening organ damage.

Diagnosis of HHC

Blood Studies

Once suspected, the diagnosis of HHC is relatively straightforward using commonly available blood studies of iron metabolism (Table 113–3). These include the serum iron and transferrin concentration, from which the percent of transferrin saturation can be calculated (serum iron ÷ transferrin × 100%), and the serum ferritin level. These studies should be obtained with the patient in the fasting state, since transferrin saturation can be falsely elevated in nonfasting individuals. In uncomplicated cases, the combination of an increased transferrin saturation (greater than 50%) and an elevated ferritin level is 86% specific and 94% sensitive for the diagnosis of HHC. More importantly, if both of these tests are normal, the chances of missing a diagnosis of HHC is less than 5%. Unfortunately, not all cases are uncomplicated, and there are many situations where the ferritin level or the transferrin saturation are elevated in the absence of hemochromatosis. For example, while serum ferritin is elevated proportionally to tissue iron stores in iron overload, it can also be elevated in patients with other types of necroinflammatory liver disease (e.g., viral hepatitis), various malignancies (e.g., lymphoma), and chronic inflammatory conditions. Conversely, occasional pa-

TABLE 113–2. CLINICAL MANIFESTATIONS OF HEREDITARY HEMOCHROMATOSIS

	%
Typical Symptoms	
Weakness, lethargy, fatigue	40–85
Apathy, lack of interest	40–85
Abdominal pain	30–60
Weight loss	30–60
Arthralgias	40–60
Loss of libido, impotence	30–60
Amenorrhea	20–60
Congestive heart failure symptoms	0–40
Common Physical Findings	
Hepatomegaly	60–85
Cirrhosis	50–95
Skin pigmentation	40–80
Arthritis (second, third metacarpophalangeal joints)	40–60
Clinical diabetes	10–60
Splenomegaly	10–40
Loss of body hair	10–30
Testicular atrophy	10–30
Dilated cardiomyopathy	0–30

TABLE 113–3. REPRESENTATIVE IRON MEASUREMENTS IN PATIENTS WITH OVERT HEREDITARY HEMOCHROMATOSIS (HHC)

	Normal	HHC
Serum iron (μg/dl)	60–180	180–300
Serum transferrin (μg/dl)	220–410	200–300
Transferrin saturation (%)	20–50	80–100
Serum ferritin (ng/ml)		
Male patients	20–200	500–6000
Female patients	15–50	500–6000
Hepatic iron concentration		
(μg/g, dry weight)	300–1200	10,000–30,000
(μmoles/g, dry weight)	5–21	175–550
Hepatic iron index		
(μmoles/g dry weight ÷ age in years)	<2	>2

tients with increased iron stores have been described with normal or very minimally elevated ferritin. Therefore, to be confident of the diagnosis once blood studies suggestive of iron overload have been obtained, the next step should be to perform a liver biopsy, both for histologic evaluation and biochemical determination of hepatic iron concentration.

Liver Biopsy

In uncomplicated HHC, iron deposition (identified by the Perls' Prussian blue stain test) is seen in a periportal distribution with virtually all the iron in hepatocytes (Fig. 113–1; see Color Plate III). In early HHC there is a periportal (Rappaport zone 1) to central (Rappaport zone 3) gradient of iron deposition, whereas in late HHC this is less apparent. Also in late HHC there may be iron deposition in Kupffer's cells and in bile duct epithelial cells. When complicated by excessive alcohol ingestion or diabetes, there may be varying degrees of hepatic steatosis. Fibrosis is typically portal, and when cirrhosis occurs, it is of the micronodular type.

Qualitative assessment of iron deposition by histologic grading (1+ to 4+) is often unreliable; thus, in all patients for whom the diagnosis of HHC is being considered, a portion of the liver biopsy sample should be submitted for biochemical determination of hepatic iron concentration. This permits an initial definitive diagnosis, can be used to roughly prognosticate the number of phlebotomies necessary for treatment, and can be used as a reference point for future assessment of therapeutic efficacy. Symptomatic patients with HHC usually have hepatic iron concentrations in excess of 10,000 µg/g, and levels may be as high as 40,000 µg/g (normal less than 1200 µg/g). In the absence of excessive alcohol consumption, fibrosis and cirrhosis are usually not seen unless the hepatic iron concentration is in excess of 20,000 µg/g. In asymptomatic individuals or in younger patients with early precirrhotic HHC, hepatic iron levels are increased but to a lesser degree, and often levels are less than 10,000 µg/g. Patients with chronic liver disease and secondary iron overload usually do not have hepatic iron concentrations in excess of 10,000 µg/g.

Differential Diagnosis

In symptomatic individuals, diagnosis of HHC requires an astute clinician with a high level of suspicion who thinks to order iron studies and, if the results of the iron studies are abnormal, follows through with a liver biopsy. Similarly, in asymptomatic individuals who are identified either by family screening or by multiphasic chemistry panels that include iron studies, the diagnosis is dependent on the recognition that iron overload is a common disorder and is best discovered and treated before symptoms or tissue damage occur. Thus, patients can range from those with no symptoms or physical findings to those with any combination of complications of chronic liver disease, diabetes, heart failure, or skin pigmentation. Diagnosis requires abnormal results from iron studies, a clinical history that excludes other causes of secondary or parenteral iron overload, and a liver biopsy specimen in which excess hepatocellular iron is demonstrated histologically and in which an elevated tissue iron concentration is confirmed.

Because hepatic iron deposition may be mildly increased histologically in other types of chronic liver disease (alcoholic, viral), discrimination between HHC and other forms of chronic liver disease with secondary iron overload is a common problem. Several recent studies have demonstrated that homozygous HHC can be clearly distinguished from heterozygous HHC or from chronic liver disease with secondary iron overload by the use of the hepatic iron index (HII). The HII is based on the concept that with age HHC homozygotes have a continued progressive increase in liver iron, whereas HHC heterozygotes and patients with chronic liver disease with secondary iron overload do not. The HII is calculated as the ratio of the hepatic iron concentration to age and thus requires biochemical determination of hepatic iron concentration. An elevated HII (greater than 1.9) is seen in patients with homozygous HHC (Table 113–4).

TABLE 113–4. HEPATIC IRON INDEX (HII) IN HEREDITARY HEMOCHROMATOSIS

STUDY	NORMAL	ALD	Hh	HH
Bassett et al[3]	<1.0	<1.4	<1.8	>2.0
Summers et al[11]	–	–	<1.5	>1.9
Olynyk et al[9]	<1.1	<1.6	–	>2.1
Bonkovsky et al[4]	<0.7	<1.1	<1.8	>2.0
Sallie et al[10]	–	<1.6	–	>2.0

Hepatic iron index is calculated by dividing the hepatic iron concentration (in µmoles per gram dry weight) by the age of the patient (in years).
ALD = alcoholic liver disease, Hh = hemochromatosis, heterozygote, HH = hemochromatosis, homozygote.

TREATMENT

Most patients with HHC can be successfully treated with regular phlebotomy. The principal goal of therapy is to remove excess tissue iron before the development of complications. If this occurs (i.e., before fibrosis or cirrhosis develops), patients should expect normal survival. At the time of diagnosis, most symptomatic patients with HHC have 15 to 30 g of excess storage iron. Typically, asymptomatic or younger individuals have less excess storage iron. Since each unit of blood contains about 250 mg of iron, these patients require extended phlebotomy regimens. During phlebotomy therapy, the goals are to remove excess iron quickly without compromising the patient's well-being. Symptoms and hematocrit are monitored weekly and dictate the speed of the phlebotomy regimen. Most patients can tolerate weekly phlebotomy of 450 to 500 ml of whole blood. Younger patients may be able to tolerate removal of 2 U (1000 ml) of blood per week, whereas some older patients can only tolerate phlebotomy of 250 ml every other week. Every 6 to 8 weeks the transferrin saturation and ferritin level can be determined; these levels predict the eventual return to normal iron stores. The ferritin level gradually decreases proportionally to the decrease in tissue iron stores, whereas the transferrin saturation remains elevated until normal iron stores are achieved. Once iron stores have reached low normal, as evidenced by a ferritin level of less than 50 ng/ml and a transferrin saturation of less than 50%, maintenance phlebotomies are required in most patients every 3 to 4 months. The rate of reaccumulation of iron varies among individuals, and some patients may not require a subsequent phlebotomy for quite some time.

The nonspecific symptoms of malaise, fatigue, and right upper quadrant abdominal pain usually improve with phlebotomy therapy; however, symptoms due to arthritis, established cirrhosis, and hypogonadism do not improve. In noncirrhotic patients who are successfully treated, the risk of hepatocellular cancer, which is increased 200-fold in patients with untreated HHC, is reduced to normal. However, treated cirrhotic patients are still at risk for hepatocellular carcinoma and should be screened at 6-month intervals with hepatic ultrasound and alpha-fetoprotein levels. Concomitant use of deferoxamine (Desferal, DFO) is only necessary in those patients who present with cardiac symptoms due to hemochromatosis.

SCREENING STUDIES

Once the diagnosis of HHC is confirmed in a proband, screening studies consisting of transferrin saturation and serum ferritin levels should be performed in all first-degree relatives. If results from either of these tests are abnormal, a liver biopsy should be performed for histologic evaluation and for biochemical determination of hepatic iron concentration. Use of HLA typing can also be helpful to study family members. If a family member has the same HLA haplotypes as the proband, that family member is highly likely to eventually develop iron overload and should be appropriately counseled, evaluated, and treated. For those family members with HLA haplotypes different from the proband, the risk of iron overload is essentially nonexistent.

SECONDARY AND PARENTERAL IRON OVERLOAD

SECONDARY IRON OVERLOAD

The various causes of secondary iron overload are usually identified by a careful history, serum iron studies, liver biopsy, and quantitative hepatic iron determination. In patients with alcoholic liver disease and secondary iron overload, phlebotomy therapy is unnecessary. The interrelationship between secondary iron overload and chronic viral hepatitis (B or C) is undetermined at the present time, but recent studies have demonstrated that patients with chronic viral hepatitis who responded to interferon alfa had lower hepatic iron concentrations than nonresponders. In patients with PCT, the role of phlebotomy therapy in ameliorating both the hepatic and dermatologic manifestations of the disease is well established. Patients with PCT usually have 3 to 4 g of excess storage iron and thus can be managed with weekly phlebotomy over a 3- to 4-month period of time.

PARENTERAL IRON OVERLOAD

Patients with chronic anemia and secondary and parenteral iron overload due to ineffective erythropoiesis and chronic RBC transfusions can develop both hepatic and cardiac disease due to iron overload. These patients cannot be treated by phlebotomy, and thus iron chelation therapy with deferoxamine is used. From the experience with thalassemic children, it has been learned that concomitant use of deferoxamine from the beginning of the transfusion regimen improves survival. Thus, all patients who are subjected to a chronic transfusion program (e.g., sickle cell anemia, sideroblastic anemia, thalassemia, pure red cell aplasia) and have an otherwise good prognosis should be considered for concomitant deferoxamine therapy. Unfortunately, iron chelation therapy is often considered in these patients only after multiple transfusions of packed RBCs have been given and patients are already grossly iron loaded, with tissue damage due to excess iron. The reluctance to begin a chronic chelation program is related to the fact that deferoxamine must be given parenterally, and there are no effective oral iron chelators available for use. Deferoxamine can be given either as an intramuscular injection or by intravenous or subcutaneous infusion. Continuous subcutaneous infusion of 2 to 4 g of deferoxamine over 12 hours using an infusion pump is the method most commonly employed. This results in urinary excretion of approximately 50 to 100 mg of iron every 24 hours. Complications of deferoxamine therapy include pain at the injection site and rarely long-term visual and auditory impairment. Ascorbic acid in dosages of 100 to 200 mg per day can be administered to enhance iron excretion with deferoxamine. This should only be given after the deferoxamine has been begun because of reported risk of enhanced cardiac toxicity when ascorbic acid is given without deferoxamine.

SUMMARY

In summary, HHC is more common than once thought, and diagnosis is reasonably straightforward. Liver biopsy with quantitative iron determination is necessary for confirmation. Treatment by means of phlebotomy has predictable results, and if the diagnosis is made prior to end-stage complications, treatment can be very successful. Clearly, the key to successful management is early diagnosis, and this requires an enhanced awareness of the disease. Secondary iron overload in patients with alcoholic liver disease does not need to be treated, whereas the role of phlebotomy therapy in PCT is well established. The role of phlebotomy prior to the use of antiviral therapy in patients with secondary iron overload and chronic viral hepatitis is still under investigation. The major cause of parenteral iron overload is that many clinicians prescribe prolonged blood transfusions without considering that the process is gradually inducing iron overload in the patient. If chelation therapy is begun at the initiation of RBC transfusion therapy, the complications of iron overload can be successfully avoided.

REFERENCES

1. Bacon BR. Causes of iron overload. *N Engl J Med.* 1992; 326:126–127.
2. Bassett ML, Halliday JW, Ferris RA, Powell LW. Diagnosis of hemochromatosis in young subjects: predictive accuracy of biochemical screening tests. *Gastroenterology.* 1984;87:628–633.
3. Bassett ML, Halliday JW, Powell LW. Value of hepatic iron measurements in early hemochromatosis and determination of the critical iron level associated with fibrosis. *Hepatology.* 1986;6:24–29.
4. Bonkovsky HL, Slaker DP, Bills EB, Wolf DC. Usefulness and limitations of laboratory and hepatic imaging studies in iron storage disease. *Gastroenterology.* 1990; 99:1079–1091.
5. Edwards CQ, Griffen LM, Goldgar D, Drummond C, Skolnick MH, Kushner JP. Prevalence of hemochromatosis among 11,065 presumably healthy blood donors. *N Engl J Med.* 1988;318:1355–1362.
6. Gordeuk V, Mukiibi J, Hasstedt SJ, et al. Iron overload in Africa: interaction between a gene and dietary iron content. *N Engl J Med.* 1992;326:95–100.
7. Nichols GN, Bacon BR. Hereditary hemochromatosis: pathogenesis and clinical features of a common disease. *Am J Gastroenterol.* 1989;84:851–862.
8. Niederau C, Fischer R, Sonnenberg A, Stremmel W, Trampisch HJ, Strohmeyer G. Survival and causes of death in cirrhotic and in noncirrhotic patients with primary hemochromatosis. *N Engl J Med.* 1985;313:1256–1262.
9. Olynyk J, Hall P, Sallie R, Reed W, Shilkin K, MacKinnon M. Computerized measurement of iron in liver biopsies: a comparison with biochemical iron measurement. *Hepatology.* 1990;12:26–30.
10. Sallie RW, Reed WD, Shilkin KB. Confirmation of the efficacy of hepatic tissue iron index in differentiating genetic haemochromatosis from alcoholic liver disease complicated by alcoholic haemosiderosis. *Gut.* 1991;32: 207–210.
11. Summers KM, Halliday JW, Powell LW. Identification of homozygous hemochromatosis subjects by measurement of hepatic iron index. *Hepatology.* 1990;12:20–25.
12. Tavill AS, Bacon BR. Hemochromatosis: iron metabolism and the iron overload syndromes. In: Zakim D, Boyer TD, eds. *Hepatology: A Textbook of Liver Disease.* 2nd ed. Philadelphia, Pa: WB Saunders Co; 1990: 1273–1299.

114
Choledochal Cysts
STUART SHERMAN

Choledochal cysts are uncommon anomalies of the biliary tree manifested by cystic dilation of the intrahepatic or extrahepatic ducts. Some authors[1,2] recommend that these anomalies be named bile duct cysts to emphasize that the dilation is not confined to the choledochus. Although Vater and Ezler are often credited with the first description of this finding in 1723, Douglas reported the first well-documented case in 1852.[3] Since that time, more than 3000 cases have been reported worldwide.[3,4] Conservative management in symptomatic patients is associated with significant morbidity and an almost uniformly fatal outcome. With appropriate surgical management, the vast majority of patients have gratifying long-term results.

EPIDEMIOLOGY

Choledochal cysts account for approximately one in 13,000 hospital admissions in the United States.[4] The exact incidence remains unknown, since many cases go unreported or undiagnosed.[5] However, worldwide estimates of incidence range from 1:13,000 to 1:2,000,000.[6] There is a female preponderance of 3:1,[3,7] as well as a predilection for Oriental races.[6] Since choledochal cysts have been observed in fetuses and neonates, they are generally considered congenital in origin.[8,9] However, choledochal cysts have been observed to develop in adulthood as well. Perhaps it is more consistent to say that affected patients have a propensity for the development of cysts.[10] Choledochal cysts are said to be primarily of concern to pediatricians and pediatric surgeons. In Flannigan's review[3] of 820 cases, 60% were diagnosed by age 10 and only 23% after age 40. However, Robertson and Raine[11] reported that 62% of their patients presented as adults. Similarly, in another series[4] choledochal cysts were diagnosed in 8 of 13 (62%) patients older than 18 years. The familial nature of choledochal cysts remains uncertain. One Japanese study suggested that they are inherited as an X-linked dominant or an autosomal dominant trait with relatively low penetrance.[12]

PATHOGENESIS

The pathogenesis of choledochal cysts remains a matter of debate and speculation. As already noted, choledochal cysts are generally considered congenital, since they occur in fetuses and neonates. Yotsuyanagi[13] postulated that there is a differential abnormality in biliary epithelial proliferation when the primitive bile ducts are still solid. Canalization of the duct then results in an abnormally dilated segment at the site of more active cellular proliferation (proximally) and a more normal or somewhat stenotic distal portion. Distal obstruction and weakness of the duct wall, either congenital or acquired, may be required to form a choledochal cyst.[14,15] Kusunoki and associates[15] suggested that intrinsic autonomic dysfunction is one of the causes of cyst formation. These investigators found a significant reduction of postcholinergic cell bodies in the narrow portion of the cyst wall compared to the dilated segment. Babbitt and associates[16] suggested that choledochal cysts arise because of an anomalous pancreaticobiliary junction (Fig. 114–1). They postulated that an unusually long common channel resulted in an extraduodenal union of the common bile duct and pancreatic duct and the loss of the normal sphincteric mechanism at the pancreaticobiliary junction. They further hypothesized that the absence of a functional sphincter would promote free reflux of pancreatic exocrine secretions into the biliary tree (this direction is favored because the pancreatic duct pressure is greater than the common duct pressure), with resultant inflammation, epithelial destruction, and obstruction and dilation

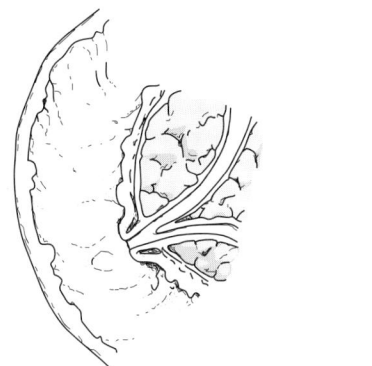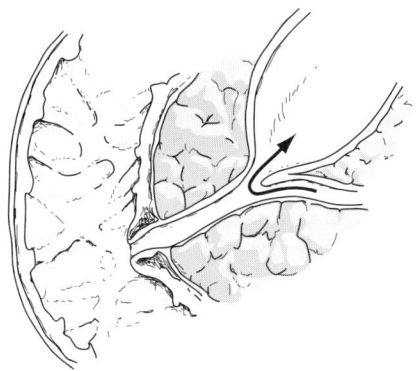

FIGURE 114–1. The normal anatomy *(left)* contrasted with the anomalous pancreaticobiliary junction *(arrow)* believed to be responsible for free reflux of pancreatic enzymes and choledochal cyst formation. (Modified from O'Neill JA. Choledochal cysts. *Curr Probl Surg.* 1992;29:365–410 with permission.)

of the bile duct.[17] In support of this theory is the frequent finding of a high amylase content in the biliary cyst aspirate and the demonstration of an anomalous pancreaticobiliary ductal union in 33% to 83% of patients with choledochal cysts.[14,18–20] Nonetheless, this theory does not necessarily explain the cause of types II, III, and V choledochal cysts (see below), which do not have an anomalous pancreaticobiliary union.[21,22] Chronic inflammation (due to reflux of pancreatic enzymes) may contribute to the increased incidence of cholangiocarcinoma and carcinoma of the gallbladder in these patients. The angle of the pancreaticobiliary union and the degree and length of the stenosis above the junction appear important in determining whether the extrahepatic dilation is cylindrical or cystic.[19] Ito and colleagues[23] emphasized the possibility that obstruction at the "narrow segment" (rather than reflux of pancreatic juice through the anomalous pancreaticobiliary junction), established in fetal life, is responsible for choledochal cyst formation. Interestingly, Suda and colleagues[24] found that the stenotic segment distal to the cyst was a branch of the ventral pancreatic duct. Thus, it appears that multiple factors may be important in the development of choledochal cysts, but in general a congenital predisposition seems necessary.

CLASSIFICATION

The classification scheme of Todani et al[25] is used most often, expanding on the earlier proposal of Alonso-Lej et al[26] by including intrahepatic cysts and further subdividing extrahepatic disease (Fig. 114–2). Type I cysts, which involve only the extrahepatic biliary tree, are the most common form, accounting for 80% to 90% of all choledochal cysts.[4] In this form of the anomaly, the cystic duct generally enters the choledochal cyst, and the right and left hepatic ducts and the intrahepatic ducts are normal in size. Type I is subdivided into type I A, cystic dilation of the common bile duct; type I B, focal segmental common duct dilation; and type I C, fusiform choledochal dilation. Type II cysts are extrapancreatic bile duct diverticula and make up 2% of reported cases.[14] Type III cysts, accounting for 1.4% to 5% of cases, are choledochoceles (Fig. 114–3) and most often involve only the intraduodenal part of the common bile duct but occasionally the intrapancreatic portion. An anatomic classification of type III cysts has been proposed (Fig. 114–4).[27] In the most common variety (type A, 67% of cases), the ampulla opens into the choledochocele, which, in turn, communicates with the duodenum via another small opening. This variety has been further subclassified as type A1 if there is a common opening of the pancreatic and common bile ducts into the cyst (33%), as type A2 if these openings are distinct (4%), and as type A3 if the choledochocele is small and entirely intramural (25%). In the less common variety (Type B, 21% of cases), the ampulla opens directly into the duodenum, with the choledochocele communicating only with the distal common duct.[27] Type IV cysts are subdvided into type IV A, multiple intrahepatic and extrahepatic cysts, and type IV B, multiple extrahepatic cysts. Type IV A cysts account for approximately 19% of reported cases, whereas type IV B cysts are much less common.[28] Finally, the type V cyst (Fig. 114–5), or Caroli's disease, consists of either single or

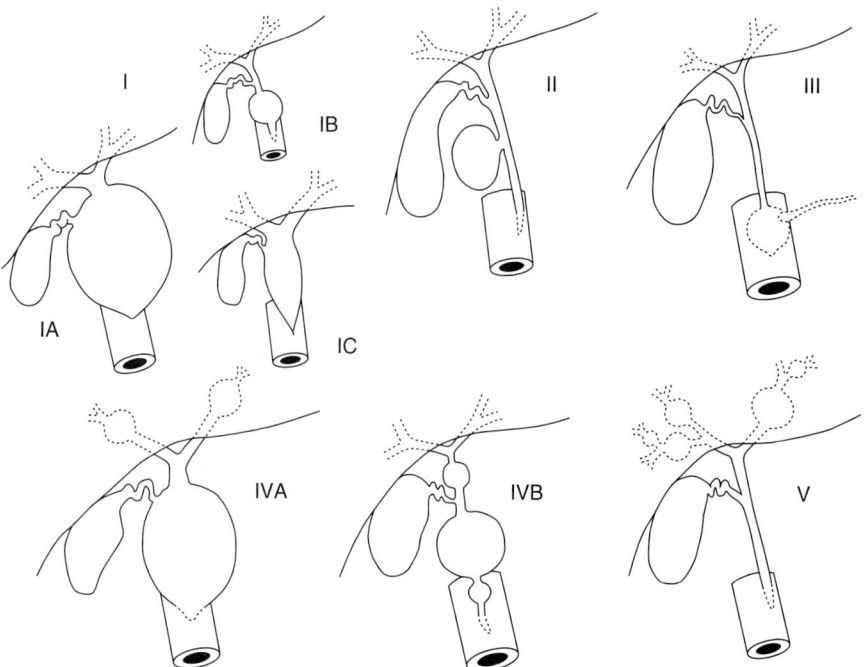

FIGURE 114-2. Classification scheme of choledochal cysts suggested by Todani et al. (Modified from Savader SJ, Benenati JF, Venbrux AC, et al. Choledochal cysts: classification and cholangiographic appearance. *AJR.* February 1991;156:328.)

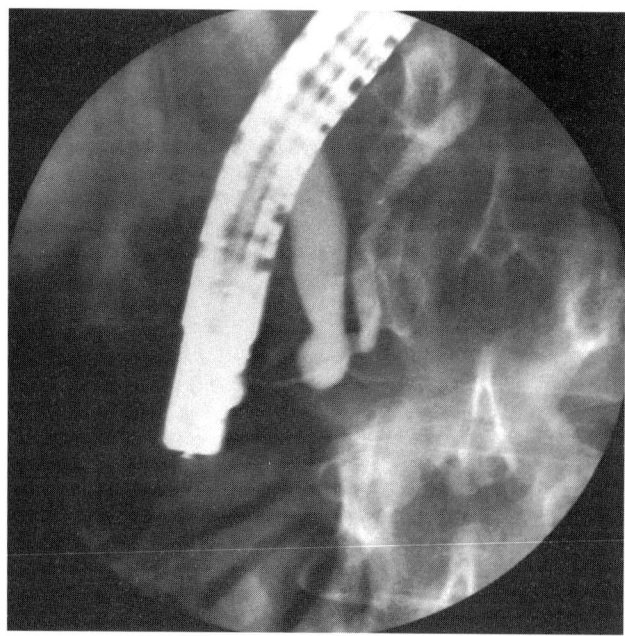

FIGURE 114-3. Choledochocele (type III choledochal cyst) demonstrated by endoscopic retrograde cholangiopancreatography.

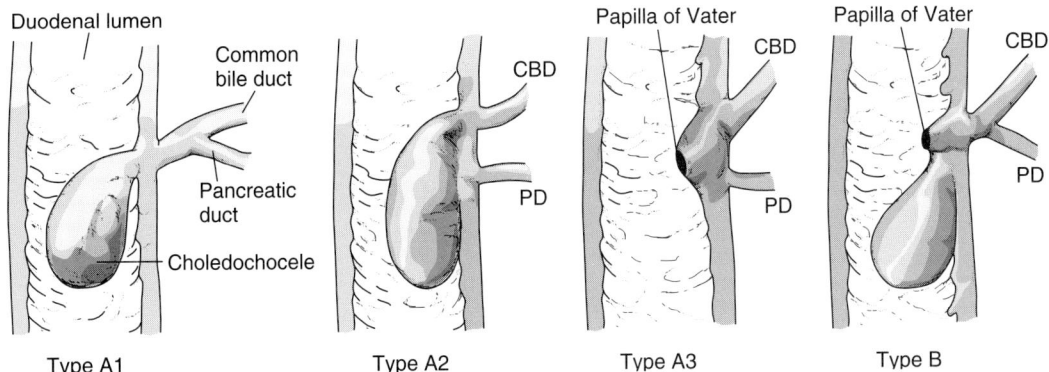

FIGURE 114–4. Proposed classification of type III choledochal cysts. In type A choledochoceles, the ampulla opens into a cyst that, in turn, empties into the duodenum via a separate opening. Type A choledochoceles may be subclassified as type A1 if there is a common opening of the pancreatic and common duct into the cyst, as type A2 if these openings are distinct, and as type A3 if the choledochocele is small and entirely intramural. In type B choledochoceles, the ampulla empties directly into the duodenum and the cyst represents a diverticulum of the distal common bile duct protruding into the duodenal lumen. CBD = common bile duct, PD = pancreatic duct. (Modified from Sarris GE, Tsang D. Choledochocele: case report, literature review and a proposed classification. *Surgery.* 1989;105:408–414 with permission.)

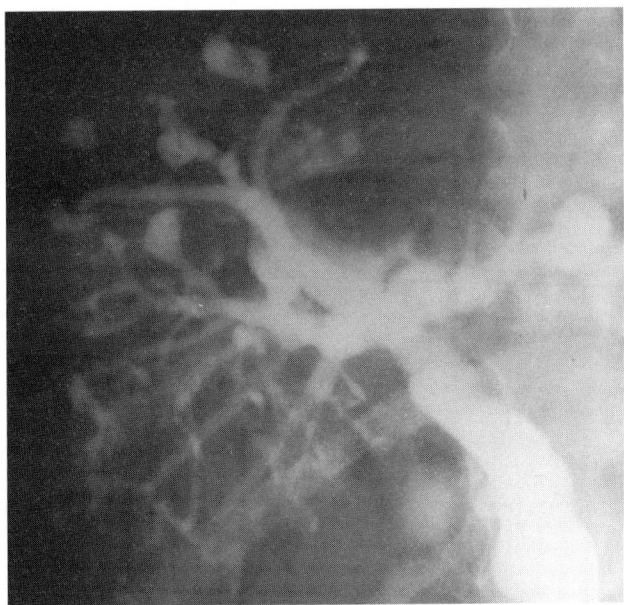

FIGURE 114–5. Endoscopic retrograde cholangiopancreatography demonstration of Caroli's disease (type V choledochal cyst).

multiple intrahepatic cysts. This is a rare disorder, with less than 200 reported cases.[29] This form of cystic disease within the liver communicates with the biliary system as opposed to fibrocystic disease in which cysts filled with bile do not.[22]

PATHOLOGY

The cyst wall varies in size from a few millimeters to 1 cm in thickness and consists of dense collagenous connective tissue with occasional elastic fibers and smooth muscle bundles.[14,30] In general, a complete epithelial lining is absent; however, scattered cuboidal or columnar cells are found (Fig. 114–6).[31] An inflammatory reaction may be present.[30] In addition, pericystic inflammation and cholangitis are frequently seen. In contrast to the other types of choledochal cysts, type III cysts are lined by either duodenal or bile duct mucosa.[32] The finding of biliary mucosal lining suggests that some choledochoceles may represent diverticula of the

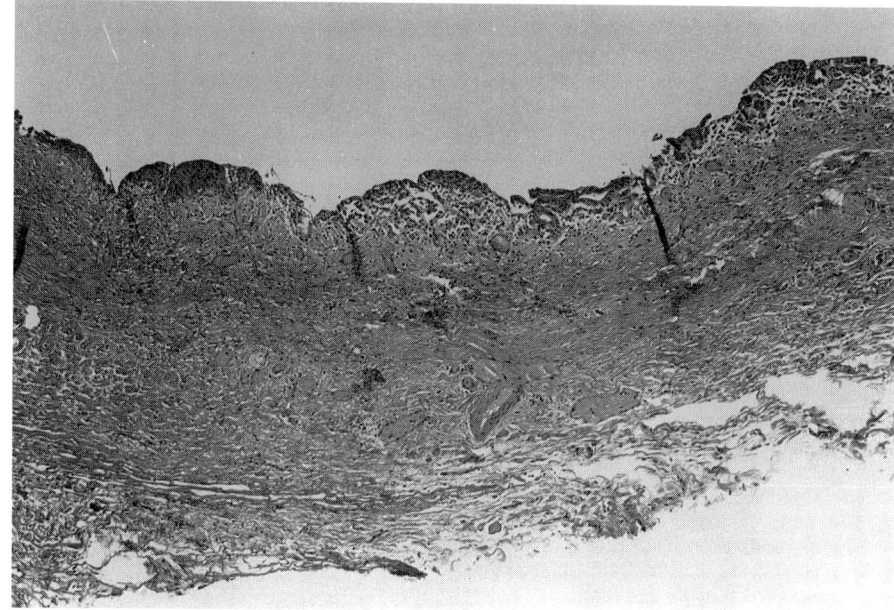
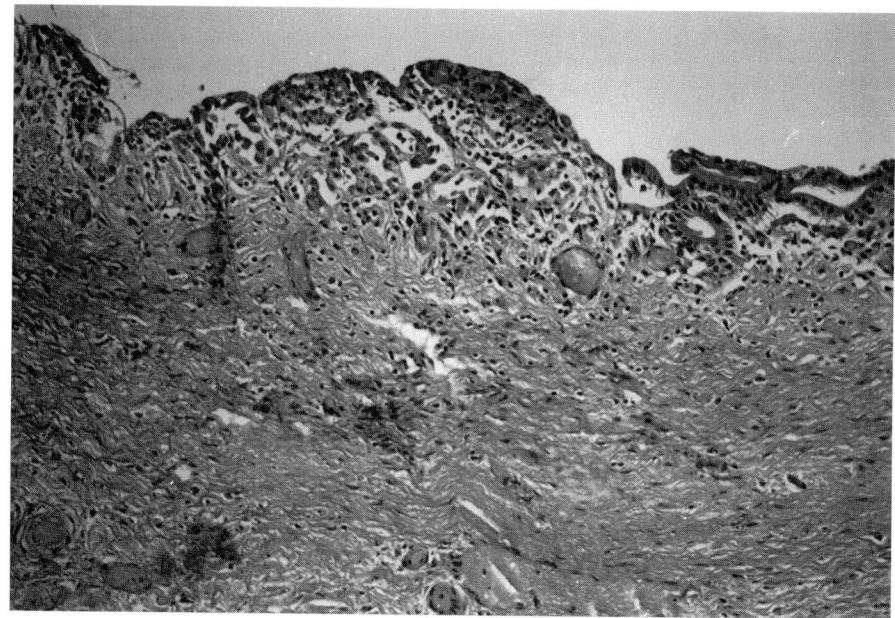

FIGURE 114-6. **A,** Histologic section of the wall of a choledochal cyst. The wall is composed of dense connective tissue with absence of a complete epithelial lining. Scattered cuboidal cells are seen. Occasional chronic inflammatory cells are present particularly in denuded areas (H&E original magnification × 65). **B,** High-power image of **A**. (H&E original magnification × 150).

distal common bile duct, whereas the presence of duodenal mucosa lining the choledochocele suggests that the lesion is in reality a duplication cyst, whether it exists within the wall of the duodenum or the head of the pancreas.[22] The capacity of the cyst may vary from a few milliliters to 8 L.[33] Interestingly, the gallbladder in patients with choledochal cysts is usually normal histologically. The liver biopsy findings are abnormal in up to 60% of patients, demonstrating biliary cirrhosis, biliary atresia, or portal fibrosis.[34]

CLINICAL FEATURES

The classic triad of right upper quadrant pain, jaundice, and abdominal mass occurs in only 13% to 62% of patients.[3,26,28] In Yamaguchi's re-

TABLE 114–1. PRESENTING SYMPTOMS IN TWO LARGE CHOLEDOCHAL CYST SERIES

Author	Number of Patients	Jaundice	Mass	Pain	Triad
Flannigan[3]	740	474	429	407	281
Yamaguchi[28]	1433	649	525	729	151
TOTAL	2173	1123 (52%)	954 (44%)	1136 (52%)	432 (20%)

view[28] of 1433 patients, 51% of patients had abdominal pain, 45% had jaundice, and 37% had an abdominal mass (Table 114–1). Similarly, Flannigan[3] reported jaundice in 64%, abdominal mass in 58%, and abdominal pain in 55% of 740 patients. Less common symptoms include fever, nausea, vomiting, acholic stool, pruritus, and weight loss.[5] In infancy, jaundice alone is the most common presenting finding, and the diagnosis of choledochal cyst disease must be considered in infants with high unexplained direct bilirubin.[14] Rarely, bile peritonitis may be the initial presentation in neonates.[26] Pancreatitis has been reported in association with all types of extrahepatic choledochal cysts, but most commonly with the choledochocele (type III).[31] In Flannigan's series,[3] the duration of symptoms prior to diagnosis was less than 5 months in 52%, 5 months to 5 years in 26%, and more than 5 years in 22%. Presumably, with the improved diagnostic capabilities that are currently available, more symptomatic patients will be discovered at an early stage.

DIAGNOSIS

Preoperative diagnosis requires a high index of suspicion. There is evidence suggesting that failure to consider choledochal cysts preoperatively is associated with poor surgical results and increased morbidity and mortality.[30,35] A variety of imaging modalities are available for assessing patients for suspected choledochal cysts. Ultrasound, computed tomography (CT), magnetic resonance imaging (MRI), technetium Tc 99m hepatobiliary scanning, endoscopic retrograde cholangiopancreatography (ERCP), and percutaneous transhepatic cholangiography (PTC) have been reported to be of benefit.[4,35–41] CT and ultrasound (Fig. 114–7,A and B) can be very helpful in demonstrating a choledochal cyst; however, occasionally a biliary origin cannot be confirmed for a cystic structure in the right upper quadrant,[36] and details such as exact ductal location, cyst morphologic features, and complicating features (e.g., stones, strictures) may not be clearly demonstrated with these modalities.[4,36] For example, in one study, 12 of 15 patients with choledochal cysts were accurately diagnosed through the use of ultrasound, but in three patients the technique was misleading.[42] Several authors have suggested that ultrasound should be the first diagnostic test performed and that interventional techniques are indicated only when this modality fails to accurately detail the lesion.[31,37]

The "classic" scintigraphic appearance of a choledochal cyst has been reported to be an early photon-deficient area that "fills in" on later (>2 hours) images.[43,44] However, Camponovo and colleagues[35] noted early appearance of cyst activity (within 1 hour) in 7 of 12 patients. In other cases, delayed images (up to 24 hours) were necessary to see cyst filling, particularly in jaundiced patients.[14,35] Unfortunately, cyst activity may not be demonstrable, and the anatomic detail may be insufficient for complete preoperative evaluation.[4]

The gold standard for choledochal cyst diagnosis is direct cholangiography. Although ERCP (Fig. 114–7C) and PTC are invasive, they can (usually) thoroughly assess the cyst anatomy, site of biliary origin, extent of intrahepatic and extrahepatic disease, and associated biliary tract anomalies and disease and shed light on possible therapeutic intervention, either definitive or for complications (e.g., cholangitis) pending surgical therapy. Savader and colleagues[4] used PTC to confirm the diagnosis of choledochal cyst disease in 13 of 13 patients. Seven patients had type I cysts (type I A, two; type I B, one; type I C, four), one had a type II cyst, four had type IV A cysts, and one had a type V cyst. Associated hepatobiliary disease was seen in six patients, including cholelithiasis (n=3), choledocholithiasis (n=2), common bile duct strictures (n=2), intrahepatic bile duct strictures (n=2), pancreatic duct strictures (n=1; contrast material refluxed into the pancreatic duct), intrahepatic abscesses (n=1), and cystolithiasis (n=1). Bile was cultured in each patient to aid in antibiotic selec-

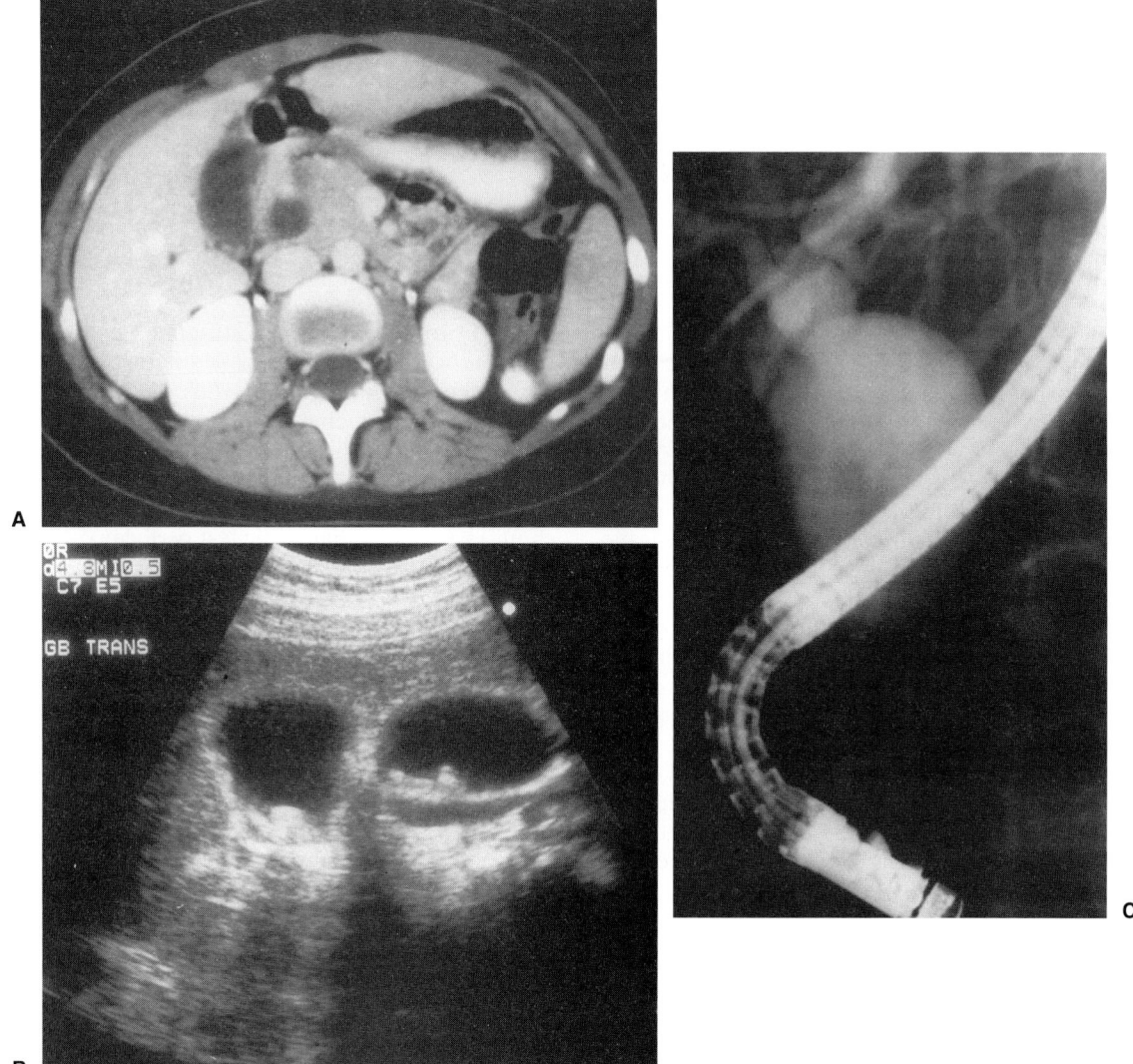

FIGURE 114–7. **A,** Computed tomography scan of a type I choledochal cyst. **B,** Abdominal ultrasound from same patient demonstrating a choledochal cyst and gallbladder containing stones. **C,** Type I choledochal cyst (containing stones) demonstrated by endoscopic retrograde cholangiopancreatography.

tion. In 11 patients, percutaneous biliary drainage procedures were successfully performed preoperatively. There were only two minor complications related to percutaneous intervention. These authors prefer preoperative percutaneous biliary drainage for several reasons:

1. Drainage relieves biliary obstruction with subsequent improvement in liver function and patients' symptoms.
2. Operative time is decreased because the biliary drains make the operation technically easier. The stents afford the surgeon physical landmarks that are easily palpated in patients with distorted and confusing anatomy. Decreased operative time may result in a lower surgical morbidity.
3. Postoperatively, the stents prevent obstruction of the hepaticojejunal anastomosis (see below).
4. Access to the biliary system is maintained for evaluation of healing or postoperative complications such as anastomotic breakdown or leaking.

In contrast to PTC, ERCP allows for detailed evaluation of the pancreatic duct and the pancreaticobiliary union. Pancreatic ductal abnormalities are common in patients with choledochal cysts. In one series five of six patients studied by ERCP were found to have abnormal pancreatographic findings consisting of pancreatic ductal stones (n=2), markedly dilated pancreatic duct (n=3), and an abnormal pancreaticobiliary junction (n=2).[45] Flannigan[46] points out that choledochal cyst patients are not only at risk for biliary tract carcinoma but also pancreatic duct carcinoma. Thus, pancreatography appears important in preoperative staging. Endoscopic techniques have also been applied for the management of patients with type III cysts (choledochocele).[39,47]

Intraoperative cholangiography should be performed to confirm the diagnosis (particularly in those patients not evaluated by cholangiographic techniques preoperatively) and to reveal unsuspected type II or III cysts in patients with biliary tract symptoms who have an acalculous gallbladder at the time of cholecystectomy.[14] Laboratory testing has not been shown to be helpful in establishing the diagnosis.[48]

COMPLICATIONS

The complications associated with choledochal cysts are summarized in Table 114-2. Stone formation within the choledochal cyst (cystolithiasis) is the most frequent complication, occurring in up to 70% of adult patients.[49] The gallbladder is commonly acalculous.[50] Cholangitis (with or without associated liver abscesses) resulting from bile duct obstruction with stasis is a common complication of choledochal cysts. Although cystolithiasis might be expected to predispose to cholangitis and pancreatitis, these entities occur just as commonly in patients with choledochal cysts but no stones.[49] In contrast, Nagorney and associates[51] suggest that acute pancreatitis is related to the anomalous pancreaticobiliary union and ductal stones. In their series, six of seven patients with pancreatitis had cystolithiasis and anomalous pancreaticobiliary anatomy. These authors hypothesize that pancreatic duct or common channel obstruction by a stone could precipitate pancreatitis. Early series suggested that cholangitis was the leading cause of death in patients who underwent the operation and in those who did not.[3] Secondary biliary cirrhosis occurs in proportion to the duration and degree of obstruction.[14] Regression of the biliary cirrhosis has been reported in a child after cyst drainage.[52] As already noted, pancreatitis has been reported in association with all types of extrahepatic choledochal cysts, but most commonly with the choledochocele (type III).[31] Among the 48 cases of type III cysts reported in the English language literature through 1987, pancreatitis occurred in 18 (38%).[27]

Carcinoma (adenocarcinoma in more than 90%) is a well-recognized complication of choledochal cysts. Bile stagnation, continual pancreatic reflux, and related chronic ulceration and regeneration of the cyst epithelium are thought to be potential etiologic factors.[53] Interestingly, Reveille and associates[54] reported an increase in secondary bile acids (most were unconjugated) within the cyst fluid from a patient with choledochal cysts previously treated by cholecystoduodenostomy. The authors attribute this change in bile acid composition to bacterial overgrowth and speculate that the change caused the patient's biliary epithelial metaplasia and could be a factor in carcinogenesis.

Tumors may develop anywhere within the biliary tree, but more than 50% occur within the cyst itself.[46] Carcinomas are most common in type I and type IV cysts but have also been reported in association with Caroli's disease (type V) and choledochoceles (type III).[49,55-57] The incidence is estimated at 2.5% to 17% compared to a 0.012% to 0.48% occurrence in the general population without choledochal cysts.[46,54] However, the lifetime risk for the individual may be as high as 50% if nonresectional surgery has been performed.[9] The incidence of carcinoma varies with the age at the initial appearance of symptoms. A child with a choledochal cyst that appears before 10 years of age carries a minimum risk (0.7%) of subsequent malignant degeneration compared to a patient in the second decade (6.8%) and older (14.3%).[58] In Flannigan's review[46] of 24 cases of malignancy in 955 patients with cysts, 50% had the cancer diagnosed at a mean time of 4 years after an internal drainage

---

TABLE 114-2. COMPLICATIONS OF CHOLEDOCHAL CYSTS

Cystolithiasis (intrahepatic and extrahepatic)
Cholangitis with or without liver abscess
Biliary cirrhosis
Acute pancreatitis
Carcinoma (gallbladder, bile duct, pancreas, duodenum)
Portal hypertension
Bile peritonitis (cyst rupture)
Pseudoaneurysm

procedure (rather than excision) was performed. Primary excision of the cyst might be expected to reduce the risk of bile duct cancer not only by removing the most vulnerable portion of the mucosa but also by providing better biliary drainage and preventing reflux of pancreatic juice.[49] However, hepatobiliary malignancy is not completely prevented by cyst excision.[51]

Preoperative diagnosis of carcinoma is very rare. The prognosis is poor, as the cancer is usually unresectable for cure because of extensive local or regional spread or multicentricity.[51]

Patients may develop portal hypertension, either due to portal vein compression by the cyst or secondary to biliary cirrhosis.[14] Cyst rupture may occur (resulting in bile peritonitis) either spontaneously, following trauma, or even during delivery in the pregnant patient.[14,59] Pseudoaneurysm with hematobilia complicating a choledochal cyst has been reported.[60]

TREATMENT

Conservative management in symptomatic patients is associated with a very high morbidity and an almost universally fatal outcome. Attar and Obeid[61] reported that 21 of 22 (95%) patients treated medically for choledochal cysts died of cyst rupture with bile peritonitis, cholangitis, or complications of secondary biliary cirrhosis. Similarly, Tsardakas and Robnett[62] stated that 29 of 30 patients treated by nonsurgical therapy died from complications of their disease. Because of the poor outcome associated with medical management and the significant risk of malignancy, surgery has become the recommended treatment.

In the past, cystoenterostomy (Fig. 114–8) represented the standard surgical procedure, since excision was felt to carry a prohibitive morbidity and mortality.[63] In 1959, Alonso-Lej and associates[26] reported a 15% to 40% mortality for operative removal of choledochal cysts. However, the operative mortality of total cyst excision steadily declined during the ensuing 15 years.[64] Simple drainage operations were largely abandoned because of the unacceptably high rate of anastomotic strictures, the major risk of recurrent cholangitis and the liability of the late occurrence of a malignant growth in the cyst.[64]

Currently, the surgical procedure of choice (when technically feasible) in the elective setting is total cyst and gallbladder excision followed by reconstruction of the extrahepatic biliary tree (Figs. 114–8 and 114–9).[65] In Flannigan's re-

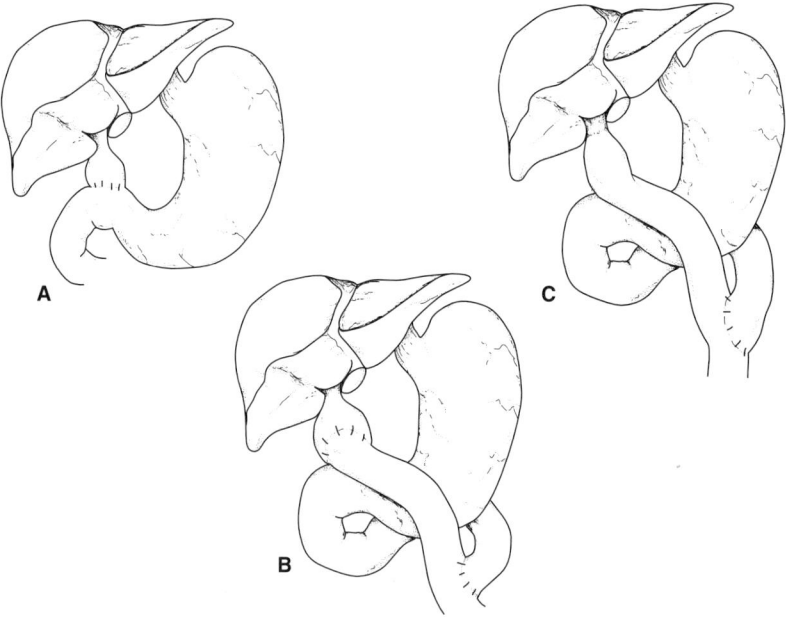

FIGURE 114–8. Surgical management of type I, II, and IV choledochal cysts **A,** Choledochocystoduodenostomy. **B,** Roux-en-Y choledochocystojejunostomy. **C,** Cyst excision with Roux-en-Y hepaticojejunostomy. This is the preferred method of operative management. (Modified from O'Neill JA. Choledochal cysts. *Curr Probl Surg.* 1992;29:365–410 with permission.)

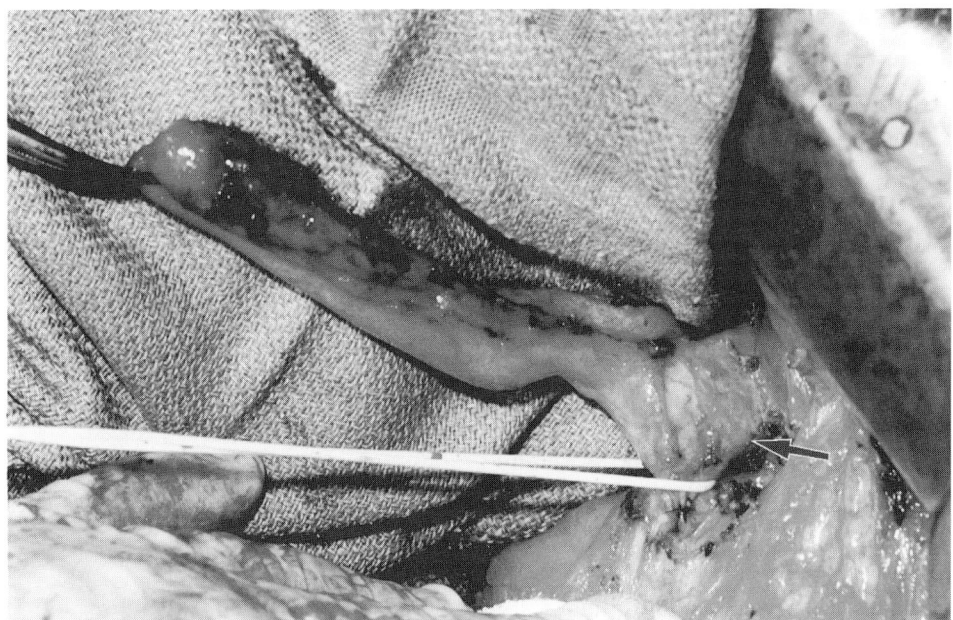

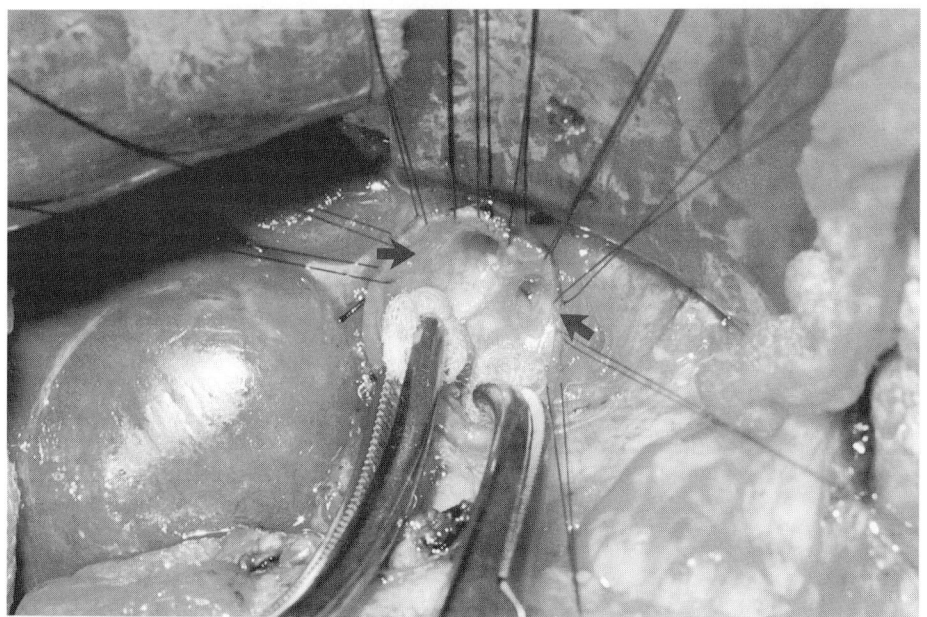

FIGURE 114-9. A, An operative photograph demonstrating a type I choledochal cyst *(arrow)*. (Courtesy of H.A. Reber, MD.) **B,** Following cyst excision, the opening of the right and left hepatic ducts are visualized *(arrows)*. (Courtesy of H.A. Reber, MD.)

view[3] (Table 114-3) of the operative treatment in 235 patients with type I choledochal cysts (mean follow-up, 5.2 years), cyst excision with Roux-en-Y hepaticojejunostomy (n=83) was associated with an 8% morbidity (includes recurrent pain, jaundice, stricture formation, or cholangitis), 7% mortality (includes operative deaths and deaths related to biliary disease or the operation performed), and 0% reoperation rate. Although the mortality in the 158 patients treated by internal drainage (Roux-en-Y choledochocystojejunostomy, choledochocystoduodenostomy, or choledochocystojejunostomy) was similar to the mortality in the group treated by excision (10% versus 7%), the morbidity (50% versus 8%) and reoperation rates (30% versus 0%) were sig-

TABLE 114-3. COMPLICATIONS OF VARIOUS SURGICAL PROCEDURES PERFORMED FOR TYPE I CHOLEDOCHAL CYSTS*

PROCEDURE	NUMBER OF PATIENTS	MORBIDITY	REOPERATION	MORTALITY
Excision	83	7 (8%)	0 (0%)	6 (7%)
Roux-en-Y choledochocystojejunostomy	53	18 (34%)	7 (13%)	9 (17%)
Choledochocystojejunostomy	12	6 (50%)	5 (42%)	1 (3%)
Choledochocystoduodenostomy	93	55 (58%)	35 (38%)	6 (5%)

*Data from Flannigan.[3]

nificantly higher. Similarly, in Powell and colleagues' review[66] of 188 patients treated surgically for type I choledochal cysts, the morbidity (2.4% versus 10%), reoperation rate (1.2% versus 22%), and mortality (2.2% versus 12%) were considerably greater in the internal drainage group. The unacceptably high morbidity and reoperation rates following internal drainage appear to be related to the abnormal cyst mucosa and the presence of an anomalous pancreaticobiliary union. Because the epithelium lining the cyst has large patches of ulceration bridged by chronically inflamed tissue, normal biliary mucosa is not available for the biliary enteric anastomosis unless the cyst is excised.[45] A 30% to 50% rate of stricture formation has been reported after choledochocystoenterostomy.[66] Cyst excision removes the diseased tissue and eliminates the reservoir for bile stasis and stone formation, thus considerably reducing the rate of cholangitis.[67] Moreover, because the pancreatic and bile ducts are disconnected, reflux of pancreatic secretions with associated complications no longer occurs in patients with an anomalous pancreaticobiliary union. Finally, although not totally eliminated, cyst excision appears to reduce the risk of developing carcinoma.[14]

Todani and associates[53] reported that patients who were undergoing internal drainage because of choledochal cysts developed carcinoma at a mean age of 35 years (mean interval between drainage and the detection of cancer was 10 years), 15 years earlier than those not operated on. The authors hypothesized that the anomalous pancreaticobiliary union allows for continued pancreatic juice reflux which can become activated by the influx of intestinal juice. Consequently, inflammatory changes of the cysts are accelerated and possibly result in carcinoma through ulceration regeneration or metaplasia of the epithelium of the retained cyst. Thus, these authors recommend early excision of the cyst retained after enteric drainage.

A variety of anastomotic[65,68] and dissection techniques[64] have been advanced, but based on the available literature, cyst excision with biliary tract reconstruction (usually Roux-en-Y hepaticojejunostomy) is the treatment of choice for patients with type I choledochal cysts.

Although limited follow-up data are available, the recommended therapy for type II choledochal cysts is excision usually with Roux-en-Y hepaticojejunostomy.[24,48,66]

Since type III choledochal cysts are so rare and long-term follow-up information sparse, there is no unified approach to management. Several authors[3,66] recommend cyst excision with reanastomosis of the pancreatic and bile duct to duodenal mucosa. Another approach would be to perform a sphincteroplasty to drain the cyst internally with or without diversion of the bile stream by Roux-en-Y choledochojejunostomy.[69] Choledochoceles that occupy a portion of the head of the pancreas can usually be excised or drained into the duodenum, but alternatively, the cyst may be drained into a Roux-en-Y limb of jejunum at the level of the head of the pancreas.[22] Rarely, a pancreaticoduodenectomy must be performed.

Recently, endoscopic therapy has been used to treat type III cysts.[39,47,48] Venu and associates[39] performed endoscopic sphincterotomy (n=5) or surgical sphincteroplasty (n=3) in eight patients with type III choledochal cysts and acute recurrent pancreatitis (n=5) or biliary colic and cholestatic jaundice (n=3). Seven of eight patients remained symptom free during a mean follow-up of 5 years (2 to 8 years). Similarly, Lopez and colleagues[48] reported symptomatic resolution in four patients treated by endoscopic sphincterotomy. Patient selection criteria for endoscopic treatment should include cyst size (large cysts are best treated surgically), anatomy of the common bile and pancreatic ducts, the suspicion of malignancy, and the overall condition of the patient.[48]

Type IV A choledochal cysts represent a management problem because of the need to provide free bile drainage from the intrahepatic cysts. Failure to achieve free drainage is associated with recurrent symptoms and a short survival.[2] Favorable results have therefore not been obtained by performing only choledochocystoenterostomy. Moreover, the risk that cancer may develop in the extrahepatic cyst following internal drainage is considerable. The current recommended therapy for patients with type IV A cysts is excision of the choledochal cyst with partial resection of the intrahepatic cyst and hepaticoenterostomy at the hilum with as wide a stoma as possible.[70] In reviewing the results of surgical therapy, Todani and associates[70] reported that five of eight patients treated by internal drainage developed late complications (cholangitis in three and cancer in two; mean follow-up time, 9.5 years) in contrast to only 6 of 32 patients (cholangitis in six; mean follow-up time, 5.5 years) treated by excision and hepaticoenterostomy. Interestingly, patients with cylindrical (in contrast to cystic) intrahepatic dilation experienced regression of the dilation following excision of the extrahepatic cyst, suggesting that the intrahepatic disease is secondary to the extrahepatic disease and not congenital. Forty-two percent of patients were found to have dilation isolated to the left lobe of the liver. Thus, left hepatic lobectomy (with excision of the choledochal cyst) has been recommended in some patients with cystic (not cylindrical) dilation confined to the left lobe of the liver.[70]

A limited number of patients with type IV B choledochal cysts have been treated. The recommended surgical approach is excision of the whole extrahepatic bile duct followed by hepaticoenterostomy at the porta hepatis.[25]

The course of Caroli's disease (type V choledochal cyst) is dominated by recurrent episodes of bacterial cholangitis. Prevention of such episodes is difficult. Transhepatic intubation and drainage of the biliary tree has been effective in a small number of patients.[71] Caroli's disease is most commonly associated with congenital hepatic fibrosis and transmitted as an autosomal recessive trait. In this situation the multifocal intrahepatic dilation is diffuse. In contrast, in the noninherited variety, the multifocal dilation is often confined to the left lobe of the liver.[72] Less than 20% of all reported cases are of the monolobar type.[29]

Patients with Caroli's disease and recurrent episodes of cholangitis are best managed surgically.[73] The anatomic configuration of the bile ducts determines the operative approach. In localized disease, partial hepatectomy is the procedure of choice, as it is often curative.[25] However, the initial absence of intrahepatic ductal dilation in other parts of the liver does not guarantee that dilation will not develop. Thus, these patients must be followed for life.[22] Partial hepatectomy should also be considered in the diffuse form, when the cystic dilation predominates in a part of the liver. Unfortunately, in such patients this therapy is usually difficult because of associated congenital hepatic fibrosis and portal hypertension.[72] Moreover, by the time these patients come to surgery, their bile ducts are often filled with sludge, stones, and mucous resulting from bile stasis and infection. Doty and Tompkins[73] recommend the following surgical approach: (1) remove all biliary debris, (2) perform biliary diversion (Roux-en-Y hepaticojejunostomy), and (3) place transhepatic stents for irrigation and future percutaneous access to the biliary tree. The transhepatic tubes are placed down a Roux-en-Y hepaticojejunostomy or brought out through the jejunum as a U-shaped tube. The patients irrigate these tubes with 20 to 30 ml of sterile saline twice a day to maintain patency and flush the biliary system. Persistent or frequent fevers suggest the need for cholangiography and tube exchange (usually every 3 to 6 months). Unfortunately, despite careful irrigation and transhepatic tube care, recurrent stones and biliary strictures recur. Most stones can be removed through the percutaneous approach via the transhepatic tract using standard stone baskets and balloons. Extracorporeal shock wave lithotripsy and a variety of other lithotripsy methods have also been used for intrahepatic stone management.[74] The strictures can be dilated through the transhepatic tube tract (using a variety of dilating catheters and Gruentzig balloon catheters), although the long-term success of this approach is not clear.[73] Alternatively, a permanent access hepaticojejunostomy allows for intermittent lavage of the affected biliary tree and endoscopic examination of the secondary and tertiary intrahepatic ducts.[75] Liver transplantation should be considered for patients with the diffuse form of disease without predominance of cysts in any part of the liver, complicated by severe recurrent bacterial cholangitis, and not amenable or responsive to more conservative surgical approaches.[67]

Because of the risk of cholangiocarcinoma in patients with Caroli's disease, careful surveillance of biliary strictures with cytologic evaluation and endoscopic biopsy seems prudent.[56,73] Although this approach may detect early cancers, the cure rate for these intrahepatic cholangiocarcinomas is dismal to date.[73]

TABLE 114–4. RECOMMENDED THERAPY FOR CHOLEDOCHAL CYSTS

Choledochal Cyst	Recommended Therapy
Type I	Cyst excision with Roux-en-Y hepaticojejunostomy
Type II	Excision usually with Roux-en-Y hepaticojejunostomy
Type III	Excision; sphincteroplasty with or without Roux-en-Y choledochojejunostomy; endoscopic sphincterotomy
Type IV A	Choledochal cyst excision with partial resection of the intrahepatic cyst and hepaticoenterostomy; left hepatic lobectomy (if isolated cystic dilation of the left intrahepatic ducts) and choledochal cyst excision
Type IV B	Excision of the entire extrahepatic bile duct with hepaticoenterostomy
Type V	Partial hepatectomy for localized disease; removal of debris, biliary diversion, and placement of a transhepatic stent or liver transplant for diffuse disease

Table 114–4 summarizes the recommended surgical therapies for choledochal cysts.

CONCLUSION

Choledochal cysts are uncommon anomalies of the biliary tree associated with a significant morbidity and a high risk for the development of a malignancy. Conservative management in symptomatic patients is almost uniformly fatal. Surgery is the recommended therapy. The operative procedure is dictated by the location of the cyst(s), but excision is preferred whenever technically feasible. Cyst excision removes the diseased tissue, eliminates the reservoir for bile stasis and stone formation, prevents pancreatic reflux, and significantly reduces the risk of developing carcinoma. With current methods of imaging and surgical management, the vast majority of patients with choledochal cysts can expect to have excellent long-term results, although observation and periodic intervention may be required.

REFERENCES

1. Nunez-Hoyo M, Lees CD, Hermann RE. Bile duct cysts: experience with 15 patients. *Am J Surg.* 1982;144:295–299.
2. Todani T, Narusue M, Watanabe Y, Tabuchi K, Okajima K. Management of congenital choledochal cyst with intrahepatic involvement. *Ann Surg.* 1978;187:272–280.
3. Flannigan DP. Biliary cysts. *Ann Surg.* 1975;182:635–643.
4. Savader SJ, Venbrux AC, Benenati JF, et al. Choledochal cysts: role of noninvasive imaging, percutaneous transhepatic cholangiography, and percutaneous biliary drainage in diagnosis and treatment. *J Vasc Interv Radiol.* 1991;2:379–385.
5. Olbourne NA. Choledochal cysts: a review of the cystic anomalies of the biliary tree. *Ann R Coll Surg Engl.* 1975;56:26–32.
6. Vanderpool D, Lane BW, Winter JW, Ettinger J. Choledochal cysts. *Surg Gynecol Obstet.* 1988;167:447–451.
7. Little KH, Loeb PM. Choledochal cysts. *South Med J.* 1989;82:255–258.
8. Dewbury KC, Aluwihare APR, Birch SJ, Freeman NV. Prenatal ultrasound demonstration of choledochal cyst. *Br J Radiol.* 1980;53:906–907.
9. Forbes A, Murray-Lyon IM. Cystic diseases of the liver and biliary tract. *Gut.* 1991;(suppl):S116–S122.
10. Witzleben CL. Cystic diseases of the liver. In: Zakim D, Boyer TD, eds. *Hepatology: A Textbook of Liver Disease.* 2nd ed. Philadelphia, Pa: WB Saunders Co; 1990:1395–1411.
11. Robertson JFR, Raine PAM. Choledochal cyst: a 33 year review. *Br J Surg.* 1988;75:799–801.
12. Iwama T, Iwata S, Murakami S, Ishida H, Mishima Y. Congenital bile duct dilatation: possibly a hereditary condition. *Jpn J Surg.* 1985;15:501–506.
13. Yotsuyanagi S. Contribution to etiology and pathology of idiopathic cystic dilatation of the common bile duct, with report of three cases. *Gann.* 1936;36:601–630.
14. Crittenden SL, McKinley MJ. Choledochal cyst: clinical features and classification. *Am J Gastroenterol.* 1985;80:643–647.
15. Kusunoki M, Saitoh N, Yamamura T, Fujita S, Takahashi T, Utsunomiya J. Choledochal cysts: oligoganglionosis in the narrow portion of the choledochus. *Arch Surg.* 1988;123:984–986.
16. Babbitt DP, Starshak RJ, Clemett AR. Choledochal cyst: a concept of etiology. *Am J Roentgenol Rad Ther.* 1973;119:57–62.
17. Weidmeyer DA, Stewart ET, Dodds WJ, Geenen JE, Vennes JA, Taylor AJ. Choledochal cysts: findings on cholangiopancreatography with emphasis on ectasia of the common channel. *AJR.* 1989;153:969–972.
18. Misra SP, Dwivedi M. Pancreatobiliary ductal union. *Gut.* 1990;31:1144–1149.
19. Todani T, Watanabe Y, Fujii T, Uemura S. Anomalous arrangement of the pancreatobiliary ductal system in patients with choledochal cysts. *Am J Surg.* 1984;147:672–676.
20. Ono J, Sakoda K, Akita H. Surgical aspect of cystic dilatation of the bile duct. *Ann Surg.* 1982;195:203–208.
21. Savader SJ, Benenati JF, Venbrux AC, Mitchell SE, Widlus DM, Cameron JL, Osterman FA. Choledochal cysts: classification and cholangiographic appearance. *AJR.* 1991;156:327–331.
22. O'Neill JA. Choledochal cysts. *Curr Probl Surg.* 1992;29:365–410.
23. Ito T, Ando H, Nagaya M, Sugito T. Congenital dilatation of the common bile duct in children: the etiologic significance of the narrow segment distal to the dilated common bile duct. *Z Kinderchir.* 1984;39:40–45.
24. Suda K, Matsumoto Y, Miyano T. Narrow duct segment distal to choledochal cyst. *Am J Gastroenterol.* 1991;86:1259–1263.

25. Todani T, Watanabe Y, Narusue M, Tabuchi K, Okajima K. Congenital bile duct cysts: classification, operative procedures, and review of thirty-seven cases including cancer arising from the choledochal cyst. *Am J Surg.* 1977;134:263–269.
26. Alonso-Lej F, Rever WB, Pessagno DJ. Congenital choledochal cyst, with a report of 2, and an analysis of 94 cases. *Int Abst Surg.* 1959;108:1–30.
27. Sarris GE, Tsang D. Choledochocele: case report, literature review and a proposed classification. *Surgery.* 1989; 105:408–414.
28. Yamaguchi M. Congenital choledochal cyst: analysis of 1,433 patients in the Japanese literature. *Am J Surg.* 1980;140:653–657.
29. Boyle MJ, Doyle GD, McNulty JG. Monolobar Caroli's disease. *Am J Gastroenterol.* 1989;84:1437–1444.
30. Spitz L. Choledochal cyst. *Surg Gynecol Obstet.* 1978; 147:444–452.
31. Mani S. Dilatation of the biliary ductal system: Choledochal cysts. *Mt Sinai J Med.* 1990;57:177–184.
32. Oldham KT, Hart MJ, White TT. Choledochal cysts presenting in late childhood and adulthood. *Am J Surg.* 1981;141:568–571.
33. Hand BH. Anatomy and embryology of the biliary tract and pancreas. In: Sivak MV, ed. *Gastroenterologic Endoscopy.* Philadelphia, Pa: WB Saunders Co; 1987;599–618.
34. Lilly JR. The surgical treatment of choledochal cyst. *Surg Gynecol Obstet.* 1979;149:36–42.
35. Camponovo E, Buck JL, Drane WE. Scintigraphic features of choledochal cyst. *J Nucl Med.* 1989;30:622–628.
36. Klein GM, Frost SS. Newer imaging modalities for the preoperative diagnosis of choledochal cyst. *Am J Gastroenterol.* 1981;76:148–152.
37. Jones SN, Lees WR, Russell RCG. Preoperative ultrasound assessment of choledochal cysts. *Acta Radiol.* 1989;30:35–37.
38. Araki T, Itai Y, Tasaka A. CT of choledochal cyst. *AJR.* 1980;135:729–734.
39. Venu RP, Geenen JE, Hogan WJ, et al. Role of endoscopic retrograde cholangiopancreatography in the diagnosis and treatment of choledochocele. *Gastroenterology.* 1984;87:1144–1149.
40. Shemesh E, Czerniak A, Klein E, Avigad I. The role of endoscopic retrograde cholangiopancreatography in the diagnosis and treatment of adult choledochal cyst. *Surg Gynecol Obstet.* 1988;167:423–426.
41. Thatcher BS, Sivak MV, Hermann RE, Esselstyn CB. ERCP in evaluation and diagnosis of choledochal cyst: report of five cases. *Gastrointest Endosc.* 1986;32:27–31.
42. Sherman P, Kolster E, Davies C, Stringer D, Weber J. Choledochal cysts: heterogeneity of clinical presentation. *J Pediatr Gastroenterol Nutr.* 1986;5:867–872.
43. Paramsothy M, Somasundram K. Technetium 99m-diethyl-IDA hepatobiliary scintigraphy in the pre-operative diagnosis of choledochal cysts. *Br J Radiol.* 1981; 54:1104–1107.
44. Huang MJ, Liaw TF. Intravenous cholescintigraphy using Tc-99m-labeled agents in the diagnosis of choledochal cyst. *J Nucl Med.* 1982;23:113–116.
45. Rattner DW, Schapiro RH, Warshaw AL. Abnormalities of the pancreatic and biliary ducts in adult patients with choledochal cysts. *Arch Surg.* 1983;118:1068–1073.
46. Flannigan DP. Biliary carcinoma associated with bile duct cysts. *Cancer.* 1977;40:880–883.
47. Siegel JH, Harding GT, Chateau F. Endoscopic incision of choledochal cysts (choledochocele). *Endoscopy.* 1981; 13:200–202.
48. Lopez RR, Pinson CW, Campell JR, Harrison M, Katon RM. Variation in management based on type of choledochal cyst. *Am J Surg.* 1991;161:612–615.
49. Hopkins NFG, Benjamin IS, Thompson MH, Williamson RCN. Complications of choledochal cysts in adulthood. *Ann R Coll Surg Engl.* 1990;72:229–235.
50. Matsumoto Y, Uchida K, Nakase A, Honjo I. Congenital cystic dilatation of the common bile duct as a cause of primary bile duct stone. *Am J Surg.* 1977;134:346–352.
51. Nagorney DM, McIlrath DC, Adson MA. Choledochal cysts in adults: clinical management. *Surgery.* 1984;96: 656–663.
52. Yeong ML, Nicholson GI, Lee SP. Regression of biliary cirrhosis following choledochal cyst drainage. *Gastroenterology.* 1982;82:332–335.
53. Todani T, Watanabe Y, Toki A, Urushihara N. Carcinoma related to choledochal cysts with internal drainage operations. *Surg Gynecol Obstet.* 1987;164:61–64.
54. Reveille RM, Steigmann GV, Everson GT. Increased secondary bile acids in a choledochal cyst: possible role in biliary metaplasia and carcinoma. *Gastroenterology.* 1990;99:525–527.
55. Pisano G, Donlon JB, Platell C, Hall JC. Cholangiocarcinoma in type III choledochal cyst. *Aust N Z J Surg.* 1991;61:855–857.
56. Dayton MT, Longmire WP, Tompkins RK. Caroli's disease: a premalignant condition? *Am J Surg.* 1983;145: 41–47.
57. Ozawa K, Yamada T, Matumoto Y, Tobe R. Carcinoma arising in a choledochocele. *Cancer.* 1980;45:195–197.
58. Voyles CR, Smadja C, Shands C, Blumgart LH. Carcinoma in choledochal cysts: age-related incidence. *Arch Surg.* 1983;118:986–988.
59. Treem WR, Hyams JS, McGowan GS, Sziklas J. Spontaneous rupture of a choledochal cyst: clues to diagnosis and etiology. *J Pediatr Gastroenterol Nutr.* 1991;13:301–306.
60. Eliscu EH, Weiss GM. Hematobilia due to a pseudoaneurysm complicating a choledochal cyst. *AJR.* 1988; 151:783–784.
61. Attar S, Obeid S. Congenital cyst of the common bile duct: a review of the literature and a report of the two cases. *Ann Surg.* 1955;142:289–295.
62. Tsardakas E, Robnett AH. Congenital cystic dilatation of the common bile duct: report of three cases, analysis of fifty-seven cases and review of the literature. *Arch Surg.* 1956;72:311–327.
63. Oweida SW, Ricketts RR. Hepatico-jejuno-duodenostomy reconstruction following excision of choledochal cysts in children. *Am Surg.* 1989;55:2–6.
64. Lilly JR. Total excision of choledochal cyst. *Surg Gynecol Obstet.* 1978;146:254–256.
65. Okada A, Nakamura T, Okumura K, Oguchi Y, Kamata S. Surgical treatment of congenital dilatation of bile duct (choledochal cyst) with technical considerations. *Surgery.* 1987;101:238–243.
66. Powell CS, Sawyers JL, Reynolds VH. Management of adult choledochal cysts. *Ann Surg.* 1981;193:666–674.
67. Tan KC, Howard ER. Choledochal cyst: a 14 year surgical experience with 36 patients. *Br J Surg.* 1988;75:892–895.
68. Gonzalez EM, Garcia IG, Pascual MH, et al. Choledochal cyst resection and reconstruction by biliary-jejuno-duodenal diversion. *World J Surg.* 1989;13:232–237.
69. Kyle S, Stubbs RS, Stewart RJ. Choledochal cyst: case reports and current concepts. *Aust N Z J Surg.* 1988;58: 855–858.
70. Todani T, Watanabe Y, Fujii T, Toki A, Uemura S, Koike

Y. Congenital choledochal cyst with intrahepatic involvement. *Arch Surg.* 1984;119:1038–1043.
71. Witlin LT, Gadacz TR, Zuidema GD, Kridelbaugh WW. Transhepatic decompression of the biliary tree in Caroli's disease. *Surgery.* 1982;91:205–209.
72. Benhamou JP. Congenital hepatic fibrosis and Caroli's syndrome. In: Schiff L, Schiff ER, eds. *Diseases of the Liver.* 6th ed. Philadelphia, Pa: JB Lippincott Co; 1987: 1461–1466.
73. Doty JE, Tompkins RK. Management of cystic diseases of the liver. *Surg Clin North Am.* 1989;69:285–295.
74. Lointier PH, Kauffmann PH, Francannet PH, Pezet D, Chipponi J. Management of intrahepatic Caroli's disease by extracorporeal shock wave lithotripsy. *Br J Surg.* 1990;77:987–988.
75. Barker EM, Kallideen JM. Caroli's disease: successful management using permanent-access hepaticojejunostomy. *Br J Surg.* 1985;72:641–643.

115

Liver Resection and Transplantation

STEFANO FAGIUOLI, AHMET GURAKAR,
TAREK HASSANEIN, HARLAN I. WRIGHT, and DAVID H. VAN THIEL

Although classically hepatology has been considered a medical rather than a surgical discipline, it is a fact that surgery currently plays a major role in the treatment of a number of hepatic diseases (Table 115–1).

As a result of its unique venous drainage, the liver can be surgically divided into eight segments. In addition, the liver has the ability to regenerate.[56] This latter feature allows a "normal" individual to undergo a 75% to 80% hepatectomy with a minimal surgical mortality of 1% to 5% if the surgery is performed by an experienced surgeon on an elective basis.[39,44] In contrast, when a resection is to be performed in a cirrhotic liver, the amount of liver that can be resected without precipitating a perioperative death declines rapidly.[3,24,46,58,88] A fascinating clinical paradox is that a total hepatic resection, namely orthotopic liver transplantation (OLT), can be performed in such cases with an 80% to 90% survival rate in patients with end-stage liver disease in whom any other hepatobiliary surgery would be contraindicated. Whenever either advanced liver disease or a metabolic dysfunction based on an enzyme deficiency isolated to the liver is no longer manageable with conventional medical therapy, liver transplantation represents an excellent life-prolonging therapeutic option.[36]

It is quite clear clinically that the severity of any underlying liver disease present in a patient anticipating a surgical procedure must be assessed accurately before the performance of the procedure.[12] Typically, a combination of clinical, biochemical, and imaging studies is used for this purpose. The most frequently used clinical criteria are those that define the individual patient's Child's class for cirrhosis and an evaluation of the presence, size, and appearance of any esophageal varices that might exist. In addition to the assessment of the severity of the confounding liver disease, the clinical status of other major organ systems, particularly the kidneys, heart, and lungs, must be ascertained in any patient with liver disease who is being considered for a surgical procedure.

Overall, the functional capacity of the liver as a whole can be assessed by the classic Child-Pugh score. If the clinician feels there is a need for a more precise quantitation of the functional reserve of the liver to predict the outcome of a hepatic resection in a patient with liver disease, the hepatic biotransformation capacity for exogenous and endogenous substances must be assessed. The evaluation of the biotransformation capacity of the liver is based on a determination of the capacity of the mixed function oxidase system to metabolize substrates. Antipyrine, aminopyrine, caffeine, and lidocaine clearance are the most frequently used substrates to assess microsomal (cytochrome P-450) activity of the liver.[60,71,96] In general, a low hepatic clearance of any of these substrates is indicative of poor he-

TABLE 115–1. INDICATIONS FOR HEPATIC RESECTION

1. Hepatic neoplasms
   a. Benign
      (1) Hepatocellular adenoma
      (2) Hemangioma
      (3) Focal nodular hyperplasia
      (4) Bile duct adenoma
      (5) Bile duct cystadenoma
      (6) Infantile hemangioendothelioma
      (7) Others: lipoma, myelolipoma
   b. Malignant
      (1) Primary malignant tumor
         (a) Hepatocellular carcinoma
         (b) Fibrolamellar carcinoma
         (c) Cholangiocarcinoma
         (d) Combined hepatocellular carcinoma and cholangiocarcinoma
         (e) Hemangioendothelioma
         (f) Hemangiosarcoma
         (g) Embryonal sarcoma
         (h) Squamous cell carcinoma
         (i) Hepatoblastoma (pediatric age)
         (j) Mesenchymal tumor (pediatric age)
      (2) Metastatic tumors
         (a) Colorectal cancer
         (b) Neuroendocrine tumors (gastrointestinal tract)
         (c) Others (contiguity or continuity)
2. Tumorlike lesions
   a. Cysts
   b. Bile duct hamartoma
   c. Mixed hamartoma
   d. Heterotopia
   e. Focal fatty change
   f. Pseudolipoma
   g. Inflammatory pseudotumor

patic function and therefore predictive of higher postoperative morbidity and mortality in a cirrhotic patient undergoing resectional surgery.

Morbidity rates and mortality after liver resection can also be correlated with the preoperative APACHE II score. It has been shown that a high score (>8) correlates with a postoperative morbidity of 80% and a mortality of 20%, compared to a morbidity rate of 34% and a mortality of 0% in patients with a low APACHE II score (<3).[23]

The most widely used biochemical method for assessing hepatic function is determination of the retention of indocyanine green (ICG) 15 minutes after it has been rapidly infused intravenously at a dose equal to 0.5 mg/kg.[28,65] The dye is removed from the circulation exclusively by the liver. It is not conjugated, and there is neither extrahepatic metabolism nor enterohepatic recirculation. It has been reported that with a 15-minute ICG retention of 0% to 10% of the infused load, two segments (or as much as 50%) of the liver can be resected safely in a subject with liver disease. With a 15-minute ICG retention of 11% to 20%, only one segment (or 15%) of the hepatic parenchyma can be resected safely. When the ICG retention at 15 minutes is above 20%, only a subsegmental (or wedge) resection can be performed safely. Even the latter becomes impossible when the retention of ICG at 15 minutes is above 30%. Less well, but more routinely, available measures of hepatic function used to assess surgical risk in patients with liver disease include the serum albumin level, serum bilirubin level, prothrombin time, and plasma factor V level. As a general principle, more than 80% of the liver can be dysfunctional before any of these parameters becomes abnormal as a consequence of a diffuse parenchymal disease. This principle is consistent with the empiric observation that a normal individual can undergo a 75% liver resection without experiencing a measurable alteration in hepatic function, as defined by these parameters.[93] This observation is particularly important when it is compared against the fact that death from hepatic failure is inevitable with a residual hepatic function of less than 12.5% to 15% of normal. Moreover, in the presence of clinical liver disease, a residual function of 12% to 15% of normal is usually sustained by a hepatic mass that is much greater than 12.5% to 15% of the normal hepatic mass. In such cases even a minor resection can be complicated by either considerable morbidity (hepatic decompensation) or death.

The ability to define the metabolic function of the liver quantitatively provides a rational means of assessing the perioperative risk of a patient. Specifically, whatever the hepatic mass may be, the residual functional activity is contained in this mass. Any resectional surgery that reduces the volume of the diseased liver below a mass containing 12.5% to 15% of normal hepatic function is doomed to cause death.

Several authors have focused on studies of the mitochondrial function of hepatocytes.[60,71,96] The phosphorylative activity of mitochondria is a necessary requirement for hepatic regeneration. Cytochrome a $(+a3)$ is an enzymatic complex (respiratory carrier) that plays a critical role in mitochondrial phosphorylation capacity. Measurement of cytochrome a $(+a3)$ content of mitochondria from liver biopsy specimens has been shown to be useful in assessing hepatic functional capacity. A reduction in cytochrome a $(+a3)$ within hepatocytes below a critical level of 0.5×10^{-10} mol/1 mg of protein is predictive of either a higher surgical morbidity or mortality.

In other studies, the hepatic mitochondrial redox state, reflected by hepatic ketone body ratio (KBR) (acetoacetate:β-hydroxybutyrate) was shown to vary in proportion to the blood glucose level after an oral glucose load. The KBR of arterial blood has been shown to correlate positively with the hepatic energy charge in jaundiced, hepatectomized, and shocked animals.[55,66] A redox tolerance index (RTI), based on a 100-fold cumulative enhancement of KBR relative to glucose level (100 × ΔKBR/ΔD-glucose) has been proposed as a method for assessing hepatic functional reserve. In cirrhotic patients, an RTI less than 1 (and even more specifically if less than 0.5) is predictive of very high risk for postoperative morbidity and mortality.[65,66]

LIVER RESECTION

The indications for hepatic resection include both benign and malignant primary tumors of the liver, isolated metastatic lesions, cysts, abscesses, and less frequently, focal nodular hyperplasia or inflammatory pseudotumor.

The initial preoperative assessment of a patient who is awaiting hepatic resection should include a careful history and physical examination of the patient, as well as a complete biochemical and hematologic investigation. If a tumor is either present or suspected, an extensive metastatic workup is mandatory. A mesenteric angiogram may be valuable in delineating a tumor mass or in defining any aberrant vasculature that may be present.

Several recent technologic developments have contributed to substantially improve patient survival after a major hepatic resection; these include intraoperative diagnostic ultrasound, which enables a clear identification and localization of hepatic mass(es) and their relationship with the adjacent biliary tree and blood vessels. Other new surgical tools include ultrasonic and microwave scalpels, infrared and argon coagulators, pressure jet dissectors, and recent modifications of conventional diathermy.[45,58,72,100] Perhaps a key factor in the increased safety of surgical procedures performed in cirrhotic and noncirrhotic patients is the management of patients by a team composed not only of surgeons but also of hepatologists, hematologists, nephrologists, microbiologists, and anesthesiologists. The combined skills of these specialists result in better overall identification and management of the many metabolic, biochemical, infectious, or systemic problems that occur in patients undergoing major hepatic surgery.

At present, the operative mortality for a major hepatic resection averages less than 10% (less than 2% to 5% in experienced hands) in noncirrhotic patients and declines to less than 4% (less than 1% in experienced hands) after a wedge or subsegmental resection. Cirrhotic patients with Child's class A can undergo as much as 50% hepatic resection and survive. A liver resection in an individual who is in Child's class B cannot exceed 25%, and patients with Child's C class cirrhotics can rarely, if ever, undergo a hepatic resection and survive.[8,24,34,39,88]

Cirrhotic patients anticipating hepatic surgery have an increased risk of postoperative morbidity because of their associated malnutrition, malabsorption, and underlying hepatic disease. The liver plays a key role in carbohydrate, fat, and protein metabolism and in vitamin storage. Nutritionally depleted patients have a significantly higher morbidity and mortality than do control patients after surgery.[37] Specifically, a reduction in total body potassium to a value less than 85% of normal or a reduction in the serum thyroxine-binding prealbumin level to a value below the normal limit appear to be predictive factors for an untoward postoperative outcome. Thus, measures to improve the nutritional status of cirrhotic patients prior to elective surgery are important in an effort to reduce the risk of a postoperative infection. In this regard, preoperative glycogen loading of the liver by means of a glucose infusion the evening and the morning before an elective surgical procedure, as well as multivitamin therapy, is advised.[37]

The absolute contraindications to liver resection other than a total hepatic resection in preparation for an immediate OLT are as follows:

1. Technical impossibility of preserving a sufficient arterial supply or venous drainage of the residual segment(s) to guarantee retention of sufficient hepatic function to maintain life
2. Inability of the residual hepatic mass to maintain minimal function required to sustain life
3. Invasion of either the inferior vena cava or the main trunk of the portal vein by a tumor
4. Extrahepatic spread of a hepatic tumor (primary or metastatic)

Essentially, the surgical options for hepatic resection can be divided into anatomic resections (lobectomy or segmentectomy) or nonanatomic resections (wedge or subsegmental resections). In Table 115–2 and Figure 115–1 the two more commonly used classification systems for describing hepatic resection are shown.

TABLE 115-2. TYPES OF LIVER RESECTION

	OPERATION	
SEGMENT EXCISED	COUINAUD	GOLDSMITH AND WOODBURNE
V, VI, VII, VIII	Right hepatectomy	Right lobectomy
II, III, IV	Left hepatectomy	Left lobectomy
IV, V, VI, VII, VIII	Right lobectomy	Extended right lobectomy (trisegmentectomy)
II, III	Left lobectomy	Left lateral segmentectomy
II, III, IV, V, VIII	Extended left hepatectomy	
Nonanatomic	Wedge resection	Wedge resection

HEPATOCELLULAR CARCINOMA

Hepatocellular carcinoma (HCC) is a malignant tumor of the liver that originates from hepatocytes. It accounts for about 90% of all primary malignant liver tumors.[14] A major clinical distinction that must be made prior to any resection of a hepatic tumor is whether the tumor arises in a normal or within a cirrhotic liver. Approximately 10% to 20% of individuals with cirrhosis eventually develop a primary hepatic malignancy. In Western countries, cirrhosis usually antedates the development of the tumor by a decade, whereas in Africa and Southeast Asia cirrhosis can occur either simultaneously or be absent. Overall, 60% to 70% of patients with HCC worldwide have cirrhosis.[24]

Grossly, the tumor can present either as a single nodular lesion with or without daughter tumors or as a diffuse hepatic lesion. The gross appearance of HCC may or may not correlate with its clinical presentation. Nonetheless, the extent of any surgical procedure and the subsequent outcome are influenced greatly by the size of the tumor. A curative hepatic resection can be performed safely only in carefully selected cirrhotic patients. Individuals with advanced, decompensated cirrhosis are not candidates for an extensive resection. The perioperative mortality of liver resections for HCC is determined by two factors: presence or absence of cirrhosis and the size of the required resection.[1] In a recent study, the operative mortality of a major hepatic resection was established to be 9.1%. It needs to be noted, however, that the reported operative mortality in a cirrhotic patient may be as high as 50%. For cirrhotic patients the actuarial 1-year survival rate after liver resection ranges between 55% and 85%, and the actuarial 3-year survival rate ranges between 26% and 58%.[8] In contrast, noncirrhotic patients have a 20% to 25% 5-year survival rate after liver resection for HCC, as compared to a rate of 4% to 8% in cirrhotic patients.[8,41] Tumor recurrence is the principal cause of late deaths and appears to be related to the presence of a high preoperative level of alpha-fetoprotein, the size of the tumor-free margin, and the presence or absence of vascular invasion by the tumor.[101] The results after liver resection for HCC are significantly better when intraoperative ultrasonography is employed to define the limits of the resection.[24] The complete removal of the intrahepatic portal vessels in which tumor is present is mandatory if tumor recurrence rates are to be minimized. Standard segmental resections can usually achieve this goal; for large lesions, however, the resection of a single segment or subsegment of the liver may not achieve this goal. An innovative method used to achieve this goal consists of clamping the portal pedicle and injecting dye into the portal vessel distal to the clamp, thereby staining the entire segment of the liver perfused by the injected portal vein.[72] With this method the critical margins of the intrahepatic portal venous unit can be identified easily and followed during the resection. Recently, it has been reported that in patients with tumors less than 4 cm in diameter the extent of the tumor-free margin is not a determinant of disease recurrence as long as some identifiable margin has been achieved. However, if the tumor exceeds 4 cm, a 1-cm tumor-free margin appears to be inadequate to achieve a cure.[101] If a wider resection is not feasible, aggressive adjuvant chemotherapy should be considered.

The presence of an intact peritumoral capsule appears to be the most reliable factor suggesting a cure after a liver resection for HCC.

The *fibrolamellar* (FLT) variant of HCC appears to be a distinct clinicopathologic entity. This indolent, monofocal, well-capsulated lesion is almost exclusively found in young adults (less than 25 years old), the majority of whom are women who are cirrhosis free. This tumor ac-

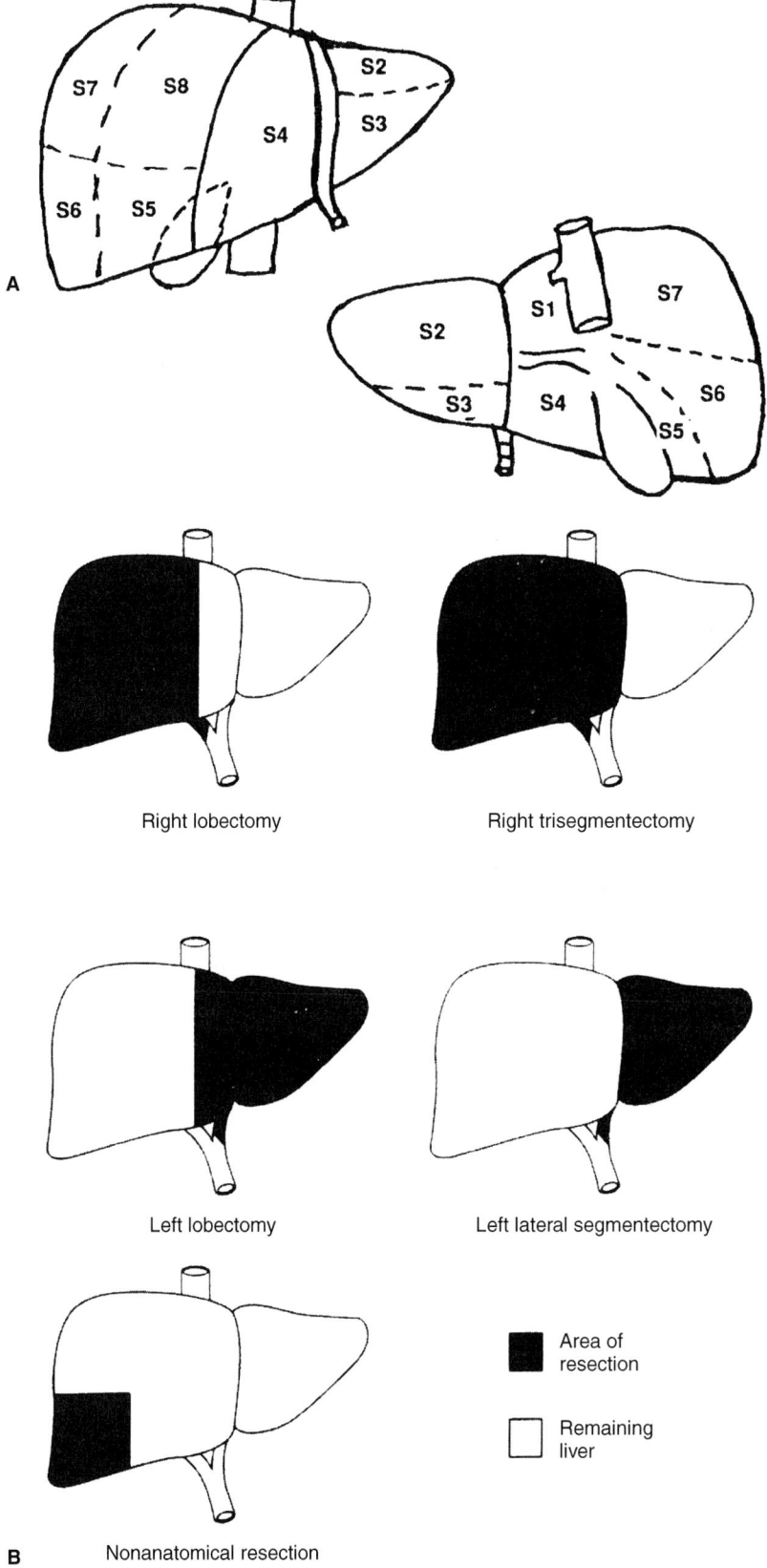

FIGURE 115–1. A, Segmental anatomy of the liver. **B,** Types of hepatic resection.

counts for 7% of all hepatocellular carcinomas. The long-term survival rate for FLT is 45% to 55% after a major hepatic resection.[84]

OTHER PRIMARY MALIGNANT TUMORS OF THE LIVER

Cholangiocarcinoma (CCa)

Cholangiocarcinoma is a malignant tumor that originates from bile ductal epithelium.[38] CCa can present either as an intraparenchymal lesion or as a central, perihilar lesion that blocks the biliary duct system ("Klatskin's tumor"). Although most CCa can be resected technically, cure is rare, and the degree of tumor palliation is uncertain. A direct surgical approach for resection of Klatskin's tumors is feasible in only 10% of the cases, where the identification of a cancer-free plane allows a resection to be done.[4,38] Typically, Klatskin's tumors grow as infiltrative masses for which a palliative biliary bypass represents the only realistic approach. Despite anecdotal reports of long-term postresection or post bypass survival, the mean survival time following surgery in such cases is less than 9 months.

Sarcomas

Sarcoma of the Liver

Hemangiosarcoma is an exceedingly rare, vascular tumor of the liver that occurs most often in older adults. In general, the prognosis for this tumor is grim. Whenever the tumor is single and localized, total resection is indicated and represents the only effective therapy.

Leiomyosarcoma, fibrosarcoma, and rhabdomyosarcoma of the liver are generally thought of as originating either from the vascular structures of the liver or from the vena cava. The prognosis for all these tumors is invariably poor, but palliation is sometimes possible.[20,47]

Epithelioid Hemangioendothelioma of the Liver (Angiosarcoma)

Epithelioid hemangioendothelioma is a very rare tumor of the liver that occurs at all ages and in both sexes. The tumor is typically multifocal and is characterized by extensive involvement of the liver. For these reasons, a total resection is rarely possible and total hepatic resection with subsequent liver transplantation represents the only realistic therapeutic option.[50]

BENIGN LIVER TUMORS

Hepatic Cell Adenoma

Hepatic cell adenoma is an uncommon benign tumor of the liver. It tends to occur most frequently in young women. Its incidence increased markedly after the introduction of oral contraceptives. Hepatic adenomas can present either as an asymptomatic or symptomatic space-occupying mass within the liver. Occasionally, it presents dramatically as an acute abdomen as a result of spontaneous rupture. Because of the strong relationship between the use of oral contraceptives and this tumor, neoplasms suspected of being adenomas need not be resected until the effect of oral contraceptive withdrawal is determined. If the tumor mass declines by at least 50%, a resection is rarely required. Absence of regression represents an indication for resection.

The differential diagnosis between an adenoma and HCC can usually be made with radioisotope scanning or magnetic resonance imaging (MRI).

Hemangiomas of the Liver

Cavernous hemangiomas are the most common benign tumors of the liver.[87] Being congenital lesions, they occur or can be recognized initially at any age and in both sexes. The prevalence of hemangioma is reported to be between 0.4% to 7.5%. The typical presentation is that of a small, asymptomatic, often incidentally identified focal lesion within the hepatic parenchyma. The diameter and number of these lesions appear to increase with age. Liver hemangiomas are almost always asymptomatic. Those less than 10 cm in diameter rarely warrant resectional surgery. Those that grow larger can produce symptoms of local compression and discomfort or even present as a cause for thrombocytopenia or hemolytic anemia as a result of cytologic injury or sequestration within the tumor. If hemorrhage, pain, or symptoms related to compression of adjacent viscera are present, resection should be considered. Enucleation of the tumor is as effective as a formal resection and can be done with less blood loss than a formal hepatic resection. The prognosis after resection of a hemangioma is excellent if no confounding liver disease is present.[87]

Focal Nodular Hyperplasia

Focal nodular hyperplasia (FNH) is a space-occupying lesion of the liver that is most often observed in young women. It is a benign, usually small, isolated lesion that rarely, if ever, ruptures or bleeds. FNH rarely if ever becomes malignant, although it has been proposed as being the benign counterpart of the fibrolamellar hepatoma.[95] On rare occasions it may regress spontaneously. FNH produces symptoms only when its mass displaces adjacent structures. For this reason FNH need not be resected unless it either rapidly or alarmingly enlarges or when a diagnosis of malignancy cannot be excluded. The prognosis is excellent whenever a resection is performed for FNH in a noncirrhotic patient.

Secondary Liver Tumors

The most common malignant neoplasm of the liver by far is metastatic tumor.[21,59] Among the tumors that represent the major causes of death, cancer of the colon, lung, stomach, pancreas, ovaries, uterus, and breast frequently produce hepatic metastases in the majority of patients with these tumors before they die. Fifty percent to 70% of all liver metastases are derived from organs drained by the portal venous system. Metastatic lesions within the liver from organs other than colon and rectum are usually part of a widespread disease process. Thus, isolated metastatic lesions of the liver are unusual. The probability of metastasis to the liver without involvement of other organs is greater in a tumor originating from an organ drained by the portal venous system than in a tumor originating elsewhere in the body by a factor of $10:1$.[52] Patients with liver metastases arising from a pancreatic or gastric cancer have a median survival of 2 months. Thus, they are not candidates for hepatic resection. The frequency of liver metastases at the time of the clinical presentation of a colorectal cancer is about 25%. An equal number of patients develop liver metastases within 3 years.[5,98] Liver metastases secondary to colon or rectal cancer or a gastrointestinal tract endocrine tumor are more often likely to be manageable with resectional surgery.[70] Nonetheless, 70% to 80% of individuals who undergo a hepatic resection for colon cancer metastases are not cured of their malignant disease.[52] Several factors have been recognized as determining, in part, the prognosis following hepatic resection. Carcinoembryonic antigen (CEA) level and the number of metastases (less than four) are significant preoperative indicators for long-term disease-free survival.[9] How the lesions are localized within the liver is only relevant for the technical feasibility of the resection. Therefore, even bilobar lesions can be treated with a hepatic resection, given that sufficient residual liver parenchyma is left to support survival. The surgical margin, amount of liver tissue resected, CEA level, and results of flow cytometry appear to be important prognostic indicators: patients with a surgical margin greater than 1 cm, resection of

TABLE 115–3. INDICATIONS FOR LIVER TRANSPLANTATION

1. Advanced chronic liver disease
    a. Cholestatic liver disease
        (1) Primary biliary cirrhosis (PBC)
        (2) Primary sclerosing cholangitis (PSC)
        (3) Secondary biliary cirrhosis
        (4) Biliary atresia
        (5) Bile duct paucity syndrome
        (6) Familial cholestatic syndromes
    b. Hepatocellular disease
        (1) Chronic viral-induced liver disease
        (2) Chronic drug-inducted liver disease
        (3) Alcoholic liver disease
        (4) Chronic autoimmune liver disease
    c. Vascular disease
        (1) Budd-Chiari syndrome
        (2) Venoocclusive disease
2. Hepatic malignancies
    a. Hepatocellular carcinoma (HCC)
    b. Cholangiocarcinoma
    c. Sarcomas of the liver
    d. Isolated metastatic disease
        (1) Neuroendocrine tumor
        (2) Colorectal cancer
        (3) Others
3. Fulminant hepatic failure
    a. Viral hepatitis: A, B, C, D, E; non-A, non-B, non-C; Epstein-Barr virus
    b. Acute alcoholic hepatitis
    c. Drug-induced or toxic acute liver disease
        (1) Halothane
        (2) Acetaminophen
        (3) Gold
        (4) Disulfiram
        (5) Amanita phalloides
        (6) Others
    d. Metabolic liver disease
        (1) Wilson's disease
        (2) Reye's syndrome
        (3) Organic acidurias
4. Metabolic liver disease
    a. α-1-Antitrypsin deficiency
    b. Wilson's disease
    c. Tyrosinemia
    d. Galactosemia
    e. Hemochromatosis
    f. Crigler-Najjar syndrome type II
    g. Erythropoietic protoporphyria
    h. Urea-cycle deficiencies
    i. Glycogen-storage disease type I and IV
    j. Homozygous type IIa hypercholesterolemia
    k. Gaucher's disease
    l. Oxalosis
    m. Protein C deficiency
    n. Protein S deficiency
    o. Antithrombin III deficiency
    p. Type A and B hemophilia

less than 1 g of liver tissue, CEA level of less than 200 ng/ml, and presence of only diploid cells on flow cytometry have an estimated 5-year disease-free survival rate greater than 50%.[9]

Contraindications to hepatic resection for colorectal cancer liver metastases include the presence of positive portal-celiac lymph nodes, extrahepatic noncontiguous disease, and four or more lesions within the liver.

Hepatic resection is curative in 30% to 35% of individuals operated on for hepatic metastases arising from a colon cancer. The best survival rates are reported as 90% at 1 year, 50% at 3 years, and 38% at 5 years.[21,34,75]

Adjuvant preoperative and postoperative chemotherapy trials are ongoing for such cases using intraperitoneal 5-fluorouracil (5-FU) or fluorodeoxyuridine (FUDR) combined with systemic intravenous chemotherapy. The average survival time for patients treated with chemotherapy alone is about 6 months compared to a figure of 60% at 2 years in patients treated with hepatic resection combined with chemotherapy.[29] Thus, the role of adjuvant chemotherapy is promising and needs to be investigated extensively with randomized trials.[87]

LIVER TRANSPLANTATION

At present, liver transplantation has undoubtedly progressed such that it must be considered an effective therapeutic option for individuals with end-stage liver disease that is no longer responsive to conventional medical therapies. The 5-year survival rate after OLT, which was 30% to 40% in the late 1970s, currently ranges from 55% to 85% in most series.[82,83] These results are particularly good when compared to the 1-year survival of 0% to 30% for the same kind of patients treated medically. The specific reasons for this dramatic improvement in results with OLT are due to refinements of both surgical and organ preservation techniques and the development of more powerful immunosuppressive drugs, such as cyclosporine and FK506.[15,18,78-80,91]

INDICATIONS AND CONTRAINDICATIONS FOR OLT

The liver diseases that can benefit from a liver transplantation can be grouped in four major groups: chronic end-stage liver diseases, hepatic malignancies, inborn errors of metabolism, and fulminant hepatic failure (Table 115–3).

Any patient who develops a complication of liver disease (Table 115–4) should be considered for early referral to a transplant center for an evaluation. Once a patient has been identified as a potential candidate for OLT, it is mandatory to stage the liver disease to more clearly define the timing of the transplant procedure. The criteria to be used for this purpose are listed in Table 115–5 and include the clinical and biochemical parameters used to assess impairments of synthetic, excretory, and metabolic function of the liver and the presence of an intolerable deterio-

TABLE 115–4. COMPLICATIONS OF END-STAGE LIVER DISEASES

COMPLICATIONS	HEPATOCELLULAR DISEASE	CHOLESTATIC DISEASE
Synthetic Failure		
Hypoalbuminemia	Typical	Late
Coagulopathy	Typical	Late
Cholestasis		
Hyperbilirubinemia	Present	Typical or important
Xanthelasma	Usually absent	Usually present
Hypercholesterolemia	Usually absent	Usually present
Portal Hypertension		
Ascites	Present	Present (late)
Variceal bleeding	Present	Late
Hepatic encephalopathy	Present	Late
Hepatomegaly	Early phase only	Present
Hypersplenism		
Anemia	Present	Present (late)
Thrombocytopenia	Present	Present (late)
Leucopenia	Present	Present (late)
Osteodystrophy	Uncommon	Common
Hepatocellular carcinoma	Present	Exceptionally rare
Cholangiocarcinoma	Exceptionally rare	Present

ration of the quality of life as a consequence of the underlying liver disease. When a patient has been identified as a potential transplant candidate, the following procedures can be used to screen for the presence of absolute and relative contraindications for OLT (Table 115–6).

The absolute contraindications for liver transplantation have been reduced progressively through the years as a result of steady improvements in technique in surgery and anesthesiology. Examples are portal vein thrombosis, previous major abdominal surgery, and advanced age (over 60 years), each of which either precluded or strongly discouraged liver transplantation only 5 to 10 years ago and are now no longer considered as being contraindications for the procedure.[18,78,91]

The cardiopulmonary function of all potential transplant recipients must be carefully evaluated not only in older potential patients but also for younger patients with specific liver diseases known to have a high incidence of certain complications (i.e., cardiomyopathy associated with alcoholism, hemochromatosis or Wilson's disease, and pulmonary hypertension in autoimmune and chronic cholestatic liver diseases).

At present, chronic renal disease is not considered as a contraindication for OLT, because combined liver-kidney transplantation can be performed successfully in such cases.

SPECIFIC DISEASE INDICATIONS FOR OLT

Virus-Related End-Stage Liver Disease

Postnecrotic cirrhosis due to hepatotropic virus infection (HBV, HCV, HDV, non-A, non-B, non-C) is the most frequent indication for liver transplantation and accounts for more than 30% of all cases in adults.[7,13,25,83,89] In evaluating patients with viral disease, it is mandatory to determine the replicative status of the virus because this factor determines the long-term outcome of the transplant procedure. It is well known that those who have evidence for viral replication have a 100% recurrence rate, which in the vast majority of the cases leads to recurrent liver disease that has a faster rate of disease progression than was seen with the original disease.[19,73] An assessment of the HBe/anti-HBe antigen-antibody system is not sufficient to define the replicative status of the HBV. An assessment of either the presence of HBV DNA or DNA polymerase activity in the serum or alternatively the demonstration of positive results from nuclear staining for the core antigen within the liver is required for a determination of the replicative state of the virus. The presence of extrahepatic reservoirs of HBV infection has been documented as being responsible for the almost inevitable recurrence of virus infection when active viral replication is present.[22,42] For this reason, the presence of active HBV replication (HBeAg + ve or HBV/DNA + ve) is considered a relative contraindication for OLT at most transplant centers.

One-year patient survival rates after liver transplantation for end-stage HBV-related liver

---

TABLE 115–5. CLINICAL AND BIOCHEMICAL INDICATIONS TO ASSESS THE TIMING FOR OLT

1. Acute liver failure
   a. Bilirubin >10–20 mg/dl and increasing
   b. Prothrombin time >10 s above normal and increasing
   c. Encephalopathy (grade 3 and progressing)
2. Chronic liver disease
   a. cholestatic liver disease
      (1) Bilirubin >15 mg/dl
      (2) Intractable pruritus
      (3) Severe bone disease
   b. Hepatocellular liver disease
      (1) Albumin <2.5 g/dl
      (2) Hepatic encephalopathy
      (3) Prothrombin time >5 s above normal
   c. Factors common to both types of liver disease
      (1) Hepatorenal syndrome
      (2) Recurrent spontaneous bacterial peritonitis
      (3) Intractable ascites
      (4) Recurrent variceal bleeding
      (5) Recurrent episodes of biliary sepsis
      (6) Development of liver malignancy

TABLE 115–6. CONTRAINDICATION FOR LIVER TRANSPLANTATION

1. Absolute
   a. Extra hepatobiliary sepsis
   b. Hepatobiliary malignancy with extrahepatic metastases
   c. Severe cardiopulmonary disease
   d. Acquired immunodeficiency syndrome
2. Relative
   a. Portal vein thrombosis
   b. Hepatitis B virus–related end-stage liver disease with active viral replication
   c. Human immunodeficiency virus positivity
   d. Marked obesity
   e. Previous major abdominal surgery
   f. Poor compliance

disease range between 45% and 55% in recipients with active infection prior to transplantation as compared to a figure of 70% to 80% in patients who do not have evidence for active viral replication.[22,83]

HCV is the major viral disease responsible for posttransfusion hepatitis. A major breakthrough in the diagnosis of HCV disease has been the availability of methods to detect antibody to structural and nonstructural proteins of the virus. However, all the current anti-HCV tests detect the patient's antibody response to the HCV and do not detect the virus itself. To define the replicative state of HCV, it is necessary to perform polymerase chain reaction (PCR) to detect both the positive and the negative strands of the virus. Such methods are highly sophisticated and are not routinely available at most centers. Without these methods, it is impossible to distinguish between viral contamination (positive strand only) and infection (positive and negative strands) due to HCV.[27] A 95% or greater recurrence rate for viremia after OLT in individuals who are HCV-RNA positive prior to transplantation has been reported.[99] Nonetheless, recent studies have demonstrated that both graft and recipient survival rates are excellent, ranging between 87% and 100% at 4 years after OLT, and only 1 in 3 develop evidence of histologic viral liver disease at 2 years.[77,99]

Alcoholic Liver Disease

Alcohol-induced cirrhosis and alcoholic hepatitis are the two most common causes of liver disease in Western societies and are likely to provide the largest number of potential candidates for OLT at most transplant centers. Because of the concerns about recidivism and the potential for a lack of compliance with the required immunosuppression by alcoholic patients, Laënnec's cirrhosis has been considered to be a relative contraindication for OLT.[2,40,85,92] However, when the alcoholic patient has been alcohol abstinent for at least 3 months, post-OLT recidivism and noncompliance are unusual, and experience has shown that patient survival for alcoholic cirrhosis after OLT does not differ at all from that observed in patients who received a liver transplant for nonalcoholic diseases. The reported recidivism rate is less than 10%. Moreover, Starzl et al,[85] have reported that alcohol consumption after OLT is less frequent in individuals who received a liver transplant for alcoholic cirrhosis than it is for patients who received a liver transplant for other disease indications.

The pretransplant evaluation of a patient with alcoholic cirrhosis requires a careful screening for the presence of alcohol-associated cardiomyopathy, chronic pancreatitis, and cerebral atrophy, conditions that increase the perioperative risks and do not allow for a maximum improvement in the quality of life following successful liver transplantation.

Primary Biliary Cirrhosis

Primary biliary cirrhosis (PBC) has been one of the more common and most successful indications for OLT worldwide. Because of the slow and progressive evolution of this liver disease, PBC has been used as a model to predict the ideal timing for transplantation. Prognostic models have been developed at several institutions, which are based on the following parameters: age, serum albumin level, serum bilirubin level, presence of cirrhosis, presence of central cholestasis, and history of previous treatment with azathioprine.[57] The score produced as a result of an analysis of these parameters can be used to predict life expectancy of the patient without OLT. As a general principle, the optimal point for timing transplantation is when a patient has less than 1 year of anticipated survival, unless other major complications such as bone demineralization, intractable itching, variceal bleeding, or ascites are present also. These additional factors should hasten rather than delay OLT.

At most centers the current 1-year survival after OLT for patients with PBC ranges between 75% and 85%.[16]

Primary Sclerosing Cholangitis

Primary sclerosing cholangitis (PSC) is a progressive cholestatic disease of the liver that has many similarities with PBC, particularly a late onset of the major complications of a chronic liver disease. Intractable itching, recurrent bleeding, osteoporosis, intractable ascites, and hepatic encephalopathy are the main indications for liver transplantation.[43] Although only a small percentage of patients with inflammatory bowel disease eventually develop PSC, the coexistence of chronic inflammatory bowel disease (particularly ulcerative colitis) is found in as much as 70% of patients with PSC.[76] For this reason, a colonoscopic examination prior to transplantation is mandatory in patients with PSC to exclude the presence of an adenocarcinoma of the colon, which is known to occur in these patients. The disease is associated also with an increased risk for CCa. Multiple percutaneous or perendoscopic brushings of the biliary tree are recommended prior to OLT in such cases. However, even with the use of both endoscopic and radiologic techniques, the detection of a CCa is difficult and the presence of a tumor is often only documented after the transplant procedure and a pathologic examination of the totally resected liver is performed.

When a patient with PSC is identified as a potential liver transplant recipient, surgical procedures such as biliary reconstructions, percutaneous biliary decompression, and partial or total colectomy should be avoided as much as possible. A reduction in the use of these procedures has led to a dramatic improvement in the survival of PSC patients with OLT. The actuarial 1-year survival for patients who receive a liver transplant for PSC ranges between 70% and 80% in patients without previous biliary surgery, compared to a figure of 50% to 60% survival in patients with prior biliary tract surgery.[51]

Chronic Active Hepatitis

Chronic active hepatitis is characterized by a highly unpredictable course, which makes the timing of transplantation particularly difficult. Such patients typically experience multiple episodes of "active hepatitis," which eventually lead to cirrhosis. Early diagnosis and aggressive immunosuppressive therapy prolong survival. Several peculiar complications of this disease contraindicate OLT. These include osteoporosis, recurrent infections, intractable steroid-induced myopathy, and marked obesity. The actuarial 1-year survival after liver transplantation ranges between 70% and 80%.[36,83]

Budd-Chiari Syndrome

This condition is characterized by hepatic vein thrombosis, which can occur either as a complication of a condition known to cause vascular thrombosis or one without any underlying disease.[54] The disease usually presents as a gradually developing liver failure with fibrosis as a result of hepatic vein thrombosis. The process of progressive vascular thrombosis and progressive hepatic failure may require months or even years before it becomes clinically evident. In rare cases, an acute syndrome characterized by a rapid onset and steady downhill course occurs. The presence of disease complications such as intractable ascites or esophageal variceal bleeding constitute clear indications for liver transplantation.[54]

The establishment of a correct specific diagnosis is mandatory when a patient with Budd-Chiari syndrome is being considered for OLT. The principal causes of the Budd-Chiari syndrome include various myeloproliferative disorders, particularly polycythemia vera, paroxysmal nocturnal hemoglobinuria, protein S or C deficiency, and antithrombin III deficiency. Some of these disorders are cured by liver transplantation; others require lifelong anticoagulation or myelotoxic therapy or both.[10] The current actuarial 1-year survival for patients who received a liver transplant for the Budd-Chiari syndrome ranges between 70% and 80%, as compared to a figure of less than 50% in patients who did not receive a transplant.

Fulminant Hepatic Failure

The management of fulminant hepatic failure (FHF) is a demanding situation that requires a high level of expertise. The prognosis for FHF is guarded and highly dependent on the ability of the intensive care unit and liver transplant teams to keep the patient alive while identifying a donor and performing a liver transplant in a very short period of time. The prognosis for FHF is greatly influenced by the cause.[61] Patients with acetaminophen intoxication are expected to have a mortality of 20% to 30%, compared to a rate of 45% to 50% in those with HAV or HBV fulminant failure, or a rate as high as 80% or more in cases of HCV or non-A, non-B, non-C or halothane hepatitis, or fulminant Wilson's disease.[6,62] These data suggest that there is no reason to delay liver transplantation in the latter disease groups. Grade III coma, a factor V level below 20%, a serum bilirubin level greater than 20 mg/dl, a serum creatinine greater than 10 mg/dl, and age greater than 10 years are indicators of a poor likelihood of survival without liver transplantation.[62] The actuarial 1-year survival rate after OLT for patients with FHF ranges between 55% and 75%.

Hepatic Malignancies

Hepatocellular Carcinoma

Patients with HCC are usually good candidates for liver transplantation because of their age and their usually well-maintained hepatic function.[32,68] As a consequence, the operative mortality is the lowest among all disease indications. Unfortunately, the rate of tumor recurrence is above 60%, which leads to a poor long-term survival rate of 63% at 1 year, 42% at 3 years, and 40% at 5 years.[83] Macroscopic vascular invasion, lymph node metastases, bilobar distribution of the tumor, presence of cirrhosis, and an infiltrative type of the tumor are factors useful in predicting disease recurrence and survival rates after liver transplantation for this indication. The median survival rate in patients without evidence of extrahepatic localization who received a liver transplant for HCC is 120 months as compared to 35 months in those with evidence of extrahepatic spread.[83] Liver transplantation appears to be the treatment of choice for HCC confined to the liver when a hepatic resection cannot be performed either because of inadequate residual hepatic function or for technical reasons.[35,63]

Recent advances in pre- and post-OLT chemotherapy protocols appear to have increased the survival of patients who receive a liver transplant for HCC.

Cholangiocarcinoma

The Klatskin variant of CCa has a high recurrence rate at 1 year after OLT (over 75%). Most patients die within 2 years after transplantation. Patients presenting with peripheral CCa or patients with an "incidental" cholangiocarcinoma found after an examination of the resected liver obtained from a patient who received a liver transplant for PSC appear to have a better prognosis with an outcome comparable to that of individuals who received a liver transplant for HCC.

Other Liver Tumors

Patients with hepatic sarcomas, leiomyosarcomas, fibrosarcomas, and rhabdomyosarcomas have an almost universal tumor recurrence rate within months after liver transplantation. The only exceptions are the patients who received a liver transplant for hemangioendothelioma; these patients usually have a longer disease-free interval.[50]

Overall, the results in patients who receive a liver transplant for hepatic metastases of primary tumors originating outside the liver have been unsatisfactory.[31] The single exception is that of patients who receive a liver transplant for liver metastases from a neuroendocrine tumor; these patients experience long-term survivals when the primary lesion is removed.[48]

Biliary Atresia

Approximately 60% of the liver transplantations performed in children are performed for biliary atresia. The survival rate after liver transplantation for biliary atresia ranges between 68% to 80% at 1 year and 68% to 75% at 5 years.[33] This represents a dramatic improvement in survival for these patients compared to a 2-year survival rate of less than 5% in the pretransplant era.

A Kasai operation for children with biliary atresia is usually required as a therapy to reestablish bile flow and allow growth of these children, thereby delaying OLT. They all eventually develop cirrhosis with portal hypertension, usually by the age of 5 years, when they can undergo a liver transplant with a much better chance of survival than that achieved when a transplant is performed in smaller children.[33]

Bile Duct Paucity Syndrome

Arteriohepatic dysplasia or Alagille's syndrome and Byler's syndrome are included in the bile duct paucity syndrome.[33] The major indications for OLT in patients with these disorders are portal hypertension, ascites, intractable itching, and presence of HCC. Congenital cardiovascular malformations are present in about 12% of these patients and may be a contraindication for liver transplantation, if severe.

Inborn Errors of Metabolism (Table 115–3)

After successful liver engraftment, the allograft retains its own metabolic specificity. Liver transplantation for inborn errors of metabolism (IBEM) that either affect the liver directly, leading to a form of acute or chronic hepatic failure, or produce liver failure as a consequence of a more widely expressed inborn error (protoporphyria or Gaucher's disease) has been performed in both adults and children. A third group of inborn errors for which an abnormality of liver metabolism exists and leads to disease in other organs includes the urea-cycle deficiencies, oxalosis, type A and B hemophilia, protein C or S deficiency, and type II lipoprotein deficiency.[17,26,74,81,97] Survival rates after liver transplantation for these indications are among the highest for any indication.

In conditions such as Wilson's disease, a-1-antitrypsin deficiency, hemochromatosis, tyrosinosis, glycogen storage disease types I and IV, galactosemia, and homozygous type IIa familial hypercholesterolemia, both the liver and other organs are damaged as a result of the metabolic disorder, and correction of the metabolic defect is coincidental with treatment of liver failure.[30,49,53,69,86,94]

REFERENCES

1. Adson MA. Primary hepatic cancers (Western experience). In: Blumgart LH, ed. *Surgery of the Liver and Biliary Tract.* New York, NY: Churchill Livingstone Inc; 1994.

2. Atterbury CE. The alcoholic in the lifeboat: should drinkers be candidates for liver transplantation? *J Clin Gastroenterol.* 1986;8:1–4.
3. Belli L, Romani F, Belli LS, et al. A reappraisal of the surgical treatment of small hepatocellular carcinomas (HCC) in cirrhosis: clinicopathological study of resection or transplantation? *Dig Dis Sci.* 1989;34:1571–1575.
4. Bengmark S, Ekberg H, Evander A, et al. Major hilar resection for hilar cholangiocarcinoma. *Ann Surg.* 1988;207:120–125.
5. Bengtsson G, Carlsson G, Hafstromm LO, Jonsson PE. Natural history of patients with untreated liver metastases from colorectal cancer. *Am J Surg.* 1981;141:586–589.
6. Bismuth H, Samuel D, Gugenheim J, et al. Emergency liver transplantation for fulminant hepatitis. *Ann Intern Med.* 1987;107:337–341.
7. Blumhardt G, Neuhaus P, Bechstein WO, et al. Liver transplantation in HBsAg positive patients. *Transplant Proc.* 1990;22:1517–1518.
8. Bozzetti F, Gennari L, Regalia P, et al. Morbidity and mortality after surgical resection of liver tumors: analysis of 229 cases. *Hepatogastroenterology.* 1992;39(3):237–241.
9. Cady B, Stone MD, McDermott WV Jr, et al. Technical and biological factors in disease-free survival after hepatic resection for colo-rectal cancer metastases. *Arch Surg.* 1992;127(5):561–568.
10. Campbell DA Jr, Rolles K, Jamieson N, et al. Hepatic transplantation with perioperative and long term anticoagulation as treatment for Budd-Chiari syndrome. *Surg Gynecol Obstet.* 1988;166:551–558.
11. Christensen E, Schlichting R, Andersen PK, et al. The Copenhagen Study Group for liver disease: updating prognosis and therapeutic effect evaluation in cirrhosis with Cox's multiple regression model for true dependent time variables. *Scand J Gastroenterol.* 1986;21:163–174.
12. Christensen E, Schlichting P, Fauerholdt L, et al. Changes of laboratory variables with time in cirrhosis: prognostic and therapeutic significance. *Hepatology.* 1985;5:843–853.
13. Colledan M, Gislon M, Doglia M, et al. Liver transplantation in patients with B viral hepatitis and delta infection. *Transplant Proc.* 1987;19:4073–4076.
14. Colombo M. Hepatocellular carcinoma. *J Hepatol.* 1992;15:225–236.
15. Dzik WH, Jenkins R. Use of intraoperative blood salvage during orthotopic liver transplantation. *Arch Surg.* 1985;120:946–948.
16. Esquivel CO, Benardos A, Demetris AJ, et al. Liver transplantation for primary biliary cirrhosis in 76 patients during the cyclosporine era. *Gastroenterology.* 1988;94:1207–1216.
17. Esquivel CO, Marino IR, Fioravanti V, Van Thiel DH. Liver transplantation for metabolic disease of the liver. In: Makowka L, Van Thiel DH, eds. *Gastroenterology Clinics of North America.* Philadelphia, Pa: WB Saunders Co; 1988;17:167–175.
18. Fagiuoli S, Gasbarrini A, Azzarone A, Francavilla A, Van Thiel DH. FK 506: a new immunosuppressive agent for organ transplantation: pharmacology, mechanism of action and clinical application. *Ital J Gastroenterol.* 1992;24:355–360.
19. Fagiuoli S, Shah G, Wright HI, Van Thiel DH. Types, causes and therapies of hepatitis occurring in a liver allograft. *Dig Dis Sci.* 1993;38:1–8.
20. Forbes A, Portmann B, Johnson P, Williams R. Hepatic sarcomas in adults: a review of 25 cases. *Gut.* 1987;28:668–674.
21. Foster JH. Surgical treatment of metastatic liver tumors. *Hepatogastroenterology.* 1990;37(2):182–187.
22. Freeman RB, Sanchez H, Lewis WD, et al. Serologic and DNA follow-up data from HBsAg positive patients treated with orthotopic liver transplantation. *Transplantation.* 1991;51:793–797.
23. Gagner M, Franco D, Vons C, et al. Analysis of morbidity and mortality rates in right hepatectomy with the preoperative APACHE II score. *Surgery.* 1991;110(3):487–492.
24. Gozzetti G, Mazziotti A, Cavallari A, et al. Clinical experience with hepatic resections for hepatocellular carcinoma in patients with cirrhosis. *Surg Gynecol Obstet.* 1988;166(6):503–510.
25. Grendele M, Gridelli B, Colledan M, et al. Hepatitis C virus infection and liver transplantation. *Lancet.* 1989;2:1221–1222.
26. Groth CG, Ringden O. Transplantation in relation to the treatment of inherited disease. *Transplantation.* 1984;38:319–327.
27. Gurakar A, Fagiuoli S, Wright HI, Van Thiel DH. Hepatitis C virus infection: when to suspect, how to detect. *J Crit Illness.* 1993;8(12):1287–1295.
28. Hemming AW, Scudamore CH, Shackleton CR, Pudek M, Erb SR. Indocyanine green clearance as a predictor of successful hepatic resection in cirrhotic patients. *Am J Surg.* 1992;163(5):515–518.
29. Hodgson WJB, Mittelman A, Kats S, et al. Treatment of colorectal hepatic metastases by intrahepatic chemotherapy alone or as an adjuvant to complete or partial removal of metastatic disease. *Ann Surg.* 1986;203:420–425.
30. Hoeg JM, Starzl TE, Brewer HB. Liver transplantation for treatment of cardiovascular disease: comparison with medication and plasma exchange in homozygous familial hypercholesterolemia. *Am J Cardiol.* 1987;59:705–707.
31. Huber C, Niederwieser D, Schonitzer D, Gratwohl A, Buckner D, Margreiter R. Liver transplantation followed by high-dose cyclophosphamide, total-body irradiation, and autologous bone marrow transplantation for treatment of metastatic breast cancer: a case report. *Transplantation.* 1984;37:311–312.
32. Ismail T, Angrisani L, Gunson BK, et al. Primary hepatic malignancy: the role of liver transplantation. *Eur J Surg Oncol.* 1990;77:983–987.
33. Iwatsuki S, Shaw BW Jr, Starzl TE. Liver transplantation for biliary atresia. *World J Surg.* 1984;8:51–56.
34. Iwatsuki S, Starzl TE. Personal experience with 411 hepatic resections. *Ann Surg.* 1988;208:421–434.
35. Iwatsuki S, Starzl TE, Sheahan DG, et al. Hepatic resection versus transplantation for hepatocellular carcinoma. *Ann Surg.* 1991;214:221–229.
36. Iwatsuki S, Starzl TE, Todo S, et al. Experience in 1000 liver transplants under cyclosporine-steroid therapy: a survival report. *Transplant Proc.* 1988;20(suppl 1):498–504.
37. Jeppson B, Halliday AW, Blumgart LH, et al. Pre- and post-operative nutrition in liver surgery. In: Bengmark S, Blumgart LH, eds. *Liver Surgery.* New York, NY: Churchill Livingstone Inc; 1986:166–181.
38. Kawarada Y, Mizumoto R. Diagnosis and treatment of cholangiocellular carcinoma of the liver. *Hepatogastroenterology.* 1990;37(2):176–181.
39. Kemeny MM. Hepatic resection: when, what kind and for which patients. *J Surg Oncol.* 1991;2:54–58.

40. Kumar S, Stauber R, Gavaler J, et al. Orthotopic liver transplantation for alcoholic liver diseases. *Hepatology.* 1990;11:159–164.
41. Lai ECS, Ng IOL, Ng MMT, et al. Long-term results of resection for large hepatocellular carcinoma: a multivariate analysis of clinicopathological features. *Hepatology.* 1990;11:815.
42. Lamelin JP, Trepo C. The hepatitis B virus and the peripheral blood mononuclear cells: a brief review. *J Hepatol.* 1990;10:120–124.
43. LaRusso NF, Wiesner RH, Ludwig J, et al. Primary sclerosing cholangitis. *N Engl J Med.* 1984;310:899–903.
44. Lin TY, Chen KM, Chen CC, et al. Role of surgery in the treatment of primary carcinoma of the liver: a 21-year experience. *Br J Surg.* 1987;74:839–842.
45. Lygidakis NJ, Makuuchi M. Clinical application of perioperative ultrasonography in liver surgery. *Hepatogastroenterology.* 1992;39(3):232–236.
46. MacIntosh EL, Minuk GY. Hepatic resection in patients with cirrhosis and hepatocellular carcinoma. *Surg Gynecol Obstet.* 1992;174:245–254.
47. Maki HS, Hubert BC, Sajjad SM, et al. Primary hepatic leimyosarcoma. *Arch Surg.* 1987;122:1193–1196.
48. Makowka L, Tzakis AG, Mazzaferro V, et al. Transplantation for the liver for metastatic endocrine tumors of the intestine and pancreas. *Surg Gynecol Obstet* 1989;168:107–111.
49. Malatack JJ, Finegold DN, Iwatsuki S, et al. Liver transplantation for type I glycogen storage disease. *Lancet.* 1983;1:1073–1075.
50. Marino IR, Todo S, Tzakis AG, et al. Treatment of hepatic epithelioid hemangioendothelioma with liver transplantation. *Cancer.* 1988;62:2079–2084.
51. Marsh JW Jr, Iwatsuki S, Makowka L, et al. Orthotopic liver transplantation for primary sclerosing cholangitis. *Ann Surg.* 1988;207:21–28.
52. Mazzaferro V, Dindzans V, Makowka L, Van Thiel DH. Approach to hepatic metastases from colorectal adenocarcinoma. *Semin Liver Dis.* 1988;8(3):247–253.
53. Mieles LA, Esquivel CO, Koneru B, et al. Liver transplantation for tyrosinemia: a review of 10 cases from the University of Pittsburgh. *Dig Dis Sci.* 1990;35:153–157.
54. Mitchell MC, Boitnott JK, Kaufman S, et al. Budd-Chiari syndrome: etiology, diagnosis and management. *Medicine.* 1982;61:199–218.
55. Mori K, Ozawa K, Yamamoto Y, et al. Response of hepatic mitochondrial redox tolerance test as a new prediction of surgical risk in hepatectomy. *Ann Surg.* 1990;211:438–446.
56. Nagasue N, Yukaya N, Ogawa Y, et al. Human liver regeneration after major hepatic resection: a study of normal livers and livers with chronic hepatitis and cirrhosis. *Ann Surg.* 1987;206:30–39.
57. Neuberger J, Altman DG, Christensen E, Tygstrup N, Williams R. Use of a prognostic index in evaluation of liver transplantation for primary biliary cirrhosis. *Transplantation.* 1986;41:713–716.
58. Noguchi T, Imai T, Mizumoto R. Preoperative estimation of surgical risk of hepatectomy in cirrhotic patients. *Hepatogastroenterology.* 1990;37(2):165–171.
59. Nudelmann LI, Cabot R, Benjamin IS, Blumgart LH. Hepatic resection for secondary tumors. *Cancer Surg.* 1989;8(1):33–48.
60. Oellerich M, Burdelsky M, Lautz HU, et al. Assessment of pretransplant prognosis in patients with cirrhosis. *Transplantation.* 1991;51:801–806.
61. O'Grady JG, Alexander GJM, Hayllan KM, Williams R. Early indicators of prognosis in fulminant hepatic failure. *Gastroenterology.* 1989;97:439–445.
62. O'Grady JG, Hamblay H, Williams R. Prothrombin time in fulminant hepatic failure. *Gastroenterology.* 1991;100:1480–1481.
63. Otte G, Heuschen UA, Hofmann WJ, et al. Primary hepatic malignancies: resection or liver transplantation? *Eur J Surg Oncol.* 1990;16:346–351.
64. Otte JB. Recent developments in liver transplantation. *J Hepatol.* 1991;12:386–393.
65. Ozawa K, Fujimoto T, Nakatani T, et al. Changes in hepatic energy charge, blood ketone body ratio and indocyanine green clearance in relation to DNA synthesis after hepatectomy. *Life Sci.* 1982;31:647–653.
66. Ozawa K, Kamiyama Y, Kimura K, et al. Relation of mitochondrial redox potential to hepatic energy charge in animals with hepatectomy, jaundice, hemorrhage and sepsis as well as patients with multiple organ failure. *Langenbecks Archi Chir.* 1982;357:204–205.
67. Peleman RR, Gavaler JS, Van Thiel DH, et al. Orthotopic liver transplantation for acute and subacute hepatic failure in adults. *Hepatology.* 1987;7:484–489.
68. Pichlmayr R, Ringe B, Wittekind C, et al. Liver grafting for malignant tumors. *Transplant Proc.* 1989;21:2403–2405.
69. Pillay P, Tzoracloeftherakis E, Tzakis AG, Kakizoe S, Van Thiel DH, Starzl TE. Orthotopic liver transplantation for hemochromatosis. *Transplant Proc.* 1991;23:1888–1889.
70. Registry of Hepatic Metastases. Resection of the liver for colo-rectal carcinoma metastases: a multi-institutional study of indications for resection. *Surgery.* 1988;278–288.
71. Renner E, Wietholtz H, Huguenin P, et al. Caffeine: a model compound for measuring liver function. *Hepatology.* 1984;4:38–46.
72. Sakairi T, Makuuchi M. Identification of the intersegmental or subsegmental plane in the liver with a surgical clip. *Surgery.* 1991;110(5):903–904.
73. Samuel D, Bismuth A, Mathieu D, et al. Passive immunoprophylaxis after liver transplantation in HBsAg-positive patients. *Lancet.* 1991;1:81.
74. Samuel D, Boboc B, Bernuau J, Bismuth H, Bernhamou JP. Liver transplantation for protoporphyria: evidence for the predominant role of the erythropoietic tissue in protoporphyrin overproduction. *Gastroenterology.* 1988;95:816–819.
75. Savage AP, Malt RA. Elective and emergency hepatic resection: determinants of operative mortality and morbidity. *Ann Surg.* 1991;214(6):689–695.
76. Schrumpf E, Fausa O, Kolmannskog F, et al. Sclerosing cholangitis in ulcerative colitis. *Scand J Gastroenterol.* 1980;15:689–697.
77. Shah G, Demetris AJ, Gavaler JS, et al. Incidence, prevalence and clinical course of hepatitis C following liver transplantation. *Gastroenterology.* 1992;103:323–329.
78. Shaw BW Jr, Iwatsuki S, Bron K, et al. Portal vein grafts in hepatic transplantation. *Surg Gynecol Obstet.* 1984;161:66–68.
79. Shaw BW Jr, Iwatsuki S, Starzl TE. Alternative methods of arterialization of the hepatic graft. *Surg Gynecol Obstet.* 1984;159:490–493.
80. Shaw BW Jr, Martin DJ, Marquez JM, et al. Venous bypass in clinical liver transplantation. *Ann Surg.* 1984;200:524–534.
81. Starzl TE. Surgery for metabolic liver disease. In: McDermott WV Jr, ed. *Surgery of the Liver.* Oxford: Blackwell Scientific Publications Inc; 1989:127–136.

82. Starzl TE, Demetris AJ, Van Thiel DH. Medical progress: liver transplantation, I. *N Engl J Med.* 1989; 321:1014–1022.
83. Starzl TE, Demetris AJ, Van Thiel DH. Medical progress: liver transplantation, II. *N Engl J Med.* 1989; 321:1092–1099.
84. Starzl TE, Iwatsuki S, Shaw BW Jr, et al. Treatment of fibrolamellar hepatoma with partial or total hepatectomy and transplantation of the liver. *Surg Gynecol Obstet.* 1986;162:145–148.
85. Starzl TE, Van Thiel DH, Tzakis AG, et al. Orthotopic liver transplantation for alcoholic cirrhosis. *JAMA* 1988;260:2542–2544.
86. Sternlieb I. Wilson's disease: indications for liver transplant. *Hepatology.* 1984;4:155–175.
87. Takagi H. Diagnosis and management of cavernous hemangioma of the liver. *Semin Surg Oncol.* 1985;1:12–22.
88. Takenaka K, Kanematsu T, Fukuzawa K, Sugimaki K. Can hepatic failure after surgery for hepatocellular carcinoma in cirrhotic patients be prevented? *World J Surg.* 1990;14(1):123–127.
89. Todo S, Demetris AJ, Van Thiel DH, et al. Orthotopic liver transplantation for patients with hepatitis B virus-related liver disease. *Hepatology.* 1991;13:619–626.
90. Tzakis AG, Gordon RD, Makowka L, et al. Clinical considerations in orthotopic liver transplantation. *Radiol Clin North Am.* 1987;25:289–297.
91. Tzakis A, Todo S, Steiber A, Starzl TE. Venous jump graft for liver transplantation in patients with portal vein thrombosis. *Transplantation.* 1989;48:530.
92. Van Thiel DH, Carr BI, Iwatsuki S, et al. Liver transplantation for alcoholic liver disease, viral hepatitis, and hepatic neoplasms. *Transplant Proc.* 1991;23:1917–1921.
93. Van Thiel DH, Hagler NG, Schade RR, et al. In vivo hepatic volume determination using sonography and computed tomography: validation and a comparison of the two techniques. *Gastroenterology.* 1985;88:1812–1817.
94. Van Thiel DH, Starzl TE. α₁Antitrypsin deficiency and liver transplantation. In: Lenfant C, ed. *Alpha 1-antitrypsin Deficiency.* Bethesda, Md: NIH Monograph; 1992.
95. Vecchio FM, Fabiano A, Ghirlanda G, et al. Fibrolamellar carcinoma of the liver: the malignant counterpart of focal nodular hyperplasia with oncocytic changes. *Am J Clin Pathol.* 1981;81:521–526.
96. Villeneuve JP, Infante-Rivard C, Ampelas M, et al. Prognostic value of the aminopyrine breath test in cirrhotic patients. *Hepatology.* 1986;6:928–931.
97. Watts RWE, Calne RY, Rolles K, et al. Successful treatment of primary hyperoxaluria type I by combined hepatic and renal transplantation. *Lancet.* 1987;2:474–475.
98. Wood CB, Gillis CR, Blumgart LH. A retrospective study of the natural history of patients with liver metastases from colorectal cancer. *Clin Oncol.* 1976;2:285–288.
99. Wright TL, Donegan E, Hsu HH, et al. Recurrent and acquired hepatitis C viral infection in liver transplant recipients. *Gastroenterology.* 1992;103:317–322.
100. Yamamoto J, Takayama T, Kosuge T, et al. An isolate caudate lobectomy by the transhepatic approach for hepatocellular carcinoma in cirrhotic liver. *Surgery.* 1992;111(6):699–702.
101. Yoshida Y, Kanematsu T, Matsumata T, Takenaka K, Sugimaki K. Surgical margin and recurrence after resection of hepatocellular carcinoma in patients with cirrhosis: further evaluation of limited hepatic resection. *Ann Surg.* 1989;209(3):297–301.

116
Neonatal Hepatitis and Cholestasis

PHILIP ROSENTHAL

The term *neonatal hepatitis* refers to a group of disorders that present with hepatic dysfunction during the perinatal period and result in a somewhat similar histologic picture. In the past, neonatal hepatitis included all causes of cholestasis or diminished bile flow in infants under 3 months of age in which extrahepatic biliary obstruction had been excluded. However, recent investigations have uncovered specific metabolic and infectious causes that can present as neonatal hepatitis. Unfortunately, in the majority of cases a specific cause cannot be found. The newborn is particularly susceptible to cholestatic insults from infections, hypoperfusion, or endocrinologic states, since the infant is in a state of "physiologic cholestasis" due to diminished synthesis, pool size, duodenal concentration, and intestinal reabsorption of bile acids. Neonatal hepatitis accounts for approximately 40% of all cases of infants with cholestasis and is the most frequently diagnosed hepatic disorder of early infancy. Some familial cases have been reported, suggesting either a recessive inheritance pattern or a maternal environmental factor.

This chapter highlights several of the known causes of neonatal hepatitis with intrahepatic cholestasis. Space limitations preclude a discussion of all known etiologic agents. It has become apparent that the term *neonatal hepatitis* is too vague and no longer clinically or therapeutically useful. A distinction between hepatitis in a neonate due to a known etiologic agent amenable to therapy must be made from idiopathic neonatal hepatitis in which etiologic agents may be multiple and therapies are currently unknown.

EVALUATION OF A JAUNDICED INFANT

The first step in the evaluation process is to determine the type of hyperbilirubinemia. Is there a conjugated or unconjugated hyperbilirubinemia? Bilirubin fractionation may be obtained using a modification of the diazo reaction, which separates bilirubin into direct and indirect reacting fractions. This fractionation is an imprecise measurement of conjugated and unconjugated bilirubins, respectively. However, for routine clinical evaluation diazo fractionation is satisfactory. Using diazo methodology, a conjugated hyperbilirubinemia is present when the direct-reacting bilirubin is greater than 30% of the total bilirubin. In cases of unconjugated hyperbilirubinemia, the direct-reacting fraction is less than 15% of the total bilirubin value. Samples with direct-reacting bilirubin fractions between 15% and 30% are indeterminate by this method. However, because diazo fractionation is imprecise, the type of hyperbilirubinemia must be carefully classified, since it will determine the type and extent of the evaluation required.

Once it has been determined that the infant has a conjugated hyperbilirubinemia, differentiation of extrahepatic from intrahepatic cholestasis becomes the challenge for the clinician. Extrahepatic obstruction may be amenable to surgical correction if performed early. Unfortunately, there is no single test that can discriminate between extrahepatic biliary atresia and neonatal hepatitis.

Infants in both groups may present with jaundice and acholic stools. Serial observation of stool pigment by an experienced observer is both inexpensive and valuable. The liver is enlarged on physical examination. Extrahepatic biliary atresia is more common in girls of normal birth weight, whereas neonatal hepatitis is more common in boys. A familial occurrence favors neonatal hepatitis. Polysplenia is more common with biliary atresia. Intermittently pigmented stools favor neonatal hepatitis, whereas consistently acholic stools favor biliary atresia. However, severe intrahepatic cholestasis results in acholic stools. With neonatal hepatitis, physiologic jaundice may directly proceed to continued jaundice during the second week of life. With extrahepatic biliary atresia, there may be a jaundice-free interval. The biochemical profile includes a conjugated hyperbilirubinemia with elevated serum transaminases, alkaline phosphatase, and γ-glutamyl transpeptidase. Unfortunately, although many attempts have been made to distinguish intrahepatic from extrahepatic cholestasis by biochemical means, significant overlap between groups has hampered this approach.

The studies performed to assess an infant with cholestatic jaundice are listed in Table 116–1. The combination of procedures performed is dependent on the individual case and the results,

---

TABLE 116–1. CONJUGATED HYPERBILIRUBINEMIA EVALUATION

Fractionated serum bilirubin
Biochemical profile: aspartate aminotransferase, alanine aminotransferase, alkaline phosphatase, γ-glutamyl transpeptidase, albumin, cholesterol
Prothrombin time
Stool color
Cultures (blood, urine, cerebrospinal fluid)
TORCH titers
VDRL test
Hepatitis A, B, and C screens
Serum α_1-antitrypsin level and phenotype
Metabolic screen: urine or serum amino acids; urine-reducing substance
Thyroid screen
Ophthalmologic examination
Sweat chloride
X-ray films: skull, long bones, abdomen, chest
Abdominal ultrasound
Duodenal intubation (string test)
Hepatobiliary scintigraphy
Endoscopic retrograde cholangiopancreatography
Percutaneous transhepatic cholangiography
Percutaneous liver biopsy

TORCH = toxoplasmosis, rubella, cytomegalovirus and herpes infections; VDRL = Venereal Disease Research Laboratory.

skills, and expertise of each institution. A complete history and physical examination are mandatory. Ophthalmologic examination by an experienced observer in congenital and pediatric eye disorders may be revealing. Cataracts, retinopathy, posterior embryotoxin, or optic nerve hypoplasia may be seen. Laboratory studies confirm a conjugated hyperbilirubinemia. Elevated serum transaminase levels reflect the degree of hepatocellular injury. Elevated alkaline phosphatase suggests hepatobiliary ductular injury. Hepatocellular synthetic function is assessed by the prothrombin time and serum albumin level. If the prothrombin time is prolonged, administration of vitamin K parenterally with a repeat prothrombin time in 24 hours aids in distinguishing between the ability of hepatocytes to synthesize vitamin K–dependent clotting factors from poor intake or absorption of vitamin K. Metabolic, infectious, and genetic disorders may be suspected from the history and physical examination. Infectious disorders may be discerned from cultures, viral titers, immunoglobulin levels, hepatitis screens, and bone radiographs. A sweat chloride determination for cystic fibrosis and serum α_1-antitrypsin level with phenotype should be obtained. Ultrasonography may reveal a choledochal cyst, abdominal mass, biliary stones, ascites, and the presence or absence of a gallbladder. Examination of duodenal bile for pigment color obtained by the string test (Enterotest Pediatric, HDC Corp, San Jose, Calif.) is simple, inexpensive, and invaluable. Yellow pigmented bile excludes complete biliary obstruction. Hepatobiliary scintigraphy after several days of phenobarbital therapy (5 mg/kg/d) may provide useful information. In neonatal hepatitis, hepatocyte uptake of the isotope may be impaired, whereas in early biliary atresia, uptake may be normal, but excretion of the isotope into the intestine is absent.

Endoscopic retrograde cholangiopancreatography (ERCP) and percutaneous transhepatic cholangiography have both recently been advocated by some investigators as useful in the diagnostic armamentarium. However, both procedures are significantly operator dependent, and a special side-viewing endoscope, which is not readily available at most institutions, is necessary for ERCP in these small infants.

Percutaneous liver biopsy may play an important role in determining the need for surgical intervention. In biliary atresia, classic histologic findings include bile duct proliferation, bile plugs, and periportal fibrosis. Giant cell proliferation may be seen in both biliary atresia and neonatal hepatitis and has no specificity. Neonatal hepatitis displays a marked infiltrate of inflammatory cells and focal hepatocellular necrosis. An adequate number of portal triads must be present on the biopsy for appropriate evaluation. Early in the course of some disorders, clas-

TABLE 116–2. DIFFERENTIAL DIAGNOSIS OF CONJUGATED HYPERBILIRUBINEMIA

Infantile obstructive cholangiopathy
  Biliary atresia
  Neonatal hepatitis
  Choledochal cyst
Other causes
  Bile plug syndrome
  Choledocholithiasis
  Spontaneous bile duct perforation
  Extrinsic bile duct compression
Genetic and metabolic disorders
  Disordered carbohydrate metabolism
    Galactosemia
    Fructosemia
    Glycogen storage disease type IV
  Disordered protein metabolism
    Tyrosinemia
  Disordered lipid metabolism
    Niemann-Pick disease
    Gaucher's disease
    Wolman's disease
    Cholesterol ester storage disease
  Chromosomal disorders
    Trisomy 18 syndrome
    Down syndrome
  Miscellaneous genetic and hereditary disorders
    α_1-Antitrypsin deficiency
    Hypopituitarism
    Cystic fibrosis
    Zellweger syndrome (cerebrohepatorenal syndrome)
    Familial hepatosteatosis
Persistent intrahepatic cholestasis
  Paucity of intrahepatic bile ducts
  Arteriohepatic dysplasia
  Benign recurrent intrahepatic cholestasis
  Byler's syndrome
  Hereditary cholestasis with lymphedema
  Trihydroxycoprostanic acidemia
Acquired intrahepatic cholestasis
  Infections
    Hepatitis A, B, and C
    Syphilis
    Toxoplasmosis
    Rubella virus
    Cytomegalovirus
    Herpes virus
    Varicella
    Echovirus
    Coxsackievirus
    Leptospirosis
    Tuberculosis
    Bacterial sepsis
  Drug-induced cholestasis
  Total parenteral nutrition–associated cholestasis

sic histologic changes may not yet be present.

The differential diagnosis of a conjugated hyperbilirubinemia is presented in Table 116–2. This list will hopefully become outdated as our understanding of the multiple causes of neonatal hepatitis improves.

ETIOLOGIC AGENTS

BACTERIAL INFECTIONS

The reticuloendothelial system in the liver and spleen is responsible for clearing bacteria from the blood. In the neonate the ability to handle bacterial infections may be impaired by diminished amounts of complement and opsonins and an immature reticuloendothelial system. Hepatic injury from bacterial infections may result from direct hepatic invasion, circulating toxins, fever, or hypoxia.

Jaundice and hepatomegaly may signal hepatic involvement in systemic sepsis. Although both gram-positive and gram-negative organisms may be involved, gram-negative organisms are more frequently isolated. *Escherichia coli* is the most common organism seen. Group B streptococci are infrequently observed. *Listeria monocytogenes* infection invariably involves the liver. Liver abscesses from umbilical catheterization are rare. *E. coli* and *Staphylococcus aureus* from the umbilical stump are the organisms usually encountered.

Liver biopsies are rarely performed in these infants because of the accompanying abnormal coagulation parameters and the nonspecific findings on biopsy. Bile stasis, hepatocyte necrosis, polymorphonuclear portal infiltrate, and giant call transformation are seen. Laboratory studies reveal leukocytosis, conjugated hyperbilirubinemia, and elevated serum transaminases and alkaline phosphatase.

URINARY TRACT INFECTIONS

Between the second and eighth weeks of life, jaundice associated with bacterial urinary tract infections is often observed. Urinary symptoms or fever are rarely observed. Instead, infants may be lethargic and irritable, feed poorly, and have vomiting or diarrhea. Boys are more frequently affected than girls. Anatomic abnormalities of the genitourinary tract are often not found. Laboratory studies reveal leukocytosis, elevated serum transaminases, and a conjugated hyperbilirubinemia. Urinalysis reveals pyuria, and urine culture often is positive for *E. coli*. Hepatic pathology is nonspecific and similar to that seen in the liver of patients with sepsis, as noted above. Treatment consists of appropriate antibiotic therapy.

CONGENITAL SYPHILIS

Congenital syphilis remains problematic in spite of penicillin therapy and routine maternal screening. Transplacental transmission of *Treponema pallidum* may result in a range of symptoms. Severe symptoms include prematurity, apnea, hepatosplenomegaly, jaundice, skin lesions, rhinitis, and bony lesions. Findings may be present at birth or appear over days to weeks. Patients with milder cases of the disease may have anicteric hepatitis, poor weight gain, or nasal discharge. Nonspecific laboratory findings include a conjugated hyperbilirubinemia with elevated serum transaminases. Hepatic pathology reveals the classic intralobular fibrosis with centrilobular mononuclear infiltration. Silver stains may reveal spirochetes. Serologic testing of serum and cerebrospinal fluid using specific treponemal antibody tests may be necessary to confirm the diagnosis. Treatment includes parenteral administration of penicillin. Erythromycin is reserved for penicillin allergy. Even after appropriate therapy, serologic examination results may remain positive for congenital syphilis for up to 2 years. Prognosis is dependent upon the extent of hepatic injury.

TOXOPLASMOSIS

Maternal infection usually results from contact with the oocytes in cat feces or from uncooked meat (lamb, beef, pork). Maternal infection may be mild and unrecognized but is necessary for congenital toxoplasmosis to occur. Infected newborns are often asymptomatic. Hepatitis may be the only sign of infection. Severe infection primarily affects the liver with hepatomegaly and the nervous system with microcephaly, chorioretinitis, intracranial calcification, meningoencephalitis, and retardation. Liver biopsy specimens show a generalized hepatitis, bile stasis intracellularly, and areas of necrosis. Fluorescent antibody staining may reveal *Toxoplasma* organisms in the tissue. Diagnostic confirmation employs *Toxoplasma* antibody tests. Treatment of infected mothers during pregnancy uses sulfadiazine and pyrimethamine or spiramycin. Infected infants may be treated with pyrimethamine and sulfadiazine with folinic acid to prevent the hematologic toxicity of therapy.

Viral Agents

Cytomegalovirus

Cytomegalovirus (CMV) may be acquired in utero, at delivery, or postnatally from maternal secretions or from transfusion of blood products. Most congenitally infected infants are asymptomatic; but if they are symptomatic, low birth weight, microcephaly, deafness, cerebral calcifications, thrombocytopenia, and retardation may result. Hepatosplenomegaly with significant extramedullary hematopoiesis may be observed. Liver biopsy specimens may reveal large intranuclear inclusion bodies in bile duct epithelium and occasionally in Kupffer's cells and hepatocytes. CMV may be confirmed by culture of the nasopharynx, saliva, and urine and by serologic testing. Treatment includes use of ganciclovir and CMV immune globulin, and hepatic transplantation has been employed in selected cases with severe hepatic involvement. Prognosis is poor for infants with severe infection, with neurologic sequelae occurring.

Herpes

Liver disease from herpes virus may be part of a generalized illness in the newborn. Congenital herpes may present with microcephaly and lesions on the mucosa or the skin. There is often hepatosplenomegaly, jaundice, and abnormal clotting, which may result in gastrointestinal tract bleeding. Liver histologic examination shows necrosis and characteristic intranuclear acidophilic inclusions in hepatocytes. Multinucleated giant cells may also be found. Treatment with acyclovir has become the drug of choice because of its ease of administration and lower toxicity compared to other drugs.

Hepatitis Viruses

Hepatitis A

Although throughout the world hepatitis A is a frequent cause of childhood hepatitis, it is infrequent in the newborn. Blood transfusion appears to be the primary route of hepatitis A acquisition in the newborn as opposed to the fecal-oral route of transmission in older children. In most reports of hepatitis A presenting in newborns, the infants were asymptomatic. However, a recent report of hepatitis A in a premature infant was fatal. Neither chronic hepatitis A or a carrier state for hepatitis A virus exists. Serologic testing for hepatitis A virus confirms the diagnosis. Treatment is supportive. Enteric precautions are advised. During the third trimester of pregnancy, icteric mothers with hepatitis A have not been shown to transmit hepatitis to their infant. However, if the mother is icteric with hepatitis A, immune globulin is recommended for the newborn infant, although the efficacy of this therapy is not proven in this situation.

Hepatitis B

Overall in the United States, hepatitis B is an uncommon cause of neonatal hepatitis. However, in certain regions of the country and parts of the world perinatal transmission of hepatitis B is common from chronic carrier mothers or mothers with acute hepatitis B during the third trimester of pregnancy. Most infants who develop hepatitis B from vertical transmission show hepatitis B surface antigen (HBsAg) positivity by 4 to 16 weeks of age and become asymptomatic carriers. However, chronic active hepatitis from hepatitis B infection can also occur. With time, some infants with hepatitis B progress to cirrhosis and hepatocellular carcinoma or may develop a superinfection with delta hepatitis (hepatitis D). Diagnosis of hepatitis B utilizes serologic tests for hepatitis B antigens, HBsAg and HBeAg, and antibodies to HBsAg, HBcAg, and HBeAg. Liver biopsy is seldom required for diagnosing acute hepatitis B. There is currently no treatment for acute hepatitis B. Most efforts in the past have been directed toward prophylaxis of hepatitis B. It has been recommended that all pregnant women be screened for HBsAg. For infants whose mothers are positive for HBsAg, immunoprophylaxis with hepatitis B immune globulin (HBIG) and hepatitis B vaccination should be instituted at birth. Recently, the Committee on Infectious Diseases of the American Academy of Pediatrics has recommended immunization with hepatitis B vaccine of all infants regardless of the hepatitis B status of the mother.

For chronic hepatitis B in childhood, there are currently limited trials using interferon therapy. In chronic hepatitis B carrier children in Taiwan, interferon was unable to clear HBsAg. In preliminary work from Spain, a small group of children with interferon therapy showed evidence of loss of HBsAg and development of antibody to HBsAg.

Hepatitis C

The introduction of serologic tests for hepatitis C and polymerase chain reaction methods have allowed for the diagnosis and treatment of this disease. Perinatal transmission of hepatitis C has been demonstrated, but the risks and consequences of this have not been well defined. Hepatitis C has been associated with a propensity to progress to a chronic infection and development of hepatocellular carcinoma. Interferon therapy in adults has demonstrated significant and sustained improvements in biochemical and histologic manifestations of hepatitis C. The effectiveness of interferon therapy in children with hepatitis C is unknown.

α_1-ANTITRYPSIN DEFICIENCY

a_1-Antitrypsin deficiency may be present in the infant with neonatal cholestasis. a_1-Antitrypsin is a potent inhibitor of many proteolytic enzymes. Many phenotypes identified by electrophoresis have been associated with liver disease in children, although the ZZ phenotype is classically seen. The diagnosis may be suspected if there is a lack of the a_1-globulin peak on protein electrophoresis, since 90% of this peak is normally due to a_1-antitrypsin. Infants usually present with a conjugated hyperbilirubinemia with jaundice, acholic stools, dark urine, and hepatomegaly. Liver histologic examination reveals characteristic periodic-acid-Schiff-positive diastase-resistant granules in periportal hepatocytes. Diagnosis is confirmed by measurement of serum a_1-antitrypsin concentration and protease-inhibitor phenotyping. Liver transplantation has been successful in many cases, with the recipient acquiring the phenotype of the donor organ.

TOTAL PARENTERAL NUTRITION–ASSOCIATED CHOLESTASIS

Total parenteral nutrition (TPN)–associated cholestasis is the most common cause of conjugated hyperbilirubinemia in the intensive care nursery. Although the exact cause is unknown, immature hepatobiliary function, lack of enteral feeding, sepsis, and amino acid toxicity may be partially responsible. Production of toxic bile acids such as lithocholic acid may mediate the injury. The disorder is manifested by a slow but progressive conjugated hyperbilirubinemia with a modest increase in serum transaminases and alkaline phosphatase. Infants are jaundiced and demonstrate hepatomegaly. If TPN is discontinued, resolution may occur within 4 months. Some infants progress to cirrhosis and liver failure. Treatment consists of discontinuation of parenteral nutrition and resumption of oral feedings. Even minimal enteral feeding during chronic TPN administration may protect against the development of a severe cholestasis.

CHROMOSOMAL DISORDERS

Trisomy 17–18 and trisomy 21 (Down's syndrome) have been associated with both neonatal hepatitis and biliary atresia. Intrahepatic cholestasis, giant cell transformation, and variable degrees of bile duct involvement have been observed. Whether the chromosomal disorder directly contributed to the hepatic lesion or predisposed to a viral agent is not known.

FAMILIAL INTRAHEPATIC CHOLESTATIC SYNDROMES

Infants with a familial intrahepatic cholestatic syndrome frequently are diagnosed in the neonatal period because of their propensity for cholestasis. Disease may be limited to the liver, or there may be abnormalities also in other organs. In this group of syndromes there are both fatal and relatively benign disorders. The most frequently encountered familial disorders in this group are highlighted below.

Alagille's Syndrome (Arteriohepatic Dysplasia)

Alagille's syndrome is the most common form of intrahepatic familial cholestasis. Most cases are first seen in infancy with jaundice or heart disease. During childhood, jaundice, pruritus, xanthomas, and hepatosplenomegaly are encountered. Laboratory studies reveal elevated serum bile acids, transaminases, cholesterol, and alkaline phosphatase. The most frequent heart lesion encountered is peripheral pulmonic stenosis, but other more serious lesions such as coarctation of the aorta may be seen. Liver biopsy specimens may reveal paucity of intrahepatic bile ducts, but a specimen obtained by needle biopsy of the liver may be insufficient to confidently allow this to be observed. The ophthalmologic finding common in patients with Alagille's syndrome is posterior embryotoxin. This is a thickening of the line formed at the junction of Descemet's membrane with the endothelium of the anterior chamber angle. Bone and joint abnormalities include butterfly vertebrae, hemivertebrae, incomplete spina bifida, shortened distal phalanges, and a short ulna. Renal anomalies include reduplication of the pelvis, renal dysfunction, focal tubular dilation, and interstitial fibrosis. The typical facial features include flattened nose, deep set and widely spaced eyes, prominent eyebrows, down-turned mouth, and a small mandible and pointed chin. Recently, the use of ursodeoxycholic acid therapy has provided biochemical improvement and relieved pruritus in some children with Alagille's syndrome.

Byler's Syndrome

Byler's syndrome is the second most common form of familial intrahepatic cholestasis that presents in infancy. A family history of an affected sibling is often encountered. Within the first year of life, there is jaundice, pruritus, and hepatomegaly. Although there is biochemical evidence of cholestasis with elevated bilirubin, bile acids, and alkaline phosphatase, there are normal or low levels for serum cholesterol during the course of the illness. Initially, liver biopsy results may be normal or may reveal giant cells or paucity of intrahepatic bile ducts. However, as the disease progresses, there is periportal fibrosis, leading to biliary cirrhosis. With time most patients develop hepatic failure, ascites, and encephalopathy, which result in death. There are rare instances of patients' surviving into adulthood with the development of Kayser-Fleischer rings from chronic copper deposition.

PROGNOSIS

Prognosis in neonatal hepatitis is variable and dependent on the extent of injury and fibrosis. In general, infants with neonatal hepatitis have a better prognosis than infants with biliary atresia or infants with metabolic disorders that are not amenable to diet therapy. Sporadic cases of neonatal hepatitis have a better prognosis than familial cases.

THERAPY

If a specific diagnosis is not determined, then treatment is empiric. Poor absorption of fat and fat-soluble vitamins in cholestatic infants is a major factor responsible for the malnutrition frequently observed in these children. The use of medium-chain triglycerides as a supplement or in special formulas may be necessary. These children are often irritable from chronic pruritus, and their appetites and oral intake may be poor, necessitating enteral or parenteral supplementation. Fat-soluble vitamin (A, D, E, K) supplementation is mandatory. Regular monitoring of these vitamins for deficiency or overdosage is required. Other micronutrients requiring monitoring and supplementation include calcium, iron, and zinc. Copper-containing foods (nuts, chocolate) should be limited because of poor copper excretion into the bile in cholestatic patients.

Drugs used to stimulate bile flow include phenobarbital (5 mg/kg/d) and cholestyramine, an anion exchange resin. Cholestyramine binds cholesterol and bile acids in the intraluminal space and increases fecal loss. Unfortunately, it is unpalatable and has the potential for the development of hyperchloremic acidosis, intestinal obstruction, and steatorrhea and can interfere with vitamin absorption. Recently, ursodeoxycholic acid (15 to 45 mg/kg/d) therapy in selected children with cholestasis has shown encouraging improvements in biochemical parameters and pruritus. The effect of early recognition and intervention with diet therapy, vitamin supplementation, choleretic agents, and hepatic transplantation awaits further studies.

117

Chronic Cholecystitis

BRET T. PETERSEN

Inflammatory disease of the gallbladder is common and usually is dealt with in a straightforward manner. Enthusiasm for the varied therapeutic alternatives recently has evolved back to surgery, following a full circle of interest in medical, mechanical, and semiinterventional approaches. The introduction of laparoscopic cholecystectomy has lowered the threshold for both physicians and patients to proceed with surgical intervention. The subsequent growth in surgical volume, with an attendant increase in cumulative costs and morbidity, prompt us to emphasize the importance of careful diagnosis.

DEFINITIONS AND PATHOGENESIS

Confusion occasionally exists regarding the terminology used to define gallbladder disease, as not all forms of cholecystitis have proportional histologic and clinical characteristics. The most common presentation of biliary disease is uncomplicated biliary colic, which has no histologic correlate per se. *Biliary colic,* as described below, is usually attributed to temporary stone impaction in the gallbladder neck with associated spasm and distension. *Chronic cholecystitis* also usually occurs in the presence of gallstones and may develop with or without prior episodes of biliary colic or acute cholecystitis. Chronic cholecystitis usually presents with biliary colic; however, symptoms and histologic findings are poorly associated, and histologic cholecystitis may be present in the absence of pain. Pathology may vary from mild round cell infiltration histologically to severe inflammatory fibrosis with gallbladder contraction and thickening evident histologically, grossly, and on imaging studies. Similar findings may be present in the absence of gallstones; however, attribution of symptoms to the gallbladder is then less reliable, particularly when results of noninvasive imaging are normal. *Chronic acalculous cholecystitis* is a poorly defined and controversial clinical entity that is idiopathic and often difficult to diagnose prospectively. Table 117–1 lists other specific pathologic entities that sometimes cause chronic or acute acalculous cholecystitis.

Acute calculous cholecystitis refers to both a clinical diagnosis and to histologic findings, which generally correlate with the severity of the clinical setting. Clinically, acute cholecystitis presents with prolonged stone obstruction and pain that lasts more than 4 to 6 hours and typically evolves from a visceral pattern to right upper quadrant parietal pain. There is often associated nausea, vomiting, fever, abdominal tenderness, and leukocytosis, with or without mild nonspecific abnormalities of liver or pancreatic enzymes. Histopathologically acute cholecystitis exhibits polymorphonuclear leukocyte infiltration, edema, and mucosal necrosis. *Acute acalculous cholecystitis* presents similarly as a complication of another illness or following trauma or major surgery.

Most complications of chronic cholecystitis

TABLE 117–1. CAUSES OF SECONDARY ACALCULOUS CHOLECYSTITIS

1. Specific infections and infestations
    a. Bacterial (typhoid, *Leptospira, Streptococcus, Staphylococcus*)
    b. Viral (hepatitis A)
    c. Helmintic *(Ascaris, Schistosoma)*
    d. Opportunistic (*Cryptosporidium*, cytomegalovirus, *Candida*)
2. Systemic diseases
    a. Collagen diseases (polyarteritis nodosa, systemic lupus erythematosus, scleroderma)
    b. Mucocutaneous lymph node syndrome
    c. Sclerosing cholangitis
    d. Sjögren's syndrome
3. Obstructive
    a. Mechanical (torsion, stent, cystic duct stenosis)
    b. Primary tumor (cystic duct, gallbladder)
    c. Secondary tumor (Hodgkin's disease, melanoma, breast carcinoma, Kaposi's sarcoma)
4. Toxic
    a. Chemotherapy
    b. Lipiodol

From Kang J-Y, Williamson RCN. Review article: cholecystitis without gallstones. *HPB Surgery.* 1990;2:83–103. © 1990 by Harwood Academic Publishers GmbH.

present after evolution to acute cholecystitis. Conditions that may develop more chronically include gallbladder cancer, hydrops of the gallbladder, and so-called "gallstone ileus." *Hydrops* describes a chronically obstructed and markedly distended gallbladder often filled with mucoid or even clear "white bile." Hydrops may present with chronic discomfort or may evolve to acute cholecystitis. *Gallstone ileus* describes overt gut obstruction in the distal small bowel or sigmoid colon occurring as a result of migration of a gallstone through an inflammatory fistula from gallbladder to duodenum or colon. Most patients are elderly women. Therapy is surgical, and morbidity is high, primarily because of delayed diagnosis and the population affected.

DIAGNOSIS OF CHRONIC CHOLECYSTTIS

A careful history is paramount in the diagnosis of chronic cholecystitis, as it is common for gallstones to be asymptomatic despite abdominal pains from other sources, and most patients do not have other imaging findings to implicate the gallbladder as the source of symptoms. Biliary colic typically occurs in the epigastrium or the right upper quadrant with radiating or concurrent pain in the back, chest, or less common abdominal locations. Contrary to the terminology, biliary colic does not wax and wane but is usually steady, with spells lasting 15 minutes to 4 to 6 hours. Fluctuating or transient pain lasting moments to minutes or continuous pain lasting days at a time is rarely due to chronic cholecystitis. Dyspepsia, bloating, isolated nausea, and specific food intolerance are not reliably attributed to the gallbladder and do not contribute to the diagnosis. Whether acalculous chronic cholecystitis presents with differing symptom patterns is not clear; however, one might anticipate varied presentations from differing pathogenetic mechanisms.

Given a history of well-defined biliary-type pain, the demonstration of gallstones strengthens the likelihood of both symptomatic biliary disease and of symptom relief by surgery. The presence of stones, however, does not clarify our understanding of an equivocal history. Asymptomatic stones and nonspecific symptoms are both widely distributed in the population, and their co-occurrence is frequent. Ultrasonography is the usual and most efficient means of diagnosing gallstones. Other static ultrasound findings include a thickened gallbladder wall or a contracted lumen despite fasting. Wall thickening may, however, be seen with ascites or hypoalbuminemia as well. Gallbladder disease can also be inferred from oral cholecystography (OCG). Although stones are somewhat less reliably identified by OCG, failure to image the gallbladder after either a sequential 2-day or a reinforced double-dose study is 95% predictive for gallbladder pathology. This may reflect cystic duct occlusion or diminished mucosal concentrating ability.

Imaging by static radionuclide hepatic iminodiacetic acid (HIDA) scanning, computed tomography (CT), or cholangiography rarely contributes to the diagnosis of chronic cholecystitis. Neither HIDA nor CT scanning reliably demonstrates gallstones. Radionuclide scanning is primarily used to clarify acute presentations, and CT has the most utility in the evaluation for possible disease complications such as abscess or in the exclusion of nonbiliary disease in those with atypical presentations. Although CT may demonstrate the changes seen by ultrasonography in chronic uncomplicated disease, it is not a cost-effective study in this setting.

Given a history strongly suggestive of biliary disease yet an initial ultrasound with no abnormal findings, stone disease can occasionally be confirmed by one of several methods. Repeated ultrasonography after several months may somewhat fortuitously detect sludge or minute stones between episodes of symptomatic stone clearance. Endoscopic cholangiography is occasionally helpful in detecting small duct or gallbladder stones. Among 195 patients referred for endoscopic retrograde cholangiopancreatography (ERCP) evaluation of biliary-type pain after no abnormal findings were demonstrated by ultrasound and OCG studies, 29 had small stones identified. This was the case for 78% of patients with a history of abnormal enzymes during prior episodes of pain, but was true for only 2.5% of those without prior abnormal laboratory values. Identification of microlithiasis, cholesterol crystals, or bilirubinate debris in duodenal bile aspirates after a cholecystokinin (CCK)-stimulated gallbladder contraction can be equated with early stone disease. This finding is highly predictive of symptom relief by cholecystectomy for recurrent biliary pancreatitis and presumably also for chronic stone-related cholecystitis.

In the absence of demonstrable stone disease, chronic biliary-type symptoms are more problematic. Dynamic evaluation of gallbladder motility has been proposed as a means of inferring biliary pathology and, presumably, symptomatology when static imaging by ultrasound or OCG are normal. Functional abnormalities of gallbladder motility have been shown to develop as a consequence of marked biliary supersaturation and are known to contribute to the pathogenesis of gallstones. Whether gallbladder dysmotility serves as a marker for undetected microlithiasis or reflects either mucosal inflammatory changes or partial cystic duct obstruction is unknown. Gallbladder contractions are assessed by either radionuclide scanning or ultrasonography following stimulation with either intravenous CCK or a defined fatty meal. No uniform approach to such studies currently exists; however, use of symptom assessment and stimulation by fatty meals or bolus CCK injections are apparently unreliable because of their lack of specificity and inconsistent reproducibility. In a recent study, cholescintigraphy performed during standardized CCK infusions accurately predicted the benefit of cholecystectomy among those with an abnormal gallbladder ejection fraction of less than 40%. Although provocative, such data require confirmation before widespread application.

MANAGEMENT

In general, cholecystectomy is advisable for those patients with demonstrated gallstones, clear biliary colic, and low surgical risk. However, healthy patients wishing to observe their clinical course before electing surgery can generally do so with acceptable risk. At issue is not the alleviation of current symptoms but rather prophylaxis against the development of future pain, biliary complications, or cancer. Following a single episode of biliary colic, 30% of patients may not have further symptoms, and only 40% to 50% have recurrent colic within 1 year. Once the condition becomes symptomatic with an established pattern of discrete episodes of biliary colic, patients can anticipate continued symptoms in a similar pattern and have a 1% to 2% annual risk of developing complications such as acute cholecystitis or pancreatitis. Although the risk of gallbladder cancer is increased by the presence of gallstones, it remains less than the risk of surgery, and hence cancer prevention alone is not an adequate indication for surgery. An exception to this rule is the presence of a calcified or so-called "porcelain gallbladder," which even in the absence of symptoms carries a somewhat greater risk for cancer and should prompt elective removal in an otherwise healthy patients.

For patients with gallstones and equivocal symptoms, plausible alternative diagnoses should be excluded including possible peptic ulcer disease, esophageal reflux, pancreatic or small bowel disease, and abdominal wall discomfort. Given the presence of gallstones, no additional biliary studies are of great utility. Although observation is reasonable, a "diagnostic cholecystectomy" is often opted in the healthy low-risk patient. If so, a careful discussion regarding the diagnostic uncertainty and potential lack of symptom resolution should take place preoperatively.

As alluded to, biliary symptoms in the absence of gallstones or gallbladder abnormality demonstrable by routine imaging are often frustrating for the physician and patient alike. Demonstration of biliary crystals or abnormally sluggish motility after provocation may provide increased confidence for symptom relief by surgery. In the absence of these findings and given the understanding of uncertain benefit, highly selected low-risk patients with prominent and typical symptoms might still be reasonably offered somewhat empiric surgery. In general, however, cholecystectomy should be reserved for those patients in whom benefit can be confidently predicted.

Although open cholecystectomy has been the gold standard of therapy for efficacy, safety, and long-term outcome, laparoscopic cholecystectomy can now be considered the optimal approach. The consistently shortened hospital stay, reduced need for analgesia, and reduced period of postoperative disability far outweigh the relative increase in bile duct injuries evident during the early experience. Based on intraoperative findings or difficulty, 2% to 5% of laparoscopic cholecystectomies are subsequently converted to open procedures. Of principal importance in selecting a surgeon is ensuring adequate training and experience in laparoscopic techniques. The risk of surgery is greater for emergent procedures, particularly in elderly patients with concurrent cardiorespiratory disease.

The practice of laparoscopic cholecystectomy has raised additional issues regarding the optimal management of associated catheter common bile duct stones. Laparoscopic approaches to the common duct are available but not yet widely practiced because of their technical difficulty. If local surgeons are skilled in the concurrent laparoscopic management of duct stones, this is the preferable approach. More commonly, duct stones are now being managed with preoperative or postoperative endoscopic extraction; 90% to 95% of duct stones can be extracted successfully by ERCP. The presence of stones that ultimately fail endoscopic extraction can usually be anticipated by preoperative studies (ultrasound and chemistry tests), thus allowing endoscopic attempts to succeed or fail before proceeding with either laparoscopic cholecystectomy alone or open cholecystectomy with duct exploration. In patients with known or probable duct stones, preoperative ERCP is thus preferable. In those patients with less certain likelihood of duct stones, the timing of ERCP should be based on the relative skills of the local endoscopist and of the surgeon in performing cholangiography. If either endoscopic or intraoperative cholangiography skills are marginal, ERCP should be performed preoperatively. Endoscopic evaluation of the duct is not indicated in patients without imaging or biochemical suggestions of possible duct stones. Ideally, the overall number of procedures and their attendant risk can be minimized by the use of intraoperative cholangiography and concurrent laparoscopic choledocholithotomy or postoperative endoscopic extraction of identified stones.

Nonoperative approaches to cholesterol gallbladder stones and associated chronic cholecystitis include oral dissolution therapy, extracorporeal shock wave lithotripsy (ESWL) plus oral dissolution of resulting debris, and rapid contact dissolution via percutaneous catheter delivery of cholesterol solvents such as methyl-tert-butyl ether (MTBE). All three therapies require a patent cystic duct, as determined by gallbladder visualization during either an OCG or HIDA scanning. Any of the nonsurgical therapies can be reasonably entertained in the symptomatic patient with eligible stone and gallbladder characteristics who is unwilling or unable to undergo general anesthesia and surgery. Currently, only oral dissolution is approved for use in the United States.

Ursodeoxycholic acid (ursodiol or Actigall) successfully dissolves 30% to 70% of radiolucent cholesterol stones when taken in adequate doses (8 to 10 mg/kg) for 1 to 2 years. Optimal candidates are those with minor or infrequent symptoms and small (≤ 5 mm) stones that are radiolucent by plain film (or preferably by CT) or float during OCG. Although side effects are minimal (diarrhea in $<5\%$), the costs are substantial and may run $1500 to $2000 per year.

ESWL has demonstrated efficacy for patients with limited stone burdens; 70% to 90% of patients with single radiolucent cholesterol stones less than or equal to 20 mm in diameter achieve gallbladder clearance after 12 to 24 months of continuous oral dissolution therapy. Patients with larger, more numerous, or calcified stones have proportionally poorer results and may require more aggressive or repeated lithotripsy. Although biliary lithotripsy remains unapproved in the United States, there is minimal postmarket oversight of renal lithotriptor use, and ESWL is occasionally applied to difficult bile duct stones on a compassionate use basis. Gallbladder lithotripsy, however, is generally not available in this country.

Rapid contact dissolution of cholesterol gallstones by MTBE is unlimited by stone size or number, and gallbladder clearance can be expected for patients with stones demonstrated to be radiolucent by CT. Therapy requires 6 to 12 hours of solvent perfusion over 1 to 3 days via a small-bore transhepatic cholecystostomy catheter. Although contact dissolution is ideal for patients with very high surgical risk and appropriate stones, it is only available as investigational therapy at a few centers.

There are no nonsurgical therapies with demonstrated efficacy for pigment stones, densely calcified cholesterol stones, or idiopathic chronic acalculous cholecystitis. Rare patients with non-soluble stones and either high surgical risk or prohibitive surgical anatomy can be palliated with stone removal via semisurgical percutaneous approaches involving dilation of cholecystostomy tracts.

The major shortcoming of all the nonsurgical therapies that leave the gallbladder in situ is the risk for recurrence of stones and symptoms. Overall, recurrent stones develop in about 10% of patients per year up to a total of 50% to 70% of patients. Recurrence is less likely in those with solitary or few index stones. The likelihood of recurrent symptoms after development of recurrent stones has not been characterized. The potential for stone recurrence is not reason to avoid nonoperative therapy in the patient at very high surgical risk.

On the whole, symptomatic chronic cholecystitis is almost always related to gallstones and can be safely and efficiently managed once a reliable diagnosis is made. Most difficult for patients and physicians alike is to avoid undeserved attribution of symptoms to otherwise asymptomatic stones with the subsequent risk of frustration or, worse, complication following unhelpful surgical management. Most complications of chronic cholecystitis evolve through stages of acute cholecystitis.

REFERENCES

1. American College of Physicians. Clinical guideline: guidelines for the treatment of gallstones. *Ann Intern Med.* 1993;119:620–622.
2. Kang J-Y, Williamson RCN. Review article: cholecystitis without gallstones. *HPB Surgery.* 1990;2:83–103.
3. Kloiber R, Molnar CP, Shaffer EA. Review article: chronic biliary-type pain in the absence of gallstones: the value of cholecystokinin cholescintigraphy. *AJR.* 1992;159:509–513.
4. Marton KI, Doubilet P. Diagnosis and treatment: how to image the gallbladder in suspected cholecystitis. *Ann Intern Med.* 1988;109:722–729.
5. National Institutes of Health Consensus Development Conference Statement on Gallstones and Laparoscopic Cholecystectomy. *Am J Surg.* 1993;165:390–396.
6. Ransohoff DF, Gracie WA. Treatment of gallstones. *Ann Intern Med.* 1993;119:606–619.

118
Acalculous Cholecystitis
DAVID P. NUNES and NEZAM H. AFDHAL

Acalculous cholecystitis accounts for approximately 10% of all cases of acute cholecystitis. It carries the highest mortality for any benign condition of the gallbladder. The prognosis depends largely on the presence of other medical or surgical conditions, but in the most severely ill patients the mortality has been reported to be as high as 90%, whereas community-acquired cases carry a mortality only slightly greater than that for calculous disease. Its importance is emphasized by recent studies suggesting that the incidence of acalculous cholecystitis is rising.

The diagnosis is frequently difficult because history, physical examination, and diagnostic studies may be inconclusive and the clinical features may be hidden by the presence of other conditions, particularly in the critically ill. The often rapidly progressive nature of the disease with a high incidence of gallbladder gangrene and perforation means that early diagnosis and treatment are necessary to reduce its high mortality and morbidity.

ACUTE ACALCULOUS CHOLECYSTITIS

PATHOGENESIS

The term *acute acalculous cholecystitis* refers to an acute necroinflammatory condition of the gallbladder, which is sometimes also known as necrotizing cholecystitis. Its pathogenesis is multifactorial and includes important roles for bile acids, systemic sepsis, and local inflammatory responses. Sepsis is associated with complement-induced injury to small vessel endothelium, activation of the clotting pathways, and thrombosis of these vessels. The resultant gallbladder ischemia leads to tissue necrosis and, when severe, progression to gangrene. Biliary stasis with high intraluminal pressures and bile salt concentrations have both been shown to predispose to acalculous cholecystitis in the clinical setting and in animal models. Both of these factors have been shown to induce an increase in proinflammatory prostaglandins (E) and a relative reduction in the antiinflammatory prostaglandins (F). Bacterial and tissue phospholipases released into the lumen of the gallbladder convert lecithin to lysolecithin, resulting in epithelial membrane injury.

The disease is seen in several clinical settings, and a number of clinically relevant predisposing factors have been identified. Dehydration is thought to be a risk factor by increasing the viscosity of bile and impairing gallbladder emptying. Prolonged fasting and intravenous hyperalimentation result in long periods of gallbladder stasis, high bile salt concentrations, and the formation of biliary sludge, which further impairs gallbladder emptying. Opiates increase the pressure in the sphincter of Oddi, resulting in an increase in the intraluminal pressure of the gallbladder and biliary tree. High intraluminal pressures can compromise gallbladder perfusion, which can be further exacerbated by systemic hypotension. The condition is therefore most commonly seen in patients with severe sepsis, following major surgery, burns, trauma, or childbirth. It was for instance commonly seen during the Vietnam war in severely injured soldiers with bacterial infections. Other predisposing factors include multiple blood transfusions, broad spectrum antibiotics, and mechanical ventilation. Patients with diabetes mellitus, ischemic heart disease, and peripheral vascular disease also appear to be at higher risk (Table 118–1).

Infection also plays an important pathogenic role in acalculous cholecystitis. Gallbladder infection may be secondary to septicemia or an ascending biliary infection. Bacterial pathogens (when present) are often the same as those found in patients with calculous cholecystitis—*Escherichia coli, Enterococcus faecalis, Klebsiella, Pseudomonas,* and *Proteus* species. Pseudomonal

TABLE 118–1. FACTORS PREDISPOSING TO ACUTE ACALCULOUS CHOLECYSTITIS

- Fasting
- Total parenteral nutrition
- Septicemia, biliary infections
- Major trauma
- Burns
- Nonbiliary surgery
- Childbirth
- Multiple blood transfusions
- Broad spectrum antibiotics
- Mechanical ventilation
- Opiates
- Immunosuppression (chemotherapy, acquired immunodeficiency syndrome)
- Diabetes mellitus
- Ischemic heart disease
- Peripheral vascular disease

infection should be considered following biliary tract instrumentation including endoscopic retrograde cholangiopancreatography (ERCP) and in patients who have been receiving broad spectrum antibiotics, particularly in patients with burns or indwelling catheters. Infection with gas-forming organisms such as *Clostridium perfringens* causes a particularly severe form of the disease referred to as emphysematous acalculous cholecystitis. When acute acalculous cholecystitis occurs in association with typhoid fever, cholecystitis normally presents in the second week of infection but may occur later. There are case reports of acalculous cholecystitis occurring in association with leptospirosis and *Campylobacter jejuni*.

Unusual opportunistic infections are increasingly being reported and are occasionally the primary cause of the disease. *Candida albicans*–associated acalculous cholecystitis has been described in severely ill postoperative patients receiving broad spectrum antibiotics. As mentioned above, immunosuppressed patients are at risk for opportunistic infections. Acalculous cholecystitis in acquired immunodeficiency syndrome (AIDS) has been associated with *Cryptosporidium* and cytomegalovirus. In cases associated with *Cryptosporidium*, it is normally possible to isolate the organism from the duodenum. More recently, a case of *Salmonella enteritidis*–associated acalculous cholecystitis has been described in a patient with AIDS. Bone marrow transplant recipients and patients receiving chemotherapy are also at increased risk.

CLINICAL PRESENTATION

The clinical presentation may be variable. Unlike calculous cholecystitis, acute acalculous cholecystitis is more common in men than women. Patients may present with the classic signs and symptoms of acute cholecystitis or insidiously with fever, leukocytosis, and vague abdominal symptoms. More significant abdominal symptoms may only develop with the onset of complications such as gallbladder gangrene or perforation. Difficulty in diagnosis is often compounded by the presence of other underlying diseases. It is therefore essential to maintain a high level of clinical suspicion to ensure early diagnosis and treatment.

Recent series have suggested that as many as 50% of cases present as outpatients with the classic features of acute cholecystitis. They present with severe right upper quadrant pain radiating to the back and right shoulder. On physical examination, the patient is usually febrile with localized tenderness and guarding in the right upper quadrant. A right upper quadrant mass is occasionally palpable. Murphy's sign can normally be elicited. Jaundice is not uncommon, probably reflecting extension of the inflammatory process to the adjacent common bile duct with partial common bile duct obstruction. Gallbladder gangrene and perforation often lead to rapid deterioration, with sepsis, shock, and features of generalized peritonitis.

The presentation of patients who develop the condition while in the hospital is often more insidious. The appearance of an unexplained fever with leukocytosis and vague abdominal complaints may be the only clue to the diagnosis. Many of the classic features may be obscured, for instance, in a patient receiving ventilation in the intensive care unit or in postoperative and severely ill medical patients who may already have causes for abdominal pain, fever, or leukocytosis. Unfortunately, the diagnosis is often missed until later in the natural history of the condition with the onset of gallbladder gangrene with or without perforation.

The differential diagnosis is often wide but includes acute calculous cholecystitis, peptic ulceration with or without perforation, acute pancreatitis, right-sided pyelonephritis, and hepatic or right subphrenic abscesses. Acute hepatic congestion may also simulate acute cholecystitis. Acute gallbladder torsion is a rare cause of severe right upper quadrant pain, and the diagnosis is not normally made until laparotomy. In patients with generalized peritonitis, ischemic injury to the bowel becomes part of the differential diagnosis. Careful clinical examination, urinalysis, and straight abdominal x-rays should help to distinguish between many of these conditions.

INVESTIGATIONS

Routine laboratory studies may be helpful, but the findings are often nonspecific. An increased white cell count with left shift is seen in about 70% to 85% of cases. Unlike acute calculous cholecystitis, the serum bilirubin is elevated in 20% to 30% of patients even in the absence of cholangitis. This may be accompanied by a mild increase in the serum alkaline phosphatase, c-glutamyl transpeptidase, and serum transaminases. Serum amylase levels should be measured to help exclude acute pancreatitis, and blood cultures should be taken before the institution of antibiotic therapy.

Plain abdominal x-ray films are normally unhelpful in making the diagnosis of acalculous cholecystitis but may be useful to exclude a perforated viscus, bowel ischemia, or renal calculi. The investigation of first choice is often ultrasonography because in addition to its being able to exclude calculous disease, ultrasound also permits assessment of the kidneys, pancreas, liver, and common bile duct. Furthermore, ultrasound can be performed at the bedside for patients in the intensive care unit. Even in the absence of gallstones, features suggestive of acute cholecystitis may be present. Positive but often nonspecific findings include thickening of the gallbladder wall (>5 mm) with pericholecystic fluid. It may be possible to elicit an ultrasound "Murphy's sign," where placement of the ultrasound probe over the gallbladder is associated with marked local tenderness. Failure to visualize the gallbladder is strongly suggestive of gallbladder disease. In this clinical setting, gallbladder disease may be due to a gallbladder filled with gallbladder sludge, a tenacious mixture of mucin bile salts and cholesterol that can be isoechogenic with the gallbladder wall. In emphysematous cholecystitis, gas bubbles may be seen arising from the fundus of the gallbladder, the so-called "champagne sign."

Where the clinical diagnosis is suggestive of acute cholecystitis disease, radioisotope studies using various iminodiacetic acid (IDA) compounds (dimethyl-IDA [HIDA], di-isopropyl-IDA [DISIDA], p-isopropyl-IDA [PIPIDA]) may be preferred as the primary investigation. Radioisotope studies require normal hepatic uptake and excretion with concentration of the radioisotope in the gallbladder, through a patent cystic duct. The studies thus give information about hepatic function as well as biliary and cystic duct patency. Failure of gallbladder opacification is the primary and most useful finding. Gallbladder opacification with excretion of the isotope into the pericystic region indicates gallbladder perforation. Failure to opacify the hepatic and common bile ducts has been associated with severe complicated acalculous cholecystitis, gallbladder gangrene, and perforation. Unfortunately, the incidence of false-positive and false-negative scans is higher in acalculous than in calculous disease. Oral cholecystography has no role in the diagnosis of acute acalculous cholecystitis. Furthermore, it should be stressed that numerous investigations should not be performed if they will delay prompt treatment of this potentially fatal emergency.

MANAGEMENT

General

The patient should be resuscitated with fluids and electrolytes as necessary. Antibiotic therapy should be instituted following blood cultures. Antibiotic cover should be aimed at covering the most likely organisms (enterococci, gram-negative organisms, and anaerobes) but may well need to be modified depending on the clinical circumstances. Hence, triple therapy with ampicillin, gentamicin, and metronidazole is satisfactory in most cases. Alternatively, a third-generation cephalosporin plus metronidazole may be used, particularly in patients with borderline or impaired renal function. It should be noted that ceftriaxone has been associated with the formation of biliary sludge and may best be avoided in these patients. Some of the newer antibiotics also give excellent coverage and have been shown to be effective in the treatment of severe biliary infections. Alternative regimens include mezlocillin with an aminoglycoside and metronidazole, imipenem, or ampicillin-sulbactam. Standard antipseudomonal regimens may be required where *Pseudomonas* is a likely pathogen (e.g., piperacillin plus an aminoglycoside).

Specific

The definitive management of acute acalculous cholecystitis is cholecystectomy. Open cholecystectomy is probably the operation of choice in these frequently complicated cases. It gives optimal visualization of the gallbladder, cystic duct, and adjacent vasculature, reducing the risk of common bile duct injury. Furthermore, the gallbladder in these patients may be encased in a large inflammatory mass that precludes other operative approaches. Some surgeons may now opt to try the laparoscopic approach initially and convert to open cholecystectomy if necessary. There are, however, no data at the present time to demonstrate the efficacy and safety of the laparoscopic approach in these patients. In the severely ill patient or where other conditions preclude open surgery, placement of a cholecystotomy tube either surgically or under radiologic control has given excellent results. Cholecystectomy can then be performed when the condition of the patient allows. At least one case of complete resorption of the gallbladder following drainage has been reported; the gallbladder could not be identified at subsequent laparotomy.

CHRONIC ACALCULOUS CHOLECYSTITIS

There has been an increasing recognition of chronic acalculous cholecystitis as a cause of abdominal pain. Recent series have demonstrated that an increasing proportion of patients undergoing cholecystectomy have chronic acalculous cholecystitis. The increased recognition of this condition has followed some advances in diagnostic techniques and together with the advent of laparoscopic surgery has led to a higher proportion of cholecystectomies being performed for this diagnosis. Despite these advances the diagnosis remains difficult, and differentiation from functional disorders remains a challenge.

ETIOLOGY

Chronic acalculous cholecystitis is a chronic inflammatory condition of the gallbladder that gives rise to signs and symptoms frequently indistinguishable from chronic calculous cholecystitis. The cause of chronic acalculous cholecystitis remains unclear in the majority of patients. Chronic cholecystitis may be seen in association with gallbladder carriage of *Salmonella typhi*, but this is not normally an indication for cholecystectomy. Gallbladder involvement in polyarteritis nodosa, Crohn's disease, sclerosing cholangitis, and systemic sclerosis are recognized, but they account for only a tiny proportion of all cases of chronic acalculous disease.

At surgery, the gallbladder may appear almost normal or may be markedly thickened and fibrosed. Histologic features include hyperplasia of the gallbladder smooth muscle with marked interstitial fibrosis and atrophy of the overlying mucosa. Cholesterosis or adenomyomatosis of the gallbladder may also be present. Cholesterosis (strawberry gallbladder) is due to deposition of cholesterol and triglycerides in the gallbladder epithelium and lamina propria, giving rise to the characteristic appearance of the mucosa. Adenomyomatosis is characterized by hyperplasia of the gallbladder mucosa with the formation of Rokitansky-Aschoff sinuses. Gallbladder polyps are occasionally discovered incidentally but may be a cause of gallbladder colic. Cholecystectomy is normally recommended in patients with polyps, as there is a risk of malignant transformation that correlates with the size of the polyp.

CLINICAL FEATURES

Patients with chronic acalculous cholecystitis may present with a variety of clinical complaints. Most characteristically, patients present with right upper quadrant or epigastric pain related to meals, which may radiate to the shoulder or back. Increased symptoms in association with fatty meals is frequently reported. In these cases the diagnosis is relatively straightforward. More nonspecific symptoms include increased flatulence, dyspepsia, and poor tolerance of fatty foods. On physical examination the patient may have right hypochondrial tenderness with a positive Murphy's sign. More frequently the physical signs are unhelpful, and other diagnostic studies are required.

The diagnosis frequently depends on the exclusion of other diseases that may present in a similar fashion. These conditions include peptic ulcer disease, chronic pancreatitis, renal calculi, chronic pyelonephritis, and functional bowel disorders. Differentiation from functional bowel disorders is probably the most difficult, and in many cases the diagnosis depends solely on clinical judgment.

INVESTIGATIONS

The increased recognition of acalculous cholecystitis as a cause of chronic abdominal pain has been associated with the development of many "diagnostic tests." Despite the development of a number of newer radiologic investigations, the diagnosis is still largely clinical. Most physicians order abdominal ultrasonography and upper gastrointestinal tract endoscopic or radiologic procedures to rule out calculous cholecystitis and peptic ulcer disease. Chronic pancreatitis is normally excluded by the absence of an etiologic factor and the quality of the pain. Occasionally it may be necessary to perform a computed tomography scan or an ERCP.

The simplest of the available direct methods is to administer cholecystokinin (CCK) as an intravenous infusion over 5 minutes. Patients with acalculous disease often report reproduction of their symptoms within 5 to 10 minutes. The injection is usually given either before or after a similar injection of normal saline to help exclude a placebo effect. Studies using this technique to select patients for cholecystectomy have shown that the early symptomatic benefit of cholecystectomy was maintained for over 12 months.

Gallbladder emptying assessed by IDA scanning, ultrasonography, or oral cholecystectomy in response to a fatty meal or CCK infusion has also been used. Demonstration of a reduced gallbladder ejection fraction on IDA following CCK infusion is taken as evidence of intrinsic gallbladder disease. The diagnosis is supported by reproduction of the patient's symptoms, but several studies have suggested that long-term symptomatic improvement occurs in patients with both positive and negative results on CCK or IDA scans.

Ultrasonography may be helpful in that a thickened gallbladder wall, nonvisualization of the gallbladder, or failure of the gallbladder to contract following a fatty meal or CCK infusion are suggestive of a diseased gallbladder. Similarly, nonopacification of the gallbladder on oral cholecystography or failure to empty the gallbladder following CCK infusion or a fatty meal are also suggestive of gallbladder pathology. It is important to remember that these investigations are likely to perform well only in highly selected patients where the clinical impression of acalculous cholecystitis is high. Furthermore, demonstration of a nonfunctioning gallbladder does not necessarily imply that the gallbladder is the source of the patient's symptoms.

TREATMENT

The treatment of acalculous cholecystitis is cholecystectomy, which is now most often performed laparoscopically. Although laparoscopic cholecystectomy has a higher patient acceptance with a shorter period away from normal activities, it should be remembered that the incidence of common bile duct injury and cystic duct leaks is higher than for open cholecystectomy, and therefore the procedure should not be performed simply as a "diagnostic test" or where the clinical suspicion is low. Long-term results are difficult to assess and clearly depend on patient selection.

REFERENCES

1. Babb RR. Acute acalculous cholecystitis: a review. *J Clin Gastroenterol.* 1992;15:238–241.
2. Johnson LB. The importance of early diagnosis of acute acalculous cholecystitis. *Surg Gynecol Obstet.* 1987;164: 197–203.
3. Pickleman J, Peiss RL, Henkin R, Salo B, Nagel P. The role of sincalide cholescintigraphy in the evaluation of patients with acalculus gallbladder disease. *Arch Surg.* 1985; 120:693–697.
4. Reed DN, Fernandez M, Hicks RD. Kinevac assisted cholescintigraphy as an accurate predictor of chronic acalculus gallbladder disease and the likelihood of symptom relief with cholecystectomy. *Am Surg.* 1993;59:273–277.
5. Williamson RCN. Acalculous disease of the gallbladder. *Gut.* 1988;29:860–872.

119

Cholelithiasis

RAHUL KUVER, MYUNG-HWAN KIM, and SUM P. LEE

Cholelithiasis is highly prevalent in Western society. In the United States alone, 20 million people are estimated to have gallstones. Indeed, for American women there is a 20% lifetime risk of developing gallstones. Although approximately two thirds of cases are asymptomatic, the sheer number of symptomatic cases has created a large burden in terms of morbidity and health care costs. Half a million cholecystectomies are performed each year in the United States, and the estimated yearly cost of gallstone disease is $5 billion.[1]

This chapter reviews the epidemiology, pathogenesis, clinical manifestations, diagnosis, and treatment of cholelithiasis. With the burgeoning knowledge regarding pathophysiology of gallstone formation and the new technologic and pharmaceutical options available, the 1990s promise to be a pivotal era in the understanding and treatment of this condition.

EPIDEMIOLOGY

The true incidence of gallstones in a given population is difficult to ascertain, as the majority of persons with cholelithiasis are asymptomatic. Nevertheless, studies based on autopsies and imaging modalities have shown a prevalence of around 10% in North America and Western Europe. Higher rates are found in Scandinavia and Chile and among the Pima Indians of Arizona.[2] Other Native American groups and Mexican-Americans also have higher prevalence rates. Lower rates are found in sub-Saharan Africa.[1] The composition of stones also differs, with Africa and Asia showing a preponderance of pigment stones, whereas in Western countries greater than 80% of stones contain cholesterol.

A number of risk factors have been associated with gallstone formation[3] (Table 119–1). Increasing age and gender show such a correlation: gallstones are rare before the age of 20; and women have a twofold to threefold higher risk of developing gallstones than men.[1] The female-male ratio is higher in younger age groups and becomes 2:1 above age 50 years. A family history of gallstones in first-degree relatives confers a doubled risk. Obesity, rapid weight loss, parity, pregnancy, ileal disease, total parenteral nutrition (TPN), medications such as clofibrate and possibly oral contraceptives and estrogens have been linked to a higher incidence of cholelithiasis. Finally, although some studies have implicated diets high in simple sugars and total fat as a risk factor, these data are inconclusive, and therefore no specific dietary recommendations are in place at this time. It must be noted, however, that vegetarians have a lower prevalence of gallstones.[4]

PATHOGENESIS

CHOLESTEROL GALLSTONES

Over the past two decades strides have been made in the elucidation of processes leading to cholesterol gallstone formation. Cholesterol in the body is maintained by de novo synthesis from acetyl coenzyme A and from dietary sources.[3,5] Cholesterol is used for the synthesis of steroids and lipoproteins. The majority of cholesterol is solubilized in bile and secreted or is converted to bile salts. The metabolic processes maintaining the total body pool of cholesterol is tightly regulated; however, defects in this regulation lead to two distinct situations that then predispose to cholesterol gallstone formation.[6]

The first is absolute biliary cholesterol hypersecretion.[7] This occurs clinically in states such as obesity, rapid weight loss, hyperlipoproteinemia, estrogen use, and clofibrate use. The second is relative bile salt hyposecretion, which is encountered with ileal disease or bypass, congenital 12a-hydroxylase deficiency, and primary biliary cirrhosis. Both situations may coexist.

TABLE 119–1. RISK FACTORS FOR CHOLESTEROL GALLSTONE FORMATION

Cholesterol Hypersecretion
Age
Obesity
Oral contraceptives
Progesterone
Clofibrate
Estrogens
Marked weight reduction
High polyunsaturated fat diet
Pima Indian descent

Relative Bile Acid Hyposecretion
Ileal disease, bypass, or resection
Congenital 12a-hydroxylase deficiency
Primary biliary cirrhosis
Chronic Cholestasis
Cholestyramine
Pima Indian descent

Free cholesterol is insoluble in aqueous solution. The solubilization of cholesterol occurs via two distinct but interdependent pathways. First, bile salts (which are amphipathic molecules, so that they are water soluble but, beyond a certain critical concentration, form micelles) form mixed micelles with cholesterol and phospholipids and thereby solubilize cholesterol.[3,6]

The second pathway of cholesterol solubilization is via the formation of unilamellar vesicles composed of cholesterol and phospholipid.[3,6,8] This occurs in the hepatocyte, and vesicles are released via the canalicular membrane into hepatic ducts. There is a dynamic interchange of cholesterol between vesicles and mixed micelles in ductules, ducts, and gallbladder. Several factors affect this interchange. For example, the fasting state and consequent low bile salt concentration favors vesicular carriage of cholesterol. The higher bile salt concentrations found in the gallbladder favor micelle formation. The amount of cholesterol and phospholipid in vesicular and mixed micelles may alter as they undergo dynamic interchange. Sometimes, multilamellar vesicles can result.

The formation of solid cholesterol crystals from saturated bile is termed nucleation.[3,6] Current understanding of this process is that within the gallbladder, concentrated bile salts preferentially remove phospholipid from vesicles, leaving thermodynamically unstable, cholesterol-rich, multilamellar vesicles. These vesicles fuse together and become nucleation prone. In addition, certain glycoproteins in bile act as both pronucleating and antinucleating agents, the relative balance of which determines whether cholesterol gallstone formation occurs. Finally, calcium complexes also play a role in nucleation, as often such complexes are found in the center of cholesterol gallstones.

The gallbladder itself plays a role in cholesterol gallstone formation, for cholecystectomy cures a person of recurrent cholesterol gallstones. Some data suggest there is a defect in acidification in gallbladder bile: a higher pH would favor precipitation of calcium salts.[9] Mucin, a high molecular weight glycoprotein that is a component of gallbladder mucus, may act as a pronucleator. Gallbladder stasis, encountered in such clinical situations as fasting, TPN, pregnancy, or long-term treatment with somatostatin analogs, also plays a role.

When cholesterol crystals have nucleated or calcium bilirubin salts have precipitated (see below), bile becomes turbid. The presence of these precipitates has been referred to as biliary sludge (microcrystalline disease, microlithiasis). Biliary sludge is believed to be a precursor for stone development.[10] Under polarized microscopy, the sediments are commonly found to be cholesterol crystals or calcium bilirubinate granules. The sediments are noted on ultrasound as echogenic material that layers in the dependent portion of the gallbladder and produces low-amplitude echoes without postacoustic shadowing. In one study, sludge developed in all patients receiving TPN over a course of 6 weeks; 40% of these patients subsequently developed stones. Restarting oral feedings resulted in sludge resolution in all patients by 4 weeks.[11] Sludge may also appear spontaneously in some patients; in 60% of such patients, the sludge disappeared and recurred.[10]

Pigment Stones

Like cholesterol, bilirubin is insoluble in water. In bile, bilirubin is therefore secreted as diglucuronide (80%), monoglucuronide (20%), or unconjugated bilirubin. Pigment stones form as a result of deconjugation of bilirubin and its resulting precipitation. There are two types of pigment stones, black and brown. These types are distinct clinically and chemically[12] (Table 119–2).

Black pigment stones have irregular and hard surfaces. They contain calcium bilirubinate, polymerized to a greater extent than in brown stones. They usually form in the gallbladder under sterile conditions. Deconjugating activity is thought to arise from epithelial cells or from hydrolytic enzymes secreted by the liver or pancreas. Stasis in the gallbladder may concentrate

TABLE 119–2. CLINICAL AND CHEMICAL CHARACTERISTICS OF PIGMENT GALLSTONES

	BLACK	BROWN
Consistency	Amorphous or powdery	Soft, laminated
Location	Gallbladder	Gallbladder, bile ducts
Geography	West, Orient	Mostly Orient
Disease associations	Hemolysis, cirrhosis	Cholangitis, ova, and parasites
Bile culture	Sterile	Usually infected
Etiology	Increased excretion or hydrolysis of conjugated bilirubin	Bacterial hydrolysis of conjugated bilirubin
X-ray appearance	Two thirds opaque	Lucent
Recurrence after removal	Uncommon	Common
Components	Pigment polymer Calcium phosphate Calcium carbonate	Calcium bilirubinate Calcium soaps of fatty acids Cholesterol

and activate these enzymes. Risk factors for the formation of black pigment stones include chronic hemolytic states (e.g., sickle cell disease), hereditary spherocytosis, thalassemia, cirrhosis of the liver, increasing age, female gender, and cardiac valvular prostheses. Cholesterol stones seldom form in the company of black pigment stones.

Brown pigment stones, in contrast, are laminated. They are often found in the bile ducts, and there is a strong association with bacterial infection, especially with enteric organisms. Infected bile exhibits bacterial β-glucuronidase activity, and this explains the pathogenesis of stone formation. Risk factors include age, female gender, pancreatitis, duodenal diverticulum, Gilbert's syndrome, and bacterial infection of bile.

NATURAL HISTORY OF CHOLELITHIASIS

New biliary pain develops at a low rate in subjects with asymptomatic gallstones (2% to 3% per year). In those who become symptomatic, the rate of complications is likewise low (10%). Complications include acute and chronic cholecystitis, pancreatitis, cholangitis, and obstructive jaundice. For symptomatic gallstones, there is a high risk of repeated attacks of pain leading to complications. Cohort studies have shown that 58% to 72% of patients continued to have symptoms once they developed.[3] Gallbladder cancer is correlated with gallstone disease, but the incidence is so low that aggressive prophylactic therapy of any patient with gallstones is unwarranted. Native Americans, however, do have a higher incidence of gallbladder cancer, so in this group prophylactic treatment may be justified.

The rate with which gallstones develop is variable. For Pima Indians, stones have been shown to develop over 5 to 10 years, whereas with TPN or rapid weight loss, stones can develop in a matter of weeks.

CLINICAL MANIFESTATIONS

BILIARY COLIC

Biliary colic is often the first and predominant symptomatic manifestation of cholelithiasis. It is a visceral pain from tonic spasm of the cystic duct due to transient obstruction by a stone. The pain often develops without precipitating events, has a sudden onset, increases sharply, and lasts 15 minutes to 3 hours. Usually located in the epigastrium, it may also localize to the right and left upper quadrants of the abdomen, the precordium, and the lower abdomen. There may be radiation to the interscapular area or to the tip of the right shoulder. The patient is often restless and diaphoretic, and vomiting is not uncommon. The interval between attacks is unpredictable and may last years.

ACUTE CHOLECYSTITIS

When biliary colic persists for longer than 3 hours, or if fever and leukocytosis ensue, obstruction of the cystic duct by a stone may have led to acute inflammation of the gallbladder. Although bacteria is often found in the gallbladder bile of patients with acute cholecystitis, this is thought to be a secondary event. The pain may shift from the epigastrium to the right upper quadrant, and localized tenderness may develop. In the elderly, pain and fever may be absent, although localized tenderness is usually present.

Murphy's sign aids in the diagnosis. In addition, in 40% of patients, the gallbladder or inflamed overlying omentum or both may be palpable. Jaundice may be seen in 15% of patients, even in the absence of choledocholithiasis.

ACALCULOUS CHOLECYSTITIS

In the setting of critical illness, such as in patients after major surgery, burns, or trauma, a difficult-to-diagnose entity known as acalculous cholecystitis may develop. Most patients are men more than 50 years old, and many are receiving TPN.[13] The pathogenesis is thought to be secondary to bile inspissation and sludge formation, with resultant stasis, chemical inflammation, and ischemia of the gallbladder. Complications are more serious, and a higher mortality is noted; this is due in part to the underlying severe illness. In one retrospective study, 70% of patients had either gangrene, empyema, or perforation of the gallbladder.[14]

CHRONIC CHOLECYSTITIS

A thickened and fibrotic gallbladder develops in patients who have had repeated attacks of biliary colic or acute cholecystitis. Histologically, evaginated mucosal pouches in the gallbladder (Rokitansky-Aschoff sinuses) are seen. These patients may present with complications of chronic cholecystitis, such as recurrent pancreatitis, choledocholithiasis, and cholangitis.

COMPLICATIONS OF CHOLECYSTITIS

Gangrenous cholecystitis is defined as severe gallbladder inflammation leading to mural necrosis. There is an increased risk of perforation of the gallbladder with this condition. Emphysematous cholecystitis is severe acute cholecystitis caused by gas-forming bacteria (one third are due to *Clostridium perfringens*).[15] This entity tends to occur in the elderly, 20% to 30% of whom are diabetic. Again, there is an increased risk of gallbladder perforation. A plain abdominal x-ray is suggested for confirmation.

Perforation of the gallbladder usually occurs in the context of chronic cholecystitis, when a gallstone erodes through the gallbladder wall and enters the small intestine. This may lead to gallstone ileus, when the gallstone causes intestinal luminal obstruction, often at the ileocecal valve. Perforation of the gallbladder is also seen in 3% to 15% of cases of acute cholecystitis. Cholescintigraphy most dramatically makes the diagnosis. Finally, Mirizzi syndrome occurs when a stone impacted in the cystic duct causes inflammation severe enough to erode into the common hepatic duct, with subsequent obstruction.[15]

CHOLEDOCHOLITHIASIS AND CHOLANGITIS

Common bile duct stones are frequently associated with infected bile. They should be removed, whether symptomatic or not. Clinically, obstructive jaundice and pruritus may be noted. Common bile duct pressure may rise because of the obstruction, distending the biliary tree and stopping bile flow. Dilation of intrahepatic and extrahepatic bile ducts may be seen on ultrasound or computed tomography (CT). Secondary biliary cirrhosis due to prolonged obstruction may develop, and the patient may present with manifestations of hepatic failure or with features of portal hypertension. Cholangitis is common in choledocholithiasis. In 70% of cases, Charcot's triad is present (biliary pain, jaundice, and chills and rigors). Results from blood cultures are often positive and show the organisms causing the biliary infection. Enteric gram-negative organisms are the most common, followed by *Pseudomonas* and *Enterococcus*.

DIAGNOSTIC STUDIES

X-ray examination of the abdomen is useful in ruling out other intraabdominal conditions. Only 15% of gallstones contain enough calcium to be radiopaque. With emphysematous cholecystitis, gas in the gallbladder wall may be seen.

Ultrasonography has both high sensitivity and specificity for the diagnosis of gallstones.[15] Signs indicative of active inflammation include thickening of the gallbladder wall (>2 mm), intramural gas, and pericholecystic fluid. The presence of sludge may be associated with biliary colic, acute cholecystitis, or acute pancreatitis.

Hepatobiliary scintigraphy is highly sensitive and specific for the diagnosis of acute cholecystitis.[15] After a 2 to 4 hour fast, the patient is given Technetium 99m-labeled iminodiacetic acid (IDA) intravenously, and sequential images with a gamma camera are taken. Images of the gallbladder, common bile duct, and small bowel appear by 30 minutes. False-negatives can occur with acalculous cholecystitis, but a scan with normal results virtually rules out a diagnosis of acute cholecystitis.

Oral cholecystography has seen a resurgence in its use as a functional study in the selection of patients for nonsurgical management of cholelithiasis (extracorporeal shock wave lithotripsy [ESWL] and oral bile acid therapy). The patient ingests a tablet of contrast orally the night before the oral cholecystography study. The agent is absorbed in the small bowel, conjugated in the liver, excreted into canaliculi, and concentrated within the gallbladder. Conditions such as gastric retention, pancreatitis, small bowel disease, hepatic dysfunction, or prolonged fasting can therefore give false-negative results.[3] As there is inadequate visualization of the gallbladder in 15% to 50% of patients, some radiologists routinely give a double dose of oral contrast. The chief advantage over ultrasonography is cholecystography's ability to assess the patency of the cystic duct and assess gallbladder function.

CT scan is useful in demonstrating dilated bile ducts and mass lesions. It is the test of choice if clinical suspicion of a tumor obstructing the common bile duct is high.

Cholangiography (percutaneous or via endoscopy) is used to visualize the biliary tract. Therapeutic maneuvers may also be performed. Endoscopic retrograde cholangiopancreatography (ERCP) is used to demonstrate the lower limit of the obstruction and has the advantage to sample tissue and perform therapeutic maneuvers. Percutaneous transhepatic cholangiography (PTC) demonstrates the upper limit of the lesion. Both modalities can introduce infection.

TREATMENT

Cholecystectomy remains the definitive treatment for cholelithiasis, and there is general agreement that asymptomatic gallstones should not be treated given the benign course.[16] Symptomatic patients, however, should be treated; the question that has arisen in recent years with the advent of nonsurgical modalities of treatment is which patients are best served with which modality. Physicians must take into account not only the clinical presentation in a particular patient but also the patient's wishes. In addition, the risk of stone recurrence with all modalities that leave the gallbladder in place must be kept in mind. Finally, the rate of stone dissolution is a factor, as it varies widely among the different nonsurgical modalities.

SURGICAL

Cholecystectomy is a safe procedure; the overall mortality from elective cholecystectomy is 0.2% to 0.9%.[17] Major systemic illnesses and age may increase the mortality, as can the extension of the procedure into a common bile duct exploration. Exceptions to the rule of not treating asymptomatic gallstones include morbid obesity, patients receiving large doses of corticosteroids long term, and patients found to have a calcified gallbladder (in whom the risk of gallbladder carcinoma is increased).[3] When cholelithiasis is encountered in children, there is usually a specific underlying factor, such as hemolytic disease; as symptoms usually develop, elective cholecystectomy is probably indicated. A similar recommendation is made for patients with sickle cell disease. Furthermore, stones in the common bile duct should be removed, even if asymptomatic. Thus, elective cholecystectomy remains the first choice in most patients with symptomatic gallstones and in those in whom complications develop.

The advent of laparoscopic cholecystectomy has meant a decrease in the length of hospital stay and higher patient acceptance of the procedure.[18] It is safe, with a mortality below 1%.[19] It can be performed electively in patients who are unlikely to have obscured anatomy due to adhesions or inflammation. In 5% of cases, the surgeon converts to an open cholecystectomy because of unexpected findings or technical considerations. The main concern is bile duct injury, which occurs at a rate of around 0.5%. The overall complication rate is 5%, caused by bile duct injury, bleeding, and bowel injury. As currently practiced, most patients who have acute cholecystitis, prior upper abdominal surgery, or biliary pancreatitis are excluded, but these exclusion criteria may evolve as more experience is gained with the technique. Training of surgeons under supervision should be enforced and monitored. It is anticipated that laparoscopic cholecystectomy will become the procedure of choice for elective cholecystectomy.[20]

NONSURGICAL

Oral Bile Acid Therapy

Chenodeoxycholic acid (CDCA) and ursodeoxycholic acid (UDCA) have been shown to gradually dissolve cholesterol gallstones by distinct physicochemical mechanisms.[20,21] This occurs via secretion of undersaturated hepatic bile, which in turn is brought about by the suppression of hepatic cholesterol synthesis via the inhibition of 3-hydroxy-3-methylglutaryl–coenzyme A (HMG-CoA) reductase activity and the enhancing of 7α-hydroxylase activity.

The efficacy of dissolution is similar for the two bile acids. Because of the marked difference in side effect profiles of the two agents (watery diarrhea, elevated serum transaminases, elevated serum cholesterol with CDCA; the absence of these side effects with UDCA), therapy with CDCA alone has been virtually abandoned. There has been a recent report of increased efficacy with combination therapy (CDCA and UDCA at a dosage of 5 mg/kg/d of each).[22] With combination therapy, the side effects of CDCA are not seen. With UDCA monotherapy, a dosage of 8 to 10 mg/kg/d is recommended.

Proper patient selection is the key to success with oral bile acid therapy.[20,21] Selected patients should have small (<1.5 cm) gallstones predominantly composed of cholesterol. Small stones that float on oral cholecystography are especially likely to yield a favorable result. Pregnant women and women likely to become pregnant are excluded because of the unknown teratogenic effects of oral bile acids. Radiolucent stones less than 15 mm in diameter in an opacifying gallbladder dissolve in 60% of patients in 2 years.[22] Stones less than 5 mm in diameter that float on oral cholecystography dissolve completely in 90% of patients in 1 year. However, if patients are restricted to this criteria, probably no more than 10% with symptomatic cholelithiasis are eligible.

Contact Dissolution

With direct access to stones, either via the percutaneous or endoscopic route, cholesterol stones have been shown to dissolve on contact with dissolving agents.[21,23] The agent most widely studied is methyl-tert-butyl ether (MTBE), an ether compound first developed as an octane enhancer for gasoline. MTBE has a high solvent capacity for cholesterol of 14 g/dl. When instilled via the percutaneous route directly into the gallbladder with stones, rapid and effective dissolution (90%) results. Usually, the substance is applied over the course of 3 to 4 days. After treatment with MTBE, UDCA is given for several months, with an overall stone dissolution rate of 50% to 90%.

Complications are related to the percutaneous access procedure, such as bleeding, bile leak, and infection, and side effects from the MTBE, such as sedation and nausea; rare cases of hemolytic anemia and renal insufficiency have been reported. Patients with an open cystic duct, an opacifying gallbladder, and radiolucent symptomatic stones are eligible. The recurrence rate after successful treatment is around 30%. Overall, the total number of patients treated with this procedure is small, and the procedure is available only in certain specialized centers; hence, it should be regarded as investigational at this time.

ESWL with Oral Bile Acid Therapy

Fragmentation of cholesterol gallstones via ESWL can be achieved in patients with symptomatic radiolucent stones and an opacifying gallbladder.[24] Patients with solitary stones have the greatest chance of success (70% with stones up to 2 cm by 8 months).[20] The success rate depends on adjuvant bile acid therapy. Adverse effects are generally related to passage of stone fragments after lithotripsy and occur in 3% to 5% of patients. In addition, local effects from the shock waves such as local pain, petechiae, and microscopic hematuria can be seen. Cholecystectomy or emergency endoscopic sphincterotomy is required in less than 5% of patients.[25] In addition, biliary pain may occur in the first 2 months in 30% to 70% of patients who are not stone free following this treatment. The recurrence rate for stones is around 10% after 1 year.

In summary, therefore, there are a number of modalities for the successful treatment of symptomatic gallstones. Surgery remains the gold standard and the definitive treatment. For patients who cannot or will not have surgery, there are nonsurgical options. The last decade has seen a remarkable increase in the understanding of biliary lipid biochemistry and physiology, the pathophysiology of stone formation, and the natural history and evolution of sludge and gallstones. The outlook for the next decade is for innovations in the prevention and treatment of this disease.

REFERENCES

1. Diehl AK. Epidemiology and natural history of gallstone disease. In: Cooper AD, ed. *Pathogenesis and Therapy of Gallstone Disease. Gastroenterology Clinics of North America.* Philadelphia, Pa: WB Saunders Co; 1991:1–19.
2. Sampliner RE, Bennett PH, Comers LJ, et al. Gallbladder disease in Pima Indians: demonstration of high prevalence and early onset by cholecystography. *N Engl J Med.* 1970;283:1358.
3. Lee SP, Sekijima J. Gallstones. In: Yamada T, Alpers DH, Owyang C, et al, eds. *Textbook of Gastroenterology.* Philadelphia, Pa: JB Lippincott Co; 1991:1966–1989.
4. Pixley F, Wilson D, McPherson K, et al. Effect of vegetarianism on development of gallstones in women. *Br Med J.* 1985;291:11–12.
5. Cooper AD. Metabolic basis of cholesterol gallstone disease. In: Cooper AD, ed. *Pathogenesis and Therapy of*

Gallstone Disease. Gastroenterology Clinics of North America. Philadelphia, Pa: WB Saunders Co; 1991: 21–46.
6. Paumgartner G, Sauerbruch T. Gallstones: pathogenesis. *Lancet.* 1991;338:1117–1121.
7. Nissel K, Angelin B, Liljequist L, et al. Biliary lipid output and bile acid kinetics in cholesterol gallstone disease: evidence for an increased hepatic secretion of cholesterol in Swedish patients. *Gastroenterology.* 1985;287:293.
8. Lee SP, Park HZ, Madani H, et al. Partial characterization of a non-micellar system of cholesterol solubilization in bile. *Am J Physiol.* 1987;252:G374.
9. Schiffman ML, Moore EW. Acidification of gallbladder bile is defective in patients with all types of gallstones: a selective defect. *Gastroenterology.* 1988;94:A591. Abstract.
10. Lee SP, Maher K, Nicholls JF. Origin and fate of biliary sludge. *Gastroenterology.* 1988;94:170.
11. Messing B, Dories C, Kunstlinger F, et al. Does total parenteral nutrition induce gallbladder sludge formation and lithiasis? *Gastroenterology.* 1983;84:1012.
12. Trotman BW. Pigment gallstone disease. In: Cooper AD, ed. *Pathogenesis and Therapy of Gallstone Disease. Gastroenterology Clinics of North America.* Philadelphia, Pa: WB Saunders Co; 1991:111–126.
13. Orlando R, Gleason E, Drezner A. Acute cholecystitis in the critically ill patient. *Am J Surg.* 1983:145–472.
14. Johndon L. The importance of early diagnosis of acute acalculous cholecystitis. *Surg Gynecol Obstet.* 1987;164:197.
15. Zeman RK, Garra BS. Gallbladder imaging. In: Cooper AD, ed. *Pathogenesis and Therapy of Gallstone Disease. Gastroenterology Clinics of North America.* Philadelphia, Pa: WB Saunders Co; 1991:127–156.
16. Schoenfield LJ, Carulli N, Dowling RH, et al. Asymptomatic gallstones: definition and treatment. *Gastroenterol Int.* 1989;2:25.
17. MacLean LD, Goldstein M, MacDonald JE, et al. Results of cholecystectomy in 1000 consecutive patients. *Can J Surg.* 1975;18:459.
18. Dubois F, Icard P, Berthelot G, et al. Coelioscopic cholecystectomy: preliminary report of 36 cases. *Ann Surg.* 1990;211:60–63.
19. The Southern Surgeons Club. A prospective analysis of 1518 laparoscopic cholecystectomies. *N Engl J Med.* 1991;324:1073–1078.
20. Sauerbruch T, Paumgartner G. Gallbladder stones: management. *Lancet.* 1991;338:1121–1124.
21. Fromm H, Albert MB. Mechanical and chemical management of gallstones. In: Yamada T, Alpers DH, Owyang C, et al. *Textbook of Gastroenterology.* Philadelphia, Pa: JB Lippincott Co; 1991:2650–2652.
22. Podda M, Zuin M, Battezzati PM, et al. Efficacy and safety of a combination of chenodeoxycholic acid and ursodeoxycholic acid for gallstone dissolution: a comparison with ursodeoxycholic acid alone. *Gastroenterology.* 1989;96:222–229.
23. Hoffmann AF, Schteingart CD, van Sonnenberg E, et al. Contact dissolution of cholesterol gallstones with organic solvents. In: Cooper AD, ed. *Pathogenesis and Therapy of Gallstone Disease. Gastroenterology Clinics of North America.* Philadelphia, Pa: WB Saunders Co; 1991:183–199.
24. Garcia G, Young HS. Biliary extracorporeal shock-wave lithotripsy. In: Cooper AD, ed. *Pathogenesis and Therapy of Gallstone Disease. Gastroenterology Clinics of North America.* Philadelphia, Pa: WB Saunders Co; 1991:201–208.
25. Sackmann M, Pauletzki J, Sauerbruch T, et al. The Munich gallbladder lithotripsy study: results of the first five years with 711 patients. *Ann Intern Med.* 1991;114:290–296.

120

Chronic Cholestatic Liver Disease

GEORGE DICKSTEIN and MARSHALL M. KAPLAN

The chronic cholestatic liver diseases (Table 120–1) comprise a group of disorders that if left untreated often progress to liver failure or cirrhosis. Clinically and histologically, primary biliary cirrhosis (PBC),[1] primary sclerosing cholangitis (PSC),[2] chronic graft-versus-host disease of the liver,[3,4] and chronic (ductopenic) liver allograft rejection[5,6] share many features, primary among which is the destruction of bile ducts by activated lymphocytes. As these bile ducts are damaged and destroyed, they either lack the capacity to regenerate or do so slowly and ineffectually. The net result is the same, an inadequate number of functioning bile ducts.[7,8]

Current evidence suggests that liver damage in PBC and PSC occurs via immunologic and non-immunologic mechanisms.[9–18] The immunologic element is mediated by activated T lymphocytes

TABLE 120-1. CHRONIC CHOLESTATIC LIVER DISEASES

- Primary biliary cirrhosis
- Primary sclerosing cholangitis
- Chronic graft-versus-host disease of the liver
- Chronic, cholestatic, or ductopenic liver transplant rejection
- Chronic drug-induced cholestasis
- Cholestasis (pruritus) of pregnancy
- Vanishing bile duct syndrome
- Intrahepatic cholestasis secondary to parenteral hyperalimentation
- Sarcoidosis?
- Secondary sclerosing cholangitis (e.g., cytomegalovirus or cryptosporidiosis in AIDS patients, cholangitis and choledocholithiasis in Southeast Asian patients, common bile duct stone or strictures with recurrent episodes of ascending cholangitis)

that are directed toward biliary epithelial cells, leading to impaired secretion and accumulation of hepatotoxic bile acids in the microenvironment of the liver and bile ductules. These bile acids may, in turn, damage hepatocyte membranes and may also exacerbate reactive immune-mediated destruction of both bile ducts and hepatic parenchyma.[19-21] Long-standing inflammation may lead to hepatic fibrosis, periductular fibrosis, intrahepatic and extrahepatic bile duct strictures (in PSC), and cirrhosis.

The medical management of PBC and PSC can be divided into three categories: (1) those treatments which attempt to control the symptoms, complications, and consequences of cholestasis; (2) treatment of the underlying disease processes; and (3) liver transplantation. Short of liver transplantation, there are as yet no proven therapies for PBC or PSC. Although preliminary results with some agents appear promising, all agents remain experimental.

CLINICAL PRESENTATIONS OF PBC AND PSC

PBC

The vast majority (90% to 95%) of patients with PBC are women.[1] The onset of disease is usually between the ages of 30 to 65, although individual patients may be older or younger.[22] Because of increased awareness of the disease and widespread biochemical screening, patients are increasingly being diagnosed earlier, and many (up to 60%) are now asymptomatic at the time of diagnosis.[23-27] Fatigue[24] and pruritus[28] are common presenting features and may be the primary symptoms in about 50% of patients with PBC or PSC.

Physical examination findings include increased skin pigmentation, which in the early stages represents melanin rather than bilirubin, excoriations from scratching, and hepatomegaly (in up to 70% of patients).[29-31] Xanthomas occur in less than 10% of patients, develop late in the course of disease, and are associated with hypercholesterolemia (with values above 1000 mg/dl).[22,25,32] As the disease becomes more advanced, muscle wasting, jaundice, splenomegaly, and complications of portal hypertension can develop, along with progressive decline in liver function.

Serum biochemical tests commonly demonstrate abnormal results in patients with PBC. The serum alkaline phosphatase is almost always elevated. Elevation of the bilirubin generally reflects advanced disease. Serum aminotransferases are moderately elevated (40 to 300 U/L) and often vary during the course of the disease.[26,32-34] Total cholesterol (with a high high-density lipoprotein fraction) is elevated in 50% of patients.[30] The antimitochondrial antibody (AMA) is positive in up to 95% of patients with PBC.[35-37] There is no correlation between the presence or titer of AMA and the severity or course of PBC. AMA-negative PBC does exist and has an identical presentation and natural history as that of AMA-positive PBC.[38] Formal diagnosis always requires liver biopsy, and characteristic findings are sought and staged (I to IV) according to well-accepted criteria.[3,39] It is important to remember that PBC is a disease that is not uniformly distributed throughout the liver, and several different stages may coexist in a single patient.

PBC is a progressive disease, but the rate of progression varies in individual patients. The insidious course of the disease and the presence of long symptom-free periods have led some to question the rationale of therapy in asymptomatic or minimally symptomatic patients. It is now clear that most asymptomatic patients develop symptoms, progress to cirrhosis, and have excess age-related mortality with shortened survival.[28,45,46] Nonetheless, a few patients with PBC do remain asymptomatic for long periods of time.

PSC

Before the diagnosis of primary sclerosing cholangitis can be established, congenital abnormalities, ischemic states, infectious processes, bile duct neoplasms, and inflammatory disorders[40-42] that cause secondary sclerosing cholangitis must be excluded. Seventy percent of patients with PSC are male, and the mean age at the time of diagnosis is 39 years; however, children, even those younger than 2 years, may be affected.[39,43] Approximately 75% of patients with PSC have inflammatory bowel disease, usually ulcerative colitis, and less often Crohn's disease, and approximately 6% of patients with ulcerative colitis have or develop PSC.[44,45]

The disease may present in two ways. In 10% to 15% of patients there is an acute presentation characterized by recurrent episodes of fever, chills, right upper quadrant pain, and jaundice, clinically indistinguishable from that of acute bacterial cholangitis. Fever and chills are usually treated with antibiotics such as amoxicillin, ciprofloxacin, or trimethoprim-sulfamethoxazole. The more typical presentation is an indolent one that is initially asymptomatic and recognized by abnormal liver function tests, typically an elevated alkaline phosphatase. Most patients also have slight increases in the aminotransferases, while serum albumin and bilirubin are normal early in the course of PSC. Evaluation of these biochemical abnormalities eventually leads to cholangiography (preferably endoscopic retrograde cholangiopancreatography, but alternatively transhepatic cholangiography) and liver biopsy. Like PBC, liver biopsy findings can be staged (I to IV).[46] However, liver biopsy findings are usually nondiagnostic of PSC. Typical onion skin lesions of bile ducts are rarely seen. It is more common to see only a paucity of bile ducts with nonspecific portal fibrosis and inflammation.[39] Symptoms of itching, fatigue, or jaundice typically indicate advanced disease. Most of these patients have cirrhosis,[47,48] and bile duct strictures are often much more extensive than suspected. Symptomatic patients, particularly those with advanced histologic stages have decreased rates of survival compared to those with early stage disease.[49] Despite the high incidence of inflammatory bowel disease in PSC, colectomy does not favorably influence the course or development of PSC.[50-53]

Given difficulties in assessing the progression of PSC (a disease characterized by slow progression and spontaneous fluctuations in liver biochemistries and bilirubin) and the fact that there is no proven totally effective medical therapy for PSC, many clinicians have chosen simply to observe patients with early disease. However, PSC is often a disease of young patients. By the time symptoms develop, the disease may be advanced, the liver cirrhotic, and survival diminished[50,51,54-57] unless liver transplantation is performed.

MANAGEMENT OF CHRONIC CHOLESTASIS AND ITS COMPLICATIONS

Pruritus

One of the more disconcerting symptoms in PSC and PBC is pruritus. Pruritus appears to present later in the course of PSC than of PBC but the manifestations and treatment are the same.[58] The itching is worse at bedtime, is exacerbated by warm or cold weather or coarse clothing, and may cause insomnia and extensive excoriations with local reactive lymphadenopathy.[58,59,unpublished observations] Itching may first develop in the third trimester of pregnancy, but unlike the pruritus in the cholestasis of pregnancy syndrome,[60] itching may persist or recur after pregnancy.[23] Symptoms are more often generalized than local but may first be sensed on the palms of the hands and the soles of the feet.[61] The exact cause of the itching is still unknown. However, pruritus is clearly more associated with cholestasis than with hepatocellular injury.[61] Although bile acids have received the most attention in the search for an etiologic agent, the pruritogenic substance is clearly not any of the naturally occurring bile acids or their major metabolites.[62,63] A recently postulated alternative view of pruritus holds that increased opioidergic neurotransmission mediates the pruritus of cholestasis.[64,65] The precise mechanism that triggers the activation of the opioid system in cholestasis is unknown.

All therapies for pruritus in liver disease are empiric, and no single agent reliably ameliorates pruritus in all patients. Table 120-2 is a list of the more effective agents and their suggested doses. Treatment of the underlying disease process (see below) may also diminish pruritus. Unfortunately, patients with high-grade cholestasis may not respond to any of these measures. Intractable, incapacitating pruritus is one indication for liver transplantation.

Fat-Soluble Vitamin Deficiency

The loss of functioning intrahepatic or extrahepatic bile ducts in PBC or PSC leads to decreased secretion of conjugated bile acids into bile and thus diminished intraluminal concen-

TABLE 120-2. MEDICATIONS AND MODALITIES EFFECTIVE IN THE TREATMENT OF PRURITUS

MEDICATION*	DRUG CLASS	DOSAGE	COMMENT
Cholestyramine	Bile acid binding resin	4 g t.i.d.	Dose may be doubled; takes 2–4 d for relief; may cause steatorrhea; can be constipating
Colestipol	Bile acid binding resin	5 g t.i.d.	Same as cholestyramine
Rifampin	Antibiotic	300–600 mg/d	Pruritus relief in 1 wk; may cause drug-induced hepatitis
Phenobarbital	Barbiturate	60–90 mg qh	Probably works as sedative; increases bile flow and induces microsomal enzymes

*Other miscellaneous medications or modalities for pruritus supported by small series or case reports: S-Adenosylmethionine, Charcoal hemoperfusion, Cimetidine, Epomediol, Flumecinol, Large-volume paracentesis, Low-dose corticosteroids, Methyltestosterone, Metronidazole, Nalmefene, Naloxone, Partial external diversion of biliary flow, Propofol, UVB light.

trations of bile acids within the small intestine. Particularly in those patients who are clinically jaundiced, in those who have long-standing disease with advanced cholestasis, and in those in whom steatorrhea is severe, maldigestion and malabsorption of dietary lipids ensues and fat-soluble vitamin (A, E, K, and D) deficiency can develop.[66–70] Pancreatic insufficiency may contribute to steatorrhea and may occur in patients with PBC and sicca syndrome[69,71] and in patients with PSC.[71]

In PBC the variables that are most predictive of a poor outcome (elevated serum bilirubin, decreased serum albumin, and advanced histologic stage of disease) correlate most closely with impaired fat-soluble vitamin nutriture.[72] Levels of aspartate aminotransferase (AST), alanine aminotransferase (ALT), and alkaline phosphatase correlate poorly or not at all.[72] In both PBC and PSC, fat-soluble vitamin deficiency may be made worse in patients receiving cholestyramine.

Vitamin A

In PSC, asymptomatic vitamin A deficiency was found in almost 50% of patients in one study.[73] Symptomatic vitamin A deficiency is rare in our experience.[58] In PBC, data on vitamin A deficiency is conflicting.[72,74] In our study of 52 patients with PBC,[72] decreased serum levels of vitamin A occurred in 17, all of whom had histologically advanced disease (i.e., stages III and IV). Only one of our patients had symptomatic vitamin A deficiency manifested as night blindness.[72] However, if vitamin A deficiency is specifically tested for by dark adaptation studies (dark adaptometry), "symptomatic" vitamin A deficiency may be more common.[75] Symptomatic vitamin A deficiency can be corrected initially with intramuscular vitamin A at a dose of 100,000 U, followed by oral vitamin A at 45,000 to 50,000 U twice a week (three times the recommended daily allowance).[76] For asymptomatic vitamin A deficiency, 15,000 U/d or 45,000 U twice a week is usually effective.[73] Replacement therapy should continue indefinitely.

Vitamin E

Vitamin E deficiency is characterized by a neuromuscular syndrome consisting of cerebellar dysfunction with truncal and appendicular ataxia, posterior column dysfunction with loss of vibratory sensation and proprioception, ophthalmoplegia, peripheral neuropathy, muscle weakness, encephalopathy, and increased erythrocyte fragility as measured by hydrogen peroxide hemolysis.[77] Both symptomatic and asymptomatic vitamin E deficiency appear to be rare in PSC.[77] The prevalence of vitamin E deficiency in adults with PBC varies considerably, but in two recent studies, serum vitamin E levels were low in 7% to 9% of patients with PBC, the vast majority of whom had advanced disease.[72,77]

Vitamin E should be given in a dosage of 400 IU/d in those with vitamin E deficiency. Because of the presence of malabsorption, prolonged therapy may be required to increase serum levels. Therapy should be continued indefinitely.

Vitamin K

Clinically important vitamin K deficiency rarely occurs in PSC unless the patient is chronically jaundiced and takes cholestyramine on a regular basis.[58] Prothrombin times are normal in most patients with PSC until late in the course of the disease when other manifestations of liver failure are present.[58] However, if easy bruising or bleeding is present, the prothrombin time should be checked, and if indicated, vitamin K should be given parenterally and continued enterally.

In our study of 52 patients with PBC,[72] seven

had serum prothrombin times that were 1 to 2 seconds above control values, and one patient had a prothrombin time 3 seconds above control values. These patients had elevated prothrombin times not as a result of serious hepatic dysfunction but primarily as a result of subclinical vitamin K deficiency.[72] Vitamin K deficiency can also result in defective skeletal synthesis of proteins that contain c-carboxyglutamic acid and contribute to hepatic osteodystrophy in PBC and PSC (see below).[78,79]

In patients with symptomatic vitamin K deficiency (i.e., easy bruising or bleeding), vitamin K should be repleted parenterally (intravenously, intramuscularly, subcutaneously) in a dose of 10 mg in consecutive dosages over 2 to 3 days.[72] Asymptomatic prolongation of the prothrombin time can be corrected with oral dosing at 5 mg every day.[72] Therapy should be continued indefinitely.

Vitamin D

In our experience in PBC, levels of 1,25-dihydroxyvitamin D (the metabolically active form of vitamin D) have been consistently normal, even in patients with advanced liver disease or symptomatic osteoporosis.[80] Levels of 25-hydroxyvitamin D, however, are more often low or low normal in PBC.[80] Since patients with low 25-hydroxyvitamin D do have an increased prevalence of bone disease,[72] we routinely supplement deficient patients with calcifediol (Calderol), 40 to 120 1g/d,[80] adjusted to maintain 25-hydroxyvitamin D levels at 35 to 55 mg/ml (high normal).[80,81]

Serum levels of vitamin D and its metabolites may be decreased in patients with PSC. However, symptomatic bone disease is not common.[50,51,73] It occurs less in PSC than it does in PBC, perhaps because the majority of patients are male and have greater baseline bone density than women at the onset of disease. As with PBC, vitamin D levels may be determined by measuring serum levels of 25-hydroxyvitamin D. If low, vitamin D replacement should be provided in doses similar to those outlined for PBC.

We recommend that fat-soluble vitamin levels be determined twice yearly in individual patients with PBC and PSC and perhaps more often in patients with symptomatic, progressive, or advanced disease. Vitamin supplements should only be given to those patients whose blood levels suggest deficiency and should be continued indefinitely or until adequate serum levels can be obtained and physiologic levels sustained without therapy. If cholestasis is severe, chronic parenteral (intramuscular) injections may be needed, as gastrointestinal tract absorption will be poor.

METABOLIC BONE DISEASE

Patients with hepatic osteodystrophy are at increased risk for bone fractures that may occur either spontaneously or with minimal trauma.[82] When more sensitive techniques such as dual photon absorptiometry, quantitative computed tomography, or dual energy x-ray absorptiometry are used on unselected patients at the time of presentation of PBC, prevalence rates average 20% or less.[82] It is important to remember, however, that although most cases of osteopenia are silent, in a few patients skeletal abnormalities, fractures, deformities, and pain can be the dominant clinical feature of the disease.[79]

Since hepatic osteodystrophy occurs with relative frequency in PBC but is rare in PSC,[58] most attention has focused on the former. Nonetheless, metabolic bone disease does occur in PSC and, like that in PBC, is osteoporosis.[83] The cause of the osteoporosis is uncertain, but it may be due to decreased osteoblast function and thus decreased bone formation and low bone turnover.[1,79] Vitamin D deficiency is not the cause of hepatic osteodystrophy in the vast majority of patients with PBC.[79] Treatment of hepatic osteodystrophy in cholestatic liver disease is problematic. Attention should be directed toward correction of any deficiencies of calcium, magnesium, phosphate, or vitamin D that are present, although there is no convincing evidence that this treatment prevents or heals the osteoporosis of PBC.[66,67,79,84] Steatorrhea, if present, should be treated with medium-chain triglycerides and a diet low in neutral triglycerides.[85] Pancreatic insufficiency, especially in patients with sicca syndrome, should be sought and corrected with pancreatic enzyme supplements. Vitamin K levels must be assessed by checking either the prothrombin time, circulating vitamin K level, or presence of abnormal prothrombin (see above)[73] and corrected promptly. Estrogen replacement therapy in postmenopausal patients with cholestatic liver disease improves lumbar spine bone mineral density without increasing clinical or biochemical cholestasis.[86] The dynamics of androgen-estrogen balance in men with advanced liver disease are less clear.[87,88] Other general measures include avoidance of corticosteroid therapy (as exogenous corticosteroids clearly accelerate bone loss),[89] avoidance of weight loss and malnutrition,[82] avoidance of immobilization,[90] and abstinence from alcohol and tobacco.[82] Finally, although liver transplantation and concomitant corticosteroid use may induce "posttransplant bone disease,"[91,92] improvements in osteoblast function are among the earliest changes seen after liver transplantation, and bone density increases 6 to 8 months after liver transplantation.[93]

RECURRENT CHOLANGITIS OR INFECTION IN PSC

Antibiotics are of no proven efficacy in slowing the progression of PSC but may be needed to treat episodes of bacterial cholangitis. Because of the rarity of PSC, there are few published studies concerning the role of antibiotics in PSC. Tetracycline was evaluated nearly 30 years ago and was ineffective.[52] Prophylactic antibiotics are often given to patients who are prone to repeated episodes of bacterial cholangitis. Although there are no published data to support this practice, anecdotal experience suggests that daily doses of amoxicillin or double strength trimethoprim-sulfamethoxazole may lower the frequency and severity of these episodes. Ciprofloxacin or other fluoroquinolones are good alternatives for patients with allergy to lactam antibiotics or sulfa.

TREATMENT OF THE UNDERLYING CAUSE OF PBC AND PSC

Table 120–3 summarizes the major categories of pharmacologic agents that have been used in the hope that they would favorably modulate inflammation and bile duct damage in PBC and PSC. In contrast to PBC, there have been few well-designed, randomized, controlled trials in PSC. At this point in time no drug has proven to be effective. Corticosteroids and D-penicillamine have been evaluated in PBC[94–100] and PSC,[48,101,102] whereas chlorambucil[103] and azathioprine[104–107] have been studied systematically only in PBC. None of these agents have been shown to favorably alter the natural history of PBC or PSC, and none of these agents are currently being widely used or systematically studied because of high toxicity rates (i.e., for chlorambucil),[103] accelerated bone loss (i.e., for corticosteroids),[99] or lack of efficacy in randomized controlled trials (i.e., D-penicillamine for PBC and PSC and azathioprine for PBC).[48,94–107]

For both PBC and PSC the most encouraging preliminary data have been obtained with ursodeoxycholic acid (UDCA)[20,21,108–134] and methotrexate (MTX).[47,135–142] Colchicine continues to maintain an important role in the treatment of PBC (but data in PSC are limited and unfavorable).[138,143–146] There is an emerging consensus that the routine use of cyclosporine (CSA) as monotherapy in PBC will be limited by high cost and unacceptable toxicity with only marginal efficacy.[147–150] No published results of the use of CSA in PSC are currently available. However, it was ineffective in a prospective, placebo-controlled trial recently conducted at the Mayo Clinic.[151]

In patients not enrolled in clinical trials, we begin treatment of both PBC and PSC with UDCA in a dosage of 13 to 17 mg/kg/d in two or three divided doses. Blood tests are repeated at monthly intervals. Biochemical improvements usually occur within several months. If blood tests become normal, we repeat the liver biopsy at 1 year. If the liver biopsy results are unchanged or improved, we continue UDCA. If the blood tests show only mild improvement after 2 to 3 months, we usually add a second agent. Here, our approach to PSC and PBC differs. With precirrhotic PSC we usually add MTX at a dosage of 0.25 mg/kg/w (usually 15 mg) in three divided doses given 12 hours apart. With cirrhotic PSC, no therapy has been of proven benefit.[135] We repeat the biopsy after 1 year of starting treatment with MTX in all patients. If the biopsy results are worse and the blood test results unchanged, we usually stop therapy with MTX. If the biopsy results are unchanged or better or the blood test results improved, we continue therapy and repeat liver biopsies at 2-year intervals. Patients on MTX should have blood count, platelet count, and liver function tests monthly for the first 3 to 6 months and every 3 months thereafter. Cholangiograms should be repeated at 2- to 4-year intervals, as they change slowly. We have seen striking improvements in the cholangiograms of a few patients, as well as gradual worsening.

Dominant strictures of the extrahepatic bile ducts cause or exacerbate symptoms in 15% to 20% of patients with PSC. Endoscopic balloon dilation of strictures with or without stent placement has relieved symptoms of jaundice, pruritus, and fever and improved the liver biochemistries in selected patients.[152] We combine endoscopic therapy with the medical regimen described above. Despite the absence of controlled trials, there appears to be little risk and much potential benefit from this approach.

TABLE 120–3. MEDICAL THERAPIES FOR PSC AND PBC

Design	Number of Patients	Dosage or Duration	Outcome	Reference
Medical Therapy for PSC				
Ursodeoxycholic Acid (UDCA)				
Controlled	80	13–15 mg/kg/d × 18 mo	Interim analysis for major treatment effects; no differences found	134
Controlled, double-blind	14	13–15 mg/kg/d × 1 y	Improved liver chemistries; improved histologic findings	131
Controlled, double-blind	20	750 mg/d × 1 y	Minimal improvement in histologic findings and LFTs; no change in symptoms; no delay in time to LTX	129
Methotrexate (MTX)				
Uncontrolled	10	15 mg/wk × 1–10 y	Improvement in symptoms, LFTs, cholangiogram, and liver histologic findings; no toxicity	142
Controlled	24	15 mg/wk × 2 y	Improvement in alkaline phosphatase; no benefit in histologic findings, cholangiogram, or LFTs; trend favoring MTX in early PSC	135
Prednisone				
Uncontrolled	10	39–23 mg/d for >6 mo	Improvement in pruritus, LFTs, liver histologic findings	102
Penicillamine				
Controlled	70	39 @ 750 mg/d × 36 mo 31 placebo	No benefit on any parameters; 21% toxicity requiring discontinuation	48
Prednisone and Colchicine				
Prospective versus historical controls	12	Prednisone 10 mg/d Colchicine 1.2 mg/d × 24 mo	No benefit on histologic findings or survival	146
Medical Therapy for PBC				
Azathioprine				
Controlled, double-blind	248	127 @ 2 mg/kg/d × 36 mo 121 placebo	Improvement in survival; no toxicity	107
Controlled, double-blind	45	22 @ 2 mg/kg/d up to 6 y 23 placebo	Improvement in AST first year only; no change in other LFTs or histologic findings	106
Chlorambucil				
Controlled, double-blind	24	13 @ 0.5–4 mg/d × 1–2 y 11 placebo	Improvement in some LFTs and histologic findings; bone marrow toxicity in 25% (4/13)	103
Colchicine				
Controlled, double-blind	57	29 @ 1.2 mg/d × 2 y 28 placebo	Improvement in LFTs; tendency toward stabilization of bilirubin; no change in histologic findings	144
Controlled, double-blind	64	32 @ 1 mg/d × 12 mo 32 placebo	Early improvement in LFTs and immunoglobulin levels; no change in histologic findings or survival	145
Controlled, double-blind	60	30 @ 1.2 mg/d × 2 y 30 placebo	Significant improvement in LFTs and survival at 4 y; no change in symptoms or histologic findings	143
Controlled, double-blind, double-dummy versus MTX	87	1.2 mg/d × 24 mo	Improvement in LFTs; stabilization of histologic findings in some patients taking colchicine	138

AST = aspartate aminotransferase, LFT = liver function test, LTX = liver transplantation, PSC = primary sclerosing cholangitis.

TABLE 120–3. MEDICAL THERAPIES FOR PSC AND PBC Continued

Design	Number of Patients	Dosage or Duration	Outcome	Reference
Prednisolone				
Controlled, double-blind	36	19 @ 30–10 mg/d × 1 y 17 placebo	Improvement in LFTs, itching, and fatigue; increased bone loss at twice expected rate	99
Controlled, double-blind	36	19 @ 30–10 mg/d × 3 y 17 placebo	Improvement only in albumin and alkaline phosphatase; better overall outcome in treated group; little evidence for increased bone loss at 3 y	98
Cyclosporine				
Controlled, double-blind	29	19 @ 4 mg/kg/d for up to 2 y 10 placebo	Improvement in symptoms, LFTs, and histologic findings; nephrotoxicity in 63%, hypertension in 47%	150
Controlled, double-blind	12	6 @ 2.5 mg/kg/d × 1 y 6 placebo	Nephrotoxicity or hypertension in 50%; improvement in LFTs	149
Controlled, double-blind	349	176 @ 3 mg/kg/d × 6 y 173 placebo	Improvement in LFTs; no difference in time to death or LTX; nephrotoxicity or hypertension in 10%	148
Methotrexate (MTX)				
Uncontrolled	9	15 mg/wk × 12–34 mo	Improvement in symptoms, LFTs, and liver histologic findings	140
Controlled, double-blind, double-dummy versus colchicine	87	15 mg/wk × 24 mo	Improvement in symptoms, LFTs, and liver histologic findings for MTX	138
Ursodeoxycholic Acid (UDCA)				
Controlled, double-blind	146	73 @ 13–15 mg/kg/d × 4 y 73 placebo	Improvement in itching, LFTs, Mayo risk score, death, and time to LTX	108, 109
Controlled, double-blind	45	22 @ 600 mg/d × 24 wk 23 placebo	No improvement in symptoms; some improvement in LFTs	122
Controlled, double-blind	20	10 @ 10 mg/kg/d × 9 mo 10 placebo	Improvement in symptoms, LFTs, and histologic findings	113
Controlled, double-blind	180	91 @ 13–15 mg/kg/d × 1–48 mo 89 placebo	Improvement in LFTs and time to treatment failure; no change in symptoms, histologic findings, survival, or time to LTX	111
Controlled, double-blind	222	111 @ 14 mg/kg/d × 2 y 111 placebo	Improvement in LFTs and some histologic features; no change in survival, symptoms, or time to LTX	110
Controlled, double-blind	153	10–12 mg/kg/d × 2 y	Improvement in LFTs, especially if bilirubin <2 μmol/L	112
Controlled, double-blind	61	13–15 mg/kg/d × 2 y	No effect on histologic findings or stage	115
Prospective open label	100	10 mg/kg/d	Improvement in symptoms and LFTs; histologic remission in 2%	126

Surgical dilation of strictures or choledochojejunostomy are rarely used today and carry the risk of postoperative infection and scarring at the porta hepatis, compounding the difficulty of liver transplantation in the future.[153] A complication unique to patients with advanced PSC who have undergone ileostomy is the development of varices at the stoma.[154] Treatment of bleeding from stomal varices is difficult and usually requires a central portosystemic shunt or liver transplantation.

In PBC, the choice of treatment is often more

difficult should UDCA fail to normalize blood tests. In older or asymptomatic patients, we usually add colchicine in dosages of 0.6 mg twice daily, follow blood tests at 3- to 4-month intervals, and repeat a liver biopsy in 1 to 2 years. If there is disease progression, we then consider MTX in dosages similar to those used in PSC. In younger patients, particularly those with advanced but precirrhotic disease, and in symptomatic patients, we add MTX, follow blood tests, and repeat liver biopsies in a regimen similar to that described above for PSC.

Although MTX therapy has had a good track record at our center for both diseases, we are concerned with the potential for bone marrow suppression; interstitial pneumonitis (which occurs in 15% of patients with PBC and 1% to 2% of patients with PSC); potential hepatotoxicity with alcohol, diabetes, and obesity; and effects on pregnancy. We counsel all patients not to drink alcohol while taking MTX, to keep their diabetes under control, to avoid excessive weight gain, to use effective birth control methods, and to report any cough or shortness of breath. If there are any signs of toxicity, MTX must be discontinued. Intravenous or oral glucocorticoids may be needed for severe pneumonitis, and they will hasten recovery.

As mentioned above, we do not use cyclosporine in PBC, as efficacy to date has been marginal at best and fraught with excessive renal toxicity and hypertension.

LIVER TRANSPLANTATION

Liver transplantation is the only proven treatment for advanced PBC and PSC. Indications for transplantation include hemorrhage from varices or portal gastropathy, intractable ascites with or without spontaneous bacterial peritonitis, recurrent episodes of bacterial cholangitis, progressive muscle wasting, severe metabolic bone disease, intractable pruritus, and hepatic encephalopathy. Most patients who require liver transplantation are jaundiced. However, jaundice alone is not an absolute indication for liver transplantation.

PBC

Some centers report up to an 80% to 90% 1-year survival after orthotopic liver transplantation for advanced PBC.[23] Patients with PBC typically fare better than most other adult patients who undergo liver transplantation.[155] The reasons for improved survival after liver transplantation are multifactorial and reflect better patient selection, improved surgical technique, and more refined immunosuppression techniques. Survival rates are higher in patients with disease that is less advanced. Patients with advanced disease (jaundice, hypoprothrombinemia, low serum albumin, and fluid retention) have decreased survival after transplantation.[23,156,157] The timing of transplantation is thus critical, and liver transplantation should be considered only when the predicted survival using clinical or mathematical models is less than 2 years,[23,32,158] so as not to subject a well patient to increased morbidity and mortality. It is unclear whether PBC recurs after liver transplantation, but if so, it is rare.[159] Recurrence of PBC is particularly difficult to assess because of histologic similarity between PBC and chronic allograft rejection.[23] Test results for AMA remain positive after liver transplantation and are not helpful in assessing disease recurrence.

PSC

Three-year survival is 85% in most centers following orthotopic liver transplantation for PSC.[160,161] A problem after liver transplantation that is common to PSC is stricturing of the transplanted bile ducts. The pattern is similar to that seen in PSC.[162,163] Possible causes include disease recurrence, ischemia, rejection, or infection. Current data favor infection. Creation of longer jejunal loops in the Roux-en-Y anastomosis and treatment with appropriate antibiotics is usually effective for this complication. Inflammatory bowel disease symptoms typically improve after liver transplantation in patients with PSC.[164] However, there are reports of colon cancer following liver transplantation in patients with PSC and ulcerative colitis.[165] Thus, it is important to continue monitoring for colon cancer in PSC patients who have ulcerative colitis and a liver transplant.

REFERENCES

1. Kaplan MM. Primary biliary cirrhosis. *N Engl J Med.* 1987;316:521–528.
2. Lee YM, Kaplan MM. Primary sclerosing cholangitis. *N Engl J Med.* 1995;332:924–933.
3. Bernau D, Feldmann G, Degott MD, Gisselbrecht C. Ultrastructural lesions and bile ducts in primary biliary cirrhosis: a comparison with the lesions observed in graft versus host disease. *Human Pathol.* 1981;12:782–793.
4. Shulman HM, Sharma P, Amos D, et al. A coded histologic study of hepatic graft-versus-host disease after human bone marrow transplantation. *Hepatology.* 1988;8:463–470.
5. Wiesner RH, Ludwig J, Krom RAI, et al. Hepatic allo-

graft rejection: new developments in terminology, diagnosis, prevention, and treatment. *Mayo Clin Proc.* 1993;68:69–79.
6. Neuberger J, Protmann B, MacDougall BRD, et al. Recurrence of primary biliary cirrhosis after liver transplantation. *N Engl J Med.* 1982;306:1–4.
7. Batts KP, Morre SB, Perkins JD, et al. Influence of positive lymphocyte crossmatch and HLA mismatching on vanishing bile duct syndrome in human liver allografts. *Transplantation.* 1988;45:376–379.
8. Wiesner RH, LaRusso NF, Ludwig J, Dickson ER. Comparison of the clinicopathologic features of primary sclerosing cholangitis and primary biliary cirrhosis. *Gastroenterology.* 1985;88:108–114.
9. Chapman RW, Varghese Z, Gaul R, et al. Association of primary sclerosing cholangitis with HLA-D8. *Gut.* 1983;24:38–41.
10. Mehal WZ, Dennis YM, Lo D, et al. HLA DR4 is a marker for rapid disease progression in primary sclerosing cholangitis. *Gastroenterology.* 1994;106:160–167.
11. Prochazka EJ, Terasaki PI, Park MS, et al. Association of primary sclerosing cholangitis with HLA-DRw52a. *N Engl J Med.* 1990;322:1842–1844.
12. Lo SK, Fleming KA, Chapman RW. Prevalence of anti-neutrophil antibody in primary sclerosing cholangitis and ulcerative colitis using an alkaline phosphatase technique. *Gut.* 1992;33:1370–1375.
13. Chapman W. The immunology of primary sclerosing cholangitis. *Semin Immunopathol.* 1990;12:121–128.
14. Lindor K, Wiesner R, Katzman J, et al. Enhanced autoreactivity of T lymphocytes in primary sclerosing cholangitis. *Hepatology.* 1987;7:884–888.
15. James SP, Hoofnagle JH, Strober W, Jones EA. Primary biliary cirrhosis: a model autoimmune disease. *Ann Intern Med.* 1983;99:500–512.
16. MacSween RN, Burt AS. The cellular pathology of primary biliary cirrhosis. *Mol Aspects Med.* 1985;3:249–267.
17. Spengler U, Pape GR, Hoffman RM, et al. Differential expression of MHC class II subregion products on bile duct epithelial cells and hepatocytes in patients with primary biliary cirrhosis. *Hepatology.* 1988;8:459–462.
18. Bahn AK, Dienstag JL, Wands JR, et al. Alterations of T-cell subsets in primary biliary cirrhosis. *Clin Exp Immunol.* 1982;47:351–358.
19. Ehrlinger S. Hypercholeretic bile acids: a clue to mechanism? *Hepatology.* 1990;11:888–890.
20. Poupon RA, Chretien Y, Poupon RE, et al. Is ursodeoxycholic acid an effective treatment for primary biliary cirrhosis? *Lancet.* 1987;11:834–836.
21. De Caestecker JS, Jazrawi RP, Petroni ML, Northfield TC. Ursodeoxycholic acid in chronic liver disease. *Gut.* 1991;32:1061–1065.
22. Christensen E, Crowe J, Doniach D, et al. Clinical pattern and course of disease in primary biliary cirrhosis based on an analysis of 236 patients. *Gastroenterology.* 1980;78:236–246.
23. Kaplan MM. Primary biliary cirrhosis. In: Schiff L, Schiff ER, eds. *Diseases of the Liver.* 7th ed. Philadelphia, Pa: JB Lippincott Co; 1993:377–410.
24. Balasubramaniam K, Grambsch PM, Wiesner RH, et al. Diminished survival in asymptomatic primary biliary cirrhosis: a prospective study. *Gastroenterology.* 1990;98:1567–1571.
25. James O, Macklon AF, Waston AJ. Primary biliary cirrhosis: a revised clinical spectrum. *Lancet.* 1981;1:1278–1281.
26. Roll J, Boyer JL, Barry D, et al. The prognostic importance of clinical and histological asymptomatic and symptomatic primary biliary cirrhosis. *N Engl J Med.* 1983;308:1–7.
27. Tournay AS. Primary biliary cirrhosis: natural history. *Am J Gastroenterol.* 1980;73:223–226.
28. Sherlock S, Scheuer PJ. The presentation and diagnosis of 100 patients with primary biliary cirrhosis. *N Engl J Med.* 1973;289:674–678.
29. Kaplan MM. Primary biliary cirrhosis. *Prac Gastroenterol.* 1987;12:64–68.
30. Dickson ER, Fleming CR, Ludwig J. Primary biliary cirrhosis. In: Popper H, Schaffner F, eds. *Progress in Liver Diseases.* Vol. 6. New York, NY: Grune & Stratton Inc; 1978:487.
31. Long RG, Scheuer PJ, Sherlock S. Presentation and course of asymptomatic primary biliary cirrhosis. *Gastroenterology.* 1977;72:1204–1207.
32. Dickson ER, Grambsch PM, Fleming TR, et al. Prognosis in primary biliary cirrhosis: model for decision making. *Hepatology.* 1989;10:1–7.
33. Sasaki H, Inoue K, Higuchi K, et al. Primary biliary cirrhosis in Japan: national survey by the subcommittee on autoimmune hepatitis. *Gastroenterol Jpn.* 1985;5:476–485.
34. Shapiro JM, Smith H, Schaffner F, et al. Serum bilirubin: a prognostic factor in primary biliary cirrhosis. *Gut.* 1979;20:137–140.
35. Frazer IH, MacKay IR, Jordan TW, et al. Reactivity of anti-mitochondrial autoantibodies in primary biliary cirrhosis: definition of two novel mitochondrial polypeptide autoantigens. *J Immunol.* 1985;135:1739–1745.
36. Lindenborn-Fotinos J, Baum H, Berg PA. Mitochondrial antibodies in primary biliary cirrhosis: species and nonspecies determinants of M2 antigen. *Hepatology.* 1985;5:763–769.
37. Mendel-Hartvig I, Nelson BD, Loof L, Totterman TH. Primary biliary cirrhosis: further biochemical and immunological characterization of mitochondrial antigens. *Clin Exp Immunol.* 1985;62:371–379.
38. Goodman ZD, McNally PR, Davis D, Ishak KG. "Autoimmune cholangitis": a variant of primary biliary cirrhosis. *Hepatology.* 1993;18:109A.
39. Klatskin G, Conn HO. *Histopathology of the Liver.* New York, NY: Oxford University Press; 1993:268–269.
40. Fiengold MJ, Carpenter RJ. Obliterative cholangitis due to cytomegalovirus: a possible precursor of paucity of intrahepatic bile ducts. *Hum Pathol.* 1982;13:662–665.
41. Ludwig J, Kim CH, Wiesner RH, Krom RAF. Floxuridine induced sclerosing cholangitis: an ischemic cholangiopathy. *Hepatology.* 1989;9:215–218.
42. Cello JP. Acquired immunodeficiency syndrome cholangiopathy: spectrum of disease. *Am J Med.* 1989;86:539–546.
43. Wiesner RH, Grambsch PM, Dickson ER, et al. Primary sclerosing cholangitis: natural history, prognostic factors and survival analysis. *Hepatology.* 1989;10:430–436.
44. Shepherd HA, Selby WS, Chapman RWG, et al. Ulcerative colitis and persistent liver dysfunction. *Q J Med.* 1983;52:503–513.
45. Schrumpf E, Fausa O, Elgjo K, Kolmannskog F. Hepatobiliary complications of inflammatory bowel disease. *Semin Liver Dis.* 1988;8:201–209.
46. Ludwig J, LaRusso NF, Wiesner RH. Primary sclerosing cholangitis. *Contemp Issues Surg Pathol.* 1986;8:193–213.
47. Knox TA, Fawaz KA, Arora S, Kaplan MM. Primary sclerosing cholangitis (PSC): improvement with metho-

trexate (MTX) treatment. *Hepatology.* 1989;10:688. Abstract.
48. LaRusso N, Wiesner R, Ludwig J, et al. Randomized trial of penicillamine in primary sclerosing cholangitis. *Gastroenterology.* 1988;95:1036–1042.
49. Dickson ER. Status of medical therapy for PBC and PSC. In: *New and Evolving Therapies for Hepatic and Biliary Diseases: AASLD Postgraduate Course Syllabus.* 1993:375–390.
50. Wiesner RH, Ludwig J, LaRusso NF, MacCarty RL. Diagnosis and treatment of primary sclerosing cholangitis. *Semin Liver Dis.* 1985;5:241–253.
51. Lindor KD, Wiesner RH, LaRusso NF. Recent advances in the management of primary sclerosing cholangitis. *Semin Liver Dis.* 1987;7:322–327.
52. Mistilis SP, Skyring AP, Goulston SJ. Effect of long term tetracycline therapy, steroid therapy and colectomy in pericholangitis associated with ulcerative colitis. *Australas Ann Med.* 1965;14:286–294.
53. Cangemi JR, Wiesner RH, Beaver SJ, et al. Effect of proctocolectomy for chronic ulcerative colitis on the natural history of primary sclerosing cholangitis. *Gastroenterology.* 1989;96:790–794.
54. Wiesner RH, LaRusso NF. Clinicopathologic features of the syndrome of primary sclerosing cholangitis. *Gastroenterology.* 1980;79:200–206.
55. Chapman RW, Arbourgh BA, Rhodes JM, et al. Primary sclerosing cholangitis: a review of its clinical features, cholangiography, and hepatic histology. *Gut.* 1980;21:870–877.
56. Lefkowitch JH. Primary sclerosing cholangitis. *Arch Intern Med.* 1982;142:1157–1160.
57. LaRusso NF, Wiesner RH, Ludwig J, MacCarty RL. Current concepts: primary sclerosing cholangitis. *N Engl J Med.* 1984;310:899–903.
58. Kaplan MM. Medical approaches to primary sclerosing cholangitis. *Semin Liver Dis.* 1991;11:56–63.
59. Sherlock S. Primary biliary cirrhosis. In: Schiff L, Schiff ER, eds. *Diseases of the Liver.* 6th ed. Philadelphia, Pa: JB Lippincott Co; 1987:979–999.
60. Knox TA, Kaplan MM. Pregnancy and liver disease. In: Taylor MB, ed. *Gastrointestinal Emergencies.* Baltimore, Md: Williams & Wilkins; 1992:510–521.
61. Bergasa NV. New therapeutic modalities for the pruritus of cholestasis. In: *New and Evolving Therapies for Hepatic and Biliary Diseases: AASLD Postgraduate Course Syllabus.* 1993:353–367.
62. Jones EA, Bergasa NV. Hypothesis: the pruritus of cholestasis: from bile salts to opiate agonists. *Hepatology.* 1990;11:884–887.
63. Murphy GM, Ross A, Billing BH. Serum bile acids in primary biliary cirrhosis. *Gut.* 1972;13:201–206.
64. Bergasa NV, Jones EA. Management of the pruritus of cholestasis: potential role of opiate antagonists. *Am J Gastroenterol.* 1991;86:1404–1412.
65. Jones EA, Bergasa NV. Hypothesis: the pruritus of cholestasis: from bile acids to opiate agonists. *Hepatology.* 1990;11:884–887.
66. Herlong HF, Recker RR, Maddrey WC. Bone disease in primary biliary cirrhosis: histologic features and response to 25-hydroxyvitamin D. *Gastroenterology.* 1982;83:103–108.
67. Matloff DS, Kaplan MM, Neer RM, et al. Osteoporosis in primary biliary cirrhosis: effects of 25-hydroxyvitamin D_3 treatment. *Gastroenterology.* 1982;83:97–102.
68. Hodgson SF, Dickson ER, Wahner HW, et al. Bone loss and reduced osteoblast function in primary biliary cirrhosis. *Ann Intern Med.* 1985;103:855–860.
69. Ros E, Garcia-Puges A, Reixach M, et al. Fat digestion and exocrine pancreatic function in primary biliary cirrhosis. *Gastroenterology.* 1984;87:180–187.
70. Lanspa SJ, Chan AT, Bell JS III, et al. Pathogenesis of steatorrhea in primary biliary cirrhosis. *Hepatology.* 1985;5:837–842.
71. Epstein O, Chapman RWG, Lake-Bakaar G, et al. The pancreas in primary biliary cirrhosis and primary sclerosing cholangitis. *Gastroenterology.* 1982;83:1177–1182.
72. Kaplan MM, Elta GH, Furie B, et al. Fat-soluble vitamin nutriture in primary biliary cirrhosis. *Gastroenterology.* 1988;95:787–792.
73. Sartin JS, Wiesner RH, LaRusso NF. Fat soluble vitamin deficiencies in primary sclerosing cholangitis. *Gastroenterology.* 1987;92:1615. Abstract.
74. Herlong HF, Russell RM, Maddrey WC. Vitamin A and zinc therapy in primary biliary cirrhosis. *Hepatology.* 1981;1:348–381.
75. Shepherd AN, Bedford GJ, Hill A, Bouchier IA. Primary biliary cirrhosis: dark adaptometry, electro-oculography and vitamin A state. *Br J Med.* 1984;289:1484–1485.
76. Nyberg A, Berne B, Nordlinger H, et al. Impaired release of vitamin A from liver in primary biliary cirrhosis. *Hepatology.* 1988;8:136–141.
77. Muñoz SJ, Heubi JE, Balistreri WF, Maddrey WC. Vitamin E deficiency in primary biliary cirrhosis: gastrointestinal malabsorption, frequency and relationship to other lipid-soluble vitamins. *Hepatology.* 1989;9:525–553.
78. Gallop PM, Lian JB, Mauschka PV. Carboxylated calcium binding proteins and vitamin K. *N Engl J Med.* 1980;302:1460–1466.
79. Rosenberg IH, Mason JB. Hepatobiliary influences on the skeletal system. In: Arias IM, et al, eds. *The Liver: Biology and Pathobiology.* 3rd ed. New York, NY: Raven Press Publishers; 1994.
80. Kaplan MM, Goldberg MJ, Matloff DS, Neer RM, Goodman DBP. Effect of 25-hydroxyvitamin D_3 on vitamin D metabolites in primary biliary cirrhosis. 1981;81:681–685.
81. Krall EA, Sahyoun N, Tannenbaum S, et al. Effect of vitamin D intake on seasonal variation in parathyroid hormone secretion in postmenopausal women. *New Engl J Med.* 1988;321:1777–1783.
82. Compston JE. Metabolic bone disease. In: Rector WG. *Complications of Chronic Liver Disease.* St Louis, Mo: Mosby-Year Book Inc; 1992:295–316.
83. Hay JE, Lindor KD, Wiesner RH, et al. The metabolic bone disease of primary sclerosing cholangitis. *Hepatology.* 1991;14:257–261.
84. Kehayoglou AK, Holdsworth CD, Agnew JE, et al. Bone disease and calcium absorption in primary biliary cirrhosis: with special reference to vitamin D therapy. *Lancet.* 1968;1:715–718.
85. Jahn CE, Schaefer EJ, Taam LA, et al. Lipoprotein abnormalities in primary biliary cirrhosis. *Gastroenterology.* 1985;89:1266–1278.
86. Crippin JS, Jorgensen RA, Dickson ER, Lindor KD. Hepatic osteodystrophy in primary biliary cirrhosis: effects of medical treatment. *Am J Gastroenterol.* 1994;89:47–50.
87. Bannister P, Oakes J, Sheridan P, et al. Sex hormone changes in chronic liver disease: a matched study of alcoholic versus non-alcoholic liver disease. *Q J Med.* 1987;63:305–313.
88. Green JRB. Mechanisms of hypogonadism in cirrhotic males. *Gut.* 1987;18:843–853.

89. Hahn TJ, Boisseau C, Avioli LV. Effect of chronic corticosteroid administration on diaphyseal and metaphyseal bone mass. *J Clin Endocrinol Metab.* 1974;39:274–282.
90. Mazess RB, Whedon GD. Immobilisation and bone. *Calcif Tissue Int.* 1983;35:265–267.
91. Weaver GA, Franck WA, Streck WF, et al. Hepatic osteodystrophy after liver transplantation in a patient with primary biliary cirrhosis. *Am J Gastroenterol.* 1983;78:102–106.
92. Haagsma EB, Thija CJP, Post CJ, et al. Value of calcium, phosphate, and alkaline phosphatase measurements in the diagnosis of histological osteomalacia. *J Clin Pathol.* 1982;35:625–630.
93. McDonald JA, Dunstan CR, Dilworth P, et al. Bone loss after liver transplantation. *Hepatology.* 1991;14:613–619.
94. Epstein O, Jain S, Lee RG, et al. D-penicillamine treatment improves survival in primary biliary cirrhosis. *Lancet.* 1981;1:1275–1277.
95. James OFW. D-penicillamine for primary biliary cirrhosis. *Gut.* 1985;26:109–113.
96. Epstein O, Cook DG, Jain S, et al. D-penicillamine and clinical trials in primary biliary cirrhosis. *Hepatology.* 1984;4:1032. Abstract.
97. Howat HT, Ralston AJ, Varley H, et al. The late results of long term treatment of primary biliary cirrhosis by corticosteroids. *Rev Int Hepatol.* 1966;16:227–238.
98. Mitchison HC, Palmer JM, Bassendine MF, et al. A controlled trial of prednisolone treatment in primary biliary cirrhosis: three year results. *J Hepatol.* 1992;15:336–344.
99. Mitchison HC, Bassendine MF, Malcolm AJ, et al. A pilot double-blind controlled one year trial of prednisolone treatment in primary biliary cirrhosis: hepatic improvement but greater bone loss. *Hepatology.* 1989;10:420–429.
100. Matloff KD, Alpert E, Resnick RH, Kaplan MM. A prospective trial of D-penicillamine in primary biliary cirrhosis. *N Engl J Med.* 1982;306:319–326.
101. Myers RN, Cooper JH, Padis N. Primary sclerosing cholangitis: complete gross and histologic reversal after long-term steroid therapy. *Am J Gastroenterol.* 1970;53:527–538.
102. Burgert SL, Brown BP, Kirkpatrick RB, La Brecque DR. Positive corticosteroid response in early primary sclerosing cholangitis. *Gastroenterology.* 1984:1037. Abstract.
103. Hoofnagle JH, David GL, Schafer DF, et al. Randomized trial of chlorambucil for primary biliary cirrhosis. *Gastroenterology.* 1986;91:1327–1334.
104. Wagner A. Azathioprine treatment in primary sclerosing cholangitis. *Lancet.* 1971;2:663–664.
105. Crowe J, Christensen E, Smith M, et al. Azathioprine in primary biliary cirrhosis: a preliminary report of an international trial. *Gastroenterology.* 1980;78:1005.
106. Heathcote J, Ross A, Sherlock S. A prospective controlled trial in azathioprine in primary biliary cirrhosis. *Gastroenterology.* 1976;70:656–660.
107. Christensen E, Neuberger J, Crowe J, et al. Beneficial effect of azathioprine and prediction of prognosis in primary biliary cirrhosis: final results of an international trial. *Gastroenterology.* 1985;89:1084–1091.
108. Poupon RE, Balkau B, Eschweger E, et al. A multicenter controlled trial of ursodiol for the treatment of primary biliary cirrhosis. *N Engl J Med.* 1991;324:1548–1554.
109. Poupon RE, Poupon R, Balkau B, UDCA-PBC Study Group. Ursodiol for the long term treatment of primary biliary cirrhosis. *N Engl J Med.* 1994;330:1342–1347.
110. Heathcote EJ, Cauch-Dudek K, Walker V, et al. The Canadian multicenter double-blind randomized controlled trial of ursodeoxycholic acid in primary biliary cirrhosis. *Hepatology.* 1994;19:1149–1156.
111. Lindor KD, Dickson ER, Baldus WP, et al. Ursodeoxycholic acid in the treatment of primary biliary cirrhosis. *Gastroenterology.* 1994;106:1284–1290.
112. Combes B, Carothers RL, Maddrey WC, et al. A randomized, double blind, placebo controlled trial of ursodeoxycholic acid (UDCA) in primary biliary cirrhosis. *Hepatology.* 1993;18:175A. Abstract.
113. Leuschner U, Fischer H, Kurtz W, et al. Ursodeoxycholic acid in primary biliary cirrhosis: results of a double blind controlled trial. *Gastroenterology.* 1989;97:1268–1274.
114. Leuschner U, Leuschner M, Sieratzki J, et al. Gallstone dissolution with ursodeoxycholic acid in patients with chronic active hepatitis and two year follow up: a pilot study. *Dig Dis Sci.* 1985;30:642–649.
115. Batts KP, Jorgensen RA, Dickson RA, et al. The effects of ursodeoxycholic acid on hepatic inflammation and histologic stage in patients with primary biliary cirrhosis. *Hepatology.* 1993;18:175A.
116. Combes B, Carothers RL, Maddrey WC, et al. A randomized, double blind, placebo controlled trial of ursodeoxycholic acid (UDCA) in primary biliary cirrhosis. *Hepatology.* 1993;18:175A. Abstract.
117. Hadziyannis SJ, Hadziyannis ES, Makris A. A randomized controlled study of ursodeoxycholic acid in primary biliary cirrhosis. *Hepatology.* 1989;10:580. Abstract.
118. Lotterer E, Stiehl A, Raedsch R, et al. Ursodeoxycholic acid in primary biliary cirrhosis: no evidence for toxicity in stages I–III. *J Hepatol.* 1990;10:284–290.
119. Matsuzaki Y, Tanaka N, Osuga T, et al. Improvement in biliary enzyme levels and itching as a result of long term administration of ursodeoxycholic acid in primary biliary cirrhosis. *Am J Gastroenterol.* 1990;85:15–23.
120. O'Brien CB, Senior JR, Sternlieb JM, et al. Ursodiol in the treatment of primary biliary cirrhosis. *Gastroenterology.* 1990;98:A617.
121. Oka H, Toda G, Ikeda Y, et al. A multicenter double-blind controlled trial of ursodeoxycholic acid for primary biliary cirrhosis. *Gastroenterol Jpn.* 1990;25:774–780.
122. Osuga T, Tanaka N, Matsuzaki Y, Aikawa T. Effect of ursodeoxycholic acid in chronic hepatitis and primary biliary cirrhosis. *Dig Dis Sci.* 1989;34(suppl):49S–51S.
123. Podda M, Battezzati PM, Crosignani A, et al. Ursodeoxycholic acid for symptomatic primary biliary cirrhosis: a double blind multicenter study. *Hepatology.* 1989;10:639. Abstract.
124. Podda M, Ghezzi C, Battezzati PM, et al. Effect of different doses of ursodeoxycholic acid in chronic liver disease. *Dig Dis Sci.* 1989;34(suppl):59S–61S.
125. Taidsch R, Stiehl A, Theilmann L, et al. Influence of ursodeoxycholic acid on primary biliary cirrhosis depending on stage of the disease. *Gastroenterology.* 1989;96:A647.
126. Wolfhagen FHJ, Van Buren GP, Van Berge H, et al. Can ursodeoxycholic acid monotherapy induce disease remission in primary biliary cirrhosis? *Hepatology.* 1993;18:220A.
127. O'Brien CB, Senior JR, Batta AK, et al. Ursodeoxycholic acid treatment produces marked clinical and bio-

chemical amelioration of primary sclerosing cholangitis. *Gastroenterology.* 1989;96:A640. Abstract.
128. O'Brien CB, Senior JR, Arora-Michandani R, et al. Ursodeoxycholic acid for the treatment of primary sclerosing cholangitis: a 30 month pilot study. *Hepatology.* 1991;14:838–847.
129. Stiehl A, and colleagues. Presented at Bile Acids and the Future. XII International Bile Acid Meeting. 1993.
130. Stiehl A, Raedsch R, Rudolph G, Thielmann L. Treatment of primary sclerosing cholangitis with ursodeoxycholic acid: first results of a controlled study. *Hepatology.* 1989;10:602. Abstract.
131. Beures U, Spengler U, Krus W, et al. Ursodeoxycholic acid for the treatment of primary sclerosing cholangitis: a placebo controlled trial. *Hepatology.* 1992;16:707–714.
132. Chazouillieres O, Poupon R, Capron JP, et al. Ursodeoxycholic acid for primary sclerosing cholangitis. *J Hepatol.* 1990;11:120–123.
133. Hayashi H, Higuchi T, Ichimiya H, Sakamoto N. Asymptomatic primary sclerosing cholangitis treated with ursodeoxycholic acid. *Gastroenterology.* 1990;99:533–535.
134. Lindor KD, and colleagues. Presented at Bile Acids and the Future. XII International Bile Acid Meeting. 1993.
135. Knox TA, Kaplan MM. A double blind controlled trial of oral-pulse methotrexate therapy in the treatment of primary sclerosing cholangitis. *Gastroenterology.* 1994;106:494–499.
136. Kaplan MM. Methotrexate treatment of chronic cholestatic liver diseases: friend or foe? *Q J Med.* 1989;72:757–761.
137. Kaplan MM, Arora S, Pincus SH. Primary sclerosing cholangitis and low dose oral pulse methotrexate therapy: clinical and histological response. *Ann Intern Med.* 1987;106:231–235.
138. Kaplan M, Schmid C, McKusick A, et al. Double blind trial of methotrexate (MTX) versus colchicine (colch) in primary biliary cirrhosis. *Hepatology.* 1993;18:176A.
139. Busher HP, Zietzschmann Y, Gerok W. Positive responses to methotrexate and ursodeoxycholic acid in patients with primary biliary cirrhosis responding insufficiently to ursodeoxycholic acid alone. *J Hepatol.* 1993;18:9–14.
140. Kaplan MM, Knox TA. Treatment of primary biliary cirrhosis with low dose weekly methotrexate. *Gastroenterology.* 1991;101:1332–1338.
141. Kaplan MM, Knox TA. Methotrexate for primary biliary cirrhosis. *Gastroenterology.* 1992;102:1824.
142. Knox TA, Kaplan MM. Treatment of primary sclerosing cholangitis with oral methotrexate. *Am J Gastroenterol.* 1991;86:546–552.
143. Kaplan MM, Alling DW, Zimmerman HJ, et al. Prospective trial of colchicine therapy in primary biliary cirrhosis. *N Engl J Med.* 1986;315:1448–1454.
144. Bodenheimer H Jr, Schaffner F, Pezzulo J. Evaluation of colchicine therapy in primary biliary cirrhosis. *Gastroenterology.* 1988;95:124–129.
145. Warnes TW, Smith A, Lee F, et al. A controlled trial of colchicine in primary biliary cirrhosis. *J Hepatol.* 1987;5:1–7.
146. Lindor KD, LaRusso NF, Wiesner RH. Prednisone and colchicine are not of benefit after two years in patients with primary sclerosing cholangitis. *Hepatology.* 1989;10:638. Abstract.
147. Kaplan MM. New strategies needed for treatment of primary biliary cirrhosis? *Gastroenterology.* 1993;104:651–653.
148. Minuk GY, Bohme CE, Burgess E, et al. Pilot study of cyclosporin A in patients with symptomatic primary biliary cirrhosis. *Gastroenterology.* 1988;95:56–63.
149. Lombard M, Portmann B, Neuberger J, et al. Cyclosporin A treatment in primary biliary cirrhosis: results of a long-term placebo controlled trial. *Gastroenterology.* 1993;104:519–526.
150. Wiesner RH, Ludwig J, Lindor KD, et al. A controlled trial of cyclosporin in the treatment of primary biliary cirrhosis. *N Engl J Med.* 1990;322:1414–1424.
151. Wiesner RH, Steiner B, LaRusso NF, et al. A controlled clinical trial evaluating cyclosporine in the treatment of primary sclerosing cholangitis. *Hepatology.* 1991;14:Suppl:63A. abstract.
152. May GR, Bender CE, LaRusso NF, Wiesner RH. Nonoperative dilation of dominant strictures in primary sclerosing cholangitis. *AJR.* 1985;145:1061–1064.
153. Cameron JL, Pitt HA, Zinner MJ, et al. Resection of hepatic duct bifurcation and transhepatic stenting for sclerosing cholangitis. *Ann Surg.* 1988;207:614–622.
154. Wiesner RH, LaRusso NF, Dozois RR, Beaver SJ. Peristomal varices after proctocolectomy in patients with primary sclerosing cholangitis. *Gastroenterology.* 1986;90:316–322.
155. Esquivel CO, Van Thiel DH, Demetris AJ, et al. Transplantation for primary biliary cirrhosis. *Gastroenterology.* 1988;94:1207–1216.
156. Markus BH, Dickson ER, Grambsch PM, et al. Efficiency of liver transplantation in patients with primary biliary cirrhosis. *N Engl J Med.* 1989;320:1709–1713.
157. Neuberger J, Altman DG, Polson R, et al. Prognosis after liver transplantation for primary biliary cirrhosis. *Transplantation.* 1989;48:444.
158. Goudie BM, Burt AS, Macfarlane GJ, et al. Risk factors and prognosis in primary biliary cirrhosis. *Am J Gastroenterol.* 1989;84:1474.
159. Polson RJ, Portmann B, Neuberger J, et al. Evidence for disease recurrence after liver transplantation for primary biliary cirrhosis: clinical and histologic follow-up studies. *Gastroenterology.* 1989;97:715.
160. Langnas AN, Grazi GL, Stratta RJ, et al. Primary sclerosing cholangitis: the emerging role for liver transplantation. *Am J Gastroenterol.* 1990;85:1136–1141.
161. Mc Entee G, Wiesner RH, Rosen C, et al. A comparative study of patients undergoing liver transplantation for primary sclerosing cholangitis and primary biliary cirrhosis. *Transplant Proc.* 1991;23:1563–1564.
162. Letourneau JG, Day DL, Hunter DW, et al. Biliary complications after liver transplantation in patients with pre-existing sclerosing cholangitis. *Radiology.* 1988;167:349–351.
163. Hunter EB, Wiesner RH, MacCarty RL, et al. Does primary sclerosing cholangitis recur after liver transplantation. *Gastroenterology.* 1989;965:610. Abstract.
164. Gavaler JS, Delemos B, Belle SH, et al. Ulcerative colitis disease activity as subjectively assessed by patient-completed questionnaires following orthotopic liver transplantation for sclerosing cholangitis. *Dig Dis Sci.* 1991;36:321–327.
165. Higashi H, Yanaga K, Marsh JW, et al. Development of colon cancer after liver transplantation for primary sclerosing cholangitis associated with ulcerative colitis. *Hepatology.* 1990;11:477–480.

121
Acute Bacterial Cholangitis
ERIC D. LIBBY and JOSEPH W. LEUNG

Acute cholangitis occurs when bacteria in bile cause inflammation of the ducts and systemic symptoms of infection. Although biliary tract inflammation can also result from parasitic infestation, chemical injury, or primary sclerosing cholangitis, this chapter focuses on cholangitis caused by acute bacterial infection.

PRESENTATION

Classically, patients with acute cholangitis present with Charcot's triad of fever, jaundice, and right upper quadrant abdominal pain. Although this presentation is highly suggestive of the diagnosis, the full triad may be observed in only 50% to 70% of patients.[1-3] Fever is the most common symptom, with pain, jaundice, chills, and nausea seen with decreasing frequency. Severe cholangitis may present additionally with hypotension and mental status changes. These symptoms, when added to those of Charcot's triad, make up Reynolds' pentad and portend a grave prognosis if not treated immediately.[4] Particularly among the elderly, cholangitis may occur without localizing signs and may present as sepsis of unclear origin. The diagnosis should be suspected in any patient with abdominal pain who has evidence of systemic infection.

PATHOPHYSIOLOGY

Bacterial cholangitis requires the presence of bacteria in bile and obstruction. Transient bacterial contamination of bile may occur frequently, but normally is without clinical consequence. Biliary defense mechanisms, including secretory IgA, bile salts, mucus production, and the flushing effect of bile flow, act to maintain bile sterility.[5] When biliary obstruction is present, however, stasis permits bacterial proliferation and the accumulation of endotoxin and other bacterial products. As biliary pressure increases, bacteria and toxins escape the ducts and enter the venous system (cholangiovenous reflux) or lymphatics, causing septicemia.[6] Hepatic dysfunction due to obstruction also contributes to impairment of the host defense mechanisms, as bacterial clearance by Kupffer cells is reduced under these conditions.[7]

Causes of biliary obstruction include choledocholithiasis, postoperative or traumatic stricture, Mirizzi's syndrome, choledochocele, and malignancy. Choledocholithiasis is the most common biliary disorder leading to cholangitis. Although neoplasia is a frequent cause of obstructive jaundice, the bile usually remains free of infection unless intervention has been attempted, and cholangitis is reported to complicate malignant jaundice in only 15% of cases.[8] However, in recent years, the increasing use of endoscopic or percutaneous biliary instrumentation has led to a much higher incidence of iatrogenic cholangitis in patients with cancer. Cholangitis may occur when drainage attempts fail or when hilar obstruction is present with multiple segment involvement. In addition, cholangitis caused by stent blockage is a major problem that complicates the subsequent management of patients with biliary malignancies.[9]

The organisms most frequently cultured from blood and bile are the enteric gram-negative bacteria such as *Escherichia coli*, *Klebsiella*, *Proteus*, and *Enterobacter* and the gram-positive *Enterococcus*. Two or more organisms are recovered in half of cases.[1,2] *Pseudomonas* may also be recovered on occasion but appears to cause cholangitis primarily following instrumentation with inadequately disinfected equipment. Anaerobic bacteria are uncommon pathogens in cholangitis and are nearly always seen as part of mixed infections with aerobes.

DIAGNOSIS

Cholangitis should be suspected in any patient with fever and abdominal pain. The differential diagnosis may include acute cholecystitis, pancreatitis, hepatitis, liver abscess, pyelonephritis, perforated peptic ulcer, appendicitis, and diverticulitis. Fever and jaundice may be prominent in the "hyperbilirubinemia of sepsis," which accompanies severe infection from sources outside of the biliary tree.

Physical findings typically include icterus, fever, and tenderness in the epigastrium or right upper quadrant of the abdomen. Frank peritonitis is uncommon and should raise the possibility of other diagnoses. Abnormal laboratory findings include leukocytosis with a shift toward neutrophil and band forms and elevations of serum bilirubin, alkaline phosphatase, aspartate aminotransferase (AST), and alanine aminotransferase (ALT). Serum amylase may also be elevated.

Ultrasonography provides the best initial radiologic evaluation. Although ultrasound detects choledocholithiasis in only 14% to 30% of cases, it does detect dilation of the bile ducts in most patients in whom common duct stones are present.[10,11] Identification of associated stones within the gallbladder is also important and further strengthens the clinical suspicion for cholangitis. It should be noted, however, that failure to visualize ductal dilation cannot be used to exclude the diagnosis of cholangitis, as this finding may be absent in a third of patients with documented choledocholithiasis.[10,11] Since infection may develop early in the course of biliary obstruction, cholangitis can occur long before ducts have had time to dilate.[12]

Computed tomography (CT) may be more accurate than ultrasonography for identifying causes of obstruction such as tumor, but CT's ability to detect ductal dilation is inferior to that of ultrasound.[12] The primary role of CT is in excluding other intraabdominal sources of infection when the diagnosis remains unclear. Direct cholangiography provides the most reliable means of demonstrating biliary obstruction and determining its cause. Cholangiography is usually required for planning the definitive treatment of obstruction and can be performed via endoscopic, percutaneous, or intraoperative techniques.

TREATMENT

Medical treatment with intravenous antibiotics and hydration successfully controls the acute attack of bacterial cholangitis in roughly 80% of patients.[2,13] For attacks of mild-to-moderate severity, single agent antibiotic therapy with a cephalosporin, quinolone, or broad spectrum penicillin to treat enteric gram-negative rods is usually sufficient. In more severe cases, antibiotic coverage should be broadened to include activity against *Enterococcus* and anaerobic bacteria. Patients should be kept nil by mouth, given vitamin K to correct coagulopathy, and observed carefully until the attack has subsided.

For those patients who respond well to initial medical management, emergent surgery, with its associated high morbidity and mortality, can be avoided. Correction of the underlying cause of obstruction can then be undertaken electively under more favorable conditions. Patients who fail to improve with initial medical treatment require urgent intervention. These patients are usually suffering from what has been termed acute suppurative cholangitis,[14] toxic refractory cholangitis,[2] or severe acute cholangitis.[15] This condition is characterized by complete biliary obstruction and the presence of frank pus within the ducts. Under the conditions of high intrabiliary pressure, cholangiovenous reflux leads to the systemic consequences of septicemia. Meanwhile antibiotic penetration is poor, allowing the infection to continue uncontrolled within the duct. Even antibiotics that are normally concentrated in bile are unable to achieve significant biliary levels under conditions of complete obstruction.[16] Thus, conservative treatment alone is inadequate to control infection under these conditions, and unless drainage is rapidly established, mortality approaches 100%.[14,17]

Historically, drainage for suppurative cholangitis has required emergency surgery. The cost of this approach is high, however, with a mortality of 20% to 60%[1-3,14,15,17,18] and a third of survivors subsequently requiring reoperation for definitive management. Establishment of initial drainage via the use of percutaneous transhepatic techniques appears to offer improved survival when compared to the surgical approach.[19] Percutaneous cholangiography may be difficult to achieve in patients with nondilated ducts or ascites, however, and complications such as bleeding can be particularly troublesome in patients who have a coagulopathy. Most patients are only temporized by percutaneous drainage, with further interventions required for definitive treatment of calculi or other causes of obstruction.

Endoscopic techniques for drainage have the advantage of gaining direct access to the biliary system without puncturing the skin or liver capsule. This factor decreases the chances of causing significant bleeding, intraperitoneal bile leakage, or contamination of other tissues with infected bile.[20] The overall complication rate of endoscopic treatment appears to be low, but vital signs must be monitored carefully during these procedures, as patients with infection may be particularly sensitive to the respiratory and hemodynamic effects of sedation. For the majority of patients, endoscopic sphincterotomy and definitive stone extraction can be performed at the same time that drainage is established. If the patient is coagulopathic or is too unstable to tolerate a prolonged procedure, a nasobiliary drain can be placed without a sphincterotomy, and elective stone removal can be performed after the patient's condition improves (Fig. 121–1). Nasobiliary drainage catheters permit monitoring of biliary drainage, provide access for repeat cholangiography, and may be used for flushing the bile ducts with saline or stone dissolution agents to aid clearance of calculi.[21] For confused or agitated patients who might dislodge a nasobiliary catheter, a large diameter (10F-gauge or greater) stent can be placed as an alternative.

Urgent endoscopic decompression has been shown to improve survival in patients with severe cholangitis. Early reports showed mortality to be only 5% to 8% when endoscopic drainage was employed for suppurative cholangitis, comparing favorably with the historical mortality for emergent surgery.[13,18,22] A randomized controlled trial recently confirmed this advantage and reported a mortality of only 10% for patients treated initially by endoscopy versus 32% among those treated by surgery.[23]

Determining which patients require urgent intervention remains problematic. Although reports in the literature frequently distinguish between cases of suppurative and nonsuppurative cholangitis, it is not possible to reliably predict the presence of pus based on the patient's clinical presentation. Some patients with severe cholangitis are not found to have frank pus in the duct at the time of drainage, whereas a number of others with suppuration follow a more indolent course.[2] Factors identified as predictive of poor outcome at the time of presentation include advanced age, concomitant medical illness, malignancy, renal insufficiency, hypoalbuminemia, thrombocytopenia, and severe hyperbiliru-

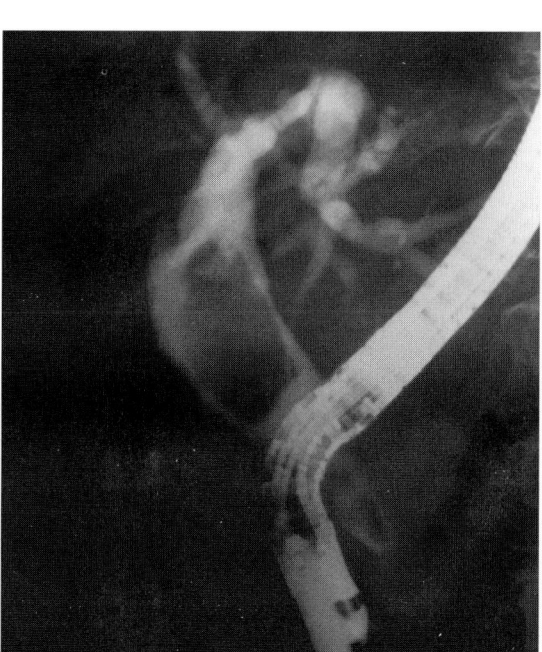
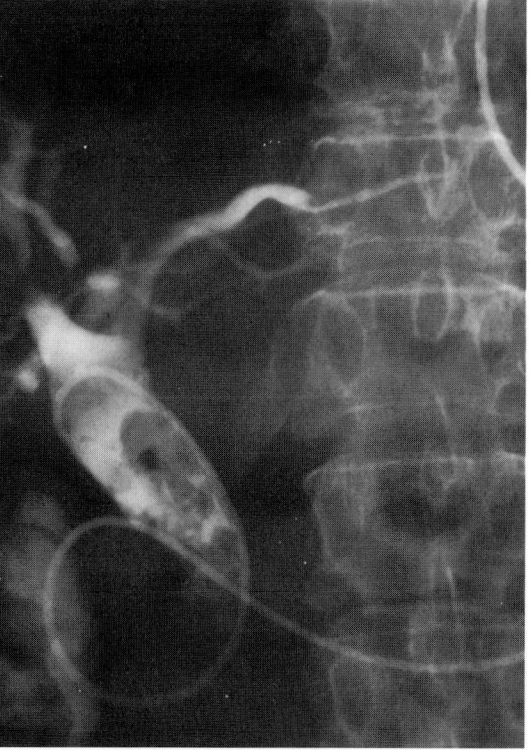

FIGURE 121–1. **A,** Endoscopic retrograde cholangiopancreatography (ERCP) demonstrates large common duct stone in patient with acute cholangitis. **B,** Nasobiliary tube placed to provide drainage. The patient returned 3 days later for ERCP with sphincterotomy, mechanical lithotripsy, and stone extraction.

TABLE 121–1. RISKS FOR MORTALITY FROM CHOLANGITIS

Risk Factor	References
Malignancy	2, 3
Renal failure	1, 3, 18, 24
Reynolds' pentad	1, 3, 24
Medical comorbidities	15, 18
Thrombocytopenia	15
Albumin <3	15, 18
Bilirubin >90 μmol/L	3, 15

binemia.[1–3,15,18,24] Shock and altered mental status are clearly associated with suppurative cholangitis but are present in only a small percentage of patients. Failure to show improvement in abdominal pain or fever despite medical therapy is a significant late sign of severe disease.

Our approach to the patient with cholangitis is to begin with medical management and monitor carefully for response. Close observation is particularly important in elderly patients or those with risk factors for poor outcome (Table 121–1). Failure to improve within 24 hours of starting antibiotics is an indication for urgent drainage. Development of hypotension or impaired mental status constitutes an emergency, requiring immediate biliary decompression. The majority of patients respond to initial conservative measures, however. Further evaluation, including cholangiography, can be performed once the infection is controlled. Definitive correction of the obstruction can then be done based on a proper study of the nature of the obstruction and of the underlying anatomy.

The goals of definitive treatment are to establish drainage and prevent recurrence of obstruction. The specific approach taken depends on the cause of obstruction and on the availability and expertise of surgeons, endoscopists, and interventional radiologists. Endoscopic treatment of choledocholithiasis typically entails sphincterotomy and stone extraction. Complete clearance of the bile ducts is achieved in 90% to 95% of patients. Large calculi may require mechanical lithotripsy prior to removal.[25] Occasionally, the duct cannot be cleared of stones, and a stent is left to prevent stone impaction and ensure drainage (Fig. 121–2).[26] Endoscopic retrograde cholangiopancreatography (ERCP) for stone extraction can be repeated after 1 or 2 months. In 10% of patients, stones are found to have fragmented, presumably because of friction against the stent. Long-term treatment with ursodeoxy-

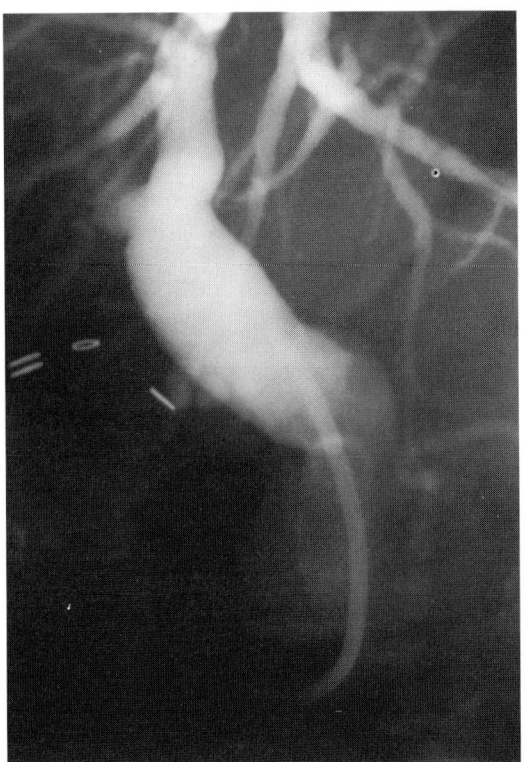

FIGURE 121–2. Biliary stent placed to ensure drainage in patient who could not be cleared of stones during first procedure. Second attempt 1 month later succeeded in removing all stones.

cholic acid has been reported to facilitate stone removal in conjunction with stenting.[27] Extracorporeal shock wave lithotripsy or intraductal stone fragmentation with electrohydraulic or laser lithotriptors can aid stone removal in selected patients, whereas other patients may be better served by traditional surgical approaches.

Surgical options for the treatment of choledocholithiasis include common duct exploration or bilienteric anastomosis. Cholecystectomy is usually performed during the same operation if the gallbladder is present. The need to perform surgery solely for cholecystectomy following successful endoscopic clearance of the duct remains an individual decision. Among patients at high risk for surgery, development of further biliary symptoms occurs in only 10% if the gallbladder is left in place; these patients are probably best managed expectantly.[28] For otherwise healthy patients, the risks associated with cholecystectomy appear to be less than the risk of further complications from gallstone disease, and cholecystectomy is usually offered.

Obstruction due to benign or malignant strictures can be treated by a variety of endoscopic, surgical, and percutaneous techniques, which may be used alone or in combination. Management of biliary strictures is described elsewhere in Chapter 124.

SUMMARY

Bacterial cholangitis results when infection of the biliary tree occurs in the setting of obstruction. Fever, pain, and jaundice are typically present but are not universal. Ultrasonography usually confirms the presence of biliary obstruction but cannot be relied on to exclude the diagnosis of cholangitis. Medical therapy with intravenous fluids and broad spectrum antibiotics aborts most acute attacks, but patients who develop shock, altered mental status, or fail to respond to initial conservative therapy require urgent biliary decompression. Endoscopic methods are preferred, but percutaneous or surgical approaches are viable alternatives when endoscopic drainage is unsuccessful or not available. Definitive correction of the problem causing obstruction is best performed after the patient's condition has been stabilized.

REFERENCES

1. Gigot JF, Leese T, Dereme T, Coutinho J, Castaing D, Bismuth H. Acute cholangitis: multivariate analysis of risk factors. *Ann Surg.* 1989;209:435–438.
2. Boey JH, Way LW. Acute cholangitis. *Ann Surg.* 1980;191:264–270.
3. O'Connor MJ, Schwartz ML, McQuarrie DG, Sumner HW. Acute bacterial cholangitis: an analysis of clinical manifestation. *Arch Surg.* 1982;117:437–441.
4. Reynolds BM, Dargan EL. Acute obstructive cholangitis: a distinct clinical syndrome. *Ann Surg.* 1959;150:299–303.
5. Sung JY, Leung JWC, Olson ME, Lundberg MS, Costerton JW. Demonstration of transient bacterobilia by foreign body implantation in feline biliary tract. *Dig Dis Sci.* 1991;36:943–948.
6. Lygidakis NJ, Brummelkamp WH. The significance of intrabiliary pressure in acute cholangitis. *Surg Gynecol Obstet.* 1985;161:465–469.
7. Sung JY, Shaffer EA, Olson ME, Leung JWC, Lam K, Costerton JW. Bacterial invasion into the biliary tract by the portal venous blood. *Hepatology.* 1991;14:313–317.
8. O'Connor MJ, Schwartz ML, McQuarrie DG, Sumner HW. Cholangitis due to malignant obstruction of biliary outflow. *Ann Surg.* 1981;193:341–345.
9. Gilbert DA, DiMarino AJ, Jensen DM, et al. Status evaluation: biliary stents. *Gastrointest Endosc.* 1992;38:750–752.
10. Cronan JJ, Mueller PR, Simeone JF, et al. Prospective diagnosis of choledocholithiasis. *Radiology.* 1983;146:467–469.
11. Laing FC, Jeffrey RB. Choledocholithiasis and cystic duct obstruction: difficult ultrasonic diagnosis. *Radiology.* 1983;146:475–479.
12. Balthazar EJ, Birnbaum BA, Naidich M. Acute cholangitis: CT evaluation. *J Comput Assist Tomogr.* 1993;17:283–289.
13. Leung JWC, Chung SCS, Sung JY, Banez VP, Li AKC. Urgent endoscopic drainage for acute suppurative cholangitis. *Lancet.* 1989;1:1307–1309.
14. Andrew DJ, Johnson SE. Acute suppurative cholangitis, a medical and surgical emergency. *Am J Gastroenterol.* 1970;54:141–154.
15. Lai ECS, Tam PC, Paterson IA, et al. Emergency surgery for severe acute cholangitis: the high risk patients. *Ann Surg.* 1990;211:55–59.
16. Leung JWC, Chan RCY, Chung SW, Sung JY, Chung SCS, French GL. The effect of obstruction on the biliary excretion of cefoperazone and ceftazidime. *J Antimicrob Chemother.* 1990;25:399–406.
17. Welch JP, Donaldson GA. The urgency of diagnosis and surgical treatment of acute suppurative cholangitis. *Am J Surg.* 1978;131:527–532.
18. Leese T, Neoptolemos JP, Baker AR, Carr-Locke DL. Management of acute cholangitis and the impact of endoscopic sphincterotomy. *Br J Surg.* 1986;73:988–992.
19. Pessa ME, Hawkins IF, Vogel SB. The treatment of acute cholangitis: percutaneous transhepatic biliary drainage before definitive therapy. *Ann Surg.* 1987;205:389–392.
20. Speer AG, Cotton PB, Russell RCG, et al. Randomized trial of endoscopic versus percutaneous stent insertion in malignant obstructive jaundice. *Lancet.* 1987;2:57–62.
21. Leung JWC, Cotton PB. Endoscopic nasobiliary catheter drainage in biliary and pancreatic disease. *Am J Gastroenterol.* 1991;86:389–394.
22. Gogel HK, Runyon BA, Volpicelli NA, Palmer RC. Acute suppurative obstructive cholangitis due to stones: treatment by urgent endoscopic sphincterotomy. *Gastrointest Endosc.* 1987;33:210–213.
23. Lai ECS, Mok FPT, Tan ESY, et al. Endoscopic biliary drainage for severe acute cholangitis. *N Engl J Med.* 1992;326:1582–1586.
24. Tai DI, Shen FH, Liaw YF. Abnormal pre-drainage serum creatinine as a prognostic indicator in acute cholangitis. *Hepatogastroenterology.* 1992;39:47–50.
25. Leung JWC, Chung SCS, Mok SD, Li AKC. Endoscopic removal of large common bile duct stones in recurrent pyogenic cholangitis. *Gastrointest Endosc.* 1988;34:238–241.
26. Cotton PB, Forbes A, Leung JWC, Dineen L. Endoscopic stenting for long-term treatment of large bile duct stones: 2- to 5-year follow-up. *Gastrointest Endosc.* 1987;33:411–412.
27. Johnson GK, Geenen JE, Venu RP, Schmalz MJ, Hogan WJ. Treatment of nonextractable common bile duct stones with combination ursodeoxycholic acid plus endoprostheses. *Gastrointest Endosc.* 1993;39:528–531.
28. Hill J, Martin DF, Tweedle DEF. Risks of leaving the gallbladder *in situ* after endoscopic sphincterotomy for bile duct stones. *Br J Surg.* 1991;78:554–557.

122

Choledocholithiasis

SIMON K. LO and JOE M. CHEN

Choledocholithiasis is the presence of gallstone(s) in the bile duct. The majority of bile duct stones are secondary in nature, originating from the gallbladder, indicating a failure of passage through the ampulla of Vater into the duodenum. In some Asian countries, de novo formation of gallstones within the bile duct is a principal cause of choledocholithiasis.

PATHOGENESIS

Treatment strategies for choledocholithiasis vary according to the types and origins of the stones. Therefore, it is important to briefly discuss the various types of gallstones: cholesterol, black pigment, and brown pigment. They are usually discussed in pure forms, but virtually all gallstones contain mixed stone substances.

Cholesterol gallstones are golden yellow stones formed within the gallbladder. In the United States, 80% of gallstones are cholesterol stones containing more than 75% cholesterol monohydrate. Structurally, these stones consist of layers of soft cholesterol crystals held tightly together by mucin glycoproteins. A prerequisite for cholesterol stone formation is the supersaturation of cholesterol, i.e., a cholesterol concentration that exceeds the ability of bile acids and phospholipids to hold it in solution. Either an excess output of biliary cholesterol or reduced synthesis of bile acids would lead to a "lithogenic bile." Cholesterol supersaturation is associated with obesity, female gender, weight loss, hyperlipidemia, American Indians, ileal disease or resection, prolonged fasting, and estrogen therapy. The relative excess of biliary cholesterol, however, does not guarantee gallstone formation. The content of biliary proteins, gallbladder emptying, and gallbladder calcium are factors that further determine the formation of stones.

Black pigment stones are composed of bilirubin polymers, mucin glycoproteins, and inorganic calcium salts (carbonate and phosphate). The calcium salts are responsible for the radiopacity. Similar to cholesterol stones, black pigment stones are also formed inside the gallbladder. The major risk factors are cirrhosis and chronic hemolysis. The mechanism for stone formation in patients with chronic hemolysis is the increased unconjugated bilirubin in the bile. Calcium, a normal constituent in bile, precipitates with unconjugated bilirubin generated from conjugated bilirubin following secretion. The mechanism for stone formation in cirrhotic patients is unknown.

Brown pigment stones are made up of calcium salts of bilirubin. They are rare in this country but are quite prevalent in some Asian countries where gastrointestinal tract parasites and recurrent pyogenic cholangitis (formerly called oriental cholangiohepatitis are common. In contrast to cholesterol and black pigment stones, they originate within the bile duct and are associated with biliary infection or stasis. Bacterial b-glucuronidase is responsible for the breakdown of conjugated bilirubin to form precipitates of calcium bilirubinate.

NATURAL HISTORY

GALLBLADDER STONES

The majority of gallbladder stones are asymptomatic and may remain unchanged for years. Of the estimated 20 million Americans with cholelithiasis, only 20% develop symptoms that require medical attention. Some stones may spontaneously dissolve within the gallbladder, but many are expelled into the duodenum via the cystic duct, common bile duct, and through the sphincter of Oddi. Symptoms may occur during the passage, particularly if the process is interrupted. Acute cholecystitis occurs when the stone is trapped within the cystic duct. Its intense pain is the result of gallbladder engorgement. Blockage beyond a few hours may lead to increased prostaglandin production, excess fluid secretion, gallbladder wall distension, gallbladder ischemia, and ultimately perforation and sepsis.

CHOLEDOCHOLITHIASIS

Choledocholithiasis is seen in 15% of cholecystectomies. Many of the calculi are found incidentally by intraoperative cholangiogram. Biliary stones, regardless of their origins, behave similarly. Many of the small common bile duct (CBD) stones are transients in the biliary tract and pass into the duodenum within a short time. Although it is not possible to study exactly how often that occurs, a substantial percentage of biliary stones are essentially asymptomatic. Anecdotally, chronic choledocholithiasis becomes symptomatic within several years of follow-up in up to 50% of cases and presents as biliary colic, acute pancreatitis, obstructive jaundice, and bacterial cholangitis. A persistent condition may also lead to biliary cirrhosis, oriental cholangiohepatitis, biliary strictures, and recurrent acute or chronic pancreatitis.

Stone passage through the ampulla of Vater may produce symptoms of biliary colic. Occasionally, acute pancreatitis occurs because of mechanical obstruction of the pancreatic sphincter or reflux of bile or gallstone into the pancreatic duct via a common pancreaticobiliary channel. Biliary pancreatitis is usually a self-limited event because the gallstone passes either through the sphincter of Oddi or retrograde into the common bile duct. On rare occasions, concomitant cholangitis, persistent biliary obstruction, and severe pancreatitis occur as a result of gallstone impaction in the ampulla.

Patients who had undergone biliary tract procedure or operation may develop a bile leak or cholangitis if a distal bile duct stone is left unattended.

PREDISPOSING CONDITIONS

Predisposing factors for choledocholithiasis are biliary stricture, sphincter stenosis, gallbladder stones, choledochoduodenostomy, congenital cystic diseases of the bile duct, biliary parasites, primary sclerosing cholangitis, recurrent cholangitis, and foreign body within the bile duct (see Table 122–1). These factors either impede the natural passage or promote de novo ductal formation of gallstones in the duct.

TABLE 122–1. CONDITIONS THAT PREDISPOSE TO CHOLEDOCHOLITHIASIS

Via cystic duct	Gallbladder stone
De novo formation	Chronic biliary obstruction
	Choledochoduodenostomy
	Congenital cystic diseases of the biliary tract
	Biliary parasites
	Recurrent cholangitis
	Primary sclerosing cholangitis
	Foreign body in the bile duct
Passage impedance	Biliary stricture
	Sphincter stenosis

SYMPTOMS

The majority of individuals with choledocholithiasis are asymptomatic; only 50% eventually develop symptoms that require medical attention. The most common symptom of gallstone disease, biliary colic, is pain associated with stone passage through the cystic or CBD. The description of biliary pain as colic is a misnomer because the painful symptom intensifies rapidly and persists for hours. Unlike colonic colic, minute-to-minute fluctuations of intensity are uncommon. Typically, the pain is located in the right upper quadrant of the abdomen, and may radiate across the entire upper abdomen or to the right back and shoulder blade. In spite of the complaints of severe pain, physical findings are usually minimal. In the patients with chronic choledocholithiasis, however, severe biliary colic is less common. Instead, patients frequently complain of a vague, deep-lying pressure or soreness in the right upper quadrant. Other common symptoms are nausea, vomiting, and intolerance to fatty meals.

Other symptoms from choledocholithiasis are dependent on the nature of the complications. Fever accompanying biliary-type pain suggests cholangitis, cholecystitis, or acute biliary pancreatitis. Charcot's triad of fever, right upper quadrant abdominal pain, and jaundice should alert the physician to the possibility of cholangitis. Although 70% of cases of cholangitis present in this classic form, the condition may be confused with cases of hepatitis or cholecystitis. It is worthwhile to keep in mind that cholangitis is most commonly associated with obstruction due to choledocholithiasis but uncommonly with malignancy unless the bile duct has been endoscopically manipulated. Jaundice and pruritus represent chronic biliary ductal or sphincter obstruction. Most acute or chronic cholecystitis cases do not manifest as jaundice. Likewise, hepaticolithiasis of a unilateral intrahepatic biliary system can maintain adequate clearance of bilirubin through the unobstructed system without causing jaundice. Borrowing experience from chronic pancreatitis-induced biliary strictures, hyperbilirubinemia occurs only in high-grade obstruction with a reduction of bilirubin clearance. Hematemesis may be due to variceal bleeding from biliary cirrhosis or hemobilia associated with CBD stones. Early postcholecystectomy bile leak is a clue to gallstone impaction of the CBD. Lastly, all of the above symptoms may be intermittent because of the ability of the gallstone to shift in position.

PHYSICAL FINDINGS

Since intense right upper quadrant abdominal or epigastric pain is a major symptom of choledocholithiasis, physicians often assume that they would be able to elicit significant local tenderness. In reality, the opposite is usually the case. A major discrepancy between symptoms and physical examination is an important clue to disease of the bile duct rather than the gallbladder or pancreas. The reason for the unimpressive physical finding in bile duct obstruction is probably because of its deep-seated location. Epigastric guarding or rebound in an icteric patient should raise the suspicion of gallstone pancreatitis or a major intraabdominal sepsis. On the other hand, a positive Murphy's sign in a jaundiced patient with an intact gallbladder should be considered for Mirizzi's syndrome (concomitant obstruction of the biliary and cystic duct from a cystic duct stone) or simultaneous choledocholithiasis and cholecystitis. Special attention should be given to patients with cholangitis and confusion and hypotension (Reynolds' pentad) because it is a life-threatening emergency. Although uncommon in this country, concomitant bacterial cholangitis and pancreatitis may occur as a result of CBD stones. In that case, the patient will have confusing symptoms and signs.

LABORATORY DIAGNOSIS

Whenever a biliary condition is suspected, the five principal serum liver enzymes should be obtained. Serum aspartate aminotransferase (AST) and alanine aminotransferase (ALT) are enzymes that rise quickly as a result of sudden increase of biliary ductal pressure. Even though they are of secondary importance in diagnosing an obstruction, their elevated levels are frequently the only detectable abnormalities within a few hours of the acute process. Since a rapid rise and fall of AST and ALT levels is the rule in an acute obstruction, their return to normalcy may not denote a resolution of the problem. Alkaline phosphatase is the most specific indicator of partial or complete biliary obstruction. It is an induced enzyme and, thus, may be elevated only after a few days of an obstructive process. Whenever a predominant elevation of hepatic alkaline phosphatase is noted, a differential of drug toxicity, hepatic infiltrative disease, or subacute or chronic biliary obstruction should be considered. Hyperbilirubinemia is very helpful in following the degree of or therapeutic progress in biliary obstruction. It is, however, much less useful in diagnosing biliary obstruction. An abnormal c-glutamyl transpeptidase (GGTP) level is useful to confirm a hepatobiliary process, particularly when there is isolated alkaline phosphatase abnormality.

It is well recognized that liver enzymes may be at normal levels in choledocholithiasis and even in cholangitis. This is particularly true in long-standing asymptomatic conditions and hepaticolithiasis. An incidental mild elevation of alkaline phosphatase is frequently the only clue to chronic choledocholithiasis.

COMPLICATIONS

BILIARY OBSTRUCTION

Liver enzymes may be normal or transiently elevated in simple cases of biliary colic. Always considered in the differential diagnosis of biliary tract disease, cholecystitis does not generally lead to liver enzyme abnormalities unless complicated by sepsis or simultaneous biliary and cystic duct obstructions (Mirizzi's syndrome). In uncomplicated gallstone obstruction of the biliary tract, liver enzyme abnormalities vary according to the degree and duration of biliary obstruction. Elevated AST and ALT levels are the first laboratory abnormalities in acute biliary obstruction. They may transiently increase by fivefold to twentyfold when the obstruction is complete. If obstruction persists, then alkaline phosphatase rises from a mild elevation to possibly 10 times the normal value. There is no strict correlation between the degree or location of biliary obstruction and the extent of alkaline phosphatase elevation. Direct bilirubin may be elevated because of either secondary biliary cirrhosis or decreased bilirubin clearance from persistent ductal obstruction. In a complete CBD obstruction, bilirubin rises approximately 1 mg/dl each day. On the other hand, in a complete obstruction of an intrahepatic duct, alkaline phosphatase levels are very high but bilirubin levels are normal. In prolonged significant biliary obstruction, the prothrombin time may be abnormal because of malabsorption of fat-soluble vitamins or cirrhosis.

BACTERIAL CHOLANGITIS

Bacterial cholangitis occurs only in the setting of biliary obstruction. Liver enzyme abnormalities are a reflection of the nature of the underlying biliary obstruction. When accompanied by prolonged prothrombin time and thrombocytopenia, suppurative cholangitis may be complicated by disseminated intravascular coagulation. On rare occasions, cholangitis may occur in patients with normal liver enzyme profiles. These are difficult cases to diagnose and may be an unusual cause of fever of unknown origin.

GALLSTONE PANCREATITIS

In acute gallstone pancreatitis, aminotransferase may be transiently elevated manyfold as in uncomplicated acute biliary obstruction. The diagnosis is based on an elevated serum amylase level, usually in the range of fivefold to twentyfold, that precipitously returns to normal within 5 days. Clinical deterioration of patients with gallstone pancreatitis, accompanied by persistent amylase elevation, suggests continuing impaction of the ampulla of Vater or the formation of pancreatic pseudocyst or abscess.

DIAGNOSTIC STUDIES

ABDOMINAL RADIOGRAPHS

A plain radiograph of the right upper abdominal quadrant is of limited value in the evaluation of biliary symptoms (see Table 122–2). Most gallstones, except for black pigment stones, do not contain sufficient amounts of inorganic calcium compounds to become radiopaque. More than 50% of black pigment stones may be detectable radiographically. An abdominal radiograph is sometimes useful in documenting biliary operation. Postoperative pneumobilia indicates patent

TABLE 122–2. UTILITY OF BILIARY IMAGING TESTS

Initial evaluation	Ultrasound
	Computed tomography
Definitive tests	Endoscopic retrograde cholangiopancreatography
	Percutaneous transhepatic cholangiogram
	(Intraoperative cholangiogram)
Special procedures	Choledochoscopy
	Peroral (endoscopic)
	Transhepatic
	Intraoperative
	Endoscopic ultrasound
	Magnetic resonance cholangiogram
	Helical computed tomographic biliary imaging
Tests of limited value	Radionuclide scan
	Abdominal plain film
	Intravenous and oral cholecystograms

biliary anastomosis. The concomitant findings of pneumobilia and distal small bowel obstruction suggest "gallstone ileus" due to passage of a large stone, usually greater than 2 cm, via a spontaneous cholecystoduodenal fistula. Scattered small calcified densities in the epigastrium may denote chronic pancreatitis. The finding of sentinel loops or the colon cutoff sign is consistent with acute pancreatitis.

RADIONUCLIDE BILIARY IMAGING

The biliary radionuclide study, commonly referred to as HIDA or PIPIDA scan, is 90% to 95% sensitive and specific for acute cholecystitis when the patient is experiencing pain. Its usefulness in choledocholithiasis is limited to the rare occasion where there is difficulty in confirming complete biliary obstruction by other means. The lack of intestinal filling in late scanning at 24 hours after intravenous injection of the radionuclide may aid in diagnosing complete biliary obstruction. PIPIDA scan is also helpful in documenting bile leak that may be associated with choledocholithiasis.

ABDOMINAL ULTRASONOGRAPHY

Ultrasound is the single most important noninvasive test in evaluating biliary-type complaints. The identification of gallbladder stones on an ultrasound performed to evaluate symptoms consistent with biliary colic implies uncomplicated gallstone passage. Cholecystitis and related complications may be readily diagnosed by ultrasound. A normal size CBD, usually less than 8 mm on ultrasound, does not exclude acute or intermittent biliary obstruction. A dilated bile duct, on the other hand, suggests subacute or chronic biliary obstruction. The level of biliary obstruction may be accurately diagnosed by identifying the lowest point of biliary dilation. A postcholecystectomy CBD of up to 12 mm is a normal physiologic response to removal of the biliary reservoir. Although it is highly accurate in detecting gallbladder stones, ultrasound is only 25% to 75% sensitive in detecting CBD stones. Therefore, a "negative" biliary ultrasound does not exclude choledocholithiasis.

COMPUTED TOMOGRAPHY

Computed tomography (CT) provides a standardized cross-sectional imaging of the biliary tract, liver, pancreas, and upper retroperitoneum. Like ultrasound, it is not sensitive in detecting choledocholithiasis except in oriental cholangiohepatitis, which has the classic appearance of multiple large stones within the markedly dilated left intrahepatic ductal system. It is helpful in diagnosing liver abscess, a frequent result of persistent biliary infection. It is also useful in excluding other processes that can mimic or predispose to biliary disease such as pancreatic carcinoma.

ENDOSCOPIC RETROGRADE CHOLANGIOPANCREATOGRAPHY

Endoscopic retrograde cholangiopancreatography (ERCP) is the most sensitive and specific study for diagnosing choledocholithiasis. In experienced hands, it is perhaps 95% sensitive in detecting a bile duct stone. In ERCP, the main differential diagnosis of a mobile filling defect in the CBD is an air bubble that has been introduced during the injection of contrast into the bile duct. Air bubbles are perfectly round filling defects that may float, change sizes, divide, and be seen in chains. Gallstones, on the other hand, are not perfectly round and usually have pointed corners and uneven borders. ERCP is also the only means to accurately define biliary and pancreatic anatomy simultaneously. During ERCP, therapy such as mechanical lithotripsy and gallstone removal can be safely performed by a skilled endoscopist. Unlike ultrasound or CT, ERCP is an invasive study and carries definite but acceptable risks. A diagnostic ERCP may encounter 1% to 2% of complications, mostly pancreatitis. Adding therapeutic maneuvers to an ERCP raises the risk of complications, usually self-limited, to 5% to 10%. Bleeding, pancreatitis, perforation, and anesthetic complications are reported complications in therapeutic ERCP procedures.

PERCUTANEOUS TRANSHEPATIC CHOLANGIOGRAM

Percutaneous transhepatic cholangiogram (PTC) is as accurate as ERCP in evaluating biliary anatomy but has some limitations. Like ERCP, many therapeutic maneuvers may be employed during a PTC to remove gallstones and dilate strictures. When compared to ERCP, it is less successful (40% to 70%) in visualizing nondilated bile duct, more likely to induce bile leak in an obstructed bile duct, and more difficult to remove gallstones that have migrated into the intrahepatic system. In addition, PTC does not visualize the entire pancreatic duct. It is also a relatively painful procedure because of repeated transhepatic punctures. As a result of these disadvantages, PTC is only employed when an ERCP is unsuccessful or in patients with difficult gastrointestinal tract anatomy.

MISCELLANEOUS

Intraoperative cholangiogram is an important study to diagnose biliary disease during a cholecystectomy. It provides adequate information about the biliary anatomy and may diagnose most cases of choledocholithiasis. Given the limitations of obtaining radiographs in an operating room, however, intraoperative cholangiography is less sensitive than ERCP and PTC in detecting bile duct stones. With the advent of ultrasound, ERCP, and nuclear scans, intravenous and oral cholecystograms (ICG and OCG) are rarely used because of their crude imaging and the risk of anaphylaxis in the case of ICG. The use of ICG or OCG in suspected choledocholithiasis is exceedingly uncommon. Upper endoscopy or upper gastrointestinal tract barium study is occasionally needed to evaluate biliary symptoms that are difficult to differentiate from those of gastroduodenal diseases. In recent years, endoscopic ultrasound has been described as a sensitive test for detecting CBD stones. However, the clinical value of this new technology for diagnosing choledocholithiasis has not been established.

TREATMENTS

Significant therapeutic advances for biliary disease have been made in surgery, endoscopy, pharmacology, and invasive radiology. It is not possible to provide a standard treatment protocol because of the lack of comparative studies among the different methods. The success in each of these modalities is operator dependent. Thus, it is crucial to be aware of the local expertise among all the disciplines before reaching a therapeutic decision.

Asymptomatic Choledocholithiasis

Given that roughly 50% of choledocholithiasis eventually gives rise to symptoms or complications, incidentally discovered CBD stones should be removed. The strategy in clearing the bile duct of these asymptomatic gallstones varies according to the manner that they are discovered. If found by an intraoperative cholangiogram during a cholecystectomy, some forms of CBD exploration or transcystic stone removal may be performed. This is true in both laparoscopic and conventional open cholecystectomy if the surgeon is trained to perform such procedures. Alternatively, the surgeon may request a postoperative ERCP for stone removal. Because of limitations in performing a thorough intraoperative cholangiogram, stones may be discovered only in postoperative T-tube cholangiogram. Depending on the location and size of the stone and on the local radiologic and endoscopic expertise, stone crushing and removal may be performed either via the T tube or by ERCP. If a stone is found incidentally on an ERCP, a transsphincteric stone removal would be appropriate. This is usually accomplished by introducing a radiologically guided basket or balloon through a 1-cm incision in the biliary sphincter (endoscopic sphincterotomy) for removal of the stones. CBD stones larger than 1.2 cm cannot be reliably removed without prior stone fragmentation by mechanical or other forms of lithotripsy. In cases of asymptomatic choledocholithiasis, documented by ultrasound or CT scans, the therapeutic decision is based on the need for a cholecystectomy. A single surgical procedure to remove the gallbladder and biliary stones or stepwise cholecystectomy and ERCP removal have been performed with equal success in our institution. The best-established indication of ERCP stone retrieval is in postcholecystectomy choledocholithiasis.

Choledocholithiasis With Biliary Colic or Obstruction

Choledocholithiasis with biliary colic or obstruction is diagnosed or suspected by ultrasound or CT scans. The management decision is the same as for asymptomatic choledocholithiasis. Antibiotic prophylaxis before a stone removing attempt is generally unnecessary, although delayed therapeutic action may allow cholangitis to develop.

Choledocholithiasis With Cholangitis

Choledocholithiasis with cholangitis is a condition that is seldom diagnosed until the classic triad of acute cholangitis becomes obvious. Management begins with broad spectrum antibiotic coverage, which results in early clinical improvement in 75% of the cases. After initial stabilization, patients with suspected cholangitis must be promptly investigated, since 90% of such cases are related to gallstone obstruction of the bile duct. In our opinion, all patients with cholangitis require ERCP during their hospitalization. In those 25% of patients who are either moribund or unresponsive to initial antibiotic therapy, emergent or urgent ERCP should be performed to identify the cause and provide a temporary but highly effective relief of sepsis. Since cholangitis always occurs in an obstructed bile duct, the provision of ductal drainage with endoscopic placement of an endoprosthesis or nasobiliary catheter should result in dramatic clinical improvement. It is preferable to use a nasobiliary drainage catheter because there is external access to the bile duct for continuous flushing and aspiration of the infected viscous content. However, it is difficult to maintain the drainage catheter for more than 3 days because of catheter kinking, luminal occlusion, and accidental dislodgement. Excessive ERCP manipulation of the bile duct must be avoided to minimize the risks of bacteremia and prolonged anesthesia. An effective endoscopic drainage procedure is usually followed by clinical improvement within 24 hours. Depending on the nature of the condition, definitive surgery or endoscopic treatment can be performed after the acute infection has subsided. In patients with mild cholangitis, a full-length ERCP including endoscopic sphincterotomy and stone clearance can be performed instead of a temporizing drainage procedure. With this management strategy, the mortality of patients with severe cholangitis has been reduced to 10%. Emergency surgical decompression of severe cholangitis, previously the treatment standard, should be reserved for patients that fail endoscopic therapy. External drainage by transhepatic puncture can also be considered if there is endoscopic failure, but caution must be taken to minimize potential peritoneal leakage of infected bile.

CHOLEDOCHOLITHIASIS WITH ACUTE PANCREATITIS

In cases of concomitant choledocholithiasis and acute pancreatitis, the severity of the pancreatitis dictates management strategy. Severe gallstone pancreatitis implies persistent stone impaction of the ampulla or pancreatic duct and deserves immediate removal, which is best accomplished by endoscopic stone extraction. Well-designed clinical trials have demonstrated that urgent endoscopic treatment of severe biliary pancreatitis reduces hospital morbidity, mortality, and duration of hospital stay. Performing ERCP in this setting, however, may worsen the pancreatitis as a result of pancreatic sphincter manipulation and pancreatic duct injections.

Patients with mild gallstone pancreatitis do not benefit from early intervention. They should be managed conservatively until symptoms and hyperamylasemia have resolved. An elective ERCP may then be performed to exclude retained stones in the bile duct. Since this condition may be complicated by pancreatic pseudocysts, it is occasionally necessary to perform an abdominal CT prior to the ERCP to prevent introduction of bacterial organisms into the pseudocysts. The role of surgery for acute gallstone pancreatitis is to remove the source of the gallstone after pancreatitis has subsided. Laparoscopic or open cholecystectomy should be performed at the end of the index hospitalization because of a 40% risk of recurrence within 6 months. In patients who do not receive an ERCP prior to cholecystectomy, intraoperative cholangiogram must be performed to exclude the possibility of retained CBD stones.

COMPLEX INTRAHEPATIC DUCT STONES

Common in Asia, complex intrahepatic duct stones have been seen in other countries where parasitic disease is common. The diagnosis is suspected on the basis of ultrasound or CT findings. ERCP should be performed to assess the extent of stone impaction and ductal anatomy. Any stricture found must be biopsied to exclude concomitant cancer, which is not uncommon in our experience. Endoscopic extraction may be attempted if the stones are mobile. These stones are rarely removable except by the most skilled endoscopists in a well-equipped endoscopy facility. If endoscopic extraction is unsuccessful, a nasobiliary or short stent should be placed proximal to the stones in the same ERCP session to prevent cholangitis. In our opinion, surgical management is the mainstay of therapy. In the patients with a contracted left liver lobe, a segmental or lobar resection is curative. In those with normal overlying liver tissue, ductal exploration may be considered, but complete stone clearance is uncommon in this type of surgery. The patients with recurrent disease should be given a subcutaneous jejunobiliary access because of the potential for further stone recurrence, stone retention, and anastomotic stricture. Likewise, patients with concomitant Caroli's disease, a condition with intrahepatic ductal dilations, and choledocholithiasis should be managed similarly. Those with choledochal cysts complicated by CBD stones should be managed by biliary resection to prevent future development of cholangiocarcinoma. Some physicians treat recurrent pyogenic cholangitis with percutaneous transhepatic choledochoscopy and stone removal with a high success rate.

SPECIAL THERAPEUTIC MODALITIES

With current advances in technology, many new methods have been developed to treat bile duct stones (see Table 122–3). Each is highly effective if applied with proper technique in the right setting. The major limitations are in the availability of the expensive devices and the individuals who are experienced in using them.

ENDOSCOPIC SPHINCTEROTOMY

Introduced 20 years ago, endoscopic sphincterotomy is one of the most common endoscopic therapies performed today. It involves cutting

TABLE 122–3. THERAPEUTIC MODALITIES FOR CHOLEDOCHOLITHIASIS

Commonly Available
Endoscopic (ERCP) sphincterotomy and stone extraction
T-tube cholangiogram and stone extraction
Common bile duct exploration and stone extraction
Endoscopic stenting with or without oral ursodeoxycholic acid therapy

Less Commonly Available
Endoscopic mechanical lithotripsy
Contact dissolution therapy with monoctanoin
Endoscopic sphincter dilation and stone extraction
Laparoscopic common bile duct exploration

Available Only at Some Referral Centers
Choledochoscopic electrohydraulic lithotripsy
Choledochoscopic laser lithotripsy
Extracorporeal shock wave lithotripsy
Endoscopic "smart laser" lithotripsy

ERCP = endoscopic retrograde cholangiopancreatography.

the biliary sphincter with a thin, heated wire inserted through the endoscope. When endoscopic sphincterotomy is performed properly by skilled biliary endoscopists, the complication rate is 8%, which is considered acceptable because prolonged hospitalization, fatality, or surgical outcome is rare. Bleeding and pancreatitis are the most commonly reported sphincterotomy-induced complications. Although sphincterotomy is considered the prerequisite to CBD stone removal, some investigators are now evaluating the success and complication rates of small stone removal by sphincter dilation without cutting.

MECHANICAL LITHOTRIPSY

The majority of CBD stones are smaller than 1.2 cm, and they can be safely removed through the biliary orifice after a sphincterotomy has been performed. Gallstones that are larger than 1.2 cm are difficult to pull through the biliary orifice even after it has been widened. Therefore, mechanical lithotripsy is developed to break the large stones into small fragments prior to removal. Mechanical lithotripsy involves grabbing a stone with a special wire "basket" and retracting the basket until the wires cut through the stone. With recent improvements, mechanical lithotripsy can be performed through the channel of a large ERCP scope. Complications are uncommon except for inadvertent basket entrapment of ductal or duodenal mucosa.

EXTRACORPOREAL SHOCK WAVE LITHOTRIPSY

Highly destructive shock waves can be generated by means of a high-voltage spark discharge that causes an explosive evaporation of the surrounding water. Since the shock waves can travel through water and tissue media, the extracorporeal shock wave lithotripsy (ESWL) devices can shatter gallstones by positioning a shock wave generator and a water cushion externally against the abdomen of a patient. The shock wave energy is then focused onto a gallstone with the guidance of an ultrasonic device. Originally intended for treatment of gallbladder stones, this device can also be used to fragment CBD stones. The use of this device has a 65% success rate, but it is limited by high cost and the low sensitivity of ultrasound in detecting bile duct stones. Even after a successful stone fragmentation, endoscopic sphincterotomy is needed to assist bile duct clearance. Mild complications such as abdominal pain, hematoma of the skin, and microhematuria occur in 29%. Severe complications including organ rupture, fever, and biliary colic occur in 8%.

ENDOSCOPIC SHOCK WAVE METHODS

Shock wave energy can be focused on a large stone by contact with a fiber probe under endoscopic guidance. There are two major types, electrohydraulic (EHL) and laser lithotriptors (LL). The EHL and LL are highly effective in fragmenting gallstones in vitro. However, their success lessen in vivo because of the biliary anatomy and the technical difficulty of using a choledochoscope. Choledochoscopy must be performed by two skilled endoscopists, with one maintaining the position of a large "mother" scope in the duodenum and another passing a small "daughter" scope through the "mother" scope into the biliary orifice. Although the applications of LL and EHL are similar, an LL is significantly more expensive than an EHL. Recently a "smart laser" that uses a feedback guidance system to control the firing of laser energy has been tested successfully for gallstone fragmentation. Theoretically, this device automatically shuts off the delivery of the laser when it senses ductal tissue. Instead of using the clumsy mother-daughter-type endoscopic setup, the smart laser is delivered by passing a laser fiber blindly through the biliary orifice. Complications from these contact lithotripsy methods may include hemobilia, perforation, cholangitis, and pancreatitis.

Infusion of a Dissolution Agent

If a nasobiliary catheter is in place a liquid solvent can be infused above the stones for dissolution. The chemical agent, usually a monoctanoin, is delivered continuously. A majority of cholesterol stones in the CBD can be cleared with this method in 7 days. The risk of cholangitis, patient discomfort, and extended duration of hospital care are some of the limitation of this technique.

Percutaneous Transhepatic Choledochoscopy and Stone Extraction

Some intrahepatic stones are difficult to reach by conventional surgical or endoscopic methods. In many instances, they are treated by surgical resection of the overlying liver segments. If that is not feasible, the only option is by transhepatic removal. This is accomplished by percutaneous puncturing of the involved bile duct, followed by sequential dilations of the fistula until a choledochoscope can be passed for stone fragmentation and removal. The main limitations of this method are the multiple treatment sessions and discomfort associated with the dilations.

Permanent Biliary Stenting

In spite of the recent surgical and endoscopic advances, some CBD stones are too difficult or risky to remove by surgery or common endoscopic methods. This is particularly true in the communities where EHL, ESWL, and percutaneous transhepatic lithotripsy methods are unavailable. A method that has gained popularity over the last few years is the endoscopic placement of a large-bore plastic stent above the stones to allow bile flow into the duodenum. As opposed to stenting for biliary strictures, stenting for refractory choledocholithiasis seems to be effective for a long duration without an obligatory stent exchange unless biliary obstruction or cholangitis becomes clinically evident. Some authors report additional benefit of extended stent effect by placing these patients on daily oral ursodeoxycholic acid.

SUMMARY

Choledocholithiasis is a condition with variable clinical presentations from no symptoms to cholangitis. Serum liver profiles and abdominal scanning may not be diagnostic of the condition. The most sensitive and specific test for choledocholithiasis is ERCP, which may allow stone removal at the same time. Treatment options include endoscopic sphincterotomy, surgical CBD exploration, and percutaneous transhepatic puncture for stone extraction. Recently, choledochoscopy and a variety of lithotripsy methods have been developed to facilitate the extraction of large bile duct stones. Local facility and expertise dictate the choice of therapy for choledocholithiasis.

123
Sclerosing Cholangitis
ELLEN C. EBERT

HISTORICAL PERSPECTIVE AND CATEGORIES OF DISEASE
(Table 123–1)

Sclerosing cholangitis (SC) is the obliterative fibrosis of intrahepatic and extrahepatic bile ducts, ultimately leading to biliary cirrhosis and definitively diagnosed by endoscopic retrograde cholangiopancreatography (ERCP). Before the introduction of ERCP in the early 1970s, the diagnosis was made, although rarely, by palpation at surgery of a fibrotic common bile duct, followed by histologic confirmation. Thereafter, the frequency of disease increased with the use of ERCP. Strict criteria for the diagnosis of primary SC (PSC) were formulated in 1964[1]:

1. No previous biliary tract surgery
2. No cholelithiasis
3. Diffuse involvement of the biliary ducts
4. Exclusion of malignancy

These criteria have been modified over the years so that patient populations included in studies have varied, resulting in different frequencies of disease. Of those with PSC, more than half have ulcerative colitis (UC), the numbers varying markedly according to the intensity of the search for colonic disease and to differences in the population studied. The incidence of PSC associated with Crohn's disease (CD) ranges from 5% to 13%, with all patients having colonic disease. The clinical features of PSC are independent of the activity of the colitis and may occur even after colectomy. In converse, patients who have received a liver transplantation for PSC are still at risk for colon cancer from UC.[2,3]

PSC, however, is relatively rare in patients with UC, occurring in 5.5% with substantial colitis and in 0.5% with distal colitis, in both cases more commonly in male than female patients.[4] It represents the most common cause of liver disease in UC if pericholangitis is considered to be part of the spectrum of PSC (see below).

Secondary SC is most commonly due to biliary obstruction, with overgrowth of enteric organisms in the upper small intestine ascending up the biliary tree. In addition, immunodeficiency diseases can lead to SC in the absence of biliary tract obstruction. The immature immune system of the neonate, for example, can predispose the biliary epithelium to infection by cytomegalovirus or reovirus, resulting in stricture formation.[5,6] In the adult, infections (usually cytomegalovirus or cryptosporidiosis) in the acquired immunodeficiency syndrome (AIDS) caused SC in 14 of 26 patients with biliary problems in one series.[7] Before AIDS, the association of immunodeficiency diseases, such as familial combined immunodeficiency or X-linked immunodeficiency syndromes, with PSC was based on occasional case reports.[8,9] The other major secondary cause of SC is ischemic necrosis of the bile ducts from damage to tributaries of the hepatic artery. For example, infusion of 5-fluorodeoxyuridine into the hepatic artery, used to treat hepatic metastases from colonic adenocarcinoma, can obstruct arterioles.[10] Injury to the hepatic artery can also occur during cholecystectomy, leading to SC. Bile duct obliteration after liver transplantation, however, may be due to one or a combination of factors: infection, damage of the hepatic artery, or graft-versus-host disease.[11]

ETIOLOGY

The cause of PSC is unknown but probably involves heredity, autoimmunity, and infectious agents. Evidence of a genetic predisposition includes an increased incidence of HLA-B8 and HLA-DR3 and a familial occurrence of PSC

TABLE 123-1. CATEGORIES OF SCLEROSING CHOLANGITIS
Primary
1. Ulcerative colitis present or absent
Secondary
1. Infections due to
a. Biliary tract obstruction
b. Immunodeficiencies, especially acquired immunodeficiency syndrome
2. Obstruction of hepatic artery due to
a. Hepatic arterial chemotherapy
b. Trauma
c. Hypercoagulation

with UC.[12,13] The association of immunodeficiency states (described above) or autoimmune events with PSC implicates the immune system in its pathogenesis. Patients with PSC have a variety of circulating autoantibodies, although the titers do not correlate with any clinical parameters of PSC.[14] Elevated circulating immune complexes have also been found with PSC, as well as with other liver diseases.[15] Whether this is an epiphenomenon or a pathogenic binding of antibody to hepatobiliary antigens is unknown. Similarly, the importance of cellular immune abnormalities (e.g., decreased CD8+ T lymphocytes and increased B lymphocytes) is unclear.[16] Expression of HLA-DR antigens on the intrahepatic biliary ducts is enhanced in PSC, as well as other hepatobiliary diseases.[17] This may enable the epithelial cells to present immunogens to T lymphocytes, triggering an inflammatory response. Alternatively, HLA-DR antigens may be induced by the disease itself.

A possible infectious cause of PSC is the entry of gut-related toxins through the leaky epithelium in patients with colitis.[18] These agents traverse the portal system to enter the liver and exit through the bile ducts, perhaps inducing an inflammatory response. If these toxic substances undergo enterohepatic recirculation, the bile ducts would be repeatedly exposed and injured. Animal models support this theory, since injection of rabbits with heat-killed *Escherichia coli* results in portal vein fibrosis, proliferation of small bile duct epithelium, and circumductal fibrosis.[19]

A likely scenario in PSC is that a group of genetically predisposed individuals, who develop damage of bile duct epithelium, will expose the immune system to epithelial cell antigens that are normally excluded from contact. The lymphocytes recognize these antigens as "foreign" and mount an autoimmune destructive process.

CLINICAL FEATURES

Two thirds of patients with PSC are male and are less than 45 years old. Although patients are often asymptomatic (despite abnormal laboratory values), progressive disease results in fatigue, nausea, pruritus, jaundice, abdominal pain, fever, and weight loss, with symptoms ranging from weeks to years before diagnosis.[20] Patients occasionally present with acute relapsing disease, with symptoms of cholangitis: fever, right upper quadrant pain, and jaundice. Although the physical examination is often normal, one may detect jaundice, hepatomegaly, or evidence of chronic liver disease. The main laboratory abnormalities are elevated alkaline phosphatase activity in most and increased total bilirubin in about half. The aminotransferases, albumin, and prothrombin times are usually normal. Although hypergammaglobulinemia often occurs (usually of the immunoglobulin M [IgM] type), the presence of antibodies to mitochondrial, nuclear, or smooth muscle antigens is rare. The lymph nodes in the porta hepatis are often enlarged, presumably a reaction to the inflammatory process. The pancreatic duct is occasionally involved in the fibrotic process, resulting in chronic pancreatitis. Gallstones are not usually found, although choledocholithiasis can occur as a result of the biliary stasis. The presenting picture, then, is consistent with a cholestatic rather than hepatocellular process. The course of disease is quite variable with some patients remaining asymptomatic for many years while others die within months from liver failure, recurrent acute cholangitis, or cholangiocarcinoma (CCa).

DIAGNOSIS AND DIFFERENTIAL DIAGNOSIS

A patient who demonstrates the signs of cholestasis should undergo an ERCP to identify any extrahepatic obstruction. This examination definitively diagnoses or excludes SC, by demonstrating short strictures of intrahepatic and extrahepatic ducts with normal or slightly dilated ducts between. The cystic duct is usually spared. Percutaneous transhepatic cholangiogram is technically difficult because of the small size of intrahepatic ducts but may be necessary to provide a complete picture. If imaging studies (ultrasound and computed tomography) reveal masses, tumor should be suspected. Liver biopsy is not diagnostic but shows a wide range of findings, classified as follows[21]:

Stage 1: The initial findings of portal inflammatory bile ductule proliferation and periductal fibrosis ("onion skin" lesions) are limited to the portal triad.
Stage 2: Inflammation then extends beyond the limiting plate ("piecemeal necrosis"), enlarging the portal triads. "Ductopenia" results from the fibrotic process around the bile ductules that eventually obliterates them.
Stage 3: Fibrous septa form bridges from one portal tract to another ("portal fibrosis").
Stage 4: Finally, nodular regeneration develops ("biliary cirrhosis"), often with accumulation of hepatic copper. Such biopsies may be interpreted as primary biliary cirrhosis, chronic active hepatitis, or Wilson's disease, whereas the underlying etiology is, in fact, PSC. Pericholangitis, frequently found in association with inflammatory bowel disease (IBD), is a disease restricted to the small bile ducts in the portal zone and is now considered by some experts to be an extension of PSC.

A major diagnostic difficulty is the exclusion of CCa. Although CCa is a rare disease, it occurs in almost 10% of patients with PSC.[22,23] The reason for this increased incidence of CCa in PSC is unknown but may be due, at least in part, to the chronic inflammation and bile stasis associated with PSC. These tumors are adenocarcinomas that occur most frequently in the extrahepatic ducts and have a poor prognosis (mean survival of 11.8 months). Radiologic features that suggest this diagnosis include excessive dilation of the ducts, polypoid mass, and progression of ductular dilation or stricturing. The diagnosis of CCa is made by pathologic examination of biliary fluid and tissue obtained through ERCP or at surgery, although the presence of active inflammation may cause difficulties in interpretation of cytologic findings. The clinical features of CCa and PSC are often identical, so that the tumor is unrecognized.

Another diagnostic difficulty may be the differentiation of PSC with primary biliary cirrhosis (PBC). However, both diseases have several distinctive features (Table 123–2). Patients with PBC, unlike those with PSC, are usually female and have pruritus as their dominant symptom. In addition, the antimitochondrial antibody is positive, and the extrahepatic ducts are normal. PBC is associated with autoimmune disorders such as thyroiditis and sicca syndrome. However, UC is not frequently seen, and there is no increased incidence of CCa.

TREATMENT

Medical management consists of treating the symptoms and complications of the disease and reducing, if possible, progression of disease. The pruritus, which occurs later in PSC than in PBC, can be treated with nonabsorbed resins as long as acholic stools (indicating inadequate bile flow) are not present. Although the substance causing pruritus has not been identified,[24] it appears to bind to these resins. Cholestyramine, starting at 12 g daily in three divided doses before meals, should relieve pruritus in 2 to 4 days. Gradually doubling the dose may provide added benefit, although the side effect of constipation may become troubling. Colestipol hydrochloride may be used for those who cannot tolerate cholestyramine. Sedatives can be administered at bedtime when the itching becomes most bothersome. Other treatments that have been used are long-term antibiotics for those who develop recurrent episodes of ascending cholangitis, phe-

TABLE 123–2. DISTINGUISHING PRIMARY SCLEROSING CHOLANGITIS (PSC) FROM PRIMARY BILIARY CIRRHOSIS (PBC)

	PSC	PBC
Sex	Male predominance	Female predominance
Symptoms	Fatigue, pain, jaundice, pruritus	Pruritus dominant, then jaundice
Antimitochondrial antibody	Negative	Positive
ERCP	Multiple strictures of intrahepatic or extrahepatic ducts	Normal extrahepatic ducts
Associated diseases	Ulcerative colitis, cholangiocarcinoma	Autoimmune diseases

ERCP = endoscopic retrograde cholangiopancreatography.

nobarbital as a sedative that may increase bile flow,[25] and ultraviolet B light or large-volume plasmapheresis for intractable pruritus.[26]

PSC leads to poor micelle formation from inadequate luminal bile salt concentrations. As a result, patients may develop deficiencies of the fat-soluble vitamins, A, D, E, and K, although patients are usually asymptomatic. If symptomatic bone disease develops, it is usually osteoporosis rather than osteomalacia.[27]

Antiinflammatory and immunosuppressive drugs have been used to halt the progression of disease, which is presumed to be immune mediated. Problems with these studies include (1) the variable inclusion criteria, (2) the fluctuations in the course of disease, and (3) the irreversibility of bile duct destruction, since unlike hepatocytes, bile ducts do not regenerate. The medications, then, must be given early in the course of disease and the patients followed for many years to determine efficacy. Although none has been definitively shown to arrest the disease process, promising preliminary results have been reported with methotrexate and ursodeoxycholic acid.[28,29] Corticosteroids and D-penicillamine[30] have been shown in several studies to be ineffective and to have toxic side effects, such as the osteoporosis induced by steroids.

All patients with PSC should initially have an ileocolonoscopy with multiple biopsies to search for UC. If the patient has combined PSC and UC with 10 or more years of colitis, colonoscopic screening for dysplasia and early colon cancer should be done. Such a patient has at least the same risk for developing colon cancer as a patient with UC alone. Proctocolectomy does not affect the course of PSC.[2,3]

If a patient has one or a few dominant strictures of the common bile duct, endoscopic dilation should be tried. The endoscopist may first perform a sphincterotomy, especially in a duct containing debris or stones, followed by dilation. For tight strictures, a stent may be placed. This approach decreases the jaundice and episodes of cholangitis, with few side effects. In addition, tissue can be retrieved by sleeved cytology brushes and intraductal "scrapers." An added advantage is that the anatomy is not altered should liver transplantation be necessary in the future.

The last alternative for a patient with PSC is surgery, either to relieve biliary obstruction or to replace a diseased liver by orthotopic liver transplantation. For patients with prolonged cholestasis, unrelieved by endoscopic techniques, a liver biopsy should be performed, since patients with advanced cirrhosis are candidates for liver transplantation. If the patient has biliary strictures without advanced cirrhosis, the narrowed bile ducts can be resected, followed by a choledochojejunostomy or hepaticojejunostomy.[31] Advantages to this approach include a more permanent solution to strictures than the endoscopic approach and the discovery of undiagnosed CCa. Portosystemic shunting, of course, has no effect on the disease process. Liver transplantation is reserved for those with progressive liver failure. In a large series from Pittsburgh, PSC was the third most common indication for liver transplantation among adults.[32] Whether PSC develops in the new organ will be difficult to answer, especially since liver transplantation, itself, can cause secondary SC.

REFERENCES

1. Holubitsky IB, McKenzie AD. Primary sclerosing cholangitis of the extrahepatic bile ducts. *Can J Surg.* 1964;7:277–283.
2. Wiesner RH, Grambsch PM, Dickson ER, et al. Primary sclerosing cholangitis: natural history, prognostic factors and survival analysis. *Hepatology.* 1989;10:430–436.
3. Rabinovitz M, Gavaler JS, Schade RR, et al. Does primary sclerosing cholangitis occurring in association with inflammatory bowel disease differ from that occurring in the absence of inflammatory bowel disease? A study of sixty-six subjects. *Hepatology.* 1990;11:7–11.
4. Olsson R, Danielsson A, Jarnerot G, et al. Prevalence of primary sclerosing cholangitis in patients with ulcerative colitis. *Gastroenterology.* 1991;100:1319–1323.
5. Finegold MJ, Carpenter RJ. Obliterative cholangitis due to cytomegalovirus: a possible precursor of paucity of intrahepatic bile ducts. *Hum Pathol.* 1982;13:662–665.
6. Morecki R, Glaser JH, Cho S, et al. Biliary atresia and reovirus type 3 infection. *N Engl J Med.* 1982;307:481–484.
7. Cello JP. Acquired immunodeficiency syndrome cholangiopathy: spectrum of disease. *Am J Med.* 1989;86:539–546.
8. Record CO, Eddleston ALWF, Shilkin KB, et al. Intrahepatic sclerosing cholangitis associated with familial immunodeficiency syndrome. *Lancet.* 1973;2:18–20.
9. Naveh Y, Mendelsohn H, Spira G, et al. Primary sclerosing cholangitis associated with immunodeficiency. *Am J Dis Child.* 1983;137:114–117.
10. Shea WJ, Demas BE, Goldberg HI, et al. Sclerosing cholangitis associated with hepatic arterial FUDR chemotherapy: radiographic-histologic correlation. *AJR.* 1986;146:717–776.
11. Vierling JM, Fennell RH Jr. Histopathology of early and late human hepatic allograft rejection: evidence of progressive destruction on interlobular bile ducts. *Hepatology.* 1985;5:1076–1082.
12. Chapman RW, Varghese Z, Gaul R, et al. Association of primary sclerosing cholangitis with HLA-B8. *Gut.* 1983;24:38–41.
13. Schrumpf E, Fausa O, Forre O, et al. HLA antigens and immunoregularity T cells in ulcerative colitis associated with hepatobiliary disease. *Scand J Gastroenterol.* 1982;17:187–191.

14. Zauli D, Schrumpf E, Crespi C, et al. An autoantibody profile in primary sclerosing cholangitis. *J Hepatol.* 1987;5:14–17.
15. Bodenheimer HC, LaRusso NF, Thayer WP Jr, et al. Elevated circulating immune complexes in primary sclerosing cholangitis. *Hepatology.* 1983;3:150–154.
16. Lindor KD, Wiesner RH, Katzman JA, et al. Lymphocyte subsets in primary sclerosing cholangitis. *Dig Dis Sci.* 1987;32:720–725.
17. Chapman RW, Kelly P, Heryet A, et al. Expression of HLA-DR antigens on bile duct epithelium in primary sclerosing cholangitis. *Gut.* 1988;29:422–427.
18. Bjarnason I, O'Morain C, Levi AJ, et al. Absorption of 51 chromium-labelled ethylcosediaminetetraacetate in inflammatory bowel disease. *Gastroenterology.* 1983;85:318–322.
19. Kono K, Ohnishi K, Omata M, et al. Experimental portal fibrosis produced by intraportal injection of killed nonpathogenic *Escherichia coli* in rabbits. *Gastroenterology.* 1988;94:787–796.
20. Chapman RWG, Arborgh BAM, Rhodes JM, et al. Primary sclerosing cholangitis: a review of its clinical features, cholangiography and hepatic histology. *Gut.* 1980;21:870–877.
21. Ludwig J, Barham SS, LaRusso NF, et al. Morphologic features of chronic hepatitis associated with primary sclerosing cholangitis and chronic ulcerative colitis. *Hepatology.* 1981;1:632–640.
22. Aadland E, Schrumpf E, Fausa O, et al. Primary sclerosing cholangitis: a long-term follow-up study. *Scand J Gastroenterol.* 1987;22:655–664.
23. Stieber AC, Marino IR, Iwatsuki S, Starzl TE. Cholangiocarcinoma in sclerosing cholangitis: the role of liver transplantation. *Int Surg.* 1989;74:1–3.
24. Jones EA, Bergasa NV. Hypothesis: the pruritus of cholestasis: from bile acids to opiate agonists. *Hepatology.* 1990;11:884–887.
25. Redinger RN, Small DM. Primate biliary physiology, VIII. The effect of phenobarbital upon bile salt synthesis and pool size, biliary lipid secretion, and bile composition. *J Clin Invest.* 1973;52:161–172.
26. Kaplan MM. Primary biliary cirrhosis. *Curr Ther Gastroenterol Liver Dis.* 1990;3–15.
27. Matloff DS, Kaplan MM, Neer RM, et al. Osteoporosis in primary biliary cirrhosis: effects of 25-hydroxyvitamin D_3 treatment. *Gastroenterology.* 1982;83:97–101.
28. Knox TA, Fawaz KA, Arora S, Kaplan MM. Primary sclerosing cholangitis (PSC): improvement with methotrexate (MTX) treatment. *Hepatology.* 1989;10:688. Abstract.
29. O'Brien CB, Senior JR, Batta AK, et al. Ursodeoxycholic acid treatment produces marked clinical and biochemical amelioration of primary sclerosing cholangitis. *Gastroenterology.* 1989;96:A640.
30. LaRusso N, Wiesner R, Ludwig J, et al. Randomized trial of penicillamine in primary sclerosing cholangitis. *Gastroenterology.* 1988;95:1036–1042.
31. Cameron JL, Pitt HA, Zinner MJ, et al. Resection of hepatic duct bifurcation and transhepatic stenting for sclerosing cholangitis. *Ann Surg.* 1988;207:614–622.
32. Marsh JW, Iwatsuki S, Makoka L, et al. Orthotopic liver transplantation for primary sclerosing cholangitis. *Ann Surg.* 1988;207:21–25.

124

Bile Duct Strictures

FRANKLIN E. KASMIN and JEROME H. SIEGEL

Stricturing of the biliary system is not an uncommon problem confronting the gastroenterologist. Several diverse disease processes account for stricture formation, but the clinical presentation is similar. Patients usually notice jaundice as a manifestation of a biliary stricture, but cholestasis—with or without pruritus, fever, chills, or pain—is also a frequent presenting symptom. The initial diagnostic approach to evaluating this condition is to identify the location of the stricture and establish its etiology and then pursue a course of therapy. One must take into account the risks and benefits of each treatment modality while considering the prognosis associated with the disease.

An important consideration in the diagnosis and treatment of these strictures is whether or not the process is due to a malignancy. Unlike other symptomatic malignancies affecting the gastrointestinal tract, malignant strictures of the biliary tree are rarely curable. Because of this, malignant strictures usually are managed palliatively. On the other hand, benign strictures should be approached with the intention to cure.

MALIGNANT STRICTURES

Malignant strictures of the biliary tree are categorized by their location: proximal, midduct, or distal. Distal lesions are the most commonly found malignant strictures affecting the biliary tree. Pancreatic carcinoma accounts for the largest number of tumors affecting the distal bile duct.

Proximal lesions, i.e., those closest to the liver, are most commonly metastatic, usually from the colon and breast. These tumors metastasize either to the hepatic parenchyma, compressing or replacing large caliber intrahepatic duct branches, or they involve lymph nodes of the porta hepatis, resulting in external compression at the hilum. The most common primary tumor of the bile duct, cholangiocarcinoma, may involve the main right or left hepatic ducts, the hilum, and branches of the right or left intrahepatic duct systems (Fig. 124–1). Cholangiocarcinoma is seen with increased frequency in patients with primary sclerosing cholangitis (PSC) or chronic parasitic infection of the biliary tree (seen predominantly in the Far East). Thorotrast, a contrast agent used in the 1950s has been attributed to an increased incidence of cholangiocarcinoma. Hepatocellular carcinoma (hepatoma) arising in the liver often encroaches on the proximal biliary tree, presenting as a mass compressing a main intrahepatic duct or, rarely, by invading the bile duct proper.

Midbile duct lesions include gallbladder carcinoma, cholangiocarcinoma, and, rarely, hepatoma. Strictures produced by these tumors mainly affect the common hepatic duct (CHD) and the proximal common bile duct (CBD).

When pancreatic cancer arises in the head of the pancreas, a compression stricture results from tumor encasement of the bile duct (Fig. 124–2). In advanced stages, the tumor actually invades the lumen of the bile duct. Ampullary carcinoma is an unusual form of adenocarcinoma arising from the duodenum in the periampullary region and may create a distal stricture. It is important to differentiate this slow-growing tumor from a pancreatic adenocarcinoma, as the cure rate for resection of ampullary carcinoma approaches 20%, and the 5-year survival may be as high as 35%, even in cases with locally invasive disease.

BENIGN STRICTURES

Benign strictures are grouped into three general categories: (1) "postinflammatory," (2) iatrogenic, and (3) "extrinsic."

Postinflammatory strictures are attributed to secondary complications of infection or to nonspecific inflammation that may be classified as autoimmune. Strictures associated with recur-

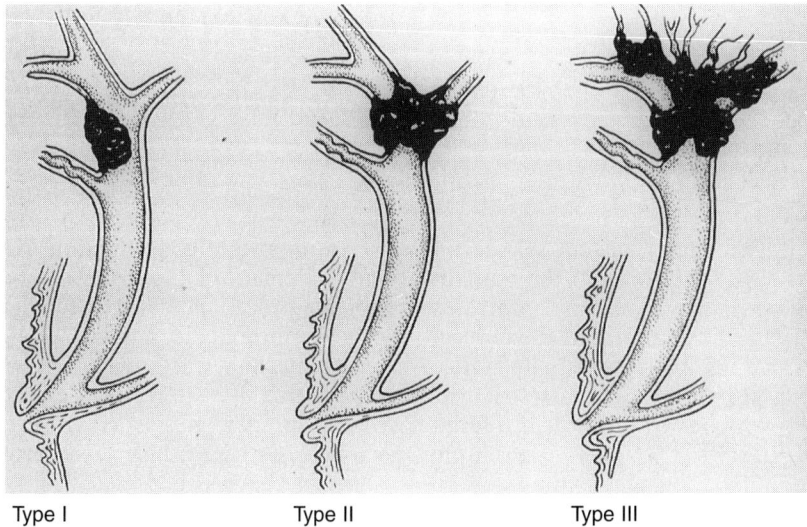

FIGURE 124–1. Bifurcation, or Klatskin's tumor, of the bile ducts. This form of cholangiocarcinoma may present as a common hepatic stricture *(type I)*, involve the main right and left hepatic ducts—either together or separately *(type II)*, or diffusely involve the hilum and the more proximal biliary tree *(type III)*. (From Siegel JH. *Endoscopic Retrograde Cholangiopancreatography.* New York, NY: Raven Press Publishers; 1992. With permission.)

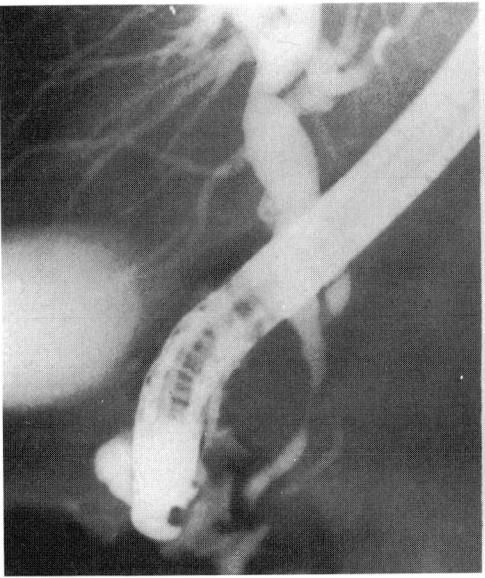 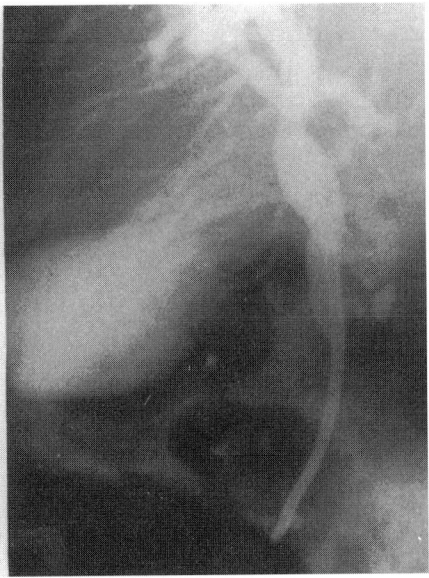

FIGURE 124–2. A distal common bile duct stricture associated with a cutoff in the pancreatic duct, suggesting pancreatic carcinoma. Following the performance of a sphincterotomy, a biliary stent is placed. (From Siegel JH. *Endoscopic Retrograde Cholangiopancreatography.* New York, NY: Raven Press Publishers; 1992. With permission.)

rent biliary tract infection are usually due to either stone disease or parasitic infestation. The latter clinical syndrome, oriental cholangiohepatitis, is seen more frequently in the Far East and is caused by bacterial colonization resulting from obstruction to the biliary tree. Byproducts from bacterial overgrowth and metabolism lead to the formation of "brown" stones.

Acute occlusion of the CBD by stones results in cholangitis or, in situations where a common channel exists at the pancreaticobiliary entrance to the duodenum, gallstone pancreatitis. Interestingly, recurrent low-grade infections attributed to stone disease lead to strictures; on the other hand, benign strictures predispose to stone formation.

PSC is the most common cause of inflammatory strictures reported in the United States. Seventy percent of patients with PSC report a coexisting history of inflammatory bowel disease. The strictures of PSC may be solitary or multiple. Usually both intrahepatic and extrahepatic biliary ducts are involved, but either system can be involved alone. Occasionally, there may be a solitary or dominant stricture affecting the extrahepatic tree, causing cholestasis, obstruction, and dilation of the proximal biliary tree (Fig. 124–3).

Iatrogenic strictures occur after injury to the duct during surgical exploration (Fig. 124–4). These injuries can be related to laceration of the duct, scarring around a T-tube site, or actual stapling or suturing of the CBD or CHD. Most commonly, stricturing results from compromise to the blood supply of the bile duct, without physical involvement of the duct itself. Stricturing of the biliary tree can occur at the site of biliary bypass, such as a choledochojejunostomy, choledochoduodenostomy, or hepaticojejunostomy. In such cases, bile flow through the bypass is impaired, resulting in increased pressure in the distal (bypassed) segment. This results in pain, and if infection is present, the "sump" syndrome occurs.

Extrinsic strictures produced by compression due to mass effect can be seen in the presence of a benign neoplasm, such as a bile duct adenoma or leiomyoma. A choledochal cyst located at the level of the ampulla, also known as a choledochocele, can produce a distal stricture. Extrinsic compression of the mid-CBD or distal CBD is commonly seen in cases of chronic pancreatitis where the head of the pancreas is prominent. In such cases, the stricture is long and smooth and is often associated with calcifications in the pancreatic parenchyma.

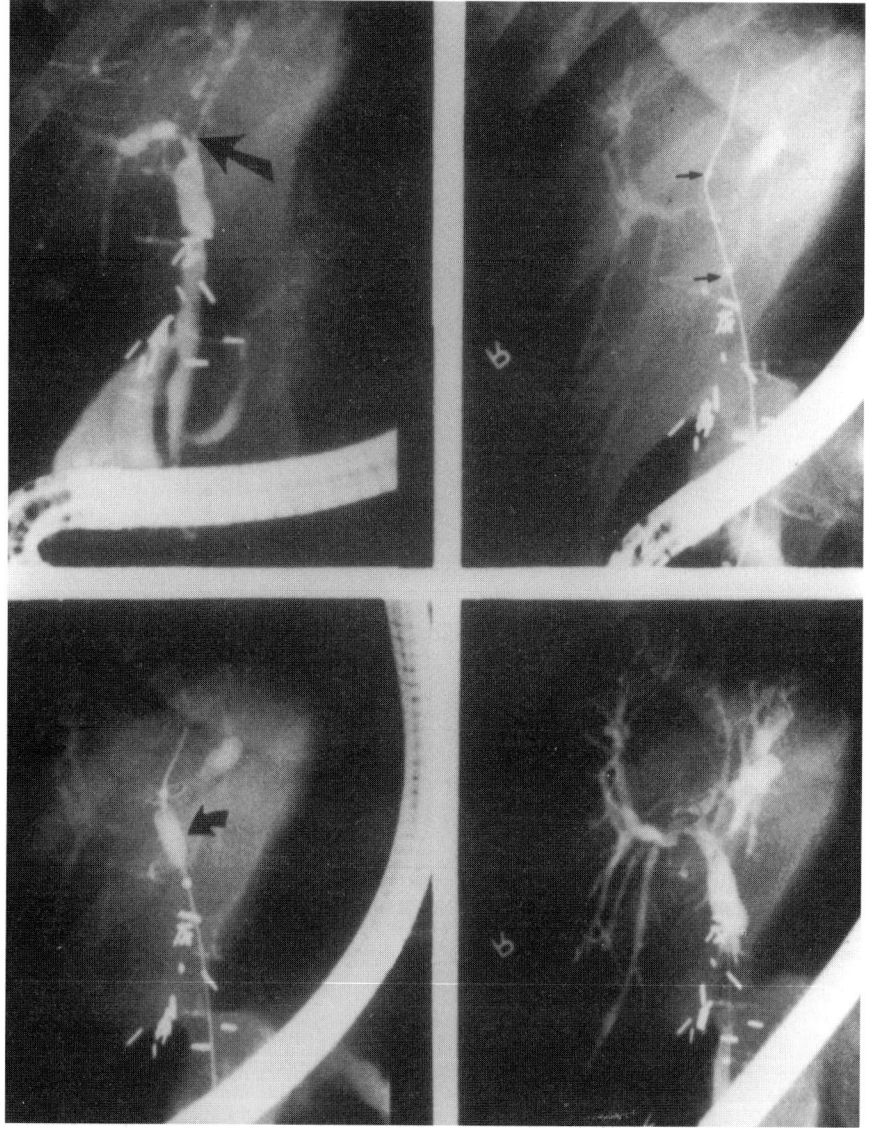

FIGURE 124–3. Balloon dilation of a dominant stricture in the hilum of a patient with primary sclerosing cholangitis. Note the diffuse changes in the intrahepatic and extrahepatic tree, with improved retrograde filling of the proximal biliary system following dilation. (From Siegel JH. *Endoscopic Retrograde Cholangiopancreatography.* New York, NY: Raven Press Publishers; 1992. With permission.)

DIAGNOSIS

Computed tomography (CT) scan and sonography are used during the initial encounter of affected patients, but the most useful modality in evaluating these lesions is direct cholangiography provided by endoscopic retrograde cholangiopancreatography (ERCP). This technique, which provides the least invasive method of obtaining a pancreatogram and cholangiogram, also offers a therapeutic option, whatever the cause, at the time of the index procedure. ERCP provides important information regarding the cause of a stricture. Defining the stricture's location and morphology, as well as identifying the presence of a coexisting pancreatic stricture ("double duct sign") or the presence of multiple strictures (as in sclerosing cholangitis), is useful in establishing a diagnosis.

Confirming malignancy of a bile duct stricture is a daunting task. Depending on the stricture's location, obtaining a biopsy specimen can

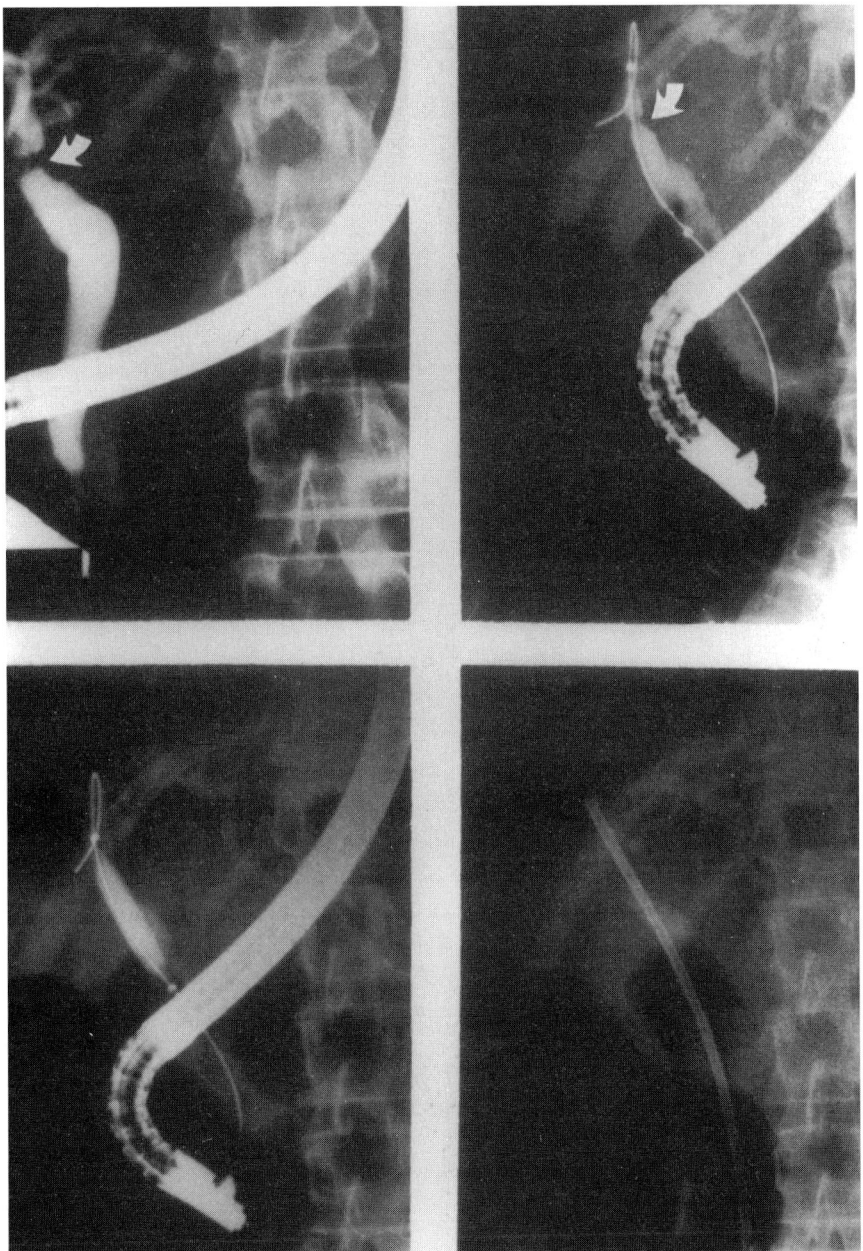

FIGURE 124–4. Balloon dilation of a postoperative stricture in the common hepatic duct. A stent is placed following dilation to maintain patency. (From Siegel JH. *Endoscopic Retrograde Cholangiopancreatography.* New York, NY: Raven Press Publishers; 1992. With permission.)

be extremely difficult, regardless of the technique employed. ERCP allows brush cytologic examination of strictures if these areas can be traversed with a brush and biopsy if there is an intraductal lesion. Because these techniques are only about 50% sensitive (despite improvement in technology), a negative result does not rule out malignancy.

The cholangiographic appearance of a stricture is useful in predicting the nature of the stricture. Long, smooth strictures with gradual tapering are more likely to be benign. The extent of these strictures indicates a slow development. Malignant strictures are more likely to be irregular and short. Often there is an abrupt transition between the contour of the normal duct and the region of the stricture, which is referred to as a "shelf." Multiple strictures are more likely to be benign, as are strictures in the area of previous surgery. Unfortunately, none of these radiographic appearances are specific.

Percutaneous transhepatic cholangiography (PTC) is useful in providing the same radiologic information regarding the biliary tree as is ERCP when the latter is unsuccessful or unavailable. Cytologic examination and biopsy, as well as therapeutic intervention, can be achieved with PTC, although the yield of malignant tissue is no greater than with the endoscopic technique.

If there is a coexisting pancreatic mass and a high index of suspicion of pancreatic carcinoma, a CT-guided needle aspiration of the pancreas can be performed. If the cytologic specimens are evaluated in the CT suite by a cytopathologist, repeated attempts can be made by the radiologist to obtain malignant cells. Even with this routine, the sensitivity remains about 70%.

Surgical exploration is employed in some patients where the diagnosis is unclear or resection is under consideration. Exploration of the bile ducts is an operation associated with significant morbidity. Simple biopsy specimens or brushings are insensitive. Usually the pancreas is evaluated at surgery by palpation and frozen section biopsy. This routine is random and is not specific for carcinoma. If there is strong suspicion of a malignant stricture, an en bloc resection of the affected area is often the only way to assure that a malignancy has not been missed.

Serum markers for malignancy are used in the evaluation of biliary strictures. Carcinoembryonic antigen (CEA) is often elevated in cholangiocarcinoma, but it is not specific for this disease. CA 19-9 is a relatively specific marker for foregut malignancies. Markedly elevated levels (>1000) in the presence of a pancreatic mass strongly suggest pancreatic cancer.

TREATMENT

The treatment strategy for a stricture varies according to the cause of the stricture. Although most strictures can be treated by any of three primary treatment modalities, namely endoscopy, surgery, and invasive radiology, the appropriate method depends on the predicted prognosis of the disease process and the likelihood of each technique's success.

ENDOSCOPIC THERAPY

ERCP is useful both in the diagnosis and the treatment of most biliary strictures. The endoscopic method begins with access to the CBD through the papilla of Vater in the second part of the duodenum. Once the location and character of the stricture has been determined, an attempt is made to traverse the stricture with a guide wire. Once this has been achieved, various accessories can be advanced over the guide wire to provide treatment. The two general techniques of endoscopic therapy are dilation and stenting.

Stricture Dilation

Once a guide wire has traversed a stricture, a variety of catheters can be passed into the area using fluoroscopic guidance. One system relies on progressively larger diameter catheters that provide direct dilation. Strictures can be dilated to 11.5F (3.8 mm) in this fashion. A more aggressive approach to stricture dilation incorporates a high-pressure cylindric balloon system. The balloon catheter is passed into the stricture, and the balloon is filled under pressure with dilute contrast material, permitting fluoroscopic monitoring of the dilation (Fig. 124–4).

Dilation is effective for short strictures resulting from surgical trauma, especially if the stricture is due to a clip. Occasionally, a clip can be seen opening or even falling off the duct during dilation. Short areas of stricturing located in the extrahepatic biliary tree, such as sclerosing cholangitis, respond well to dilation, especially if the stricture is dominant or solitary (Fig. 124–3).

Following dilation of a stricture, a transpapillary plastic stent is often placed into the stricture to prevent early restenosis. These stents can be removed several months after therapy during another ERCP session. At that time, a second cholangiogram is performed to assess the luminal patency.

Malignant strictures and those due to external compression of the duct from a mass generally are not amenable to dilation therapy. In these situations, there is immediate recoil by the disease process, and luminal occlusion recurs.

Stenting

Palliation of strictures can be provided by endoprostheses or "stents." These tubes are inserted through a stricture over a guide wire, generally following a sphincterotomy, and permit the reestablishment of a normal flow of bile (Fig. 124–2). Stents are available in a variety of outer diameters, from 5F to 12F. They are usually made of polyethylene, but a newer design incorporates the use of a mesh or interlocking link structure made of stainless steel, with inner diameters that reach 30F.

The most significant limitation of internal stents is occlusion resulting from an accumulation of bacterial debris and cholesterol stone material, which occurs in 3 to 6 months when large plastic stents are used, or by tumor ingrowth and sludge accumulation, which occur in 6 to 12 months when the wire stents are used. Once occlusion occurs, plastic stents can be changed, but the metal stents, which are permanent, must be stented with a plastic stent. The primary advantage to stents is that they can be placed quickly with a minimal degree of invasiveness and little postprocedure recuperation time. In patients with advanced malignant disease, the stent often remains patent up to the time of death, eliminating the need for surgical therapy.

ERCP with sphincterotomy, stent placement, and stricture dilation remain techniques requiring advanced skill and experience. In addition, there is a predictable morbidity and mortality associated with the endoscopic procedures; namely, pancreatitis, bleeding, cholangitis, and bile duct or bowel perforation. The complications can occur in up to 10% of procedures. Although most complications are mild, there is a 1% mortality reported in many large series. Although these figures compare favorably with other techniques (surgery, percutaneous drainage) employed to deal with bile duct strictures, therapeutic ERCP should be attempted only by those endoscopists with extensive experience.

SURGERY

Surgical management of biliary strictures was the rule prior to the introduction of ERCP in the 1970s. Stricture surgery can be viewed as an attempt at resection versus bypass; alternatively, the surgical approach is one of palliation versus attempted cure. The approach to a specific problem depends on the presumed diagnosis, the severity of the condition, and the general condition of the patient.

Palliation of strictures includes a biliary-enteric bypass, which drains a proximal (closer to the liver) portion of the biliary tree into the intestine. Alternatively, strictureplasty can be attempted for benign disease such as sclerosing cholangitis or postoperative strictures, but this approach is fraught with a high restenosis rate. Generally, when biliary-enteric bypasses are performed for malignant disease and especially for pancreatic carcinoma, a gastrojejunostomy is also performed to prevent or treat gastric outlet obstruction due to duodenal invasion by tumor.

Aggressive surgical therapy of strictures generally involves resection. The Whipple procedure, or pancreatoduodenectomy, when performed for pancreatic carcinoma, provides palliation of biliary obstruction by creating a hepaticojejunostomy, and it is designed to treat or avert gastric outlet obstruction by creating a gastrojejunostomy. In expert hands the mortality for this procedure is less than 5%. Unfortunately, the 5-year survival is usually also less than 5%; but if patients are carefully preselected for resectability, the 5-year survival may approach 20%. Ampullary carcinoma is treated with a similar resection approach. Cholangiocarcinoma can be palliated with a resection of the tumor and subsequent bypass, but the cure rate is also low. Benign strictures secondary to complications of surgery or pancreatitis are generally not treated by resection because of the extensive nature of the resection often required, the incidence of postoperative scar formation and recurrent stricturing, and the satisfactory results achieved with bypass.

INVASIVE RADIOLOGY

The invasive radiologist can do much of what the endoscopist can accomplish, namely dilation and stenting, via percutaneous access of the biliary tree. Plastic or the larger metal mesh stents can be placed, and drainage can be either transpapillary to the duodenum (internal) or to a bag on the skin (external). In cases where ERCP is unsuccessful because of a failure to achieve selective cannulation of the CBD, a combined approach, or "rendezvous procedure," can be used, allowing the radiologist to pass a guide wire through the bile duct into the duodenum, while the endoscopist retrieves the wire, permitting endoscopic treatment as described above.

The primary limitations of PTC are its failure rate in patients without dilated ducts and its high postprocedural infection rate. The success of the procedure, like ERCP, is highly operator dependent.

RECOMMENDATIONS

The approach to strictures of the biliary tree has changed since the advent of therapeutic ERCP. The therapy of malignant strictures should be nonsurgical unless a careful workup in a fit person reveals the strictures are resectable. A caveat regarding ampullary carcinoma is that this disease should be treated surgically, if the patient's clinical condition permits, because of the higher cure rates for this disease, even in cases with local invasion.

Therapy of benign strictures can begin with the less invasive endoscopic approach in most situations. Surgery is reserved for patients in whom endoscopic or percutaneous treatment failed, in healthy patients with mass lesions, or in patients in whom the severity of the disease process indicates that ERCP or PTC would only result in short-term palliation.

REFERENCES

1. Dowsett JF, Vaira D, Hatfield ARW, et al. Endoscopic biliary therapy using the combined percutaneous and endoscopic technique. *Gastroenterology.* 1989;96:1180–1184.
2. Gaing AA, Geders JM, Cohen SA, Siegel JH. Endoscopic management of primary sclerosing cholangitis: review, and report of an open series. *Am J Gastroenterol.* 1993;89:2000–2008.
3. Geenen DJ, Geenen JE, Hogan WJ, et al. Endoscopic therapy for benign bile duct strictures. *Gastrointest Endosc.* 1989;35:367–371.
4. Parsons L, Palmer CH. How accurate is fine-needle biopsy in malignant neoplasia of the pancreas? *Arch Surg.* 1989;124:681–683.
5. Preece PE, Cuschieri A, Rosin RD, eds. *Cancer of the Bile Ducts and Pancreas.* Philadelphia, Pa: WB Saunders Co; 1989.
6. Ryan ME. Cytologic brushings of ductal lesions during ERCP. *Gastrointest Endosc.* 1991;37:139–142.
7. Siegel JH. *Endoscopic Retrograde Cholangiopancreatography.* New York, NY: Raven Press Publishers; 1992.
8. Siegel JH, Snady H. The significance of endoscopically placed prostheses in the management of biliary obstruction due to carcinoma of the pancreas: results of nonoperative decompression in 277 patients. *Am J Gastroenterol.* 1986;81:634–641.
9. Steinberg W. The clinical utility of the CA 19-9 tumor-associated antigen. *Am J Gastroenterol.* 1990;85:350–355.
10. Warshaw AI, Fernandez-Del Castillo C. Pancreatic carcinoma. *N Engl J Med.* 1992;326:455–465.

125

Tumors of the Gallbladder and Biliary Tract

SOROYA M. RAHAMAN and GLEN A. LEHMAN

Tumors of the gallbladder and biliary tract are uncommon malignancies of the gastrointestinal tract. Symptoms are initially similar to those of cholelithiasis. Metastases are commonly present when the cancer is diagnosed. Thus, these tumors often represent a difficult challenge in early detection and palliative management.

NEOPLASMS OF THE GALLBLADDER

INCIDENCE AND ASSOCIATIONS

Although a variety of neoplasms occur in the gallbladder, carcinoma is the main clinically significant tumor and is the fifth most common malignancy of the gastrointestinal tract, resulting in over 6000 new cases per year in the United States. It is the most common malignancy of the biliary tract, usually occurs in the seventh decade, and has a significant female preponderance. The higher incidence of gallbladder cancer in women is ascribed to an increased prevalence of gallstone disease. Among patients undergoing surgery for biliary tract disease or cholelithiasis, the reported incidence is 1% to 2%. Autopsy studies indicate an incidence of 0.2% to 0.8%.

Although cancer is identified in only a small fraction of patients with gallstones, nearly 80% of patients with gallbladder cancers have concomitant cholelithiasis (Table 125–1). Evidence suggests that the chronic presence of gallstones induces metaplastic changes in the mucosal epithelium, resulting in hyperplasia and atypia. Gallstone size greater than 3 cm has been associated with an increased incidence of gallbladder cancer. Dysplasia or atypia have been noted adjacent to carcinoma in situ, suggesting a dysplasia-carcinoma sequence.

A significant number of gallbladder cancers occur in the absence of gallstones. Thus, a number of other etiologic agents have been proposed and include chemical carcinogens such as nitrosamines and methylcholanthrene as encountered in the automotive and rubber industries. In addition, the high incidence of gallbladder cancer in Hispanics and Native Americans beyond the expected increase due to gallstones may indicate genetic susceptibility. Calcification of the wall of the gallbladder (porcelain gallbladder) has also been noted to be a factor in the development of cancer and may be a dysplasia-inducing factor. Anomalous junction of the pancreatobiliary ducts (AJPBD) as defined by union of the pancreatic and bile duct outside the duodenal wall has been identified as a risk factor for gallbladder cancer. This anomaly can only be detected by invasive cholangiography. In a review of 34 patients with gallbladder cancer associated with this congenital abnormality, Tanaka et al[1] found a high rate of unresectable cancers and low incidence of associated gallstones. Proliferative activity of premalignant gallbladder mucosa is increased with AJPBD, and this may be secondary to mutations of p53 and k-*ras* genes.[2]

CLINICAL PRESENTATION AND INITIAL MANAGEMENT

The clinical diagnosis of gallbladder cancer is a difficult endeavor. Patients often present with signs or symptoms similar to cholelithiasis. Most commonly, patients complain of epigastric or right upper quadrant abdominal pain, with or without associated nausea, vomiting, jaundice, or weight loss. The physical examination generally reveals only mild abdominal tenderness. A palpable abdominal mass is rare. Serum liver chemistries are usually not specific, with mild-to-moderate alkaline phosphatase elevations, and one third of patients have elevated bilirubin. In one series of 71 patients, none had a preoperative diagnosis of cancer; 50% were positively identified by the surgeon at cholecystectomy or laparotomy, 40% were identified by the pathologist, and 10% were diagnosed at autopsy.[3] Plain film of the abdomen may reveal porcelain gallbladder; ultrasound examination may identify an intraluminal mass or wall thickening; and computed tomography (CT) scan may in addition reveal a hilar mass or metastases. In jaundiced patients, cholangiography via percutaneous transhepatic cholangiography (PTC) or endoscopic retrograde cholangiopancreatography (ERCP) may reveal obstruction of the biliary tract (most typically at the level of the common hepatic duct) or multiple biliary strictures, reflecting both direct invasion and a propensity to spread via the periductal lymphatics. Laparoscopy may be a useful adjuvant diagnostic tool, particularly in identifying patients with unresectable cancer, obviating the need for laparotomy. In general, preoperative diagnosis of gallbladder cancer is made in less than 20% of patients. The diagnosis is often made at the time of pathologic examination following a cholecystectomy for gallstone disease.

Benign gallbladder tumors are mainly discovered via ultrasound during evaluation of upper abdominal pain. The tumors appear as a focal wall mass or mucosal polypoid lesions. Resection for such lesions is generally recommended, as current imaging studies do not differentiate benign from malignant polypoid lesions.

HISTOLOGY

Benign tumors of the gallbladder are of epithelial (adenoma) and mesenchymal (leiomyoma, hemangioma, lipoma) origin. Benign adenomas may be papillary or tubular types. Other changes in gallbladder epithelium that do not have malignant potential include inflammatory polyps, cholesterol polyps, and adenomatous hyperplasia, which may, however, give rise to benign adenomas. Premalignant conditions of the gallbladder mucosa include dysplasia and squamous

TABLE 125–1. CARCINOMA OF THE BILIARY TREE

FACTOR	GALLBLADDER		BILE DUCTS			AMPULLARY
	FOUND ONLY HISTOLOGICALLY	FOUND BY SURGEON, CT, OR ULTRASOUND	HILAR	MIDDLE	DISTAL	
Clinical presentation	Biliary colic (due to stones or cholecystitis)	Biliary colic (due to stones or cholecystitis)	Obstructive jaundice	Obstructive jaundice	Obstructive jaundice	Obstructive jaundice Gastrointestinal tract bleeding
Gallstone association	Yes	Yes	No	No	No	No
Special risk factors	Native American Hispanic Porcelain gallbladder AJPBD 100%	Native American Hispanic Porcelain gallbladder AJPBD 10%	Choledochal cyst AJPBD Southeast Asia Sclerosing cholangitis 10%	Choledochal cyst AJPBD Southeast Asia Sclerosing cholangitis 40%	Choledochal cyst AJPBD Southeast Asia Sclerosing cholangitis 75%	Gardner's syndrome 75%
Patients resectable for attempted cure						
Palliative therapies		Chemotherapy EBXRT	Chemotherapy EBXRT Brachytherapy 2%	Chemotherapy EBXRT Brachytherapy 15%	Chemotherapy EBXRT Brachytherapy 40%	Chemotherapy EBXRT Brachytherapy 30%
5-year survival of all such cancer patients	80%	3%	15%*	25%	50%	50%
5-year survival of patients having resection for curative attempt	80%	10%				

AJPBD = anomalous junction of the pancreatobiliary ducts, EBXRT = external beam radiation therapy.
*Includes Asian series of patients, who may have better prognosis than European or American patients.

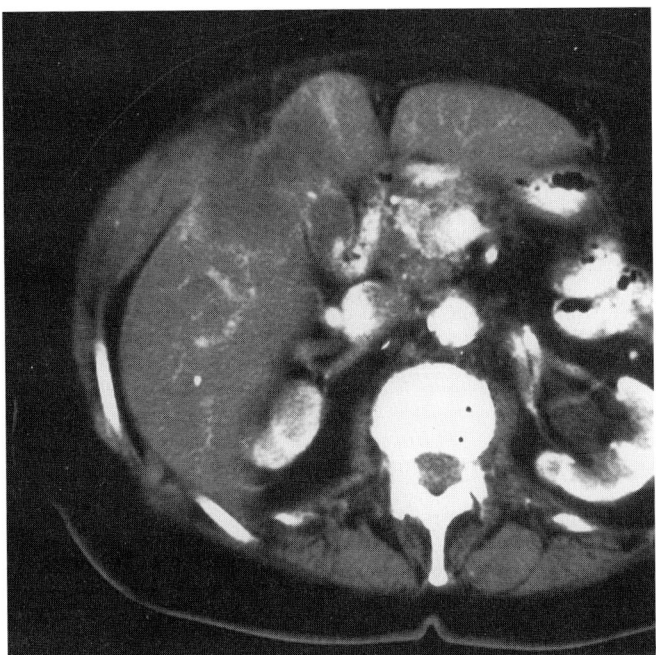

FIGURE 125–1. Carcinoma of the gallbladder with local infiltration into the right lobe of the liver, as seen on computed tomography scan. Calcified stone is present in the shrunken gallbladder. The diagnosis was made by percutaneous fine needle aspirate that showed adenocarcinoma. Only symptomatic treatment was given to this 83-year-old patient who lived an additional 6 months.

metaplasia, the latter giving rise to squamous cell carcinoma.

Adenocarcinoma is the most common histopathologic type of gallbladder cancer and occurs most commonly as a diffuse infiltrating process (Fig. 125–1). Papillary tumors occur in 20% of cases, are the type most frequently reported as an incidental finding, and tend to be less invasive and thus have a better postoperative survival rate. Other histologic types include squamous cell carcinoma (more common in the Native American population), undifferentiated carcinoma, adenoacanthoma, mucinous cystadenomas, and mesodermal tumors. Spread of these tumors is by local invasion of the liver and adjacent organs, via the bloodstream and lymphatics. Regional lymph node and liver involvement is present in 30% to 50% of patients at surgical exploration. Peritoneal carcinomatosis occurs in approximately 20% of patients, whereas pulmonary metastases are seen in 10%.

THERAPY

Surgery

Curative therapy of benign and malignant gallbladder tumors is cholecystectomy. Cancer cures usually occur in the setting of intramucosal lesions coincidentally discovered by the pathologist. As noted above, the majority of patients present with unresectable disease. The surgical approaches proposed for cancer identified intraoperatively include cholecystectomy with or without regional lymphadenectomy, adjacent wedge resection of the liver, and the more radical resection of the right hepatic lobe and the medial segment of the left hepatic lobe. There is little evidence to suggest improved life span with these more radical interventions, and a high perioperative mortality makes these interventions difficult to recommend. Prophylactic cholecystectomy has been advocated in high-risk populations such as Native American and Hispanic women with gallstones, anomalous pancreatobiliary junction without bile duct dilation, and porcelain gallbladder. In addition, oral bile salt therapy has been advocated as a metaplasia-arresting agent, but the long-term effects of this therapy are unknown.

Radiation and Chemotherapy

Radiation and chemotherapy have not yet been proven beneficial in the treatment of neoplasms of the gallbladder. Most chemotherapeutic regimens include 5-fluorodeoxyuridine. The Eastern Cooperative Oncology Group reported a 10% response rate to chemotherapy.[4] Silk et al[3] describe a modest increase in median survival (8.4 months in the group treated with chemotherapy compared to 5.3 months in the nonchemotherapy group) in a nonrandomized review of 71 patients. This improvement in survival may be due to patient selection alone and included patients with stage II through V disease with previous surgical resection. The median survival of all patients in this series from the time of diagnosis was 6 months, and the estimated 5-year survival was 3%. The most clinically important determinant of survival was the stage of disease, with patients with stage II disease surviving a median of 24 months and those with stage V disease surviving 6 months. The 5-year survival for patients with tumors confined to the wall of the gallbladder and found incidentally by the pathologist has previously been reported as 65% to 70%.

NEOPLASMS OF THE BILE DUCTS

INCIDENCE AND ASSOCIATIONS

Cholangiocarcinoma is an uncommon malignancy with approximately 5000 cases per year in the United States. It is found in less than 0.5% of all autopsies. There are a number of risk factors felt to predispose to the development of cholangiocarcinoma, but the cause of most of these tumors is not determined. Unlike gallbladder cancer, gallstones do not have a known association with cholangiocarcinoma. As outlined in Table 125–1, there are a number of risk factors, but no definitive causative agents have been identified.

PATHOLOGY

Benign tumors of the bile ducts are unusual and are most often adenomas, cystadenomas, or granular cell tumors. These most commonly occur in the extrahepatic bile ducts, and their malignant potential is not known. Papillomatosis is a very rare premalignant condition occurring as multiple papillary lesions of the extrahepatic bile ducts.

Ninety percent of bile duct tumors are adenocarcinomas. Squamous cell carcinoma is the second most common malignancy. Like gallbladder cancer, the papillary form has a better prognosis but occurs less commonly than the scirrhous, infiltrating type. Invasion of the liver or metastases to regional lymph nodes is common and present at diagnosis in up to 35% of patients. In addition, invasion of vascular structures (such as the portal vein or hepatic artery) and neural invasion are common. Distant metastases are uncommon, particularly at the time of diagnosis.

The proximal biliary tract, or upper third, is the most common site of bile duct tumors, accounting for 40% to 50%. The middle third accounts for approximately 20%, and the lower third accounts for the remainder. Tumors of the common hepatic duct bifurcation are known as Klatskin's tumors.

CLINICAL PRESENTATION

Nearly all patients with cholangiocarcinoma present with obstructive jaundice. Other symptoms include pruritus (occasionally preceding jaundice), weight loss, nausea, vomiting, and occasionally abdominal pain. Hepatomegaly is infrequently present.

DIAGNOSIS

Serum liver chemistries typically reveal an elevated total and direct bilirubin (usually 10 to 25 mg/dl), indicating obstructive jaundice, elevation of alkaline phosphatase, and smaller increases in serum aminotransferases. Mild serum albumin depression, coagulopathy, and anemia are also frequently encountered. The tumor-associated antigens carcinoembryonic antigen (CEA) and CA 19-9 are often elevated but are not specific. Transabdominal ultrasound and CT scan of the abdomen nearly always show biliary tract dilation down to the level of the tumor. Recently, endoscopic ultrasound has proven to be more accurate than CT or ultrasound in the staging of these lesions, i.e., assessing regional nodal involvement and invasion of vascular structures such as the portal vein. Angiography is rarely needed as a diagnostic tool, but may be helpful in planning surgical resection.

Cholangiography should be undertaken in all patients with suspected obstructive jaundice to define the cause and level of obstruction. Cholangiography can be performed via PTC or via ERCP. PTC requires less technical expertise, especially if intrahepatic bile duct dilation is present. Cholangiograms typically show a shelved narrowing of 1 to 3 cm length with upstream ductal dilation. Both techniques are suitable for obtaining diagnostic cytologic and histopathologic specimens, and in capable hands, drainage of the biliary tract can be achieved. Both procedures may cause cholangitis. PTC has greater risks of bile leakage and bleeding. ERCP has the added risk of pancreatitis. If ERCP is undertaken, the endoscopist must be prepared and able to accomplish drainage of the biliary tract to prevent cholangitis subsequent to contrast injection. An additional benefit of ERCP is the ability to evaluate the papilla of Vater and the pancreas.

TABLE 125–2. BILIARY ENDOLUMINAL HISTOLOGIC OR CYTOLOGIC TECHNIQUES FOR PANCREATOBILIARY MALIGNANCY DIAGNOSIS

	EASE OF USE	COMPLICATION RATE	CANCER DETECTION SENSITIVITY
Bile Aspiration	Easy	Very low	Low
Brush	Easy	Very low	Low-moderate
Fine needle aspiration	Moderately difficult	Low	Low-moderate
Forceps	Difficult	Low	Moderate
Stent*	Easy	Very low	Low-moderate
Combination of above	–	Low	Moderate-high

*Stent removed after 3 to 4 months and adherent debris analyzed for cytologic examination.

Ideally, all obstructing bile duct tumors would be managed after histologic confirmation is obtained (Table 125–2). Sampling may be done via PTC, ERCP, or percutaneous fine-needle aspirate (FNA). Single brush cytology detects 40% of malignancies. Repeated brushings can increase sensitivity to 65%.[5] An exfoliative cytologic specimen obtained by bile aspiration has a sensitivity of only 30%.[6] Forceps biopsy via ERCP has a 50% to 60% sensitivity. Preliminary intraductal FNA cytology has been shown to be highly specific with sensitivity reported up to 62%.[7] At our institution, a combination of brush cytology, FNA cytology, and intraductal biopsy detects malignant bile duct tumors in 73% of cases. Cholangioscopic forceps biopsy via percutaneous or endoscopic routes is technically demanding but has also been shown to have a high degree of accuracy (85%) in the diagnosis of cancer. It should be noted that in patients less than 60 years old who are otherwise healthy, exploratory laparotomy may be the most reasonable diagnostic approach if initial evaluation does not reveal unresectable disease. Aggressive attempts to prove unresectable lesions may be better reserved for elderly or debilitated patients in whom palliative therapy is more appropriate.

TREATMENT

Surgery

The role of surgery in hilar cholangiocarcinoma is controversial. Recent reports have extolled aggressive curative resection. The rationale for major liver resection and right or left hepatic lobectomy for hilar cholangiocarcinoma is based on the knowledge that local recurrence is the most common cause of death in these patients. Improved expertise in major hepatic resection and orthotopic liver transplantation has also influenced more aggressive surgical methods.

Bismuth and colleagues[8] reported that the operative mortality was 0% in 23 of 112 patients who underwent curative resection for hilar cholangiocarcinomas with histologic negative margins. Nimura et al,[9] using a rigorous preoperative diagnostic evaluation, performed curative resection in 66 patients with an operative mortality of 6.4% and a 5-year survival of 40.5%. Of 11 patients not resected, the median survival was less than 9 months. More importantly, this study reported an operative morbidity of 41%. A review of 40 papers, including 581 resections, by Boerma[10] emphasizes the still significant operative mortality of extensive hepatic resection (15% in those described from 1980 to 1989) but improvement in 5-year survival (17%) in those treated after 1980 as compared to those treated before 1980 (0%). Improvement in operative mortality is largely due to improved perioperative management of sepsis, coagulopathy and renal failure.

Curative surgical resection of tumors located in the mid and lower third of the bile duct is technically easier than in tumors located in the proximal third of the bile duct; curative surgical resection is recommended for patients of reasonable operative risk who have no evidence of unresectable lesions (by CT scan with or without endoscopic ultrasound or angiography). Pancreatoduodenectomy (Whipple's procedure) is usually employed; however, resection of the bile duct with choledochojejunostomy is possible for midduct tumors.

Palliative surgical biliary-enteric bypass procedures should be reserved for patients who already have undergone laparotomy for attempted cure, patients with duodenal obstruction, and those intolerant of endoscopic or percutaneous manipulation.

Liver transplantation has a limited role in the treatment of cholangiocarcinoma. Median survival is 16 months, and recurrence of tumor nearly always occurs.

Palliative Biliary Decompression (Stenting)

Palliative biliary decompression should generally be undertaken in patients who are expected to live at least 30 to 60 more days and whose lesions are deemed to be unresectable. Relief of jaundice is associated with improvement in quality of life. Biliary drainage can be accomplished by percutaneous, endoscopic, or surgical means. Each method has relative advantages and disadvantages (Fig. 125–2). ERCP is least invasive and generally the procedure of choice. Although success rates vary with the expertise of the endoscopists, stents can be successfully placed in 85% to 90% of mid and distal bile duct lesions, whereas hilar lesions can be passed in only 70% to 75%.[11] Percutaneous assistance can increase this to 95% to 100%. High-grade, tortuous, and

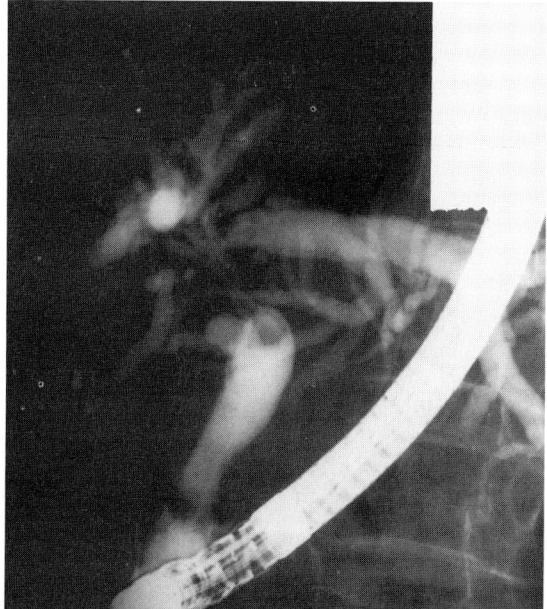
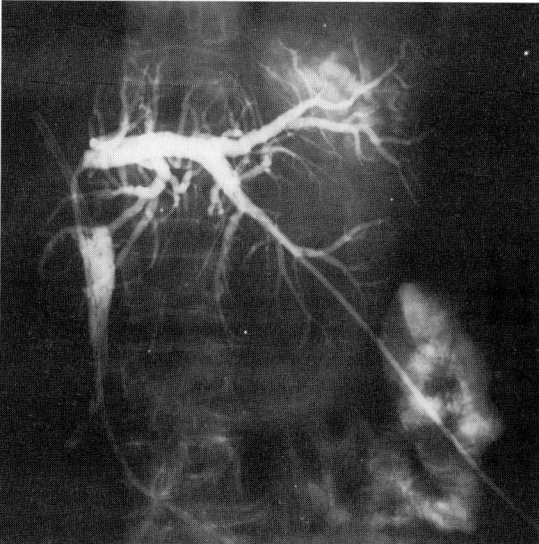
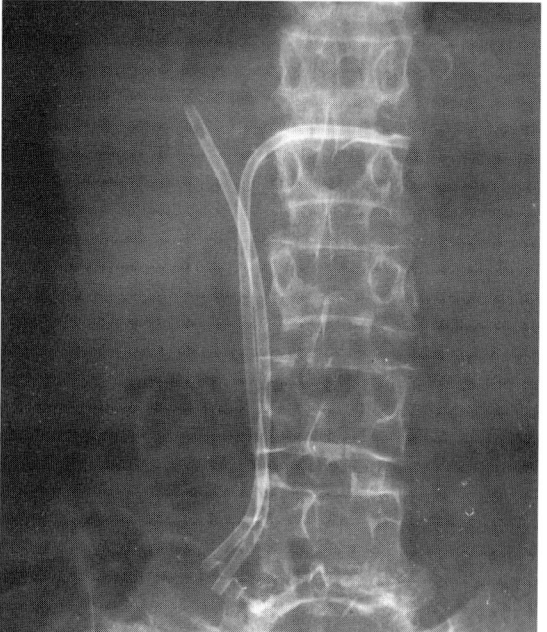

FIGURE 125–2. A, Typical cholangiocarcinoma involving the entire common hepatic duct and the confluence of the right and left hepatic ducts. B, A 10F, 12-cm long polyethylene stent has been placed endoscopically in the right lobe, but continued fever required percutaneous entry into the left lobe to decompress the left lobe. C, A left lobe 10F, 15-cm long polyethylene stent has been placed endoscopically via combined endoscopic-percutaneous technique. To date, the patient has survived 4 years without use of chemotherapy or radiation therapy. Multiple stent exchanges have been required in this interval.

long segment obstructions are most problematic. Percutaneous biliary drainage is recommended for endoscopic failures and patients without endoscopic access (Roux-en-Y) and may be used in combined percutaneous and endoscopic procedures.

Most biliary endoprostheses are polyethylene tubes of 10F- to 11.5F-gauge diameter and of straight or single pigtail design. Obstruction of plastic biliary endoprostheses is clearly a limiting factor in the use of these devices. Stent occlusion with subsequent cholangitis results from bacterial contamination and growth that leads to the development of an adherent biofilm.

Recurrent jaundice or cholangitis occurs as a complication of stent occlusion in at least 50% of patients with cholangiocarcinoma who survive 6 to 9 months. Initial occlusion commonly causes flulike symptoms (malaise and low-grade fever) before frank cholestasis occurs. Patients should be warned of such symptoms and seek medical attention. We recommend that patients have oral antibiotics (ciprofloxacin or cephalexin) at home to initiate at the onset of such symptoms. This may prevent serious cholangitis or sepsis and need for hospitalization. Various methods to limit stent occlusion (silver impregnation, ultraslick stent surface, elimination of side holes, placement of downstream tip in the bile duct, and administration of systemic antibiotics) are being evaluated but are yet of no proven efficiency. There are generally two stent occlusion or prevention schemes: (1) prophylactically replace plastic stents at 3- to 4-month intervals and (2) replace stents at the earliest sign of occlusion. We favor the latter because fewer total stent exchanges are probably needed.

Additional clinically significant complications of endoscopic biliary stent placement include bleeding (1%) and retroduodenal perforation (1%) (usually due to preceding papillotomy), acute pancreatitis (2%), and migration of the stent (5%). Direct procedure-related mortality is approximately 1% and is most commonly related to biliary sepsis.

Because of the high rates of plastic stent occlusion, self-expanding metal mesh stents (Wallstent [Schneider] and Gianturco Z stent [Wilson Cook]) have been developed recently for percutaneous and endoscopic use (Fig. 125–3). These stents can be deployed as 8F catheters but expand to a 24F to 30F diameter once they are placed. They cost $600 to $1000 in contrast to less than $100 for plastic endoprostheses.

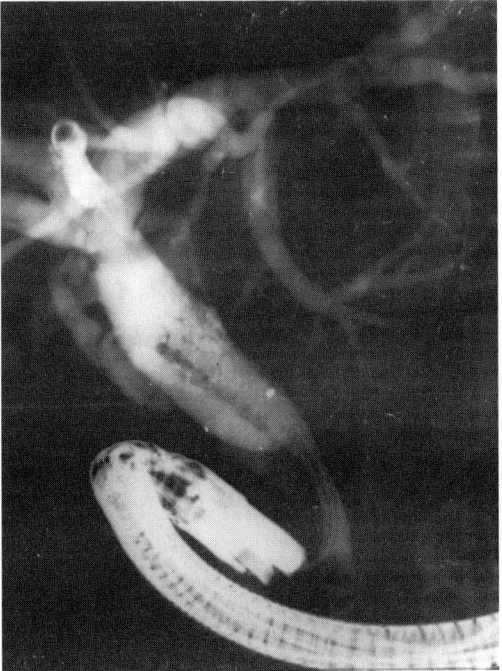
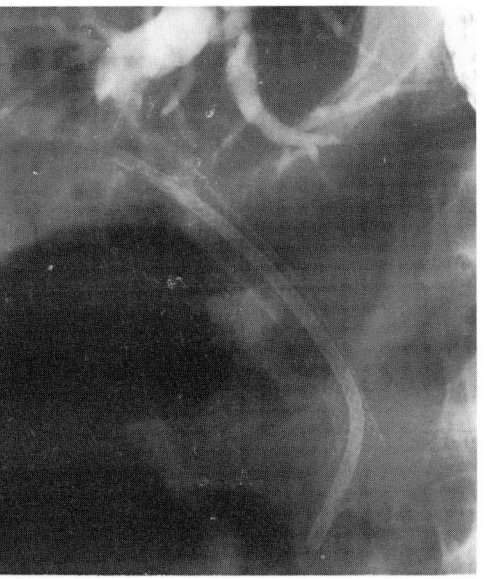

FIGURE 125–3. A, A 67-mm long, 10-mm diameter Wallstent has been placed in the distal bile duct in this patient with distal bile duct carcinoma. He was not an operative resection candidate because of heart and lung disease. **B,** Metal stent occlusion occurred 4 months later. A 10F plastic stent has been placed within the metal stent for further biliary decompression.

Four prospective randomized controlled trials have shown that metal stents occlude less frequently and less quickly than plastic stents. Despite the high initial costs, most studies show ultimate cost savings for the metal stents. Since one third to one half of patients with stents die before the plastic stent occludes, the challenge is to selectively place metal stents in patients who have anticipated longevity greater than 6 to 9 months. Alternatively, some authorities use metal stents for patients in whom the first plastic stent occludes (Table 125–3).[12–15]

Approximately 25% of metal stents occlude. This is generally from tumor ingrowth through the spaces between the struts of the stent. These occlusions are generally best managed by placement of a plastic stent within the metal stent. The role of membrane-coated metal stents looks promising in preliminary evaluations.

Surgical biliary-enteric bypass procedures are as equally effective in relieving common bile duct obstruction as are stents, but early morbidity and mortality are higher from surgery. However, stent occlusion and cholangitis, recurrent jaundice, and the need for repeated procedures make surgical bypass an option for a more prolonged palliation.

Radiation and Chemotherapy

The efficacy of chemotherapy in the palliative treatment of cholangiocarcinoma remains poorly defined. Small patient numbers have limited the evaluation to date. Most current regimens contain 5-fluorodeoxyuridine and mitomycin, as do other regimens for gastrointestinal tract malignancies. There have been no convincing data regarding chemotherapy's effect on prolonging survival.

As previously noted, the most frequent cause of death in patients with cholangiocarcinoma is local recurrence of disease. Therefore, radiation therapy has been used as both primary and adjuvant therapy. Using radiation therapy alone, both for short-term and long-term local control, has been reported in patients with unresectable disease.[16] More recently, intraoperative radiation therapy combined with noncurative resection has been reported to result in a 2-year survival of 17% compared to 9% for noncurative resection alone.[16] There is a high complication rate, however, with external beam radiation therapy. Complications include hepatic failure secondary to hepatic and biliary fibrosis, sepsis, cholangitis, and late gastrointestinal tract bleeding occurring in up to 40% of patients. Intracavitary radiotherapy can be delivered through endoscopically or percutaneously[17,18] placed catheters. The mean survival in patients receiving brachytherapy is reported at 10 to 14 months. A multicenter prospective randomized trial is needed to assess the efficacy of brachytherapy in the treatment of unresectable cholangiocarcinoma.

TABLE 125–3. RANDOMIZED CONTROLLED TRIALS OF EXPANDABLE METAL STENTS VERSUS PLASTIC STENTS FOR MALIGNANT BILIARY STRICTURES

	Davids et al[12] (1992)	Carr-Locke et al[13] (1993)	Knyrim et al[14] (1993)	Wagner et al[15] (1993)
Placement method	Endoscopy	Endoscopy	Endoscopy	Percutaneous
Type metal stent (diameter)	Wallstent (30F)	Wallstent (30F)	Wallstent (30F) Strecker (21F)	Wallstent (24F) Strecker (21F)
n = Number of patients	n=49	n=94	n=21	n=11 (bilateral)
Plastic stent (diameter)	10F	10/11.5F	11.5/14F	14F
n = Number of patients	n=56	n=89	n=31	n=9 (bilateral)
Tumor type by Bismuth classification	I	I, II, III	I	II, III
Median stent patency				
Metal	273 d } p = .006	185 d } Not significant	Not given	Not given
Plastic	126 d	175 d		
First stent occlusion rate				
Metal	33% } p = .03	16% } p < .05	22% } p = .004	18% } p = .2
Plastic	54%	31%	43%*	55%
More cost effective	Metal	Metal	Metal	Metal
Percent of patients living at time of report	36%	19%	5%	Not given

*Includes patients with stent migration.

AMPULLARY TUMORS

INCIDENCE AND ASSOCIATIONS

Tumors of the ampulla are unusual, with approximately 3000 cases per year in the United States. Tumors of the ampulla are reported in 0.2% of autopsies. These tumors present earlier in their clinical course than other bile duct tumors and periampullary tumors and thus have a better prognosis. There are no definitive etiologic factors, although there is a known association with Gardner's syndrome and familial adenomatous polyposis (FAP).

CLINICAL FEATURES AND PATHOLOGY

Malignant tumors of the ampulla are almost exclusively adenocarcinoma. These may be characterized as papillary (villous) or tubular and are usually well differentiated. A variety of benign tumors occur at the ampulla and include benign adenoma, lipoma, neurogenic tumors, fibroma, and neuroendocrine tumors. Benign adenomas (villous and tubular), the most common benign tumor, are considered premalignant lesions based on the frequency with which benign adenomatous tissue is found within malignant tumors and on the foci of carcinoma found within largely benign adenomas. Yamaguchi et al[19] described 18% of carcinomas of the ampulla with definite evidence of an adenoma at the tumor margin in 109 patients. Thus, a polyp-cancer sequence, as occurs with colonic adenomas and carcinoma, is proposed.

The classic symptom triad of fluctuating painless jaundice, anemia with or without symptoms of gastrointestinal tract bleeding, and a palpably enlarged gallbladder is relatively specific for ampullary tumors but is seen rarely. More commonly, patients present with jaundice or weight loss, abdominal pain, and anemia. Overt gastrointestinal tract bleeding is uncommon, and cholangitis is rare. Coincident cholelithiasis and choledocholithiasis, found in up to 40% of patients, are likely due to bile stasis.

DIAGNOSIS

Upper gastrointestinal tract series may identify a duodenal mass, but there is a high frequency of false-negative studies. CT scan and ultrasound identify biliary obstruction with dilation down to the ampullary region. Endoscopy, with a side-viewing duodenoscope, is the most sensitive and specific method of diagnosing carcinoma of the papilla of Vater. The endoscopic appearance of the papilla is variably enlarged, polypoid, smooth, or ulcerated.[20] Tumors arising within the ampulla usually mimic an impacted distal bile duct stone. Contrast injection usually reveals a dilated bile duct or main pancreatic duct associated with a 1- to 3-cm long strictured zone. An irregular filling defect of the distal bile duct is visualized in 10% to 15% of cases. Histologic examination is mandatory in the diagnostic evaluation. Standard forceps biopsy yields a cancer diagnosis in 75% of cases. Many authors now advocate standard forceps biopsy of the papilla following endoscopic sphincterotomy. Biopsies should be taken at the time of sphincterotomy; if biopsy results are negative for cancer, the biopsy should be repeated in 2 to 3 weeks if suspicion of cancer is high. Delayed forceps biopsies plus needle aspiration cytologic examination give positive results from tissue diagnosis in nearly all patients with tumors of the ampulla. Endoscopic ultrasound is an effective method of tumor staging, showing with high sensitivity the depth of tumor invasion and nodal involvement.

TREATMENT

The optimal therapy for carcinoma of the ampulla is surgical resection. However, 25% of carcinomas are not resectable. Two types of operation may be performed: pancreatoduodenectomy (Whipple's procedure) or local excision with reimplantation of the bile and pancreatic ducts. The choice of procedure depends on the size and extent of tumor and the patient's ability to undergo extensive surgery. Although surgical morbidity and mortality following pancreatoduodenectomy has improved in recent years, 5-year survival remains only moderate (37% to 55%) for lesions that do not involve the lymph nodes. As expected, lower rates of survival (23% to 40%) but also lower morbidity and mortality postoperatively are reported with local excision. For patients with widely disseminated carcinoma of the ampulla, treatment is palliative and directed toward relief of pain and jaundice. The preferred treatment for benign villous adenomas is by local excision, although endoscopic snare resection of papillary tumors is gaining acceptance.

Endoscopic palliation is appropriate for patients in poor general condition with a short life expectancy. Sphincterotomy alone has been described with effective relief of jaundice lasting 4 to 12 months in the majority of patients. Endoscopically or percutaneously placed plastic biliary endoprostheses can be placed with relief of jaundice in 95%. Stent obstruction and recurrence of jaundice or cholangitis occurs within 6 to 9 months in more than 50% of patients who survive prosthesis placement. Late complications include duodenal obstruction and recurrent obstructive jaundice, occasionally requiring surgical biliary-enteric bypass. Endoscopic debulking of tumor to prevent duodenal obstruction or ongoing hemorrhage may be needed.

In summary, biliary tree tumors are uncommon. Several risk factors for their development have been identified. Early recognition is difficult. The possibility of cancer cure is influenced by site, and early detection and palliative stenting are commonly needed.

REFERENCES

1. Tanaka K, Nishimura A, Yamada K, et al. Cancer of the gallbladder associated with anomalous junction of the pancreatobiliary duct system without bile duct dilation. *Br J Surg.* 1993;80:622–624.
2. Hanada K, Itoh M, Hiraoha M, et al. Assessment of proliferative activity and carcinogenesis in gallbladder mucosa with an anomalous junction of the pancreatobiliary tract. *DTW.* 1994. Abstract.
3. Silk Y, Douglass H, Nava H, et al. Carcinoma of the gallbladder: the Ronuell Park experience. *Ann Surg.* 1989;210(6):751–757.
4. Eastern Cooperative Oncology Group Report. Chemotherapy of gallbladder, bile duct and primary liver cancer: more bad news. *Cancer.* 1984;54:965–969.
5. Rabinovitz M, Zajko A, Hassanein T, et al. Diagnostic value of brush cytology in the diagnosis of bile duct carcinoma: a study in 65 patients with bile duct strictures. *Hepatology.* 1990;12(4):747–752.
6. Davidson B, Varsamidakas N, Dooley J. Value of exfoliative cytology for investigating bile duct strictures. *Gut.* 1992;33:1408–1411.
7. Howell DA, Beveridge RP, Bosco J. Endoscopic needle aspiration biopsy at ERCP in diagnosis of biliary strictures. *Gastrointest Endosc.* 1992;38:531–535.
8. Bismuth H, Nakache R, Diamond T. Management strategies in resection for hilar cholangiocarcinoma. *Ann Surg.* 1992;215:31–38.
9. Nimura Y, Hayakawa N, Kamiya J, et al. Hepatic segmentectomy with caudate lobe resection for bile duct Ca of the hepatic hilus. *World J Surg.* 1990;14:525–544.
10. Boerma EJ. Research into the results of resection of hilar bile duct cancer. *Surgery.* 1990;108:572–580.
11. Polydorou AA, Carns SR, Dowsett JF, et al. Palliation of proximal malignant biliary obstruction by endoscopic endoprosthesis insertion. *Gut.* 1991;32:685–689.
12. Davids PHP, Groen AK, Rauws EA, Tytgat GNJ, Huibregtse K. Randomized trial of self-expanding metal stents versus polyethylene stents for distal malignant biliary obstruction. *Lancet.* 1992;340:1488–1492.
13. Carr-Locke DL, Ball TJ, Connors PJ, et al. Multicenter, randomized trial of Wallstent biliary endoprosthesis versus plastic stents. *Gastrointest Endosc.* 1993;39:310A.
14. Knyrim K, Wagner J, Pausch J, Vakil N. A prospective, randomized, controlled trial of metal stents for malignant obstruction of the common bile duct. *Gastrointest Endosc.* 1993;39:321A.
15. Wagner HJ, Knyrim K, Vakil N, Klose KJ. Plastic endoprostheses versus metal stents in the palliative treatment of malignant hilar biliary obstruction: a prospective and randomized trial. *Endoscopy.* 1993;25:207–212.
16. Iwasaki Y, Todoroliu T, Fuka OK, et al. The role of intraoperative radiation therapy in the treatment of bile duct cancer. *World J Surg.* 1988;12:91–98.
17. Venu R, Geenen J, Johanson J, et al. A modified technique of endoscopic intraluminal radiation therapy (ILRT) for treatment of cholangiocarcinoma: comparison with stent therapy alone. *Gastroenterology.* 1991;100:A343.
18. Chang LF, Morphis JG, Lehman GA, et al. Iridium 192 intraluminal brachytherapy for cholangiocarcinoma. *Int J Radiat Oncol Biol Phys.* 1994. In press.
19. Yamaguchi K, Enjoji M. Carcinoma of the ampulla of Vater: a clinicopathologic study and pathogenic staging of 109 cases of carcinoma and 5 cases of adenoma. *Cancer.* 1987;59:506.
20. Hawes RH, Jamidar PA. Endoscopic diagnosis and treatment of ampullary tumors. *Gastrointest Endosc Clin North Am.* 1992;2:529–542.

Index

Note: Page numbers in *italics* refer to illustrations; page numbers followed by t refer to tables.

A

Abdominal abscess, 117–121. See also *Abscess, abdominal.*
Abdominal bloating, 70–74, *71*. See also *Gas, intestinal.*
Abdominal pain, functional, 61–68, 62t
    antidepressants in, 65, 65t
    ascertainment bias in, 67
    cognitive behavior therapy in, 67
    diagnosis of, 63–64, 63t
    dicyclomine hydrochloride in, 65
    dietary management in, 64–65
    diphenoxylate in, 65
    drug therapy in, 65–66, 65t
    hypnotherapy in, 66–67
    loperamide in, 65
    physiologic mechanisms of, 62
    placebo effects in, 67–68
    progressive muscle relaxation training in, 67
    psychologic factors in, 62
    psychotherapy in, 66
    tranquilizers in, 65–66
    treatment of, 64–66, 65t
  in acute appendicitis, 464
  in carcinoid syndrome, 306
  in collagenous colitis, 595
  in hereditary pancreatitis, 614–615
  in intestinal obstruction, 492
  in irritable bowel syndrome, 498, 500
  in pancreatic cancer, 639
  in porphyria, 732
Abdominopelvic pain, 573
Abetalipoproteinemia, malabsorption in, 83t, 84
Abscess, abdominal, 117–121
  clinical manifestations of, 117–118
  development of, 117
  diagnosis of, 118–119, *119, 120*
  organisms in, 117
  subphrenic, 118
  treatment of, 119–121
  amebic, 768–771
    diagnosis of, 769–770
    percutaneous aspiration in, 769–770
    presentation of, 768–769
    rupture of, 669, 770
    serologic confirmation of, 769
    treatment of, 770–771
  anorectal, 560–565
    anatomy of, 560, *561*

Abscess *(Continued)*
    clinical features of, 560, 562, 562t
    Crohn's disease and, 564–565
    diagnosis of, 562
    HIV disease and, 565, 565t
    intersphincteric, *563*, 564
    ischiorectal, 563–564, *563*
    leukemia and, 565
    management of, 562–564, *563*
    of postanal space, 562
    pathogenesis of, 560, *561,* 561t
    perianal, 563, *563*
    supralevator, *563*, 564
    surgical management of, 563–564, *563*
  appendiceal, 466
  in diverticulosis coli, 513
  pancreatic, in acute pancreatitis, 627–628
  periappendiceal, 466
  subphrenic, 118
Acetaminophen, hepatotoxicity of, 648–649, 677, 679–680
Acetylcysteine, in bezoar therapy, 281
5-Acetylsalicylic acid (5-ASA), in ulcerative colitis, 520
Achalasia, 186–193
  barium esophagram in, 187, *188*
  chest pain in, 186–187
  clinical presentation of, 186–187, 187t
  complications of, 192–193
  cricopharyngeal, 179–182, *179–181*
    secondary, 182
  diagnosis of, 187–189, *188*
  esophageal carcinoma and, 192–193
  esophageal manometry in, 188–189
  idiopathic, belch reflex in, 184
  infectious esophagitis and, 192
  malignancy in, 187, 187t
  rapid gastric emptying in, 260
  secondary, 187, 187t
  treatment of, 189–192
    botulinum toxin injection in, 192
    bougienage in, 189
    esophagomyotomy in, 192
    medication in, 189
    pneumatic dilation in, 189–192, *190,* 190t, *191*
    upper endoscopy in, 189
Achlorhydria, drug-induced, 27
Acid ingestion, 30–35, 31t, 33t, 34t
  gastritis with, 320

Acid ingestion *(Continued)*
    management of, 32–35, 33t, 34t
    pathophysiology of, 31–32, 31t
Acid posterior laryngitis, in gastroesophageal reflux disease, 206
Acid-base balance, in fulminant hepatic failure, 679
Acidosis, lactic, in fulminant hepatic failure, 682
    metabolic, in acute pancreatitis, 624
Acquired immunodeficiency syndrome (AIDS), acute acalculous cholecystitis in, 854
    anal fissure in, 558–559
    anorectal abscess in, 565, 565t
    coccidioidomycosis in, 764
    hepatic function in, 784, 785t
    hepatic granulomas in, 765–766, 765t
    in diarrhea, 538
    liver disease in, 784, 784t
    malabsorption in, 82, 83t
    Salmonella infection in, 384
Acute tubular necrosis, diagnosis of, 700, 701t
Acyclovir (Zovirax), in herpes simplex virus esophagitis, 241
Adenocarcinoma, ampullary, 911–912
    anal, 572
    Barrett's esophagus and, 206–207, 219
    choledochal cysts and, 821–822, 824
    esophageal, 224–226
    gastric, 289–294. See also *Gastric adenocarcinoma.*
    taste alteration and, 47–48
Adenoma, hepatic, 778
    drug-induced, 648
    resection in, 833
    of Brunner's gland, 420
    of small bowel, 419, 421–422
Adriamycin (doxorubicin), in hepatocellular carcinoma, 774
Aeromonas, toxigenic diarrhea with, 378–379
Aeromonas hydrophila, invasive infection with, 383t, 387
Aflatoxin B_1, hepatocellular carcinoma with, 648
African iron overload, 809
Aganglionosis, gastrointestinal lesions in, 443t
Air insufflation test, in endometriosis, 576
Air swallowing, 72
Air-fluid level, in intestinal obstruction, 493
Alagille's syndrome, liver transplantation in, 839
Alanine aminotransferase, in alcoholism, 708t
    serum, 781, 781t
Albumin, serum, 780–781, 781t
Alcohol, acetaminophen interaction with, 649
Alcoholic gastritis, 135, 318
Alcoholic liver disease, 707–713, 782t, 788, *789*
    acute hepatitis in, 710–712, 710t
    anabolic steroids in, 711–712
    cirrhosis in, 712
    colchicine in, 712
    corticosteroids in, 711
    fatty liver in, 709, 784
    insulin in, 712
    liver transplantation in, 712, 837
    nutritional supplementation in, 710–711
    D-penicillamine in, 712
    prognosis for, 713
    propylthiouracil in, 711
    treatment of, 709–713
Alcoholism, in porphyria, 737
    management of, 707–709, 708t

Alcoholism *(Continued)*
    urinary coproporphyrin in, 740
Aldactone (spironolactone), in ascites, 723
Alkali ingestion, 30–35
    gastritis with, 320
    management of, 32–35, 33t, 34t
    pathophysiology of, 31–32, 31t
    squamous cell carcinoma and, 35
Alkaline phosphatase, serum, 781, 781t
    in primary biliary cirrhosis, 751, 790
Allergic gastroenteropathy, 86
Allergy, in eosinophilic gastroenteritis, 360
$Alpha_1$-antitrypsin, accumulation of, 796
    structure of, 793–795
    upregulation of, 798
$Alpha_1$-antitrypsin clearance, in protein-losing gastroenteropathy, 86
$Alpha_1$-antitrypsin deficiency, 791–801
    clinical manifestations of, 792, 792t
    diagnosis of, 792–793, *793, 794*
    emphysema in, 799
    gene replacement therapy in, 800
    liver injury in, 795–799, *797*
    model of, 796–798, *797*
    pathophysiology of, 793–795
    prognosis for, 792
    replacement therapy in, 799–800
    synthetic peptides in, 798, 800
    treatment of, 798, 799–801
Alpha-fetoprotein, in hepatocellular carcinoma, 772
ALT (alanine aminotransferase), in alcoholism, 708t
    serum, 781, 781t
Amanita phalloides, hepatotoxicity of, 677, 680
Amantadine, in hepatic encephalopathy, 658
Amebic abscess, 768–771. See also *Abscess, amebic.*
Amenorrhea, in eating disorders, 11
American Endoscopy dilator, 227, *227*
Amino acids, essential, 17t
    in alcoholic patient, 711
    in fulminant hepatic failure, 682
γ-Aminobutyric acid (GABA), in hepatic encephalopathy, 654
Aminoglycosides, in hepatorenal syndrome, 702
Aminosalicylates, in Crohn's disease, 411
    in ulcerative colitis, 515–516
5-Aminosalicylic acid (5-ASA), in Crohn's disease, 411
Aminotransferases, serum, 781, 781t
Amiodarone, steatonecrosis with, 647
Amitriptyline, in functional abdominal pain syndromes, 65t
Ammonia, neurotoxicity of, 654
Amphotericin B (Fungizone), in *Candida* esophagitis, 240
Ampulla, tumors of, 911–912
    clinical features of, 911
    diagnosis of, 911
    treatment of, 911–912
Amyloidosis, gastrointestinal lesions in, 442t
Anabolic steroids, in alcoholic patient, 711–712
Anacobon (flucytosine), in *Candida* esophagitis, 240
Anal encirclement, in fecal incontinence, 99
Anal fissure, 555–559
    atypical, 557
    etiology of, 555–556
    in children, 151
    in HIV-positive patient, 558–559

Anal fissure *(Continued)*
    pathogenesis of, 555–556
    physiology of, 555–556
    site of, 555
    symptoms of, 556–557
    treatment of, 557–558
Anal sphincter, anatomy of, 560, *561,* 586
    artificial, in fecal incontinence, 99
    external, 95
        in fecal incontinence, 96
    internal, 95
    stretch of, in anal fissure, 558
    surgical repair of, in fecal incontinence, 99–100
Anal wink, 95
Androgens, hepatotoxicity of, 650
    in α_1-antitrypsin deficiency, 799
Anemia, iron deficiency, in ulcerative colitis, 519
Aneurysm, cirsoid (Dieulafoy's vascular malformation), 137, 165, 428
Angina, microvascular, 172
Angiodysplasia, 425–427
    bleeding from, 137, 140–141, *141,* 160–162, 161t
Angiography, in angiodysplasia, 426
    in bleeding peptic ulcer, 130–131
    in diverticulosis coli, 512
    in gastrointestinal tract bleeding, 158
    in hepatocellular carcinoma, 773
    in lower gastrointestinal tract bleeding, 142–143
    in pancreatic cancer, 636
    in pediatric gastrointestinal tract bleeding, 149
Angioma, bleeding from, 140–141, 160–162
        treatment of, 161–162, 161t
        injection therapy for, 161
        of small bowel, 420
        thermal coagulation of, 161, 161t
Angiosarcoma, hepatic, 777–778
        resection of, 833
        toxin-induced, 648
Anorectal abscess, 560–565. See also *Abscess, anorectal.*
Anorectal angle, 529
Anorectal electromyography, in fecal incontinence, 97
Anorectal manometry, in fecal incontinence, 97
Anorectum, physiology of, 95
Anorexia nervosa, 9–15. See also *Eating disorders.*
    gastric emptying in, 248, 261
Anoscopy, in anal fissure, 557
Antacids, in esophageal stricture, 35
    in gastroesophageal reflux disease, 204
Anterior nerves of Laterjet, 345–346, *346*
Anthropometric measurements, in malnutrition, 18
Antiandrogens, in hepatocellular carcinoma, 774
Antibiotics, in abdominal abscess, 120
    in acute acalculous cholecystitis, 855
    in esophageal stricture, 34
    in intestinal obstruction, 114
    in peridiverticulitis, 512–513
    in spontaneous bacterial peritonitis, 728–729
    in toxic megacolon, 536
    in ulcerative colitis, 517
Anticholinergic agents, in esophageal motility disorders, 173
    in irritable bowel syndrome, 505, 506–507, 507t
    in noncardiac chest pain, 176
    in Zollinger-Ellison syndrome, 328

Anticolon antibodies, in primary sclerosing cholangitis, 743
Antidepressants, in eating disorders, 14
    in irritable bowel syndrome, 507t, 508
Antidiarrheal agents, 83t
    in infectious diarrhea, 540–542
    in irritable bowel syndrome, 505
    in ulcerative colitis, 517
Antiemetic agents, 52t—53t
    in delayed gastric emptying, 250–251, 276
Antiinflammatory agents, in infectious diarrhea, 542
Antimicrobial agents, in infectious diarrhea, 542–544, 543t
Antimitochondrial antibodies, in primary biliary cirrhosis, 751, 789–790
Antimotility agents, in infectious diarrhea, 541
Antisecretory agents, in infectious diarrhea, 541–542
Antispasmodic agents, in irritable bowel syndrome, 507, 507t
Antrectomy, in delayed gastric emptying, 257
    in peptic ulcer disease, 343
    in pyloric stenosis, 341
Antrum, in eosinophilic gastroenteritis, 360
Anus, basal cell carcinoma of, 570–571
    Bowen's disease of, 571
    motility of, 529
    Paget's disease of, 571
    squamous cell carcinoma of, 571–572
    trauma to, 151
    tumors of, 570–572, 571t
    verrucous cancer of, 571
Anxiolytic agents, in irritable bowel syndrome, 507t, 508
Aortoenteric fistula, bleeding from, 137–138
Aortography, in chronic mesenteric ischemia, 434, *434*
Aortomesenteric bypass, in chronic mesenteric ischemia, 435–436, *436*
Aphthous ulcers, in ulcerative colitis, 518
Appendectomy, laparoscopic, 466–467
Appendicitis, 462–469
    acute, 463–467
        antibiotics for, 465
        appendiceal mass with, 465–466
        clinical manifestations of, 463–464
        differential diagnosis of, 464–465
        etiology of, 463
        laboratory findings in, 464
        laparoscopic appendectomy in, 466–467
        pathophysiology of, 463
        radiographic findings in, 464
        surgical management of, 465
    chronic, 467–469
        clinical manifestation of, 468, 468t
        etiology of, 468
        incidence of, 468
        pathology of, 469
        treatment of, 469
    recurrent, 467–469
        clinical manifestation of, 468, 468t
        etiology of, 468
        incidence of, 468
        pathology of, 469
        treatment of, 469
Appendix, abscess of, 466
    anatomy of, 462–463
    mass in, 465–466

Apresoline (hydralazine), in esophageal motility disorders, 173, 176
    vitamin deficiency with, 25t
Arteriography, in pancreatic cancer, 638
Arteriohepatic dysplasia, liver transplantation in, 839
Arteriovenous malformation, bleeding from, 137, 140–141, *141,* 153, 160–162, 161t
    classification of, 425, 425t
    of small bowel, 420
Artery, caliber-persistent, of stomach, 137, 165, 428
Arthritis, colitic, 518
    collagenous colitis and, 596
    in primary biliary cirrhosis, 751, 751t
5-ASA (acetylsalicylic acid), in ulcerative colitis, 520
Asacol, in ulcerative colitis, 520
Ascites, 721–724. See also *Peritonitis, bacterial.*
    diagnosis of, 721–722
    etiology of, 721, 721t
    in eosinophilic gastroenteritis, 359
    laboratory analysis of, 722, 728
    management of, 723–724
    neutrocytic, 726
    pancreatic, in acute pancreatitis, 627
        in hereditary pancreatitis, 616
    pathophysiology of, 722–723
    protein concentration of, 725
    symptoms of, 721
    vs. spontaneous bacterial peritonitis, 722
Ascorbic acid, in parenteral iron overload, 813
Aspartate aminotransferase, in alcoholism, 708t
    in ischemic hepatitis, *692,* 693, 694
    serum, 781, 781t
Aspergillus, esophageal, 240
Aspiration, gastric, in fulminant hepatic failure, 685
Aspirin, in gastric ulcer, 312–313
    in gastritis, 319
    vitamin deficiency with, 25t
Atrial natriuretic peptide, in hepatorenal syndrome, 703
Atrophic gastritis, 320
    delayed gastric emptying in, 249
    vitamin deficiencies with, 27
Autoantibodies, in primary biliary cirrhosis, 751–752, 789–790
    in primary sclerosing cholangitis, 743
Autoimmune chronic active hepatitis, 678, 785
    in ulcerative colitis, 519
    primary sclerosing cholangitis and, 746
    vs. primary biliary cirrhosis, 755
Azathioprine, in primary biliary cirrhosis, 756
    in ulcerative colitis, 516, 521
    nodular regenerative hyperplasia with, 648

B

Bacille Calmette-Guérin (BCG), hepatic granulomatosis with, 764
Bacillus, esophageal, 243
Back pain, in pancreatic cancer, 639
Backwash ileitis, ileal pouch—anal anastomosis in, 526
Bacteremia, in salmonellosis, 382t, 384
Bacteria, overgrowth of, 398–402. See also *Blind loop syndrome.*
Bacterial peritonitis, 724–730. See also *Peritonitis, bacterial.*
Bacteriascites, 726–727, *727.* See also *Ascites.*

BAL (British antilewisite), in Wilson's disease, 807
Balloon dilation, of pyloric stenosis, 341
Balloon distension test, of esophageal dysfunction, 198, *199*
Balloon tamponade, in variceal bleeding, 716
Band ligation, in variceal bleeding, 134, 716–717, 719
Barbiturates, in fulminant hepatic failure, 684
Barium study, in achalasia, 187, *188*
    in acute appendicitis, 464
    in intestinal obstruction, 113–114, 494
    in pediatric gastrointestinal tract bleeding, 149
Barrett's esophagus, 225
    adenocarcinoma and, 206–207, 219
    in gastroesophageal reflux disease, 206–207
Basal cell carcinoma, anal, 570–571
BCG (bacille Calmette-Guérin), hepatic granulomatosis with, 764
Beanase (Beano), 74
Behavior therapy, in functional abdominal pain syndromes, 67
    in irritable bowel syndrome, 500–501
Belching, upper esophageal sphincter in, 183–184
Bentiromide (Chymex) test, in malabsorption syndromes, 78
Bentyl (dicyclomine hydrochloride), in functional abdominal pain syndromes, 65
    in irritable bowel syndrome, 506–507, 507t
Benzodiazepines, in alcohol withdrawal, 708
    in irritable bowel syndrome, 507t, 508
Beriberi, postgastrectomy, 26–27
Bernstein test, in gastroesophageal reflux disease, 203
Bethanechol (Urecholine), in chronic constipation, 104
    in delayed gastric emptying, 255, 278
    in gastroesophageal reflux disease, 203t, 204
    in pediatric gastroesophageal reflux, 209–210
Bezoars, 280–283, 281t
    acetylcysteine in, 281, 281t
    cellulase in, 281, 282t
    clinical manifestation of, 280–281
    endoscopic treatment of, 282
    laser therapy of, 282
    lithotripsy for, 282
    papain in, 281–282, 281t
    surgery for, 282
    treatment of, 281–282, 281t, 282t
Bile acid malabsorption, 93
Bile acid therapy, in gallstones, 862–863
Bile duct(s), 788–790
    bleeding from, 138
    cysts of, 814–826. See also *Choledochal cysts.*
    gallstones in, 882–890. See also *Choledocholithiasis.*
    in acute pancreatitis, 634
    infection of, 876–881. See also *Cholangitis, bacterial.*
    strictures of, 895–902
        benign, 896–897, *898, 899*
        diagnosis of, 989–900
        dilation in, 900
        dilation of, 900
        endoscopic therapy in, 900–901
        iatrogenic, 897, *899*
        in primary sclerosing cholangitis, 746, 869, 894, 897, *898*
        malignant, 895–896, *896, 897*
        mass effect in, 897
        stenting in, 900–901
        treatment of, 900–902

Bile duct(s) *(Continued)*
  tumors of, 904t, 906–910
    chemotherapy in, 910
    clinical presentation of, 906
    diagnosis of, 906–907, 907t
    in primary sclerosing cholangitis, 746
    incidence of, 906
    palliative biliary decompression in, 908–910, *908, 909,* 910t
    pathology of, 906
    radiation therapy in, 910
    treatment of, 907–910
Bilharziasis, 388–393, 763t, 765. See also *Schistosomiasis.*
Biliary colic, 849
Biliary sclerosis, drug-induced, 647
Biliary stent, in acute bacterial cholangitis, 880, *880*
  in bile duct strictures, 900–901
  in cholangiocarcinoma, 777, 908–910, *908, 909,* 910t
  in choledocholithiasis, 890
Biliary-enteric bypass, in bile duct strictures, 901
Bilirubin, serum, 781–782, 781t
Billroth I operation, for gastric ulcer, 348–349
Binge eating disorder, 10. See also *Eating disorders.*
Biofeedback, in fecal incontinence, 98–99, 99t
Biotin, deficiency of, 26t
Bismuth subsalicylate (Pepto-Bismol), in infectious diarrhea, 541–542, 545
Blastomycosis, esophageal, 241
Bleeding, from esophageal varices, 714–720. See also *Esophageal varices, bleeding of.*
  from lower gastrointestinal tract, 139–144. See also *Gastrointestinal tract bleeding, lower.*
  from upper gastrointestinal tract, 126–139, *127,* 128t. See also *Gastrointestinal tract bleeding, upper.*
Blind loop syndrome, 398–402
  ^{14}C-cholylglycine breath test in, 400
  clinical features of, 399–400
  diagnosis of, 400–401, *401*
  malabsorption in, 82, 83t
  pathophysiology of, 399
  treatment of, 401–402
  [^{14}C]-*d*xylose breath test in, 400–401
Bloating, intestinal, 70–74, *71.* See also *Gas, intestinal.*
β-Blockers, for portal pressure reduction, 134
Blood transfusion, in upper gastrointestinal tract bleeding, 128–129
Blood urea nitrogen, in ischemic hepatitis, 693
Body mass index, 3
Boerhaave's syndrome, vs. Mallory-Weiss tear, 136
Bone disease, metabolic, in primary biliary cirrhosis, 753–754
Boric acid, vitamin deficiency with, 25t
Botulinum toxin, in achalasia, 192
Bougienage, in achalasia, 189
  in esophageal foreign bodies, 44
  in esophageal stricture, 35
Boutonneuse fever, hepatic granuloma in, 759
Bowel. See *Intestine.*
Bowel cleanings, in hepatic encephalopathy, 657
Bowel retraining, in irritable bowel syndrome, 500
Bowel sounds, in abdominal abscess, 117
  in intestinal obstruction, 111, 113
Bowen's disease, 571
Bradydysrhythmia, in fulminant hepatic failure, 685

Bradygastria, 250
Brain, schistosomiasis of, 392
Brainerd diarrhea, 92
Breast cancer, primary biliary cirrhosis and, 751, 751t
Breath test, in blind loop syndrome, 400
  in lactose intolerance, 363–364
British antilewisite (BAL), in Wilson's disease, 807
Bromocriptine, in hepatic encephalopathy, 658
Bronchopulmonary dysplasia, intestinal pseudoobstruction and, 449
Brooke ileostomy, 530–531, *530*
Brown bag maneuver, 786
Brucellas, 764
Brucellosis, granulomas of, 762t
  hepatic, 762t, 764
Brunner's gland, abnormalities of, 421
Budd-Chiari syndrome, drug-induced, 647
  in hepatic sarcoidosis, 763
Bulimia nervosa, 9–15. See also *Eating disorders.*
  delayed gastric emptying in, 248
  laxative use in, 103
  rapid gastric emptying in, 261
Bulking agents, in irritable bowel syndrome, 506, 507t
Burns, esophageal, 30–35, 31t, 33t, 34t
Buschke-Löwenstein tumor, anal, 571
Button battery ingestion, 32, 45
Butyric acid, colonocyte utilization of, 591
Byler's syndrome, liver transplantation in, 839

C

CA 19-9, in pancreatic cancer, 636–637
CA 125, in endometriosis, 577
Calcification, pancreatic, in hereditary pancreatitis, 615, *616*
Calcium, in lactose malabsorption, 365–366
  replacement therapy with, 79t
Calcium channel blockers, in esophageal motility disorders, 173
  in hepatorenal syndrome, 703
  in irritable bowel syndrome, 507t, 508
  in noncardiac chest pain, 176
Calcium infusion test, in Zollinger-Ellison syndrome, 324, *325, 326*
Caliber-persistent artery of the stomach, 137, 165, 428
Calicivirus, 662
Camplobacteriosis, 385–386
Campylobacter, in diarrhea, 538, 543t, 544
  in proctitis, 602t, 605
  invasive infection with, 385–386
Campylobacter fetus, invasive infection with, 383t, 385–386
Campylobacter jejuni, invasive infection with, 383t, 385–386
  toxigenic diarrhea with, 379–380
Candida albicans, esophageal, 238–241, 239t
  complications of, 238–239
  diagnosis of, 238–239
  treatment of, 239–240, 239t
  in acute acalculous cholecystitis, 854
  in pruritus ani, 568
Cap polyps, 548
Carafate (sucralfate), bezoar with, 280
  in gastroesophageal reflux disease, 203t, 204
Carbohydrate infusion, in fulminant hepatic failure, 682
Carcinoembryonic antigen (CEA), 307
  in hepatic metastases, 835

Carcinoid crisis, 310
Carcinoid heart disease, 310–311
Carcinoid syndrome, 305, 307
  crisis of, 310
Carcinoid tumor, 305–311
  biologic markers for, 306–307
  chemotherapy for, 309–310
  diarrhea with, 93
  hepatic artery embolization for, 308–309
  octreotide acetate for, 308
  pharmacologic treatment of, 307–308
  presentation of, 305–306, 360t
  surgery for, 309
Carcinoma, anal, 571–572
  choledochal cysts and, 821–822, 824
  esophageal, 219–223. See also *Esophageal carcinoma.*
  gastric, 289–294. See also *Gastric adenocarcinoma.*
  hepatic, 771–777. See also *Cholangiocarcinoma; Hepatocellular carcinoma.*
  pancreatic, 635–639. See also *Pancreatic carcinoma.*
  ulcerative colitis and, 520, 525
Cardiac output, decrease in, liver in, 782–783
Caries, dental, in eating disorders, 11
Caroli's disease, 821, 824
Cathartic agents, in chronic constipation, 103–104
Cathartic colon, 103
Catheters, central venous, in intestinal obstruction, 114
  in fulminant hepatic failure, 679
Caustic ingestion, 30–35, 31t, 33t, 34t, 320
  endoscopic evaluation of, 33–34, 33t, 34t
  management of, 32–33, 33t, 34t
  pathophysiology of, 31–32, 31t
Cavernous hemangioma, of small bowel, 420
Cecum, distension of, 112
  volvulus of, in intestinal obstruction, 110
Celiac compression syndrome, in chronic mesenteric ischemia, 435
Celiac sprue, 81, 82t, 83t, 367–371. See also *Sprue, celiac.*
Cellulase, in bezoar therapy, 281, 282t
Central nervous system, schistosomiasis of, 392
Central venous catheter, in intestinal obstruction, 114
Cephalosporin, vitamin deficiency with, 25t
Cercarial dermatitis, 389–390
Cerebral edema, in acute hepatitis, 663
  in fulminant hepatic failure, 683–684
Cerebral palsy, intestinal pseudoobstruction in, 449
Cerebral perfusion pressure, in fulminant hepatic failure, 683
Ceruloplasmin, serum, 803
Chagas' disease, gastrointestinal lesions in, 443t
Chemoembolization, in hepatocellular carcinoma, 774
Chemoreceptor trigger zone, in vomiting, 48
Chemotherapy, in carcinoid syndrome, 309–310
  in cholangiocarcinoma, 777, 910
  in esophageal cancer, 222–223, 225
  in gallbladder cancer, 905–906
  in gastric cancer, 293, 294t
  in gastric lymphoma, 298, 299
  in hepatocellular carcinoma, 774
  in pancreatic cancer, 639
  in radiation colitis, 430
  in Zollinger-Ellison syndrome, 331–333, 332t
  vomiting with, 55–56, 55t

Chenodeoxycholic acid, in gallstones, 862–863
  in protoporphyrin, 740
Chest pain, noncardiac, 171–176, 186–187. See also *Achalasia.*
  antireflux therapy in, 173
  diagnosis of, 172
  gastroesophageal reflux in, 171–172
  management of, 174–176, *175*
  tests for, 172–174, 197–198, *199*
  visceral nociception in, 172, 197–198, *199*
Childhood visceral myopathy, gastrointestinal lesions in, 442t
  intestinal pseudoobstruction syndrome in, 441, 441t, 445
Children, anal fissures in, 151
  anal trauma in, 151
  antibiotic-associated enterocolitis in, 152
  arteriovenous malformation in, 153
  coagulopathy in, 146–147
  Crohn's disease in, 153
  fecal incontinence in, 98
  foreign bodies in, 41–46, *42*
    algorithm for, *45*
    complications of, 46
    diagnosis of, 42–43
    metal detector evaluation of, 43
    radiographic examination for, 42–43
    rectal, 46
    signs of, 42
    swallowed, 43–46, *44, 45,* 46t
    symptoms of, 42
  gastroesophageal reflux disease in, 207–210
    clinical presentation of, 208
    diagnosis of, 208–209
    treatment of, 209–210
  gastrointestinal tract bleeding in, 145–154
    diagnosis of, 145–149, 146t, *147*
    esophagogastroduodenoscopy in, 147–148
    lower, 151–153, 151t
    upper, 149–151, 150t
  hemangioma in, 153
  hemolytic-uremic syndrome in, 153
  Henoch-Schönlein purpura in, 153
  infectious diarrhea in, 152
  inflammatory bowel disease in, 153
  intestinal pseudoobstruction in, 448–456
    diagnosis of, 450–454, 451t, *453, 454*
    etiology of, 449
    pathology of, 449–450
    treatment of, 454–456
  intestinal tract duplication in, 152
  intussusception in, 109, 115, 152
  Meckel's diverticulum in, 152
  midgut malrotation in, 151
  milk intolerance in, 151–152
  necrotizing enterocolitis in, 151
  nodular lymphoid hyperplasia in, 153
  peptic ulcer in, 145–146, 150
  polyps in, 152–153
  rapid gastric emptying in, 261
  telangiectasias in, 153
  visceral myopathy in, 441, 442t, 445
Chlamydia trachomatis, in proctitis, 602t, 603
Chlorambucil, in primary biliary cirrhosis, 756
Chlordiazepoxide, in alcohol withdrawal, 708t

Chlormethiazole, in alcohol withdrawal, 708t
Chlorpromazine, in porphyria, 735
    vitamin deficiency with, 25t
Cholangiocarcinoma, 775–777, 906–910
    clinical presentation of, 775
    diagnosis of, 906–907, 907t
    epidemiology of, 775
    growth of, 775
    hepatic resection in, 833
    hilar, 776
    histology of, 775
    in Caroli's disease, 821
    liver transplantation for, 777
    palliation for, 777
    pathology of, 906
    radiologic assessment of, 775–776
    resection of, 776
    risk factors for, 775
    toxin-induced, 648
    treatment of, 776–777, 907–910
Cholangiography, in choledocholithiasis, 886
    in gallstones, 850, 862
Cholangitis, bacterial, 877–881
        diagnosis of, 878
        in primary sclerosing cholangitis, 746
        pathophysiology of, 877
        presentation of, 877
        treatment of, 878–881, *879, 880,* 880t
    choledochal cysts and, 821
    choledocholithiasis with, 887–888
    destructive, nonsuppurative, chronic. See *Primary biliary cirrhosis.*
Cholecystectomy, diarrhea after, 91
    in acute acalculous cholecystitis, 855–856
    in chronic acalculous cholecystitis, 857
    in gallstone disease, 850–851
Cholecystitis, 848–857
    acalculous, 853–857, 861
        acute, 849, 853–856
            clinical presentation of, 854–855
            evaluation of, 855
            management of, 855–856
            pathogenesis of, 853–854, 854t
        chronic, 849, 849t, 856–857
        emphysematous, 854
    acute, 849, 860–861
    chronic, 848–852, 861
        definition of, 849
        diagnosis of, 849–850
        management of, 850–852
        pathogenesis of, 849, 849t
    emphysematous, 861
    necrotizing. See *Cholecystitis, acalculous, acute.*
Cholecystography, oral, in gallstones, 850, 861–862
Cholecystokinin (CCK) test, in chronic acalculous cholecystitis, 857
Cholecystokinin receptor antagonists, in delayed gastric emptying, 256
Choledochal cysts, 814–826
    classification of, *186,* 815–817
    clinical features of, 818–819, 819t
    complications of, 821–822, 821t
    diagnosis of, 819–821, *820*

Choledochal cysts *(Continued)*
    epidemiology of, 814
    pathogenesis of, 814–815, *815*
    pathology of, 817–818, *818*
    treatment of, *822,* 822–825, *823,* 824t, 826t
Choledochocele, 897
Choledochocystoduodenostomy, in choledochal cysts, 822, *822*
Choledochocystojejunostomy, in choledochal cysts, 822, *822*
Choledochoduodenostomy, in primary sclerosing cholangitis, 747
Choledochojejunostomy, in primary sclerosing cholangitis, 747
Choledocholithiasis, 882–890
    abdominal radiographs in, 885
    abdominal ultrasonography in, 885–886
    acute pancreatitis with, 888
    bacterial cholangitis in, 885
    biliary colic in, 887
    biliary obstruction in, 884–885, 887
    biliary stenting in, 890
    cholangitis with, 887–888
    complications of, 884–885
    computed tomography in, 886
    endoscopic retrograde cholangiopancreatography in, 886
    endoscopic shock wave methods in, 889
    endoscopic sphincterotomy in, 888–889
    endoscopic ultrasound in, 887
    extracorporeal shock wave lithotripsy in, 889
    gallstone pancreatitis in, 885
    intrahepatic duct stones with, 888
    intraoperative cholangiogram in, 886
    laboratory diagnosis in, 884
    liquid dissolution in, 890
    mechanical lithotripsy in, 889
    natural history of, 882–883
    pathogenesis of, 882
    percutaneous transhepatic cholangiogram in, 886
    percutaneous transhepatic choledochoscopy in, 890
    physical findings in, 884
    predispositions to, 883, 883t
    radionuclide biliary imaging in, 885
    stone extraction in, 890
    symptoms of, 883–884
    treatment of, 887–888
Cholelithiasis, 858–863
    acalculous cholecystitis in, 861
    acute cholecystitis in, 860–861
    bile acid therapy in, 862–863
    biliary colic in, 860
    black, 859–860, 860t, 882
    brown, 860, 860t, 882
    cholecystectomy in, 862
    cholesterol, 858–859, 858t, 882
    chronic cholecystitis in, 861
    clinical manifestations of, 860–861
    contact dissolution in, 863
    diagnosis of, 861–862
    diagnostic studies in, 861–862
    epidemiology of, 858, 859t
    extracorporeal shock wave lithotripsy in, 863
    imaging of, 850
    in bile duct, 882–890. See also *Choledocholithiasis.*
    in short bowel syndrome, 458
    inflammatory bowel disease and, 748

Cholelithiasis (Continued)
    natural history of, 860
    pathogenesis of, 858–860
    pigment, 859–860, 860t, 882
    recurrent, 853
    treatment of, 862–863
Cholera toxin, 372–374, 373t
Cholestasis, 864–872, 865t. See also *Primary biliary cirrhosis; Primary sclerosing cholangitis.*
    drug-induced, 646, 647
        vs. primary biliary cirrhosis, 754
    familial, intrahepatic, 847–848
    in hepatic sarcoidosis, 763
    neonatal, α_1-antitrypsin deficiency in, 847
    total parenteral nutrition—induced, 460–461
Cholesterol, gallstone formation from, 858–859, 858t, 882
    serum, in primary biliary cirrhosis, 751, 755
Cholestyramine, 755
    in infectious diarrhea, 540–541
    in neonatal cholestasis, 848
    in primary biliary cirrhosis, 790
    in primary sclerosing cholangitis, 893
    in protoporphyrin, 740
    vitamin deficiency with, 25t
^{14}C-Cholylglycine breath test, in blind loop syndrome, 400
Chronic intestinal ischemic syndrome, 433–437
    aortomesenteric bypass in, 435–436
    clinical presentation of, 433
    diagnosis of, 434–435, *434*
    percutaneous transluminal angioplasty in, 435
    recurrence of, 437
    transaortic endarterectomy in, 435, 436, *436*
Chronic intestinal pseudoobstruction, 438–447
    biopsy in, 446
    blood tests in, 445
    childhood, 448–456
        diagnosis of, 450–451, 451t
        etiology of, 449
        manometry in, 451–454, *453, 454*
        misdiagnosis of, 451
        pathology of, 449–450
        treatment of, 454–456
        visceral myopathies in, 441, 441t, 442t—443t, 445
    clinical manifestations of, 438–439, *438*
    connective tissue disease in, 445
    diagnosis of, 439, *439,* 440t
    etiology of, 440–445, 441t, 442t—443t
    extragastrointestinal manifestations of, 439
    familial visceral myopathies in, 440–441, 441t, 442t—443t
    familial visceral neuropathies in, 441, 441t, 442t—443t, 445t
    manometry in, 446
    prognosis for, 446–447
    radiologic tests in, *444*, 445
    treatment of, 446–447
    vs. mechanical obstruction, 440t
Chronic nonsuppurative destructive cholangitis. See *Primary biliary cirrhosis.*
Chronic obstructive pulmonary disease, pneumatosis cystoides intestinalis with, 582
Chubby cheeks, in eating disorders, 11
Churg-Strauss syndrome, 321
Chymex (bentiromide) test, in malabsorption syndromes, 78

Cigarette smoking, in α_1-antitrypsin deficiency, 799
Ciguatoxin, 380
Cimetidine, in fulminant hepatic failure, 686
    in gastric ulcer, 315
    in pediatric peptic ulcer, 150
    in Zollinger-Ellison syndrome, 326–327, 327t
    vitamin deficiency with, 25t
Cirrhosis, alcoholic, 712–713. See also *Alcoholic liver disease.*
    biliary, primary, 749–757. See also *Primary biliary cirrhosis.*
    in hepatocellular carcinoma, 772
    vitamin deficiencies in, 29, 29t
Cirrhotic ascites, 721–724. See also *Ascites.*
    spontaneous bacterial peritonitis in, 725
Cirsoid aneurysm (Dieulafoy's vascular malformation), 137, 165, 428
Cisapride (Propulsid), in childhood intestinal pseudoobstruction, 456
    in chronic constipation, 104
    in delayed gastric emptying, 253–254, 277
    in dyspepsia, 58
    in gastroesophageal reflux disease, 203t, 204, 210
    in irritable bowel syndrome, 500
    in pediatric gastroesophageal reflux, 210
    side effects of, 254
Clam-diggers' itch, 389
Clonazepam, in porphyria, 735
Clostridium difficile, characteristics of, 404
    culture of, 405
    diarrhea with, 89–90, 403–408, 538, 543t
        diagnosis of, 405–406, *406, 407*
        historical perspective on, 403–404
        pathogenesis of, 405
        prevention of, 408
        treatment of, 406–408
    identification of, 405–406, *406, 407*
    in proctitis, 602t, 606
    toxins of, 404
Clostridium perfringens, in acalculous cholecystitis, 854
    in acute cholecystitis, 861
    in pneumatosis cystoides intestinalis, 581
    toxigenic diarrhea with, 379
Clotrimazole, in *Candida* esophagitis, 239, 239t
Coagulation, in acute pancreatitis, 625
    in children, 146–147
    in fulminant hepatic failure, 687
    in ulcerative colitis, 519
Cobalamin, replacement therapy with, 29t
Cocaine, hepatotoxicity of, 651
Coccidioidomycosis, granulomas of, 763t
Codeine, in fecal incontinence, 98
Coffee-bean sign, 493
Cognitive behavior therapy, in functional abdominal pain syndromes, 67
Coins. See *Children, foreign bodies in.*
Colchicine, in alcoholic cirrhosis, 712
    in primary biliary cirrhosis, 756, 869, 870t
    vitamin deficiency with, 25t
Colectomy, in chronic constipation, 105–106
    in toxic megacolon, 536–537
Colestipol, in primary sclerosing cholangitis, 893
    vitamin deficiency with, 25t

Colitis, antibiotic-associated, *Clostridium difficile* in, 404, 407
  collagenous, 92, 595–599
    celiac sprue with, 369
    clinical features of, 595
    colonoscopy in, 596
    differential diagnosis of, 597–598, 597t
    etiology of, 598–599
    illnesses associated with, 596, 596t
    laboratory features of, 595–596
    pathogenesis of, 598
    pathology of, 596–597
    radiology of, 596
    treatment of, 599
    vs. celiac sprue, 596
  diversion, 590–594, 593t
    clinical presentation of, 591
    differential diagnosis of, 591–592, 593t
    pathogenesis of, 590–591
    pathology of, 592
    radiographic features of, 591–592
    treatment of, 592–594
  granulomatous. See *Crohn's disease*.
  indeterminate, ileal pouch—anal anastomosis in, 525
  infectious, 537–545, 593t. See also *Diarrhea, infectious*.
  ischemic, 593t
  lymphocytic, 599
    celiac sprue with, 369–370
  microscopic, 92, 599
  pseudomembranous, 593t
    Clostridium difficile in, 404–405
    Clostridium perfringens in, 379
    Hirschsprung's disease—associated, 472, 472t
    sigmoidoscopy in, 405–406, *406*
  radiation, 430–432, 593t
  ulcerative, 514–532, 593t. See also *Ulcerative colitis*.
Colitis cystica profunda, 548
Collagen, in rectal ulcers, 586
Collagen band, in collagenous colitis, 596–597
Collagen vascular disease, esophageal, 185
  liver in, 785
Collagenous colitis, 595–599. See also *Colitis, collagenous*.
Collagenous sprue, 370
Colon, cancer of, diarrhea with, 93
    in ulcerative colitis, 520
  cathartic, 103
  diverticular disease of, 510–513. See also *Diverticulosis coli*.
  dysplasia of, in ulcerative colitis, 520
  foreign bodies in, 39–40
  hemangiomatosis of, 427
  hemorrhoids of, bleeding from, 165
  in irritable bowel syndrome, 498
  in short bowel syndrome, 458
  motility of. See *Constipation, chronic*.
  polyps of, 547–548
    in schistosomiasis, 391
  pseudoobstruction of (Ogilvie's syndrome), 106, 116
  transit study of, in irritable bowel syndrome, 498
  ulcers of, 588
    Hirschsprung's disease—associated, 472, 472t
Colonoscopy, in diverticulosis coli, 512
  in lower gastrointestinal tract bleeding, 142
  in pediatric gastrointestinal tract bleeding, 148
  in tropical sprue, 396

Colostomy, in fecal incontinence, 100
CoLyte, in chronic constipation, 104
Computed tomography, in abdominal abscess, 118–119, *119*
  in achalasia, 189
  in acute bacterial cholangitis, 878
  in choledochal cysts, 819, *820*
  in choledocholithiasis, 886
  in endometriosis, 576
  in hepatocellular carcinoma, 773
  in pancreatic cancer, 636
  in pneumatosis cystoides intestinalis, 583
Condyloma acuminata, in proctitis, 604
Condyloma latum, 602
Congenital megacolon. See *Hirschsprung's disease*.
Connective tissue disease, gastrointestinal lesions in, 442t
  intestinal pseudoobstruction syndrome in, 445
Constipation, 100–106, 499–500
  chronic, 100–106, 101t
    cathartics for, 103–104
    diagnosis of, 101–102
    dietary fiber for, 102–103
    drug-induced, 101, 101t
    enemas for, 105
    etiology of, 100–101, 101t
    exercise in, 102
    laxatives for, 103–104
    primary, 100–101, 101t
    prokinetic agents for, 104–105
    rectoanal inhibitor reflex impairment in, 105
    secondary, 101, 101t
    surgical approaches to, 105–106
  differential diagnosis of, 477
  in Hirschsprung's disease, 470, 471
  in irritable bowel syndrome, 499–500. See also *Irritable bowel syndrome, constipation-predominant*.
Continence, fecal, 95. See also *Fecal incontinence*.
Continuous arteriovenous hemofiltration, in hepatorenal syndrome, 704
Contraceptives, hepatic adenoma with, 648
  hepatic vein thrombosis with, 647
Controlled mandatory ventilation, in fulminant hepatic failure, 686
Copper, hepatic accumulation of, 802–808. See also *Wilson's disease*.
  urinary, 803–804
Coronary artery disease, gastroesophageal reflux in, 176
Corticosteroids, in acute hepatitis, 663
  in alcoholic patient, 711
  in Crohn's disease, 411
  in eosinophilic gastroenteritis, 361
  in esophageal stricture, 34–35
  in primary biliary cirrhosis, 756
  in ulcerative colitis, 516, 520, 521
Corynebacterium minutissimum, in pruritus ani, 568
Cotazyme, 81t
Cough, in gastroesophageal reflux disease, 206
Courvoisier's gallbladder, 788
Creatinine, in hepatorenal syndrome, 696
  in ischemic hepatitis, 693
Creon, 81t
CREST (calcinosis cutis, Raynaud's phenomenon, esophageal dysfunction, sclerodactyly, and telangiectasia) syndrome, primary biliary cirrhosis in, 425, 751, 751t

Cricopharyngeal achalasia, 179–182, *179–181*
Cricopharyngeal bar, 182
Cricopharyngeal muscle, 177
    dysfunction of, 179–182, *179–181*
        CNS disorders and, 183
        secondary, 182
    electromyography of, 181, *181*
Crohn's disease, 408–413, 593t
    anal fissure in, 557
    anorectal abscess with, 564–565
    antibiotics in, 410–411
    antiinflammatory drug therapy in, 411
    diet in, 409–410
    gallstones in, 748
    gastric outlet obstruction and, 265
    gastrointestinal tract bleeding with, 153
    immunomodulatory drugs in, 411–412
    immunosuppressive drugs in, 411–412
    malabsorption in, 81, 83t
    patient education in, 409
    Pentasa in, 515
    symptomatic therapy of, 410, 410t
    vitamin deficiencies in, 28, 29t
    vs. collagenous colitis, 597
Cronkhite-Canada syndrome, 423
Cryptosporidium, in acute acalculous cholecystitis, 854
    in infectious diarrhea, 544
    in proctitis, 606
Cullen sign, in hereditary pancreatitis, 615
Current jelly stool, in intussusception, 109
Cushing's disease, vs. Cushing's syndrome, 331
Cutaneous hypersensitivity, in malnutrition, 18
Cyanoacrylate, for gastric varices, 163
Cycloserine, vitamin deficiency with, 25t
Cyclosporine, in Crohn's disease, 412
    in primary biliary cirrhosis, 756, 869, 871t
    in ulcerative colitis, 516–517, 521
Cyst, choledochal, 814–826. See also *Choledochal cysts.*
Cystic fibrosis, malabsorption in, 80
Cystoenterostomy, in choledochal cysts, 822, *822*
Cystolithiasis, in choledochal cysts, 821
Cytomegalovirus, esophageal, 241–242
    in proctitis, 602t, 606
    neonatal, 846
Cytotoxin, 372

D

Danazol, in α_1-antitrypsin deficiency, 799
Defecography, in fecal incontinence, 97
    in rectal ulcers, 585
Deferoxamine, in parenteral iron overload, 813
Deglutition, upper esophageal sphincter in, 178, *178*, 178t
Dehydration, in acute acalculous cholecystitis, 853
    in infectious diarrhea, 539–540, 540t
Delayed cutaneous hypersensitivity, in malnutrition, 18
Delayed gastric emptying, 54, 54t, 247–250, 248t. See also
        Gastroparesis.
    gastritis and, 249
    gastroenteritis and, 249
    idiopathic, 249–250
    in diabetes mellitus, 247–248, 249
    in eating disorders, 248

Delayed gastric emptying *(Continued)*
    in gastric smooth muscle disorders, 248–249
    in gastroesophageal reflux disease, 250
    in hyperthyroidism, 249
    in neuropathic disorders, 249
    in nonulcer dyspepsia, 250
    in peptic ulcer disease, 250
    ischemic, 249
    mechanical obstruction in, 247
    medication-induced, 249, 249t
    postoperative gastric stasis and, 248
    treatment of, 250–257
        antiemetics in, 250–251
        bethanechol in, 255
        cholecystokinin receptor antagonists in, 256
        cisapride in, 253–254
        domperidone in, 252–253
        erythromycin in, 255
        hydration in, 250
        5-hydroxytryptamine receptor antagonists in, 256
        leuprolide acetate in, 255–256
        metoclopramide in, 251–252
        nutrition in, 250, 256–257
        opiate receptor antagonists in, 256
        prokinetics in, 251–256, 251t
        surgery in, 256–257
Demeclocycline, in hepatorenal syndrome, 702
Depression, in eating disorders, 12
    in obesity, 8
Dermatitis, cercarial, 389–390
Dermatitis herpetiformis, jejunal mucosal lesions in, 371
Dermatomyositis, gastrointestinal lesions in, 442t
Desipramine, in functional abdominal pain syndromes, 65t
Desmopressin (DDAVP), in variceal bleeding, 714
Dextrose, in fulminant hepatic failure, 683
Diabetes mellitus, delayed gastric emptying in, 247–248, 270
    fecal incontinence in, 96–97
    gastrointestinal lesions in, 443t
    in hereditary pancreatitis, 616
    rapid gastric emptying in, 261
Diarrhea, 87–94
    acute, 89–90, 89t
    Brainerd, 92
    chronic, 90–94, 90t, 91t
        physical examination in, 88–89
    classification of, 87
    Clostridium difficile in, 403–408, *406, 407*
    diabetic, malabsorption in, 83t
    drug-induced, 92
    evaluation of, 87–89, 88t
    hormonal, vs. collagenous colitis, 598
    iatrogenic, 91
    idiopathic, 93–94
    in blind loop syndrome, 401
    in carcinoid syndrome, 307–308
    in Crohn's disease, 410, 410t
    in fecal incontinence, 96–97
    in inflammatory bowel disease, 92–93
    in irritable bowel syndrome, 502–508, *503.* See also
        Irritable bowel syndrome, diarrhea-prone.
    in malabsorption syndromes, 75, 93
    in malignancy, 93

Diarrhea *(Continued)*
  in systemic diseases, 92
  infectious, 92, 381–387, 537–545
    Aeromonas in, 383t, 387
    Campylobacter in, 383t, 385–386
    Escherichia coli in, 383t, 386–387
    Plesiomonas in, 387
    Salmonella in, 382t, 384–385
    Shigella in, 381, 382t, 384
    Vibrio in, 383t, 387
    Yersinia in, 383t, 386
  laxative abuse and, 92
  medical history in, 88
  pharmacologic treatment of, 83t
  physical examination in, 88–89
  postsurgical, 91
  radiation-induced, 92
  social history in, 88
  toxigenic, 372–380
    Aeromonas in, 378–379
    Campylobacter in, 379–380
    Clostridium in, 379
    Escherichia coli in, 374–376, 374t, 375t
    host factors in, 372
    Plesiomonas shigelloides in, 376
    Salmonella in, 377–378, 377t
    seafood consumption in, 380
    Shigella in, 377
    Staphylococcus in, 378
    Vibrio cholerae in, 372–374, 373t
    Vibrio parahaemolyticus in, 374
    Yersinia in, 378
  traveler's, 543–544, 543t, 545t
Dicyclomine hydrochloride (Bentyl), in functional abdominal pain syndromes, 65
  in irritable bowel syndrome, 506–507, 507t
Diet, after endorectal ileal pullthrough procedure, 552
  gluten-free, 82t, 368–369
  in bezoar prevention, 282–283
  in blind loop syndrome, 402
  in celiac sprue, 368–369
  in chronic constipation, 102–103
  in Crohn's disease, 409–410
  in diarrhea, 88
  in dyspepsia, 59
  in esophageal carcinoma, 219
  in fecal incontinence, 98, 98t
  in gastroesophageal reflux disease, 203
  in hepatic encephalopathy, 655–656, 656t
  in hereditary pancreatitis, 618
  in irritable bowel syndrome, 64–65, 506, 507t
  in porphyria, 733–734
  in pruritus ani, 568
  in short bowel syndrome, 459–460, 460t
  in ulcerative colitis, 517
  in undernutrition, 19
  restrictive, vitamin deficiency and, 23–24, 23t
Dietary history, in malnutrition, 17–18
Dieulafoy's vascular malformation, 137, 165, 428
Diffuse esophageal spasm, dysphagia with, 188
  manometric evaluation of, 196
Diflucan (fluconazole), in *Candida* esophagitis, 239t, 240
Diiodohydroxyquin (iodoquinol), in amebic abscess, 771

Dilation, esophageal, balloon, 227–228
  contraindications to, 229–230
  hazards of, 229–230
  Maloney mercury-filled bougies in, 228–229, 229t
  wire-guided, 226–227, *226*, *227*
  pneumatic, in achalasia, 189–192, *190*, 190t, *191*
  vs. esophagomyotomy, 191
Diloxanide, in amebic abscess, 771
Dimercaprol, in Wilson's disease, 807
16,16-Dimethyl prostaglandin E_2, in fulminant hepatic failure, 680–681
Diphenoxylate (Lomotil), in fecal incontinence, 98
  in functional abdominal pain syndromes, 65
  in infectious diarrhea, 541
  in irritable bowel syndrome, 505, 506, 507t
  in ulcerative colitis, 517
Disaccharidase assay, in lactose intolerance, 364
Disodium cromoglycate, in irritable bowel syndrome, 507t, 508
Disseminated intravascular coagulation, in acute pancreatitis, 625
Distension, intestinal, 70–74, *71*. See also *Gas, intestinal.*
  in dyspepsia, 58, *59*
  in functional abdominal pain syndromes, 62
  in intestinal obstruction, 111, 112
Disulfiram, in alcohol abstinence, 709
Diversion colitis, 590–594, 593t. See also *Colitis, diversion.*
Diverticulosis coli, 510–513
  abscess in, 513
  bleeding from, 141
  classification of, 510, 511t
  diarrhea with, 92–93
  epidemiology of, 510
  fistula in, 513
  hemorrhage in, 511–512
  inflammation in, 512–513
  obstruction in, 513
  peritonitis in, 513
  treatment of, 510–513
  uncomplicated, 510–511
Diverticulum, Meckel's, 149, 152
  Zenker's, 182–183, *183*
    perforation of, 229
Docusate sodium, in chronic constipation, 104
Domperidone (Motilium), in chronic constipation, 104
  in delayed gastric emptying, 252–253, 278
  in Parkinson's disease, 253
Doughnut granuloma, 764
Down's syndrome, hepatic involvement in, 847
  intestinal pseudoobstruction in, 449
Doxorubicin (Adriamycin), in hepatocellular carcinoma, 774
Drug(s), bezoar with, 280–283, 281t
  delayed gastric emptying with, 249, 249t, 271
  gastrointestinal bleeding and, 138
  hepatic granulomas with, 760t, 765
  in porphyria, 735, 735t
  in pruritus ani, 568
  vitamin deficiencies with, 25, 25t
  vomiting with, 55–56, 55t
Duchenne's muscular dystrophy, gastrointestinal lesions in, 442t
  intestinal pseudoobstruction in, 449
Duct of Wirsung, dilation of, in hereditary pancreatitis, 615, *616*

Duhamel procedure, in Hirschsprung's disease, 475, *476,* 476t
Dumping syndrome, 259–260
Duodenal ulcer, perforation of, 350–351
  rapid gastric emptying with, 250, 260
Duodenum, adenoma of, 421
  bleeding from, 165
  obstruction of, in pancreatic cancer, 638–639
  varices of, 164
Dyspepsia, 57–61
  algorithm for, 60, *60*
  altered gastrointestinal motility and, 57–58, *58,* 58t
  categories of, 57
  definition of, 57
  delayed gastric emptying in, 250
  diagnosis of, 60, *60*
  diet and, 59–60
  environmental factors and, 59–60
  gastric acid and, 59
  Helicobacter pylori and, 59
  increased visceral perception and, 58, *59*
  mechanisms of, 57–60, *58,* 58t
  motility in, 57–58, *58*
  psychologic factors and, 59–60
  stress and, 59–60
  treatment of, 60–61, *61*
Dysphagia, in achalasia, 186
  in diffuse esophageal spasm, 188
  in esophageal cancer, 225
Dysrhythmia, antral, 250

E

Eating disorders, 9–15
  assessment of, 13–15
  clinical features of, 9–11, 10t
  cultural factors in, 13
  diagnosis of, 9–11, 10t
  epidemiology of, 9
  etiology of, 12–13
  family factors in, 13
  gastric emptying in, 248, 261
  gastrointestinal findings in, 11–12, 11t
  laxative use in, 14
  management of, 13–15
  medical findings in, 11
  pathogenesis of, 12–13
  prognosis for, 13
  psychiatric conditions in, 12
  psychiatric consultation in, 14
  psychological factors in, 12–13
  social factors in, 13
  symptoms of, 10–11, 14
  tricyclic antidepressants in, 14
Ectasia, vascular, bleeding from, 137, 160–162, 161t
  treatment of, hormone therapy in, 162
    injection therapy in, 161
    surgical, 162
    thermal coagulation in, 161, 161t
Edema, cerebral, in fulminant hepatic failure, 683–684
Electrocautery, in peptic ulcer disease—associated hemorrhage, 337–338
Electroencephalography, in hepatic encephalopathy, 654
Electrogastrography, in delayed gastric emptying, 271, 273

Electrolytes, in fulminant hepatic failure, 679
  in infectious diarrhea, 539–540, 540t
  in intestinal obstruction, 111
Electromyography, in fecal incontinence, 97
Embolization, in gastric ulcer, 349
Emphysema, elastase-antielastase model for, 798–799
Encephalopathy, hepatic, 653–658. See also *Hepatic encephalopathy.*
  pancreatic, 625
Endamoeba histolytica, in proctitis, 604–605
Endarterectomy, transaortic, in chronic mesenteric ischemia, 435, *436*
Endometriosis, 573–578
  air insufflation test in, 576
  appendiceal, 578
  CA 125 marker in, 577
  computed tomography in, 576
  embryonic theory of, 574
  immunologic therapy of, 574
  magnetic resonance imaging in, 576
  metaplasia theory of, 574
  rectosigmoid, 575–576, 578
  transport theory of, 574
  treatment of, 577–578
  ultrasound in, 576
  vs. irritable bowel syndrome, 574–575
Endorectal ileal pullthrough procedure, 548–553
  clinical experience with, 550
  complications of, 551–552, 551t
  evaluation of, 552–553
  indications for, 548–549
  reservoir configuration for, 550, *550,* 552–553
  stages of, 549–550
Endoscopic retrograde cholangiopancreatography (ERCP), in cholangiocarcinoma, 776
  in cholangitis, 878–879, *879,* 880
  in choledochal cysts, 819, *820,* 820–821
  in choledocholithiasis, 886
  in gallstones, 862
  in pancreatic cancer, 636
  in pancreatitis, 622
  in ulcerative colitis, 519
Endoscopy, in achalasia, 189
  in angiodysplasia, 426–427
  in bezoar therapy, 282
  in caustic ingestion, 33–34, 33t, 34t
  in foreign body removal, 44
  in gastric ulcer evaluation, 313–314
  in gastric volvulus, 288
  in gastroesophageal reflux disease, 202
  in peptic ulcer disease—associated hemorrhage, 337–338
  in small bowel tumors, 416, *417,* 418, *418*
Endotoxin, in hepatorenal syndrome, 702
Enema, in chronic constipation, 105
  in fecal incontinence, 98
Energy balance, in obesity, 3, *4*
Energy metabolism, liver function in, 784
Energy requirements, in fulminant hepatic failure, 682
Entamoeba histolytica, 768–771. See also *Abscess, amebic.*
  in infectious diarrhea, 543t
Enteral nutrition, in childhood intestinal pseudoobstruction, 455
  in gastrointestinal fistula, 124
  in short bowel syndrome, 459–460, 460t

Enteral nutrition *(Continued)*
    in undernutrition, 19–20, 20t
Enterectomy, in childhood intestinal pseudoobstruction, 455
Enteric fever, 382t, 384–385
Enteritis, after Kock continent ileostomy, 554
Enterobius vermicularis, in pruritus ani, 568
Enteroclysis, in gastrointestinal tract bleeding, 158
Enterocolitis, antibiotic-associated, 152
    Hirschsprung's disease—associated, 470, 471–472, 472t
    Salmonella, 384
Enterohepatic cycle, 22
Enterokinase, deficiency of, 81
Enteroptosis, 55–56
Enteroscopy, in gastrointestinal tract bleeding, 157, 158–159
Enterotoxin, 372
Enzymes, pancreatic, replacement therapy with, 81t
Eosinophilia, peripheral, 359–360
    tissue, 361
Eosinophilic gastroenteritis, 359–361. See also
        Gastroenteritis, eosinophilic.
Episcleritis, in ulcerative colitis, 518–519
Epithelioid granuloma, hepatic, 758–759
Epstein-Barr virus, 661t
Ergotamine tartrate suppositories, rectal ulcers and, 587
Erosive gastritis, bleeding from, 134–135
Erythema nodosum, in ulcerative colitis, 518
Erythrocyte PBG deaminase, in porphyria, 736
Erythromycin, in childhood intestinal pseudoobstruction, 456
    in delayed gastric emptying, 255, 277–278
Escherichia coli, enteroadherent, 376
    enterohemorrhagic, 375, 386–387
    enteroinvasive, 375, 386–387
    enteropathogenic, 376
    heat-labile enterotoxins of, 374–375
    heat-stable enterotoxins of, 375
    in diarrhea, 538
    in infectious diarrhea, 543–544, 543t, 545t
    in proctitis, 602t, 605–606
    invasive infection with, 383t
    toxigenic diarrhea with, 374–376, 374t, 375t
Esophageal carcinoma, 219–226, 220t, *221, 222*
    achalasia and, 192–193
    cell biology of, 219
    complications of, 220
    diagnosis of, 220
    epidemiology of, 219
    fistulae with, 233–235, *234*
    lye ingestion and, 35
    management of, 220–223, *221, 222*
        adjuvant, 222–223
        palliative, 223
    prognosis for, 219
    screening for, 220
    spread of, 219
    staging of, 220, 220t
    symptoms of, 220
Esophageal rings, 184, *184*
Esophageal sphincter, lower, basal pressure of, 194, 195t
    cisapride effect on, 254
    domperidone effects on, 253
    manometric evaluation of, 194, 195t
    relaxation of, 194, 195t
    spasm of, 174

Esophageal sphincter *(Continued)*
    upper, components of, 177
        cricopharyngeal bar of, 182
        disorders of, 177–184
        in deglutition, 178, *178,* 178t
        opening mechanism of, 179
            CNS disorders and, 183
            disorders of, 179–182, *179–181*
            in belching in, 183–184
            Zenker's diverticulum of, 182–183, *183*
Esophageal strictures, caustic ingestion and, 30–35, 31t, 33t, 34t
    in achalasia, 189
    malignant, 185
    prevention of, 34–35
    proximal, 185
Esophageal varices, bleeding of, 131–134, *132,* 133t, 714–720
    liver transplantation for, 720
    management of, balloon tamponade in, 716
        band ligation in, 716–717
        initial, 714
        pharmacologic therapy in, 715–716, 717, 719
        prophylactic, 718–719
        sclerotherapy in, 715, 717, 719
        shunting procedures in, 716, 718
    mortality with, 714–720
    recurrent, prevention of, 717–718
    in fulminant hepatic failure, 687
    in primary biliary cirrhosis, 754, *754*
    liver transplantation in, 720
    prophylactic management of, 718–719
Esophageal webs, 184–185, 224
Esophagectomy, in esophageal carcinoma, 222, *222*
Esophagitis, infectious, 237–243, 238t
    achalasia and, 192
    bacterial, 242
    Candida, 238–241, 239t
    cytomegalovirus, 241–242
    herpes simplex virus, 241
    mycobacterial, 242
    varicella-zoster virus, 242
    viral, 241–242
    peptic, benign esophageal stricture with, 224
        bleeding from, 136
Esophagogastrectomy, Ivor-Lewis, in esophageal carcinoma, 221–222, *221*
Esophagogastroduodenoscopy, in pediatric gastrointestinal tract bleeding, 147–148
    in peptic ulcer disease, 335–336, 337t
    in pyloric stenosis, 341
Esophagomyotomy, in achalasia, 192
    vs. pneumatic dilation, 191
Esophagram, barium, in achalasia, 187, *188*
Esophagus, 184–185, *184*
    acid perfusion test of, in gastroesophageal reflux disease, 203
    balloon dilation of, 227–228
    Barrett's, adenocarcinoma and, 206–207, 219
        in gastroesophageal reflux disease, 206–207
    bleeding from, 136
    button battery in, 45
    carcinoma of, 219–226, 220t, *221, 222.* See also
            Esophageal carcinoma.
    caustic burns of, 30–35, 31t, 33t, 34t

Esophagus *(Continued)*
    collagen vascular disease of, 185
    contraction wave of, 194, 195t
    dilation of, 226–230, *226, 227*
        balloon, 227–228
        contraindications to, 229–230
        hazards of, 229–230
        Maloney mercury-filled bougies for, 228–229, 229t
        wire-guided, 226–227, *226, 227*
    drug-induced irritation of, 205, 205t
    fistulae of, 233–235, *234*
    foreign bodies in, 42, *42*
        bougienage removal of, 43–44
        esophagoscope removal of, 44
        flexible endoscopic removal of, 44
        Foley balloon catheter removal of, 43–44
        in children, 43–44
    24-hour ambulatory monitoring of, 174
    infection of, 237–243, 238t. See also *Esophagitis.*
    intubation of, in esophageal carcinoma, 223
    leiomyosarcoma of, 223
    Maloney mercury-filled bougie dilation of, 228–229, 229t
    manometry of, 193–200
        clinical implications of, 198–200
        diagnoses from, 195–196, 196t
        interpretation of, 196–198, *197–199*
        normal values for, 194–195, 195t
    melanoma of, 223
    motor disorders of, 173–174, 193–200, 195t, 196t, *197–199*
        in gastroesophageal reflux disease, 202–203
        in noncardiac chest pain, 173–174
    nutcracker, 171, 173
    oat cell carcinoma of, 223
    obstruction of, 224–236
        benign, 224
        dilation for, 226–230, *226, 227,* 229t
        malignant, 224–226
        stents for, 230–235, *232–236*
    perforation of, by stent, 231
        management of, 191
        pneumatic dilation-associated, 190–191, *190, 191*
        vs. Mallory-Weiss tear, 136
    peristalsis of, 194, 195t
    rings of, 184, *184*
    safety pins in, 45
    sensory dysfunction of, 198, *199*
    spasm of, dysphagia with, 188
        manometric evaluation of, 196
    stents for, 230–235
        complications of, 231, 233
        contraindications to, 230
        evaluation for, 230
        manufacture of, *234, 235, 236, 236*
        placement of, 231, *232*
        removal of, 233, *233*
        selection of, 230–231
    stricture of, 185
        caustic ingestion and, 30–35, 31t, 33t, 34t
        in achalasia, 189
        malignant, 185
        prevention of, 34–35
        proximal, 185
    transection of, in variceal bleeding, 718

Esophagus *(Continued)*
    webs of, 184–185
    wire-guided dilation of, 226–227, *226, 227*
Estrogen, hepatotoxicity of, 650
Estrogen-progesterone therapy, for vascular ectasia, 137, 162
Ethanol injection, in hepatocellular carcinoma, 774
Exercise, gastroesophageal reflux and, 176
    in chronic constipation, 102
Extracorporeal shock wave lithotripsy, in choledocholithiasis, 889
    in gallstone disease, 851–852, 863
Exulceratio simplex (Dieulafoy's vascular malformation), 137, 165, 428

F

Familial adenomatous polyposis, 153, 421–422, *422*
Familial visceral myopathy, classification of, 444t
    gastrointestinal lesions in, 442t
    intestinal pseudoobstruction syndrome in, 440–441, 441t, 442t—443t, 444t, 445t
Familial visceral neuropathy, 445t
    classification of, 445t
    gastrointestinal lesions in, 443t
    intestinal pseudoobstruction syndrome in, 441, 441t, 443t, 444t, 445t
Famotidine, in gastric ulcer, 315
    in Zollinger-Ellison syndrome, 326–327, 327t
Fasting, fatty liver in, 784
Fasting hypergastrinemia, in Zollinger-Ellison syndrome, 324, 324t
Fat, in acute hepatitis, 660
    in rapid gastric emptying, 262
Fatty acids, essential, 17t
Fatty liver, 783–784
Fecal impaction, 100–106, 101t. See also *Constipation, chronic.*
    Hirschsprung's disease—associated, 472, 472t
Fecal incontinence, 91, 95–100
    anal sphincter dysfunction in, 96
    anorectal electromyography in, 97
    anorectal manometry in, 97
    biofeedback for, 98–99, 99t
    colostomy in, 100
    defecography in, 97
    diagnosis of, 97
    diarrhea in, 96–97
    diet in, 98, 98t
    in diabetic patient, 96–97
    pathophysiology of, 95–96, 96t
    patient history of, 97
    pharmacologic agents for, 98
    physical examination in, 97
    polyurethane sponge plugs in, 100
    proctography in, 97
    rectal compliance in, 96
    rectal sensation in, 96
    surgery for, 99–100
    treatment of, 98–100, 98t
Feedings, in pediatric gastroesophageal reflux, 209
Fiber, dietary, in chronic constipation, 102–103
    in irritable bowel syndrome, 499, 505
Fibrinolysis, in fulminant hepatic failure, 687

INDEX 927

Fibroma, of small bowel, 421
Fibrosis, pipestem, 391
Fish, toxin-containing, 380
Fish oil, in ulcerative colitis, 517
Fissure, anal, 555–559. See also *Anal fissure.*
Fissurectomy, in anal fissure, 558
Fistula (fistulae), aortoenteric, bleeding from, 137–138
    in esophageal carcinoma, 220
  biliary, 125
  esophageal, 233–235, *234*
  esophagopleural, 242
  esophagotracheal, 242
  gastrointestinal, 121–125
    acquired, 121
    classification of, 122, 122t
    complicated, 122
    congenital, 121
    etiology of, 121–122
    external, 122
    internal, 122
    management of, 123–125
      investigation phase of, 124
      stabilization phase of, 123–124
      surgical phase of, 124–125
    mortality with, 122–123
    prognosis for, 122–123, 123t
    sequelae of, 122–123, 123t
    simple, 122
  in blind loop syndrome, 399
  in diverticulosis coli, 513
  with ileal pouch—anal anastomosis, 527
Fistulogram, in gastrointestinal fistula, 124
Fistuloscopy, in gastrointestinal fistula, 124
FK506, in Crohn's disease, 412
Flatus, 72–74
  pathophysiology of, 72, *72, 73*
  treatment of, 73–74, *73*
Flora, intestinal, 398, *399*
Fluconazole (Diflucan), in *Candida* esophagitis, 239t, 240
Flucytosine (Ancobon), in *Candida* esophagitis, 240
Fluid overload, in acute pancreatitis, 623
Fluids, in acute pancreatitis, 622–623
  in delayed gastric emptying, 250
  in infectious diarrhea, 539–540, 540t
  in intestinal obstruction, 114
  in perforated peptic ulcer, 339
  in upper gastrointestinal tract bleeding, 128
  peripancreatic, in acute pancreatitis, 625–627
  third spacing of, in acute pancreatitis, 622–623
Flumazenil, in hepatic encephalopathy, 654, 656t, 657–658, 685
5-Fluorouracil, biliary sclerosis with, 647
  in pancreatic cancer, 639
Fluoxetine (Prozac), in functional abdominal pain, 65t
Flushing, in carcinoid syndrome, 306
Focal nodular hyperplasia, hepatic, 778–779
Folate, deficiency of, in ulcerative colitis, 519
    postgastrectomy, 26
    small bowel resection and, 27
  in tropical sprue, 397
  replacement therapy with, 79t
Foley balloon catheter, for swallowed foreign bodies, 43–44
Folic acid, deficiency of, 26t
  in Crohn's disease, 409

Folic acid *(Continued)*
  in tropical sprue, 397
  replacement therapy with, 29t
Food. See also *Eating disorders.*
  decreased intake of, vitamin deficiency and, 23–24, 23t
  flatugenic, in irritable bowel syndrome, 500
  lactose content of, 367
  regurgitation of, 15, 47
Food poisoning. See *Diarrhea, toxigenic.*
Foreign bodies, colonic, 39, 40
  colorectal, 40
  esophageal, 42–44, *42.* See also *Esophagus, foreign bodies in.*
  in children, 41–46, *42.* See also *Children, foreign bodies in.*
  pharyngeal, 42, *42*
  rectal, 37–40, 37t. See also *Rectum, foreign bodies in.*
Foscarnet, in cytomegalovirus esophagitis, 242
Fulminant hepatic failure, 675–690. See also *Hepatic failure, fulminant.*
Functional gastrointestinal disease, 57. See also *Abdominal pain, functional; Dyspepsia; Irritable bowel syndrome.*
Fundoplication, in childhood intestinal pseudoobstruction, 455
  in gastroesophageal reflux disease, 205–206
  in pediatric gastroesophageal reflux, 209, 210
Fungizone (amphotericin B), in *Candida* esophagitis, 240
Fungus, in pruritus ani, 568
Furosemide, in ascites, 723

G

GABA (¦-aminobutyric acid), in hepatic encephalopathy, 654
Gallbladder, Courvoisier's, in hepatic tumor, 788
  inflammation of, 848–857. See also *Cholecystitis.*
  perforation of, in cholecystitis, 861
  porcelain, 851, 903
  tumors of, 902–906
    clinical presentation of, 903
    disease associations with, 903, 904t
    histology of, 903, 905, *905*
    incidence of, 902–903
    management of, 903
    treatment of, 905–906
Gallstone ileus, 109, *109,* 849
Gallstones, 848–852. See also *Cholelithiasis.*
Ganciclovir (Cytovene), in cytomegalovirus esophagitis, 242
Gardner's syndrome, 421–422
  gastrointestinal tract bleeding with, 153
Gas, intestinal, 70–74, *71, 580*–583. See also *Pneumatosis cystoides intestinalis.*
  composition of, 72, *72*
  excess passage of, 72–74, *73*
  in irritable bowel syndrome, 500
  in toxic megacolon, 536
Gastrectomy, dumping syndrome after, 259–260
  gastric cancer after, 353
  in delayed gastric emptying, 256–257, 278
  vitamin deficiencies after, 26–27
Gastric acid, in dyspepsia, 59
  in Zollinger-Ellison syndrome, 326–328, 327t
Gastric adenocarcinoma, 289–294
  after ulcer disease surgery, 353
  biopsy in, 290

Gastric adenocarcinoma *(Continued)*
   diagnosis of, 290
   gastric ulcer and, 313–314, 353
   lymphadenectomy in, 292
   pathophysiology of, 289–290
   polyps and, 301
   screening for, 290
   spread of, 291, 292t
   staging of, 290–291, 290t, *291*
   treatment of, 292–294, 293t
      chemotherapy in, 293, 294t
      radiation in, 293–294
      surgery in, 292–293, 293t
Gastric antral vascular ectasia, 164, 321, 428
Gastric artery, 345, *346*
Gastric aspiration, in fulminant hepatic failure, 685
Gastric bypass, vitamin deficiencies after, 27
Gastric emptying, delayed. See *Delayed gastric emptying.*
Gastric epithelial dysplasia, gastric adenocarcinoma and, 290
Gastric erosions, in fulminant hepatic failure, 687
Gastric lavage, in peptic ulcer disease, 335
Gastric lymphoma, 296–299
Gastric outlet obstruction, 264–268
   diagnosis of, 267, 267t
   etiology of, 265–267, 266t
   gastric surgery and, 266–267
   in peptic ulcer disease, 352
   inflammation in, 265
   neoplasm in, 266
   peptic ulcer and, 268
   peptic ulcer disease in, 265
   signs of, 265
   symptoms of, 264–265, 265t
   treatment of, 267–268
Gastric ulcer, 312–316. See also *Ulcer(s), gastric.*
Gastric varices, 136, 163–164, 714. See also *Esophageal varices.*
Gastrinoma, 322–334. See also *Zollinger-Ellison syndrome.*
Gastritis, 317–321
   alcoholic, 318
   aspirin-induced, 319
   atrophic, 320
      delayed gastric emptying in, 249
      vitamin deficiencies with, 27
   caustic, 320
   eosinophilic, 321
   erosive, bleeding from, 134–135
   ethanol-induced, 135
   graft-versus-host, 321
   granulomatous, 321
   Helicobacter pylori-induced, 319
   hypertrophic, 320
   in immunocompromised host, 321
   ischemic, 320–321
   NSAID-induced, 319
   phlegmonous, 321
   postgastrectomy, 320
   radiation-induced, 321
   stress-induced, 320
Gastrocolic ligament, *284*
Gastroenteritis. See also *Diarrhea.*
   eosinophilic, 321, 359–361
      biopsy in, 360

Gastroenteritis *(Continued)*
   clinical features of, 359
   diagnosis of, 360
   diarrhea with, 92
   differential diagnosis of, 359–360
   malabsorption in, 82, 83t
   pathophysiology of, 360–361
   prognosis for, 361
   sites of, 360
   treatment of, 361
   Salmonella, 384
   viral, intestinal pseudoobstruction after, 449
Gastroenterostomy, gastric outlet obstruction after, 266
   in delayed gastric emptying, 256–257
Gastroepiploic artery, 345, *346*
Gastroesophageal junction, in hiatal hernia, 216, 216t
Gastroesophageal reflux disease, 201–207
   Barrett's esophagus and, 206–207
   delayed gastric emptying in, 250, 271
   diagnosis of, 201–203, 202t
   exercise and, 176
   in children, 207–210
   in coronary artery disease, 176
   in noncardiac chest pain, 171–172
   laryngeal disease and, 206
   lung disease and, 206
   metoclopramide in, 251
   treatment of, 203–205, 203t
      surgical, 205–206
Gastrointestinal fistula, 121–125. See also *Fistula (fistulae), gastrointestinal.*
Gastrointestinal tract bleeding, in children, 145–154, 146t, *147,* 150t, 151t
   lower, 139–144, 140t
      angiography in, 142–143
      colonoscopy in, 142
      diagnosis of, 141–142
      from angiodysplasia, 140–141, *141*
      from angioma, 140–141
      from arteriovenous malformation, 140–141, *141*
      from diverticular disease, 141
      in children, 145–149, 146t, 151–153, 151t
      management of, 141–142, 142t
      occult, 140
      radionuclide scan in, 142
      treatment of, 143–144
      vs. upper gastrointestinal tract bleeding, 141
   unknown origin of, 155–166
      angioma in, 160–162, 161t
      classification of, 155–156, 156t
      clinical features of, 155
      colonic lesions in, 165–166
      diagnosis of, 156–159, 157t
         angiography in, 158
         barium studies in, 157–158
         endoscopy in, 158–159
         intraoperative enteroscopy in, 159
         push enteroscopy in, 158–159
         radionuclide examination in, 158
         Ropeway enteroscopy in, 159
         Sonde enteroscopy in, 159
      Dieulafoy's lesion in, 165
      duodenal lesions in, 165

Gastrointestinal tract bleeding *(Continued)*
    esophagogastric lesions in, 164–165, 165t
    gastric varices in, 163–164
    hiatal hernia in, 164–165
    small intestine sources in, 159–163, 161t, 162t
    small intestine tumors in, 162
    small intestine ulcerations in, 162–163, 162t
    submucosal masses in, 164
    watermelon stomach in, 164
  upper, 126–139, *127*, 128t
    clinical presentation of, 128–130, 129t
    drug-induced, 138
    endoscopy of, 129
    from aortoenteric fistula, 137–138
    from Dieulafoy's lesion, 137
    from erosive gastritis, 134–135
    from hypertensive gastropathy, 136
    from Mallory-Weiss tear, 136
    from neoplasm, 136–137, 138
    from peptic esophagitis, 136
    from peptic ulcer, 130–131
    from varices, 131–134, *132*, 133t
    from vascular ectasia, 137
    in acute pancreatitis, 625
    in children, 145–149, 146t, 149–151, 150t
    in fulminant hepatic failure, 686–687
Gastrojejunostomy, in peptic ulcer disease, 352
Gastroparesis, 269–279. See also *Delayed gastric emptying.*
  definition of, 269–270
  diabetic, 270
  diagnosis of, 271–273, *282–275*
  etiology of, 270–271, 270t
  gastric ulcer and, 271
  gastroesophageal reflux and, 271
  idiopathic, 271
  medication-induced, 271
  postoperative, 270
  symptoms of, 269–270
  treatment of, 273, 276–279, 276t, 277t
Gastroplasty, gastric outlet obstruction after, 266–267
Gastropyloroduodenal manometry, in delayed gastric emptying, 271
Gastrosplenic ligament, *284*
Gentamicin, in hepatorenal syndrome, 702
Giant condylomata, anal, 571
Giant hypertrophic gastritis, 86
Giant pseudopolyps, 548
Gianturco Z-stent, 233, 235
Giardia lamblia, in infectious diarrhea, 543t
Glénard's disease, 55–56
Glomerular filtration rate, 696
Glucagon, in alcoholic patient, 712
  in fulminant hepatic failure, 688
Glucagonlike peptide-1 (GLP-1), in dumping syndrome, 260
Glucose, in fulminant hepatic failure, 679
Glucose-regulated proteins, 795
¦-Glutamyltranspeptidase, in alcoholism, 708t
Gluten-sensitive enteropathy, 367–371. See also *Sprue, celiac.*
GoLytely, in chronic constipation, 104
Gonadotropin-releasing hormone, in endometriosis, 577
Gonorrhea, 600–601, 602t
Graft-versus-host gastritis, 321

Granuloma, doughnut, 764
  hepatic, 758–766. See also *Hepatic granuloma.*
Granulomatous gastritis, 321
Granulomatous hepatitis, drug-induced, 647
Grey Turner sign, in hereditary pancreatitis, 615

H

H_2 (histamine-2) receptor antagonists, in gastroesophageal reflux disease, 203t, 204
  in pediatric peptic ulcer, 150
Hamartoma, of Brunner's gland, 420
  of small bowel, 421
Hands, scarring of, in eating disorders, 11
Head injury, rapid gastric emptying after, 261
Heart, carcinoid disease of, 310–311
  in hepatorenal syndrome, 698–699
  iron accumulation in, 808–813. See also *Hemochromatosis.*
Heater probe, in peptic ulcer disease—associated hemorrhage, 338
Helicobacter pylori, antibiotic treatment for, 315–316
  in dyspepsia, 59
  in gastric disease, 289–290, 312, 319
  in peptic ulcer, 131, 342
Hemangioendothelioma, epithelioid, hepatic resection in, 833
Hemangioma, 427
  gastrointestinal tract bleeding with, 153
  hepatic, resection in, 833
  of small bowel, 420
Hemangiosarcoma, hepatic resection in, 833
Hematemesis, 145
Hematin, in porphyria, 733–734
Hematochezia, 145
Hemigastrectomy, in perforated duodenal ulcer, 350–351
Hemochromatosis, 808–813, 809t
  hereditary, 808–812, 810t
    blood studies in, 810–811, 810t
    clinical manifestations of, 808–810, 810t
    diagnosis of, 810–812, 810t
    differential diagnosis of, 811, 811t
    liver biopsy in, 811
    screening for, 812
    treatment of, 812
  secondary, 812–813
Hemodialysis, in hepatorenal syndrome, 703–704
Hemofiltration, in Wilson's disease, 807
Hemoglobin, in fulminant hepatic failure, 687
Hemolytic-uremic syndrome, gastrointestinal tract bleeding with, 153
  in infectious diarrhea, 543–544
Hemorrhage. See also *Gastrointestinal tract bleeding.*
  diverticular, 511–512
  gastric ulcer—associated, 349–350
  peptic ulcer disease—associated, 335–339, *336,* 337t
    endoscopic management of, 337–338
    medical management of, 336–337
    surgery for, 338–339
  pseudocyst, in acute pancreatitis, 626
Hemorrhoids, bleeding from, 165
  injection sclerotherapy of, 557
Henoch-Schönlein purpura, gastrointestinal tract bleeding with, 153

Hepatic adenoma, 778
  drug-induced, 648
  resection in, 833
Hepatic angiosarcoma, 777–778
Hepatic artery, embolization of, in carcinoid syndrome, 308–309
  ligation of, in hepatocellular carcinoma, 774
Hepatic coma, 653
Hepatic encephalopathy, 653–658, 684–685
  clinical manifestations of, 653–654, 653t, 654t
  definition of, 653–654
  differential diagnosis of, 684–685
  pathogenesis of, 654–655, 655t
  stages of, 653–654, 653t, 654t
  treatment of, 655–658
    antibiotics in, 656t, 657
    bowel cleansing in, 657
    diet in, 655–656, 656t
    flumazenil in, 656t, 657–658
    lactulose in, 656–657, 656t
    sodium benzoate in, 656t, 657
    surgical, 658
    zinc in, 656t, 657
Hepatic failure. See also *Hepatorenal syndrome.*
  fulminant, 675–690
    acetaminophen-induced, 677
    autoimmune chronic active hepatitis and, 678
    cardiorespiratory complications of, 685–686
    cerebral edema in, 683–684
    chronic active hepatitis and, 680
    clinical features of, 676–678, 676t
    coagulopathy in, 687
    definition of, 675
    etiology of, 675–676, 676t
    fatty liver of pregnancy and, 677, 680
    gastrointestinal tract bleeding in, 686–687
    hepatic encephalopathy in, 653–658, 684–685. See also *Hepatic encephalopathy.*
    hepatic vascular congestion and, 680
    herpes hepatitis and, 680
    HSV-induced, 678
    liver transplantation in, 689–690, 689t
    management of, 678–682
      assessment studies in, 678–679
      catheters in, 679
      N-acetylcysteine in, 679–680
      tubes in, 679
    metabolic complications of, 688
    mushroom poisoning and, 677, 680
    nutritional deficiencies in, 682–683
    prognosis for, 688–689
    renal failure in, 687
    sepsis in, 688
    treatment of, cytoprotection in, 680–681
      hepatic regeneration in, 681
      support systems in, 681–682
    vascular hepatic congestion and, 677
    viral hepatitis and, 676–677
    Wilson's disease and, 677–678, 680
  late onset, 664
Hepatic fibrin ring granuloma, 759
Hepatic granuloma, 758–766
  clinical features of, 760–761, 762t

Hepatic granuloma *(Continued)*
  definition of, 758–759
  diagnosis of, 761
  drug-related, 760t, 765
  epithelioid, 758–759
    in primary biliary cirrhosis, 765
    in sarcoidosis, 761–763, 762t
  etiology of, 759–760, 760t
  fibrin ring, 759
  idiopathic, 760
  in acquired immunodeficiency syndrome, 765–766, 765t
  infectious, 759–760, 760t
  inflammatory, 759
  noninfectious, 759, 760t
  pathogenesis of, 759
  radiographic studies of, 761
  treatment of, 766
Hepatic iron index, in hereditary hemochromatosis, 811, 811t
Hepatic vein, thrombosis of, 838. See also *Budd-Chiari syndrome.*
  drug-induced, 647
Hepaticojejunostomy, in choledochal cysts, 822, *822,* 824
Hepatitis, 788
  acute, 659–665
    alcohol-associated, 662
    clinical course of, 663–664
    clinical features of, 659
    diagnosis of, 660–661, 661t
    differential diagnosis of, 660
    drug-induced, 662–663, 663t
    etiology of, 661–663, 663t
    extrahepatic manifestations of, 659
    histology of, 659–660
    in alcoholic liver disease, 710–712, 710t
    prevention of, 664–665
    treatment of, 663
  alcoholic, liver transplantation in, 837
  autoimmune, vs. primary sclerosing cholangitis, 746
  chronic, 664
    definition of, 666
    differential diagnosis of, 666, 666t
    drug-induced, 646–647
    histopathology of, 667
    in ulcerative colitis, 519
    inflammatory bowel disease and, 748
    interferon therapy of, 669–673
      administration of, 670, 672
      contraindications to, 669, 671
      indications for, 669–670, 670t, 671–672
      results of, 670–671, 672
      side effects of, 672–673
  fulminant, 663, 664. See also *Hepatic failure, fulminant.*
    Wilsonian, 804–805
  granulomatous, 761
    drug-induced, 647
  HSV-induced, 678, 680
  ischemic, 690–694
    aspartate aminotransferase in, *692,* 693, 694
    biochemical changes of, 691–693, *692*
    definition of, 690
    diagnosis of, 691
    differential diagnosis of, 693, 694t
    histology of, 691

Hepatitis (Continued)
    prognosis for, 693–694
    treatment of, 693–694
        vs. acute viral hepatitis, 693, 694t
        vs. drug hepatotoxicity, 693, 694t
    lupoid, 785
    neonatal, 843, 843t, 848
Hepatitis A, 661–662, 661t
    neonatal, 846
Hepatitis A vaccine, 665
Hepatitis B, 661t, 662
    in hepatocellular carcinoma, 772
    interferon therapy for, 669–673, 670t
    liver transplantation in, 836–837
    neonatal, 846
Hepatitis B immune globulin (HBIG), 664
Hepatitis B vaccine, 664–665
Hepatitis C, 661t, 662, 666–668, 668t
    ELISA assay for, 667–668
    in hepatocellular carcinoma, 772
    in porphyria, 737, 738
    interferon therapy for, 669–673, 670t
    liver transplantation in, 836–837
    neonatal, 846–847
    polymerase chain reaction assay for, 668
    RIBA assay for, 668
Hepatitis D, 661t, 662
Hepatitis E, 662
Hepatocellular carcinoma, 771–775
    chemoembolization for, 774
    chemotherapy for, 774
    clinical presentation of, 772
    epidemiology of, 771–772
    ethanol injection for, 774
    external beam radiation for, 774
    fibrolamellar, 772
        hepatic resection in, 833
    hepatic resection in, 773, 831, 833, *833, 833*
    histology of, 772
    hormonal therapy for, 774
    laboratory assessment of, 772
    liver transplantation for, 773–774
    radiologic assessment of, 772–773
    recurrence of, 773
    screening for, 775
    toxin-induced, 648
    treatment of, 773–775
Hepatocytes, mitochondrial function of, 829
Hepatoduodenal ligament, *284*
Hepatogastric ligament, *284*
Hepatorenal syndrome, 695–705
    afferent events in, 698–699
    blood volume in, 698
    cardiovascular function in, 698–699
    definition of, 696–697, *697*
    diagnosis of, 700–701, *701*, 701t
    differential diagnosis of, 695–696
    efferent events in, 699–700
    nephrotoxic drug avoidance in, 702
    pathogenesis of, 697, *697*
    prevention of, 701–702
    Starling forces in, 698
    treatment of, 701–705

Hepatorenal syndrome (Continued)
    dialysis in, 703–704, 704t
    liver transplantation in, 704–705, 705t
    pharmacologic, 703
    volume expansion in, 702–703
    urinary sodium in, 700, 701t
    volume contraction in, 701–702
Hepatotoxicity, drug-induced, acute, 645–646, *645*
    chronic, 646–648
    vs. ischemic hepatitis, 693, 694t
Hepatotoxins, classification of, 644–645, *645*
    idiosyncratic, 644–645, *645*
    intrinsic, 644–645, *645*
Hereditary hemochromatosis, 808–812. See also
        Hemochromatosis, hereditary.
Hereditary hemorrhagic telangiectasia, 427–428
Hernia, hiatal, 211–217, *212, 213*
    benign esophageal stricture with, 224
    bleeding with, 164–165
    diagnosis of, 214–215, *214, 215*
    esophageal pH in, 216, 216t
    gastroesophageal junction in, 216, 216t
    in esophageal dilation, 229
    incidence of, 211
    pathophysiology of, 215–216, 216t, *217*
    rolling, 211, *212,* 213–214, *213, 215,* 216, *217*
    sliding, 211, *212,* 214, *215,* 216, *217*
    sliding-rolling, 211, *212, 215*
    symptoms of, 213–214
    treatment of, 216–217
    in intestinal obstruction, 108, 110, *110*
Herpes simplex virus, esophageal, 241
    hepatitis with, 678, 680
    in proctitis, 602t, 603–604
    in pruritus ani, 568
    neonatal, hepatic involvement in, 846
5-HIAA (5-hydroxyindoleacetic acid), in carcinoid heart
        disease, 310
    in carcinoid syndrome, 306–307
Hirschsprung's disease, 470–477
    biopsy in, 473–474, *475*
    clinical presentation of, 470–471, 471t
    complications of, 471–472, 472t
    differential diagnosis of, 475, 476t, 477
    etiology of, 470, 471t
    evaluation of, 472–474, 472t
    gastrointestinal lesions in, 443t
    genetic anomalies in, 470
    historical perspective on, 470
    in chronic constipation, 105
    treatment of, 474–475, *476*
    variants of, 471
    vs. acquired megacolon, 473
Histamine (H_2) receptor antagonists, in gastroesophageal reflux
        disease, 203t, 204
    in pediatric peptic ulcer, 150
Histoplasma capsulatum, 764
Histoplasmosis, esophageal, 241
    granulomas of, 763t
    hepatic, 763t, 764, 766
HLA-DR haplotype, in α_1-antitrypsin deficiency, 795–796
Hoarseness, in gastroesophageal reflux disease, 206
Hodgkin's disease, hepatic granuloma in, 765

Hoesch test, in porphyria, 733, *733*
Hollow viscus myopathy, delayed gastric emptying in, 248
Hormones, for vascular ectasia, 137, 162
　in angiodysplasia, 426
　in hepatorenal syndrome, 699–700
Human immunodeficiency virus (HIV), anorectal abscess and, 565, 565t
Human papillomavirus, in proctitis, 602t, 604
Hunger, in eating disorders, 12
Hurst dilator, *227*
Hydralazine (Apresoline), in esophageal motility disorders, 173, 176
　vitamin deficiency with, 25t
Hydrops, 849
5-Hydroxyindoleacetic acid (5-HIAA), in carcinoid heart disease, 310
　in carcinoid syndrome, 306–307
5-Hydroxytryptamine receptor agonists, in delayed gastric emptying, 256
5-Hydroxytryptamine receptor antagonists, in delayed gastric emptying, 256
Hyperbaric oxygen, in pneumatosis cystoides intestinalis, 582–583
　in radiation colitis, 432
Hyperbilirubinemia, neonatal, 842–848
　　etiology of, 845–848
　　evaluation of, 843–845, 843t, 844t
　　in Alagille's syndrome, 847–848
　　in α_1-antitrypsin deficiency, 847
　　in bacterial infections, 845
　　in Byler's syndrome, 848
　　in chromosomal disorders, 847
　　in congenital syphilis, 845
　　in cytomegalovirus infection, 846
　　in familial intrahepatic cholestatic syndromes, 847–848
　　in hepatitis virus infection, 846–847
　　in herpes virus infection, 846
　　in total parenteral nutrition, 847
　　in toxoplasmosis, 845
　　in urinary tract infections, 845
　　treatment of, 848
　unconjugated, 843
Hypercalcemia, in carcinoid syndrome, 307
Hypercholesterolemia, in primary biliary cirrhosis, 755
Hypercoagulation, in ulcerative colitis, 519
Hypergastrinemia, fasting, in Zollinger-Ellison syndrome, 324, 324t
Hyperglycemia, delayed gastric emptying and, 270
　in acute pancreatitis, 624
Hyperlipidemia, in acute pancreatitis, 624
Hyperplastic polyps, 547
Hypertension. See *Portal hypertension.*
Hyperthyroidism, delayed gastric emptying in, 249
Hypertriglyceridemia, in acute pancreatitis, 623
Hypertrophic disease, 86, 320
Hyperventilation, in fulminant hepatic failure, 684
Hypnotherapy, in functional abdominal pain syndromes, 66–67
Hypoalbuminemia, in acute pancreatitis, 623
　in blind loop syndrome, 400
Hypocalcemia, in acute pancreatitis, 624
Hypoglycemia, in dumping syndrome, 260
　in fulminant hepatic failure, 682
Hypoparathyroidism, gastrointestinal lesions in, 442t

Hypoperfusion, hepatic, 782–783
Hypotension, in fulminant hepatic failure, 686
Hypothyroidism, gastrointestinal lesions in, 442t
Hypovolemia, in acute pancreatitis, 622–623
Hypoxemia, in acute pancreatitis, 623

I

Ileal pouch—anal anastomosis, 524–530
　defecation after, 528–529
　failure of, 528
　fistula with, 527
　in backwash ileitis, 526
　in indeterminate colitis, 525
　in primary sclerosing cholangitis, 525–526
　in toxic megacolon, 525
　indications for, 524–526
　physiologic changes after, 528–529
　pouchitis with, 527–528
　quality of life after, 529–530
　results of, 527–528, 527t
　stricturing of, 527
　technique of, 526–527, *526*
Ileal pouch—distal rectal anastomosis, 532
Ileal ulcers, celiac sprue and, 370
Ileitis, after Kock continent ileostomy, 554
　backwash, ileal pouch—anal anastomosis in, 526
Ileocecal valve, in short bowel syndrome, 458
　incompetent, 493
Ileocolectomy, gallstones after, 748
Ileocolic resection, diarrhea after, 92
Ileocolonoscopy, in primary sclerosing cholangitis, 894
Ileorectostomy, 531–532, *531*
Ileus, gallstone, 109, *109*, 849
　vs. intestinal obstruction, 108, 116
Immune globulin, in hepatitis prevention, 664
Immune system, in malnutrition, 18
Immunodeficiency, gastritis in, 321
Immunoglobulin A (IgA) deficiency, celiac sprue and, 370
Immunoproliferative small intestinal disease, vs. in tropical sprue, 397
Immunorepressive malnutrition, 19, 19t, 20
Imodium. See *Loperamide.*
Incontinence, fecal, 91, 95–100. See also *Fecal incontinence.*
Infection. See also specific types, e.g., *Abscess.*
　esophageal, 237–243. See also *Esophagitis, infectious.*
　in acute acalculous cholecystitis, 853–854
　in primary sclerosing cholangitis, 869
　rectal, 567–568. See also *Proctitis, infectious.*
　with esophageal dilation, 229
Inflammatory bowel disease. See also *Crohn's disease; Ulcerative colitis.*
　cholelithiasis in, 748
　chronic hepatitis in, 748
　diarrhea in, 92–93
　gastrointestinal tract bleeding in, 153
　hepatobiliary complications of, 740–748
　primary sclerosing cholangitis in, 742–748, 744–745. See also *Primary sclerosing cholangitis.*
INH (isoniazid), hepatotoxicity of, 649–650, 783
　vitamin deficiency with, 25t
Insulin, in alcoholic patient, 712

Interferon, in carcinoid syndrome, 307
  in Zollinger-Ellison syndrome, 333
Interferon alfa, in chronic viral hepatitis, 665–673, 666t, 668t, 670t
  side effects of, 673
Interferon beta, in hepatitis C, 663
Intestinal ischemic syndrome, 433–437. See also *Chronic intestinal ischemic syndrome.*
Intestine, compression of, 110, *110*
  congenital duplication of, gastrointestinal tract bleeding with, 152
  flora of, 398, *399.* See also *Blind loop syndrome.*
  gas in, 70–74, *71,* 580–583. See also *Pneumatosis cystoides intestinalis.*
    composition of, 72, *72*
    excess passage of, 72–74, *73*
    in dyspepsia, 58, *59*
    in functional abdominal pain syndromes, 62
    in intestinal obstruction, 111, *112*
    in irritable bowel syndrome, 500
    in toxic megacolon, 536
  intubation of, in intestinal obstruction, 114, 116
  lumen of, obturation of, 109, *109*
  motility of, in intestinal obstruction, 111
  obstruction of, 108–116, 490–495
    clinical presentation of, 492–494, 492t
    definition of, 108
    diagnosis of, 112–114
    etiology of, 491, 491t, 492t
    extrinsic, 491, 491t
    extrinsic lesions in, 110, *110*
    fluid resuscitation in, 114–115
    functional, 491, 491t
    hernia in, 108, 110, *110*
    incidence of, 108–109
    intestinal wall lesions in, 109–110
    intraluminal, 491, 491t
    laboratory findings in, 113, 493
    lumen obturation in, 109, *109*
    management of, 114–116, 494–495, *494*
    motility in, 111
    mural, 491, 491t
    pathophysiology of, 110–112, 491–492
    patient history in, 112
    physical examination in, 112–113, 493
    pneumatosis cystoides intestinalis and, 583
    postoperative, 116
    radiologic studies in, 113–114, 493–494
    surgical approaches to, 115
    symptoms of, 492
    tumor in, 108
    types of, 109–110, *109,* 490–491, 491t
    volvulus in, 110, *111*
    vs. ileus, 108, 116
    vs. pseudoobstruction (Ogilvie's syndrome), 116
  pseudoobstruction of, 438–456. See also *Chronic intestinal pseudoobstruction.*
    idiopathic, delayed gastric emptying in, 248–249
  resection of, in gastrointestinal fistula, 125
    in intestinal obstruction, 115
    vitamin deficiencies after, 27
  schistosomiasis of, 391
  small, 415

Intestine *(Continued)*
  adenoma of, 419, 421–422, *422*
  benign tumors of, 414–423
    diagnosis of, 416–418, *416,* 416t, *417, 418*
    etiology of, 414–415
    pathogenesis of, 414–415
    polyposis syndromes with, 421–423, *422*
    symptoms of, 415–416
    treatment of, 418
  diameter of, 113
  fibroma of, 421
  hamartoma of, 421
  hemangioma of, 420
  in malabsorption syndromes, 78, 78t, 81–84, 82t
  leiomyoma of, 418–419
  lipoma of, 419–420
  lymphangioma of, 421
  neurogenic tumors of, 420–421
  resection of, 457–458, 458t
  short, 457–461. See also *Short bowel syndrome.*
  transplantation of, in childhood intestinal pseudoobstruction, 455–456
    in short bowel syndrome treatment, 461
  wall of, in eosinophilic gastroenteritis, 360
    lesions of, 109–110
Intracranial pressure, in fulminant hepatic failure, 679, 683–684
Intraluminal agents, in infectious diarrhea, 540–541
Intraluminal gastropyloroduodenal manometry, in delayed gastric emptying, 271
Intubation, in esophageal carcinoma, 223
  in fulminant hepatic failure, 685–686
  in intestinal obstruction, 114, 116
Intussusception, pediatric, 109
  gastrointestinal tract bleeding with, 152
  treatment of, 115
Inverse ratio ventilation, in fulminant hepatic failure, 686
Iodoquinol (Diiodohydroxyquin), in amebic abscess, 771
Iron, in hereditary hemochromatosis, 810–811
  in porphyria, 737
  replacement therapy with, 79t
Iron deficiency anemia, in ulcerative colitis, 519
Iron overload, African, 809
  hereditary, 808–813. See also *Hemochromatosis, hereditary.*
  parenteral, 809, 812–813
  secondary, 809, 812
Irritable bowel syndrome, 70–74, *71*
  anticholinergic compounds in, 65
  antidepressants in, 65, 65t
  biopsy in, 506
  cognitive behavior therapy in, 67
  constipation-predominant, 496–501
    abdominal pain in, 500
    behavioral therapy in, 500–501
    bloating in, 500
    definition of, 497, 497t
    diagnosis of, 497–498, 497t
    gas in, 500
    pathophysiology of, 496–497
    patient history in, 497–498
    physical examination in, 497–498
    psychologic therapy in, 500–501
    treatment of, 498–501

Irritable bowel syndrome *(Continued)*
  diarrhea-prone, 502–508
    anticholinergics in, 506–507, 507t
    antidepressants in, 507t, 508
    antispasmodics in, 507, 507t
    anxiolytics in, 507t, 508
    biogenic amines in, 507t, 508
    calcium channel blockers in, 507t, 508
    diagnosis of, 504t, 505
    diet in, 506, 507t
    differential diagnosis of, 502, 502t
    disodium cromoglycate in, 507t, 508
    laboratory evaluation of, 504t, 505
    management of, *503,* 505–508, 507t
    opiates in, 506, 507t
    patient history in, 502, 504, 504t
    peppermint oil in, 507–508, 507t
    peptides in, 507t, 508
    physical findings in, 504
  diet in, 64–65
  distention perception in, 62
  hypnotherapy in, 66–67
  motility in, 496
  opiate analogs in, 65
  progressive muscle relaxation training in, 67
  psychotherapy in, 66
  tranquilizers in, 65–66
  treatment of, 71–72, *71*
  vs. collagenous colitis, 597
  vs. endometriosis, 574–575
Ischemia, 433–437. See also *Chronic intestinal ischemic syndrome.*
  delayed gastric emptying with, 249
  intestinal, in intestinal obstruction, 111–112
  rectal ulcers and, 587
Ischemic colitis, 593t
Ischemic gastritis, 320–321
Isoniazid (INH), hepatotoxicity of, 649–650, 783
  vitamin deficiency with, 25t
Isosorbide-5-mononitrate, in variceal bleeding, 718
Isospora belli, in infectious diarrhea, 543t
Ivor-Lewis esophagogastrectomy, in esophageal carcinoma, 221–222, *221*

J

Jaundice, in abdominal abscess, 118
  in cholangiocarcinoma, 777
  in hereditary pancreatitis, 616
  in pancreatic cancer, 638
  infection-related, 783
  neonatal, 842–848. See also *Hyperbilirubinemia, neonatal.*
Jejunal aspirate, in blind loop syndrome, 400
Jejunal ulcers, celiac sprue and, 370
Jejunitis, ulcerative, diarrhea with, 92
Jejunoileal bypass, vitamin deficiencies and, 27
Jejunostomy tube, in childhood intestinal pseudoobstruction, 455
  in delayed gastric emptying, 256
Jet ventilators, in fulminant hepatic failure, 686
Juvenile polyposis, generalized, 422–423
Juvenile polyps, 548

K

Kaolin, in infectious diarrhea, 541
Katayama fever, 390, 390t
Kayser-Fleischer rings, 803
Ketoconazole, in *Candida* esophagitis, 239–240, 239t
Ketotifen, in eosinophilic gastroenteritis, 361
Kidney, failure of, chronic, cutaneous porphyria-like lesions in, 738
  in ascites, 722
  in fulminant hepatic failure, 687
Klatskin's tumor, 839, 896, *896*
  hepatic resection in, 833
Kock continent ileostomy, 532, 553–554, *554*
  complications of, 553–554
Kwashiorkor, 19, 19t, 20, 784
  malabsorption in, 80

L

Lactase deficiency, 82, 83t, 364
  congenital, 365
  in irritable bowel syndrome, 500
Lactase substitutes, 366, 366t
Lactate dehydrogenase, in ischemic hepatitis, *692,* 693
Lactic acidosis, in fulminant hepatic failure, 682
Lactose, colonic salvage of, 363
  digestion of, 362–363
Lactose absorption test, 363
Lactose breath test, 78
Lactose intolerance, 362–366, 363
  developmental, 365
  evaluation of, 363–365, 364t, 365t
  in Crohn's disease, 409
  secondary, 365
  signs of, 363
  symptoms of, 363
  treatment of, 365–366, 366t
Lactulose, in chronic constipation, 104
  in hepatic encephalopathy, 655, 656–657, 656t
  in hepatorenal syndrome, 702
  pneumatosis cystoides intestinalis and, 582
Lamina propria, 415
Lansoprazole, in Zollinger-Ellison syndrome, 327, 327t
Laparoscopic appendectomy, 466–467
Laparoscopic cholecystectomy, in gallstone disease, 851, 862
Laparoscopy, in peptic ulcer disease, 354
Laparotomy, in foreign body removal, 44
  in gastrointestinal tract bleeding, 157
Laprascopic cholecystectomy, in chronic acalculous cholecystitis, 857
Large bowel. See *Intestine.*
Laryngitis, in gastroesophageal reflux disease, 206
Laser, in bezoar therapy, 282
  in esophageal carcinoma, 223
  in peptic ulcer disease—associated hemorrhage, 338
  in vascular ectasia therapy, 137
Laxatives, adverse effects of, 103–104
  in chronic constipation, 103–104
  in eating disorders, 14
  use of, diarrhea with, 92
    vs. collagenous colitis, 598
L-Dopa, vitamin deficiency with, 25t

Lecithin bezoar, 280–283, 281t
Leiomyoma, 418–419
  bleeding from, 164
Leiomyosarcoma, esophageal, 223
Leishmaniasis, visceral, hepatic granuloma in, 759
Leprosy, granulomas of, 763t
  hepatic, 763t, 764
  treatment of, 766
Leukemia, anorectal abscess and, 565
Leuprolide acetate (Lupron), in delayed gastric emptying, 255–256
  in irritable bowel syndrome, 508
LeVeen peritoneovenous shunt, in hepatorenal syndrome, 702–703
Levodopa, in hepatic encephalopathy, 658
Ligation, in gastric ulcer, 350
Linton tube, in variceal hemorrhage, 133
Linton-Nachlas tube, in variceal bleeding, 716
Lipids, in fulminant hepatic failure, 683
  in rapid gastric emptying, 262
Lipogranuloma, hepatic, 759
Lipoma, of small bowel, 419–420
Lipoproteins, in alcoholism, 708t
  in primary biliary cirrhosis, 751
Lithotripsy, in bezoar therapy, 282
  in choledocholithiasis, 889
  in gallstone disease, 851–852, 863
  mechanical, in choledocholithiasis, 889
Liver. See also at *Hepatic*.
  acetaminophen-induced injury to, 648–649
  alcohol-induced disease of, 707–713, 708t, 710t. See also *Alcoholic liver disease*.
  androgenic steroid—induced injury to, 650
  α_1-antitrypsin deficiency effects on, 791–801. See also *Alpha$_1$-antitrypsin deficiency*.
  bioartificial support for, 681
  biopsy of, in conjugated hyperbilirubinemia, 844
    in hepatocellular carcinoma, 773
    in hereditary hemochromatosis, 811
    in neonatal cytomegalovirus infection, 846
    in porphyria, 737
    in primary sclerosing cholangitis, 743–744, *744*
    in Wilson's disease, 804
  cholestatic disease of, 864–872, 865t. See also *Primary biliary cirrhosis; Primary sclerosing cholangitis*.
    malabsorption in, 80, 83t
    vitamin deficiencies in, 28–29, 29t
  circulation of, 690–691
  cocaine-induced injury to, 651
  copper accumulation in, 802–808. See also *Wilson's disease*.
  drug metabolism of, 643–645, *644, 645*
  drug-induced injury to, 643–651, 783
    acute, 645–646, *645*
      cholestasis in, 646
      microvesicular steatosis in, 646
      parenchymal necrosis in, 645–646
      phospholipidosis in, 646
    chronic, *645*, 646–648
      cholestasis in, 647
      hepatitis in, 646–647, 648
      neoplasms in, 648
      parenchymal injury in, 646–647

Liver *(Continued)*
      steatonecrosis in, 647
      steatosis in, 647
      vascular disease in, 647
    mechanisms of, 643–645, *644, 645*
    patterns of, 645–648, *645*
  estrogen-induced injury to, 650
  evaluation of, 786–788, 786t, *787*
  failure of, 675–690. See also *Hepatic failure*.
  fatty, 783–784
  focal nodular hyperplasia of, 778–779
    resection in, 833–834
  hypoperfusion of, 782–783
  in acquired immunodeficiency syndrome, 784, 784t
  in collage-vascular disease, 785
  in malabsorption syndromes, 75–76, 76t, 77t, 80, 83t
  in porphyria cutanea tarda, 736–738, *738*
  in protoporphyria, 738–740
  in systemic disease, 780–790, 781t, 782t, *787, 789*
  in systemic infections, 783
  in ulcerative colitis, 519
  inflammation of. See *Hepatitis*.
  iron accumulation in, 808–813. See also *Hemochromatosis*.
  isoniazid-induced injury to, 649–650
  methotrexate-induced injury to, 651
  passive congestion of, 677, 680
  phenytoin-induced injury to, 650
  protoporphyrin deposition in, 739
  pseudotumor of, 763
  regeneration of, 681
  resection of, 829t, 830–835, 831t, *832*
    contraindication to, 830
    in adenoma, 833
    in angiosarcoma, 833
    in cholangiocarcinoma, 776, 833
    in focal nodular hyperplasia, 833–834
    in hemangioma, 833
    in hemangiosarcoma, 833
    in hepatocellular carcinoma, 773, 831, 833, *833*
    mortality for, 830
  schistosomiasis of, 391
  tests of, 780–782, 781t
    abnormalities of, 786–788, *787, 789*
    preresection, 829–830
  transplantation of, 134, 835–839
    contraindications to, 836, 836t
    in acute hepatitis, 663
    in alcoholic cirrhosis, 712
    in alcoholic liver disease, 837
    in α_1-antitrypsin deficiency, 799
    in bile duct paucity syndrome, 839
    in biliary atresia, 839
    in Budd-Chiari syndrome, 838
    in cholangiocarcinoma, 776, 839
    in chronic active hepatitis, 838
    in fulminant hepatic failure, 689–690, 689t, 838
    in hepatic encephalopathy, 658
    in hepatic metastases, 839
    in hepatocellular carcinoma, 773–774, 838–839
    in hepatorenal syndrome, 704–705, 705t
    in inborn errors of metabolism, 839
    in primary biliary cirrhosis, 757, 837, 872
    in primary sclerosing cholangitis, 747–748, 837–838, 872

Liver *(Continued)*
  in protoporphyrin, 740
  in virus-related end-stage liver disease, 836–837
  in Wilson's disease, 807
  indications for, 834t, 835–836, 835t, 836t
  spontaneous bacterial peritonitis and, 729
  tumors of, 771–779. See also *Cholangiocarcinoma; Hepatocellular carcinoma.*
    metastatic, 788
    secondary, hepatic resection in, 834–835
  variceal hemorrhage with, 131–134, *132,* 133t
Liver function tests, 780–782, 781t
  abnormalities of, 786–788, *787,* 789
  preresection, 829–830
Lomotil. See *Diphenoxylate.*
Loperamide (Imodium), in fecal incontinence, 98
  in functional abdominal pain syndromes, 65
  in infectious diarrhea, 541
  in irritable bowel syndrome, 505, 506, 507t
Lord procedure, in anal fissure, 558
Loxiglumide, in gastric emptying, 260
Lungs, schistosomiasis of, 392
Lupoid hepatitis, 785
Lye ingestion, 30–35. See also *Alkali ingestion.*
Lymphangiectasia, intestinal, in protein-losing gastroenteropathy, 85
  malabsorption in, 83–84, 83t
Lymphangioma, 421
Lymphocytes, in malnutrition, 18
Lymphocytic colitis, 599
  celiac sprue with, 369–370
Lymphoid polyps, 548
Lymphoma, gastric, 296–299
    celiac sprue and, 370
    clinical presentation of, 296
    diagnosis of, 297
    diarrhea with, 93
    etiology of, 296
    pathogenesis of, 296
    prognosis for, 297
    treatment of, 297–298
  hepatic, 765

M

M2 autoantibodies, in primary biliary cirrhosis, 752
Macrolides, in Crohn's disease, 412
Macronutrients, 17t
Magnesium, replacement therapy with, 79t
Magnesium citrate, in chronic constipation, 104
Magnesium hydroxide, in chronic constipation, 104
Magnetic resonance imaging, in endometriosis, 576–577
  in pancreatic cancer, 636
Malabsorption syndromes, 75–84
  abetalipoproteinemia in, 84
  acquired immunodeficiency syndrome in, 82
  bacterial overgrowth in, 82
  cholestatic liver disease in, 80
  chronic pancreatitis in, 80
  clinical presentation of, 75–76, 76t
  Crohn's disease in, 81
  cystic fibrosis in, 80
  diarrhea with, 93

Malabsorption syndromes *(Continued)*
  enterokinase deficiency in, 81
  eosinophilic gastroenteritis in, 82
  etiology of, 77t
  evaluation of, 77t
  gluten-sensitive enteropathy in, 81, 82t
  in eosinophilic gastroenteritis, 359
  Kwashiorkor in, 80
  lactase deficiency in, 82
  lactose, 362–366. See also *Lactose intolerance.*
  liver in, 76–77, 77t, 80, 83t
  lymphangiectasia in, 82–83
  management of, 78–80, 79t
  nutrient replacement in, 78–80, 79t
  pancreas in, 77–78, 77t, 80–81, 83t
  pancreatic carcinoma in, 80
  pathophysiology of, 76t
  postsurgical, 80
  short bowel syndrome in, 82
  small intestine in, 78, 78t, 81, 83t
  stomach in, 76, 77t, 80, 83t
  treatment of, 83t
  tropical sprue in, 82
  trypsinogen deficiency in, 81
  vs. collagenous colitis, 597–598
  Whipple's disease in, 81
Mallory-Weiss tear, 136
Malnutrition, 16–22
  anthropometric measurements in, 18
  biochemical tests in, 18
  categories of, 18–19, 19t
  delayed gastric emptying in, 248
  dietary history in, 17–18
  enteral nutrition for, 19–20, 20t
  immunologic tests in, 18
  immunorepressive, 19, 19t, 20
  in anorexia nervosa, 10
  in blind loop syndrome, 400
  in gastrointestinal fistula, 123, 124
  medical history in, 16–17
  mixed, 19, 19t
  parenteral nutrition for, 20
  physical examination in, 16–17, *17*
  primary, 16
  screening for, 16, 17t
  secondary, 16
  treatment of, 19–20, 20t
    support teams in, 21
  weight history in, 16
Maloney dilator, *227*
Mannitol, in fulminant hepatic failure, 684
Manometry, anorectal, in fecal incontinence, 97
    in Hirschsprung's disease, 472t, 473, *474*
    in rectal ulcers, 586–587
  antroduodenal, in childhood intestinal pseudoobstruction, 452, *453, 454*
  colonic, in childhood intestinal pseudoobstruction, 453–454
  esophageal, evaluation of, 199
    in achalasia, 188–189
    in childhood intestinal pseudoobstruction, 452
    of upper esophageal sphincter, *180*
  gastropyloroduodenal, in delayed gastric emptying, 271
  in intestinal pseudoobstruction, 446, 451–454, *453, 454*

Marasmus, 18–19, 19t, 20
Mean corpuscular volume, in alcoholism, 708t
Meckel's diverticulum, diagnosis of, 149
　gastrointestinal tract bleeding with, 152
Meckel's scan, in gastrointestinal tract bleeding, 158
Megacolon, 472
　acquired, vs. Hirschsprung's disease, 473
　congenital, 470–477. See also *Hirschsprung's disease.*
　toxic, 534–537. See also *Toxic megacolon.*
Megacystis microcolon—intestinal hypoperistalsis syndrome, 441, 445, 450
　treatment of, 454–455
Megaduodenum, 446
　in familial visceral myopathy, *444*
Megarectum, in fecal incontinence, 96
Melanoma, anal, 572
　esophageal, 223
Melanosis coli, cathartic-induced, 103
Melena, 145
Ménétrier's disease, 86, 87, 320
Meningitis, *Plesiomonas shigelloides* in, 376
6-Mercaptopurine, in ulcerative colitis, 516, 521
Mesalamine (5-ASA), in ulcerative colitis, 515
Mesenteric angiography, in diverticulosis coli, 512
Mesenteric ischemia, chronic, 433–437. See also *Chronic intestinal ischemic syndrome.*
Metabolic acidosis, in acute pancreatitis, 624
Metabolic rate, in obesity, 4–5, 8
Metaraminol, in hepatorenal syndrome, 703
Metformin, vitamin deficiency with, 25t
Methotrexate, in Crohn's disease, 412
　in primary biliary cirrhosis, 756, 869, 870t, 871t, 872
　in primary sclerosing cholangitis, 747, 869, 870t, 871t, 872
　macrovesicular steatosis with, 646, 651
　vitamin deficiency with, 25t
α-Methyldopa, in carcinoid syndrome, 307
Methyl-tert-butyl ether (MTBE), in gallstone disease, 853
　in gallstones, 863
Metoclopramide (Reglan), in chronic constipation, 104
　in delayed gastric emptying, 251–252, 277
　in gastroesophageal reflux disease, 203t, 204, 251
　in irritable bowel syndrome, 500
　in pediatric gastroesophageal reflux, 210
　in variceal bleeding, 716
　side effects of, 252, 277
Metolazone, in ascites, 723
Metronidazole, in amebic abscess, 770
　in *Clostridium difficile* diarrhea, 407
　in Crohn's disease, 410–411
　in hepatic encephalopathy, 656t, 657
Microbial agents, in infectious diarrhea, 542
Micronutrients, 17t
Microscopic colitis, 599
Microscopy, in tropical sprue, 396–397
Midgut malrotation, in children, 151
Migrating motor complex, in bacterial overgrowth, 399
　in childhood intestinal pseudoobstruction, 452, *453*
Milk intolerance, in children, 151–152
Milroy's disease, in protein-losing gastroenteropathy, 85
　malabsorption in, 83–84, 83t
Mineral oil, in chronic constipation, 104
　vitamin deficiency with, 25t

Minnesota multiphasic personality inventory, in chronic nausea, 50–51
Minnesota tube, in variceal bleeding, 133, 716
Mirizzi's syndrome, 884
Mixed connective tissue disease, gastrointestinal lesions in, 442t
Mixed malnutrition, 19, 19t
Morphine, in irritable bowel syndrome, 506, 507t
Motilium. See *Domperidone.*
Multiple endocrine neoplasia type 1 (MEN-1), diagnosis of, 329
　genetics of, 331
　in Zollinger-Ellison syndrome, 322–323, 329–330
　treatment of, 331
Multiple juvenile polyposis, gastrointestinal tract bleeding with, 153
Multiple sclerosis, gastrointestinal lesions in, 443t
Munchausen syndrome by proxy, chronic childhood intestinal pseudoobstruction in, 451, 451t
Murphy's sign, 884
　in acute acalculous cholecystitis, 855
Muscular dystrophy, gastrointestinal lesions in, 442t
Mushroom poisoning, hepatotoxicity of, 677, 680
Mycobacterium avium-intracellulare, 766
Mycoses, hepatic, 763t, 764, 766
Myopathy, visceral, 440–441, 444t, 445t
　childhood, 441, 442t, 445

N

Naloxone, in chronic constipation, 105
Nasal gastric feedings, in pediatric gastroesophageal reflux, 209
Nasogastric suction, in perforated peptic ulcer, 339
Nasogastric tube, in acute pancreatitis, 621–622
　in fulminant hepatic failure, 679
　in intestinal obstruction, 494–495
Nausea, 47–56, 48t
　anticipatory, 56
　clinical approach to, 50–53, 51t, 52t—53t
　Minnesota multiphasic personality inventory in, 50–51
　of pregnancy, 54
　postoperative, 54–55
　treatment of, 52t—53t
Necrosis, caustic ingestion and, 31–32, 31t
　hepatocellular, drug-induced, 645–646, *645*
Necrotizing enteritis, *Clostridium perfringens* in, 379
Necrotizing enterocolitis, 151
Needle ingestion, 44–45, *44*
Negative expressed emotion, in eating disorders, 12
Neisseria gonorrhoeae, in proctitis, 600–601, 602t
　in pruritus ani, 568
Neomycin, in hepatic encephalopathy, 656t, 657
　vitamin deficiency with, 25t
Neostigmine, in chronic constipation, 104
Nephrogenic hepatic dysfunction syndrome, 785
Neurofibroma, 420
Neurogenic tumor, 420
Neurologic disorders, in pruritus ani, 568
Neuropathy, visceral, 441, 443t, 445t
Niacin, deficiency of, 26t
　replacement therapy with, 79t
Nifedipine, in esophageal motility disorders, 173

Nitric oxide, in hepatorenal syndrome, 698
Nitroglycerin, in esophageal motility disorders, 173
　in variceal bleeding, 133, 715
Nociception, visceral, in noncardiac chest pain, 172, 197–198, *199*
Nodular lymphoid hyperplasia, gastrointestinal tract bleeding with, 153
Nodular regenerative hyperplasia, azathioprine-induced, 648
Non-A, non-B, non-C hepatitis, 662
Non-Hodgkin's lymphoma, hepatic granuloma in, 765
Nonneoplastic polyps, 547–548
Nonsteroidal anti-inflammatory drugs (NSAIDs), in gastric ulcer, 312–313
　in gastritis, 319
　in hepatorenal syndrome, 702
Norfloxacin, in spontaneous bacterial peritonitis, 730
Nortriptyline, in functional abdominal pain syndromes, 65t
Norwalk agent virus, in infectious diarrhea, 544
Nuclide scan, in abdominal abscess, 118, *120*
Nulyte, in chronic constipation, 104
Nutrients, 17t
Nutrition, assessment of, 17t
　in delayed gastric emptying, 250, 256, 276
　in fulminant hepatic failure, 682–683
　in hereditary pancreatitis, 617
　in irritable bowel syndrome, 499
　in toxic megacolon, 536
　in ulcerative colitis, 517
　in undernutrition, 19
Nystatin, in *Candida* esophagitis, 239, 239t

O

Oat cell carcinoma, of esophagus, 223
Obesity, 3–9
　complications of, 3, 3t
　conservative management of, 5–6, 5t
　depression in, 8
　diagnosis of, 5
　diet composition and, 4
　drugs and, 4
　eating habits and, 4
　environmental influences on, 4
　etiology of, 3–5, *4*
　fenfluramine for, 6–7
　genetic influences on, 3
　health risks of, 3, 3t
　low-calorie diet in, 21
　metabolic rate in, 4–5, 8
　morbid, 21
　pharmacologic therapy in, 6–7, 21
　phenylpropanolamine for, 6–7
　prevalence of, 3
　psychologic influences on, 3–4
　rapid gastric emptying in, 261
　reduced-calorie diet for, 5–6, 5t
　self-help programs for, 6
　social influences on, 4
　surgical treatment of, 6, 6t, 21
　sympathetic nervous system in, 4
　treatment of, 5–9, 21
　　guidelines for, 7–8, 7t, 8t
　　risks of, 8–9

Obesity *(Continued)*
　types of, 5–7, 5t, 6t
　very low calorie diet for, 6, 6t, 21
　weight loss goals in, 8
Obsessive-compulsive disorder, in eating disorders, 12
Obstipation, in intestinal obstruction, 112
Octapressin, in hepatorenal syndrome, 703
Octreotide acetate (Sandostatin), in angiodysplasia, 426
　in carcinoid syndrome, 307, 308
　in infectious diarrhea, 542
　in irritable bowel syndrome, 508
　in rapid gastric emptying, 262
　in short bowel syndrome treatment, 461
　in variceal hemorrhage, 133
　in Zollinger-Ellison syndrome, 328, 333
Octylonium, in irritable bowel syndrome, 507, 507t
Ogilvie's syndrome, 106
　vs. intestinal obstruction, 116
Omental patch, in perforated peptic ulcer, 339–340
Omeprazole (Prilosec), in gastric ulcer, 315
　in gastroesophageal reflux disease, 203t, 204
　in noncardiac chest pain, 174
　in perforated peptic ulcer, 340
　in short bowel syndrome treatment, 461
　in upper gastrointestinal tract hemorrhage, 336–337
　in Zollinger-Ellison syndrome, 327, 327t, 331
Ondansetron (Zofran), in delayed gastric emptying, 251
　in dyspepsia, 61
　in irritable bowel syndrome, 508
　in porphyria, 735
　in Zollinger-Ellison syndrome, 332–333, 332t
Opiate receptor antagonists, in delayed gastric emptying, 256
Opiates, in acute acalculous cholecystitis, 853
　in infectious diarrhea, 541
　in irritable bowel syndrome, 506, 507t
Oral contraceptives, hepatic adenoma with, 648
　hepatic vein thrombosis with, 647
Oral replacement fluid, in infectious diarrhea, 539–540, 540t
Ornipressin, in hepatorenal syndrome, 703
Osteomalacia, small bowel resection and, 27
Osteopenia, 755
Osteoporosis, in primary biliary cirrhosis, 753–754, 868–869
　in primary sclerosing cholangitis, 868–869
Overnutrition, 16, 21. See also *Obesity*.
Overweight, 5. See also *Obesity*.
Oxamniquine, in schistosomiasis, 393
Oxygen therapy, in pneumatosis cystoides intestinalis, 582–583

P

P-450 enzymes, 643
Paget's disease, 571
Pain, chest, noncardiac, 171–176, *175*. See also *Chest pain, noncardiac*.
　in intestinal obstruction, 112
　in porphyria, 735–736
Pancolonoscopy, in pediatric gastrointestinal tract bleeding, 148
Pancreas, bleeding from, 138
　calcification in, in hereditary pancreatitis, 615, *616*
　cancer of, 635–639, 896, *897*. See also *Pancreatic carcinoma*.

Pancreas *(Continued)*
    in malabsorption syndromes, 77–78, 77t, 80
    inflammation of. See *Pancreatitis.*
    iron accumulation in, 808–813. See also *Hemochromatosis.*
Pancrease MT, 81t
Pancreatic ascites, in hereditary pancreatitis, 616
Pancreatic carcinoma, 635–639
    adjuvant therapy in, 639
    angiography of, 636
    biopsy in, 637
    biopsy of, 637
    clinical presentation of, 635–636
    computed tomography of, 636
    duodenal obstruction in, 638–639
    endoscopic retrograde cholangiopancreatography of, 636
    in hereditary pancreatitis, 616
    magnetic resonance imaging of, 636
    malabsorption in, 80
    metastases from, 635
    obstructive jaundice in, 638
    pain relief in, 639
    palliative treatment of, 638–639
    serum markers of, 636–637
    treatment of, 637–638
    ultrasound of, 636
Pancreatic encephalopathy, in acute pancreatitis, 625
Pancreatic insufficiency, celiac sprue and, 370–371
    malabsorption in, 83t
    rapid gastric emptying in, 261
    vitamin deficiencies in, 28, 29t
Pancreatic pseudocysts, in acute pancreatitis, 625–627
    in hereditary pancreatitis, 616, *617*
Pancreatic rests, 547
Pancreaticobiliary junction, in choledochal cysts, 814–815, *815*
Pancreatitis, acute, 620–628
    abscess with, 627–628
    acute renal insufficiency with, 623
    ascites with, 627
    choledocholithiasis with, 888
    coagulation abnormalities with, 625
    complications of, 622–628
    diagnosis of, 620
    fluid collections with, 625–627
    gastrointestinal tract bleeding with, 625
    grade of, 621
    hemodynamic complications of, 622–623
    hyperglycemia with, 624
    hyperlipidemia with, 624
    hypocalcemia with, 624
    neurologic complications with, 625
    phlegmon with, 625
    pseudocysts with, 625–627
    respiratory failure with, 623–624
    treatment of, 620–622, 621t
  choledochal cysts and, 821
  chronic, 630–634
    bile duct obstruction with, 634
    complications of, 633–634
    diagnosis of, 631
    etiology of, 630–631
    pain in, 632–633, *633*
    pathophysiology of, 630–631

Pancreatitis *(Continued)*
    pseudocysts with, 633–634
    splenic vein thrombosis with, 634
    steatorrhea in, 631–632, 632t
    treatment of, 631–634
  gallstone, 885
  hereditary, 613–618
    abnormalities with, 614
    clinical manifestations of, 614–615, 615t
    complications of, 615–616, 616t, *617*
    definition of, 613
    diagnosis of, 615, *616*
    etiology of, 613–614
    incidence of, 613
    management of, 616–618
    pathology of, 614
    pattern of, 613, *614*
  in Crohn's disease, 412
  in malabsorption syndromes, 80
Pancreatobiliary duct, anomalous, in gallbladder cancer, 903
Pancreatoduodenectomy, in bile duct strictures, 901
Papain, in bezoar therapy, 281–282
Paracentesis, in ascites, 722, 723
    in spontaneous bacterial peritonitis, 727–728, 729
Paracholoro-phenylalanine, in carcinoid syndrome, 307
Paraneoplastic visceral neuropathy, gastrointestinal lesions in, 443t
Parenteral iron overload, 809, 812–813
Parenteral nutrition, in childhood intestinal pseudoobstruction, 454–455
  in short bowel syndrome, 459–460, 460t
Parietal cell vagotomy, in duodenal ulcer, 353–354
  in peptic ulcer, 352
Parkinson's disease, domperidone in, 253
  gastrointestinal lesions in, 443t
Paromomycin, in amebic abscess, 771
Paterson-Brown-Kelly syndrome, 184–185
Pectenosis, in anal fissure, 556
Pectin, in rapid gastric emptying, 262
Pediculosis pubis, in pruritus ani, 568
Peliosis hepatis, drug-induced, 647
D-Penicillamine, in alcoholic patient, 712
  in primary biliary cirrhosis, 756
  in Wilson's disease, 805
  side effects of, 805–806
  vitamin deficiency with, 25t
Pentasa, in ulcerative colitis, 515, 520
Pentobarbital, in fulminant hepatic failure, 684
Peppermint oil, in irritable bowel syndrome, 507–508, 507t
Peptic ulcer disease. See *Ulcer(s), gastric.*
Percutaneous endoscopic gastrostomy, in gastric volvulus, 288, *288*
Percutaneous transhepatic cholangiogram, in choledocholithiasis, 886
Percutaneous transhepatic choledochoscopy, in choledocholithiasis, 890
Percutaneous transhepatic stenting, in pancreatic cancer, 638
Percutaneous transluminal angioplasty, in chronic mesenteric ischemia, 435
Pericholangitis, 744
Peridiverticulitis, 512
Peripheral eosinophilia, 359–360
Peripheral neuropathy, in porphyria, 732

Peritoneal cavity, fluid accumulation in, 721–724, 722t, 727. See also *Ascites*.
Peritoneal lavage, in acute pancreatitis, 622
Peritoneovenous shunt, in hepatorenal syndrome, 702–703
Peritoneum, hemangiomatosis of, 427
Peritonitis, bacterial, secondary, 728
  spontaneous, 724–730
    antibiotic therapy for, 728–729
    clinical features of, 725–726
    diagnosis of, 726–728, 727
    differential diagnosis of, 728
    liver transplantation for, 729
    mortality with, 729
    pathogenesis of, 725
    prevention of, 729–730
    treatment of, 728–729
    vs. ascites, 722
  in diverticulosis coli, 513
Persimmon bezoar, 280–283, 281t
Peutz-Jeghers syndrome, 146–147, 422, 548
  gastrointestinal tract bleeding with, 153
pH, in gastroesophageal reflux, 202, 208–209
Pharyngoesophageal diverticulum, 182–183, *183*
  perforation of, 229
Pharynx, foreign bodies of, 42, *42*
Phenergan (promethazine), in delayed gastric emptying, 250
Phenobarbital, in neonatal cholestasis, 848
  vitamin deficiency with, 25t
Phenolphthalein, ingestion of, vs. collagenous colitis, 598
  vitamin deficiency with, 25t
Phenothiazine, visceral neuropathy with, gastrointestinal lesions in, 443t
Phenytoin, hepatotoxicity of, 650
  vitamin deficiency with, 25t
Phlebotomy, in hereditary hemochromatosis, 812
  in porphyria, 737
Phlegmon, pancreatic, 625
  periappendiceal, 466
Phlegmonous gastritis, 321
Phosphate enema, in fecal incontinence, 98
Phospholipidosis, drug-induced, 646
Photofluorography, in gastric cancer, 290
Photosensitivity, in protoporphyria, 738–739
Phrenicoesophageal membrane, in hiatal hernia, 211, 213, *213*
Phytobezoar, 280–283, 281t
Pigmentation, in malignant carcinoid syndrome, 306
  in primary sclerosing cholangitis, 743
Pilling dilator, 227
Pinworms, in pruritus ani, 568
Pipestem fibrosis, 391
Plasmapheresis, in Wilson's disease, 807
Plesiomonas shigelloides, invasive infection with, 387
  meningitis with, 376
  toxigenic diarrhea with, 376
Pleural effusion, in acute pancreatitis, 623
Plummer-Vinson syndrome, 184–185
Pneumatic dilation, in achalasia, 189–192, *190,* 190t, *191*
  vs. esophagomyotomy, 191
Pneumatosis coli, 548
Pneumatosis cystoides intestinalis, 580–583
  complications of, 583, 583t
  development of, 581
  diagnosis of, 580

Pneumatosis cystoides intestinalis *(Continued)*
  idiopathic, 581
  oxygen in, 582–583
  secondary, 581–582, 581t
  symptoms of, 580
  treatment of, 582–583, 582t
Pneumoperitoneum, pneumatosis cystoides intestinalis and, 583
Polyethylene glycol saline lavage, in chronic constipation, 104
Polymyositis, gastrointestinal lesions in, 442t
Polypectomy, endoscopic, 302–303
Polyps, colonic, 547–548
  in schistosomiasis, 391
  duodenal, gastric outlet obstruction and, 266
  gastric, 300–304, 547
    adenomatous, 300
      follow-up for, 304
      management of, 302
    carcinoma and, 301
    clinical presentation of, 300–301
    diagnosis of, 301
    endoscopic removal of, 302–303
    follow-up for, 303–304
    gastric outlet obstruction and, 266
    Helicobacter pylori in, 303
    hyperplastic, 300
      follow-up for, 304
      management of, 301–302
    incidence of, 300
    management of, 301–302
    pathology of, 300–301
  juvenile, gastrointestinal tract bleeding with, 152–153
    generalized, 422–423
  nonneoplastic, 547–548
Polyurethane sponge plug, in fecal incontinence, 100
Porcelain gallbladder, 851, 903
Porphyria, 731–741
  acute, 731–735, *732,* 732t, *733, 734,* 735t
  chronic pain in, 735–736
  gene for, 736
  prevention of, 736
  classification of, 732t
Porphyria cutanea tarda, liver disease in, 736–738, *738*
  clinical features of, 736–737
  management of, 737–738, *738*
  relapse in, 737–738
Porphyrinuria, secondary, 740–741
Portacaval shunt, in α_1-antitrypsin deficiency, 799
Portal hypertension. See also *Esophageal varices, bleeding of.*
  choledochal cysts and, 822
  in hepatic sarcoidosis, 762–763
  in hepatosplenic schistosomiasis, 391
  rapid gastric emptying and, 261
Portal hypertensive gastropathy, 136
Portasystemic encephalopathy. See *Hepatic encephalopathy.*
Portosystemic shunt, in hepatic encephalopathy, 658
  in variceal bleeding, 716, 718
Postgastrectomy dumping, 259–260
Postgastrectomy gastritis, 320
Postpyloric feeding, in pediatric gastroesophageal reflux, 209
Potassium chloride, vitamin deficiency with, 25t
Potassium hydroxide ingestion, 32
Pouchitis, after Kock continent ileostomy, 554
  with ileal pouch—anal anastomosis, 527–528

Praziquantel, in schistosomiasis, 392–393
Prednisone, in ulcerative colitis, 521
Pregnancy, fatty liver of, 677, 680
    ulcerative colitis in, 521–522
    vomiting of, 54
Premature infant, intestinal pseudoobstruction in, 449, 450
Prepyloric ulcer, 347
Prerenal azotemia, 700, 701t
Pressure support ventilation, in fulminant hepatic failure, 686
Prilosec. See *Omeprazole.*
Primary biliary cirrhosis, 749–757
    alkaline phosphatase in, 790
    asymptomatic, 751
    autoantibodies in, 751–752, 789–790
    azathioprine in, 756
    biliary tree evaluation in, 752
    blood chemistries in, 751
    breast cancer and, 751, 751t
    chlorambucil in, 756
    cirrhotic stage (stage IV) of, 753
    clinical features of, 750–751, 750t, 751t, 865
    colchicine in, 756
    complications of, 753–754, *754*
    corticosteroids in, 756
    cyclosporine in, 756
    decompensated, 755–756
    diagnosis of, 751–752
    differential diagnosis of, 754–755
    disease association of, 751, 751t
    epidemiology of, 749
    esophageal varices in, 754, *754*
    etiology of, 750, 750t
    fat-soluble vitamin deficiency in, 754, 755, 866–868
    genetics of, 749–750
    granulomas in, 765
    hepatic granulomas in, 765
    hepatic pathology in, 752–753, *752*
    hypercholesterolemia in, 755
    lipid profile in, 751
    liver transplantation in, 757, 872
    metabolic bone disease in, 753–754, 868–869
    methotrexate in, 756
    natural history of, 753, *753*
    osteopenia in, 755
    osteoporosis in, 753–754, 868–869
    D-penicillamine in, 756
    periportal hepatitis (stage II) of, 752–753
    physical examination in, 750–751
    portal hepatitis (stage I) of, 752
    protal hypertension in, 754
    pruritus in, 755, 866, 867t
    septal stage (stage III) of, 753
    steatorrhea in, 753
    survival with, 753, *753, 754*
    symptomatic, 750–751, 750t, 751t
    treatment of, 755–757, 869–872, 870t—871t
    ursodeoxycholic acid in, 756–757
    vitamin A deficiency in, 754, 755, 867
    vitamin D deficiency in, 755, 868
    vitamin E deficiency in, 754, 755, 867
    vitamin K deficiency in, 754, 755, 867–868
    vs. autoimmune chronic active hepatitis, 755

Primary biliary cirrhosis *(Continued)*
    vs. drug-induced cholestasis, 754
    vs. primary sclerosing cholangitis, 754, 893, 893t
Primary sclerosing cholangitis, 741–748, 790
    adenocarcinoma with, 746
    anticolon antibodies in, 743
    autoantibodies in, 743
    autoimmune chronic active hepatitis and, 746
    bacterial cholangitis in, 746
    bile duct strictures in, 869, 897, *898*
    biliary tree evaluation in, 743, *743*
    blood chemistries in, 743
    classic, 744
    clinical features of, 742–743, 743t, 865–866, 892
    complications of, 745–746
    diagnosis of, 743–744, *743, 744,* 892–893, 893t
    differential diagnosis of, 746
    etiology of, 742, 891–892
    fat-soluble vitamin deficiency in, 866–868
    hepatic histology in, 743–744, *744*
    ileal pouch—anal anastomosis in, 525–526
    in ulcerative colitis, 519
    infection in, 869
    inflammatory bowel disease and, 744–745
    large duct, 744
    liver transplantation in, 747–748, 872
    metabolic bone disease in, 868–869
    natural history of, 745
    osteoporosis in, 868–869
    physical examination in, 743
    proctocolectomy in, 747
    pruritus in, 866, 867t
    recurrent, 869
    small duct, 744
    strictures with, 746–747
    treatment of, 746–748, 747t, 869–872, 870t—871t, 893–894
    vitamin A deficiency in, 867
    vitamin D deficiency in, 868
    vitamin E deficiency in, 867
    vitamin K deficiency in, 867–868
    vs. adenocarcinoma, 893
    vs. primary biliary cirrhosis, 754, 893, 893t
Prochlorperazine (Compazine), in delayed gastric emptying, 250–251
Proctitis, infectious, 600–608, 601t
    biopsy in, 607
    Campylobacter in, 602t, 605
    Chlamydia trachomatis in, 602t, 603
    Clostridium difficile in, 602t, 606
    Cryptosporidium in, 602t, 606
    cytomegalovirus in, 602t, 606
    Entamoeba histolytica in, 602t, 604–605
    Escherichia coli in, 602t, 605–606
    evaluation of, 606–608, *607*
    Herpes simplex virus in, 602t, 603–604
    human papillomavirus in, 602t, 604
    Neisseria gonorrhoeae in, 600–601, 602t
    Salmonella in, 602t, 605
    Shigella in, 602t, 604
    treatment of, 606–608, *607*
    Treponema pallidum in, 601–603, 602t
    Yersinia enterocolitica in, 602t, 606
    symptoms of, 600, 601t

Proctocolectomy, in primary sclerosing cholangitis, 747
Proctocolitis, 600, 601t
Proctography, in fecal incontinence, 97
Proctosigmoidoscopy, for foreign bodies, 38, 39
    in pediatric gastrointestinal tract bleeding, 148
Progressive muscle relaxation training, in functional abdominal pain syndromes, 67
Prokinetics, in delayed gastric emptying, 251–256, 251t, 276–278, 277t
    in gastric outlet obstruction, 268
    in irritable bowel syndrome, 500
Promethazine (Phenergan), in delayed gastric emptying, 250
Propranolol, in variceal bleeding, 717–718, 719
Propulsid. See *Cisapride*.
Propylthiouracil, in alcoholic patient, 711
Prostaglandins, in fulminant hepatic failure, 680–681
    in hepatorenal syndrome, 700
    in infectious diarrhea, 542
Protein(s), dietary, in hepatic encephalopathy, 655–656
    glucose-regulated, 795
    stone, in hereditary pancreatitis, 613–614
    stress, 795
        in α_1-antitrypsin deficiency, 795, 797
Protein malnutrition, in blind loop syndrome, 400
Protein-calorie malnutrition, in alcoholic patient, 710–711
Protein-losing gastroenteropathy, 84–87
    diagnosis of, 86
    etiology of, 85
    intestinal lymphatic obstruction in, 85, 85t
    nonulcerative diseases in, 86
    treatment of, 87
    ulcerative diseases in, 85t, 86
Prothrombin time, 781t, 782
Proton-pump antagonists. See *Omeprazole (Prilosec)*.
Protoporphyria, liver disease in, 738–740
    clinical features of, 738–739
    management of, 739–740
Prozac (fluoxetine), in functional abdominal pain, 65t
Pruritus, 755
    in primary biliary cirrhosis, 790, 866
    in primary sclerosing cholangitis, 866
Pruritus ani, 567–569
    bowel dysfunction and, 567
    clinical features of, 567
    dermatologic disease and, 569
    diet and, 568
    drug ingestion and, 568
    infections and, 567–568
    mechanical irritants and, 568
    neurologic illness and, 569
    systemic illness and, 569
    treatment of, 569
Pseudoachalasia, 187, 187t
Pseudocysts, pancreatic, in acute pancreatitis, 625–627
    in hereditary pancreatitis, 616, *617*
    infection of, 626–627
    rupture of, 626
Pseudomembranous colitis, 593t
    Clostridium difficile in, 404–405
    Clostridium perfringens in, 379
    Hirschsprung's disease—associated, 472, 472t
    sigmoidoscopy in, 405–406, *406*
Pseudomonas aeruginosa, esophageal, 243
Pseudoobstruction, intestinal, chronic. See *Chronic intestinal pseudoobstruction*.
Pseudopolyp, 548
Psychologic disorders, in endometriosis, 577
    in irritable bowel syndrome, 496, 498, 499, 500–501
    in pruritus ani, 568
    in ulcerative colitis, 517
Psychologic testing, in noncardiac chest pain, 174
Psychotherapy, in functional abdominal pain syndromes, 66–67
    in irritable bowel syndrome, 500–501
Puborectalis muscle, 95
    in fecal incontinence, 96
    in rectal ulcers, 586
Puestow dilator, *227*
Purine analogs, in Crohn's disease, 411–412
Purple pigmentation, in malignant carcinoid syndrome, 306
Push enteroscopy, in gastrointestinal tract bleeding, 158–159
Pyloric stenosis, 340–341
Pyloroplasty, in delayed gastric emptying, 257
    in gastric ulcer, 350
    in peptic ulcer disease, 343
    in perforated duodenal ulcer, 350–351
    in pyloric stenosis, 341
Pyoderma gangrenosum, in ulcerative colitis, 518
Pyridoxine, deficiency of, 26t
    jejunoileal bypass and, 27
    replacement therapy with, 79t
Pyrimethamine, vitamin deficiency with, 25t

Q

Q fever, granulomas of, 762t
    hepatic, 762t, 764, 766
    hepatic granuloma in, 759
    treatment of, 766
Q-Tip examination, of anus, 557

R

Radiation colitis, 430–432, 593t
    acute, 430
    chronic, 431–432
    diagnosis of, 431
    prevention of, 432
    treatment of, 431, 432
Radiation enteritis, malabsorption in, 83t
Radiation gastritis, 321
Radiation therapy, diarrhea with, 92
    in cholangiocarcinoma, 777, 910
    in esophageal cancer, 225
    in gallbladder cancer, 905–906
    in gastric cancer, 293–294
    in hepatocellular carcinoma, 774
    in pancreatic cancer, 639
Radiocopper loading tests, in Wilson's disease, 804
Radionuclide scan, in acute acalculous cholecystitis, 855
    in choledocholithiasis, 885
    in gastroesophageal reflux disease, 203
    in gastrointestinal tract bleeding, 158
    in lower gastrointestinal tract bleeding, 142
    in pediatric gastrointestinal tract bleeding, 148–149

Ranitidine, in fulminant hepatic failure, 686
    in gastric ulcer, 315
    in pediatric peptic ulcer, 150
    in Zollinger-Ellison syndrome, 326–327, 327t
    vitamin deficiency with, 25t
Rapamycin, in Crohn's disease, 412
Rapid gastric emptying, 259–262
    treatment of, 261–262
Rapunzel syndrome, 280
Razor blade ingestion, 45
Rectal prolapse, 99, 587
Rectoanal inhibitor reflex, in chronic constipation, 105
Rectosigmoid balloon distension, in irritable bowel syndrome, 496
Rectosigmoid carcinoma, vs. diverticulosis coli, 513
Rectum, compliance of, in fecal incontinence, 96
    examination of, in acute appendicitis, 464
        in Hirschsprung's disease, 470
    foreign bodies in, 37–40, 37t
        anal nerve block for, 38
        high-lying, 39
        in children, 46
        low-lying, 37–39
        management of, 37–41
        perforation with, 39
        presentation of, 37–38
        proctosigmoidoscopy for, 38, 39
        transanal retrieval of, 38
    in diversion colitis, 591
    infection of, 567–568
    inflammation of, 586, 600–608. See also *Proctitis, infectious.*
    motility of, 529
    sensation of, in irritable bowel syndrome, 496, 498
    stretch receptors of, in fecal incontinence, 96
    ulcers of, 584–588
        clinical features of, 584
        diagnosis of, 584–585, *585*
        histopathology of, 586
        pathophysiology of, 586–587
        treatment of, 587
    varices of, 164
    viscoelasticity of, in fecal incontinence, 96
Refeeding syndrome, 20
Reflux. See *Gastroesophageal reflux disease.*
Reglan. See *Metoclopramide.*
Regurgitation, 47
    in achalasia, 186
Rehydration therapy, in cholera, 373, 373t
Renal insufficiency, in acute pancreatitis, 623
Renal tubular acidosis, in primary biliary cirrhosis, 751, 751t
Rendu-Osler-Weber syndrome, 427–428
Respiratory failure, in acute pancreatitis, 623–624
Resuscitation, in infectious diarrhea, 539–540, 540t
    in variceal bleeding, 714
Retention polyps, 548
Reynolds' pentad, 884
Rheumatoid arthritis, hepatomegaly in, 785
Riboflavin deficiency, 26t, 79t
Rice paddy itch, 389
Rigiflex achalasia dilator, 190–191, *190*
Ring, esophageal, 184, *184*
    Schatzki's, 224
Ringer's lactate, in cholera, 373, 373t

Ropeway enteroscopy, in gastrointestinal tract bleeding, 159
Rotavirus, in infectious diarrhea, 544
Roux-en-Y gastrojejunostomy, in peptic ulcer disease, 352
Rubber band ligation, for gastric varices, 163
Rumination, 15, 47

S

Saccharomyces boulardii, in infectious diarrhea, 542
Safety pin ingestion, 45
Saline load test, in gastric outlet obstruction, 267
    in peptic ulcer disease, 352
    in pyloric stenosis, 340
Salmonella, carrier of, 385
    extraintestinal, 384
    in diarrhea, 538
    in infectious diarrhea, 543t, 544
    in proctitis, 602t, 605
    invasive infection with, 382t, 384–385
    toxigenic diarrhea with, 377–378, 377t
Salmonella enteritidis, in acute acalculous cholecystitis, 854
Salmonella typhi, 382t, 384–385
Salmonellosis, 384–385
Sandostatin. See *Octreotide acetate.*
Sarcoidosis, hepatic, 761–762, 762t, 766
Sarcoma, hepatic, resection in, 833
Sarcoptes scabiei, in pruritus ani, 568
Savary-Guillard dilator, 227, *227*
Saxitoxin, 380
Schatzki's ring, 224
Schilling test, in malabsorption syndromes, 78
Schistosoma, life cycle of, 388–389
Schistosoma haematobium, 388, 392
Schistosoma intercalatum, 388
Schistosoma japonicum, 388, 765
Schistosoma mansoni, 388, 765
Schistosoma mekongi, 388
Schistosomiasis, 388–393
    acute, 390, 390t
    asymptomatic stage of, 391
    cercarial dermatitis in, 389–390
    chronic, 390–391, *391*
    diagnosis of, 392
    epidemiology of, 388
    granulomas of, 763t
    hepatic, 763t, 765
    hepatosplenic, 391
    intestinal, 391
    of urinary tract, 391–392
    treatment of, 392–393, 766
Scintigraphy, in acute cholecystitis, 861
    in delayed gastric emptying, 271, *272–275*
    in gastrointestinal tract bleeding, 158
Scleroderma, gastrointestinal lesions in, 442t
    primary biliary cirrhosis in, 751, 751t
Sclerosing cholangitis, 891–894. See also *Primary sclerosing cholangitis.*
    secondary, 891–894
Sclerosis, biliary, drug-induced, 647
Sclerotherapy, in gastric varices, 163–164
    in peptic ulcer disease—associated hemorrhage, 338
    in variceal bleeding, 715, 717, 719
    in varices, 133–134

Scombroid fish poisoning, 380
Scopolamine (Transderm Scop), in delayed gastric emptying, 251
Secretin stimulation test, in malabsorption syndromes, 78
　in Zollinger-Ellison syndrome, 324, 324t, *325*
Sengstaken-Blakemore tube, in variceal bleeding, 133, 716
Sepsis, in abdominal abscess, 121
　in fulminant hepatic failure, 679
　in gastrointestinal fistula, 122
　liver function in, 783
　neonatal, 845
Septicemia, *Yersinia enterocolitica* in, 378
Serpin-enzyme complex receptors, 798
Severe compulsive overeating, 10. See also *Eating disorders.*
Shiga toxin, 372
Shigella, in diarrhea, 538
　in infectious diarrhea, 543t
　in proctitis, 602t, 604
　invasive infection with, 381, 382t, 384
　toxigenic diarrhea with, 377
Shigellosis, 381, 384
Shock, in fulminant hepatic failure, 686
　in ischemic hepatitis, 691
Shock wave lithotripsy, endoscopic, in choledocholithiasis, 889
Short bowel syndrome, 457–461
　colon in, 458
　complications of, 458t
　enteral nutrition in, 459–460, 460t
　ileocecal valve in, 458
　malabsorption in, 82
　motility in, 458–459
　parenteral nutrition in, 459–460, 460t
　pathophysiology of, 457–459, 458t
　pediatric, 459
　pharmacologic therapy in, 461
　surgical therapy in, 461
　treatment of, 459–461, 460t
Short chain fatty acid enema, in diversion colitis, 592–594
Shunt, for varices, 134, *135*
Sickle cell anemia, hepatic function in, 785–786
Sigmoid, volvulus of, in intestinal obstruction, 110, *111*
　treatment of, 115
Sigmoidoscopy, in proctitis, 607
　in pseudomembranous colitis, 405–406, *406*
　in rectal ulcers, 585
Skin, in porphyria, 736
　in pruritus ani, 568
SLAP (serum alkaline phosphatase), 781, 781t
　in primary biliary cirrhosis, 751, 790
Small bowel. See *Intestine, small.*
Smoking, in gastroesophageal reflux disease, 203
Soave procedure, in Hirschsprung's disease, 475, *476*, 476t
Sodium, urinary, in hepatorenal syndrome, 700, 701t
Sodium benzoate, in hepatic encephalopathy, 656t, 657
Sodium bicarbonate, vitamin deficiency with, 25t
Sodium cromoglycate, in eosinophilic gastroenteritis, 361
Sodium hydroxide ingestion, 32
Solitary rectal ulcer syndrome, 584. See also *Rectum, ulcers of.*
Somatization, chronic childhood intestinal pseudoobstruction in, 451, 451t
Somatoform disorder, chronic childhood intestinal pseudoobstruction in, 451, 451t

Somatostatin, in gastrointestinal fistula, 124
　in infectious diarrhea, 542
　in short bowel syndrome treatment, 461
　in upper gastrointestinal tract hemorrhage, 337
　in variceal bleeding, 715–716
Sonde endoscopy, in angiodysplasia, 426–427
　in gastrointestinal tract bleeding, 159
Soya bean oil, in rapid gastric emptying, 262
Spastic pelvic floor syndrome, in chronic constipation, 105
Sphincter. See *Anal sphincter; Esophageal sphincter.*
Sphincterotomy, in anal fissure, 558
　in choledochal cysts, 824
　in choledocholithiasis, 888–889
Spinal cord, injury to, gastrointestinal lesions in, 443t
　schistosomiasis of, 392
Spironolactone (Aldactone), in ascites, 723
Splanchnoptosis, 55–56
Splenorenal shunt, in α_1-antitrypsin deficiency, 799
Spontaneous bacterial peritonitis, 724–730
　antibiotic therapy for, 728–729
　clinical features of, 725–726
　diagnosis of, 726–728, *727*
　differential diagnosis of, 728
　liver transplantation for, 729
　mortality with, 729
　pathogenesis of, 725
　prevention of, 729–730
　treatment of, 728–729
　vs. ascites, 722
Sprue, celiac, 81, 82t, 83t, 367–371
　biopsy in, 367, 370
　collagenous colitis with, 369
　complications of, 370–371
　diagnosis of, 367–368
　genetics of, 371
　lymphocytic colitis with, 369–370
　lymphoma with, 370
　pancreatic insufficiency and, 370–371
　steatorrhea in, 371
　treatment of, 368–369
　ulcers and, 370
　vs. collagenous colitis, 596
　collagenous, 370
　tropical, 394–397
　　biopsy in, 396
　　clinical history of, 394
　　histology of, 396–397
　　laboratory findings in, 396
　　malabsorption in, 82, 83t
　　physical examination in, 394–395
　　radiology in, 396–397
　　treatment of, 397
　　vs. immunoproliferative small intestinal disease, 397
ST segment elevation, in fulminant hepatic failure, 685
Stagnant loop syndrome, after Kock continent ileostomy, 554
Standard meal test, in Zollinger-Ellison syndrome, 326
Stanozolol, in α_1-antitrypsin deficiency, 799
Staphylococcus, esophageal, 243
　toxigenic diarrhea with, 378
Staphylococcus aureus, in pruritus ani, 568
Starling forces, in hepatorenal syndrome, 698
Stauffer's syndrome, 785
Steatonecrosis, nonalcoholic, drug-induced, 647

Steatorrhea, in blind loop syndrome, 400
  in celiac sprue, 371
  in malabsorption syndromes, 75
  in primary biliary cirrhosis, 753
Steatosis, 783–784
  drug-induced, 646, 647
  methotrexate-induced, 651
Stenosis, pyloric, 340–341
Stents, esophageal, 230–235
    complications of, 231, 233
    contraindications to, 230
    endoscopic evaluation for, 230
    esophageal perforation with, 231
    follow-up for, 231
    for fistulae, 233–235, *234*
    for stricture, 35
    indications for, 230
    manufacture of, *234, 235,* 236, *236*
    migration of, 231
    placement of, 231, *232*
    pressure necrosis with, 231
    removal of, 233, *233*
    selection of, 230–231
    slippage of, 231, 233
Stercoral ulcer, Hirschsprung's disease—associated, 472, 472t
Steroids, anabolic, in alcoholic patient, 711–712
  hepatotoxicity of, 650
  in toxic megacolon, 536
Stomach, adenocarcinoma of, 289–294. See also *Gastric adenocarcinoma.*
  anatomy of, 283–284, *284*
  bezoars of, 280–283, 281t, 282t
  blood supply of, 345, *346*
  caliber-persistent artery of, 137, 165, 428
  emptying, delayed, 247–250, 248t
  emptying of, 264, 264t
    delayed. See also *Delayed gastric emptying.*
    electrogastrographic measurement of, 271, 273
    manometric measurement of, 271
    measurement of, 271–273
    obstruction to, 264–268, 265t, 266t, 267t
    radiographic measurement of, 271
    rapid, 259–262
    scintigraphic evaluation of, 271, *272–275*
  in malabsorption syndromes, 76, 76t, 77t, 80
  lymphoma of, 296–299
  motor disorders of, 247–256. See also specific disorders, e.g., *Delayed gastric emptying.*
  needle in, 44–45, *44*
  paresis of, 269–279. See also *Gastroparesis.*
  polyps of, 300–304. See also *Polyps, gastric.*
  rotation of, 283–288. See also *Volvulus, gastric.*
  safety pins in, 45
  ulcers of, 312–316
  watermelon, 321, 428
    bleeding from, 164
Stone protein, in hereditary pancreatitis, 613–614
Stool softeners, in chronic constipation, 104
Streptococcus viridans, esophageal, 243
Streptozocin, in Zollinger-Ellison syndrome, 332–333, 332t
Stress, in diarrhea, 88
  in dyspepsia, 59–60

Stress *(Continued)*
  in gastritis, 320
  in irritable bowel syndrome, 62
Stress proteins, 795
  in α_1-antitrypsin deficiency, 795, 797
Stricture, esophageal. See *Esophageal strictures.*
  in blind loop syndrome, 399
  with ileal pouch—anal anastomosis, 527
Strictureplasty, in bile duct strictures, 901
Subcutaneous fat necrosis, in acute pancreatitis, 624
Substance P, in carcinoid heart disease, 311
Sucralfate (Carafate), bezoar with, 280
  in gastroesophageal reflux disease, 203t, 204
Sulfasalazine, during pregnancy, 522
  in collagenous colitis, 599
  in Crohn's disease, 411
  in ulcerative colitis, 514–515, 520, 521
  side effects of, 515
  vitamin deficiency with, 25t
Suppositories, rectal ulcers and, 587
Supraventricular tachycardia, in fulminant hepatic failure, 685
Swallowing, upper esophageal sphincter in, 178, *178,* 178t
Swan Ganz catheter, in intestinal obstruction, 114
Swenson procedure, in Hirschsprung's disease, 475, *476,* 476t
Swimmers' itch, 389
Syphilis, 601–603, 602t
  congenital, hepatic involvement in, 845
Systemic lupus erythematosus, gastrointestinal lesions in, 442t
  hepatomegaly in, 785

T

Tabes dorsalis, 602
Tachygastria, 250
Tachypnea, in fulminant hepatic failure, 685
Taste, adenocarcinoma-associated alteration in, 47–48
Telangiectasias, bleeding from, 137
  gastrointestinal tract bleeding with, 153
Temperature, in acute appendicitis, 464
Tetracycline, vitamin deficiency with, 25t
Tetrathiomolybdate, in Wilson's disease, 807
Tetrodotoxin, 380
Theophylline, bezoar with, 280
Thermal coagulation, in peptic ulcer disease—associated hemorrhage, 337–338
Thiamine deficiency, 26t, 79t
  jejunoileal bypass and, 27
  postgastrectomy, 26–27
Thiazide, in ascites, 723
Thoracic duct drainage, in acute pancreatitis, 622
Thorium dioxide, cholangiocarcinoma with, 648
Thrombosis, in acute pancreatitis, 634
  in hereditary pancreatitis, 616
Thyroid gland, disease of, in primary biliary cirrhosis, 751, 751t
    rapid gastric emptying with, 261
  dysfunction of, interferon alfa therapy and, 673
Thyrotoxicosis, rapid gastric emptying with, 261
Tigan (trimethobenzamide), in delayed gastric emptying, 251
TIPS (transjugular intrahepatic portosystemic shunt), for varices, 134, *135*
Tissue eosinophilia, 361
Toilet articles, in pruritus ani, 568

Tooth (teeth), caries of, in eating disorders, 11
Toothpick ingestion, 45
Total parenteral nutrition, cholestasis with, 460–461
    in esophageal stricture, 35
    in gastrointestinal fistula, 124
    in toxic megacolon, 536
Toxic megacolon, 534–537
    clinical features of, 535
    diagnosis of, 535–536
    ileal pouch—anal anastomosis in, 525
    in ulcerative colitis, 519–520
    management of, 536
    radiography of, 535
    surgery for, 536–537
    treatment of, 520
Toxoplasmosis, neonatal, 845
Tranexamic acid, in upper gastrointestinal tract hemorrhage, 337
Transaortic endarterectomy, in chronic mesenteric ischemia, 435, *436*
Transferrin, in alcoholism, 708t
Transfusion, blood, in upper gastrointestinal tract bleeding, 128–129
Transhepatic stenting, in pancreatic cancer, 638
Transhiatal esophagectomy, in esophageal carcinoma, 222, *222*
Transition zone, in Hirschsprung's disease, 472, *473*
Transjugular intrahepatic portosystemic shunt (TIPS), for varices, 134, *135*
    in ascites, 723–724
    in primary biliary cirrhosis, 755–756
    in variceal bleeding, 720
Transpapillary stenting, endoscopic, in pancreatic cancer, 638
    in pancreatic cancer, 638
Trauma, rectal ulcers and, 587
Traveler's diarrhea, 374–376, 374t, 375t, 543–544, 543t, 545t
Treponema pallidum, in proctitis, 601–603, 602t
    transplacental transmission of, 845
Triamterene, vitamin deficiency with, 25t
Trichloroethylene, pneumatosis cystoides intestinalis and, 582
Trichobezoar, 280–283, 281t
Trichophagia, 280
Trichophyton, in pruritus ani, 568
Trichotillomania, 280
Tricyclic antidepressants, visceral neuropathy with, 443t
Trientine, in Wilson's disease, 806
Triglycerides, in fulminant hepatic failure, 683
    medium-chain, 79t
Trimethobenzamide (Tigan), in delayed gastric emptying, 251
Trimethoprim, vitamin deficiency with, 25t
Trimipramine, in functional abdominal pain syndromes, 65t
Trisomy 17-18, hepatic involvement in, 847
Trisomy 21, hepatic involvement in, 847
Tropical sprue, 394–397. See also *Sprue, tropical.*
Trypsinogen deficiency, 81
Tube feeding, in undernutrition, 19–20, 20t
Tuberculosis, esophageal, 242
    hepatic, 762t, 763–764
    treatment of, 766
Tucker dilator, *227*
Tumor(s), achalasia with, 187, 187t
    anal, 570–572, 571t
    bleeding from, 136–137, 138, 162
    diarrhea with, 93

Tumor(s) *(Continued)*
    esophageal, 218–223
        benign, 218
        malignant, 219–223. See also *Esophageal carcinoma.*
    gastric outlet obstruction and, 266
    hepatic, 771–779. See also Hepatocellular carcinoma; *specific tumors, e.g.,* Cholangiocarcinoma.
    metastatic, 788
    in achalasia, 189
    neuroendocrine, vs. collagenous colitis, 598
Turcot's syndrome, 421–422
Typhoid fever, 382t, 384–385

U

Ulcer(s), aphthous, in ulcerative colitis, 518
    colonic, 588
    duodenal, perforation of, 350–351
        rapid gastric emptying with, 250, 260
    gastric, 312–316
        antibiotic therapy in, 342
        bleeding with, 127, 130–131
        chronic, 353–354
        delayed gastric emptying with, 250, 271
        endoscopy of, 348
        esophagogastroduodenoscopy in, 335–336, 337t
        etiology of, 312–313
        gastric lavage in, 335, *336*
        gastric obstruction with, 352
        gastric outlet obstruction with, 265, 268
        Helicobacter pylori in, 342
        hemorrhage with, 349–350
        in Zollinger-Ellison syndrome, 323
        laparoscopic treatment of, 354
        malignancy and, 313–314
        natural history of, 313
        pathogenesis of, 348
        pathology of, 312–313
        pediatric, 145–146, 150
        perforation with, 339–340
            surgery for, 350–351
        pyloric stenosis with, 340–341
        rapid gastric emptying in, 260
        recurrence of, 342–343, 348, 353–354
        surgery for, 342–343, 345–354
            anatomy for, 345–347, *346*
            complications of, 352–353
            incidence of, 347
        symptoms of, 313
        treatment of, 314–316, 316t, 348–349
        types of, 347
    ileal, celiac sprue and, 370
    rectal, 584–587, 584–588, *585*
        clinical features of, 584
        diagnosis of, 584–585, *585*
        histopathology of, 586
        pathophysiology of, 586–587
        treatment of, 587
    stercoral, Hirschsprung's disease—associated, 472, 472t
Ulcerative colitis, 593t
    carcinoma and, 520, 525
    complications of, 519–520
    distal, 520

Ulcerative colitis *(Continued)*
  dysplasia with, 520
  extraintestinal manifestations of, 518–519
  hematologic manifestations of, 519
  hepatic manifestations of, 519
  hepatitis and, 519, 748
  in pregnancy, 521–522
  management of, diet in, 517
    endorectal ileal pullthrough procedure for, 548–554, *550*, 551t, *554*
    Kock pouch for, 553–554, *554*
    medical, 514–522
      aminosalicylates in, 515–516
      antibiotics in, 517
      antidiarrheal agents in, 517
      corticosteroids in, 516
      immunosuppressives in, 516–517
      sulfasalazine in, 514–515
    nutrition in, 517
    psychosocial aspects of, 517
    surgical, 524–532, 548–554
      Brooke ileostomy for, 530–531, *530*
      ileal pouch—anal anastomosis for, 524–530, *526*, 527t
        failure of, 528
        indications for, 524–526
        physiologic changes after, 528–529
        quality of life after, 529–530
        results of, 527–528, 527t
        technique of, 526–527, *526*
      ileal pouch—distal rectal anastomosis for, 532
      ileorectostomy for, 531–532, *531*
      Kock pouch for, 532
  mucocutaneous manifestations of, 518
  musculoskeletal manifestations of, 518
  ophthalmologic manifestations of, 518–519
  primary sclerosing cholangitis and, 519, 742–748, 790. See also *Primary sclerosing cholangitis*.
  proximal, 521
  severe, 521
  toxic megacolon with, 519–520
  treatment of, 520–521
  vitamin deficiencies in, 28, 29t
Ultrasonography, in abdominal abscess, 118
  in acute acalculous cholecystitis, 855
  in acute bacterial cholangitis, 878
  in acute hepatitis, 660
  in anorectal abscess, 562
  in choledocholithiasis, 885–886
  in chronic acalculous cholecystitis, 857
  in endometriosis, 576
  in esophageal carcinoma, 220
  in gallstones, 861
  in gastric cancer, 291, *291*
  in pancreatic cancer, 636
  in small bowel tumors, 418, *418*
Undernutrition, 16. See also *Malnutrition*.
Urecholine. See *Bethanechol*.
Uric acid, in alcoholism, 708t
Urinary sodium, in hepatorenal syndrome, 700, 701t
Urinary tract, infection of, hepatic involvement in, 845
  schistosomiasis of, 391–392
Ursodeoxycholic acid, in gallstone disease, 852
  in gallstones, 862–863

Ursodeoxycholic acid *(Continued)*
  in neonatal cholestasis, 848
  in primary biliary cirrhosis, 756–757, 869, 870t, 871t
  in primary sclerosing cholangitis, 747, 869, 870t, 871t
  in short bowel syndrome treatment, 460–461
Uveitis, in ulcerative colitis, 518–519

V

Vaccine, cholera, 374
  hepatitis A, 665
  hepatitis B, 664–665
Vagotomy, gastric outlet obstruction and, 266
  in gastric ulcer, 350
  in peptic ulcer disease, 343, 352
  in perforated duodenal ulcer, 350–351
  in pyloric stenosis, 341
Vagus nerve, 345–346, *346*
  in gastric emptying, 270
Valvular heart disease, in carcinoid syndrome, 306
Vancomycin, in *Clostridium difficile* diarrhea, 407
  in hepatic encephalopathy, 657
Vapreotide, in infectious diarrhea, 542
Varicella-zoster virus, esophageal, 242
Varix (varices), duodenal, 164
  esophageal, 131–134, 714–720. See also *Esophageal varices*.
  gastric, 136, 163–164, 714
  rectal, 164
Vascular ectasia, bleeding from, 137, 160–162, 161t
  treatment of, hormone therapy in, 162
    injection therapy in, 161
    surgical, 162
    thermal coagulation in, 161, 161t
Vascular malformations, 424–429
  bleeding from, 137
  classification of, 425, 425t
Vascular occlusive disease, in radiation colitis, 430
Vasoactive intestinal peptide, in dumping syndrome, 260
Vasodilators, in hepatorenal syndrome, 698, 703
Vasopressin, in upper gastrointestinal tract hemorrhage, 337
  in variceal bleeding, 133, 715
Veneral warts, in proctitis, 602t, 604
Venoocclusive disease, drug-induced, 647
Ventilation, in fulminant hepatic failure, 685–686
Ventricular function, in hepatorenal syndrome, 699
Verrucous cancer, anal, 571
Vibrio, in infectious diarrhea, 544
Vibrio alginolyticus, 387
Vibrio cholerae, 372–374, 373t, 387, 543t
Vibrio parahaemolyticus, 374, 383t, 387, 544
Vibrio vulnificus, 387
Viokase, 81t
Viral gastroenteritis, intestinal pseudoobstruction after, 449
Viruses, in pruritus ani, 568
Visceral leishmaniasis, hepatic granuloma in, 759
Visceral myopathy, 440–441, 442t, 444t, 445t
  childhood, 441, 442t, 445
Visceral neuropathy, 441, 443t, 445t
Viscerovisceral reflex response, in dyspepsia, 58, *59*
Vital signs, in fulminant hepatic failure, 678
Vitamin(s), 17t
  absorption of, 24

Vitamin(s) *(Continued)*
  deficiency of, 22–30
    atrophic gastritis and, 27
    cholestatic liver disease and, 28–29
    cirrhosis and, 29
    Crohn's disease and, 28
    drug-induced, 23t, 25, 25t
    gastric bypass and, 26–27
    gastrointestinal disorders with, 26–30, 27t, 29t
    impaired metabolism in, 23t, 24
    in neonatal cholestasis, 848
    in primary biliary cirrhosis, 754, 755
    in primary biliary sclerosis, 866–868
    in primary sclerosing cholangitis, 866–868
    inadequate food intake in, 23–24, 23t
    intestinal malabsorption syndromes and, 27–28, 27t
    malabsorption in, 23t, 24
    pancreatic exocrine insufficiency and, 28
    pathogenesis of, 23–25, 23t
    postgastrectomy state and, 26–27
    recognition of, 25, 26t
    small bowel resection and, 27
    treatment of, 29–30, 29t
    ulcerative colitis and, 28
Vitamin A, deficiency of, 26t
  in primary biliary cirrhosis, 754, 755, 867
  in primary sclerosing cholangitis, 867
  jejunoileal bypass and, 27
  replacement therapy with, 29t, 30, 79t
Vitamin B_1 (thiamine), deficiency of, 26t
  jejunoileal bypass and, 27
  postgastrectomy, 27
  replacement therapy with, 79t
Vitamin B_2 (riboflavin), deficiency of, 26t
  replacement therapy with, 79t
Vitamin B_3 (niacin), replacement therapy with, 79t
Vitamin B_6 (pyridoxine), deficiency of, 26t
  replacement therapy with, 79t
Vitamin B_{12}, deficiency of, 26t
  atrophic gastritis and, 27
  in blind loop syndrome, 400
  in Crohn's disease, 28
  in tropical sprue, 397
  replacement therapy with, 79t
Vitamin D, deficiency of, 26t
  in cholestatic liver disease, 28–29
  in primary biliary cirrhosis, 868
  in primary sclerosing cholangitis, 868
  postgastrectomy, 26
  small bowel resection and, 27
  replacement therapy with, 29t, 30, 79t
Vitamin E, deficiency of, 26t
  in primary biliary cirrhosis, 754, 755, 867
  in primary sclerosing cholangitis, 867
  jejunoileal bypass and, 27
  in protoporphyrin, 740
  replacement therapy with, 29t, 30, 79t
Vitamin K, deficiency of, 26t
  in Crohn's disease, 28
  in primary biliary cirrhosis, 754, 755, 867–868
  in primary sclerosing cholangitis, 867–868
  in ulcerative colitis, 28
  replacement therapy with, 29t, 30, 79t

Volume contraction, in hepatorenal syndrome, 701–702
Volume expansion, in hepatorenal syndrome, 702–703
Volvulus, gastric, 283–288
  acquired, 284–285, 284t
  classification of, 285, 285t
  clinical presentation of, 286–287
  combined, 286
  congenital, 284, 284t
  diagnosis of, 287
  differential diagnosis of, 287
  mesenteroaxial rotation in, 286, *286*
  organoaxial rotation in, 285–286, *286*
  surgery for, 287–288, *288*
  in intestinal obstruction, 110, *111*, 112
  midgut malrotation with, 151
  treatment of, 115
Vomiting, 47–56, 48t
  anticipatory, 56
  chemotherapy-induced, 55–56, 55t
  clinical approach to, 50–53, 51t, 52t—53t
  complications of, 48, 48t
  emotion and, 51–52
  etiology of, 48–49, 49t, *50*
  in intestinal obstruction, 112, 492
  mechanisms of, 49–50
  of motion sickness, 54
  of pregnancy, 54
  pharmacologic treatment of, 52t—53t
  postoperative, 54–55
  psychologic factors in, 51–52
  treatment of, 52t—53t

W

Warfarin, vitamin deficiency with, 25t
Watermelon stomach, 321, 428
  bleeding from, 164
Watson-Schwartz test, in porphyria, 733, *733*
Webs, esophageal, 184–185, 224
Weight loss. See also *Obesity*.
  in achalasia, 187
  in gastroesophageal reflux disease, 203–204
Wernicke-Korsakoff syndrome, postgastrectomy, 27
Wheezing, in gastroesophageal reflux disease, 206
Whipple procedure, in bile duct strictures, 901
  in pancreatic cancer, 637
Whipple's disease, malabsorption in, 81, 83t
Wilson-Cook balloon cuff prosthesis, 233, *234*
Wilson's disease, 677–678, 680, 802–808
  British Antilewisite in, 807
  diagnosis of, 802–805, 803t
  fulminant hepatitis with, 804–805
  hemofiltration in, 807
  Kayser-Fleischer rings in, 803
  liver biopsy in, 804
  liver transplantation in, 807
  molecular genetic analysis in, 804
  D-penicillamine in, 805–806
  plasmapheresis in, 807
  radiocopper loading tests in, 804
  serum ceruloplasmin in, 803
  tetrathiomolybdate in, 807
  treatment of, 805–807

Wilson's disease *(Continued)*
    monitoring of, 807–808
    trientine in, 806
    urinary copper in, 803–804
    zinc in, 806–807
World Health Organization oral replacement fluid, in infectious diarrhea, 539–540, 540t

X

D-Xylose absorption test, in malabsorption syndromes, 78
[^{14}C]-*d*Xylose breath test, in blind loop syndrome, 400–401

Y

Yersinia, in infectious diarrhea, 543t, 544
    in proctitis, 602t, 606
Yersinia enterocolitica, invasive infection with, 383t, 386
    toxigenic diarrhea with, 378
Yersinia pseudotuberculosis, invasive infection with, 386
Yogurt, in *Clostridium difficile* diarrhea, 407

Z

Zenker's diverticulum, 182–183, *183*
    perforation of, 229
Zinc, in Wilson's disease, 806–807

Zinc *(Continued)*
    replacement therapy with, 79t
Zinc acetate, in hepatic encephalopathy, 656t, 657
Zinc sulfate, in hepatic encephalopathy, 656t, 657
Zofran. See *Ondansetron.*
Zollinger-Ellison syndrome, 322–334, *333*
    basal acid output in, 324t, 325, *325*
    calcium infusion test in, 324, *325,* 326
    chemotherapy in, 331–333, 332t
    diagnosis of, 323–326, 323t, 324t, 325t, 328–329, 328t
    disease extent in, 328–329, 328t
    gastrectomy in, 151
    gastric acid hypersecretion of, 326–328, 327t
    interferon in, 333
    malabsorption in, 80, 83t
    maximal acid output in, 324t, 325, *325*
    multiple endocrine neoplasia-1 syndrome and, 329–330
    octreotide in, 333
    onadansetron in, 332–333, 332t
    rapid gastric emptying in, 261
    secretin stimulation test in, 324, 324t, *325*
    standard meal test in, 326
    streptozocin in, 332–333, 332t
    surgery in, 328, 330, 333, 350
    symptoms of, 323, 323t
    treatment of, 330–333, 332t
Zovirax (acyclovir), in herpes simplex virus esophagitis, 241

ISBN 0-7216-4670-0